ENCYCLOPEDIA OF VIROLOGY

SECOND EDITION

Volume 3

Edited by

ALLAN GRANOFF

St. Jude Children's Research Hospital, Memphis, USA

and

ROBERT G. WEBSTER

St. Jude Children's Research Hospital, Memphis, USA

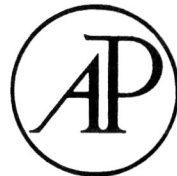

ACADEMIC PRESS
A Harcourt Science and Technology Company
San Diego   San Francisco   New York   Boston
London   Sydney   Tokyo

This book is printed on acid-free paper ∞

Copyright © 1999 by ACADEMIC PRESS LIMITED

All Rights Reserved
No part of this publication may be reproduced or transmitted in any form or by any means, electronic or mechanical, including photocopying, recording, or any information storage and retrieval system, without permission in writing from the publisher.

Academic Press
A Harcourt Science and Technology Company
525 B Street, Suite 1900, San Diego, California 92101-4495, USA
http://www.apnet.com

Academic Press
24–28 Oval Road, London NW1 7DX, UK
http://www.hbuk.co.uk/ap/

ISBN 0-12-227030-4

A catalogue for this book is available from the British Library

Access for a limited period to an on-line version of the Encyclopedia of Virology Second Edition is included in the purchase price of the print edition.

This on-line version has been uniquely and persistently identified by the Digital Object Identifier (DOI)

10.1006/rwvi.1999
By following the link
http://dx.doi.org/10.1006/rwvi.1999
from any Web Browser, buyers of the Encyclopedia of Virology Second Edition will find instructions on how to register for access

Typeset by Page Bros, Norwich, UK
Printed in Great Britain by The Bath Press, Bath, Avon, UK

99 00 01 02 03 04 BP 9 8 7 6 5 4 3 2 1

EDITORIAL ADVISORY BOARD

JEFFREY A ALMOND
Pasteur Merieux Connaught
1541 Avenue Marcel Merieux
69280 Marcy-L'Etoile
France

L ANDREW BALL
Department of Microbiology
University of Alabama at Birmingham
BBRB 373/17
845 19th Street South, Birmingham,
AL 35294, USA

Y BECKER
Department of Molecular Virology
Institute of Microbiology, Faculty of Medicine
The Hebrew University of Jerusalem
POB 12272, 91120 Jerusalem
Israel

DLH BISHOP
St Cross College
Oxford University
Oxford
UK

TO DIENER
USDA ARS
Beltsville Agricultural Research Center
Beltsville
MD 20705
USA

WALTER H DOERFLER
Institut für Genetik
Universität zu Köln
121 Weyertal
D-50931 Köln
Germany

CLAUDE FAUQUET
Division of Plant Biology - BCC 206
The Scripps Research Institute
10550 North Torrey Pines Road
La Jolla, CA 92037
USA

E PETER GEIDUSCHEK
Center for Molecular Genetics, 0634
University of California, San Diego
9500 Gilman Drive
La Jolla, CA 92093-0634
USA

ROB GOLDBACH
Department of Virology
Wageningen Agricultural University
Binnehaven 11/ 6709 PD Wageningen
The Netherlands

WK JOKLIK
Department of Microbiology
Duke University Medical Centre
E Jones Building, Room 410, PO Box 3020
Research Drive, Durham, NC 27710
USA

LA KING
Oxford Brookes University
School of Biological & Molecular Sciences
Gipsy Lane Campus
Headington, Oxford OX3 OBP
UK

MIKE A MAYO
Scottish Crop Research Institute
Invergowrie
Dundee
DD2 5DA
Scotland
UK

LK MILLER
Department of Entomology and Genetics
University of Georgia
Athens
GA 30602
USA

LUC MONTAGNIER
Institut Pasteur
Viral Oncology Unit
75724 Paris Cedex 15
France

G MOSIG
Department of Molecular Biology
Vanderbilt University
Nashville
TN 37235
USA

BERNARD MOSS
NIAID, NIH
LVD, Bldg 4, Room 229
9000 Rockville Pike
Bethesda, MD 20892-0455
USA

A NOMOTO
Department of Microbiology
The Institute of Medical Science
The University of Tokyo
4-6-1, Shirokanedai, Mionato-ku
Tokyo 108-8639, Japan

E NORRBY
MTC, Karolinska Institutet
PO Box 280
S-171 77 Stockholm
Sweden

MBA OLDSTONE
Department of Neuropharmacology
Scripps Clinic and Research Foundation
La Jolla
CA 92037
USA

B ROIZMAN
Marjorie B Kovler Viral Oncology Laboratories
University of Chicago
Chicago
IL 60637
USA

MARGARITA SALAS
Centro de Biologica Molecular (CSIC-VAM)
Universidad Autonoma de Madrid
Canto Blanco
28049 Madrid
Spain

PK VOGT
Department of Molecular & Experimental Medicine, SBR-7
The Scripps Research Institute
10666 N Torrey Pines Road
La Jolla, CA 92037
USA

RR WAGNER
Department of Microbiology
University of Virginia School of Medicine
Charlottesville
VA 22908
USA

G WERTZ
University of Alabama School of Medicine
Microbiology-BBRD 17/366
BBRB 17/366, 845 19th Street South
Birmingham, AL 35294
USA

MILTON ZAITLIN
Cornell University
334 Plant Science Building
Ithaca, New York 14853-4203
USA

GUIDE TO USE OF THE ENCYCLOPEDIA

Structure of the Encyclopedia

The material in the Encyclopedia is arranged as a series of entries in alphabetical order. Most of the entries comprise a single article, while entries on the most common or widely studied viruses and important aspects of virology consist of two or more articles. These combined articles are arranged in a logical sequence within the entry, with a summary contents list at the beginning.

In the entry titles common names are followed in parentheses by the taxonomic family of the virus or viruses addressed. For example:

> African swine fever virus (*Asfarviridae*).

Entry titles for viruses that have not been assigned to a family have no information in parentheses, but the genus is specified in the text.

The Contents List

Your first point of reference will probably be the Contents list. The complete Contents list appears in all three volumes.

Dummy entries

You will find "dummy entries" where related topics have been grouped together. Dummy entries appear in both the Contents list and the body of the text. For example:
if you wished to locate the entry which discusses Bovine Parvovirus in the Contents list you would find the following:

> Bovine parvovirus **See** Parvoviruses – rodents, pigs, cattle and waterfowl

Further use of the Contents list would lead you to the following:

Parvoviruses: (*Parvoviridae*)
General features	Caroline R Astell	1151
Molecular biology	Caroline R Astell	1155
Cats, dogs and mink	Colin R Parrish	1159
Rodents, pigs, cattle and waterfowl	Peter Tijssen, Mohamed Laakel, Zoltán Zádori and Benoît Hébert	1167

Scanning Through the Text

Alternatively if you were to try to locate the material by browsing through the text in the B section of Volume 1 you would find:

BOVINE PARVOVIRUS

See Parvoviruses (*Parvoviridae*): Rodents, pigs, cattle and waterfowl

This would lead you to the P section in Volume 2 to find:

PARVOVIRUSES (*Parvoviridae*)

Contents
General features
Molecular biology
Cats, dogs and mink
Rodents, pigs, cattle and waterfowl

The running headline at the top of each page helps locate the correct page.

To direct the reader to other entries on related topics, the section before the References entitled "See also" in most articles lists related entry titles. For example, the entry *Parvoviruses: Rodents, pigs, cattle and waterfowl* includes the following cross-references:

See also: **Parvoviruses (*Parvoviridae*): Cats, dogs and mink, General features, Molecular biology**

To further aid the reader to locate material the Contents list is followed by:

- **an alphabetical listing of the subset of entries covering general topics**

  A number of entries address general subjects related to specific viruses or viral diseases. For example, the effects of viruses on the immune system, the role of viruses in disease, oncology and gene therapy.

  If you were looking up immune response via this listing you would find the following:

  Immune response –
General features	Gordon Ada	812
Cell mediated immune response	Janice Riberdy and Peter Doherty	818

- **a listing of entries dealing with individual viruses arranged alphabetically by taxa**

  For example, by looking up *Siphoviridae* the reader can locate all entries which discuss viruses in the taxonomic family *Siphoviridae*. A list of relevant entries is provided as follows:

  Siphoviridae
Coliphage lambda	Alan M Campbell	281
T1-like phages	JR Christensen	1701
T5-like phages	D James McCorquodale	1716

Index

The complete index for the three volumes is provided at the back of each volume. Further guidance on the use of the index is supplied with the index.

Colour Plates

The colour figures for each volume have been grouped together in a plate section. The location of this section is cited at the end of the Contents list.

Appendix

A complete list of all virus names from the VIIth ICTV Meeting Report is provided. Also included are abbreviated virus names and family names. Further explanation of the Appendix is supplied at its location.

Contributors

A full list of Contributors is supplied at the beginning of each volume.

CONTENTS

Table of Contents ix
General Entries: alphabetical listing of entries covering general topics xxvii
Virus Entries: alphabetical listing by taxa of entries covering individual viruses xxxiii
Virus and Taxa Name changes xliii
Contributors xlv
Preface lxxiii
Acknowledgments lxxv
Forewords:
   100 Years of Contributions to Virology lxxvii
   100 Years of Foot and Mouth Disease lxxxi

VOLUME 1

A

Adenoviruses (*Adenoviridae*)		
General features	Göran Wadell	1
Molecular biology	Jörg Schröer, Stefan Kochanek, Marianna Hösel and Walter Doerfler	7
Animal viruses	William C Russell and Mária Benko	14
Malignant transformation and oncology	Margaret P Quinlan	21
African swine fever virus (*Asfarviridae*)	Maria L Salas	30
Aleutian mink disease virus **See** Parvoviruses		
Alfamovirus and ilarviruses (*Bromoviridae*)	JF Bol	38
Algal viruses (*Phycodnaviridae*)	James L Van Etten	44
Alpha 3 bacteriophage **See** Coliphage φX174 and related phages		
Amphibian herpesviruses (*Herpesviridae*)	Allan Granoff	51
Antivirals	A Kirk Field and Catherine A Laughlin	54
Apoptosis and virus infection	Margaret Quinlan	68

Archaeal phages	Hans Peter Arnold, Kenneth Stedman and Wolfram Zillig	76
Arteriviruses (*Arteriviridae*)	Margo Brinton	89
Ascoviruses (*Ascoviridae*)	Brian A Federici	97
Astroviruses (*Astroviridae*)	Stephan S Monroe	104
Autoimmunity	Robert S Fujinami	108
Avian type C retroviruses (*Retroviridae*)	John M Coffin	112

B

Baboon herpesvirus **See** Herpesvirus – baboon and chimpanzee		
Bacillus phage φ29 (*Podoviridae*)	Margarita Salas	119
Bacillus subtilis phages	H Ernest Hemphill	130
Bacterial identification – use of phages	Michael S DuBow	137
Baculoviruses (*Baculoviridae*)		
Granuloviruses	Doreen Winstanley and David O'Reilly	140
Nucleopolyhedrovirus	George F Rohrmann	146
Barnaviruses (*Barnaviridae*)	C Peter Romaine	152
Benyviruses	Tetsuo Tamada	154
BF23 phage **See** T5-like phage and related phages		
Birnaviruses – animal (*Birnaviridae*)	Hermann Becht	160
BK virus **See** JC and BK viruses		
Border disease virus **See** Bovine diarrhea virus and Border disease virus		
Borna disease virus (*Bornaviridae*)	Lothar Stitz and Rudolf Rott	167
Bovine diarrhea virus and border disease virus (*flaviviridae*)	Edward J Dubovi	173
Bovine herpesvirus (*Herpesviridae*)	Michael J Studdert	180
Bovine immunodeficiency virus (*Retroviridae*)	Matthew A Gonda	184
Bovine leukemia virus (*Retroviridae*)	Kathryn Radke	191
Bovine papilloma virus **See** Bovine Diarrhea Virus and Border Disease Virus		
Bovine parvovirus **See** Parvoviruses – rodents, pigs, cattle and waterfowl		
Bovine spongiform encephalopathy **See** Prions		
Bromoviruses (*Bromoviridae*)	Paul Ahlquist	198
Bunyaviruses (*Bunyaviridae*)		
General features	Neal Nathanson and Francisco González-Scarano	204
Replication	Richard M Elliott	212

C

Caliciviruses (*Caliciviridae*)	Michael J Studdert	217
Canine distemper virus **See** Rinderpest and canine distemper viruses		
Canine parvoviruses **See** Parvoviruses		
Capilloviruses	Luis Falipe Salazar	222
Caprine arthritis encephalitis virus	Gilles Quérat and Robert Vigne	223
Cardioviruses (*Picornaviridae*)	Douglas G Scraba and Ann C Palmenberg	229
Carlaviruses	Sergei K Zavriev	238
Carmoviruses (*Tombusviridae*)	Feng Qu and T Jack Morris	243
Cell structure and function in virus infections	Samuel Dales	247
Central European encephalitis virus **See** Encephalitis viruses		
Chandipura, Piry and Isfahan viruses (*Rhabdoviridae*)	P De Bishnu and Amiya K Banerjee	257
Channel catfish virus **See** Fish herpesviruses		
Chicken herpesvirus **See** Marek's disease virus		
Chickenpox virus **See** Varicella-zoster virus		
Chikungunya, O'nyong nyong and Mayaro viruses (*Togaviridae*)	Charles H Calisher	261
Chilo iridescent virus **See** Tipula iridescent virus		
Chimpanzee herpesvirus **See** Herpesvirus – baboon and chimpanzee		
Chlorella virus **See** Algal viruses		
Closteroviruses (*Closteroviridae*)	Sylvie German-Retana, Giovanni Martelli and Thierry Candresse	266
Coltiviruses **See** Orbiviruses and coltiviruses		
Coliphage ϕX174 and related phages (*Microviridae*)	David T Denhardt	274
Coliphage lambda (*Siphoviridae*)	Allan M Campbell	281
Comoviruses (*Comoviridae*)	G George P Lomonossoff and Michael Shanks	285
Coronaviruses (*Coronaviridae*)	Kathryn V Holmes	291
Cowpox virus (*Poxviridae*)	Derrick Baxby and M Bennett	298
Coxsackieviruses (*Picornaviridae*)	Bruno Pozzetto and Odette G Gaudin	305
Creutzfeld-Jakob disease **See** Prions		

Cricket paralysis virus **See** Picornaviruses – insect
Cryptoviruses (*Partitiviridae*) — Robert G Milne and Cristina Marzachi — 312

Cucumoviruses (*Bromoviridae*)
  General features — Marilyn Roossinck — 315
  Molecular biology — Marilyn Roossinck — 320
Cyanophages — Eugene L Martin and Tyler A Kokjohn — 324

Cypoviruses (*Reoviridae*) — Serge Belloncik — 332
Cytokines and chemokines — Diane E Griffin — 339
Cytomegaloviruses (*Herpesviridae*)
  General features (human) — Edward S Mocarski, Jr — 344
  Molecular biology (human) — Wade Gibson — 351
  Animal cytomegaloviruses — Donald J Alcendor and Gary S Hayward — 357
  Murine cytomegaloviruses — John Staczek — 363

D

Defective interfering viruses — Laurent Roux — 371
Dengue viruses (*Flaviviridae*) — Duane J Gubler — 375
Densonucleosis viruses (*Parvoviridae*) — Jacov Tal — 384
Diagnostic techniques
  Detection of viral antigens, nucleic acids and specific antibodies — Aloys CM Kroes and Linda FF Kox — 388
  Isolation and identification by culture and microscopy — Marie L Landry and GD Hsiung — 395
Dianthoviruses (*Tombusviridae*) — Steven A Lommel — 403
Drosophila C virus **See** Picornaviruses – insect
Drosophila Melanogaster Gypsy Virus **See** Retroviruses of Drosophila: The Gypsy Paradigm

E

Eastern equine encephalitis virus **See** Equine encephalitis viruses
Ebola virus **See** Marburg and Ebola viruses
Echoviruses (*Picornaviridae*) — Helena Kopecka — 411
Ectromelia virus **See** Mousepox and rabbitpox
Emerging and re-emerging virus diseases — Frederick A Murphy — 418

Encephalitis viruses (*Flaviviridae*)
   Encephalitis viruses and related viruses causing hemorrhagic disease — James S Porterfield — 424
   Tick-borne encephalitis and Wesselsbron viruses — EA Gould — 430
Endogenous viruses — Bernard F Benkel — 437
Enteric viruses — Ruth F Bishop — 441
Enterobacteria phage N4 (*Podoviridae*) — Lucia B Rothman-Denes — 450
Enterobacteria phage P1 (*Myoviridae*) — Hansjörg Lehnherr and Jürg Meyer — 455

Enteroviruses (*Picornaviridae*)
   Animal and related viruses — Elizabeth M Hoey and Samuel J Martin — 461
   Human enteroviruses (serotypes 68–71) — Jeffrey W Almond and Margeruite Yin-Murphy — 468

Entomopoxviruses (*Poxviridae*) — Richard W Moyer — 474
Epidemiology of viral diseases — Frederick A Murphy — 482
Epstein-Barr virus (*Herpesviridae*)
   General features — Lawrence S Young — 487
   Molecular biology — Jeffrey T Sample and Clare E Sample — 494

Equine arteritis virus **See** Arteriviruses
Equine encephalitis viruses (*Togaviridae*) — Diane E Griffin — 501
Equine herpesviruses (*Herpesviridae*) — Dennis J O'Callaghan and Nikolaus Osterrieder — 508
Equine infectious anemia virus (*Retroviridae*) — Ronald C Montelaro — 515
Eye infections — James Chodosh — 522

F

Fabaviruses (*Comoviridae*) — JI Cooper — 531
Feline calicivirus **See** Caliciviruses
Feline immunodeficiency virus (*Retroviridae*) — Janet K Yamamoto — 535
Feline leukemia and sarcoma viruses (*Retroviridae*) — James C Neil and David Onions — 541
Feline panleukopenia virus **See** Parvoviruses
Feline sarcoma virus **See** Feline leukemia and sarcoma viruses
Filamentous phages (*Inoviridae*) — Robert E Webster — 547
Fish herpesviruses (*Herpesviridae*) — Andrew J Davison — 553
Fish viruses — Carol H Kim and Jo-Ann Leong — 558
Foot and mouth disease viruses (*Picornaviridae*) — David J Rowlands — 568
Fowlpox virus (*Poxviridae*) — Deoki N Tripathy and William M Schnitzlein — 576

Frog virus 3 (*Iridoviridae*)	Rakesh M Goorha and Allan Granoff	582
Furoviruses	Yukio Shirako and T Michael A Wilson	587

G

G4 bacteriophage **See** Coliphage φX174 and related phages		
Geminiviruses (*Geminiviridae*)	KW Buck	597
Genetics of animal viruses	Frank Fenner	606
Giardiaviruses (*Totiviridae*)	Alice L Wang and Ching C Wang	613
Gibbon ape leukemia virus (*Retroviridae*)	Marvin S Reitz, Jr	617
Goat pox virus **See** Poxviruses		
Gonometa virus **See** Picornaviruses – insect		
Goose parvovirus **See** Parvoviruses		
Granuloviruses **See** Baculoviruses		
Guanarito virus **See** Lassa, Junin, Machupo and Guanarito viruses		

H

Hantaviruses (*Bunyaviridae*)	Connie S Schmaljohn	621
Hare fibroma virus **See** Poxviruses		
Hepatitis A virus (*Picornaviridae*)	Michael R Beard and Stanley M Lemon	631
Hepadnaviruses (*Hepadnaviridae*) Human hepatitis B virus		
General features	William S Robinson	640
Molecular biology	Christopher Seeger	645
Avian hepatitis B virus	William Mason and Patricia Marion	650
Hepatitis C virus (*Flaviviridae*)	Robert H Purcell	657
Hepatitis delta virus	Michael MC Lai	664
Hepatitis E virus	Albert W Tam, Patrice O Yarbough and Daniel W Bradley	669

VOLUME 2

Herpes simplex viruses (*Herpesviridae*)		
General features	Laure Aurelian	677
Molecular biology	Edward K Wagner	686

Herpesviruses 6 and 7 – human (*Herpesviridae*)	Takuya Shimamoto and Koichi Yamanishi	697
Herpesvirus sylvilagus (*Herpesviridae*)	Peter G Medveczky	703
Herpesviruses – baboon and chimpanzee (*Herpesviridae*)	SS Kalter and RL Heberling	707
Herpesviruses saimiri and ateles (*Herpesviridae*)	Julia K Hilliard	714
History of virology		
General	Frank Fenner	718
Bacteriophages	Donna H Duckworth	725
Polio, coxsackie, echo and other enteroviruses	Joseph L Melnick	730
Hog cholera virus (*Flaviviridae*)	Jan T Van Oirschot	738
Honey bee viruses	Brenda V Ball and Leslie Bailey	743
Hordeiviruses (*Hordeivirus*)	Dianne M Lawrence and Andrew O Jackson	749
Host genetic resistance	David G Brownstein	753
Host-controlled modification and restriction	Deklev H Krüger and Monika Reuter	758
Human immunodeficiency viruses (*Retroviridae*)		
General features	Luc Montaginer	763
Molecular biology	Leon F García Martínez and L Victor García-Martínez	774
Antiretroviral agents	Ranga V Srinivas and Arnold Fridland	778
Human T-cell leukemia viruses (*Retroviridae*)		
HTLV-1	Mitsuaki Yoshida	788
HTLV-2	Bobbie J Rimel, Joseph D Rosenblatt and Vincente Planelles	794
Hypoviruses (*Hypoviridae*)	Donald L Nuss	804

I

Idaeoviruses	MA Mayo and AT Jones	809
Ilarviruses **See** Alfamoviruses and ilarviruses		
Immune response		
General features	Gordon L Ada	812
Cell mediated immune response	Janice Riberdy and Peter Doherty	818
Infectious pancreatic necrosis virus **See** Birnaviruses – animal		

Influenza viruses (*Orthomyxoviridae*)
   General features — Robert G Webster — 824
   Molecular biology — Peter Palese and Adolfo Garcia-Sastre — 830
   Structure of antigens — Jonathan W Yewdell, Jack R Bennink and W Graeme Laver — 836

Insect pest control by viruses — Davin Miller, David R O'Reilly and David Dall — 842

Interference — Julius S Youngner and Patricia Whitaker-Dowling — 850

Interferons – General features — Philip I Marcus — 854

Iridoviruses – invertebrate — Richard Webby and James Kalmakoff — 862

Isfahan virus **See** Chandipura, Piry and Isfahan viruses

J

Japanese encephalitis virus (*Flaviviridae*) — Akira Igarashi — 871

JC and BK viruses (*Polyomaviridae*) — Richard J Frisque — 876

Junin virus **See** Lassa, Junin, Machupo and Guanarito viruses

K

Killer virus system **See** Totiviruses and yeast RNA viruses

Kyasanur forest disease **See** Encephalitis viruses

L

Lassa, Junin, Machupo and Guanarito viruses (*Arenaviridae*) — Joseph B McCormick — 887

Latency — Jack G Stevens — 897

Lelystad virus **See** Arteriviruses

Lumpy skin disease **See** Poxviruses

Luteoviruses — W Allen Miller — 901

Lymphocystis disease virus (*Iridoviridae*) — Christian A Tidona and Gholamreza Darai — 908

Lymphoproliferative disease virus of turkeys (*Retroviridae*) — Arona Gazit and Abraham Yaniv — 911

Lymphocytic choriomeningitis virus (*Arenaviridae*)
    General features — Raymond M Welsh — 915
    Molecular biology — Peter J Southern and Barbara J Meyer — 920

Lysogeny and prophage — Max E Gottesman and Arnos Oppenheim — 925

M

Machlomoviruses (*Tombusviridae*) — Steven A Lommel — 935
Machupo virus **See** Lassa, Junin, Machupo and Guanarito viruses
Mammalian hepadnaviruses **See** Hepatitis B viruses
Marburg and Ebola viruses (*Filoviridae*) — Hans-Dieter Klenk, Werner Slenczka and Heinz Feldmann — 939
Marek's disease virus (*Herpesviridae*) — LN Payne — 945
Mayaro virus **See** Chikungunya, O'nyong nyong and Mayaro viruses
Measles virus (*Paramyxoviridae*) — Sibylle Schneider-Schaulies and Volker ter Meulen — 952
Mink enteritis virus **See** Parvoviruses
Molluscum contagiosum virus (*Poxviridae*) — LC Archard, BA Soteriou and CD Porter — 960
Monkeypox virus **See** Smallpox and monkeypox viruses
Morbilliviruses **See** Rinderpest and distemper viruses
Mouse mammary tumor virus (*Retroviridae*) — Jackie P Dudley — 965
Mousepox and rabbitpox viruses (*Poxviridae*) — Frank Fenner — 973
Mu-like phages (*Myoviridae*) — Michael S DuBow — 981
Mumps virus (*Paramyxoviridae*) — Bertus K Rima — 988
Murine leukemia viruses (*Retroviridae*) — Hung Fan — 995
Murine parvoviruses **See** Parvoviruses
Murray Valley encephalitis **See** Encephalitis viruses
Myxoma virus **See** Poxviruses

N

Necroviruses (*Tombusviridae*) — Frank Meulewaeter — 1003
Nepoviruses (*Comoviridae*) — Mike A Mayo and AT Jones — 1007
Nervous system viruses — Richard T Johnson — 1013
Newcastle disease virus (*Paramyxoviridae*) — Peter T Emmerson — 1020
Nodaviruses (*Nodaviridae*) — L Andrew Ball — 1026

Nonoccluded baculoviruses — John P Burand — 1031
Norwalk and related viruses (*Caliciviridae*) — Mary K Estes and Isabelle Leparc-Goffart — 1035

Nucleopolyhedrosis viruses **See** Baculoviruses

O

Omsk hemorrhagic fever virus **See** Encephalitis viruses

O'nyong-nyong virus **See** Chikungunya, O'nyong-nyong and Mayaro viruses (*Togaviridae*)

Orbiviruses and coltiviruses (*Reoviridae*)
   General features — PPC Mertens — 1043
   Molecular biology — Polly Roy and Peter PC Mertens — 1062

Organ system infections — Jangu E Banatvala and Felicity Nicholson — 1074

P

P2, 186 and related phages (*Myoviridae*) — Ian B Dodd and J Barry Egan — 1087

P4 phage (Satellites) — Gianni Deho and Daniela Ghisotti — 1094

Papillomaviruses – human (*Papillomaviridae*)
   General features — Gérard Orth — 1105
   Molecular biology — Paul Lambert, Elsa Flores, Pirkko Heino and Shiyu Song — 1115

Papillomaviruses – animal — William C Phelps, Gary L Bream and Alison A McBride — 1121

Parainfluenza viruses (*Paramyxoviridae*)
   Human — Allen Portner — 1130
   Animal — Kailash C Gupta — 1134

Parapoxviruses (*Poxviridae*) — Andrew Mercer and David Haig — 1140

Partitiviruses – fungal (*Partitiviridae*) — Said A Ghabrial and Bradley I Hillman — 1147

Parvoviruses (*Parvoviridae*)
   General features — Caroline R Astell — 1151
   Molecular biology — Caroline R Astell — 1155
   Cats, dogs and mink — Colin R Parrish — 1159
   Rodents, pigs, cattle and waterfowl — Peter Tijssen, Mohamed Laakel, Zoltán Zádori and Benoît Hébert — 1167

Pathogenesis
   Animal viruses — Kenneth L Tyler — 1175
   Plant viruses — James Culver — 1184

Pea enation mosaic virus (*Luteoviridae*) — Jihad S Skaf, Steven A Denler and Gustaaf A de Zoeten — 1191

Pecluviruses — DVR Reddy, P Delfosse and Mike A Mayo — 1196

Persistent viral infection — Maryann T Puglielli and Rafi Ahmed — 1200

Peste des petits ruminants virus **See** Rinderpest and distemper viruses

Phage φ6 (*Cystoviridae*) — Dennis H Bamford — 1205

Phage ecology, evolution and speciation — Allan M Campbell — 1208

Phage PRD1 (*Tectiviridae*) — Dennis H Bamford — 1210

Phage homologous recombination — Kenneth N Kreuzer — 1213

Phage taxonomy and classification — Jack Maniloff, Hans-Wolfgang Ackermann and Audrey Jarvis — 1221

Phage toxins and disease — Randall K Holmes, Michael G Jobling and Michael P Schmitt — 1228

Phage transduction — Werner Arber — 1234

Phages as cloning vehicles — Noreen E Murray — 1240

Phages in industrial fermentations — Mary Ellen Sanders — 1244

Phages in soil — Stanley T Williams, Martin A Mortimer and Jackie Parry — 1248

Phages of *Streptococcus thermophilus* — Harold Brüssow — 1253

Phocid distemper virus **See** Rinderpest and distemper viruses

Phytoreoviruses (*Reoviridae*) — Bradley I Hillman and Donald L Nuss — 1262

Picornaviruses – insect (*Picornaviridae*) — Paul D Scotti and Peter D Christian — 1267

Piry virus **See** Chandipura, Piry and Isfahan viruses

Plant pararetroviruses *(Caulimoviridae)*
    Caulimoviruses: general features   James E Schoelz and June E Bourque   1275
    Caulimoviruses: molecular biology   Thomas Hohn   1281
    Cassava vein mosaic virus   Alexandre de Kochko   1285
    Legume caulimoviruses   DVR Reddy and Richard D Richins   1289

Plant pararetroviruses
    Rice tungro bacilliform virus   Roger Hull   1292
    Badnaviruses   Benham E Lockhart and Neil E Olszewski   1296

Plant resistance to viruses
    Natural resistance   RSS Fraser   1300
    Engineered resistance   C Michael Deom   1307
Plant retroelements   Roger Hull   1314
Plant virus disease – economic aspects   OW Barnett and Charles E Main   1318

Polioviruses *(Picornaviridae)*
    General features   Philip D Minor   1326
    Molecular biology   Thomas Pfister, Caroline Mirzayan and Eckard Wimmer   1330

Polydnaviruses *(Polydnaviridae)*   Don Stoltz   1349
Polyomaviruses – murine *(Polyomaviridae)*
    General features   James M Pipas   1352
    Molecular biology   Walter Eckhart   1356

VOLUME 3

Pomoviruses   L Torrance   1361
Potexviruses   Mounir AbouHaidar and Duncan Gellatly   1364
Potyviruses   Juan José López-Moya and Juan-Antonio Garcia   1369

Poxviruses *(Poxviridae)*
    Capripoxviruses   R Paul Kitching   1376
    Leporipoviruses and suipoxviruses   Grant McFadden   1381
Prions
    Human and Animal   Stanley B Prusiner   1388
    Kuru   Carlo Masullo   1398
    Yeast and Fungi   Marie-Lise Maddelein, Herman Edskes, Kim Taylor and Reed B Wickner   1402

Propagation of viruses
   Animal — Steffen Faisst — 1408
   Bacteria — Gail E Christie — 1413
   Plant — William M Wintermantel — 1418
Pseudorabies virus *(Herpesviridae)* — Saul Kit — 1421

Q

Quasispecies — Esteban Domingo — 1431

R

Rabbit fibroma virus **See** Poxviruses
Rabbit hemorrhagic disease virus **See** Caliciviruses
Rabbitpox virus **See** Mousepox and rabbitpox viruses and poxviruses
Rabies virus *(Rhabdoviridae)* — George M Baer and Noël Tordo — 1437
Rabies-like viruses *(Rhabdoviridae)* — Robert E Shope — 1442
Recombination of viruses — Jozef J Bujarski — 1446
Reoviruses *(Reoviridae)*
   General features — Kenneth L Tyler — 1454
   Molecular biology — WK Joklik — 1464
Replication of viruses — V Gregory Chinchar — 1471
Respiratory syncytial virus – human *(Paramyxoviridae)* — Peter L Collins — 1479
Respiratory viruses — David O White and Lorena E Brown — 1488
Reticuloendotheliosis viruses *(Retroviridae)* — Radmila Hrdlickova, Jiri Nehyba and Henry R Bose — 1496
Retrotransposons of fungi — Jef D Boeke — 1503
Retroviral oncogenes — Paula J Enrietto, Gabriela Maldonado-Codina and Michael Hayman — 1507
Retroviruses – type D *(Retroviridae)* — Maja A Sommerfelt and Eric Hunter — 1518
Retroviruses of Drosophila: The gypsy paradigm — Alain Bucheton, Alain Pélisson and Christophe Terzian — 1526

Rhabdoviruses (*Rhabdoviridae*)
   Plant rhabdoviruses   Andrew O Jackson, Michael Goodin, Ignacio Moreno, Jennifer Johnson and Diane M Lawrence   1531

   Ungrouped mammalian, bird and fish rhabdoviruses   P De Bishnu and Amiya K Banerjee   1541

Rhinoviruses (*Picornaviridae*)   Glyn Stanway   1545

Ribozymes   Robert H Symons   1551

Rinderpest and distemper viruses (*Paramyxoviridae*)   Tom Barrett   1559

Ross River virus and Barmah Forest virus (*Togaviridae*)   Lyn Dalgarno and Ian D Marshall   1570

Rotaviruses (*Reoviridae*)
   General features   Robert D Shaw and Harry B Greenberg   1576

   Molecular biology   Mary K Estes   1583

Rubella virus (*Togaviridae*)   Terly K Frey and Jerry S Wolinsky   1592

Russian spring summer encephalitis virus **See** Encephalitis viruses

S

Salmonella phage P22 (*Podoviridae*)   Anthony R Poteete   1603

Satellite RNAs and satellite viruses   ME Taliansky and PF Palukaitis   1607

S13m bacteriophage **See** Coliphage ϕX174 and related phages (*Microviridae*)

San Miguel sea lion virus **See** Caliciviruses

Scrapie **See** Prions

Semliki Forest virus **See** Sindbis and Semliki Forest viruses

Sendai virus (*Paramyxoviridae*)   Mario Homma and Masato Tashiro   1616

Sequiviruses (*Sequiviridae*)   Mike A Mayo and AF Murant   1622

Sheep poxvirus **See** Poxviruses

Shrimp viruses   Philip C Loh   1625

Shope fibroma virus **See** Poxviruses

Shope papilloma and bovine viruses **See** Papillomaviruses – animal

Sigma rhabdoviruses *(Rhabdoviridae)*	Danielle Teninges	1635
Simian hemorhagic fever virus **See** Encephalitis viruses and arteriviruses		
Simian herpesvirus **See** Herpesvirus saimiri and ateles		
Simian immunodeficiency viruses *(Retroviridae)*	Vito G Sasseville, Ronald C Desrosiers and Hillary G Morrison	1640
Simian virus 40	Janet S Butel	1647
Sindbis and Semliki Forest viruses *(Togaviridae)*	Miton J Schlesinger	1656
Single-stranded RNA phages *(Leviviridae)*	J van Duin	1663
Smallpox and monkeypox viruses *(Poxviridae)*	Keith Dumbell and Geoffrey L Smith	1668
Sobemoviruses	OP Sehgal	1674
SPO1 phage *(Myoviridae)*	Charles R Stewart	1681
Spongiform encephalopathies **See** Prions		
Spumaviruses *(Retroviridae)*	Mel Campbell, Ayalew Mergia, Philip C Loh and Paul A Luciw	1685
Squirrel fibroma virus **See** Poxviruses		
St. Louis encephalitis virus **See** Encephalitis viruses		
Swine herpesvirus 1 **See** Pseudorabies virus		
Swine vesicular exanthema virus **See** Caliciviruses		
Swinepox virus **See** Poxvirus		
Synergism – Plant viruses	Vicki Bowman Vance	1694

T

T1-like phages *(Siphoviridae)*	JR Christensen	1701
T4-like phages *(Myoviridae)*	Gisela Mosig	1706
T5-like phages *(Siphoviridae)*	D James McCorquodale	1716
T7-like phages *(Podoviridae)*	Ian J Molineux	1722
Tanapox virus **See** Yabapox viruses		
Taxonomy, classification and nomenclature of viruses	Claude M Fauquet	1730
Tenuiviruses	Bryce W Falk	1756
Tetraviruses *(Tetraviridae)*	Terry N Hanzlik and Karl HJ Gordon	1764
Theiler's viruses *(Picornaviridae)*	Howard L Lipton	1773
Tick-borne encephalitis virus **See** Encephalitis viruses		

Tobamoviruses	Dennis J Lewandowski and William O Dawson	1780
Tobraviruses	Peter B Vissler, Alexander Mathis and Hubb JM Linthorst	1784
Tombusviruses	D'Ann Rochon	1789
Toroviruses *(Coronaviridae)*	Marian C Horzinek	1798
Tospoviruses *(Bunyaviridae)*	James W Moyer	1803
Totiviruses *(Totiviridae)*		
General features	Said A Ghabrial and Jean L Patterson	1808
Ustilago maydis viruses	Jeremy Bruenn	1812
Transformation – Animal viruses	Ron Wisdom and Inder M Verma	1817
Transplantation and virus infections	Robert A Krance, Helen E Heslop and Malcolm Brenner	1823
Transportable bacteriophages **See** Mu-like phages		
Tree shrew herpesviruses *(Herpesviridae)*	Christian A Tidona and Gholamreza Darai	1834
Trichoviruses	Sylvie German-Retana and Thierry Candresse	1837
Tumor viruses – human	Herbert Pfister and Bernard Fleckenstein	1842
Turkey herpesvirus **See** Marek's disease virus		
Tymoviruses	Adrian Gibbs	1850
Ty elements **See** Retrotransposons of fungi		

U

Umbraviruses	DJ Robinson and AF Murant	1855
Ustilago maydis viruses **See** Totiviruses		

V

Vaccines and immune response	Gordon L Ada	1861
Vaccinia virus *(Poxviridae)*	Riccardo Wittek	1865
Varicella-zoster virus *(Herpesviridae)*		
General features	Jeffrey I Cohen and Stephen E Straus	1872
Molecular biology	William T Ruyechan and John Hay	1878
Variola virus **See** Smallpox and monkeypox viruses		

Vectors		
Animal viruses	Geoffrey Kitchingman and J Victor Garcia	1885
Plant viruses	Thomas Hohn and Rob Goldbach	1892
Vector transmission of plant viruses	Stewart M Gray and D'Ann Rochon	1899
Venezuelan equine encephalitis virus **See** Equine encephalitis viruses		
Vesicular exanthema virus **See** Caliciviruses		
Vesicular stomatitis viruses (*Rhabdoviridae*)	Luis L Rodriguez and Stuart T Nichol	1910
Viral membranes	John Lenard	1920
Viral receptors	Horacio U Saragovi, Gordon J Sauvé and Mark I Greene	1926
Viroids	Robert A Owens	1928
Virus species	Marc HV Van Regenmortel	1937
Virus structure		
Atomic structure	Ming Luo	1943
Principles of virus structure	John E Johnson and Jeffrey A Speir	1946
Virus-host cell interactions	Patricia Whitaker-Dowling and Julius S Youngner	1957
Visna-Maedi viruses (*Retroviridae*)	Opendra Narayan	1961

W

Waikaviruses (*Sequiviridae*)	Donald T Gordon	1965
Wesselbron virus **See** Encephalitis viruses		
West Nile encephalitis virus **See** Encephalitis viruses		
Western equine encephalitis virus **See** Equine encephalitis viruses		

Y

Yabapox and Tanapox viruses (*Poxviridae*)	HA Rouhandeh	1971
Yeast RNA viruses (*Totiviridae*)	Lionel Bernard, Herman Edskes, Juan Carlos Ribas and Reed B Wickner	1974
Yellow fever virus (*Flaviviridae*)	Thomas P Monath	1979

Z

Zoonoses　　　　　　　　　　　　　Thomas M Yuill　　　　　　1987

Color Plate Sections
  in Volume 1　　　　　　　　　　　　　　　between pages　366–367
  in Volume 2　　　　　　　　　　　　　　　between pages　1043–1044
  in Volume 3　　　　　　　　　　　　　　　between pages　1694–1695
Appendix　　　　　　　　　　　　　　　　　　　　　　　　　　　　Ai
Index　　　　　　　　　　　　　　　　　　　　　　　　　　　　　　Ii

GENERAL ENTRIES: ALPHABETICAL LISTING OF ENTRIES COVERING GENERAL TOPICS

A

Antivirals	A Kirk Field	54
Apoptosis and virus infection	Margaret Quinlan	68
Archaeal phages	Hans Peter Arnold, Kenneth Stedman and Wolfram Zillig	76
Autoimmunity	Robert S Fujinami	108

B

Bacillus subtilis phages	H Ernest Hemphill	130
Bacterial identification – use of phages	Michael S DuBow	137

C

Cell structure and function in virus infections	Samual Dales	247
Cyanophages	Eugene L Martin and Tyler A Kokjohn	324
Cytokines and chemokines	Diane E Griffin	339

D

Defective interfering viruses	Laurent Roux	371
Diagnostic techniques		
Detection of viral antigens, nucleic acids and specific antibodies	Aloys CM Kroes and Linda FF Kox	388
Isolation and identification by culture and microscopy	Marie L Landry and GD Hsiung	395

E

Emerging and re-emerging virus diseases	Frederick A Murphy	418
Endogenous viruses	Bernard F Benkel	437

Enteric viruses	Ruth F Bishop	441
Epidemiology of viral diseases	Frederick A Murphy	482
Eye infections	James Chodash	522

F

Fish viruses	Carol H Kim and Jo-Ann Leong	558

G

Genetics of animal viruses	Frank Fenner	606

H

History of virology		
General	Frank Fenner	718
Bacteriophages	Donna H Duckworth	725
Polio, coxsackie, echo and other enteroviruses	Joseph L Melink	730
Honey bee viruses	Brenda V Ball and Leslie Bailey	743
Host genetic resistance	David G Brownstein	753
Host-controlled modification and restriction	Deklev H Krüger and Monika Reuter	758

I

Immune response		
General features	Gordon Ada	812
Cell mediated immune response	Janice Riberdy and Peter Doherty	818
Insect pest control by viruses	Davin Miller, David R O'Reilly and David Dall	842
Interference	Julius S Youngner and Patricia Whitaker-Dowling	850
Interferons – General features	Philip I Marcus	854

L

Latency	Jack G Stevens	897
Lysogeny and prophage	Max E Gottesman and Arnos Oppenheim	925

N

Nervous system viruses	Richard T Johnson	1013

O

Organ system infections	Jangu E Banatvala and Felicity Nicholson	1074

P

Pathogenesis		
Animal viruses	Kenneth L Tyler	1175
Plant viruses	James Culver	1184
Persistent viral infection	Maryann T Puglielli and Rafi Ahmed	1200
Phage ecology, evolution and speciation	Allan M Campbell	1208
Phage homologous recombination	Kenneth N Kreuzer	1213
Phage taxonomy and classification	Jack Maniloff, Hans-Wolfgang Ackermann and Audrey Jarvis	1221
Phage toxins and disease	Randall K Holmes, Michael G Jobling and Michael P Schmitt	1228
Phage transduction	Werner Arber	1234
Phages as cloning vehicles	Noreen E Murray	1240
Phages in industrial fermentations	Mary Ellen Sanders	1244
Phages in soil	Stanley T Williams, Martin A Mortimer and Jackie Parry	1248
Phages of *Streptococcus thermophilus*	Harold Brüssow	1253
Plant resistance to viruses		
Natural resistance	RSS Fraser	1300
Engineered resistance	C Michael Deom	1307
Plant retroelements	Roger Hull	1314
Plant virus disease – economic aspects	OW Barnett and Charles E Main	1318
Prions		
Human and Animal	Stanley B Prusiner	1388
Kuru	Carlo Masullo	1398
Yeast and Fungi	Marie-Lise Maddelein, Herman Edskes, Kim Taylor and Reed B Wickner	1402
Propagation of viruses		
Animal	Steffan Faisst	1408
Bacteria	Gail E Christie	1413
Plant	William M Wintermantel	1418

Q

Quasispecies	Esteban Domingo	1431

R

Recombination of viruses	Jozef J Bujarski	1446
Replication of viruses	V Gregory Chinchar	1471
Respiratory viruses	David O White and Lorena E Brown	1488
Retrotransposons of fungi	Jef Boeke	1503
Retroviral oncogenes	Paula J Enrietto, Gabriela Maldonado-Codina and Michael Hayman	1507
Retroviruses of Drosophila: The gypsy paradigm	Alain Bucheton, Alain Pélisson and Christophe Terzian	1526
Ribozymes	Robert H Symons	1551

S

Shrimp viruses	Philip C Loh	1625
Synergism – Plant viruses	Vickie Bowman Vance	1694

T

Taxonomy, classification and nomenclature of viruses	Claude M Fauquet	1730
Transformation – Animal viruses	Ron Wisdom and Inder M Verma	1817
Transplantation and virus infections	Robert A Krance, Helen E Heslop and Malcolm Brenner	1823
Tumor viruses – human	Herbert Pfister and Bernard Fleckenstein	1842

V

Vaccines and immune response	Gordon L Ada	1861
Vectors		
Animal viruses	Geoffrey Kitchingham and J Victor Garcia	1885
Plant viruses	Thomas Hohn and Rob Goldbach	1892
Vector transmission of plant viruses	Stewart M Gray and D'Ann Rochon	1899
Viral membranes	John Lenard	1920

Viral receptors	Horacio U Saragovi, Gordon J Sauvé and Mark I Greene	1926
Virus species	Marc HV Van Regenmortel	1937
Virus structure		
Atomic structure	Ming Luo	1943
Principles of virus structure	John E Johnson and Jeffrey Speir	1946
Virus–host cell interactions	Patricia Whitaker-Dowling and Julius S Youngner	1957

Z

Zoonoses	Thomas M Yuill	1987

VIRUS ENTRIES: ALPHABETICAL LISTING BY TAXA OF ENTRIES COVERING INDIVIDUAL VIRUSES

Adenoviridae	Adenoviruses		
	General features	Göran Wadell	1
	Molecular biology	Jörg Schröer, Stefan Kochanek, Marianna Hösel and Walter Doerfler	7
	Animal adenoviruses	William C Russell and Mária Benko	14
	Malignant transformation and oncology	Margaret R Quinlan	21
Arenaviridae	Lassa, Junin, Machupo and Guanarito viruses	Joseph B McCormick	887
	Lymphocytic chorio-meningitis virus		
	General features	Raymond M Welsh	915
	Molecular biology	Peter J Southern and Barbara J Meyer	920
	Arteriviruses	Margo Brinton	89
Ascoviridae	Ascoviruses	Brian A Federici	97
Asfarviridae	African swine fever virus	Maria L Salas	30
Astroviridae	Astroviruses	Stephan S Monroe	104
Baculoviridae	Baculoviruses		
	Granuloviruses	Doreen Winstanley and David O'Reilly	140
	Nucleopolyhedrovirus	George F Rohrmann	146
	Nonoccluded baculoviruses	John P Burand	1031
Barnaviridae	Barnaviruses	C Peter Romaine	152
Benyvirus	Benyviruses	Tetsuo Tamada	154
Birnaviridae	Birnaviruses – animal	Hermann Becht	160

Bornaviridae	Borna disease virus	Lothar Stitz and Rudolf Rott	167
Bromoviridae	Alfamovirus and ilarviruses	JF Bol	38
	Bromoviruses	Paul Ahlquist	198
	Cucumoviruses		
	General features	Marilyn Roossinck	315
	Molecular biology	Marilyn Roossinck	320
Bunyaviridae	Bunyaviruses		
	General features	Neal Nathanson and Francisco González-Scarano	204
	Replication	Richard M Elliott	212
	Hantaviruses	Connie S Schmaljohn	621
	Tospoviruses	James W Moyer	1803
Caliciviridae	Caliciviruses	Michael J Studdert	217
	Norwalk and related viruses	Mary K Estes and Isabelle Leparc-Goffart	1035
Capillovirus	Capilloviruses	Luis Falipe Salazar	222
Carlavirus	Carlaviruses	Sergei K Zavriev	238
Caulimoviridae	Plant pararetroviruses		
	Calimoviruses: general features	James E Schoelz and June E Bourque	1275
	Caulimoviruses: molecular biology	Thomas Hohn	1281
	Cassava vein mosaic virus	Alexandre de Kochko	1285
	Legume caulimoviruses	DVR Reddy and Richard D Richins	1289
	Rice tungro bacilliform virus	Roger Hull	1292
	Badnaviruses	Benham E Lockhart and Neil E Olszewski	1296
Closteroviridae	Closteroviruses	Sylvie German-Retana, Giovanni Martelli and Thierry Candresse	266
Comoviridae	Comoviruses	G George P Lomonossoff and Michael Shanks	285
	Fabaviruses	JI Cooper	531
	Nepoviruses	Mike A Mayo and AT Jones	1007
Coronaviridae	Coronaviruses	Kathryn V Holmes	291
	Toroviruses	Marian C Horzinek	1798
Cystoviridae	Phage $\phi6$	Dennis H Bamford	1205

Deltavirus	Hepatitis delta virus	Michael MC Lai	664
Filoviridae	Marburg and Ebola viruses	Hans-Dieter Klenk, Werner Slenczka and Heinz Feldmann	939
	Bovine diarrhea virus and Border disease virus	Edward J Dubovi	173
Flaviridae	Dengue viruses	Duane J Gubler	375
	Encephalitis viruses		
	Encephalitis viruses and related viruses causing hemorrhagic disease	James S Porterfield	424
	Tick-borne encephalitis and Wesselsbron viruses	EA Gould	430
	Hepatitis C virus	Robert H Purcell	657
	Hog cholera virus	Jan T Van Oirschot	738
	Japanese encephalitis virus	Akira Igarashi	871
	Yellow fever virus	Thomas P Monath	1979
Furovirus	Furoviruses	Yukio Shirako and T Michael A Wilson	587
Geminiviridae	Geminiviruses	KW Buck	597
Hepadnaviridae	Hepadnaviruses – Human hepatitis B virus		
	General features	William S Robinson	640
	Molecular biology	Christopher Seeger	645
	Hepadnaviruses – Avian hepatitis B virus	William Mason and Patricia Marion	650
Herpesviridae	Amphibian herpesviruses	Allan Granoff	51
	Bovine herpesvirus	Michael J Studdert	180
	Cytomegaloviruses		
	General features (human)	Edward S Mocarski, Jr	344
	Molecular biology (human)	Wade Gibson	351
	Animal cytomegaloviruses	Donald J Alcendor and Gary S Hayward	357
	Murine cytomegaloviruses	John Staczek	363
	Epstein-Barr virus		
	General features	Lawrence S Young	487
	Molecular biology	Jeffrey T Sample and Clare E Sample	494

Herpesviridae (cont.)	Equine herpesviruses	Dennis J O'Callaghan and Nikolaus Osterrieder	508
	Fish herpesviruses	Andrew J Davison	553
	Herpes simplex viruses		
	General features	Laure Aurelian	677
	Molecular biology	Edward K Wagner	686
	Herpesviruses 6 and 7 – human	Takuya Shimamoto and Koichi Yamanishi	697
	Herpesvirus sylvilagus	Peter G Medveczky	703
	Herpesviruses – baboon and chimpanzee	SS Kalter and RL Heberling	707
	Herpesviruses saimiri and ateles	Julia K Hilliard	714
	Marek's disease virus	LN Payne	945
	Pseudorabies virus	Saul Kit	1421
	Tree shrew herpesviruses	Christian A Tidona and Gholamreza Darai	1834
	Varicella-zoster virus		
	General features	Jeffrey I Cohen and Stephen E Straus	1872
	Molecular biology	William T Ruyechan and John Hay	1878
HEV-like viruses	Hepatitis E virus	Albert W Tam, Patrice O Yarbough and Daniel W Bradley	669
Hordeivirus	Hordeiviruses	Dianne M Lawrence and Andrew O Jackson	749
Hypoviridae	Hypoviruses	Donald L Nuss	804
Idaeovirus	Idaeoviruses	MA Mayo and AT Jones	809
Inoviridae	Filamentous phage	Robert E Webster	547
Iridoviridae	Frog virus 3	Rakesh M Goorha and Allan Granoff	582
	Iridoviruses – invertebrate	Richard Webby and James Kalmakoff	862
	Lymphocystis disease virus	Christian A Tidona and Gholamreza Darai	908
Leviviridae	Single-stranded RNA phages	J van Duin	1663
Luteoviridae	Luteoviruses	W Allen Miller	901
	Pea enation mosaic virus	Jihad S Skaf, Steven A Denler and Gustaaf A de Zoeten	1191

Microviridae	Coliphage φX174 and related phages	David T Denhardt	274
Myoviridae	Enterobacteria phage P1	Hansjörg Lehnherr and Jürg Meyer	455
	Mu-like phages	Michael S DuBow	981
	P2, 186 and related phages	Ian B Dodd and J Barry Egan	1087
	SPO1 phage	Charles R Stewart	1681
	T4-like phages	Gisela Mosig	1706
Nodaviridae	Nodaviruses	L Andrew Ball	1026
Orthomyxoviridae	Influenza viruses		
	General features	Robert G Webster	824
	Molecular biology	Peter Palese and Adolfo Garcia-Sastre	830
	Structure of antigens	Jonathan W Yewdell, Jack R Bennick and W Graeme Laver	836
Papillomaviridae	Papillomaviruses – human (*Papovaviridae*) –		
	General features	Gérard Orth	1105
	Molecular biology	Paul Lambert, Elsa Flores, Pirkko Heino and Shiyu Song	1115
	Papillomaviruses – animal	William C Phelps, Gary L Bream and Alison A McBride	1121
Paramyxoviridae	Measles virus	Sibylle Schneider-Schaulies and Volker ter Meulen	952
	Mumps virus	Bertus K Rima	988
	Newcastle disease virus	Peter T Emmerson	1020
	Parainfluenza viruses		
	Human	Allen Portner	1130
	Animal	Kailash C Gupta	1134
	Respiratory syncytial virus – human	Peter L Collins	1479
	Rinderpest and distemper viruses	Tom Barrett	1559
	Sendai virus	Mario Homma and Masato Tashiro	1616
Partitiviridae	Cryptoviruses	Robert G Milne and Cristina Marzachi	312
	Partitiviruses – fungal	Said A Ghabrial and Bradley I Hillman	1147
Parvoviridae	Densonucleosis viruses	Jacov Tal	384

Parvoviridae (cont.)	Parvoviruses		
	General features	Caroline R Astell	1151
	Molecular biology	Caroline R Astell	1155
	Cats, dogs and mink	Colin R Parrish	1159
	Rodents, pigs, cattle and waterfowl	Peter Tijssen, Mohamed Laakel, Zoltán Zádori and Benoît Hébert	1167
Pecluvirus	Pecluviruses	DVR Reddy, P Delfosse and Mike A Mayo	1196
Phycodnaviridae	Algal viruses	James L Van Etten	44
Picornaviridae	Cardioviruses	Douglas G Scraba and Ann C Palmenberg	229
	Coxsackieviruses	Bruno Pozzetto and Odette G Gaudin	305
	Echoviruses	Helena Kopecka	411
	Enteroviruses		
	Animal and related viruses	Elizabeth M Hoey and Samuel J Martin	461
	Human enteroviruses (serotypes 68–71)	Jeffrey W Almond and Margeruite Yin-Murphy	468
	Foot and mouth disease viruses	David J Rowlands	568
	Hepatitis A virus	Michael R Beard and Stanley M Lemon	631
	Picornaviruses – insect	Paul D Scotti and Peter D Christian	1267
	Polioviruses		
	General features	Philip D Minor	1326
	Molecular biology	Thomas Pfister, Caroline Mirzayan and Eckard Wimmer	1330
	Rhinoviruses	Glyn Stanway	1545
	Theiler's viruses	Howard L Lipton	1773
Podoviridae	Bacillus phage $\phi 29$	Margarita Salas	119
	Enterobacteria phage N4	Lucia Rothman-Denes	450
	Salmonella phage P22	Anthony R Poteete	1603
	T7-like phages	Ian J Molineux	1722
Polydnaviridae	Polydnaviruses	Don Stoltz	1349
Polyomaviride	JC and BK viruses	Richard J Frisque	876

Polyomaviride (cont.)	Polyomaviruses murine		
	General features	James M Pipas	1352
	Molecular biology	Walter Eckhart	1356
	Simian virus 40	Janet S Butel	1647
Pomovirus	Pomoviruses	L Torrance	1361
Potexvirus	Potexviruses	Mounir AbouHaidar and Duncan Gellatly	1364
Potyviridae	Potyviruses	Juan José López-Moya and Juan-Antonio Garcia	1369
Poxviridae	Cowpox virus	Derrick Baxby and M Bennett	298
	Entomopoxviruses	Richard W Moyer	474
	Fowlpox virus	Deoki N Tripathy and William M Schnitzlein	576
	Molluscum contagiosum virus	LC Archard, BA Soteriou and CD Porter	960
	Mousepox and rabbitpox viruses	Frank Fenner	973
	Parapoxviruses	Andrew Mercer and David Haig	1140
	Poxviruses		
	Capripoxviruses	R Paul Kitching	1376
	Leporipoviruses and suipoxviruses	Grant McFadden	1381
	Smallpox and monkeypox viruses	Keith Dumbell and Geoffrey L Smith	1668
	Vaccinia virus	Riccardo Wittek	1865
	Yabapox and Tanapox viruses	HA Rouhandeh	1971
Reoviridae	Cypoviruses	Serge Belloncik	332
	Orbiviruses and coltiviruses		
	General features	PPC Mertens	1043
	Molecular biology	Polly Ray and Peter PC Mertens	1062
	Phytoreoviruses	Bradley I Hillman and Donald L Nuss	1262
	Reoviruses		
	General features	Kenneth L Tyler	1454
	Molecular biology	WK Joklik	1464

VIRUS ENTRIES LISTED ACCORDING TO TAXA

Reoviridae (cont.)	Rotaviruses		
	General features	Robert D Shaw and Harry B Greenberg	1576
	Molecular biology	Mary K Estes	1583
Retroviridae	Avian type C retroviruses	John M Coffin	112
	Bovine immunodeficiency virus	Matthew A Gonda	184
	Bovine leukemia virus	Kathryn Radke	191
	Caprine arthritis encephalitis virus	Gilles Quérat and Robert Vigne	223
	Equine infectious anemia virus	Ronald C Montelaro	515
	Feline immunodeficiency virus	Janet K Yamamoto	535
	Feline leukemia and sarcoma viruses	James C Neil and David Onions	541
	Gibbon ape leukemia virus	Marvin S Reitz, Jr	617
	Human immunodeficiency viruses		
	General features	Luc Montaginer	763
	Molecular biology	Leon F García-Martínez and L Victor García-Martínez	774
	Anti-retroviral agents	Ranga V Srinivas and Arnold Fridland	778
	Human T-cell leukemia viruses		
	HTLV-1	Mitsuaki Yoshida	788
	HTLV-2	Bobbie J Rimel, Joseph D Rosenblatt and Vincente Planelles	794
	Lymphoproliferative disease virus of turkeys	Arona Gazit and Abraham Yaniv	911
	Mouse mammary tumor virus	Jackie P Dudley	965
	Murine leukemia viruses	Hung Fan	995
	Reticuloendotheliosis viruses	Radmila Hrdlickova, Jiri Nehyba and Henry R Bose	1496

Retroviridae (cont.)	Retroviruses – type D	Maja A Sommerfelt and Eric Hunter	1518
	Simian immunodeficiency viruses	Vito G Sasseville, Ronald C Desrosiers and Hillary G Morrison	1640
	Spumaviruses	Mel Campbell, Ayalew Mergia, Philip C Loh and Paul A Luciw	1685
	Visna-Maedi viruses	Opendra Narayan	1961
Rhabdoviridae	Chandipura, Piry and Isfahan viruses	P De Bishnu and Amiya K Banerjee	257
	Rabies virus	George M Baer and Noël Tordo	1437
	Rabies-like viruses	Robert E Shope	1442
	Rhabdoviruses		
	Plant rhabdoviruses	Andrew O Jackson, Michael Goodin, Ignacio Moreno, Jennifer Johnson and Diane M Lawrence	1531
	Ungrouped mammalian, bird and fish rhabdoviruses	P De Bishnu and Amiya K Banerjee	1541
	Sigma rhabdoviruses	Danielle Teninges	1635
	Vesicular stomatitis viruses	Luis L Rodriguez and Stuart T Nichol	1910
Satellites	P4 phage	Gianni Deho and Daniela Ghisotti	1094
	Satellite RNAs and satellite viruses	ME Taliansky and PF Palukaitis	1607
Sequiviridae	Sequiviruses	Mike A Mayo and AF Murant	1622
	Waikaviruses	Donald T Gordon	1965
Siphoviridae	Coliphage lambda	Allan M Campbell	281
	T1-like phages	JR Christensen	1701
	T5-like phages	D James McCorquodale	1716
Sobemovirus	Sobemoviruses	OP Sehgal	1674
Tectiviridae	Phage PRD1	Dennis H Bamford	1210
Tenuivirus	Tenuiviruses	Bryce W Falk	1756

Tetraviridae	Tetraviruses	Terry N Hanzlik and Karl HJ Gordon	1764
Tobamovirus	Tobamoviruses	Dennis J Lewondowski and William O Dawson	1780
Tobravirus	Tobraviruses	Peter B Vissler, Alexander Mathis and Hubb JM Linthorst	1784
Togaviridae	Chikungunya, O'nyong nyong and Mayaro viruses	Charles H Calisher	261
	Equine encephalitis viruses	Diane G Griffin	501
	Ross River virus and Barmah Forest virus	Lyn Dalgarno and Ian D Marshall	1570
	Rubella virus	Terly K Frey and Jerry S Wolinsky	1592
	Sindbis and Semliki Forest viruses	Miton J Schlesinger	1656
Tombusviridae	Carmoviruses	Feng Qu and T Jack Morris	243
	Dianthoviruses	Steven A Lommel	403
	Machlomoviruses	Steven A Lommel	935
	Necroviruses	Frank Meulewaeter	1003
	Tombusviruses	D'Ann Rochon	1789
Totiviridae	Giardiaviruses	Alice L Wang and Ching C Wang	613
	Totiviruses General features	Said A Ghabrial and Jean L Patterson	1808
	Ustilago maydis viruses	Jeremy Bruenn	1812
	Yeast RNA viruses	Lionel Bernard, Herman Edskes, Juan Carlos Ribas and Reed B Wickner	1974
Trichovirus	Trichoviruses	Sylvie German-Retana and Thierry Candresse	1837
Tymovirus	Tymoviruses	Adrian Gibbs	1850
Umbravirus	Umbraviruses	DJ Robinson and AF Murant	1855

VIRUS AND TAXA NAME CHANGES

Due to time constraints some, but not all, of the new virus and taxa names published in the 1999 Seventh ICTV Report[1] have been incorporated into the Encyclopedia entries.
New virus names, along with former names and the entries in which these viruses are discussed, are listed below.

New virus names	Former virus names	Entry title in the Encyclopedia	Page No.
Alpharetroviruses (*Retroviridae*)	Avian type C retroviruses	Avian type C retroviruses (*Retroviridae*)	112
Bacillus phage SPO1 (*Myoviridae*)	SPO1 phage	SPO1 phage (*Myoviridae*)	1681
Enterobacteria phage φX174 (*Microviridae*)	Coliphage φX174	Coliphage φX174 and related phages (*Microviridae*)	274
Enterobacteria phage lambda (*Siphoviridae*)	Coliphage lambda	Coliphage lambda (*Siphoviridae*)	281
Enterobacteria phage P2 (*Myoviridae*)	P2 phage	P2, 186 and related phages (*Myoviridae*)	1087
Enterobacteria phage 186 (*Myoviridae*)	186 phage	P2, 186 and related phages (*Myoviridae*)	1087
Enterobacteria phage P4 (*Satellites*)	P4 phage	P4 phage (*Satellites*)	1094
Enterobacteria phage PRD1 (*Tectiviridae*)	Phage PRD1	Phage PRD1 (*Tectiviridae*)	1210
Enterobacteria phage α3 (*Microviridae*)	Alpha 3 bacteriophage	Coliphage φX174 and related phages (*Microviridae*)	274
Enterobacteria phage BF23 "T5-like phages"	BF23 phage	T5-like phages (*Siphoviridae*)	1716
Enterobacteria phage G4 (*Microviridae*)	G4 bacteriophage	Coliphage φX174 and related phages (*Microviridae*)	274
Enterobacteria phage S13m (*Microviridae*)	S13m bacteriophage	Coliphage φX174 and related phages (*Microviridae*)	274
Pseudomonas phage φ6 (*Cystoviridae*)	Phage φ6	Phage φ6 (*Cystoviridae*)	1205

Additional Changes

The family *Papovaviridae* has been separated into two families: *Papillomaviridae* and *Polyomaviridae*.
The genera names of the family *Retroviridae* have been redefined as follows:

New names	Type Species	Former names
Alpharetrovirus	Avian leukosis virus	"Avian type C retroviruses"
Betaretrovirus	Mouse mammary tumor virus	"Mammalian type B retrovirus"
Gammaretrovirus	Murine leukemia virus	"Mammalian type C retrovirus"
Deltaretrovirus	Bovine leukemia virus	"BLV-HTLV retrovirus"
Epsilonretrovirus	Walleye dermal sarcoma virus	new
Lentivirus	Human immunodeficiency virus	Lentivirus
Spumavirus	Chimpanzee foamy virus	Spumavirus

[1] van Regenmortel et al, 1999. *Virus Taxonomy Seventh ICTV Report*. Academic Press, London.

CONTRIBUTORS

AbouHaidar, Mounir
Department of Botany
University of Toronto
25 Willcocks Street
Toronto, Ontario M5S 3B2
Canada

Ackerman, Hans-Wolfgang
Department de Biologie Medicale
Universite Laval, Faculte de Medicine
Cite Universitaire
Quebec PQ, G1K 7P4
Canada

Ada, GL
Division of Immunology and Cell Biology
John Curtin School of Medical Research
The Australian National University
Canberra, ACT 2601
Australia

Ahlquist, Paul
Institute for Molecular Virology
University of Wisconsin
Madison
Wisconsin, WI 53706-1596
USA

Ahmed, R
GRA Chair in Vaccine Research
Emroy University School of Medicine
Emroy Vaccine Center
1510 Clifton Road
Atlanta, Georgia GA 30322, USA

Alcendor, Donald J
Departments of Pharmacology and Oncology
Johns Hopkins School of Medicine
Baltimore
MD 21205
USA

Almond, Jeffrey W
School of Animal and Microbial Sciences
University of Reading
Whiteknights
Reading RG6 6AJ
UK

Arber, Werner
Biocentrum der Universitut, Basel
Abteilung Mikrobiologie
CH 4056
Basel
Switzerland

Archard, LC
Department of Biochemistry
Charing Cross and Westminster Medical School
London
W6 8RF
UK

Arnold, Hans Peter
Max-Planck-Institut fur Biochemie
Am Klopferspitz 18a
D-82152 Martinsried bei Munchen
Germany

Astell, Caroline R
Biochemistry of Molecular Biology
University of British Colombia
2146 Health Science Mall
Vancouver, BC V6T 1Z3
Canada

Aurelian, Laure
Virology/Immunology Laboratories
Dept of Pharmacology and Experimental
Therapeutics, University of Maryland
School of Medicine, Baltimore
Maryland MD 21201
USA

Baer, George M
Laboritoris Baer, SA
Cuautla 150
Col. Condesa
Mexico, 06140 DF
Mexico

Bailey, Leslie
20 West Common Grove
Harpenden
Hertfordshire, AL5 2AT
UK

Baker, James A
Institute for Animal Health
College of Veterinary Medicine
Cornell University
Ithica
USA

Ball, BV
Department of Entomology and Nematology
IACR-Rothamsted Experimental Station
Harpenden
Hertfordshire, AL5 2JQ
UK

Ball, L Andrew
Department of Microbiology
University of Alabama at Birmingham
BBRB 373/17
845 19th Street South, Birmingham,
Alabama AL 35294, USA

Bamford, DH
Institute of Biotechnology & Bioscience
Biocenter 2 (Room 6002)
PO Box 56 (Viikinkaari 5), 00014 University of Helsinki
Finland

Banatvala, Jangu E
Department of Virology
United Medical and Dental Schools
St Thomas's Hospital
London SE1 7EH
UK

Banerjee, Amiya K
Department of Molecular Biology
The Cleveland Clinic Foundation
9500 Euclid Avenue, NC20
Cleveland, Ohio OH 44195
USA

Barnett, OW
Department of Plant Pathology
North Carolina State University
Raleigh
North Carolina NC 27695
USA

Barrett, T
Molecular Biology Department
AFRC Institute for Animal Health
Pirbright Laboratory
Woking GU24 0NF
UK

Baxby, Derrick
Department of Medical Microbiology
University of Liverpool
PO Box 147
Liverpool L69 3BX
UK

Beard, Michael R
Department of Medicine, Microbiology and Immunology
The University of North Carolina at Chapel Hill
Chapel Hill
North Carolina NC 27599-7030
USA

Becht, Hermann
Institut fur Virologie
Tannenweg 12
35440 Linden
Germany

Belloncik, Serge
Centre de Recherche en Virologie
University du Quebec
Institute Armand Frappier
Laval, Quebec H7V 1B7
Canada

Bemoit, Herbert
Institut Armand-Frappier
Universite du Quebec
Laval
Quebec H7V 1B7
Canada

Benkel, Bernard
Agriculture and Agri-Food
Lethridge Research Centre
Livestock Sciences Section
Lethridge, Alberta T1J 4B1
Canada

Benko, Mária
Veterinary Research Institute
Hungarian Academy of Sciences
Budapest H-1581
Hungary

Bennett, M
Department of Medical Microbiology
University of Liverpool
PO Box 147
Liverpool L69 3BX
UK

Bennink, Jack R
Laboratory of Viral Diseases
NIAID-NIH
Bethesda
Maryland MD 20892
USA

Bernard, Lionel
Laboratory of Biochemistry and Genetics
NIDDK, NIH,
8 Centre Drive, MSC 0830
Bethesda, Maryland MD 20892-0830
USA

Bishop, Ruth F
Department of Gastroenterology
Royal Children's Hospital
Parkville
Victoria 3052
Australia

Boeke, JD
Department of Molecular Biology and Genetics
The Johns Hopkins University School of Medicine
Baltimore
Maryland MD 21205
USA

Bol, JF
Gorlaeus Laboratories
Leiden University
Einsteinweg 55, 2333 CC Leiden
P O Box 9502, 2300 RA Leiden
The Netherlands

Bose, Henry R
Department of Microbiology
University of Texas at Austin
2402 Speedway, ESB Room 226
Austin, Texas TX 78712-1095
USA

Bourque, June E
Plant Pathology
University of Missouri–Columbia
108 Waters Hall
Columbia, Missouri MO 65211
USA

Bradley, Daniel W
Virology Laboratory Section
Hepatitis Branch
Centers for Disease Control
Atlanta, Georgia GA 30333
USA

Bream, Gary L
Lineberry Research Associates
Research Triangle Park, PO Box 14626
North Carolina, NC 27709
USA

Brenner, M
Department of Hematology and Oncology
St Jude Children's Research Hospital
Memphis
Tennessee TN 38101
USA

Brenner, Malcolm K
Stem Cell Transplantation Program
Shell Center for Cell and Gene Therapy, Baylor
College of Medicine
Houston
Texas TX 77030
USA

Brinton, Margo A
Department of Biology
Georgia State University
Atlanta
Georgia GA 30302-4010
USA

Brown, Lorena
Department of Microbiology
University of Melbourne
Parkville, Victoria 3052
Australia

Brownstein, David G
Yale University School of Medicine
New Haven
Connecticut, CT-06510
USA

Bruenn, Jeremy
Department of Biological Sciences
663 Cooke
SUNY/Buffalo
Buffalo, New York NY 14260
USA

Brüssow, Harold
Nestlé Research Center Lausanne
PO Box 44
CH-1000
Lausanne 26
Switzerland

Bucheton, Alain
Institut de Genetique Humaine
CNRS 34396
Montpellier, Cedex
France

Buck, KW
Department of Biology
Imperial College of Science, Technology & Medicine
London SW7 2BB
UK

Bujarski, JJ
Plant Molecular Center
Northern Illinois University
Montgomery Hall
DeKalb, Illinois IL 60115
USA

Burand, John
Department of Entomology
University of Mass at Amherst
Fenald Building
Amherst, Massachusetts MA 01113
USA

Butel, JS
Division of Molecular Virology
Baylor College of Medicine
Houston
Texas TX 77030-3998
USA

Calisher, Charles H
Arthropod-borne Infectious Diseases Laboratory
Department of Microbiology
Foothills Campus, Colorado State University
Fort Collins, Colorado CO 80523-1682
USA

Campbell, Allan M
Department of Biological Science
Stanford University
Stanford
California CA 94305
USA

Campbell, Mel
Department of Medical Pathology
University of California
Davis
California CA 95016
USA

Candresse, Thierry
Station De Pathologie Végétalie
Institut National de la Recherche Agronomique
BP 81
3383 Villenave
D'Ornon, Cedex
France

Chinchar, V Gregory
Department of Microbiology
University of Mississippi
Medical Center, 2500 North State Street
Jackson, Mississippi MS 39216-4505
USA

Chodosh, James
Dean McGee Eye Institute
608 Stanton L. Young Blvd.
Oklahoma City, Oklahoma OK 73190
USA

Christensen, JR
105 Greenaway Road
Rochester
New York NY 14610
USA

Christian, Peter D
CSIRO Division of Entomology
PO Box 1700
Canberra, ACT 2601
Australia

Christie, Gail E
Department of Microbiology and Immunology
Virginia Commonwealth University
Richmond
VA 23298
USA

Coffin, John M
Department of Molecular Biology and Microbiology
Tufts University School of Medicine
136 Harrison Avenue
Boston, Massachusetts MA 02111
USA

Cohen, Jeffrey I
Medical Virology Section
Laboratory of Clinical Investigation
NIAID-NIH
Bethesda, Maryland MD 20892,
USA

Collins, PL
Laboratory of Infectious Diseases
NIAID-NIH
Bethesda
Maryland MD 20892
USA

Cooper, JI
Department of Plant Virology
Natural Environment Research Council
Institute of Virology and Environmental
Microbiology
Oxford OX1 3SR
UK

Culver, Jim
Center for Agricultural Biotechnology
University of Maryland
Room 6139, Plant Science Building #36
College Park, Maryland MD 20742
USA

Dales, Samuel
Pro.Bono Humani Generis
The Rockefeller University
1230 York Avenue
New York NY 10021-6399
USA

Dalgarno, L
Division of Biochemistry and Molecular Biology
School of Life Sciences
The Australian National University
Canberra ACT 2601
Australia

Dall, David
Division of Entomology
CSRIO
PO Box 1700
Canberra ACT 2601
Australia

Darai, Gholamreza
Institut fur Medizinisch Virologie
der Universitat Heidelberg
Im Neuenheimer Feld 324
D-6900 Heidelberg
Germany

Davison, Andrew J
MRC Virology Unit
Institute of Virology
Glasgow G11 5JR
Scotland, UK

Dawson, WO
University of Florida
Citrus Research and Education Center
Lake Alfred
Florida FL 33850
USA

De Bishnu, P
Department of Molecular Biology
The Cleveland Clinic Foundation
9500 Euclid Avenue, NC20
Cleveland, Ohio OH 44195
USA

De Kochko, Alex
ILTAB/TSRI-ORSTOM
TSRI, BCC206
10550N. Torrey Pines Road
La Jolla, California CA 92037
USA

De Zoeten, GA
Department of Botany and Plant Pathology
Michigan State University
East Lansing
Michigan MI 4882-4131
USA

Deho, PG
Dipartimento di Genetica e di Biologia
dei Microrganismi
Universita degli Studi di Milano
Via Celoria 26, 20133 Milan
Italy

CONTRIBUTORS

Delfosse, P
ICRISAT
Patancheru 502 324
Andhra Pradesh
India

Denhardt, David T
Department of Biological Sciences
Rutgers University
Piscataway
New Jersey NJ 08855-1059
USA

Denler, Steven A
Department of Botany and Plant Pathology
Michigan State University
East Lansing
Michigan MI 4882-4131
USA

Deom, Carl Michael
Department of Plant Pathology
College of Agricultural & Environmental Sciences
Julian H. Miller Plant Sciences Bldg
Athens, Georgia GA 30602-7274
USA

Desrosiers, RC
New England Regional Primate Research Center
Harvard Medical School
Southborough
Massachusetts MA 01772
USA

Dodd, Ian B
Department of Biochemistry
The University of Adelaide
Adelaide
South Australia 5000
Australia

Doerfler, Walter H
Institute für Genetik
Universität zu Köln
121 Weyertal
50931 Köln
Germany

Doherty, Peter
Department of Immunology
St Jude Children's Research Hospital
332 North Lauderdale Street, Memphis
Tennessee TN 38105-2794
USA

Domingo, Esteban
Centro de Biologia Molecular
Univ. Autonoma de Madrid
Canto Blanco
28049 Madrid
Spain

Dubovi, Edward J
Department of Population Medicine and
Diagnostic Science
College of Veterinary Medicine
Cornell University
Ithaca, New York NY 14853
USA

DuBow, Michael S
Department of Microbiology and Immunology
McGill University
Montreal
Quebec H3A 2B4
Canada

Duckworth, DH
Department of Immunology & Medical Microbiology
University of Florida
College of Medicine
Gainesville, Florida FL 32610
USA

Dudley, Jackie
Department of Microbiology, ESB 226
University of Texas at Austin
Austin, Texas TX 78712
USA

Dumbell, K
Department of Medical Microbiology
University of Cape Town Medical School
Cape 7925
South Africa

Eckhart, W
Arm and Hammer Center for Cancer Biology
The Salk Institute
San Diego
California CA 92186
USA

Edskes, Herman
Laboratory of Biochemistry and Genetics
NIDDK, NIH, Building 8, Room 225
8 Centre Drive, MSC 0830
Bethesda, Maryland MD 20892-0830
USA

Egan, JBM
Department of Biochemistry
The University of Adelaide
Adelaide
South Australia 5000
Australia

Elliott, Richard M
Institute of Virology
University of Glasgow, Church Street
Glasgow
G11 5JR
Scotland

Emmerson, PT
Department of Biochemistry and Genetics
Medical School
University of Newcastle upon Tyne
Newcastle upon Tyne NE2 4HH
UK

Enrietto, Paula J
Genomica Corporation
4100 Discovery Drive
Boulder
Colorado CO 80027
USA

Estes, MK
Division of Molecular Virology
Baylor College of Medicine
Houston
Texas TX 77030
USA

Faisst, S
Novo Nordisk AIS
Building SMH
Moerkhoej Bygade 28
DK-2860 Soeborg
Denmark

Falk, Bryce
Department of Plant Pathology
College of Agricultural & Environmental Sciences
University of California
Davis, California CA 95616
USA

Fan, H
Department of Molecular Biology and Biochemistry
University of California
Cancer Research Institute
Irvine, California CA 92717-3905
USA

Fauquet, Claude M
Division of Plant Biology BCC 206
The Scripps Research Institute
10550 North Torrey Pines Road
La Jolla, California CA 92037
USA

Federici, Brian A
Department of Entomology and Interdepartmental
Graduate Programme in Genetics
University of California
Riverside, California CA 92521
USA

Feldman, Heinz
Institut fur Virologie
der Philipps-Universitat
Robert-Koch-Str. 17
35037 Marburg
Germany

Fenner, Frank
John Curtin School of Medical Research
The Australian National University
Canberra
ACT 2601
Australia

Field, A Kirk
Department of Pharmacology and Toxicology
Umass Medical Centre
Worcester
Massachusetts, MA 01695
USA

Fleckenstein, B
Institut fur Klinische und Molekulare Virologie
Universitat Erlangen-Nurnberg
Schloßgarten 4
91054 Erlangen
Germany

Flores, Elsa
McArdle Cancer Center
University of Wisconsin
1400 University Avenue
Madison, Wisconsin WI 53706
USA

Fraser, RSS
Society for General Microbiology
Marlborough House
Basingstoke Road, Spencers Wood
Reading RG7 1AE
UK

Frey, Teryl K
Department of Biology
Georgia State University
PO Box 4010
Atlanta, Georgia GA 30302-4010
USA

Fridland, Arnold
Infectious Diseases
St Jude Children's Research Hospital
332 N. Lauderdale Street
Memphis, Tennessee TN 38105
USA

Frisque, Richard J
Department of Biochemistry & Molecular Biology
The Pennsylvania State University
University Park
Pennsylvania PA 16802
USA

Fujinami, Robert S
Department of Neurology
3R330 School of Medicine
University of Utah, 50 North Medical Drive
Salt Lake City, Utah UT 84132
USA

Garcia, Juan-Antonio
Centro National de Biotecnologia, CSIC
Campus Universidad Autonoma
28049 Cantoblanco
Madrid
Spain

Garcia-Martinez, J Victor
Virology & Molecular Biology
St Jude Children's Research Hospital
332 N Lauderdale Street
Memphis, Tennessee TN 38105
USA

Garcia-Martinez, Leon F
Virology & Molecular Biology
St Jude Children's Research Hospital
332 N Lauderdale Street
Memphis, Tennessee TN 38105
USA

Garcia-Sastre, Adolfo
Department of Microbiology
Mount Sinai School of Medicine
New York
NY 10029
USA

Gaudin, Odette G
Laboratoire de Bactériologie-Virologie
Université Jean Monnet Saint-Etienne
15 rue Ambroise Paré
42023 St Etienne Cedex 2
France

Gazit, Arnona
Department of Human Microbiology
Sackler School of Medicine
Tel Aviv University
Tel Aviv 69778
Israel

Gellatly, Duncan
Department of Botany
University of Toronto
25 Willcocks Street
Toronto, Ontario M5S 3B2
Canada

German-Retana, Sylvie
Station De Pathologie Végétalie
INRA, BP 81
3383 Villenave d'Ornon
Cedex 33883
France

Ghabrial, Said A
Department of Plant Pathology
University of Kentucky College of Agriculture
S-305 Agricultural Science Building – North
Lexington, Kentucky 40546-0091
USA

Ghisotti, Daniela
Dipartimento di Genetica e di Biologia
dei Microrganismi
Universita degli Studi di Milano
Via Celoria 26, 20133 Milan
Italy

Gibbs, A
Research School of Biological Sciences
The Australian National University
P.O. Box 475, ACT 2601
Canberra
Australia

Gibson, Wade
Department of Pharmacology and Molecular Sciences
Johns Hopkins University School of Medicine
Baltimore
Mississippi MS 21205
USA

Goldbach, Rob
Wageningen Agricultural University
Birnehaven 11/6709 PD
Wageningen
The Netherlands

Gonda, Matthew A
Program Resources, Inc./DynCorp
National Cancer Institute – Frederick Cancer
Research and Development Center
Frederick
Maryland MD 21702
USA

Gonzalez-Sarano, Francisco
Department of Microbiology
University of Pennsylvania
School of Medicine
Philadelphia, Pennsylvania PA 19104
USA

Goodin, Michael
Department of Plant Pathology
University of California Berkeley
College of Natural Resources
Berkeley, California CA 94720
USA

Goorha, Rakesh M
Department of Virology and Molecular Biology
St Jude Children's Research Hospital
Memphis
Tennessee TN 38101
USA

Gordon, Donald T
Department of Plant Pathology
Ohio State University
Ohio Agricultural Research Development Center
(OARTC)
1680 Madison Avenue
Wooster, Ohio OH 44691, USA

Gordon, Karl HJ
Division of Entomology
CSIRO
Box 1700
Canberra ACT 2601
Australia

Gottesman, Max E
Institute of Cancer Research
Columbia University
College of Physicians and Surgeons
701 West 168th Street, New York NY 10032
USA

Gould, EA
Institute of Virology and Environmental
Microbiology
Mansfield Road
Oxford OX1 3SR
UK

Granoff, Allan
Department of Virology and Molecular Biology
St Jude Children's Research Hospital
Memphis
Tennessee TN 38101
USA

Gray, Stewart M
USDA, ARS and Department of Plant Pathology
Cornell University
334 Plant Science Bldg.
Ithaca, New York NY 14853-4203
USA

Greenberg, Harry B
Division of Gastroenerology
Stanford University Medical School
Stanford, California CA 94305-5900
USA

Greene, Mark I
University of Pennsylvania School of Medicine
Philadelphia
Pennsylvania, PA-19104
USA

Griffin, Diane E
Department of Molecular Microbiology &
Immunology
Johns Hopkins University School of Hygiene
and Public Health, 615 N Wolfe Street
Baltimore, Maryland 21205
USA

Gubler, Duane J
Division of Vector-Borne Infectious Diseases
Centers for Disease Control
PO Box 2087
Fort Collins, California CA 80522
USA

Gupta, Kailash C
Laboratory of Molecular Microbiology
NIAID, NIH, Bldg 4, Room 315
4 Center Drive, MSC 0460
Bethesda, Maryland MD 20892-0460
USA

Haig, David
Moredun Research Institute
Edinburgh
UK

Hanzlik, Terry
Division of Entomology
CSIRO
Box 1700
Canberra ACT 2601
Australia

Hay, J
Department of Microbiology
State University of New York at Buffalo
138 Farber Hill, 3435 Main Street
Buffalo, New York NY 14214,
USA

Hayman, Mike
Molecular Genetics & Microbiology
University of New York at Stoneybrook
Stoneybrook
New York NY 11794-5222
USA

Hayward, Gary S
Departments of Pharmacology and Oncology
Johns Hopkins School of Medicine
Baltimore
Maryland MD 21205-2185
USA

Heberling, RL
Virus Reference Laboratories Inc.
7540 Louis Pasteur
San Antonio
Texas TX 78229
USA

Hébert, Benoît
Institut Armand-Frappier
Universite du Quebec
Lavel
Quebec H7N 4Z3
Canada

Heino, Pirkko
McArdle Cancer Center
University of Wisconsin
1400 University Avenue
Madison, Wisconsin WI 53706
USA

Hemphill, H Ernest
Department of Biology
Syracuse University
Syracuse
New York NY 13244
USA

Heslop, Helen E
Stem Cell Transplantation Program
Shell Center for Cell and Gene Therapy
Baylor College of Medicine
Houston
Texas TX 77030
USA

Hilliard, Julia K
Virology & Immunology
Southwest Fdn. for Biomed. Res.
7620 Northwest Loop 410
San Antonio, Texas TX 78228
USA

Hillman, Bradley I
Rutgers University, Cook College
Plant Pathology Department
339 Foran Hall
New Brunswick, New Jersey NJ 08901-8520
USA

Hoey, Elizabeth M
School of Biology and Biochemistry
The Queen's University of Belfast
Medical Biology Centre
Belfast BT9 7BL
Northern Ireland

Hohn, Thomas
Frederick Miescher Institute
PO Box 2543
Basel
CH 4002
Switzerland

Holmes, Kathryn V
University of Colorado
School of Medicine
4200 E. 9th Avenue, Campus Box B175
Denver, Colorada CO 80262
USA

Holmes, Randall K
University of Colorado Health Science Center
4200 E., 9th Avenue
Campus Box B175
Denver
Colorado, CO 80262
USA

Homma, M
Kobe Women's University
2-1, Aoyama Higashi-Suma
Suma-Ku,
Kobe 654
Japan

Horzinek, MC
Vakgroep Infectieziekten en Immunologie
Faculteit Diergeneeskunde
Rijksuniversitateit te Utrecht
PO Box 80.165, 3508 TD Utrecht
The Netherlands

Hösel, Marianna
Institute für Genetik
Universität zu Köln
121 Weyertal
50931 Köln
Germany

Hrdlickova, Radmila
Department of Microbiology
University of Texas at Austin
2402 Speedway, ESB Room 226
Austin, Texas TX 78712-1095
USA

Hsiung, GD
Virology Laboratory/113C
Veterans Administration Medical Center
Yale University
West Haven, Connecticut CT 06520
USA

Hull, Roger
Department of Virus Research
John Innes Institute
Colney Lane
Norwich, NR4 7UH
UK

Hunter, Eric
Department of Microbiology
University of Alabama at Birmingham
Birmingham, Alabama, AL 35294
USA

Igarashi, A
Department of Virology
Institute of Tropical Medicine
Nagasaki University
Nagasaki
Japan

Jackson, AO
Department of Plant Pathology
University of California Berkeley
College of Natural Resources
Berkeley, California CA 94720
USA

Jarvis, Audrey
New Zealand Dairy Research Institute
Microbia Genetics Section
Palmerston North
New Zealand

Jobling, Michael G
University of Colorado Health Science Center
Denver
Colorado, CO 80262
USA

Johnson, JE
Department of Biological Sciences
Purdue University
West Lafayette
Indiana IN 47907
USA

Johnson, RT
Department of Neurology
Johns Hopkins University School of Medicine
600 Wolfe Street, Meyer 6-181
Baltimore, Maryland MD 21287-7609
USA

Johnson, Jennifer
Department of Plant Pathology
University of California Berkeley
College of Natural Resources
Berkeley, California CA 94720
USA

Joklik, WK
Department of Microbiology
Duke University Medical Centre
E Jones Building, Room 410, PO Box 3020
Research Drive,
Durham, North Carolina NC 27710
USA

Jones, AT
Scottish Crop Research Institute
Invergowrie
Dundee
DD2 5DA
Scotland

Kalmakoff, James
Department of Microbiology
University of Otago
PO Box 56
Dunedin
New Zealand

Kalter, SS
Virus Reference Laboratories Inc.
7540 Louis Pasteur
San Antonio
Texas TX 78229
USA

Kim, Carol H
Department of Microbiology
Oregon State University
Corvillis
Oregon OR 97331-3804
USA

Kit, Saul
Novagene Inc
11935 Wink Road
Houston
Texas TX 77024
USA

Kitching, RP
World Reference Laboratory for Foot and Mouth Disease
Pirbright Laboratory
BAFRC Institute for Animal Health
Pirbright GU24 0NF
UK

Kitchingman, Geoffrey
Virology & Molecular Biology
St Jude Children's Research Hospital
332 N Lauderdale Street
Memphis, Tennessee TN 38105
USA

Klenk, H-D
Institut fur Virologie
der Philipps-Universitat
Robert-Koch-Str. 17
35037 Marburg
Germany

Kochko, Alexandre de
International Laboratory for Tropical Agricultural Biotechnology
La Jolla
California
USA

Kochanek, Stefan
Institute für Genetik
Universität zu Köln
121 Weyertal
50931 Köln
Germany

Kokjohn, Tyler A
Department of Biological Sciences
University of Nebraska
Lincoln
Nebraska NB 68588
USA

Kopecka, Helena
Unit de Virologie Moleculaire
Institut Pasteur
75724 Paris-Cedex
France

Kokjoh, Tyler A
Department of Biological Sciences
University of Nebraska
Lincoln
Nebraska N6 68588
USA

Kox, Linda FF
Clinical Virology Laboratory, Department of
Virology
University Hospital Leiden
PO Box 9600
2300 RC Leiden
The Netherlands

Krance, Robert A
Stem Cell Transplantation Program
Shell Center for Cell and Gene Therapy
Baylor College of Medicine
Houston
Texas TX 77030
USA

Kreuzer, Kenneth N
Department of Microbiology
Duke University Medical Center
Durham
North Carolina NC 27710
USA

Kroes, Aloys CM
Clinical Virology Laboratory, Department of
Virology
University Hospital Leiden
PO Box 9600
2300 RC Leiden
The Netherlands

Krüger, DH
Institüt für Med. Virologie
Universitätsklinikum Charité
Medizinische Fakultät der Humboldt-Universität zu Berlin
D-10098 Berlin
Germany

Laakel, Mohamed
Institut Armand-Frappier
Universite du Quebec
Laval
Quebec H7V 1B7
Canada

Lai, Michael MC
Howard Hughes Medical Institute
Department of Molecular Microbiology and
Immunology
University of Southern California School of Medicine
2011 Zonal Avenue, HMR-401
Los Angeles, CA 90033, USA

Lambert, Paul
McArdle Cancer Center
University of Wisconsin
1400 University Avenue
Madison, Wisconsin WI 53706
USA

Landry, Marie L
Virology Reference Laboratory
VA Connecticut Healthcare System
West Haven
Connecticut CT 06520
USA

Laughlin, Catherine A
NIAID
Bethesda
Maryland MD 20892
USA

Laver, W Graeme
Influenza Research Unit
John Curtin School of Medical Research
The Australian National University
Canberra
Australia

Lawrence, Dianne M
Department of Plant Pathology
University of California Berkeley
College of Natural Resources
Berkeley, California CA 94720
USA

Lehnherr, Hansjörg
Odense Universitet
Institut fur Molekylaer Biologi
Campusvej 55
DK-5230 Odense M
Denmark

Lemon, Stanley M
Department of Medicine, Microbiology and
Immunology
The University of North Carolina at Chapel Hill
Chapel Hill
North Carolina NC 27599-7030
USA

Lenard, J
Department of Physiology and Biophysics
Robert Wood Johnson Medical School
University of Medicine and Dentistry of New Jersey
Piscataway, New Jersey NJ 08854
USA

Leong, Jo-Ann
Department of Microbiology
Oregon State University
Corvillis
Oregon OR 97331-3804
USA

Leparc-Goffart, Isabelle
Division of Molecular Virology
Baylor College of Medicine
Houston
Texas TX 77030
USA

Lewandowski, Dennis J
University of Florida
Citrus Research and Education Center
Lake Alfred
Florida FL 33850
USA

Linthorst, HJM
Institute of Molecular Plant Sciences
Gorlaeus Laboratories
PO Box 9502
2300 RA Leiden
The Netherlands

Lipton, HL
Division of Neurology
Evanston Hospital
Evanston
Illinois IL 60201
USA

Lockhart, Benham E
Department of Plant Biology
University of Minnesota
220 Biological Sciences Center
145 Gortner Avenue, Minnesota MN 55108-1095
USA

Loh, Philip C
Department of Microbiology
University of Hawaii at Manoa
Honolulu
Hawaii HI 96822
USA

Lommel, Steven A
Department of Plant Pathology
North Carolina State University
College of Agriculture and Life Sciences
Raleigh, North Carolina NC 27675
USA

Lomonossoff, G George P
Department of Virus Research
John Innes Institute
Norwich
NR4 7UH
UK

Lopez-Moya, Juan José
Centro National de Biotecnologia, CSIC
Campus Universidad Autonoma
Cantoblanco
28049 Madrid
Spain

Luciw, PA
Department of Medical Pathology
University of California
Davis
California CA 95616
USA

Luo, M
Center for Macromolecular Crystallography
The University of Alabama at Birmingham
Birmingham
Alabama AL 35127
USA

Maddelein, Marie-Lise
Laboratory of Biochemistry and Genetics, National Institute of Diabetes, Digestive and Kidney Diseases
National Institutes of Health
Building 8 Room 225
8 Center Drive MSC 0830, Bethesda
Maryland MD 20802-0830
USA

Main, Charles E
Department of Plant Pathology
North Carolina State University
Campus Box 7616
Raleigh
North Carolina NC 27695-7616
USA

Maldonado-Codina, Gabriela
Genomica Corporation
4100 Discovery Drive
Boulder
Colorado CO 80027
USA

Maniloff, Jack
Department of Microbiology and Immunology
University of Rochester Medical Center
601 Elmwood Avenue, Box 672
Rochester, New York NY 14642
USA

Marcus, Philip I
Department of Molecular and Cell Biology
The University of Connecticut
75 North Eagleville Road, Rm. TLS 265
Storrs, Connecticut CT 06269-3044
USA

Marion, Patricia
Division of Gastroenterology
Stanford University Medical Centre
Stanford
California CA 94305
USA

Marshall, Ian D
Division of Biochemistry and Molecular Biology
School of Life Sciences
The Australian National University
Canberra ACT 2601
Australia

Martelli, Giovanni
Dipartimento di Protezione delle Piante dalle Malatie
Universita degli Studi and Centro di Studi del CNR
sui Virus delle Colture
Mediteranee, Via Amendola 165/A
Bari 70126
Italy

Martin, Eugene L
Department of Biological Sciences
University of Nebraska
Lincoln
Nebraska NB 68588
USA

Martin, Samuel J
School of Biology and Biochemistry
The Queen's University of Belfast
Medical Biology Centre
Belfast BT9 7BL
Northern Ireland

Marzachi, Cristina
Consiglio Nazionale delle Ricerche
Istituto di Fitovirologia Applicata
Strada delle Cacce, 73
10135 Torino
Italy

Mason, William
Institute for Cancer Research
Fox Chase Cancer Center, 7701 Burholme Avenue
Philadelphia
PA 19111
USA

Masullo, Carlo
Institute of Neurology
Catholic University School of Medicine
00168 Roma
Italy

Mathis, Alexander
Institute of Molecular Plant Sciences
Gorlaeus Laboratories
PO Box 9502
2300 RA Leiden
The Netherlands

Mayo, Mike A
Scottish Crop Research Institute
Invergowrie
Dundee
DD2 5DA
Scotland

McBride, Alison A
National Institute of Allergy and Infectious Diseases,
Laboratory of Viral Diseases,
Building 4 Room 137
Bethesda
Maryland MD20892
USA

McCormick, JB
Institut Pasteur
28 Rue du Roux
75015 Paris
France

McCorquodale, DJ
858 Balton Court
Naperville
Illinois IL 60563
USA

CONTRIBUTORS

McFadden, G
Department of Biochemistry
University of Alberta
Edmonton
Alberta T6G 2H7
Canada

Medveczky, Peter G
Department of Medical Microbiology and Immunology
College of Medicine, University of South Florida
12901 Bruce B Downs Blvd
Tampa, Florida FL 33620
USA

Melnick, JL
Division of Molecular Virology
Baylor College of Medicine
Houston
Texas TX 77030
USA

Mercer, Andrew
Virus Research Unit
Department of Microbiology
University of Otago
PO Box 56, Dunedin
New Zealand

Mergia, Ayalew
Department of Medical Pathology
University of California
Davis
California CA 95616
USA

Mertens, PPC
Division of Molecular Biology
Pirbright Laboratory
AFRC Institute for Animal Health
Pirbright, Woking, Surrey GU24 0NF
UK

Meulen, Volker ter
University Professor
Institut fuer Virologie und Immunbiologie
Universitat Wurzburg
Versbatcher Str.7, D-97078 Wuerzburg
Germany

Meulewaeter, Frank
Plant Genetic Systems
University of Gent
Josef Plateaustraat 22-B
9000 Gent
Belgium

Meyer, Barbara J
Department of Microbiology
University of Minnesota
Minneapolis
MN 55455
USA

Meyer, Jürg
Dental Center
University of Basel
Detersplatz 14, CH-4051
Basel
Switzerland

Miller, Davin
Department of Biology
Imperial College of Science, Technology and Medicine
Prince Consort Road
London SW7 2AZ
UK

Miller, WA
Department of Plant Pathology
Iowa State University
Ames
Iowa IA 50011-1020
USA

Milne, Robert G
Consiglio Nazionale delle Ricerche
Istituto di Fitovirologia Applicata
Strada delle Cacce, 73
10135 Torino
Italy

Minor, PD
Division of Virology
National Institute for Biological Standards and Control
Blanche Lane, South Mimms
Potters Bar, Herts EN6 3QG
UK

Mirzayan, Caroline
Department of Microbiology
State University of New York Stony Brook
Stony Brook
New York, NY 11794-5222
USA

Mocarski Jr, Edward S
Department of Microbiology and Immunology
Stanford University School of Medicine
Stanford
California CA 94305-5402
USA

Molineux, IJ
Department of Microbiology
The University of Texas at Austin
Austin
Texas TX 78712-1095
USA

Monath, Thomas P
OraVax, Inc.
38 Sidney Street
Cambridge
Massachusetts MA 02139
USA

Monroe, Stephan S
DVRD
CDC & Prevention
1600 Clifton Road, GO4
Atlanta, Georgia GA 30333
USA

Montagnier, Luc
Institut Pasteur
Viral Oncology Unit
75724 Paris Cedex 15
France

Montelaro, Ronald C
Department of Molecular Genetics and Biochemistry
University of Pittsburgh
Biomedical Science Tower, Room W1144
Pittsburgh, Pennsylvania PA 15261
USA

Moreno, Ignacio
Department of Plant Pathology
University of California Berkeley
College of Natural Resources
Berkeley, California CA 94720
USA

Morris, T Jack
School of Biological Sciences
University of Nebraska
Lincoln
Nebraska NE 68588-0118
USA

Morrison, Hillary G
Marine Biological Laboratory
Woods Hole
Massachusettes MA 02543
USA

Mortimer, A Martin
School of Biological Sciences
University of Liverpool
PO Box 147
Liverpool L69 3BX
UK

Mosig, G
Department of Molecular Biology
Vanderbilt University
Nashville
Tennessee TN 37235
USA

Moyer, JW
Plant Pathology
North Carolina State University
2506 Gardner
Campus Box 7616
Raleigh, North Carolina NC 27695, USA

Moyer, Richard W
Department of Molecular Genetics and Microbiology
University of Florida
College of Medicine
Gainesville, Florida FL 32610-0266
USA

Murant, AF
Scottish Crops Research Institute
Invergowrie
Dundee DD2 5DA
Scotland

Murphy, Frederick A
School of Veterinary Medicine
University of California
Davis, California
CA 95616-8734
USA

Murray, Noreen E
Division of Biological Sciences, Institute of Cell and Molecular Biology
The University of Edinburgh
King's Buildings
Mayfield Road, Edinburgh
EH9 3JR, UK

Narayan, O
Johns Hopkins School of Medicine
Baltimore
Maryland MD 21287
USA

Nathanson, Neal
Department of Microbiology
University of Pennsylvania
School of Medicine
Philadelphia, Pennsylvania PA 19104
USA

Nehyba, Jiri
Department of Microbiology
University of Texas at Austin
2402 Speedway, ESB Room 226
Austin, Texas TX 78712-1095
USA

Neil, James C
Department of Veterinary Pathology
University of Glasgow Veterinary School
Bearsden Road
Glasgow G61 1QH
Scotland

Nichol, Stuart T
Special Pathogens Branch
Division of Rickettsial Diseases, National Center for Infectious Diseases and Prevention
Atlanta
Georgia, GA 30333
USA

Nicholson, Felicity
Trailfinders Travel Clinic
Kensington
London
UK

Nuss, Donald L
Center for Agricultural Biotechnology
University of Maryland
2115 Agricultural Life Sciences Bldg
College Park, Maryland MD 20742-1582
USA

O'Callaghan, Dennis J
Department of Microbiology and Immunology
Louisiana State University Medical Center
1501 Kings Highway
Shreveport, Los Angeles LA 71130
USA

Olszewski, Neil E
Department of Plant Biology
University of Minnesota
220 Biological Sciences Center
145 Gortner Avenue, Minnesota MN 55108-1095
USA

Onions, David
Department of Veterinary Pathology
University of Glasgow Veterinary School
Bearsden Road
Glasgow G61 1QH
Scotland

Oppenheim, Arnos
Department of Medical Genetics
Hebrew University
Hadassah Medical School
Jerusalem
Israel

O'Reilly, David R
Department of Biology
Imperial College of Science, Technology and Medicine
Prince Consort Road
London SW7 2AZ
UK

Orth, Gerard
Unite des Papillomavirus, INSERM U.190
Institut Pasteur
75015 Paris
France

Osterrieder Nikholas
Federal Research Centre for Virus Diseases of Animals
Friedrich-Loeffler-Institutes
Insel Rimes
Germany

Owens, RA
Molecular Plant Pathology Laboratory
Beltsville Agricultural Research Center
Bldg. 011A, 252, BARC-West
Beltsville, Maryland MD 20705-2350
USA

Palese, Peter
Department of Microbiology
Mount Sinai School of Medicine
New York
NY 10029
USA

Palmenberg, Ann C
Institute for Molecular Virology
Department of Biochemistry
University of Wisconsin-Madison
1655 Linden Drive
Madison, Wisconsin WI 53706
USA

Palukaitis, PF
Virology Department
Scottish Crop Research Institute
Invergowie
Dundee, DD2 5DA
UK

Paoletti, Euzo
297 Murray Avenue
Delmar
NY 12054
USA

Parrish, CR
James A Baker Institute
New York State College of Veterinary Medicine
Cornell University
Ithaca, NY 14853
USA

Parry, Jackie
Division of Biological Sciences
Lancaster University
Lancaster
LA1 4YQ
UK

Patterson, Jean L
Department of Virology and Immunology
Southwest Foundation for Biomedical Research
PO Box 760549
San Antonio
Texas TX 78245-0549
USA

Payne, LN
Institute for Animal Health
Compton
Nr Newbury
Berks. RG20 7NN
UK

Pélisson, Alain
Institut de Genetique Humaine
CNRS 34396
Montpellier, Cedex
France

Pfister, Herbert
Institute for Virology
University of Koln
50935 Koln
Germany

Pfister, Thomas
State University of New York Stony Brook
Stony Brook
New York, NY 11794-5222
USA

Phelps, WC
Department of Virology
Glaxo Welcome
Five Moore Drive
RTP, North Carolina NC 27709
USA

Pipas, JM
Department of Biological Sciences
University of Pittsburgh
Pittsburgh
PA 15260
USA

Planelles, Vincente
Division of Hematology Oncology
University of Rochester
601 Elmwood Avenue, Box 704
Rochester, New York NY 14642
USA

Porter, CD
Institute for Cancer Research
London WG1N 1EH
UK

Porterfield, James S
"Green Valleys"
Goodleigh
Barnstaple
Devon EX32 7NH
UK

Portner, A
Department of Virology and Molecular Biology
St Jude Children's Research Hospital
Memphis
Tennessee TN 38101
USA

Poteete, Anthony R
Molecular Genetics & Microbiology Department
University of Massachusetts Medical Center
55 Lake Avenue North
Worcester, Massachusetts MA 01655
USA

Pozzetto, Bruno
Laboratoire de Bactériologie-Virologie
Université Jean Monnet Saint-Etienne
15 rue Ambroise Paré
42023 St Etienne Cedex 2
France

Prusiner, Stanley B
Department of Neurology
University Cal-San Francisco
P.O. Box 0518
HSE 781
San Francisco, California CA 94143-0518
USA

Puglielli, Maryann T
Emory University Vaccine Center
1510 Clifton Road
Atlanta
Georgia GA 30322
USA

Purcell, Robert H
Hepatitis Viruses Section
Laboratory of Infectious Diseases
NIAID-NIH
Bethesda, Maryland MD 20892
USA

Qu, Feng
School of Biological Sciences
University of Nebraska
Lincoln
Nebraska NB 68588-0118
USA

Quérat, Gilles
INSERM U372
Campus de Luminy
13276 Marseille Cedex 9
France

Quinlan, Margaret
Department of Microbiology and Immunology
University of Tennessee
858 Madison Avenue
Memphis, Tennessee TN 38163
USA

Radke, Kathryn
Avian Sciences Department
University of California
Davis
California CA 95616-8532
USA

Reddy, DVR
ICRISAT
Patancheru PO
Pradesh 502 324
Andhra Pradesh
India

Reitz Jr, Marvin S
Division of Basic Sciences
Institute of Human Virology
University of Maryland
725 W. Lombard Street
Baltimore, Maryland MD 71201, USA

Reuter, Monica
Institüt für Med. Virologie
Universitätsklinikum Charité
Medizinische Fakultät der Humboldt-Universität zu Berlin
D-10098 Berlin
Germany

Ribas, Juan Carlos
Laboratory of Biochemistry and Genetics
NIDDK, NIH,
8 Centre Drive, MSC 0830
Bethesda, Maryland MD 20892-0830
USA

Riberdy, Janice
Department of Immunology
St Jude Children's Research Hospital
332 North Lauderdale Street, Memphis
Tennessee TN 38105-2794
USA

Richins, Richard D
Department of Plant Pathology
University of California
Riverside
California, CA 92521
USA

Rima, BK
Division of Molecular Biology
School of Biology & Biochemistry
The Queen's University of Belfast
Medical Biology Centre
Belfast BT9 7BL
Northern Ireland

Rimel, Bobbie J
Division of Hematology Oncology
University of Rochester
601 Elmwood Avenue, Box 704
Rochester, New York NY 14642
USA

Robinson, DJ
Scottish Crops Research Institute
Invergowrie
Dundee DD2 5DA
Scotland

Robinson, William S
Department of Medicine, Division of
Infectious Diseases
Stanford University Medical Center
Stanford
California CA 94305
USA

Rochon, D'Ann
Agriculture & Agri-food Canada
Pacific Agri-food Research Centre
Summerlard, B.C.
V0H 1Z0
Canada

Rodriguez, Luis L
Plum Island Animal Disease Center
ARS/USDA
PO Box 848
Greenport, New York NY 11944-0848
USA

Rohrmann, George F
Department of Microbiology
Oregon State University
Corvallis
Oregon OR 97331-3804
USA

Romaine, C Peter
Pennsylvania State University
Department of Plant Pathology
215 Buckholt Lab.
University Park
Pennsylvania PA 16802
USA

Roossinck, Marilyn
Plant Biology Division, The Samuel Roberts
Noble Foundation
2510 Sam Noble Parkway
PO Box 2180
Ardmore, Oklahoma OK 73402
USA

Rosenblatt, Joseph D
Division of Hematology Oncology
University of Rochester
601 Elmwood Avenue, Box 704
Rochester, New York NY 14642
USA

Rothman-Denes, Lucia B
Department of Molecular Genetics and Cell Biology
University of Chicago
Chicago
Illinois IL 60637
USA

Rott, Rudolf
Institut fur Virologie
Justus-Liebig-Universitat Giessen
D-35392 Giessen
Germany

Rouhandeh, HA
Torrey Pines Cancer and Aids Research Institute, Inc.
9853 Pacific Heights Blvd, Suite G
San Diego
California CA 92121
USA

Roux, Laurent
Department of Genetics and Microbiology
University of Geneva Medical School
Geneva 4
Switzerland

Rowlands, David J
Department of Microbiology
University of Leeds
Leeds LS 29JT
UK

Roy, Polly
NERC Institute of Virology and Environmental Microbiology
Mansfield Road
Oxford
OX1 3SR
UK

Russell, William C
Division of Cell and Molecular Biology
School of Biological and Medical Sciences
University of St Andrews, Irvine Bldg., North St.
St Andrews, Fife, KY16 9AL
Scotland

Ruyechan, William T
Department of Microbiology
State University of New York at Buffalo
138 Farber Hill, 3435 Main Street
Buffalo, New York NY 14214,
USA

Salas, Margarita
Centro de Biologica Molecular (CSIC-VAM)
Universidad Autonoma de Madrid
Canto Blanco
28049 Madrid
Spain

Salazar, Luis Falipe
Centro International de la Papa
Department of Pathology
International Potato Center (CIP), A.P. Postal 1558
Lima 100
Peru

Sample, Clare E
Department of Virology and Molecular Biology
St Jude Children's Research Hospital
332 North Lauderdale
Memphis, Tennessee TN 38105
USA

Sample, Jeffery T
Department of Virology and Molecular Biology
St Jude Children's Research Hospital
332 North Lauderdale
Memphis, Tennessee TN 38105
USA

Sanders, Mary Ellen
Dairy and Food Culture Technologies
7119 South Glencoe Court
Littleton, Colorado CO 80122
USA

Saragovi, Horacio U
University of Pennsylvania School of Medicine
Philadelphia
Pennsylvania, PA-19104-6082
USA

Sasseville, Vito G
New England Regional Primate Research Center
Harvard Medical School
Southborough
Massachusetts MA 01772
USA

Sauvé, Gordon J
University of Pennsylvania School of Medicine
Philadelphia
Pennsylvania, PA-19104-6082
USA

Schlesinger, MJ
Department of Molecular Microbiology
Washington University School of Medicine
660 South Euclid
St Louis, Missouri MO 63110-1093
USA

Schmaljohn, Connie S
Department of Molecular Virology, Virology Division
USAMRIID Annex
1301 Ditto Avenue
Ft Detrick, Maryland MD 21701-5011
USA

Schmidt, Michael P
Laboratory of Bacterial Toxins, Center for Biologics Evaluation and Research
Food and Drug Administration
Building 29 Room 108
8800 Rockville Pike, Bethesda,
Maryland, MD 20892
USA

Schneider Schaulies, Sibylle
Institut fur Virologie und Immunbiologie
Universitat Wurzburg
Versbatcher Str.7, D-97078 Wuerzburg
Germany

Schitzlein, William M
Department of Veterinary Pathology
College of Veterinary Medicine
University of Illinois
Urbana, Illinois IL 61802
USA

Schoelz, James E
Plant Pathology
University of Missouri
108 Waters Hall
Columbia, Missouri MO 65211
USA

Schröer, Jörg
Institute für Genetik
Universität zu Köln
121 Weyertal
50931 Köln
Germany

Scraba, Douglas G
Department of Biochemistry
4–55 Medical Sciences Building
University of Alberta
Edmonton T6G 2H7
Canada

Scotti, PD
The Horticulture and Food Research Institute of New Zealand
Private Bag 92169
Mt Albert Research Centre
Auckland
New Zealand

Seeger, Christopher
Institute for Cancer Research
Fox Chase Cancer Center
Philadelphia
Pennsylvania PA 19111
USA

Sehgal, OP
Department of Plant Pathology, Plant Sciences Unit
University of Missouri-Columbia
College of Agriculture, Food & Natural Resources
108 Waters Hall, Columbia
Missouri MO 65211
USA

Shanks, Michael
Department of Virus Research
John Innes Institute
Norwich
NR4 7UH
UK

Shaw, RD
Research Service (151)
Northport VA Medical Center
Research Service
Northport, New York NY 11768
USA

Shimamoto, Yakayua
Department of Microbiology
Faculty of Medicine
Osaka University
Osaka 565
Japan

Shirako, Y
University of Tokyo
1-1-1 Yayoi
Bunkyo-ku
Tokyo 113-8657
Japan

Shope, Robert E
Center for Tropical Diseases
University of Texas Medical Branch
301 University Boulevard
Texas TX 77555-0609
USA

Skaf, Jihad S
Department of Botany and Plant Pathology
Michigan State University
East Lansing
Michigan MI 4882-4131
USA

Slenczka, Werner
Institut fur Virologie
der Philipps-Universitat
Robert-Koch-Str. 17
35037 Marburg
Germany

Smith, Geoffrey L
Sir William Dunn School of Pathology
University of Oxford
South Parks Road
Oxford OX1 3RE
UK

Sommerfelt, Maja A
Department of Microbiology and Immunology
Gades Institute
University of Bergen
N-5020 Bergen
Norway

Song, Shiyu
McArdle Cancer Center
University of Wisconsin
1400 University Avenue
Madison, Wisconsin WI 53706
USA

Soteriou, BA
Division of Biomedical Sciences
Imperial College, School of Medicine
London W6 8RF
UK

Southern, PJ
Department of Microbiology
University of Minnesota
Minneapolis
MN 55455
USA

Srinivas, Ranga V
Infectious Diseases
St Jude Children's Research Hospital
332 N. Lauderdale Street
Memphis, Tennessee TN 38105
USA

Staczek, John
Department of Microbiology and Immunology
Louisiana State University Medical Center
1501 Kings Highway
Shreveport, Los Angeles LA 71130
USA

Stanway, G
Department of Biological Sciences
University of Essex
Wivenhoe Park
Colchester CO4 3SQ
UK

Stedman, Kenneth M
Max-Planck-Institut fur Biochemie
Am Klopferspitz 18a
D-82152 Martinsried bei Munchen
Germany

Stevens, Jack G
Department of Microbiology and Immunology
University of California
Los Angeles
California, CA-90024
USA

Stewart, Charles R
Department of Biochemistry and Cell Biology
Wiess School of Natural Sciences
Rice University
Houston, Texas TX 77005
USA

Stitz, Lothar
Institut fur Virologie
Justus-Liebig-Universitat
D-35392 Giessen
Germany

Stoltz, D
Department of Microbiology
Dalhousie University
Halifax
Nova Scotia, B3H 4H7
Canada

Straus, Stephen E
Medical Virology Section
Laboratory of Clinical Investigation
NIAID-NIH
Bethesda, Maryland MD 20892,
USA

Studdert, Michael J
The University of Melbourne
School of Veterinary Science
Flemington Road, Parkville
Victoria 3052
Australia

Symons, Robert
Department of Plant Science
Waite Institute
University of Adelaide
Glenn Osmond SA 5064
Australia

Tal, Jacov
Department of Virology
Faculty of Health Sciences
Ben-Gurion University of the Negev
Beer-Sheva 84105
Israel

Taliansky, ME
Virology Department
Scottish Crop Research Institute
Invergowie
Dundee, DD2 5DA
UK

Tam, Albert W
Genelabs Technology, Inc.
505 Penobscot Drive
Redwood City
California CA 94063
USA

Tamada, Tetsuo
Research Institute for Bioresources
Okayama University
Kurashiki, 710
Japan

Tashiro, Masato
Department of Viral Diseases and Vaccine Control
National Institute of Infectious Diseases
Toyama 1-23-1, Shinjuku-Ku
Tokyo 102
Japan

Taylor, Kim
Laboratory of Biochemistry and Genetics, National
Institute of Diabetes, Digestive and Kidney Diseases
National Institutes of Health
Building 8, Room 225
8 Center Drive MSC 0830, Bethesda
Maryland MD 20802-0830
USA

Teninges, D
Centre de Genetique Moleculaire – CNRS
Institut de Genetique humaine
91198 Gif sur Yvette Cedex 5
Montpellier
France

Terzian, Christophe
Institut de Genetique Humaine
CNRS 34396
Montpellier, Cedex
France

Tidona, Christian A
Institut fur Medizinisch Virologie
Universitat der Heidelberg
Im Neuenheimer Feld 324
D-6900 Heidelberg
Germany

Tijssen, Peter
Institut Armand-Frappier
Universite du Quebec
Laval
Quebec H7N 4Z3
Canada

Tordo, Noël
Laboritoris Baer, SA
Cuautla 150
Col. Condesa
Mexico, DF
Mexico 06140

Torrance, L
Scottish Crop Research Institute
Invergowrie
Dundee DD2 5DA
UK

Tripathy, Deoki N
Department of Veterinary Pathology
College of Veterinary Medicine
University of Illinois
Urbana, Illinois IL 61802
USA

Tyler, Kenneth L
Department of Veterans Affairs Medical Center
Neurology Service (127), V A Medical Center
1055 Clermont Street
Denver, Colorado CO 80220
USA

Van Duin, J
Department of Chemistry
Leiden University
2300 RA Leiden
PO Box 9502
The Netherlands

Van Etten, James L
Department of Plant Pathology
University of Nebraska
Lincoln
Nebraska NB 68583-0722
USA

Van Oirschot, JT
Central Veterinary Institute
PO Box 65, Edelhertweg 15
NL 8200
AB Lelystad
The Netherlands

Van Regenmortel, MHV
Centre National de la Recherche Scientifique
IBMC
I.B.M.C. 15, Rue Descartes
Strasbourg, Cedex 67084
France

Vance, Vicki Bowman
Biology
University of South Carolina
Columbia, South Carolina SC 29208
USA

Verma, Inder M
Molecular Biology and Virology Laboratory
The Salk Institute
San Diego
California CA 92186
USA

Vigne, Robert
INSERM U372
Campus de Luminy
13276 Marseille Cedex 9
France

Vissler, Peter B
Institute of Molecular Plant Sciences
Gorlaeus Laboratories
PO Box 9502
2300 RA Leiden
The Netherlands

Wadell, Göran
Department of Virology
University of Umea
S-901 85 Ume
Sweden

Wagner, Edward K
Program in Animal Virology
Department of Molecular Biology and Biochemistry
University of California
Irvine, California CA 92717
USA

Wang, Alice L
Department of Pharmaceutical Chemistry
University of California
San Francisco School of Pharmacy
California CA 94143
USA

Wang, Ching C
Department of Pharmaceutical Chemistry
University of California
San Francisco School of Pharmacy
California CA 94143
USA

Webby, Richard
Department of Microbiology
University of Otago
PO Box 56
Dunedin
New Zealand

Webster, Robert E
Department of Biochemistry
Duke University Medical Center
Box 3711
Durham, North Carolina NC 27710
USA

Webster, Robert G
Department of Virology and Molecular Biology
St Jude Children's Research Hospital
Memphis
Tennessee TN 38101
USA

Welsh, Raymond M
Department of Pathology
University of Massachusetts
Medical Center
Worcester, Massachusetts MA 01655
USA

Whitaker-Dowling, Patricia
University of Pittsburgh School of Medicine
Pittsburgh
Pennsylvania, PA-15261
USA

White, David O
Department of Microbiology
University of Melbourne
Parkville, Victoria 3052
Australia

Wickner, Reed B
Laboratory of Biochemistry and Genetics
NIDDK, NIH, Bldg. 8, Room 225
8 Centre Drive, MSC 0830
Bethesda, Maryland MD 20892-0830
USA

Williams, Stanley T
School of Biological Sciences
University of Liverpool
Liverpool L69 3BX
UK

Wilson, T Michael A
Scottish Crop Research Institute
Invergowrie
Dundee
DD2 5DA
Scotland

Wimmer, E
C/o Connie Rafferty
Department of Molecular Genetics and Microbiology
State University of New York at Stony Brook
Health Sciences Center
Stony Brook, New York NY 11794-5222
USA

Winstanley, Doreen
Horticulture Research International
Wellesbourne
Warwick, CV35 9EF
UK

Wintermantel, William M
USDA-ARS
1636 E Alisal Street
Salinas
California CA 93905
USA

Wisdom, Ron
The Salk Institute
San Diego
California
USA

Wittek, R
Institut de Biologie Animale
Batiment de Biologie
Universit de Lausanne
CH-1015, Lausanne
Switzerland

Wolinsky, Jerry S
Department of Neurology
The University of Texas Health Science Center at Houston
Houston, Texas TX 77225
USA

Yamamoto, Janet K
University of Florida College of Veterinary Medicine
PO Box 100145
Gainsville
Florida FL 32610
USA

Yamanishi, Koichi
Department of Microbiology
Faculty of Medicine
Osaka University
Osaka 565
Japan

Yaniv, A
Department of Human Microbiology
Sackler School of Medicine
Tel Aviv University
Tel Aviv 69778
Israel

Yarbough, Patrice O
Genelabs Technology, Inc
505 Penobscot Drive
Redwood City
California CA 94063
USA

Yewdell, JW
Laboratory of Viral Diseases
NIAID-NIH
Bethesda
Maryland MD 20892
USA

Yin-Murphy, M
#4 Jalan Pandan
Raffles Park
Singapore 288789

Yoshida, M
Department of Cellular and Molecular Biology
Institute of Medical Science
The University of Tokyo
Tokyo 108
Japan

Young, Lawrence S
CRC Laboratories
Department of Cancer Studies
The University of Birmingham Medical School
Birmingham B15 2TJ
UK

Youngner, Julius S
University of Pittsburgh School of Medicine
Pittsburgh
Pennsylvania, PA-15261
USA

Yuill, TM
Institute for Environmental Studies
University of Wisconsin
550 North Park Street, Room 40
Madison, Wisconsin WI 53706
USA

Zádori, Zoltán
Institut Armand-Frappier
Universite du Quebec
Laval
Quebec H7V 1B7
Canada

Zavriev, Sergei K
Laboratory of Molecular Virology
Institute of Agricultural Biotechnology
Timiryazevskaya st. 42
Moscow 127550
Russia

Zillig, Wolfram
Max-Planck-Institut fur Biochemie
Am Klopferspitz 18a
D-82152 Martinsried bei Munchen
Germany

PREFACE

The *Encyclopedia of Virology*, now in its second edition, continues to assemble the basic and practical aspects of virology in a concise form, providing a rapidly accessible synopsis of each subject for the use of both professional and interested lay readers. The number of subjects (including animal, insect, plant, and bacterial viruses) and the number of illustrations have been significantly increased, and the contents have been revised and updated. Although it is not possible to cover all members of taxonomic families or genera, important examples of each are discussed by acknowledged experts in those fields. Articles that address general subjects related to specific viruses or viral diseases help to synthesize the relevant biomedical and economic issues. Thus, the encyclopedia addresses a large number of topics that are of interest to experimentalists, clinical virologists, and students, as well as to scientists and educators in related fields. The format of the book readily lends itself both to casual reading of articles on general subjects and to use as a primary reference source. As the Foreword to this edition, we are pleased to present two articles that describe 100 years of research on Tobacco Mosaic Virus and Foot and Mouth Disease Virus. Studies of these two viruses have contributed many conceptual and practical advances to the field of virology.

Although the report of the Seventh International Committee on Taxonomy of Viruses (ICTV) will not be published until the summer of 1999, we were provided preliminary information about prospective revisions of the scheme of virus classification. The editing and production deadlines prevented the comprehensive incorporation of these changes into the encyclopedia and we include a table listing the changes in taxa which follows the Table of Contents. This information was provided by Claude M. Fauquet who is the author of the *Taxonomy, Classification and Nomenclature of Viruses* entry and is also a member of our Advisory and ICTV Committees.

To accommodate the anticipated broad readership of the encyclopedia, we have provided a comprehensive Table of Contents that allows readers to locate any topic quickly. First, all entries are listed alphabetically by title. In the titles, common virus names are followed by the taxonomic family of the virus or viruses addressed. When viruses have not been assigned to a family, the genus is specified in the text. After the list of titles is an alphabetized list of general topics, followed by a list of all virus entries alphabetized by taxa.

The encyclopedia is presented in three volumes. Volume 1 covers *Adenoviruses* to *Hepatitis E Virus*, Volume 2 covers *Herpes Simplex Viruses* to *Polyomaviruses*, and Volume 3 covers *Pomoviruses* to *Zoonoses*. A complete Table of Contents appears at the beginning of each volume. When multiple viruses or subjects are addressed in a single entry, each is listed in the Table of Contents. Our aim is to allow the reader to locate quickly any topic that does not have its own separate entry by referring to the Table of Contents or the Index. The Guide to Use of the encyclopedia provides detailed information about locating subjects of interest. We have also included, as an Appendix, the complete list of all virus names from the Seventh ICTV meeting report, kindly provided by Claude M. Fauquet.

The individual articles are written by researchers who are widely acknowledged as experts in their fields. Because each entry is complete in itself, some overlap is inevitable. Redundancy has been minimized where possible, but some repetition is needed to ensure that readers can locate information without repeated reference to the index. Because the size of entries had to be limited, the information supplied is not exhaustive. Our aim was to provide the most relevant information in as concise a manner as possible. Readers should consider each entry an introduction to the specific topic addressed; the updated reading list at the end of each provides ample direction for more detailed study. Further, each entry contains a 'See Also' list that directs readers to related sections in the encyclopedia.

New developments will obviously continue to emerge in the rapidly advancing field of virology, but we expect the fundamental information offered by the encyclopedia to remain valid. Contributors were asked to project their fields into the future and to anticipate progress that can be expected at the beginning of the new millenium. Our colleagues in the subspecialties of virology have consistently found the *Encyclopedia of Virology* a valuable source of quick information and a useful teaching aid. Our goal has been to maintain and to improve that usefulness.

Allan Granoff
Robert G. Webster

ACKNOWLEDGMENTS

Like the first edition, the second edition of the *Encyclopedia of Virology* represents the work of many people. Its success rests most significantly on the expertise of the individual contributors, who are preeminent in their fields. We thank each of them for their willingness to take part in this endeavor and for the quality of their contributions. Our task as editors was eased enormously by the help of our outstanding editorial advisory board, which identified potential contributors and provided advice, especially in the areas of the insect, plant, and bacterial viruses, as the project progressed. We are pleased to acknowledge Ms. Valerie Audino at St. Jude Children's Research Hospital who provided expert editorial assistance in the production stage of publication. Special thanks are also due to Dr. Martha Howe, who was particularly helpful in identifying prospective authors for the bacteriophage sections and to Dr. Milton Zaitlin for his help in identifying appropriate authors for plant virus entries. We greatly appreciate Dr. Claude M. Fauquet's extensive contribution to the updated taxonomic organization of viruses and to his providing the ICTV's virion icons for use in the book. We also wish to acknowledge Lorraine Parry's contributions in bringing the second edition of the *Encyclopedia of Virology* to completion. As associate editor at Academic Press, she had the considerable task of seeing that this work was published on schedule.

FOREWORD: TMV – 100 YEARS OF CONTRIBUTIONS TO VIROLOGY

Tobacco mosaic virus (TMV) has played a prominent role in the development of the concept of viruses as pathological agents and in unraveling the composition and structure of these unique agents. It also is the virus with which many concepts and phenomena unique to plant virology have been discovered. The mosaic disease which afflicted tobacco was known in Europe since tobacco was introduced there in the 17th century. It causes light and dark green areas on infected plants, accompanied by considerable stunting and loss of yield. The first person to transmit it experimentally was Adolph Mayer who in 1886 reported that when he took juice from diseased plants, it was infectious to healthy plants; he also gave the disease its name. The capacity to transmit the disease experimentally facilitated the studies which ultimately resulted in depicting the new class of infectious agents, the viruses.

Attribution for the discovery of the virus concept is in dispute, ascribed by some to Dmitrii Ivanowski in 1892, but by others, to Martinus Beijerinck in 1898. The basis for the dispute lies in the interpretation of the results both workers obtained when tobacco sap was passed through a porcelain, bacteria-retaining filter; the agent had retained its infectivity. Ivanowski found it difficult to accept that the agent was something new, even after he was aware of Beijerinck's conclusions. Ivanowski was concerned that the filter might have had a crack, or that some small spore of the bacterial causal organism had passed through. Beijerinck, on the other hand (1898) concluded that he had a unique pathogen, which he termed a *'contagium vivum fluidum'* – a contagious living fluid. Animal virologists will also argue that early work on foot-and-mouth disease also should be considered for attribution for the virus concept (see foreword by Fred Brown in this volume).

In the years before the agent was purified and characterized, several findings were made using TMV that had important ramifications for plant virology. In 1929, McKinney discovered the phenomenon of 'cross protection', i.e., that infection of a plant with a mild strain of a virus would protect the plant from disease when inoculated subsequently with a severe form of that virus, but would not protect it against unrelated viruses. This phenomenon was used for many years to determine virus relationships, and in a few cases it was used to protect crops against disease. Additionally, in 1929 Holmes developed a quantitative bioassay for the virus using host plants that developed necrotic local lesions in response to infection, thereby potentiating experiments where virus quantification was important.

Prior to the ultimate isolation of the infectious agent in the 1930s, a number of studies gave clues to its nature and pointed the direction for its isolation. By injecting sap from infected plants into rabbits, Purdy (1929) demonstrated that the agent was immunogenic; others found that the infectious agent could be precipitated from tobacco sap with protein precipitants, both findings hinting at a proteinaceous agent. Further, birefringence experiments suggested it was elongate. Purification was being actively pursued in the United States by several groups, and by scientists in Australia and England. Wendell Stanley, then at the Rockefeller Institute in Princeton, New Jersey, was the first to publish that he had purified the virus (1935), and he received the principal recognition, most notably the Nobel Prize in 1946. However, he incorrectly thought the virus to be composed of only protein, missing the fact that it contained both phosphorus and carbohydrate. Bawden and Pirie, who were one step behind Stanley in the purification, set the record straight in 1936, by showing that the virus contained RNA.

TMV was the first virus seen in the electron microscope (1939) and in 1941 it was the first to have its structure revealed by X-ray crystallographic analysis. Further investigations in the 1950s revealed the position of the RNA in the particle, and defined its structure.

The 1950s saw an intense rivalry between workers in Tübingen, Germany (Schramm, Melchers, Gierer, Wittmann and others) and the group in Berkeley directed by Fraenkel-Conrat at the Virus Laboratory established by Wendell Stanley. Many of the findings outlined here were made almost simultaneously in both laboratories, although partisans might not agree with such attribution. The work was greatly facilitated because TMV, unlike any other virus known at the time, was easy to purify, and because of the large quantities which could be obtained. (In my own laboratory we isolated 60 grams of highly purified virus for one of our studies.) Also, TMV – at least the common 'strain' – is very stable, and will maintain its infectivity for decades at refrigerated temperatures if a little chloroform is added to inhibit growth of microorganisms.

In the 1950s both groups discovered that the RNA of the virus was infectious, that the virus could be reconstituted from isolated coat protein and RNA, determined the sequence of amino acids in the coat protein, and found that chemical agents could mutate the virus. The latter studies were particularly meaningful in the confirmation of the universality of the genetic code, in that directed mutational changes induced in the RNA led to predictable changes in the viral coat protein. Additionally, mixed reconstitution experiments, utilizing proteins from one strain and RNA from another, demonstrated conclusively that the RNA was indeed the genetic material of the virus, as some had questioned that the infectivity of 'naked' RNA was really a reflection of a small amount of a protein contaminant. These studies demonstrated conclusively that the coat protein was coded for by the RNA component of the mixed reconstituted virus.

In 1969 Takebe and Otsuki published a paper which revolutionized plant virology when they demonstrated that cell wall-free protoplasts isolated from tobacco leaves could be infected by TMV and that TMV would replicate in those cells. Thus, plant virologists now had a system to enable single cycle analysis of virus replication, previously not possible in inoculated leaf tissues involving only a few initial infections, followed by subsequent sequential replication in surrounding layers of cells.

In 1970 my colleague V. Hari and I ascertained that TMV-infected tissues contained at least four viral proteins. Subsequent events showed these to be the 126-kDa and 183-kDa proteins of the replicase complex, the 30-kDa movement protein, and the 17.6-kDa coat protein. There is also an open reading frame for a 54-kDa protein within the read-through portion of the 126-kDa replicase protein, coincident with sequences in the 183-kDa protein. This protein has not been detected in diseased tissues, however.

Plant viruses are now known to potentiate their passage from cell-to-cell in their hosts. The 30-kDa protein of TMV was shown to be involved in this process, deduced from studies with a temperature sensitive mutant of the related tomato mosaic virus, which was defective in cell-to-cell movement. In 1987 the movement protein was shown to modify the size exclusion limit of plant plasmodesmata to allow for cell-to-cell movement, by some elegant microinjection studies from the laboratories of William Lucas and Roger Beachy. Movement proteins have now been found in most plant viruses in which they have been sought, and have been shown to have RNA binding properties.

The concept that translation of some proteins in many RNA viruses is controlled by the production of subgenomic mRNAs was first demonstrated with TMV. Virus-infected tissues were shown to contain small, virus related RNAs, and *in vitro* translation demonstrated their mRNA capacities.

Other phenomena of particular significance to plant virology were the detailed analysis of how the virus assembles *in vivo*, and the phenomenon of co-translational disassembly in which it was demonstrated that cytoplasmic ribosomes remove the coat protein from the virion, thus exposing the RNA, which is also being translated during the process to synthesize the replicase subunits. TMV was the first plant virus to be completely sequenced (1982), and was the first virus to be shown to have at least one ubiquitinated subunit in the virion. In 1996, Barbara Baker reported the first isolation of a plant gene conferring resistance to a virus. This was the *N gene*, utilized in the aforementioned bioassay developed by Holmes in 1929.

The important discoveries in which transformation of plants with viral sequences to induce resistance or tolerance to disease were all pioneered with TMV. The widely-adopted coat protein-mediated protection concept was developed in 1983–84 in the laboratory of Roger Beachy, then at Washington University, in collaboration with scientists at the Monsanto Company who had developed technology for plant transformation. They found that the gene for the TMV coat protein, when transformed into tobacco plants gave significant delay of symptom development, and in some cases led to complete resistance. This concept has now been widely applied to at least 30 different viruses, representing at least 15 genera. Squash plants have been marketed which are resistant to several viruses, and currently there are plantings of papaya trees in Hawaii resistant to the devastating papaya ringspot virus.

The use of replicase genes for resistance was also first shown with TMV in my laboratory in work started in 1988. We found that a portion of the 183-kDa replicase gene gave near immunity to TMV disease. This phenomenon, known as 'replicase-mediated resistance' has also found application with a number of other viruses in other genera. Potato plants with the replicase gene of potato leaf roll virus are in commercial production.

TMV movement protein was also the first to be used in plant transformation experiments, seeking resistance. The laboratories of Beachy, Allan Dodds, and Josef Atabekov were pioneers in this technology. Interestingly, transformation with a defective movement protein from TMV was able to provide some measure of resistance to TMV, other tobamoviruses, and to several unrelated viruses.

A recently-published anthology on TMV contains reprints of the original papers with commentaries on the discoveries described above (Scholthof, K-B.G., Shaw, J.G., and M. Zaitlin (1999) *Tobacco Mosaic Virus: One Hundred Years of Contributions to Virology*. American Phytopathological Society Press, St. Paul, Minnesota, USA).

Milton Zaitlin
Department of Plant Pathology,
Cornell University, Ithaca, New York 14853, USA

FOREWORD: ONE HUNDRED YEARS OF FOOT-AND-MOUTH DISEASE

Foot-and-mouth disease (FMD) is a highly contagious disease of cattle, goats, pigs and sheep which often leads to great losses in productivity. Consequently, as an understanding of infectious diseases began to emerge during the last two decades of the nineteenth century, stemming from the pioneering work of Pasteur and Koch, FMD became the subject of intensive study in Germany because of the many outbreaks that were occurring there. The problem was so great that it led to the offer in 1893 by the Prussian Ministry of Agriculture of a prize of 3000 Reichmarks for the person who "identified and, if possible, isolated the contagious matter causing foot-and-mouth disease and demonstrated its effectiveness by means of decisive experiments on animals". Ten applicants worked unsuccessfully on the problem until 1895. A year later a motion was submitted to the Reichstag "to request the Imperial Chancellor to take account of the need for the immediate establishment of experimental institutions for the thorough investigation of FMD on behalf of the Empire and in the individual Federal States". This led to the allotment of 55,000 Reichmarks and to the establishment of a commission for research into the disease. Loeffler, who was Professor in the Institute of Hygiene at the University of Greifswald, started experiments on the disease in 1897, working with Frösch in Berlin, and in their third Report to the Prussian Minister of Culture in 1898 they described their landmark studies which established the causal agent as a virus. This was an historic event because it was the first demonstration that an animal disease could be caused by a virus and, remarkably, was made in the same year as Beijerink's description of the nature of tobacco mosaic virus. Loeffler continued the work at Greifswald but the highly contagious nature of the disease resulted in pressure from farmers in the area to stop the studies until they could be done in a safe place. This led eventually to the move in 1909 to Insel Riems, a small island in the Baltic Sea just north of Greifswald.

Clearly vaccination against the disease was the major target and methods to provide effective vaccines dominated research for the first 60 years of this century. One of the problems was the expense and difficulties associated with working with the natural hosts and led to the search for a susceptible laboratory animal. This search did not succeed until 1920 when Waldmann and Pape produced the disease in guinea pigs. This animal has been particularly useful in assessing the potency of experimental vaccines because the immunized animal can be challenged for its ability to resist infection. It was not until Skinner's work in 1951 that the suckling baby mouse was added to the repertoire of experimental animals that could be used for FMD research. The baby mouse was used extensively for the titration of the virus in the days before tissue culture cells became generally available. Moreover, it was the species used extensively by Skinner in attempts to produce strains of the virus which would be useful as attenuated vaccines.

A major step in the study of the disease and its control by vaccination took place in the early 1920s when Vallée and Carré in France and Waldmann in Germany showed that the virus occurs as multiple serotypes. The two groups discovered three serotypes now known as O, A and C. The nomenclature caused some confusion until it was resolved by discussion at the Office International des Epizooties in Paris. Vallée and Carré had first recognized the occurrence of two serotypes and named them after their place of origin, O for the Department of Oise in France and A for Allemagne. Their observation was confirmed by Waldmann and Trautwein in Germany who called them A and B. The latter group then discovered a third serotype which they called C. It was eventually decided to name them Vallée O, Vallée A and Waldmann C, which have now been reduced to O, A and C. The antigenic differences were such that an animal that had been infected with a virus of one serotype was still susceptible to the other serotypes. Clearly this was to have considerable importance in the control of the disease by vaccination and the problem was exacerbated by the demonstration of sub-types within the major serotypes in the late 1920s, a problem which can cause havoc in the control of the disease because antigenic variants continue to emerge.

To add to the problem, four further serotypes were identified later by the Pirbright triumvirate of Galloway, Brooksby and Henderson, three in the Southern African Territories (SAT1, SAT2 and SAT3) in the 1940s and Asia 1 in 1954. Interestingly, no other major serotypes have been identified in the past 45 years. Nevertheless the wide antigenic spectrum within each serotype and the new variants which are constantly emerging means that vaccines have to correspond closely to these emerging variants if they are to be effective in controlling outbreaks. Many devastating outbreaks in vaccinated animals provide evidence of the importance of this issue.

Consequently the composition of vaccines remains important in FMD. The first experimental vaccines were prepared in 1925, using formaldehyde-inactivated vesicular fluid from infected calves. However, large-scale field trials did not take place until 1948 when Rosenbusch and his colleagues successfully vaccinated more than two million cattle in Argentina. It was clear, however, that the necessary large-scale production of the virus would require its *in vitro* cultivation. Work in the early 1930s by Hecke in Germany and the Maitlands in England had shown that this could be achieved. It was Frenkel who showed in 1947 that *in vitro* cultivation of the virus on a large scale could be achieved by using surviving bovine tongue epithelial fragments. This was a major step in the provision of vaccines for the control of the disease and it was Holland, where Frenkel worked, which introduced the first comprehensive vaccination programme. Germany and France soon followed and these vaccination programmes have led to the eradication of the disease from Western Europe.

There have been minor hiccups on the way. One of the problems was the uncertainty surrounding the use of formaldehyde as the inactivant. This reagent had been used by Glenny and Ramon to detoxify diphtheria and tetanus toxins and it was probably the influence of Ramon on the French workers Vallée, Carré and Rinjard which persuaded them to use formaldehyde in their experimental vaccine studies in 1925. However, the suspicion that formaldehyde-inactivated vaccines were not innocuous, first expressed by Moosbrugger, led to studies with alternative reagents. From these studies, first N-acetylethyleneimine and then ethyleneimine were introduced and the latter compound is now used exclusively for the preparation of FMD vaccines.

The comprehensive vaccination programmes introduced have gradually led to the control of the disease and its elimination from many countries. Western Europe and several countries in South America which formerly had tens of thousands of outbreaks each year are now free from the disease.

The development of molecular techniques during the past 50 years has enabled us to study the virus and its nucleic acid and proteins in great detail. The structure of the virus at a resolution of 2.8 Å has been described and its mode of replication is known in the most intimate detail. From these fundamental studies have emerged two important practical issues. The first is the demonstration that protective immunity can be achieved by the inoculation of a 20-mer peptide corresponding to the highly immunogenic epitope located on the surface of the virus particle. Moreover, the important antigenic variation of the virus is almost certainly related to the amino acid sequence in the surface epitope. The second practical issue is the ability to identify animals that have been infected with the virus. Many of these animals become persistently infected for as long as three years and are consequently potential sources of further outbreaks of the disease. These animals can be identified by the presence in their sera of antibodies against non-structural proteins which are not present in naive or vaccinated animals. This information has emerged from the finding that certain of the non-structural proteins are not secreted from the cells in which the virus is grown and are consequently not included in the medium from which the vaccine is prepared.

Consequently, eradication of the disease could be accomplished worldwide because the scientific knowledge and means are available. It would be an appropriate ending to a century of FMD research if this goal were placed high on the agenda of the Food and Agricultural Organisation.

Fred Brown
Department of Agriculture,
Agricultural Research Service,
Greenport, New York 11944-0848, USA.

POMOVIRUSES

L. Torrance, Scottish Crop Research Institute, Invergowrie, Dundee, UK

Copyright © 1999 Academic Press

History

Fungus-transmitted, tubular rod-shaped viruses were classified as furoviruses in 1987 based on the properties of particle shape, transmission by zoosporic Plasmodiophorid 'fungi' and the possession of a divided genome. However, as more nucleotide sequences became available, it was apparent that the *Furovirus* genus contained species with different genome organizations and sequence relatedness. The classification was revised in 1998 and three new genera (*Pomo-*, *Peclu-* and *Benyvirus*) were established in addition to the genus *Furovirus* with no assignment to families.

Taxonomy and Classification

Pomovirus is a siglum derived from *po*tato *mo*p-top virus (PMTV), the type species. There are four member species in the genus *Pomovirus*: PMTV, beet soil-borne virus (BSBV), beet virus Q (BVQ) and broad bean necrosis virus (BBNV). Pomoviruses have genomes comprising three species of linear positive-sense single-stranded RNA of c. 5.8–6.5 kb, 2.9–3.5 kb and 2.5–3 kb, respectively. The RNA is not polyadenylated, and the genome encodes a triple block of proteins thought to be involved in virus movement.

Physical Properties of Particles

Pomovirus particles have helical symmetry, and are 18–20 nm in diameter comprising multiple copies of the major coat protein (c. 19–20 kDa). The stop codon of the coat protein gene can be suppressed to produce a larger readthrough protein. The readthrough domain of PMTV is expressed as a fusion with the coat protein and remains attached to one extremity of some virus particles. Virus particles are fragile and preparations contain large numbers of short fragments; the protein helix is sometimes uncoiled at one end in particles of PMTV. The particle size distribution is reported to be 100–150 nm and 250–310 nm. Measurements of PMTV particles gave predominant lengths of 125 nm, 137 nm and 283 nm. Virus particles sediment as three components and sedimentation coefficients ($s_{20,w}$) of PMTV are reported to be 126, 171 and 236S.

Genome Properties

The complete sequence has been determined for the genomes of BSBV (**Fig. 1**) and BVQ, and for RNA 2 and 3 of PMTV. Partial sequence information is available for PMTV RNA 1 and the three RNA species of BBNV.

RNA 1 contains a single large open reading frame (ORF) that is interrupted by a UAA codon followed in phase by an additional coding region. The ORF encodes putative proteins of c. 145–149 kDa and c. 204–207 kDa (readthrough protein). The smaller protein contains methyltransferase and helicase motifs, and the readthrough protein also contains a RNA-dependent RNA polymerase (RdRp) motif suggesting that these proteins are involved in virus replication.

RNA 2 (RNA 3 of PMTV) encodes the coat protein gene which is terminated by a UAG stop codon and followed in phase by an additional coding region of variable size. Suppression of the UAG stop codon produces a readthrough protein of 54–104 kDa. The molecular mass of the readthrough protein of a glasshouse-maintained isolate of PMTV (PMTV-T) is 67 kDa, but is c. 82 kDa in several field isolates. The shorter size of PMTV-T is caused by internal sequence deletion in the 3' half of the gene.

RNA 3 (RNA 2 of PMTV) contains three or four ORFs. The first three ORFs partially overlap and

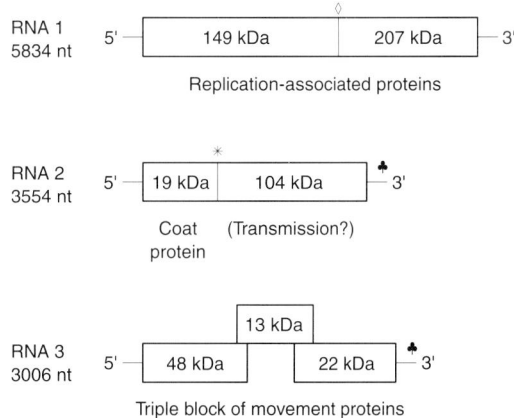

Figure 1 Diagram of BSBV genome organization showing the molecular mass of predicted protein products and their putative functions. * represents an UAG stop codon; ◇ represents a UAA stop codon; ♣ represents a tRNA-like structure.

share some characteristics with the triple gene block (TGB) found in the genomes of other rod-shaped viruses such as barley stripe mosaic hordeivirus and beet necrotic yellow vein benyvirus (BNYVV). By analogy they are thought to encode proteins that are involved in virus movement. The pomovirus-encoded proteins share the greatest sequence identity with each other in the second TGB protein (68–75%), and share 53–58% and 35–41% identity in the first and third TGB proteins, respectively. Also, the dNTP binding site motif in the first TGB protein is conserved. Pomovirus TGBs share some sequence identity with the respective TGB proteins of furo-, peclu-, beny- and hordeiviruses, but fewer identical amino acids when compared with those of other TGB containing viruses. PMTV (RNA 2) and BBNV (RNA 3) contain a fourth ORF which in PMTV encodes a putative 8 kDa cysteine-rich protein and in BBNV a putative 6 kDa protein. The RNA 3 of BVQ is shorter than the equivalent RNA in the other pomoviruses mainly because of the shorter lengths of its 5' and 3' untranslated regions. The three prime ends of the BSBV and BVQ RNAs and of PMTV RNA 2 can be folded into tRNA-like structures which contain an anticodon for valine.

Serological Relationships

The viruses are serologically distinct. PMTV particles contain an immunodominant epitope at the extreme N-terminus of the coat protein which is exposed along the entire length of the particles and reacts with monoclonal antibody SCR 69 (**Fig. 2**). The coat proteins of PMTV, BSBV and BVQ contain a conserved sequence of amino acids (SALNVAHQL) which are not exposed in the assembled particles but which react with a monoclonal antibody SCR 70 (raised to PMTV) in western immunoblotting tests. Distant serological relationships have been reported between BSBV and BVQ, and between soil-borne wheat mosaic furovirus and tobamoviruses with PMTV or BBNV.

Host Range and Geographical Distribution

The host range of pomoviruses is narrow, and restricted to dicotyledonous plants principally in the families Aizoaceae, Solanaceae, Chenopodiaceae and Leguminosae (only BBNV). The principal hosts of PMTV, BSBV and BBNV are potato, sugar beet and broad bean, respectively. PMTV occurs in Europe, South and North America and Asia in regions that have a cool, wet potato growing season. BSBV is widespread in sugar beet growing areas in Europe and

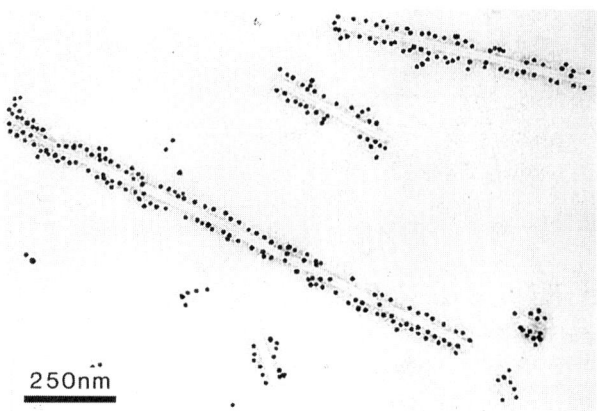

Figure 2 Electron micrograph of PMTV particles labelled with monoclonal antibody SCR 69/gold conjugate.

North America. BVQ has been reported to occur only in sugar beet crops in Europe and BBNV has been reported only from Japan.

Cytopathology

Virus-induced inclusions are seen in thin sections of virus-infected plants. Sheaves of PMTV particles have been found in thin sections of all cell types including vascular tissues. In addition, microtubules have been seen in the cytoplasm, apoplast and vacuole of most cell types, sometimes associated with membranes of the endoplasmic reticulum and tonoplast. Enlarged endoplasmic reticulum and distorted membranes are seen in thin sections of plants infected with BSBV and BVQ.

Transmission

Pomovirus vectors are zoosporic protozoans in the family *Plasmodiophoridae*. They are obligate parasites with a complex life cycle, producing resting spores that survive in soil for long periods and biflagellate zoospores that swim in soil water and infect plant roots. The viruses are acquired during infection of root cells by the vector, and virus particles are thought to be carried within the zoospores and resting spores. Soil remains infective after air-drying. PMTV is transmitted by the potato powdery scab pathogen *Spongospora subterranea* f. sp. *subterranea*. *Polymyxa betae* is thought to be the vector of BSBV and BVQ. The viruses can also be transmitted by mechanical inoculation.

By analogy with BNYVV, the readthrough domain of the coat protein may play a role in vector transmission of virus. A correlation has been found between the deletion of amino acids in the C-terminal portion of the readthrough domain and lack of transmission of PMTV by *S. subterranea*.

Ecology and Control

BBNV causes spots, streaks and veinal necrosis on the leaves of broad bean and pea and severely affected plants are stunted and defoliated. BSBV is widespread in sugar beets, it has been found in mixed infections with BNYVV, but no distinct symptoms have been attributed to infection by BSBV alone.

PMTV induces internal brown lines (spraing) and raised surface lines on potato tubers of sensitive cultivars infected directly from infested soil (**Fig. 3**). The spraing symptoms can be confused with those induced by the nematode-transmitted tobacco rattle tobravirus. Potato plants grown from infected tubers display yellow chevrons or markings on leaves or the mop-top dwarfing symptom caused by shortened internodes. PMTV decreases the quality of tubers produced for processing and consumption, and decreases the yield of tubers produced from plants of sensitive cultivars. Not every stem on an infected plant displays symptoms, and PMTV is erratically distributed in plants. The virus infects only a small proportion of plants grown from infected tubers, and it can be eliminated from stocks of cultivars that display obvious symptoms by removing infected plants. However, this method of control is limited to sensitive cultivars, and it carries the risk of establishment of PMTV at new sites. Haulm and tuber symptoms vary greatly with potato cultivar and environmental conditions especially temperature.

Resting spores of viruliferous vectors can be spread to new sites on contaminated farm vehicles or equipment, by planting contaminated tubers, by wind-blown surface soil or contaminated drainage water. Once the soil is infested by the viruliferous vector it is very difficult to control virus incidence. The Plasmodiophorid resting spores are resistant to chemical and environmental stresses and can remain viable in soil for many years, constituting an important reservoir of infection. The viruses are transmitted by the motile zoospores that swim in soil water, and their spread is favored by wet conditions. Soil fumigants such as methyl bromide are effective in controlling the Plasmodiophorids but it is environmentally damaging and its use is being restricted. Other chemical methods can provide partial control, e.g. decreasing soil pH to 5.0, by the application of sulphur, inhibits the spread of *S. subterranea* zoospores but the resting spores are not affected. At present there are no effective and environmentally safe chemical control methods. The best prospect for control of these soil-borne viruses is the development of virus-resistant

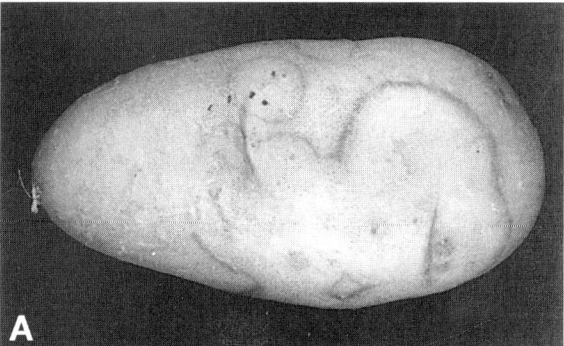
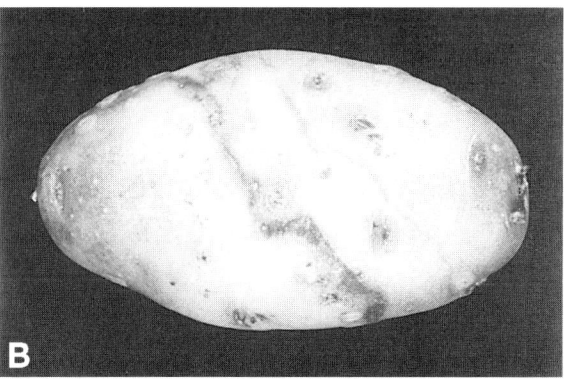
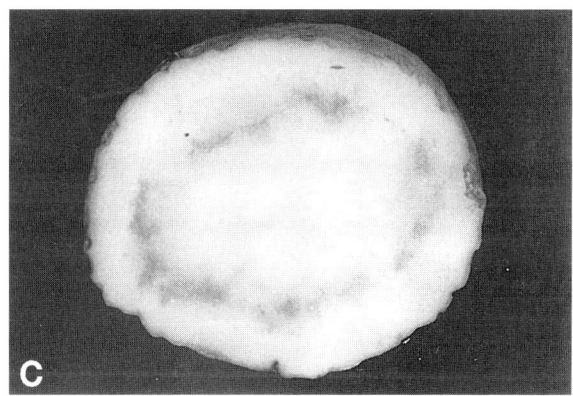

Figure 3 PMTV symptoms on potato tubers. Surface lines on **A** cv. Pentland Marble and **B** cv. Arran Pilot; **C** internal spraing on cv. Arran Pilot.

cultivars. There are no sources of natural resistance in potato to PMTV but plants transformed with the PMTV coat protein gene have shown high levels of resistance to virus infection by manual or fungal inoculation. This form of resistance may provide effective control if incorporated into potatoes.

See also: **Benyviruses; Furoviruses; Pecluviruses; Tobamoviruses.**

Further Reading

Arif M, Torrance L and Reavy B (1995) Acquisition and transmission of potato mop-top furovirus by a culture of

Spongospora subterranea f. sp. subterranea derived from single cystosorus. *Ann. Appl. Biol.* 126: 493.

Jones RAC (1988) Epidemiology and control of potato mop-top virus. In: Cooper JI and Asher MJC (eds). *Applied Biology II. Viruses with Fungal Vectors*, p. 225. Wellesbourne, UK: Association of Applied Biologists.

Kashiwazaki S, Scott KP, Reavy B and Harrison BD (1995) Sequence analysis and gene content of potato mop-top virus RNA 3: further evidence of heterogeneity in the genome organization of furoviruses. *Virology* 206: 701.

Koenig R and Loss S (1997) Beet soil-borne virus RNA1: genetic analysis enabled by a starting sequence generated with primers to highly conserved helicase-encoding domains. *J. Gen. Virol.* 78: 3161.

Koenig R, Pleij CWA, Beier C and Commandeur U (1998) Genome properties of beet virus Q, a new furo-like virus from sugar beet, determined from unpurified virus. *J. Gen. Virol.* 79: 2027–2036.

Reavy B, Arif M, Kashiwazaki S, Webster KD and Barker H (1995) Coat protein-mediated immunity to potato mop-top virus in *Nicotiana benthamiana* is effective against fungal inoculation. *Mol. Plant–Microbe Interact.* 8: 286.

Reavy B, Arif M, Cowan GH and Torrance L (1998) Association of sequences in the coat protein/readthrough domain of potato mop-top virus with transmission by *Spongospora subterranea*. *J. Gen. Virol.* 79: 2343–2347.

POTEXVIRUSES

Mounir G AbouHaidar and **Duncan Gellatly**, University of Toronto, Toronto, Ontario, Canada

Copyright © 1999 Academic Press

General Features

Potexviruses consist of a genus (no family) of about 30 definite and possible member viruses, with the prototype member being potato virus X (PVX). The potexviruses share common properties with the carlavirus genus of plant viruses. The two genera are now being considered for merger into a single family. All potexviruses are morphologically similar, flexuous, filamentous viruses with virions ranging in size from 470 to 580 nm in length and about 14 nm in width. The central canal of the particle is about 3 nm in diameter. Infectious potexvirus particles typically consist of 1000–1500 subunits of a single species of capsid protein (CP) wrapped around one single-stranded, messenger-sense genomic RNA (gRNA) that ranges in size from 5845 to 7057 nucleotides (nt) (**Table 1**). These viruses have a broad geographic range reflecting the distribution of their hosts. Although any one potexvirus member has a limited number of hosts, many dicotyledonous and monocotyledonous plant species are susceptible to infection when the group is considered together. Unlike many other plant viruses that are transmitted by insect vectors, potexviruses are apparently spread via a mechanical mode of transmission. Seed transmission has been reported in a few cases, but it is not confirmed. Systemically infected plants usually display chlorotic mosaic or mottle symptoms. Yield losses due to potexvirus infection of crops can be as high as 30%.

Virion Structure and Assembly

Potexvirus particles are highly hydrated particles that have molecular weights ranging in the order of 35×10^6 kDa and sediment from 100 to 130 S. The single species of CP, which ranges in size from 21 to 29 kDa, coats the genomic RNA in a helical fashion giving rise to a flexible rod. Optical and x-ray diffraction studies of virus particles have shown that there are $8\frac{3}{4}$ subunits per turn of the helix, which repeats one every four turns and exhibits a pitch of 3.3–3.6 nm, depending on the degree of hydration of the particle. The RNA is localized to a position about 3.5 nm radius (in contrast to tobacco mosaic virus (TMV)-RNA which is located at about 4 nm radius). The tendency for viral RNA to be encapsidated at a low radius may afford the RNA better protection and allow for bending (flexibility) of the particle. There are approximately five nucleotides of the RNA which interact with the protein subunit. A considerable degree of variability (40–65%) in the amino acid sequences of the CPs of potexviruses, much of which is localized to the amino terminus (located on the outside of the virus particle), results in low serological cross-reactivity between different potexvirus members. The gRNA comprises 6.5–7.5% of the viral mass and ranges from 5845 to 7057 nt in size.

Self-assembly of purified CP monomers and gRNA to produce reconstituted virion particles resistant to ribonuclease A can occur *in vitro* in low ionic-strength buffers (e.g. pH 8.0). The assembly process

Table 1 Propagation host species, complete and partial nucleotide sequences of some potexviruses

Potexviruses	Propagation species	gRNA[a] (nucleotides)	Capsid protein[b] (kDa)
Bamboo mosaic (BaMV)	Hordeum vulgare	6366	25
Cactus X (CVX)	Chenopodium quinoa		
Cassava common mosaic (CCMV)	Euphorbia prunifolia	6376	24.3
Clover yellow mosaic (CYMV)	Vicia faba	7015	23.5
Cymbidium mosaic (CybMV)	Datura stramonium	6227	23.5
Dioscorea latent (DLV)	Nicotiana megalosiphon		
Foxtail mosaic (FMV)	H. vulgare		
Hippeastrum latent (HsLV)	Hippeastrum hybridum		
Hydrangea ringspot (HRSV)	Hydrangea macrophylla		
Lily virus X (LVX)	Lilium hybrid		21.6
Nandina mosaic (NdMV)	Nicotiana benthamiana		
Narcissus mosaic (NMV)	Narcissus tazetta	6955	26.1
Nerine virus X (NVX)	Nerine sarniensis		
Papaya mosaic (PMV)	Carica papaya	6656	23
Pepino mosaic (PpMV)	Nicotiana glutinosa		
Plantago asiatica mosaic (P1AMV)	Plantago asiatica	6128	22
Potato aucuba mosaic (PAMV)	Nicotiana tabacum cv. Xanthi nc	7057	27
Potato X (PVX) (strain X 3)	N. tabacum	6435	25.1
Strawberry mild yellow edge-associated (SMYEAV)	Rubus rosifolius	5966	25.7
Viola mottle (VMV)	C. quinoa		
White clover mosaic (WC1MV)	Phaseolus vulgaris	5846	22.5
Wineberry latent (WbLV)	C. quinoa		
Zygocactus X (zvx)	C. quinoa		

[a] Genomic RNA (gRNA) size is determined from nucleotide sequence of cDNA of viral RNA.
[b] Molecular mass is calculated from the nucleotide sequence of cloned viral cDNA.

occurs in two stages: initiation and elongation. The initiation step is rapid (less than 20 s) and independent of temperature. Initiation occurs at a specific sequence (packaging signal, 38 to 47 nt in size) at the 5' end of the gRNA. In papaya mosaic virus (PMV), this sequence contains several repeats (of the type GCAAA) which are postulated to interact with $8\frac{3}{4}$ protein subunits of the 14S double disk (or helix) to specifically initiate assembly. Particles approximately 50 nm in length are formed. Synthetic poly(A) and poly(C) can also be specifically recognized and packaged at pH 8.0 by PMV protein. The elongation phase is a slower, temperature-driven process in which small polymers of CP are added, with growth toward the 3' end. Elongation, unlike the initiation process, seems to be non-specific. Any RNA can be packaged by PMV protein provided that the initiation sequence (packaging signal) is present at the 5' end. At lower pH values, the specificity of PMV protein for its RNA is lost. Any viral and non-viral RNAs may be packaged by the PMV CP but no complete particles are formed because initiation simultaneously starts at several sites of the RNA, resulting in multi-initiated 'kinky' particles. In the absence of RNA, CP monomers will assemble to form helical or stacked disk structures at low pH. Assembly of potexviruses is unlike that of tobamoviruses because it is unidirectional (starts at the 5' end of RNA) and no site of internal initiation is present.

Genome Organization

The monopartite genome of potexviruses consists of a messenger-sense, single-stranded RNA that is 5' capped (m^7GpppG) and 3' polyadenylated. An A-C-rich 5' noncoding region, from 80 to 107 nt in length, occurs upstream of five open reading frames (ORFs) which are well conserved in sequence and position among different potexviruses. The largest ORF, ORF 1, codes for a protein that has two motifs of amino acid sequences that are present in the conserved domains of NTP-binding helicases and RNA-dependent RNA polymerases. Mutation of PVX ORF 1 in one of the conserved glycine-lysine-serine (GKS) sequence, a motif that is present among the replicating enzymes of many RNA viruses, eliminates PVX replication. The product of ORF 1 thus appears to represent a component of a replicase complex that directs, together with host proteins, and possibly other viral proteins, the synthesis of viral RNA

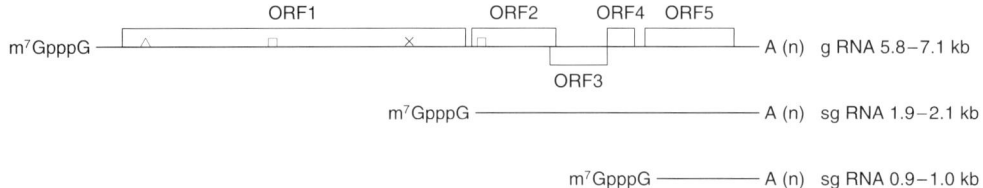

Figure 1 Organization of a potexvirus genome (gRNA). The diagram represents genomic organization of PVX, the type member of potexviruses. Five open reading frames (ORF) encoding the viral proteins with the following molecular weights: 166 kDa (ORF 1/putative RNA polymerase), 25 kDa (ORF 2), 12 kDa (ORF 3), 8 kDa (ORF 4) (ORF 2–4/triple gene block involved in viral transport) and 25 kDa (ORF 5/capsid protein). The sizes of the viral proteins vary among the other potexviruses of which the genomes have been sequenced. The sizes are: 147–191 kDa, 24–26 kDa, 11–14 kDa, 6–11 kDa and 21–26 kDa for ORF 1 to ORF 5, respectively. The two most abundant subgenomic RNAs (sgRNA) are also depicted. m⁷GpppG represents the cap structure. $A_{(n)}$ represents the poly(A) tail. Triangle depicts the methyltransferase motif. Squares represent the NTPase/helicase motif (GSK). × depicts the GDD polymerase motif.

(Fig. 1). ORFs 2, 3 and 4 slightly overlap, and are commonly referred to as the 'triple gene block'. Products of the triple gene block function in cell-to-cell movement, being required for infectivity in a host plant but not in protoplasts. The amino acid sequences of ORF 2 from various potexviruses indicate an ATPase–helicase function, and the ORF 2 product of PVX has been shown to bind nucleic acids *in vitro*. Hydrophobic sequences in the products of ORFs 3 and 4 suggest an association with host cell membranes. Immunological localization has demonstrated the product of PVX ORF 4 to be associated with the cell wall. There are some apparent exceptions to the organization of ORFs 2–4. The genome of lily virus X (LVX) lacks the initiation codon for ORF 4, strawberry mild yellow edge-associated potexvirus (SMYEAV) lacks one for ORF 2. However, the rest of the coding sequences of these ORFs are present and are similar to other potexviruses. The exact role(s) of these ORFs in the potexvirus life cycle is not fully determined at present. ORF 5 codes for the CP. In two potexviruses, clover yellow mosaic (CYMV) and foxtail mosaic virus (FoMV), ORF 5 is contained within a larger ORF that appears to encode a 'readthrough' protein. Various potexviruses also contain other small putative ORFs that are embedded in, and often out of frame from, the five major ORFs. Other putative ORFs found on the negative (complement) strand have also been described. The *in vivo* significance of such ORFs remains speculative. The 3′ noncoding region ranges from 43 to 138 nt in length and precedes a poly(A) tail that varies in length. A U-rich 8-nt sequence within the 3′ noncoding region of PVX is required for virus replication by binding two host proteins (28 and 32 kDa in tobacco) of unknown function. A consensus polyadenylation sequence (5′-AAUAAA-3′) occurs at different distances from the 3′ end of the gRNA.

During potexvirus replication, capped and poly(A)-tailed subgenomic RNAs (sgRNAs) are produced. The two most abundant sgRNAs are 1.9–2.1 kilobase (kb) and 0.9–1.0 kb in size. These have 5′ ends which correspond to internal regions of the gRNA, and are coterminal with the gRNA at their 3′ ends. The formation of sgRNAs was previously thought to alleviate the problem of translation of polycistronic mRNAs by eukaryotic ribosomes, which follow the Kozak scanning model. However, recent work has demonstrated that the PVX CP gene can be expressed in transgenic plants from an internal ribosome binding site. Consequently, the formation of sgRNAs in this group of viruses (and probably in other viruses) is merely for amplification (and not for initiation of translation) purposes. A 1.2-kb sgRNA in CYMV has been isolated, consisting of 757 and 415 nt segments from the 5′ and 3′ ends, respectively, joined so that the N-terminus of ORF 1 and C-terminus of ORF 5 are fused in frame. This sgRNA is clearly defective and requires the full-length genome as a helper for replication. Furthermore, this CYMV 1.2-kb sgRNA appears to be the only defective-interfering (DI)-like RNA seen among potexviruses.

Replication

The essential potexvirus replication strategy is believed to involve an RNA intermediate, in which the messenger-sense gRNA is initially copied to produce a full-length antisense complement. This antisense complement is then used as a template for the synthesis of full-length messenger-sense gRNA. Detection of double-stranded gRNA in infected tissue supports this model. The full-length antisense complement also serves as a template for the synthesis of sgRNAs. These sgRNAs are 3′ coterminal with the gRNA, and function as mRNAs for viral products coded for in the 3′-half of the gRNA. It is believed the sgRNAs are produced from the full-length antisense complement via internal initiation. Membrane-containing extracts isolated from PVX-infected tobacco plants have been shown to support synthesis of all viral RNA types, both single and double stranded. Several conserved sequence motifs, identified at the 5′ and 3′ ends of the gRNA as well as regions immediately 5′ to the initiation sites of sgRNAs synthesis, may act as promoter elements for a replicase complex. The putative promoter sequence at the 5′ end of all potexvirus gRNAs is 5′-GAAAACAAAAC-3′ and at the 3′ end is 5′-ACUUAA-3′. PVX mutants in the 5′ noncoding region have demonstrated that sequence elements in this region also play a crucial role in the synthesis of both gRNA and sgRNA. The presence of a conserved octanucleotide sequence, and the spacing between this sequence and the 5′ start site of sgRNA synthesis initiation, has been shown to be essential for accumulation of the two major sgRNAs in PVX replication. The RNA-dependent RNA polymerase (RdRp) of PVX (ORF 1) contains a glycine-lysine-serine (GKS), a glycine-aspartate-aspartate (GDD) and a methyltransferase (for capping) motif which are also found in many RdRps of RNA viruses. The GKS motif is thought to be required for the binding of nucleoside triphosphates. Mutation of GKS to GNS or GES rendered that virus unable to replicate in plants or protoplasts. Substitution of glycine to alanine had only a minor effect on the replication of PVX. However, mutation of any of the three amino acids GDD rendered the viral genome noninfectious.

The function of the triple gene block products appears to be that of cell-to-cell movement, as mutations in ORFs 2, 3 or 4 prevent the development of systemic infection in plants but not of viral replication in protoplasts. Systemic spread of a transport-defective PVX ORF 2 mutant was restored by transformation of host cells with transport proteins from either a tobamovirus, dianthovirus, or bromovirus. Mutations to the conserved elements of ORF 2 (ATPase-helicase domain) and ORF 3 (hydrophobic domain) also inhibited viral spread in intact hosts. In PVX, the ORF 2 product has been localized to complex lamellar structures and inclusion bodies in the cytoplasm and possibly the nucleus, whereas in bamboo mosaic potexvirus, the ORF 2 product is found in electron-dense crystalline bodies in both the cytoplasm and nucleus. From studying size-exclusion limits of plasmodesmata, the 25-kDa protein (ORF 2) of PVX was shown to be required for full plasmodesmatal modification. A nucleotide triphosphate/helicase consensus sequence (GSGKS/T), similar to that found in ORF 1, has also been found in the ORF 2 of some potexviruses. The ORF 4 product of PVX has been localized to the cell wall. An intact product of ORF 5, the CP, is essential for systemic infection with PVX as well as for replication of PVX gRNA and packaging of this RNA to form complete virus particles.

The messenger-sense gRNA of potexviruses can be translated directly after uncoating in the plant cell. *In vitro* translation of gRNAs isolated from virions typically generates products that correspond to the putative replicase protein encoded by ORF 1 at the 5′ end of the gRNA. Only small and variable amounts of CP, encoded by ORF 5 at the 3′ end, are produced. Production of any CP is likely a result of internal initiation of translation. Efficient *in vitro* synthesis of CP can be achieved by using the smaller (0.9–1.0 kb) of the two major sgRNAs as template. *In vitro* translation of the larger (1.9–2.1 kb) major sgRNA yields product corresponding to ORF 2. The mechanism of expression of the products of ORFs 3 and 4 is less clear, apparently involving internal initiation or the presence of less abundant sgRNAs.

The 5′ cap structure, present on all potexvirus gRNAs and sgRNAs, is essential for infectivity. For instance, infectious *in vitro* RNA transcripts of white clover mosaic potexvirus (WCMV) are only 4% as infectious as capped viral gRNA. Similarly, the length of the 3′ poly(A) tail is critical; shortening the tail length from 71 to 24 nt of *in vitro* RNA transcripts of papaya mosaic virus reduced infectivity from 43% to 16% of native viral gRNA. Mutations to the polyadenylation signal of WCMV reduced both transcript infectivity and the average length of the poly(A) tail in progeny virus.

Fusion of a 27-kDa reporter gene (*Aequorea victoria* green fluorescent protein) to the amino terminus of PVX ORF 5 (CP) resulted in assembly of intact virions that were over twice the diameter of wild-type PVX virions. However, free CP was also required. Efficient functioning of the reporter-gene product was observable, and the assembled virus was capable of both local and systemic movement. The further potential of the use of potexviruses as vectors for the production of high levels of foreign proteins in plants remains to be seen.

Pathology

Symptoms on systemically infected hosts range from undetectable to moderate, depending on the individual potexvirus. Generally, systemic symptoms include chlorotic mottle or mosaic patterns, with stunting also being common. Potexviruses are capable of infecting most host tissues. Both primary and systemic cytopathology can occur in a single host. *Gomphrena globosa* is the most common local lesion host among members of the potexvirus group.

Inclusion bodies, composed of potexvirus particles

packed in parallel arrays, often form in the cytoplasm and sometimes in the nucleus of infected cells. These aggregates often vary in size and have irregular shapes, but can form spindle-shaped structures in some potexviruses. Another type of inclusion, laminated inclusion components (LIC), are thin proteinaceous sheets associated with bead-like structures. LICs display no viral antigens. A third type, the amorphous inclusions, occur in the cytoplasm and vacuoles. Amorphous inclusions contain viral antigens.

Co-infecting a single host with a potexvirus and another virus (e.g. a potyvirus) can have a synergistic effect on symptoms. For instance, mixed infections with PVX and potato virus Y (PVY) produces a dramatic increase in the severity of PVX symptoms, pathogenicity and accumulation, compared to that observed by infection with PVX alone. Other potyviruses such as tobacco vein mottling virus (TVMV), tobacco etch virus (TEV) and pepper mottle virus are also capable of the synergistic effect on PVX replication and symptom severity. The replication of the entire potyviral genome is not increased nor required for PVX/potyviral synergism. The synergistic response is mediated by expression of the 5′-proximal third of the genomic potyviral RNA (i.e. protease-1, helper component protease (HC-Pro) and protein-3 gene). The exact molecular basis for PVX/PVY synergism is not presently well understood.

Host Resistance

The product of the N gene in tobacco confers resistance to PVX. Similarly, three genes in potato have been identified which are associated with potexvirus resistance: Nx and Nb are involved in hypersensitivity, and Rx with immunity. Rx1 has been mapped to the distal end of potato chromosome XII. PVX is recognized to comprise five subgroups (i.e. I, II, III, IV and HB) based on the ability to infect hosts of different resistance genotypes. For instance, group III is the largest PVX subgroup, which systemically infects Nb hosts. Within a group, sequence conservation and host susceptibility are difficult to correlate. In PVX, the CP has been shown to be a strain-specific elicitor of Rx-mediated resistance in potato. Amino acids 121 and 127 may interact with cellular components involved in spread of the virus and with products of Rx resistance gene. The PVX CP also harbors at least two types of virulence determinants, X and B, which differ by only 14 amino acids. Type X CPs are avirulent on potato cultivars carrying the Nx resistance gene, whereas type B CPs are capable of overcoming Nx resistance. Resistance 'breaking' strains of PVX have emerged by minor sequence changes in both the CP and other regions of the viral genome. Expression of the PVX CP or mutant movement proteins in transgenic plants can result in a delay in the onset of symptoms upon subsequent challenge with PVX virus or gRNA. It has been shown recently that a replicating viral RNA (i.e. PVX) is a potent trigger of 'gene silencing', a phenomenon characterized by a genetic control mechanism implicated in virus resistance. Gene silencing is associated with the induced natural defense response of plants against viruses. The signal may move ahead of the inducing virus and result in delaying the spread of the infectious front. The exact molecular mechanisms involved in this phenomenon are currently not well understood.

This work is dedicated to the memory of Duncan Gellatly (1969–1998).

See also: **Carlaviruses; Plant resistance to viruses: Natural resistance, Engineered resistance; Synergism: Plant viruses; Virus structure: Atomic structure, Principles of virus structure.**

Further Reading

AbouHaidar MG and Erickson JW (1985) Structure and *in vitro* assembly of papaya mosaic virus. In: Davies JW (ed.) *Molecular Plant Virology*, Vol. I. Boca Raton, Florida: CRC Press.

Commonwealth Mycological Institute/Association of Applied Biologists (CMI/AAB) Description of Plant Viruses, No. 200, August 1978 (Potexvirus Group) and No. 354, December 1989 (potato virus X).

Francki RIB, Milne RG and Hatta T (1985) Potexvirus Group. In: *Atlas of Plant Viruses*, Vol. II. Boca Raton, Florida: CRC Press.

White KA, Rouleau M, Bancroft JB and Mackie GA (1995) Potexviruses. In: *Encyclopedia of Virology* 1st edn, p. 1142. London: Academic Press.

POTYVIRUSES (*POTYVIRIDAE*)

Juan José López-Moya and Juan Antonio García, Centro Nacional de Biotecnologia, CSIC, Campus UAM, Cantoblanco, Madrid, Spain

Copyright © 1999 Academic Press

History, Taxonomy and Classification

The *Potyvirus* genus (type species potato virus Y) of the *Potyviridae* family currently contains the largest group of plant viruses – up to 30% of the total number of plant viruses. The family *Potyviridae* includes five other genera: *Rymovirus*, *Macluravirus*, *Ipomovirus*, *Bymovirus* and *Tritimovirus*. Historically, several viruses later classified in the family *Potyviridae* were known for a long time; some were reported as early as the beginning of the twentieth century, some during the 1930s and the number has increased further from the 1960s to the present day. Viruses of the *Potyviridae* family are among the most damaging plant viruses and a considerable literature has been devoted to them. Since the mid-1980s, complete genome sequences of potyviruses have become available, and genetic studies were made possible by the production of full-length directly infectious cDNA clones, or from infectious transcripts. This technique has also become available for a bymovirus.

The taxonomic standards currently in use for classification into the family *Potyviridae* include properties of the virus particles (long flexuous, as shown in **Fig. 1A**), their genome structure (positive sense single-stranded (ss) RNA, with a 5′ terminal protein and a 3′ poly(A) tail), their expression strategy (polyprotein containing several gene products, separable by proteolysis) and their cytopathological manifestations (particularly the formation of pinwheel- or scroll-shaped cylindrical cytoplasmic inclusions in infected plant cells, as shown in **Fig. 1B**).

Potyviruses can be differentiated from other genera in the family because they are aphid-transmissible and possess a monopartite genome. Bymoviruses are transmitted by fungi and have a genome composed of two molecules of ssRNA which are encapsidated separately. Rymoviruses and Tritimoviruses have monopartite genomes, and their natural vectors are eriophyd mites. Ipomoviruses and Macluraviruses also have monopartite genomes, and they are whitefly and aphid transmitted, respectively.

Although an extensive review of taxonomic issues exceeds the purpose of this entry, recent molecular information has essentially confirmed the classification shown in **Table 1**. Relationships between members of the family should be further examined when more complete sequences become available.

Geographic Distribution, Host Range, Epidemiology and Propagation

Members of the *Potyviridae* family are distributed throughout the world. Some of them have restricted natural and experimental host ranges; others may infect a considerable number of plant species distributed in many families. In general, there are members that are able to infect the most economically important crops, including grain, legumes, forage, vegetables, fruits and ornamentals.

Severity of outbreaks is commonly related to the abundance of initial foci of infection, vector populations and other factors. Vector organisms are mainly involved in the propagation of viruses within a localized region, although they might also have a role in initiation of epidemics at long distance. Human intervention is responsible in many cases for the spread of diseases in larger areas, and the introduction of new diseases. Seed transmission is also important in some potyviruses, and weeds can act as reservoirs of viruses. A typical example of well-documented spread of a potyvirus over a territory and over time is the progressive emergence of plum pox virus (PPV) in European countries during the twentieth century, and its recent spread to other continents.

Properties of Virions

Virion particles of potyviruses are long and flexuous (**Fig. 1A**), 680–900 nm long and 11–15 nm wide. They comprise protein (95%) and RNA (5%). Viruses belonging to other genera in the family possess particles with similar properties. Ipomovirus particles are around 900 nm long, while macluravirus ones are shorter (around 650 nm). The two bymovirus particles are about 250–300 and 500–600 nm in length.

Around 2000 subunits of a single protein (CP) compose the capsid of potyviruses. The molecular weight of each subunit ranges between 30 and 47 kDa, and they are disposed helicoidally around the nucleic acid. Variations in CP size are due mainly to

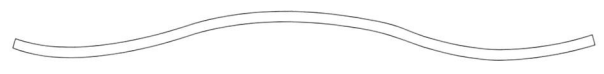

Table 1 Classification of members of the family *Potyviridae* into genera, with indication of the number of members, transmission vectors and number of genomic RNAs

Genus	Members[a]		Transmission	Genome
	Definite	Possible		
Potyvirus	75	93	Aphids	Monopartite
Bymovirus	5	—	Fungi	Bipartite
Rymovirus	3	2	Mites	Monopartite
Tritimovirus	2	—	Mites	Monopartite
Ipomovirus	1	1	Whiteflies	Monopartite
Macluravirus[a]	2	—	Aphids	Monopartite

[a] Number of members according to the International Committee on Taxonomy of Viruses.

differences in the length of the variable N-terminal region, while the internal core (of about 220 amino acids) is more conserved, as expected for its involvement in particle architecture. Although the structure of the potyvirus virions has not yet been determined, Shukla and others have established some structural characteristics (**Fig. 2**). It is known that both N- and C-termini of CP are surface exposed on the particle, the N-terminus being the immunodominant region. In addition, superficially located residues in this region play a role during aphid transmission and are involved in other important functions such as long distance movement in the host plant. A nonspecific nucleic acid binding-domain has been characterized recently in the CP of barley yellow mosaic bymovirus (BaYMV).

Serologic Relationships

Relationships among members of the *Potyviridae* family, based on serology, have been problematic because of their extreme complexity. Virus particles are strongly immunogenic as a general rule, but for many years antisera had limited application in taxonomy. Nonstructural proteins had even more restricted use in serological identification.

The unexpected serological crossreactivities between viruses, and inconsistent relationships derived from virion-based serology, may be due to the fact that group-specific epitopes are mainly located in the conserved internal core region of CP, while the virus-specific ones map in the variable N-terminus, a region that is surface-exposed and prone to undergo degradation. Once the origin of the problem has been identified, solutions have been proposed to obtain virus-specific antibodies by targeting towards the N-terminal epitopes. In addition, the highly conserved CP core may be used to generate *Potyviridae*-specific

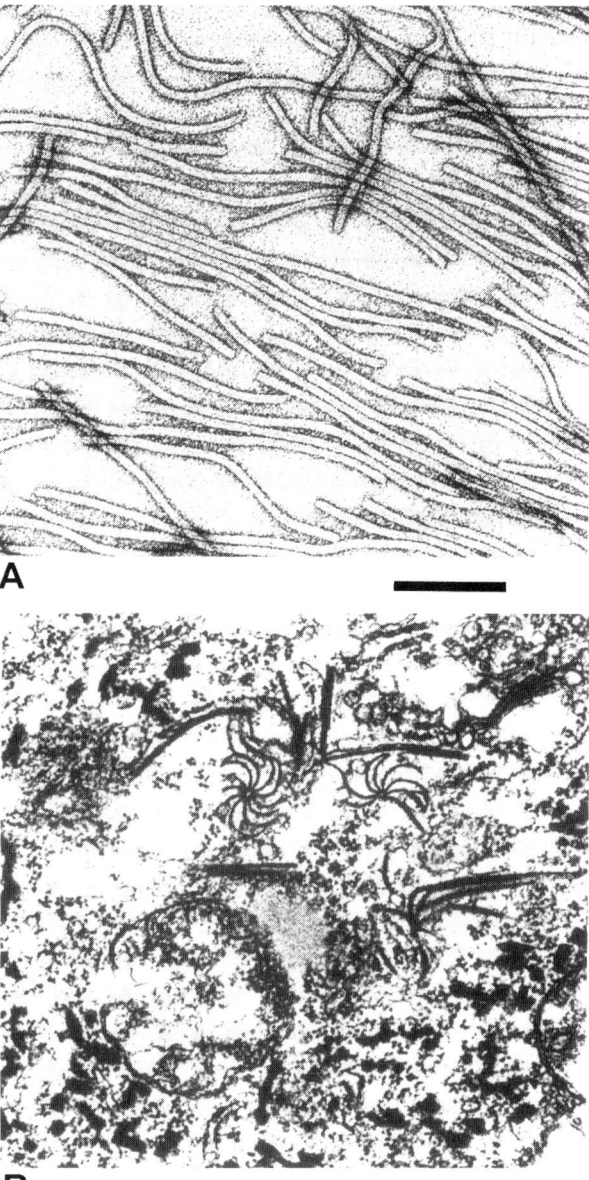

Figure 1 (**A**) Negative stain preparation of purified tobacco etch potyvirus particles. (**B**) Thin section showing the typical pinwheel shaped cytoplasmic inclusions present in cells of a *Nicotiana benthamiana* plant infected with plum pox potyvirus. Bar = 200 nm. (Courtesy of D. López-Abella, CIB, CSIC.)

antibody probes, useful in detecting numerous viruses.

Properties of the Genome

The nucleic acid of potyviruses is an ssRNA molecule of 9.4–10.3 kb, messenger (positive) sense, with a 5′ terminal protein (VPg), and polyadenylated at its 3′ end. It comprises a single open reading frame (ORF) coding for a long polyprotein (340–370 kDa) that

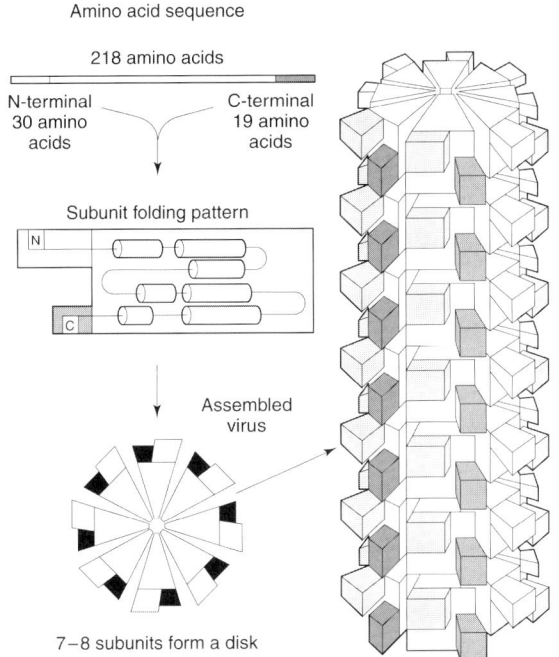

Figure 2 Structural model of potyvirus particles. The predicted folding of individual CP subunits is shown. CP cores unite together to build the virion, leaving both N- and C-termini superficially exposed. (Reproduced with permission from Shukla DD and Ward CW (1989) *Adv. Virus Res.* 36: 273.)

rymo- and ipomoviruses are similar in size and organization. In contrast, bymoviruses have their genome divided into two RNAs: the long RNA1 is analogous to the 3′ three-quarters portion of potyvirus genome, and the short RNA2 includes sequences corresponding to others in the 5′ portion of potyviruses, not having in the rest of the molecule clearly matching counterparts in the potyvirus genome. The majority of molecular data available have been obtained with potyviruses. Unless otherwise noted, the following sections describe characteristics of potyviruses.

Three potyvirus-encoded proteinases are involved in the proteolytic cleavage of gene products. The processing events have been studied in depth *in vitro*, and the present figure includes probable cotranslational and autocatalytic cleavages, followed by *trans* cleavages. Processing is dependent on the sequences surrounding each particular cleavage site. A review of this process can be found in the article by Riechmann and coworkers cited in the further reading section.

A typical potyvirus genome starts at the 5′ end with a noncoding region (NCR), usually less than 200 bp long. Studies performed with PPV showed that most of this region is dispensable for infectivity, although it contributes to viral competitiveness and pathogenesis. Although there is some controversy about the existence of internal ribosome entry sites in the 5′ NCR of potyviruses, recent results seem to indicate that translation takes place by a cap-independent leaky scanning mechanism. The 5′ NCR of poty-

generates mature products (**Fig. 3**) after initiating an autoproteolysis processing cascade. Genomes of

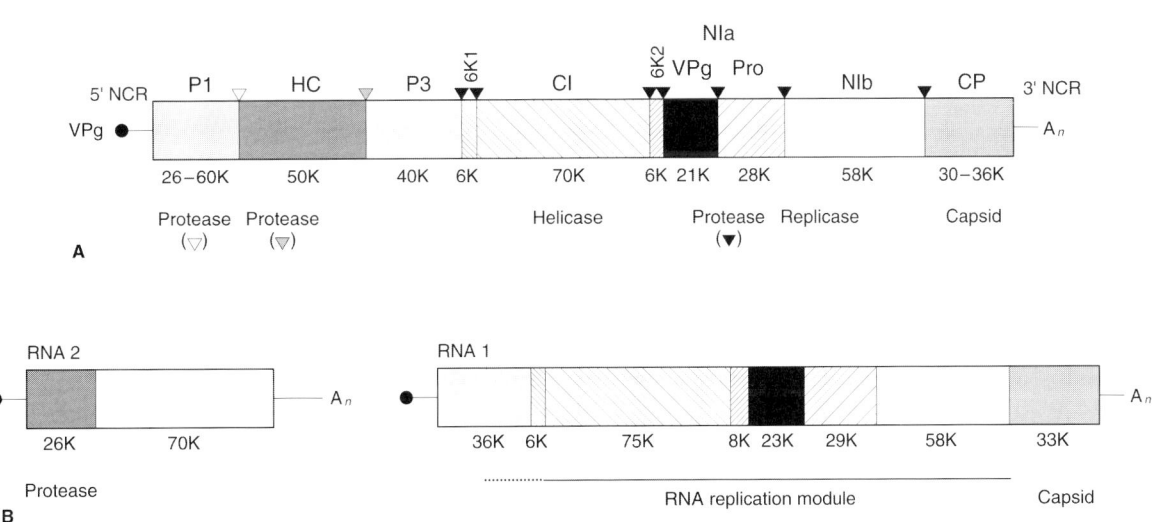

Figure 3 Genomic maps of (**A**) potyviruses and (**B**) bymoviruses. The ssRNA genomes are shown with boxes representing ORFs flanked by NTRs as lines. VPgs are represented by solid circles at each 5′ end, and poly(A) tails are located at each 3′ end. Names of gene products are indicated, as well as some of their known functions and their approximate size K (kDa). The three protease-specific cleavage sites (rendering functional proteins or regulating their activity) are also indicated by triangles above the potyvirus polyprotein. Genomic structures of rymo-, ipomo-, tritimo- and macluraviruses are similar to that of potyviruses.

viruses has been used as an enhancer of translation in transgenic plants.

Another NCR of about 200 bp is located at the 3′ end of the genome, before a variable-length poly(A) tail. Putative RNA structures in this region confer pathogenic properties, as shown in tobacco vein mottling virus (TVMV). In addition, work performed with tobacco etch virus (TEV) has demonstrated the existence of a *cis*-acting element necessary for infectivity near the 3′ end of the genomic RNA, including sequences contained in the last cistron of the ORF.

Properties and Functions of Gene Products

The polyprotein coded in the genome of a potyvirus comprises the following gene products. The first N-terminal protein, named P1, is a protease (similar to chymotrypsin-like serine proteinases) responsible for cleavage at its C-terminus. This region accounts for the largest sequence differences among potyviruses, being extremely variable in size (26–60 kDa) and sequence. Its functions have not yet been established. In TEV, it acts in *trans* as an accessory factor for genome amplification, and experiments suggest that it must be separated from the next gene product to restore debilitated infectivity caused by inactivation of its proteolytic activity. It also has RNA-binding activity.

After P1, the next gene product is the helper component, HC (about 50 kDa), a protein implicated in aphid transmission. Its N-terminal region, which includes a cysteine-rich portion with a putative zinc-finger-type structure, seems to be essential for transmission but is also needed for efficient RNA replication. The carboxy half of the protein is a papain-like cysteine protease, which serves to cleave at its own C-terminus. It has been reported that, like P1, HC is able to interact with RNA *in vitro*. Other functions have been assigned to this protein, such as a factor for long-distance transport and genome amplification. HC also forms amorphous-type inclusions in the cytoplasm of several potyviruses.

All other gene products are excised from the polyprotein by the action of the NIa protease (see below). The third gene product in the ORF is known as P3 (about 40 kDa), and there is little information regarding its role during infection. Immunocytological studies have found P3 associated with cylindrical inclusions in TVMV, and nuclear inclusions in TEV. A small protein $6K_1$ is located next. However in potyviruses such as TEV cleavage between P3 and $6K_1$ has not been observed *in vitro*, and in PPV excision seems not to be required for virus viability. Immunological data suggest that both P3 and P3+$6K_1$ products are present in infected cells. The region contains hydrophobic domains which might result in association to membranes. It has been hypothesized that the functional product of this genome region is P3+$6K_1$, whose activity would be modulated by cleaving off the $6K_1$ fragment.

The next protein, CI, is the largest potyvirus gene product in size (around 70 kDa). It forms very distinctive cylindrical inclusions in the cytoplasm of infected cells, with a high taxonomic value because they are unique to members of the *Potyviridae* family (**Fig. 1B**). CI includes domains peculiar to RNA helicases, and this activity has been proved experimentally. Two domains have been shown to bind RNA. Functionally, CI is believed to act during unwinding of RNA chains in replication. In addition, it has been found associated to the plasma membrane and plasmodesmata in early stages of infection and it is required for cell-to-cell spread.

A second small peptide, $6K_2$, is involved in virus replication, and its role seems to be related to its membrane-anchoring properties, maintaining the replication complex in place. Separation of $6K_2$ from NIa by autoproteolysis regulates localization of the latter in the nucleus.

The next protein, NIa, of about 49 kDa, may undergo a further cleavage in an internal suboptimal processing site, giving origin to NIaVPg (21 kDa) and NIaPro (27 kDa). VPg is found covalently attached to the 5′ end of genomic RNAs, and it may act as a protein primer during initiation of replication. However, parental VPg is not needed for infectivity (RNA synthesized *in vitro* without VPg is infectious). Recently, a role for VPg during long-distance movement has been identified. In addition to forming VPg, NIa is the protease responsible for the majority of proteolytic events leading to the appearance of final gene products, acting in *cis* and *trans* at processing sites mainly defined by characteristic heptapeptides. Although NIa is structurally related to serine proteases, it has a cysteine at the active site. Moreover, the protease domain of NIa resembles P1 and HC in having nonspecific RNA-binding activity. The complete NIa forms inclusion bodies in the nucleus, where it is translocated by a bipartite signal sequence.

NIb (58 kDa), the second component of nuclear inclusions, is located next. It is the RNA-dependent RNA polymerase (RdRp). NIb contains domains distinctive of polymerases, including a highly conserved GDD motif. Recruitment for the replication complex is postulated to occur via its interaction with NIa. As well as NIa, it is directed to the nucleus by signals in its sequence.

The last product in the ORF is CP. Many roles have been assigned to this protein. First, it forms the virus

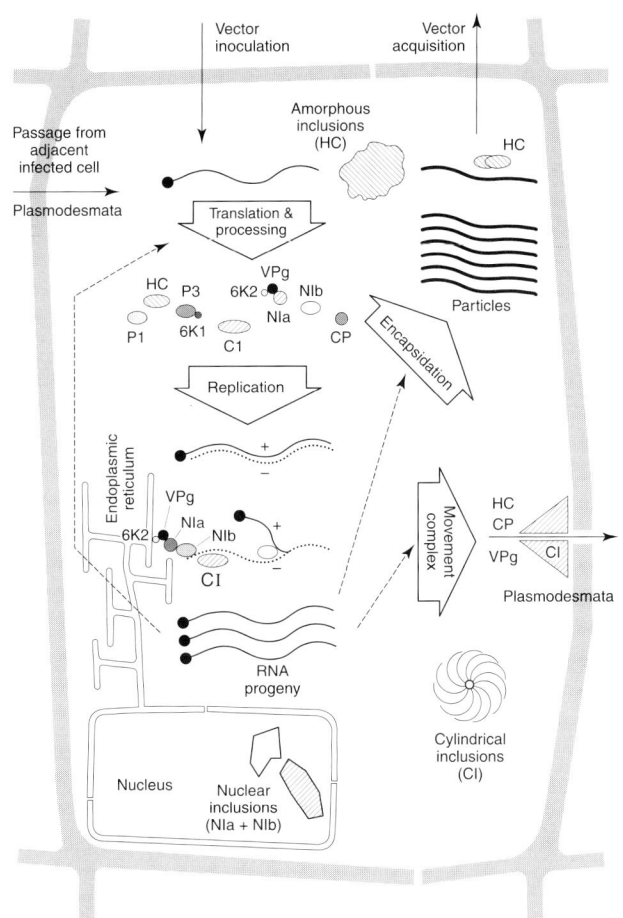

Figure 4 Different events during potyvirus infection of a plant cell. The eventual accumulation of viral proteins as inclusions in different compartments is also indicated.

particles, acting as protection for the genomic RNA. It is implicated in aphid transmission by interaction with HC (see Transmission). CP also participates in cell-to-cell and long-distance movement.

Gene products of viruses belonging to other genera in the family are believed to have equivalent functions. In the case of bymovirus RNA2, the large gene product has no sequence similarity with any potyvirus protein, and it has been postulated to play a role in fungus transmission.

Replication

Potyviruses replicate in the cytoplasm of infected cells. A scheme, based on works done by many researchers, is given in **Fig. 4**. After entering into a cell and undergoing desencapsidation, the genomic RNA must first be translated to give origin to the replication complex, which is composed of several viral products and probably host factors. The replication complex uses the genomic RNA (+ sense) as a template to generate a complementary chain (− sense), which serves as a template for the synthesis of numerous genomic RNAs. Translation of these genomic molecules results in accumulation of viral proteins, including the structural CP which encapsidates RNA to generate viral progeny particles. Movement to adjacent cells in the plant occurs via passage of the RNA through the plasmodesmata, in a form not totally identified, with the involvement of many products such as HC, CI, VPg and CP, and in the newly infected cell the replication cycle is repeated. Proteins involved could vary depending on cell type. Movement has been thoroughly studied by J. C. Carrington.

As a result of the potyvirus expression strategy using a polyprotein, the generation of many copies of CP needed to encapsidate progeny genomes implies the production of equimolar amounts of all other gene products. Some of them accumulate in inclusion bodies in different cellular compartments, while others might be secreted, degraded or remain in a nonnoticeable pattern. It is interesting that, whereas in all potyviral infections cylindrical inclusions (made by CI) are formed in the cytoplasm of infected cells, amorphous or nuclear inclusions (made by HC or NIa and NIb, respectively) are formed by some, but not all, potyviruses.

Potyvirus RNA replication takes place in membranous structures, probably derived from endoplasmic reticulum. NIb forms the core of the viral RNA replicase. NIb protein from TVMV shows *in vitro* RdRp activity, as recently proved. All NIb functions essential for RNA amplification may be provided *in trans*, as free protein supplied in transgenic plants complement TEV deletion mutants. Other proteins probably involved in viral RNA replication are the RNA helicase CI, the putative replication primer VPg, and the membrane anchoring factor $6K_2$. On the other hand, NIa interacts with NIb and RNA, serving perhaps to recruit products during the process. Other factors such as P3 might be involved as found by mutagenesis studies. P1 is also believed to play a role in replication, although it is the only nonessential potyvirus protein. Host factors also might be involved. In this regard, turnip mosaic virus (TuMV) VPg is able to interact with the translational eukaryotic initiation factor (iso) 4E, which may be involved in virus replication or/and translation.

A novel approach for the study of potyvirus replication and its effects on host cells has been developed by Maule. Using pea seed-borne mosaic virus (PSbMV) synchronous infection of cotyledon tissue and *in situ* hybridization, early events during infection have been studied. An infectious front can be identified, which involves active synthesis of minus-strand

RNA and subsequent later accumulation of genomic forms. Along with the presence of the viral RNAs in newly infected cells, a shutoff mechanism of translation of many host proteins was observed, as well as upregulation of other products (interestingly heat shock-related proteins or ubiquitin). These findings have been extended to other viruses and tissues, suggesting common molecular processes which might be significant in pathogenesis.

Evolution

Members of the family *Potyviridae* were considered within the Picorna-like supergroup of viruses, due to a fairly conserved set of proteins with replication-related functions present in analogous placement in the genome.

Genera in the family show a close relationship, indicated by gene product order in the polyprotein, strategy of expression and protein homologies. Each genus within the family seemed to be adapted to specific vector organisms. Cassette evolution has been proposed as the means used by viruses to incorporate new functions in their genomes, and this must have been the case for members of the family *Potyviridae*.

One intriguing issue is the shocking number of aphid-transmitted potyviruses. A combination of a very efficient transmission system and adaptation to new hosts must have contributed to this large expansion. In particular, vector transmission acting as bottlenecks might lead to broad speciation in the highly variable quasispecies structure of RNA genomes. Indications of recombination events, partial duplications, point mutations which confer different host responses, as well as other facts, might help to explain the extraordinary variability observed among potyviruses.

Transmission

As mentioned above, viruses in the *Potyviridae* family have different vector organisms. Bymoviruses are believed to be present and travel in the zoospores of their fungus vector. Rymoviruses and tritimoviruses are transmitted by eriophyd mites through a little known mechanism. Similarly, relationships between ipomoviruses and their whitefly vectors have not been clearly established. In contrast, the process of aphid transmission of potyviruses has been intensely studied in several aspects, specially in Pirone's laboratory. Transmission occurs in a nonpersistent manner, with the involvement of two viral proteins, CP and HC. There are nontransmissible variants of potyviruses exhibiting defects in either of these proteins, and by mutagenesis analysis alterations responsible for these phenotypic effects have been identified in TVMV and other potyviruses. The integrity of a highly conserved DAG motif near the N-terminus of CP has proved to be essential for transmission. In HC, mutations in several domains, mainly located in its N-terminal portion, result in failure of transmission.

The hypothesis currently suggested for the mechanism of aphid transmission involves a function for HC serving as a bridge to retain virus particles to internal structures in the aphid stylets. Using radioactively-labeled virions, it has been found that they are retained mainly in the distal part of the stylets. An *in vitro* interaction between HC and CP has been shown recently to correlate with transmissibility of CP variants of TVMV, and the domain of CP involved in the interaction includes the DAG motif. Recent results show that a PTK domain identified in the HC of zuchini yellow mosaic virus (ZYMV) is likely to be related to this binding to CP. Presumably other motifs in the HC might be involved in the interaction with the vector. In addition, specificity for each virus–vector combination is probably determined by compatibility between HC and the aphid.

Pathogenicity

The information about how potyviruses cause diseases in their host plants is limited. Recent research has begun to identify sequences and products in the genome of potyviruses that are directly implicated in the production of symptoms. As mentioned above, symptom alteration determinants have been identified in the 3' NCR of TVMV, and sequences in the 5' NCR of PPV, not essential for infectivity, contribute to pathogenesis. Chimeras between variants of viruses differing in their pathogenic responses have been generated, and thus used to identify the differences accounting for their phenotypic behavior. Single products are not always responsible for the effects. For instance, two separate domains have been identified in TEV implicated in the specific wilting response of Tabasco pepper.

VPg seems to be an important determinant of pathogenicity in potyviruses. Thus, sequence variations in the VPg are involved in resistance-breaking of TVMV and TEV in tobacco, and VPg determines pathotype-specificity of PSbMV in pea.

Sequences of the P1/HC region are involved in a synergistic effect in the case of mixed infections with other viruses. It has been proposed that HC is a broad-range pathogenicity enhancer that seems to transactivate viral replication by interfering with a plant defense response.

For bymoviruses, determinants for pathogenicity

and symptomatology have been found in the RNA1 of barley mild mosaic virus (BaMMV).

Control

Strategies considered for potyvirus control are diverse, from culture practices to the use of genetic resistance. Insecticide treatment of vectors has limited use because of the transmission type. The knowledge currently available about potyvirus replication, movement and transmission will eventually allow design strategies directed at interfering with these key roles during the virus life cycle.

Presently, a considerable effort (with not always equally gratifying results) has been placed in the exploitation of pathogen-derived resistance. Transgenic plants have been generated incorporating viral sequences. Since the early reports of CP-mediated resistance to plant viruses, this approach has been tried with several potyviruses. Results show that expression of one potyvirus CP in transgenic plants might confer resistance to other unrelated potyviruses. Nonstructural genes of viruses have been tested as sources of resistance, with promising results. Replicase sequences, for instance, create several resistant phenotypes, considered to be RNA-mediated. Elucidation of the mechanisms involved in resistance has been initiated after works done by Dougherty with potyvirus-derived transgenic lines, which pointed out the relationship of resistance and the cellular phenomenon known as cosuppression or gene silencing.

Future Perspectives

Analysis of potyvirus molecular biology using full-length cDNA clones has been extraordinarily successful in many respects, and it is likely to continue to provide interesting data. In particular, new control strategies might be developed after much better understanding of the potyvirus life cycle is achieved. Virus–host relationships involved in virus multiplication and pathogenesis, as well as in virus resistance, must be further characterized. Transgenic plants will provide information at this level, and even extend beyond, to be used as tools in plant molecular biology studies.

In addition, biotechnological uses of potyviruses has begun. The junction of P1–HC has been manipulated as a potential insertion site for foreign genes, allowing applications of potyviruses as expression vectors in plants, and it is likely that this or similar strategies will be further exploited.

See also: **Comoviruses (*Comoviridae*); Nepoviruses (*Comoviridae*); Plant virus disease – economic aspects; Pathogenesis: Plant viruses.**

Further Reading

Carrington JC, Kasschau KD, Mahajan SK and Schaad MC (1996) Cell-to-cell and long-distance transport of viruses in plants. *Plant Cell* 8: 1669.

Dougherty WG and Dawn Parks T (1995) Transgenes and gene suppression: telling us something new? *Curr. Opin. Cell Biol.* 7: 399.

Maia IG, Haenni A-L and Bernardi F (1996) Potyviral HC-Pro: a multifunctional protein. *J. Gen. Virol.* 77: 1335.

Riechmann JL, Lain S and Garcia JA (1992) Highlights and prospects of potyvirus molecular biology. *J. Gen. Virol.* 73: 1.

Shukla DD, Ward CW and Brunt AA (1994) *The Potyviridae*. CAB International, Oxon, UK.

Wang D and Maule AJ (1995) Inhibition of host gene expression associated with plant virus replication. *Science* 267: 229.

POXVIRUSES (*POXVIRIDAE*)

Contents

Capripoxviruses

Leporipoxviruses and Suipoxvirus

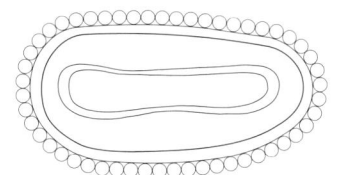

Capripoxviruses

R Paul Kitching, World Reference Laboratory for Foot and Mouth Disease, Pirbright Laboratory, BBSRC Institute for Animal Health, Pirbright, UK

Copyright © 1999 Academic Press

History

Sheeppox and goatpox are malignant pox diseases of sheep and goats easily recognizable by their characteristic clinical signs, and described in the earliest texts on animal diseases. Lumpy skin disease (Neethling) of cattle (LSD), however, was first described in 1929 in Northern Rhodesia (Zambia), having apparently been absent from domestic cattle until that time. From Zambia LSD spread south to Botswana and Zimbabwe and by 1944 the disease appeared in South Africa, where it caused a major epizootic, affecting over 6 million cattle. In 1957 LSD was first diagnosed in Kenya, and was thought at the time to be associated with the introduction of a flock of sheep affected with sheeppox on to the farm. Since then LSD has been present in most of the countries of sub-Saharan Africa, often associated with large epizootics followed by periods in which the disease is only rarely reported. In 1988 LSD caused a major outbreak in Egypt and in 1989 spread from Egypt to a village in Israel. This was the first time that a diagnosis of LSD outside of Africa had been supported by laboratory confirmation.

Taxonomy and Classification

The viruses that cause sheeppox, goatpox and LSD are all members of the genus *Capripoxvirus*, in the *Chordopoxvirinae* subfamily of the *Poxviridae* family, and have morphological, physical and chemical properties similar to vaccinia virus. Originally the viruses were classified according to the species from which they were isolated, but comparisons of their genomes indicate that the distinction between them is not so clear, and that recombination events occur naturally between isolates from different species. This is reflected in the ability of some strains to cause disease in both sheep and goats and in experimental results which show that all the sheep isolates examined could infect goats, and that goat isolates could infect sheep. The epidemiological relationship between sheeppox and goatpox isolates and cattle isolates is less clear, apparent in differences in the geographical distribution of sheeppox and goatpox and LSD (see later). However, some isolates recovered from sheep and goats in Kenya have genome characteristics very similar to cattle isolates. It has been proposed that confusion can be reduced by referring to the malignant pox diseases of sheep, goats and cattle, including Indian goat dermatitis and Kenyan sheep and goatpox, as capripox. It is envisaged that when sufficient isolates have been examined biochemically, no clear distinction will be possible between sheep, goat and cattle isolates, but a spectrum will emerge in which some strains have clear host preferences while others will be less defined and will naturally infect the host with which they come into contact.

Geographical and Seasonal Distribution

Capripox of sheep and goats is enzootic in Africa north of the equator, the Middle East and Turkey, Iran, Afghanistan, Pakistan, India, Nepal and parts of the People's Republic of China, and in 1986, Bangladesh. Sheeppox was eradicated from Britain in 1866, and from France, Spain and Portugal in 1967, 1968 and 1969 respectively. Sporadic outbreaks still occur in Europe, for instance in Italy in 1983 and Greece and Bulgaria both in 1995 and 1996, and Greece in 1997 and 1998.

LSD is enzootic in the sub-Saharan countries of Africa and is possibly still present in Egypt. The single outbreak in Israel was eradicated by slaughter of affected and in-contact cattle.

There is no clear seasonality to outbreaks of capripox in sheep and goats. In enzootic areas lambs and kids are protected against infection with capripoxvirus for a variable time dependent on the immunity of the mother. However, the spread of LSD is related to the density of biting flies and consequently major enzootics have been associated with humid weather when fly activity is greatest.

Host Range and Virus Propagation

Amongst domestic species, capripoxvirus is restricted to cattle, sheep and goats. Experimentally it is possible to infect cattle, sheep or goats with isolates derived from any of these three species, although clinically the reaction following inoculation may be indiscernible. Viral genome analysis using restriction endonucleases has identified fragment size characteristics by which it is possible to classify strains into cattle, sheep or goat isolates. However, the identification of strains that have intermediate characteristics between typical sheep and goat isolates does suggest the movement of strains between these species. Analysis of some Kenyan isolates derived from sheep and goats shows very close homology with cattle LSD isolates.

The involvement of the African buffalo (*Syncerus caffer*) in the maintenance of LSD has not been clearly established. Some surveys have shown the presence of capripoxvirus antibody in buffalo, while others have failed to show its presence. Buffalo clinically affected with LSD have not been described. Experimental infection of giraffe (*Giraffe calemopardelis*), impala (*Aepyceros melampus*) and gazelle (*Gazella thomsonii*) has resulted in the development of clinical disease.

Bos indicus cattle are generally less susceptible to LSD and develop milder clinical disease than *B. taurus*, of which the fine-skin Channel Island breeds are particularly susceptible. Similarly, breeds of sheep and goats indigenous to capripoxvirus enzootic areas appear less susceptible to severe clinical capripox than do imported European or Australian breeds.

Capripoxvirus will grow on the majority of primary and secondary cells and cell lines of ruminant origin. Primary lamb testes cells are considered the most sensitive system for isolation and growth of capripoxvirus. The virus produces a characteristic cytopathic effect (cpe) on these cells which can take up to 14 days for field isolates, but can be as short as 3 days for well-adapted strains.

Isolates of capripoxvirus derived from cattle have been adapted to grow on the chorioallantoic membrane of embryonated hens' eggs, although attempts to grow isolates from sheep and goats in eggs have been unsuccessful. Vaccine strains of capripoxvirus have been adapted to grow on Vero cells. Capripoxvirus will not grow in any laboratory animals.

Genetics

Less is known concerning the specific genetics of capripoxvirus than is known about the orthopoxvirus genome. Studies on field isolates taken from cattle suggest that the virus is very stable, as *Hin*d III restriction endonuclease digest patterns of isolates from the 1959 Kenya outbreak of LSD are identical to those obtained from 1986 LSD isolates. However, recombination has been shown to occur between cattle and goat isolates and this could be the natural method by which the virus evolves. By analogy with the orthopoxviruses, it is also likely that sequences are deleted or repeated within the genome in the normal replicative cycle.

Comparisons between the genomes of the different poxvirus genera show a relatively low level of nucleotide sequence homology. In common with other poxviruses, capripoxviruses contain a gene coding for thymidine kinase. Genes which code for attachment, fusion, interferon γ receptor and chemokine receptor proteins have also been identified, and sequenced, and shown to be highly conserved between isolates. Within the capripoxvirus genus, nucleotide divergence values suggest that the typical sheep and cattle isolates are more closely related to each other than to goat isolates. There is, however, less divergence between capripoxvirus genomes than seen in orthopoxvirus genomes, particularly in the near-terminal regions, which in the orthopoxvirus is considered to account for the considerably larger host range of this genus.

The usual technique for developing capripox vaccines has been to serially passage virulent isolates in tissue culture. This has been shown to reduce the virulence of the strain, although the mechanism by which it occurs is not known.

Evolution

The capripoxviruses have evolved into specific cattle, sheep and goat lines, but, as has been described above, intermediate strains exist, particularly those with cattle and goat genome characteristics. In Kenya there is evidence of movement of strains between all three species, but the absence of sheeppox or goatpox in LSD enzootic areas in Southern Africa, and the absence of LSD outside of Africa, would suggest that host-specific strains are being maintained and presumably are continuing to evolve.

Serologic Relationships and Variability

Polyclonal sera fail to distinguish in the virus neutralization test between any of the isolates of capripoxvirus so far examined. Sheep, goats or cattle that have been infected with any of the isolates are totally resistant to challenge with any of the other isolates. On this basis it has been possible to use the same vaccine strain to protect all three species. No monoclonal antibodies are yet available against capripoxvirus, but it can be expected that differences will emerge between strains using these reagents.

Capripoxviruses share a precipitating antigen with parapoxviruses, but no crossimmunity has been shown between these two genera, or between capripoxvirus and any other pox virus genera.

Epidemiology

In sheeppox and goatpox enzootic areas the distribution of disease is frequently a reflection of the traditional form of husbandry. For instance, in the Yemen Arab Republic, the sheep and goat flocks kept on the grassland of the central plateau and better irrigated regions of the coastal plain move about in search of food, frequently mixing with flocks from neighboring villages at water holes, and in this situation disease is restricted to the young stock. Animals over 1 year of age have a solid immunity. The animals belonging to villages in the more mountainous regions and the arid areas of the coastal plain are isolated by terrain or semidesert from mixing with animals from other villages. It is not known what is the critical number of animals required to maintain capripoxvirus within a single population but it is over a thousand adult animals, which is the approximate village sheep and goat populations. In these villages disease is usually only seen following the introduction of new animals, typically from market, and generally affects animals of all age groups. The disease spreads through the village, usually within 3–6 months, and then disappears in the absence of more susceptible animals. Occasionally, even within areas of high sheep and goat density, it is possible to encounter animals that have been kept totally isolated in the confines of a domestic residence, and these may remain susceptible to infection until adult.

In Sudan, large numbers of sheep and goats are trekked from the west to the large collecting yards and markets of Omdurman, outside Khartoum. Here also it is possible to see capripox infection in adult animals. Many of the flocks originate in villages which, like in the Yemen, are isolated from their neighbors. Capripoxvirus does not persist in these villages, and as a result the animals acquire no resistance, and are fully susceptible when they first encounter disease on the long journey across Sudan. Animals being exported from countries that are free of capripoxvirus may suffer a similar fate when they arrive in a capripoxvirus enzootic area, as often seen in Australian or New Zealand sheep imported into the Middle East.

In a study of 49 outbreaks of capripox in the Yemen, only eight were reported to affect both sheep and goats, the remaining 41 causing clinical disease in either sheep or goats. It is possible that both sheep and goats could have been involved in more than the eight outbreaks, but that the disease was inapparent in one species; whether, therefore, the species in which the disease was inapparent could transmit virus and become a vector for disease has not been determined. In Kenya, capripox is frequently encountered in both sheep and goats within the same flock, and there is the possibility that the same strain of capripoxvirus could also cause LSD in cattle.

The epidemiology of sheeppox, goatpox and LSD is similar; the severity of outbreaks depends on the size of the susceptible population, the virulence of the strain of capripoxvirus, the breed affected (indigenous animals tending to be less susceptible to clinical disease than imported), and, with LSD, the presence of suitable insect vectors. Morbidity rates vary from 2 to 80%, and mortality rates may exceed 90%, particularly if the infection is in association with other disease or bad management.

Transmission and Tissue Tropism

Under natural conditions capripoxvirus is not transmitted very readily between animals, although there are circumstances when transmission appears very rapid; for example, in association with factors that damage the mucosae, such as peste des petits ruminants infection or feeding on abrasive forage. Animals are most infectious soon after the appearance of papules and during the 10 day period before the development of significant levels of protective antibody. High titres of virus are present in the papules, and those papules on the mucous membranes quickly ulcerate and release virus in nasal, oral and lachrymal secretions, and into milk, urine and semen. Viremia may last up to 10 days, or in fatal cases until death. Those animals that die of acute infection before the development of clinical signs and those that develop only very mild signs or single lesions rarely transmit infection, while those that develop generalized lesions produce considerable virus and are highly infectious. Aerosol infection over a few meters only, as with other poxvirus infections, is probably the usual form of transmission. Contact transmission of LSD virus under experimental conditions in the absence of insect vectors has only rarely been reported. Biting flies are significant in the mechanical transmission of LSD, and *Stomoxys calcitrans* and *Biomyia fasciata* have been implicated. There are probably a number of insects capable of mechanically transmitting LSD virus, but insects such as mosquitoes, which preferentially feed on hyperaemic sites such as papules and if interrupted inoculate a new host intravenously, are considered the most likely to be involved in outbreaks characterized by large numbers of affected animals with generalized infections. Experimentally, *S. calci-*

trans has also been shown to be capable of transmitting sheeppox and goatpox.

During the recovery phase following infection, the papules on the skin become scabs. It is relatively easy to demonstrate virions in the scab, but difficult to isolate virus on tissue culture, probably because of the complexing of antibody and virus within the scab. Capripoxvirus is reported to remain viable in wool for 2 months and in contaminated premises for 6 months, and is reported to remain infectious in skin lesions of cattle for 4 months. The true epidemiological significance of the virus within the scab, and ultimately the environment, is not clear. It has been suggested that the protein material that envelops the virus within the type A intracytoplasmic inclusion bodies of infected cells protects the virus in the environment.

There is no evidence for the existence of animals persistently infected with capripoxvirus. Transplacental transmission of capripoxvirus may be possible in association with simultaneous pestivirus infection, as may occur with pestivirus-contaminated capripox vaccine.

Capripoxvirus can be isolated from the leukocytes during viremia, and has been isolated from lesions in the liver, urinary tract, testes, digestive tract and lungs; however, the cells of the skin and skin glands and the internal and external mucous membranes appear to be the major sites of virus replication.

Pathogenicity

There is considerable variation in the pathogenicity of strains of capripoxvirus. Nothing is known concerning the genes responsible in the capripoxvirus genome for virulence or host restriction.

Clinical Features of Infection

The incubation period of capripox infection, from contact with virus to the onset of pyrexia, is approximately 12 days, although it frequently appears longer as transmission is often not immediate between infected and susceptible animals. Following experimental inoculation of virus the incubation period is approximately 7 days, and this is similar to that shown experimentally using biting flies to transmit virus.

The clinical signs of malignant disease are similar in sheep, goats and cattle. Twenty-four hours after the development of pyrexia of between 40 and 41°C, macules (2–3 cm diameter areas of congested skin) can be seen on the white skin of sheep and goats, particularly under the tail. Macules are not seen on the thicker skin of cattle, and are frequently missed on

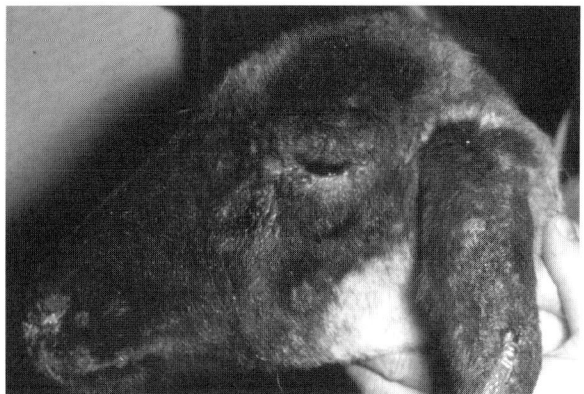

Figure 1 Sheep pox showing rhinitis and conjunctivitis.

skin of pigmented sheep and goats. After a further 24 h the macules swell to become hard papules of between 0.5 and 2 cm diameter, although they may be larger in cattle. In the generalized form of capripox, papules cover the body, being concentrated particularly on the head and neck, axilla, groin and perineum, and external mucous membranes of the eyes, prepuce, vulva, anus and nose. In cattle these papules may exude serum, and there may be considerable edema of the brisket, ventral abdomen and limbs. The papules on the mucous membranes quickly ulcerate, and the secretions of rhinitis and conjunctivitis become mucopurulent (**Fig. 1**). Keratitis may be associated with the conjunctivitis.

All the superficial lymph nodes, particularly the prescapular, are enlarged. Breathing may become labored as the enlarged retropharyngeal lymph nodes put pressure on the trachea. Mastitis may result from secondary infection of the lesions on the udder.

The papules do not become vesicles and then pustules, typical of orthopoxvirus infections. Instead they become necrotic, and if the animal survives the acute stage of the disease, change to scabs over a 5–10

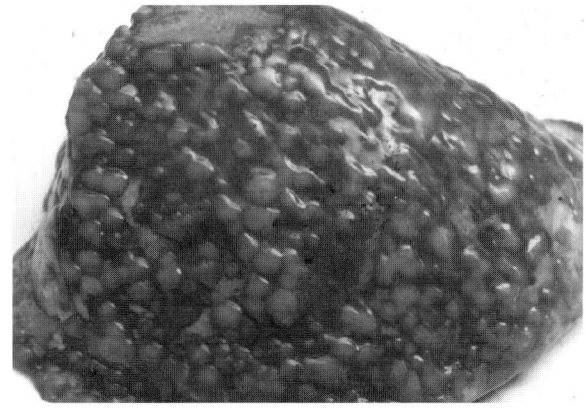

Figure 2 Sheep pox showing severe lung lesions.

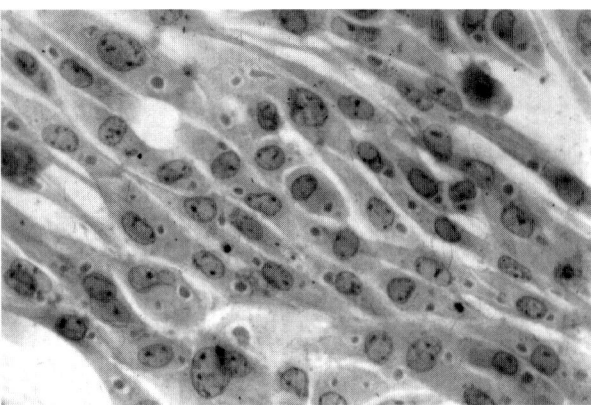

Figure 3 Capripoxvirus growing in lamb testis cells showing many intracytoplasmic inclusion bodies. ×400.

day period from the first appearance of papules. The scabs can persist for up to a month in sheep and goats, whereas in cattle the necrotic papules which penetrate the thickness of the skin may remain as 'sitfasts' for up to a year.

Severe disease is accompanied by significant loss of condition, agalactia, possibly secondary abortion and pneumonia. Eating, drinking and walking may become painful, and death from dehydration is not uncommon. Secondary myiasis is also a major problem in tropical areas.

Pathology and Histopathology

The lesions of capripox are not restricted to the skin, but also may affect any of the internal organs, in particular the gastrointestinal tract from the mouth and tongue to the anus, and the respiratory tract. In generalized infections papules are prominent in the abomasal mucosa, trachea and lungs. Those in the lungs are approximately 2 cm in diameter, and papules may coalesce to form areas of gray consolidation (**Fig. 2**).

In affected skin there is an initial epithelial hyperplasia followed by coagulation necrosis as thrombi develop in the blood vessels supplying the papules. Histiocytes accumulate in the areas of the papules, and the chromatin of the nuclei of infected cells marginates. The cells appear stellate as their boundaries become poorly defined, and many undergo hydropic degeneration with the formation of microvesicles. Intracytoplasmic inclusion bodies are present in infected cells of the dermis and also in the columnar epithelial cells of the trachea where frequently gross lesions may not be apparent. These are initially type B inclusions at the sites of virus replication (**Fig. 3**), but later in infection they are replaced by type A inclusions (see earlier). The maximum titer of virus is obtained from papules approximately 6 days after their first appearance.

Immune Response

Capripoxvirus, like orthopoxvirus, is released from an infected cell within an envelope derived from modified cellular membrane. The enveloped form of the virus is more infectious than the nonenveloped form, which can be obtained experimentally by freeze–thawing infected tissue culture. By analogy with orthopoxvirus, antigens on the envelope and on the tubular elements of the virion surface may stimulate protective antibodies. Animals immune to nonenveloped virus are still fully susceptible to the enveloped form. Passively transferred antibody, either colostral or experimentally inoculated, will protect susceptible animals against generalized infection; however, in the vaccinated or recovered animal there is no direct correlation between serum levels of neutralizing antibody and immunity to clinical disease. Antibody may limit the spread of capripoxvirus within the body, but it is the cell-mediated immune response which eliminates infection. In sheep, major histocompatibility complex (MHC)-restricted cytotoxic T lymphocytes are required in the protective immune response to orthopoxvirus infection, and therefore probably also capripoxvirus infection.

Immune animals challenged with capripoxvirus by intradermal inoculation develop a delayed-type hypersensitivity reaction at the challenge site. This may not be apparent in animals with high levels of circulating antibody. It has been suggested that the very severe local response shown by some cattle at the site of vaccination against LSD may be a hypersensitivity reaction due to previous contact with the antigens of parapoxvirus.

There is total crossimmunity between all strains of capripoxvirus, whether derived from cattle, sheep or goats.

Prevention and Control

In temperate climates capripox can be effectively controlled by slaughter of affected animals, and movement control of all susceptible animals within a 10 km radius for 6 months. In tropical climates, particularly in humid conditions when insect activity is high, movement restrictions are not sufficient and vaccination of all susceptible animals should be considered. In outbreaks of LSD it is not considered necessary to vaccinate sheep and goats, although theoretically cattle strains of virus could infect them. Similarly, in outbreaks of capripox in sheep and goats, cattle are not normally vaccinated.

Countries in which capripoxvirus is absent can maintain freedom by preventing the importation of animals from infected areas. There is always a possibility that skins from infected animals could introduce infection into a new area, although there have been no proven examples of this. The insect transmission of capripoxvirus into Israel from Egypt over a distance of between 70 and 300 km would indicate that it is impossible for countries neighboring enzootic areas totally to secure their borders.

In enzootic areas annual vaccination of susceptible animals with a live vaccine will control the disease. Calves, kids and lambs up to 6 months of age may be protected by maternal antibody, but this would only occur if the mother had recently been severely affected with capripox. Although maternal antibody will inactivate the vaccine, it is advisable to vaccinate all stock over 10 days of age. No successful dead vaccines have been developed for immunization against capripoxvirus infection, other than those that give only very short-term immunity.

Future Perspectives

Capripox of sheep and goats is present in most of Africa and Asia, whereas LSD is restricted to Africa. There is no good explanation as to why LSD has not spread into the Middle East and India, carried by the considerable trade in live cattle. Unless there is a reservoir host in Africa which is required for the maintenance of the cattle-adapted capripoxvirus, it can be anticipated that LSD will spread out of Africa, with major economic consequences.

While considerable attention has been given to vaccinia virus as a vector of other viral genes for development as a recombinant vaccine, little attention has been given to capripoxvirus as a potential vector vaccine. Although its use would be restricted to the not inconsiderable capripoxvirus enzootic area, it would have the advantage of not being infectious to humans, and being a useful vaccine in its own right.

See also: **Cowpox virus (*Poxviridae*); Fowlpox virus (*Poxviridae*); Immune response: Cell mediated immune response, General features; Mousepox and rabbitpox viruses (*Poxviridae*); Yabapox and Tanapox viruses (*Poxviridae*); Vaccinia virus (*Poxviridae*); Vectors: Animal viruses, Plant viruses.**

Further Reading

Black DN, Hammond JM and Kitching RP (1986) Genomic relationship between capripoxviruses. *Virus Res*. 5: 277.
Carn VM and Kitching RP (1995) An investigation of possible routes of transmission of lumpy skin disease (Neethling). *Epidemiol. Infect*. 114: 219.
Gershon PD, Ansell DM and Black DN (1989) A comparison of the genome organization of capripoxviruses with that of the orthopoxviruses. *J. Virol*. 63: 4703.
Gershon PD, Kitching RP, Hammond JM and Black DN (1989) Poxvirus genetic recombination during natural virus transmission. *J. Gen. Virol*. 70: 485.
Kitching RP, Hammond JM and Taylor WP (1987) A single vaccine for the control of capripox infection in sheep and goats. *Res. Vet. Sci*. 42: 53.
Kitching RP, Bhat PP and Black DN (1989) The characterization of African strains of capripoxvirus. *Epidemiol. Infect*. 102: 335.

Leporipoxviruses and Suipoxviruses

Grant McFadden, The John P. Robarts Research Institute, University of Western Ontario, London, Ontario, Canada

Copyright © 1999 Academic Press

History

Poxviruses of leporids and swine cause a broad range of symptoms varying from mild lesions of the skin right up to lethal systemic diseases (**Table 1**). The agent of myxomatosis, a virulent disease of domestic rabbits described originally by G. Sanarelli in 1896, was in fact the first viral pathogen discovered for a laboratory animal. The close similarity of myxoma virus (MYX) with other members of the poxvirus family, such as variola and fowlpox, was first recognized by Aragão in 1927. MYX is notable because, although it causes rather benign lesions in the native *Sylvilagus* rabbit (the brush rabbit in North America and the tropical forest rabbit in South America), when introduced to the European (*Oryctolagus*) rabbit it causes an invasive disease syndrome with up to 100% mortality. MYX was the first viral agent ever introduced into the wild for the purpose of eradicating a vertebrate pest, namely the feral European rabbit population in Australia in 1950 and, two years later, in Europe. The resulting genetic selection of virus isolates with lesser pathogenicity and upsurgence of rabbits with greater resistance to the viral disease was studied intensively by Frank Fenner and his colleagues as a model system to investigate the ecological consequences of virus/host evolution in an outbred population.

Also of interest to the history of animal virology is the fact that the first DNA virus associated with

Table 1 Members of the Leporipoxvirus and Suipoxvirus Genera

Member	Abbreviation	Natural host	Major arthropod vector	Natural host disease	Disease in domesticated European rabbit (Oryctolagus cuniculus)
Leporipoxvirus					
Myxoma	MYX	California brush rabbit[a] S. American tapeti[b] (*Sylvilagus* sp.)	Mosquito, flea	Localized benign fibroma	Systemic lethal myxomatosis
Rabbit fibroma (Shope fibroma)	SFV	N. American cottontail rabbit (*Sylvilagus floridans*)	Mosquito, flea	Localized benign fibroma	Localized benign fibroma
Malignant rabbit fibroma[c]	MRV	Lab. rabbit[d] (*Oryctolagus cuniculus*)	—	Not observed in wild	Systemic lethal syndrome similar to myxomatosis
Squirrel fibroma	SqFV	Gray squirrel (*Sciurus* sp.)	Probably mosquito	Localized or multiple fibromas	Occasional nodular dermal lesions
Hare fibroma	HFV	Wild hares (*Lepus* sp.)	Probably mosquito	Localized benign fibroma	Localized benign fibroma
Suipoxvirus					
Swinepox	SPV	Domestic pigs (*Suidae* sp.)	Hog lice	Localized cutaneous lesions	Intradermal lesions but no serial propagation

[a] Also called Marshall–Regnery myxoma.
[b] Also called Aragão's (or Brazilian) myxoma.
[c] Laboratory recombinant between MYX and SFV.
[d] MRV has been propagated only by serial inoculation of lab. rabbits and in cultured cells.

transmissible tumors was Shope fibroma virus (SFV), described in 1932 by Richard Shope as an infectious agent of fibroma-like hyperplasia in cottontail rabbits (*Sylvilagus floridanus*) in eastern USA. It is likely that the agent of 'hare sarcoma', described first in Germany in 1909, was also a poxvirus, now called hare fibroma virus (HFV). HFV remains the only leporipoxvirus to have arisen outside the Americas but its biology closely resembles that of SFV.

Very little is known about the remaining leporipoxviruses. Subcutaneous fibromatosis in gray squirrels of eastern USA and western gray squirrels in California, caused by poxviruses now collectively called squirrel fibroma virus (SqFV), have been observed since 1936, but their rigorous classification within the MYX–SFV family was not made until 1951 by L. Kilham. Similarly, HFV, described first in 1959 in the European hare (*Lepus europaeus*), was also shown to be a closely related poxvirus in 1961. In 1983, an outbreak of a disease resembling myxomatosis in laboratory rabbits in San Diego was caused by a novel leporipoxvirus later shown to be a genetic recombinant between SFV and a still-undefined strain of MYX. This virus, called malignant rabbit fibroma virus (MRV), has never been observed in wild rabbit populations but is of interest as an experimental model for poxvirus-induced immunosuppression and tumorigenesis. In most respects, MRV can be considered to be a substrain of MYX.

Based on landmark experiments with pneumococcus in the 1920s, the very first example of what was believed to be genetic interaction between viruses was reported in 1936 with the discovery that heat-inactivated myxoma could be reactivated with live SFV ('Berry-Dedrick' transformation), but later work showed this to be a genome rescue phenomenon rather than true recombination.

The only known member of the *Suipoxvirus* genus, swinepox virus (SPV), has been observed sporadically in pig populations throughout the world, but is not considered a serious pathogen because infected animals usually have only moderate symptoms and recover completely.

Taxonomy and Classification

The *Leporipoxvirus* and *Suipoxvirus* genera are in the subfamily *Chordopoxvirinae* of the family *Poxviridae*. The name lepori- comes from Latin *lepus* or *leporis* ('hare') and sui- from Latin *sus* ('swine'), to denote the relatively restricted host range of these viruses. All the viruses in the genus *Leporipoxvirus* can be shown to be closely related to each other by serology, immunodiffusion and fluorescent antibody tests although antigenic differences can be detected in strains of MYX. SPV (genus *Suipoxvirus*) is antigenically unique and is not known to have any closely related members. In terms of broad features, all are typical poxviruses, with characteristic brick-shaped virions containing a double-stranded (ds) DNA genome with covalently closed hairpin termini and terminal inverted repeat (TIR) sequences. Like other poxviruses, viral macromolecular synthesis takes place exclusively in the cytoplasm of infected cells.

Properties of the Virion

Like all members of the poxvirus family, the virions have a characteristic brick-shaped morphology with dimensions of approximately 250–300 nm × 250 nm × 200 nm. The leporipoxviruses are uniquely sensitive to ether and chloroform but otherwise the virions are very stable at ambient temperatures and in skin lesions. In all other respects, such as chemical composition and physical properties, the virus particles are very similar to those of vaccinia.

Properties of the Viral DNA and Protein

Detailed information about the viral DNA is available only for SFV, MYX and SPV. The leporipoxviruses have dsDNA genomes of 160–163 kb, with hairpin termini and TIR sequences of 10–13 kb. SPV DNA is somewhat larger (175 kb) and the TIR is only 4–5 kb but otherwise the genome has similar characteristics. It is believed that each virus encodes in excess of 200 genes. Restriction cleavage maps have been deduced for these viral genomes and generally the profiles are unique for each genus member but relatively well conserved amongst substrains and variants. Viral DNAs of leporipoxviruses crosshybridize at moderate stringencies only with other members of the genus, and SPV DNA is unique and is not known to crosshybridize with any other poxvirus DNA. The MRV DNA genome is 95% identical to MYX, except that it encodes five genes derived from SFV plus three SFV/MYX fusion genes.

The GC content of the leporipoxviruses (40% for SFV) is higher than that of the orthopoxviruses (35% for vaccinia) but there is evidence that many of the viral genes important for replication, gene expression and viral assembly are conserved between the genera. These essential genes for viral replication are clustered near the central regions of the viral genome. In contrast, viral genes mapping near the termini show considerable variability, and are believed to encode many of the specific determinants of pathogenesis that dictate host range and disease characteristics.

The protein complexities of these viruses as determined by one-dimensional gel electrophoresis are comparable to that of vaccinia virus, although the profiles are unique for each member. In the cases where specific genes involved in viral propagation have been sequenced, such as thymidine kinase and topoisomerase, the proteins have been shown to be highly homologous to their counterparts from other poxviruses. Leporipoxviral proteins involved in virulence and pathogenesis, such as growth factors and serine proteinase inhibitors, tend to diverge more extensively from homologues in other poxviruses.

DNA Replication, Transcription and Translation

All of the major features of macromolecular synthesis by these viruses are very analogous to those deduced for the prototype poxvirus, vaccinia. DNA synthesis is restricted to cytoplasmic sites, although replication tends to be initiated somewhat more slowly than for vaccinia. The virus-encoded transcriptional apparatus is well conserved between the poxvirus genera, and many of the important regulatory signals that are utilized by vaccinia, such as promoters and transcription termination sequences, are also utilized with comparable efficiency in the leporipoxviruses. Thus, viral genes from one genus can be introduced to another by recombination or by DNA transfection technologies to generate chimeric virus constructs that maintain the correct regulation of the new genetic information. As in the case of vaccinia, transcriptional units can be of different kinetic classes (early/intermediate/late) and there is no splicing of viral mRNA.

The leporipoxviruses replicate in cytoplasmic factories that appear by microscopic analysis as eosinophilic B-type inclusion bodies. These factories, also called virosomes, can also be visualized by Feulgen, Giemsa or fluorescent antibody staining. SPV produces nuclear inclusions and vacuolations in addition to cytoplasmic bodies but these nuclear alterations are not believed to be sites of viral replication.

Molecular Mechanisms of Pathogenesis

Since these viruses are of only minor veterinary importance, recent research has focused on the elucidation of the determinants for viral virulence, particularly with respect to the cellular hyperplasia associated with viral replication in affected tissue and the mechanism(s) underlying the immune dysfunction caused by MYX in *Oryctolagus* rabbits. To date, at least two classes of leporipoxvirus gene products have been directly implicated in viral pathogenesis.

1. 'Virokines' are secreted virus-encoded proteins that are targeted to host-specific pathways outside the infected cell. For example, SFV and MYX encode growth factors related to epidermal growth factor and transforming growth factor alpha that participate in stimulating fibroblastic proliferation at primary and secondary tumors.
2. 'Viroceptors' are viral proteins that mimic cellular receptors and function by sequestering important host cytokines that normally participate in the antiviral immune response. Leporipoxviral-encoded receptor-like molecules have been discovered for tumor necrosis factor (TNF) and interferon γ (IFN-γ), and may exist for other antiviral lymphokines as well. Swinepox virus encodes a novel homologue of cellular chemokine receptors, and the leporipoxviruses express secreted chemokine binding proteins that are important for virus pathogenesis.

Interference with antigen presentation by MYX is believed to play a role in circumventing T-cell recognition during early stages of virus infection. One MYX gene product responsible for evading immune clearance, designated Serp1, is an extracellular inhibitor of cellular serine proteinases but its precise target remains to be identified.

Geographic and Seasonal Distribution

All three major species of *Sylvilagus* rabbits in the Americas have endemic fibroma-like poxviruses, and myxomatosis is now established in wild *Oryctolagus* rabbit populations of South America, Europe and Australia. SqFV and HFV have been reported to date only in North America and Europe, respectively. The leporipoxviruses in the wild undergo seasonal fluctuations that correlate well with increased populations of arthropod vectors in summer and autumn, most prominently mosquitoes. An exception to this is found in Britain, where the major vector of MYX is the flea, which is not as seasonally variable.

In the case of SPV, outbreaks are not tied to seasonal cycles but are generally associated with the degree of hog lice infestation.

Host Range and Virus Propagation

These viruses demonstrate a very restricted host range in terms of ability to cause disease, although viral replication can also occur in cultured cells from some nonsusceptible hosts as well. In some cases viral replication in tissue culture monolayers or chicken chorioallantoic membranes produces 'foci' in which infected cells manifest minimal cytopathic effects, thus permitting macroscopic cell aggregations to develop. The extent of cytopathology is markedly influenced by both the cell type and the virus strain and in some instances the infected cells may detach from the monolayer to produce visible plaques. When viral replication is relatively slow and the toxicity to the target cell sufficiently moderate, a chronically infected carrier culture can be established in which progeny virus production persists for extended passages. Although poxviruses cannot permanently transform primary cells into an immortalized state, cells persistently infected with the fibroma-inducing leporipoxviruses assume many of the phenotypic characteristics associated with the transformed phenotype, such as novel morphology, growth in reduced serum and ability to form colonies in soft agar. It is likely that some of these phenotypic characteristics are facilitated by secreted poxviral proteins which mimic cellular mitogens, such as epidermal growth factor, and trigger neighboring cells into excessive proliferation.

In the cases of the benign leporipoxviruses and SPV, replication is restricted to dermal and subcutaneous sites, with occasional involvement of draining lymph nodes. However, MYX and MRV are unique in that they also replicate efficiently in lymphoid cells, such as macrophages, B cells and T cells. MYX, like HIV-1, replicates in either resting or stimulated T cells, and can be readily isolated from splenocyte cultures. The molecular basis for the uniquely permissive nature of MYX replication in lymphocytes is unknown, but is unquestionably an important factor in the extreme virulence of myxomatosis. Several MYX genes have been identified (M-T2, M-T5 and M11L) which function as host range determinants in infected lymphocytes by blocking the apoptosis response to infection.

Evolution and Genetic Variability

The deliberate release of MYX into rabbit populations of Australia, France and Britain in the early 1950s provided a unique opportunity to study the natural selection pressures exerted on a particularly virulent virus/host interaction. There is an extensive literature on the ecological consequences of this eradication program and the rapid evolution of myxomatosis in the wild is well documented. Although the original South American MYX virus strain that was introduced left very few survivors in selected populations, within a few years attenuated viral strains with reduced virulence took over and more resistant rabbits became predominant.

In terms of the categories of viral virulence, some strains of MYX are classified as highly virulent (e.g. Moses and Lausanne), and attenuated variants exist down to relatively nonpathogenic (e.g. neuromyxoma and the Nottingham strains). Little is known about the extent of genetic variation in other leporipoxviruses, although different isolates of SFV show marked variations in tumorigenicity. Generally, leporids which recover from infection with one member either become resistant or undergo partial protection from infection by another member.

SPV shares some antigenic crossreactivity with vaccinia, but neutralizing antibody does not confer crossprotection for secondary infections by members of different genera.

Transmission and Tissue Tropism

The principal mode of transmission is by biting arthropod vectors, and the major inoculation route is dermal. Since these viruses do not replicate in the vector, the transmission is purely mechanical and hence virus spread can be readily accomplished by alternative routes as well. Thus, mosquitoes, fleas, blackflies, ticks, lice, mites, and even thistles and the claws of predatory birds, have all been implicated in leporipoxvirus transmission. The efficiency of transmission by arthropods is quite variable, and is related to viral titers in skin lesions as well as the size of the vector populations. There are no known respiratory or oral routes of infection with members of either genus, but in some infections, such as MYX in domestic rabbits, the disease can be transmitted by direct contact with ocular discharges or open cutaneous lesions.

The sui- and leporipoxviruses in their native hosts are specific for the epidermis or subdermis and usually do not progress to secondary sites, although draining lymph nodes can be affected. However, in the case of MYX infection of the domestic rabbit the virus can propagate efficiently in lymphocytes and migrates via infected leukocytes through lymphatic channels to establish secondary sites of infection.

Pathogenicity

The leporipoxviruses are restricted to rabbits, squirrels and hares and swinepox is found only in domestic pigs. For SFV infection of *Sylvilagus* rabbits, tumors can last for many months before regressing, whereas in *Oryctolagus* rabbits recovery is usually complete within a few weeks. Only MYX manifests dramatic alterations in pathogenicity when the European rabbit is infected. For all of these viruses the immune status of the host rabbit plays a critical role; for example, in adult rabbits SFV rarely causes disease symptoms except for the primary fibroblastic lesion but in newborn or immunocompromised animals the infection can lead to invasive tumors and much higher titers of infectious virus in infected tissues. Agents such as cortisone, x-rays or immunosuppressants can dramatically increase SFV tumor development, and chemical promoters like 3,4-benzopyrene or methylcholanthrene can predispose progression to invasive fibromatosis or even metastatic fibrosarcoma.

The ability to evade the host immune response, replicate in lymphocytes and spread efficiently to secondary sites is a unique property of MYX in *Oryctolagus* rabbits. The myxomatosis syndrome can be associated with multiple external signs (e.g. South American MYX) or may have relatively fewer gross symptoms (e.g. California MYX) and mortalities can range up to 100%. Supervening Gram-negative bacterial infections in the respiratory tract and conjunctiva are often observed concomitantly with MYX, particularly by the adventitious pathogens *Pasteurella multocida* and *Bordetella bronchoseptica*, and contribute to the lethality of the disease.

SPV is only mildly pathogenic in pigs although it can cause a minor level of mortality, usually associated with milk feeding reduction in younger animals.

Clinical Features of Infection

The cutaneous tumors induced by the different leporipoxviruses in their natural hosts are clinically very similar to each other. The fibromas are rarely associated with any other symptoms, such as fever or appetite loss, and invariably regress as long as the animal is not otherwise immunocompromised. In the case of MYX in *Oryctolagus* rabbits, however, the symptoms rapidly become severe as the tumors fail to regress and the concomitant immunosuppression contributes to the lethal myxomatosis syndrome. The clinical features of myxomatosis are influenced by the genetic background of both the virus strain and the rabbit host. In the preacute form of the disease caused by California MYX the rabbits succumb in less than a week, and often have only minor external symptoms, such as inflammation and edema of the eyelids. Skin hemorrhages can be observed in some cases and convulsions often precede death. In the acute form caused by South American strains of MYX, the rabbits survive 1–2 weeks and develop more distinctive symptoms. The primary tumor can be either flat and diffuse or protuberant, and secondary site tumors around the nose, eyes and ears become prominent by 6–7 days, at which time purulent exudates from the nose and eyes frequently develop. The cutaneous tumors often become necrotic and a generalized immune dysfunction exacerbates the progressive secondary bacterial infestation of the respiratory tract. In the case of the more attenuated MYX isolates, such as neuromyxoma, the disease course is less severe and may be associated with little or no mortality.

The disease course of SPV in pigs is rather different, and resembles vaccinia in humans. Inoculation results in localized dermal papules, which progress on to vesicles and pustules, after which the lesions crust and scab over. The only clinical symptom is occasional minor fever and the animals recover completely within three weeks.

Pathology and Histopathology

The primary tumors caused by leporipoxviruses in *Sylvilagus* rabbits, squirrels and hares all closely resemble proliferant fibromas. Following inoculation, an acute inflammatory reaction occurs with infiltration of polymorphonuclear and mononuclear cells and proliferation of fibroblast-like cells of uncertain origin. The 'tumor' consists of pleomorphic cells imbedded in a matrix of intercellular fibrils of collagen. Unlike the transformed cells induced by other DNA tumor viruses, cells from poxviral tumors are not immortalized and cannot be propagated independently. Instead they appear to require secreted virus-encoded proteins in order to sustain the hyperproliferative state. Inclusion bodies characteristic of poxviral replication can be observed in the cytoplasms of epithelial and some fibroma cells. As the tumor develops, mononuclear leukocyte cuffing of adjacent vessels is observed and at the base of the tumor there is accumulation of lymphocytes, plasma cells, macrophages and neutrophils. The ratio between influx of inflammatory cells and fibroblast proliferation is variable but generally there is little or no necrosis. The speed with which immune cells clear the viral infection and reverse the hyperproliferation can range from 1–2 weeks up to 6 months, depending on both the virus and the host.

The principal difference between the benign fibroma syndrome described above and the devastating disease caused by MYX in *Oryctolagus* rabbits is that the latter viruses efficiently propagate in host lymphocytes and are able to circumvent the cell-mediated immune response to the viral infection. The subcutaneous tumors consist of proliferating undifferentiated mesenchymal cells which become large and stellate with prominent nuclei ('myxoma' cells). In surrounding tissue there can be extensive proliferation of endothelial cells of the local capillaries and venules, often to the point where complete occlusion leads to extensive necrosis of the infected site. The overlying epithelial cells can show hyperplasia or degeneration, depending on the virus strain, and poxviral inclusion bodies are frequently observed in the prickle-cell layer. In some MYX strains primary and secondary skin tumors can undergo extensive hemorrhage and internal lesions may be found in the stomach, intestines and heart. The virus readily migrates to secondary sites within infected immune cells and concomitant cellular proliferation can be detected in the reticulum cells of lymph nodes and spleen, as well as the conjunctival and pulmonary alveolar epithelium. The nasal mucosa and conjunctiva overlying secondary tumors undergo squamous metaplasia such that the epithelia become nonciliated and nonkeratizing. Disruption of the ciliary architecture may be one of the factors which facilitate the extensive Gram-negative bacterial infections of the eyes, nose and respiratory tract. Varying degrees of inflammatory cell infiltration by polymorphonuclear heterophils occur soon after infection but there is only a limited effective cellular immune response. The lymph nodes and spleen show evidence of aberrant T-cell activation and hyperplasia and infectious virus can be isolated from all lymphoid organs except the thymus. Death is believed to be caused by a combination of tissue damage from the increasing tumor burden, generalized immunosuppression and debilitating bacterial colonization of the respiratory tract.

Little is known about SPV pathogenesis but gross features closely resemble those of the noninvasive orthopoxviruses in their native hosts.

Immune Response

The benign fibromas caused by SFV/SqFV/HFV regress, albeit slowly, due to a combined cellular and humoral immune response. These viruses are excellent antigens and neutralizing antibody produced during recovery will also crossreact with other members of the genus. All of the leporipoxviruses are strongly cell-associated and cell-mediated immunity is probably the single most important mechanism of viral clearance. Other immune mechanisms are also activated, including interferon production, antibody-mediated cell lysis, sensitized macrophages and natural killer (NK) cells. Neutralizing antibody can last for many months after viral clearance and immunity is usually crossprotective to the other leporipoxviruses.

In the case of MYX in *Oryctolagus* rabbits the picture is very different. Although circulating antibody can be detected against virions, as determined by neutralization or agglutination, and against soluble antigens, as determined by complement fixation and precipitin tests, the antibody provides little protection against the disease progression. Instead, cellular immunity is severely compromised, and by day 6–7 lymphocytes (especially splenocytes) are demonstrably dysfunctional in their response to mitogens and lose the ability to secrete critical cytokines such as interleukin-2. Unlike the case of SFV, there is a notable absence of virus-specific T-cells in either the spleen or draining lymph nodes. Immune dysfunction is common in viruses that replicate in lymphocytes, but the precise levels at which MYX intervenes in cellular immunity remain to be clarified. There is some evidence that these viruses interfere with the function of cell surface MHC class I molecules, which could prevent proper viral antigen presentation and hence interfere with immune recognition of infected cells. Also, several virus-specific gene products have been shown to be secreted homologues of the cellular receptors for TNF and IFN-γ that are believed to bind and sequester these extracellular ligands in the vicinity of virus-infected cells and thus short-circuit immune pathways dependent on TNF and IFN-γ.

SPV-infected pigs generally recover from the infection and become immune to secondary challenge. There are few data on the nature of this immunity, but it bears close resemblance to that of vaccinia immunization in humans.

Prevention and Control

Since these viruses are spread principally by biting arthropods, vector control is the single most effective method of disease prevention. The viruses are susceptible to standard anti-poxvirus chemical agents, such as phosphonoacetic acid, arabinosyl cytosine and rifampicin, but these are of limited utility in infected animals. Immunization against myxomatosis can be accomplished with live SFV or attenuated strains of MYX.

Future Perspectives

Now that DNA sequencing studies have been initiated for many different poxviruses, it is likely that more viral genes which determine the clinical characteristics of their diseases will be discovered. Studies on viral gene products which stimulate fibroblastic and endothelial cells to proliferate will likely provide information on how mitogenesis is regulated by surface receptors on these target cells. The ability of MYX to replicate in lymphocytes offers an important system in which to elucidate the mechanisms of cellular tropism by which these viruses suppress the innate apoptosis response to virus infection. Furthermore, the analysis of virus-induced immunosuppression should shed light on the various immune strategies used by the host to combat viral infections in general. Finally, the restricted host ranges of the lepori- and suipoxviruses suggests the potential for the genetic manipulation of these viruses such that heterologous foreign antigen genes can be expressed for the purpose of developing novel vaccines against important pathogens of domestic leporids and swine.

See also: **Cowpox virus (*Poxviridae*); Fowlpox virus (*Poxviridae*); History of virology: General; Immune response: Cell mediated immune response, General features; Molluscum contagiosum virus (*Poxviridae*); Mousepox and rabbitpox viruses (*Poxviridae*); Pathogenesis: Animal viruses; Smallpox and monkeypox viruses (*Poxviridae*); Vaccinia virus (*Poxviridae*); Yabapox and Tanapox viruses (*Poxviridae*).**

Further Reading

DiGiacomo RF and Maré CJ (1994) Viral diseases. In: Manning P, Ringler DH and Newcomer CE (eds) *The Biology of the Laboratory Rabbit*, 2nd edn, p. 171. San Diego: Academic Press.

Fenner F and Ratcliffe FN (1965) *Myxomatosis*. Cambridge, UK: Cambridge University Press.

McFadden G and Graham K (1994) Modulation of cytokine networks by poxviruses: the myxoma virus model. *Semin. Virol.* 5: 421.

McFadden G (ed.) (1995) *Viroceptors, Virokines and Related Immune Modulators Encoded by DNA Viruses*. Austin: R. G. Landes.

Robinson AJ, Jackson R, Kerr P et al. (1997) Progress towards using recombinant myxoma virus as a vector for fertility control in rabbits. *Reprod. Fertil. Dev.* 9: 77.

Tripathy DN, Hanson LE and Crandall RA (1981) Poxviruses of veterinary importance: diagnosis of infections. In: Kurstak E and Kurstak C (eds) *Comparative Diagnosis of Viral Diseases III. Vertebrate Animal and Related Viruses. Part A – DNA Viruses*. p. 268. New York, London, Toronto, Sydney, San Francisco: Academic Press.

PRIONS

PrP

Contents
Human and Animal
Kuru
Yeast and Fungi

Human and Animal

Stanley B Prusiner, Departments of Neurology and Biochemistry and Biophysics, University of California, San Francisco, California, USA

Copyright © 1999 Academic Press

Introduction

Prions are novel transmissible pathogens causing a group of invariably fatal neurodegenerative diseases that present as genetic, infectious or sporadic disorders, all of which involve modification of the prion protein (PrP). This unprecedented spectrum of disease presentations demanded a new mechanism; prions provide a conceptual framework within which this remarkably diverse spectrum can be accommodated.

Prion diseases of humans are referred to as Creutzfeldt–Jakob disease (CJD), Gerstmann–Sträussler–Scheinker disease (GSS), fatal familial insomnia (FFI), fatal sporadic insomnia (FSI) and kuru (**Table 1**). In animals the prion diseases are called scrapie of sheep and goats, bovine spongiform encephalopathy (BSE), chronic wasting disease (CWD) of mule deer and elk, feline spongiform encephalopathy (FSE) and transmissible mink encephalopathy (TME).

Because prions and the mechanism of disease pathogenesis are without precedent, classification of the prion diseases has been quite varied. For many years, the human prion diseases were classified as neurodegenerative disorders of unknown etiology based upon pathologic changes being confined to the central nervous system (CNS). With the transmission of kuru and CJD to apes, investigators began to view these diseases as CNS infectious illnesses caused by slow viruses. Even though the familial nature of a subset of CJD cases was well described, the significance of this observation became more obscure with the transmission of CJD to animals. Eventually, the meaning of heritable CJD became clear with the discovery of mutations in the PrP gene of these patients.

Table 1 The prion diseases

Disease	Host	Mechanism of pathogenesis
A. Kuru	Fore people	Infection through ritualistic cannibalism
iCJD	Humans	Infection from prion-contaminated hGH, dura mater grafts, etc.
vCJD	Humans	Infection from bovine prions?
fCJD	Humans	Germline mutations in PrP gene
GSS	Humans	Germline mutations in PrP gene
FFI	Humans	Germline mutation in PrP gene (D178N, M129)
sCJD	Humans	Somatic mutation or spontaneous conversion of PrP^C into PrP^{Sc}?
FSI	Humans	Somatic mutation or spontaneous conversion of PrP^C into PrP^{Sc}?
B. Scrapie	Sheep	Infection in genetically susceptible sheep
BSE	Cattle	Infection with prion-contaminated MBM
TME	Mink	Infection with prions from sheep or cattle
CWD	Mule deer, elk	Unknown
FSE	Cats	Infection with prion-contaminated beef
Exotic ungulate encephalopathy	Greater kudu, nyala, oryx	Infection with prion-contaminated MBM

BSE, bovine spongiform encephalopathy; CJD, Creutzfeldt–Jakob disease; sCJD, sporadic CJD; fCJD, familial CJD; iCJD, iatrogenic CJD; vCJD, (new) variant CJD; CWD, chronic wasting disease; FFI, fatal familial insomnia; FSE, feline spongiform encephalopathy; FSI, fatal sporadic insomnia; GSS, Gerstmann–Sträussler–Scheinker disease; hGH, human growth hormone; MBM, meat and bone meal; TME, transmissible mink encephalopathy.

The Prion Concept

Prions are unprecedented infectious pathogens that are devoid of nucleic acid and seem to be composed exclusively of a modified isoform of PrP designated PrP^{Sc}. The normal, cellular PrP, denoted PrP^C, is converted into PrP^{Sc} through a process whereby a portion of its α-helical and coil structure is refolded into a β sheet. This structural transition is accompanied by profound changes in the physicochemical properties of the PrP. The amino acid sequence of PrP^{Sc} corresponds to that encoded by the PrP gene of the mammalian host in which it last replicated. In contrast to pathogens with a nucleic acid genome that encode strain-specific properties in genes, prions encipher these properties in the tertiary structure of PrP^{Sc}. Transgenetic studies argue that PrP^{Sc} acts as a template upon which PrP^C is refolded into a nascent PrP^{Sc} molecule through a process facilitated by another protein.

Perhaps the best current working definition of a prion is a proteinaceous infectious particle that lacks nucleic acid. Because prions appear to be composed entirely of a protein that adopts an abnormal conformation, it is not unreasonable to think of prions as infectious proteins. Although PrP^{Sc} is the only *known* component of the infectious prion particles, these unique pathogens share several phenotypic traits with other infectious entities such as viruses.

In a broader view, prions are elements that impart and propagate variability through multiple conformers of a normal cellular protein. The species of a particular prion is encoded by the sequence of the chromosomal PrP gene of the mammal in which it last replicated. In contrast to pathogens with a nucleic acid genome that encode strain-specific properties in genes, prions seem to encipher these properties in the tertiary structure of PrP^{Sc}.

The discovery that mutations of the PrP gene caused dominantly inherited prion diseases in humans linked the genetic and infectious forms of prion diseases and presented another hurdle for investigators who continued to argue that prion diseases are caused by viruses. More than 20 mutations of the PrP gene are now known to cause the inherited human prion diseases and significant genetic linkage has been established for five of these mutations. The prion concept readily explains how a disease can manifest as a heritable as well as an infectious illness. Moreover, the hallmark common to all of the prion diseases, whether sporadic, dominantly inherited or acquired by infection, is that they involve the aberrant metabolism of the prion protein.

Prion Protein Isoforms

PrP^C and PrP^{Sc} have the same covalent structure and each consists of 209 amino acids in Syrian hamsters (**Fig. 1**). The N-terminal sequencing, the deduced

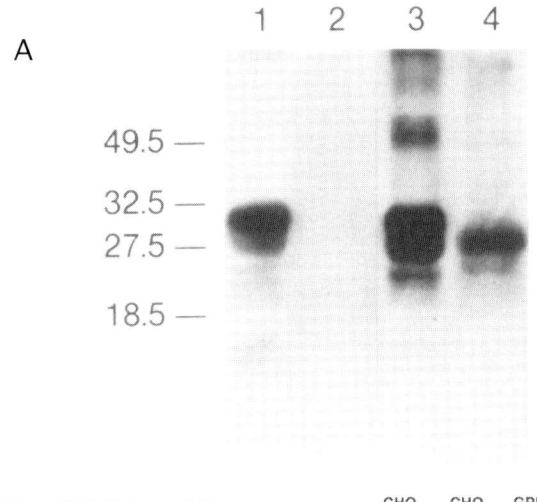

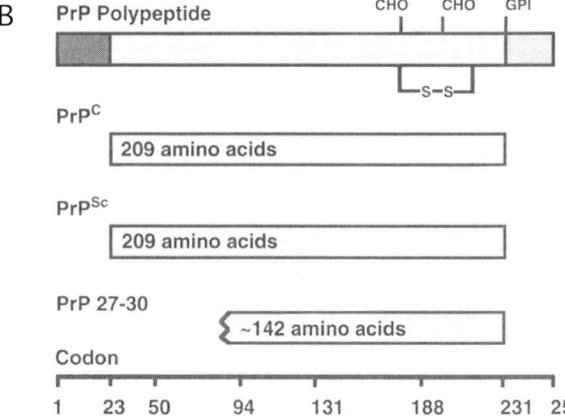

Figure 1 Prion protein isoforms. (**A**) Western immunoblot of brain homogenates from uninfected (lanes 1 and 2) and prion-infected (lanes 3 and 4) Syrian hamsters. Samples in lanes 2 and 4 were digested with 50 μg ml^{-1} of proteinase K for 30 min at 37°C. PrP^C in lanes 2 and 4 was completely hydrolyzed under these conditions, whereas approximately 67 amino acids were digested from the N-terminus of PrP^{Sc} to generate PrP 27–30. After polyacrylamide gel electrophoresis (PAGE) and electrotransfer, the blot was developed with anti-PrP R073 polyclonal rabbit antiserum. Molecular size markers are in kilodaltons (kDa). (**B**) Bar diagram of SHaPrP which consists of 254 amino acids. After processing of the N- and C-termini, both PrP^C and PrP^{Sc} consist of 209 residues. After limited proteolysis, the N-terminus of PrP^{Sc} is truncated to form PrP 27–30 which is composed of approximately 142 amino acids. (Reprinted with permission from *Molecular Neurology*, pp 175–204. Copyright 1998 Scientific American, Inc.)

amino acid sequences from PrP cDNA and immunoblotting studies argue that PrP 27–30 is a truncated protein of about 142 residues that is derived from PrP^{Sc} by limited proteolysis of the N-terminus.

In general, $\sim 10^5$ PrP^{Sc} molecules correspond to one ID$_{50}$ unit of prions, using the most sensitive bioassay. PrP^{Sc} is probably best defined as the abnormal isoform of the prion protein that stimulates conversion of PrP^C into nascent PrP^{Sc}, accumulates and causes disease. Although resistance to limited proteolysis has proved to be a convenient tool for detecting PrP^{Sc}, not all PrP^{Sc} molecules possess protease resistance.

The prion diseases are caused by the accumulation of PrP^{Sc}. In accord with the autosomal dominant inheritance of familial prion diseases caused by mutations of the PrP gene, PrP^{Sc} represents a gain of dysfunction.

Human Prion Diseases

Most humans afflicted with prion disease present with rapidly progressive dementia, but some manifest cerebellar ataxia. Although the brains of patients appear grossly normal upon postmortem examination, they usually show spongiform degeneration and astrocytic gliosis under the light microscope (**Fig. 2**). In all cases of GSS and variant (v) CJD, PrP amyloid plaques are found. Before PrP immunostaining was available, histochemical staining was used to examine brains from kuru patients where $\sim 70\%$ of cases were thought to have amyloid plaques. The presence or absence of PrP amyloid plaques in sporadic and inherited CJD is quite variable.

Human prion disease should be considered in any patient who develops a progressive subacute or chronic decline in cognitive or motor function. Typically, adults between 40 and 80 years of age are affected. The young age of more than 30 people who have died of vCJD in Britain and France has raised the possibility that these individuals were infected with bovine prions that contaminated beef products. Over 100 young adults have also been diagnosed with iatrogenic CJD between 4 and 30 years after receiving human growth hormone (hGH) or gonadotropin derived from cadaveric pituitaries. The longest incubation periods (20–30 years) are similar to those associated with more recent cases of kuru.

Sporadic CJD

Sporadic forms of prion disease comprise most cases of CJD and possibly a few cases of GSS (**Table 1A**). In these patients, mutations of the PrP gene are not found. How prions causing disease arise in patients with sporadic forms is unknown; hypotheses include horizontal transmission of prions from humans or animals, somatic mutation of the PrP gene, and spontaneous conversion of PrP^C into PrP^{Sc}. Since numerous attempts to establish an infectious link between sporadic CJD and a pre-existing prion disease in animals or humans have been unrewarding,

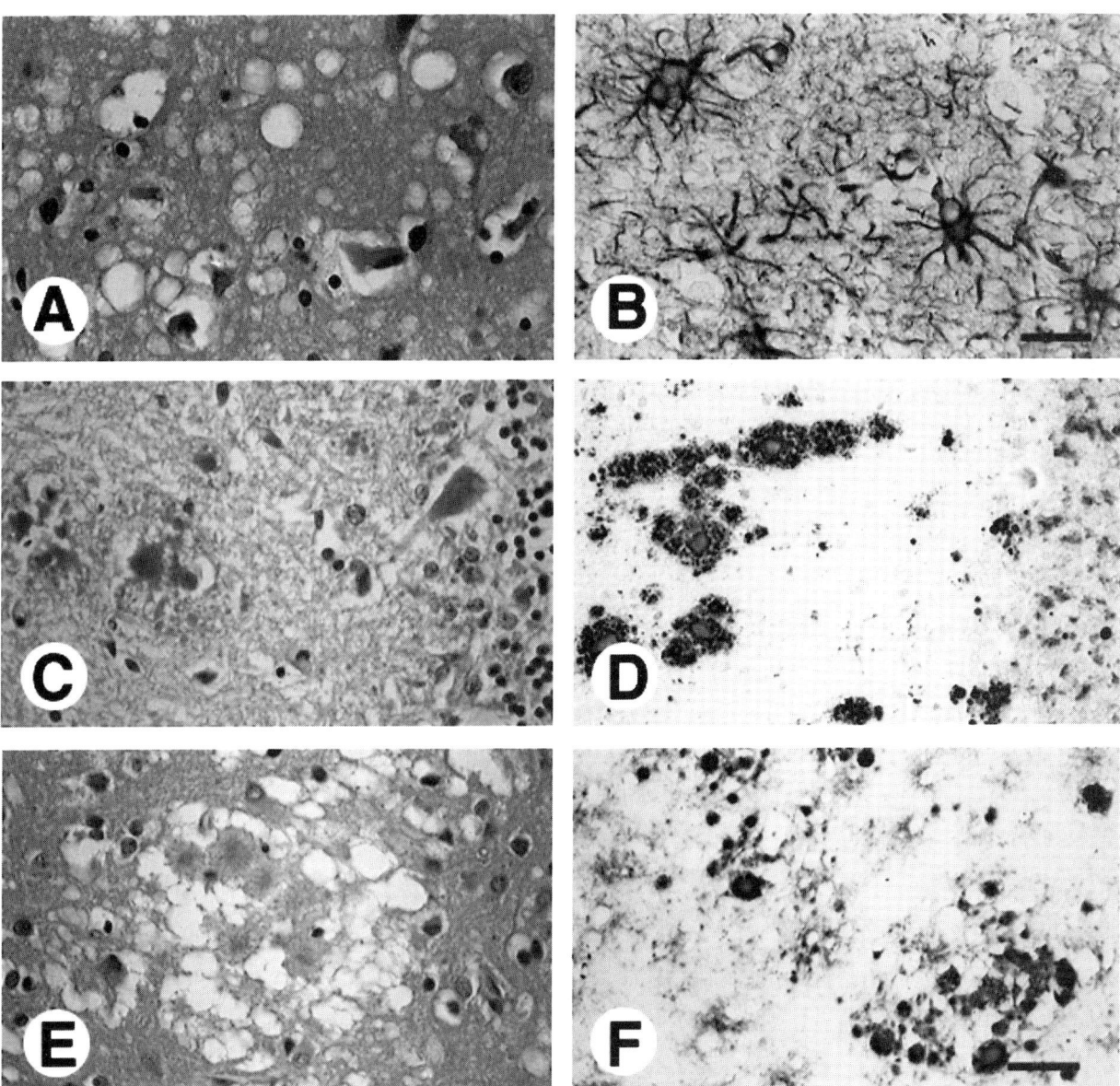

Figure 2 Neuropathology of human prion diseases. Sporadic CJD is characterized by vacuolation of the neuropil of the gray matter, by exuberant reactive astrocytic gliosis, the intensity of which is proportional to the degree of nerve cell loss, and, rarely, by PrP amyloid plaque formation (not shown). The neuropathology of familial CJD is similar. GSS(P102L), as well as other inherited forms of GSS (not shown), is characterized by numerous deposits of PrP amyloid throughout the CNS. New variant CJD (vCJD) has clinical and epidemiological features that suggest it was acquired by infection with prions. The neuropathological features of vCJD are unique among CJD cases because of the abundance of PrP amyloid plaques that are often surrounded by a halo of intense vacuolation. (**A**) Sporadic CJD, cerebral cortex stained with hematoxylin and eosin showing widespread spongiform degeneration. (**B**) Sporadic CJD, cerebral cortex immunostained with anti-GFAP antibodies demonstrating the widespread reactive gliosis. (**C**) GSS, cerebellum with most of the GSS-plaques in the molecular layer (left 80% of micrograph) and many but not all are periodic acid Schiff (PAS) reaction positive. Granule cells and a single Purkinje cell are seen in the right 20% of the panel. (**D**) GSS, cerebellum at the same location as panel C with PrP immunohistochemistry after the hydrolytic autoclaving reveals more PrP plaques than seen with the PAS reaction. (**E**) Variant CJD, cerebral cortex stained with hematoxylin and eosin shows that the plaque deposits are uniquely located within vacuoles. With this histology, these amyloid deposits have been referred to as 'florid plaques'. (**F**) Variant CJD, cerebral cortex stained with PrP immunohistochemistry after hydrolytic autoclaving reveals numerous PrP plaques often occurring in clusters as well as minute PrP deposits surrounding many cortical neurons and their proximal processes. Bar in B = 50 μm and applies also to panels A, C, and D. Bar in F = 100 μm and applies also to panel D. (**For color references see Color Plate 27.**)

it seems unlikely that transmission features in the pathogenesis of sporadic prion disease.

Inherited prion diseases

To date, 20 different mutations in the human PrP gene resulting in nonconservative substitutions have been found that segregate with the inherited prion diseases (**Fig. 3**). Familial (f) CJD cases suggested that genetic factors might influence pathogenesis, but this was difficult to reconcile with the transmissibility of fCJD and GSS. The discovery of genetic linkage between the PrP gene and scrapie incubation times in mice raised the possibility that mutation might feature in the hereditary human prion diseases. The P102L mutation was the first PrP mutation to be genetically linked to CNS dysfunction in GSS (**Fig. 3**) and has since been found in many GSS families throughout the world. Indeed, a mutation in the protein coding region of the PrP gene has been found in all reported kindred with familial human prion disease; besides the P102L mutation, genetic linkage has been established for four other mutations.

Tg mouse studies confirmed that mutations of the PrP gene can cause neurodegeneration. The P102L mutation of GSS was introduced into the MoPrP transgene, and five lines of Tg(MoPrP-P101L) mice expressing high levels of mutant PrP developed spontaneous CNS degeneration consisting of widespread vacuolation of the neuropil, astrocytic gliosis and numerous PrP amyloid plaques similar to those seen in the brains of humans who die from GSS(P102L). Brain extracts prepared from spontaneously ill Tg(MoPrP-P101L) mice transmitted CNS degeneration to Tg196 mice but contained no protease-resistant PrP. The Tg196 mice do not develop spontaneous disease, but express low levels of the mutant transgene MoPrP-P101L and are deficient for mouse PrP ($Prnp^{0/0}$). These studies, combined with the transmission of prions from patients who died of GSS to apes and monkeys or to Tg(MHu2M-P101L) mice, demonstrate that prions are generated *de novo* by mutations in PrP. Additionally, brain extracts from patients with some other inherited prion diseases, fCJD(E200K) or FFI, transmit disease to Tg(MHu2M) mice.

Infectious prion diseases

The infectious prion diseases include kuru of the Fore people in New Guinea, where prions were transmitted by ritualistic cannibalism. With the cessation of cannibalism at the urging of missionaries, kuru began to decline long before it was known to be transmissible. Sources of prions causing infectious CJD on several different continents include impro-

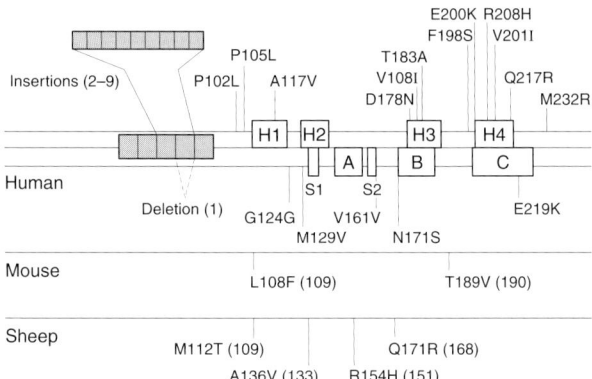

Figure 3 Mutations and polymorphisms of the prion protein gene. Mutations causing inherited human prion disease and polymorphisms in human, mouse and sheep. Above the line of the human sequence are mutations that cause prion disease. Below the lines are polymorphisms, some but not all of which are known to influence the onset as well as the phenotype of disease. Data were compiled by Paul Bamborough and Fred E Cohen. (Reprinted with permission from *Science* 278: 245–251. Copyright 1997 American Association for the Advancement of Science.)

perly sterilized depth electrodes, transplanted corneas, hGH and gonadotropin derived from cadaveric pituitaries, and dura mater grafts. As noted above, many young adults have developed CJD after treatment with cadaveric hGH. Dura mater grafts implanted during neurosurgical procedures seem to have caused more than 60 cases of CJD; these incubation periods range from 1 to more than 14 years.

Studies of the prion diseases have taken on new significance with the recent reports of ∼30 cases of an atypical vCJD in teenagers and young adults. To date, all of these cases have been reported in Great Britain, with the exception of one case from France. It now seems possible that bovine prions passed to humans through the consumption of tainted beef products. How many cases of vCJD caused by bovine prions will occur in the years ahead is unknown. Until more time passes, we shall be unable to assess the magnitude of this problem. These tragic cases have generated a continuing discourse concerning mad cows, prions and the safety of human and animal food supplies throughout the world. Untangling politics and economics from the science of prions seems to have been difficult in disputes between Great Britain and other European countries over the safety of beef and lamb products.

Strains of Prions

The existence of prion strains raises the question of how heritable biological information can be enci-

Table 2 Distinct prion strains generated in humans with inherited prion diseases and transmitted to transgenic mice

Inoculum	Host species	Host PrP genotype	Incubation time (days ± SEM) (n/n_o)	PrP^{Sc} (kDa)
None	Human	FFI(D178N, M129)		19
FFI	Mouse	Tg(MHu2M)	206 ± 7 (7/7)	19
FFI → Tg(MHu2M)	Mouse	Tg(MHu2M)	136 ± 1 (6/6)	19
None	Human	fCJD(E200K)		21
fCJD	Mouse	Tg(MHu2M)	170 ± 2 (10/10)	21
fCJD → Tg(MHu2M)	Mouse	Tg(MHu2M)	167 ± 3 (15/15)	21

phered in any molecule other than nucleic acid. Strains or varieties of prions have been defined by incubation times and the distribution of neuronal vacuolation. Subsequently, the patterns of PrP^{Sc} deposition were found to correlate with vacuolation profiles and these patterns were also used to characterize strains of prions.

The typing of prion strains in C57Bl, VM and F1(C57Bl × VM) inbred mice began with isolates from sheep with scrapie. The prototypic strains, called Me7 and 22A, gave incubation times of ~150 and ~400 days in C57Bl mice, respectively. The PrPs of C57Bl and I/Ln (and later VM) mice differ at two residues and control incubation times (**Fig. 3**).

Until recently, support for the hypothesis that the tertiary structure of PrP^{Sc} enciphers strain-specific information was minimal, except for the DY strain isolated from mink with transmissible encephalopathy. PrP^{Sc} in DY prions showed diminished resistance to proteinase K digestion as well as an anomalous site of cleavage. The DY strain presented a puzzling anomaly as other prion strains exhibiting similar incubation times did not show this altered susceptibility to proteinase K digestion of PrP^{Sc}. Also notable was the generation of new strains during passage of prions through animals with different PrP genes.

PrP^{Sc} conformation enciphers variation in prions

Persuasive evidence that strain-specific information is enciphered in the tertiary structure of PrP^{Sc} comes from transmission of two different inherited human prion diseases to mice expressing a chimeric MHu2M PrP transgene. In FFI, the protease-resistant fragment of PrP^{Sc} after deglycosylation has an M_r of 19 kDa, whereas in fCJD(E200K) and most sporadic prion diseases it is 21 kDa. This difference in molecular size was shown to be due to different sites of proteolytic cleavage at the NH_2-termini of the two human PrP^{Sc} molecules, reflecting different tertiary structures. These distinct conformations were not unexpected because the amino acid sequences of the PrPs differ.

Extracts from the brains of FFI patients transmitted disease into mice expressing a chimeric MHu2M PrP gene about 200 days after inoculation and induced formation of the 19 kDa PrP^{Sc}, whereas fCJD(E200K) and sporadic (s) CJD produced the 21 kDa PrP^{Sc} in mice expressing the same transgene. On second passage, Tg(MHu2M) mice inoculated with FFI prions showed an incubation time of ~130 days and a 19 kDa PrP^{Sc}, while those inoculated with fCJD(E200K) prions exhibited an incubation time of ~170 days and a 21 kDa PrP^{Sc} (**Table 2**). The experimental data demonstrate that $MHu2MPrP^{Sc}$ can exist in two different conformations based on the sizes of the protease-resistant fragments, yet the amino acid sequence of $MHu2MPrP^{Sc}$ is invariant.

The results of our studies argue that PrP^{Sc} acts as a template for the conversion of PrP^{C} into nascent PrP^{Sc}. Imparting the size of the protease-resistant fragment of PrP^{Sc} through conformational templating provides a mechanism for both the generation and propagation of prion strains.

Interestingly, the protease-resistant fragment of PrP^{Sc} after deglycosylation with an M_r of 19 kDa has been found in a patient who died after developing a clinical disease similar to FFI. Since both PrP alleles encoded the wt sequence and a Met at position 129, we labeled this case fatal sporadic insomnia (FSI). At autopsy, the spongiform degeneration, reactive astrogliosis, and PrP^{Sc} deposition were confined to the thalamus. These findings argue that the clinicopathologic phenotype is determined by the conformation of PrP^{Sc}, in accord with the results of the transmission of human prions from patients with FFI to Tg mice.

Interplay between the species and strains of prions

Studies on the role of the primary and tertiary structures of PrP in the transmission of disease have given new insights into the pathogenesis of the prion diseases. The amino acid sequence of PrP encodes the species of the prion, and the prion derives its PrP^{Sc}

sequence from the last mammal in which it was passaged. While the primary structure of PrP is likely to be the most important, or even sole, determinant of the tertiary structure of PrP^C, existing PrP^{Sc} seems to function as a template in determining the tertiary structure of nascent PrP^{Sc} molecules as they are formed from PrP^C. In turn, prion diversity appears to be enciphered in the conformation of PrP^{Sc}, and prion strains may represent different conformers of PrP^{Sc}.

Evidence for different conformations of PrP^{Sc} in eight prion strains

Using a highly sensitive conformation-dependent immunoassay for measurement of PrP^{Sc} in tissue homogenates, eight different prion strains passaged in Syrian hamsters were examined. Brains from Syrian hamsters were collected when the animals displayed signs of neurologic dysfunction; the incubation times for the prion strains varied from 70 to 320 days. Most of the PrP in the brains of Syrian hamsters with signs of neurologic disease was PrP^{Sc} as defined by the β-sheet conformation. The level of PrP^{Sc} in the brains of these clinically ill animals exceeded that of PrP^C by 3- to 10-fold. The highest levels of PrP^{Sc} were found in the brains of Syrian hamsters infected with the Me7-H strain; in contrast, the lowest levels were found in the brains of Syrian hamsters inoculated with the SHa(Me7) strain. Interestingly, the Me7-H and SHa(Me7) strains were both derived from Me7 passaged in mice, but they accumulated PrP^{Sc} to quite different levels.

Using this conformation-dependent immunoassay, each strain was found to initiate formation of PrP^{Sc} molecules with a distinct conformation. When the incubation times of the eight strains were plotted as a function of the concentration of either PrP^{Sc} or PrP 27–30, no relationship could be discerned.

To assess the fraction of PrP^{Sc} that is sensitive to proteolysis during limited digestion with proteinase K, we subtracted the protease resistant PrP 27–30 fraction from the total PrP^{Sc} for each of the eight prion strains. It was asked whether the proteinase K-sensitive fraction of PrP^{Sc} ([PrP^{Sc}] − [PrP 27–30]) might reflect those PrP^{Sc} molecules that are most readily cleared by cellular proteases. The clearance of PrP^{Sc} is of considerable interest with respect to control of the length of the incubation time and other phenotypic features of prion strains. When the [PrP^{Sc}] − [PrP 27–30] fraction was plotted as a function of the incubation time, a linear relationship was found with an excellent correlation coefficient ($r = 0.94$) (**Fig. 4**).

The above results demonstrate that eight different

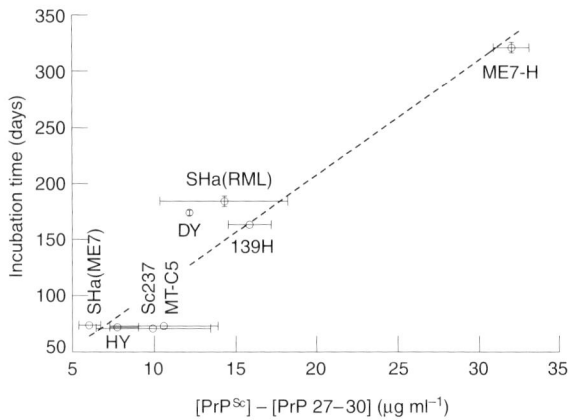

Figure 4 Eight prion strains distinguished by the conformation-dependent immunoassay. Brain homogenates of Syrian hamsters (LVG/LAK) inoculated with different scrapie strains were either undigested or digested with 50 µg ml^{-1} of proteinase K for 2 h at 37°C prior to the conformation-dependent immunoassay. The immunoassay was used to measure the concentration of PrP^{Sc} and PrP 27–30 for each strain. Incubation time plotted as a function of the concentration of the proteinase K-sensitive fraction of PrP^{Sc} ([PrP^{Sc}] − [PrP 27–30]). (Reprinted with permission from *Nature Medicine*, in press. Copyright 1998 Nature America, Inc.)

strains possess at least eight different conformations. Additional data argue that each strain is composed of a spectrum of conformations as revealed by limited protease digestion and GdnHCl denaturation studies. These findings contrast with the until recently held notion that the primary structure of a protein determines a single tertiary structure.

How many formations can PrP^{Sc} adopt? The conformation-dependent immunoassay described here provides a rapid tool capable of discriminating the secondary and tertiary structures of a substantial number of PrP^{Sc} molecules.

As noted above for studies of strains passaged from humans with fCJD(E200K) and FFI, PrP^{Sc} must act as a template in the replication of nascent PrP^{Sc} molecules. Also as discussed above, it seems likely that the binding of PrP^C or a metastable intermediate PrP* to protein X is the initial step in PrP^{Sc} formation and that this is the rate-limiting step in prion replication. PrP^{Sc} interacts with PrP^C but not protein X in the PrP^C–protein X complex. When PrP^C or PrP* is converted into a nascent PrP^{Sc} molecule, protein X is released.

It also follows from these observations that the different incubation times of various prion strains should arise predominantly from distinct rates of PrP^{Sc} clearance rather than from different rates of PrP^{Sc} formation. Thus, prion strains that are readily cleared should have prolonged incubation times, while those that are poorly cleared should display abbreviated incubation periods. This hypothesis was investigated by relying upon the difference in brain PrP^{Sc} concentrations before and after proteinase K treatment as a surrogate for *in vivo* clearance of each prion strain. When clearance, as approximated by $[PrP^{Sc}] - [PrP\ 27–30]$, was plotted as a function of the incubation time for eight strains, a linear relationship was found (**Fig. 4**). It is important to recognize that proteinase K sensitivity is an imperfect model for *in vivo* clearance and that only one strain with a long incubation time exceeding 300 days has been studied.

It has been suggested that Asn-linked carbohydrates (CHOs) specify prion strains, but this proposal is difficult to reconcile with the addition of high mannose oligosaccharides to Asn-linked consensus sites on PrP in the endoplasmic reticulum and subsequent remodeling of the sugar chains in the Golgi. Modification of the complex CHOs attached to PrP^C is clearly completed prior to the PrP^C trafficking to the cell surface, which indicates that the Asn-linked CHOs of PrP^{Sc} do not instruct the addition of such complex-type sugars to PrP^C.

Mutagenesis of the complex-type sugar attachment sites seemed to increase PrP^{Sc} formation in cultured cells, but resulted in prolonged incubation times in Tg mice and differences in the patterns of PrP^C distribution and PrP^{Sc} deposition in mice expressing mutant PrPs. These studies suggest that Asn-linked glycosylation might alter the stability of PrP, and in particular PrP^{Sc}, which results in various patterns of PrP^{Sc} deposition. Thus, different clearance rates of PrP^{Sc} may be important in determining not only strain-specific neuropathology but also the length of the incubation time.

Mechanism of selective neuronal targeting?

In addition to incubation times, neuropathologic profiles of spongiform change have been used to characterize prion strains. However, recent studies with PrP transgenes argue that such profiles are not an intrinsic feature of strains. The mechanism by which prion strains modify the pattern of spongiform degeneration was perplexing, as earlier investigations had shown that PrP^{Sc} deposition precedes neuronal vacuolation and reactive gliosis. When FFI prions were inoculated into Tg(MHu2M) mice, PrP^{Sc} was confined largely to the thalamus (**Fig. 5A**), as is the case for FFI in humans. In contrast, fCJD(E200K) prions inoculated into Tg(MHu2M) mice produced widespread deposition of PrP^{Sc} throughout the cortical mantel and many of the deep structures of the CNS (**Fig. 5B**), as is seen in fCJD(E200K) of humans. To examine whether the diverse patterns of

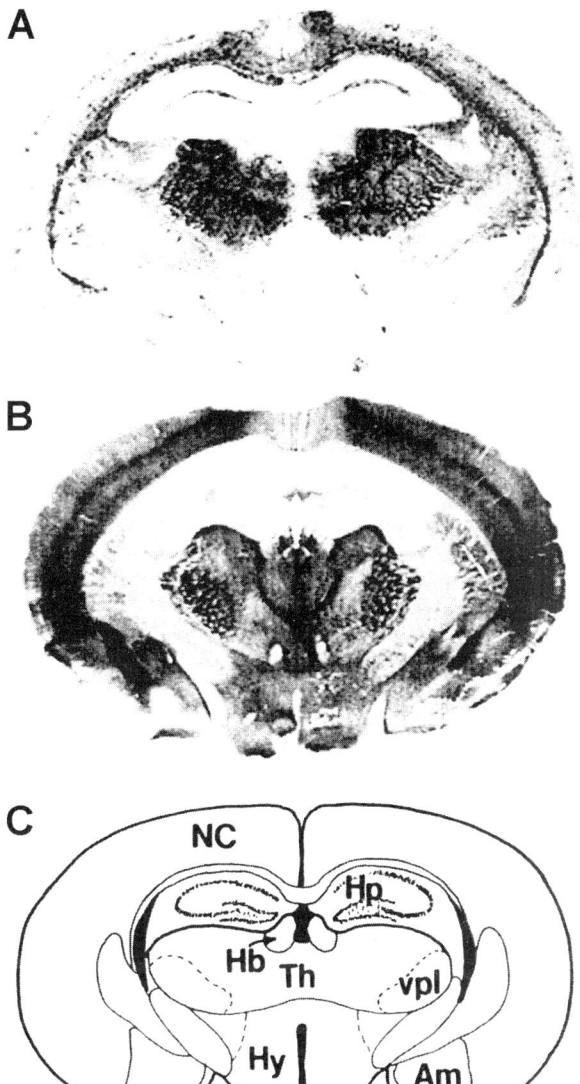

Figure 5 Regional distribution of PrP^{Sc} deposition in Tg(MHu2M)Prnp$^{0/0}$ mice inoculated with prions from humans who died of inherited prion diseases. Histoblot of PrP^{Sc} deposition in a coronal section of a Tg(MHu2M)Prnp$^{0/0}$ mouse through the hippocampus and thalamus. (**A**) The Tg mouse was inoculated with brain extract prepared from a patient who died of FFI. (**B**) The Tg mouse was inoculated with extract from a patient with fCJD(E200K). Cryostat sections were mounted on nitrocellulose and treated with proteinase K to eliminate PrP^C. To enhance the antigenicity of PrP^{Sc}, the histoblots were exposed to 3-guanidinium isothiocyanate before immunostaining using α-PrP 3F4 mAb. (**C**) Labeled diagram of a coronal section of the hippocampus/thalamus region. NC, neocortex; Hp, hippocampus; Hb, habenula; Th, thalamus; vpl, ventral posterior lateral thalamic nucleus; Hy, hypothalamus; Am, amygdala. (Reprinted with permission from *Cell* 93: 337–348. Copyright 1998 Cell Press.)

PrP^{Sc} deposition are influenced by Asn-linked glycosylation of PrP^C, we constructed Tg mice expressing PrPs mutated at one or both of the Asn-linked glycosylation consensus sites. These mutations resulted in aberrant neuroanatomic topologies of PrP^C within the CNS, whereas pathologic point mutations adjacent to the consensus sites did not alter the distribution of PrP^C. Tg mice with mutation of the second PrP glycosylation site exhibited prion incubation times of >500 days and unusual patterns of PrP^{Sc} deposition. As noted above, glycosylation can modify the conformation of PrP and affect either the turnover of PrP^C or the clearance of PrP^{Sc}. Regional differences in the rate of deposition or clearance would result in specific patterns of PrP^{Sc} accumulation.

Prion Diseases of Animals

The prion diseases of animals include scrapie of sheep and goats, bovine spongiform encephalopathy, transmissible mink encephalopathy, chronic wasting disease of mule deer and elk, feline spongiform encephalopathy and exotic ungulate encephalopathy (Table 1B).

Sheep and cattle PrP gene polymorphisms

Parry argued that host genes were responsible for the development of scrapie in sheep. He was convinced that natural scrapie is a genetic disease that could be eradicated by proper breeding protocols. He considered its transmission by inoculation of importance primarily for laboratory studies and communicable infection of little consequence in nature. Other investigators viewed natural scrapie as an infectious disease and argued that host genetics only modulates susceptibility to an endemic infectious agent.

In sheep, polymorphisms at codons 136, 154 and 171 of the PrP gene that produce amino acid substitutions have been studied with respect to the occurrence of scrapie (Fig. 3). Studies of natural scrapie in the USA have shown that ~85% of the afflicted sheep are of the Suffolk breed. Only those Suffolk sheep homozygous for Gln (Q) at codon 171 developed scrapie, although healthy controls with QQ, QR and RR genotypes were also found. These results argue that susceptibility in Suffolk sheep is governed by the PrP codon 171 polymorphism. In Cheviot sheep, the PrP codon 171 polymorphism has a profound influence on susceptibility to scrapie, as in the Suffolk breed, and codon 136 seems to play a less pronounced role.

In contrast to sheep, different breeds of cattle have no specific PrP polymorphisms. The only polymorphism recorded in cattle is a variation in the number of octarepeats: most cattle, like humans, have five octarepeats but some have six; however, the presence of six octarepeats does not seem to be overrepresented in BSE.

Bovine spongiform encephalopathy

Prion strains and the species barrier are of paramount importance in understanding the BSE epidemic in Britain, in which it is estimated that almost one million cattle were infected with prions. The mean incubation time for BSE is about 5 years. Therefore, most cattle did not manifest disease because they were slaughtered between 2 and 3 years of age. Nevertheless, more than 170 000 cattle, primarily dairy cows, have died of BSE over the past decade. BSE is a massive common source epidemic caused by meat and bone meal (MBM) fed primarily to dairy cows. The MBM was prepared from the offal of sheep, cattle, pigs and chickens as a high-protein nutritional supplement. In the late 1970s, the hydrocarbon-solvent extraction method used in the rendering of offal began to be abandoned, resulting in MBM with a much higher fat content. It is now thought that this change in the rendering process allowed scrapie prions from sheep to survive rendering and to be passed into cattle. Alternatively, bovine prions were present at low levels prior to modification of the rendering process and, with the processing change, survived in sufficient numbers to initiate the BSE epidemic when inoculated back into cattle orally through MBM. Against the latter hypothesis is the widespread geographical distribution throughout England of the initial 17 cases of BSE, which occurred almost simultaneously. Furthermore, there is no evidence of a pre-existing prion disease of cattle, either in Great Britain or elsewhere.

Origin of BSE prions?

The origin of the bovine prions causing BSE cannot be determined by examining the amino acid sequence of PrP^{Sc} in cattle with BSE, as the PrP^{Sc} in these animals has the bovine sequence, whether the initial prions in MBM came from cattle or sheep. The bovine PrP sequence differs from that of sheep at seven or eight positions. In contrast to the many PrP polymorphisms found in sheep, only one PrP polymorphism has been found in cattle. Though most bovine PrP alleles encode five octarepeats, some encode six. PrP alleles encoding six octarepeats do not seem to be overrepresented in BSE, as noted above (Fig. 3).

Brain extracts from BSE cattle cause disease in cattle, sheep, mice, pigs and mink after intracerebral inoculation, but prions in brain extracts from sheep with scrapie fed to cattle produced illness substantially different from BSE. However, no exhaustive effort has been made to test different strains of sheep prions or to examine the disease following bovine to bovine passage. The annual incidence of sheep with scrapie in Great Britain over the past two decades has remained relatively low. In July 1988, the practice of feeding MBM to sheep and cattle was banned. Recent statistical analysis argues that the epidemic is now disappearing as a result of this ruminant feed ban, reminiscent of the disappearance of kuru in the Fore people of New Guinea.

Monitoring cattle for BSE prions

Although many plans have been offered for the culling of older cattle in order to minimize the spread of BSE, it seems more important to monitor the frequency of prion disease in cattle as they are slaughtered for human consumption. No reliable, specific test for prion disease in live animals is available, but immunoassays for PrP^{Sc} in the brainstems of cattle might provide a reasonable approach to establishing the incidence of subclinical BSE in cattle entering the human food chain. Determining how early in the incubation period PrP^{Sc} can be detected by immunological methods is now possible because a reliable bioassay has been created by expressing the BoPrP gene in Tg mice. Prior to development of Tg(BoPrP)Prnp$^{0/0}$ mice, non-Tg mice inoculated intracerebrally with BSE brain extracts required more than 300 days to develop disease. Depending on the titer of the inoculum, the structures of PrP^C and PrP^{Sc} and the structure of protein X, the number of inoculated animals developing disease can vary over a wide range. Some investigators have stated that transmission of BSE to mice is quite variable, with incubation periods exceeding 1 year, while others report low prion titers in BSE brain homogenates compared to rodent brain scrapie.

Have bovine prions been transmitted to humans?

In 1994, the first cases of CJD in teenagers and young adults that were eventually labelled new variant (v) CJD occurred in Great Britain. In addition to the young age of these cases, the brains of these patients showed numerous PrP amyloid plaques surrounded by a halo of intense spongiform degeneration. These unusual neuropathologic changes have not been seen in CJD cases in the USA, Australia or Japan. Both macaque monkeys and marmosets developed neurologic disease several years after inoculation with bovine prions, but only the macaques exhibited numerous PrP plaques similar to those found in vCJD.

The restricted geographical occurrence and chronology of vCJD have raised the possibility that BSE prions have been transmitted to humans. That only ~30 vCJD cases have been recorded and the incidence has remained relatively constant make establishing the origin of vCJD difficult. No set of dietary habits distinguishes vCJD patients from apparently healthy people. Moreover, there is no explanation for the predilection of vCJD for teenagers and young adults. Why have older individuals not developed vCJD-based neuropathologic criteria? It is noteworthy that epidemiological studies over the past three decades have failed to find evidence for transmission of sheep prions to humans. Attempts to predict the future number of cases of vCJD, assuming exposure to bovine prions prior to the offal ban, have been uninformative because so few cases of vCJD have occurred. Are we at the beginning of a human prion disease epidemic in Britain like those seen for BSE and kuru, or will the number of vCJD cases remain small, as seen with iatrogenic (i) CJD caused by cadaveric hGH?

Strain of BSE prions

Was a particular conformation of bovine PrP^{Sc} selected for heat resistance during the rendering process, and then reselected multiple times as cattle infected by ingesting prion-contaminated MBM were slaughtered and their offal rendered into more MBM? Recent studies of PrP^{Sc} from brains of patients who died of vCJD show a pattern of PrP glycoforms different from those found for sCJD or iCJD. But the utility of measuring PrP glycoforms is questionable in trying to relate BSE to vCJD because PrP^{Sc} is formed after the protein is glycosylated and enzymatic deglycosylation of PrP^{Sc} requires denaturation. Alternatively, it may be possible to establish a relationship between the conformations of PrP^{Sc} from cattle with BSE and those from humans with vCJD by using Tg mice, as was done for strains generated in the brains of patients with FFI or fCJD. A relationship between vCJD and BSE has been suggested, based on the finding of similar incubation times in non-Tg RIII mice of ~310 days after inoculation with human or bovine prions.

Summation

Although prions were originally defined in the context of an infectious mammalian pathogen, it is now becoming widely accepted that prions are elements that impart and propagate variability through multiple conformers of a normal cellular protein. Such a mechanism must surely not be restricted to a single class of transmissible pathogens. Indeed, proteins that act like prions have recently been reported in fungi. It is likely that the original definition will need to be extended to encompass other situations where a similar mechanism of information transfer occurs.

The study of prions has taken several unexpected directions over the past three decades; a novel and fascinating story of prion biology is emerging. Investigations of prions have elucidated a previously unknown mechanism of disease in humans and animals. While learning the details of the structures of PrPs and deciphering the mechanism of PrP^C transformation into PrP^{Sc} will be important, the fundamental principles of prion biology have become reasonably clear. Though some investigators prefer to view the composition of the infectious prion particle as unresolved, such a perspective denies an enlarging body of data, none of which refutes the prion concept. Moreover, the discovery of prion-like phenomena mediated by proteins unrelated to PrP in yeast and other fungi serves not only to strengthen the prion concept but also to widen it.

The discovery that prion diseases in humans are uniquely both genetic and infectious greatly strengthened and extended the prion concept. To date, 20 different mutations in the human PrP gene, all resulting in nonconservative substitutions, have been found either to be linked genetically to or to segregate with the inherited prion diseases (**Fig. 3**). Yet the transmissible prion particle is composed largely, if not exclusively, of an abnormal isoform of the prion protein designated PrP^{Sc}.

The wealth of data establishing the essential role of PrP in the transmission of prions and the pathogenesis of prion diseases has provoked consideration of how many biological processes are controlled by changes in protein conformation. The extreme radiation-resistance of the scrapie infectivity suggested that the pathogen causing this disease and related illnesses would be different from viruses, viroids and bacteria. Indeed, an unprecedented mechanism of disease has been revealed where an aberrant conformational change in a protein is propagated. The future of this emerging area of biology should prove even more interesting and productive as many new discoveries emerge.

See also: **Prions: Kuru.**

Acknowledgements

I thank Drs Fred Cohen, Stephen DeArmond, Jiri Safar and Michael Scott for helpful discussions. This research was supported by grants from the National Institute of Aging and the National Institute of Neurologic Diseases and Stroke of the National Institutes of Health, International Human Frontiers of Science Program and American Health Assistance Foundation, as well as by gifts from the Sherman Fairchild Foundation, Keck Foundation, G Harold and Leila Y Mathers Foundation, Bernard Osher Foundation, John D French Foundation and Centeon.

Further Reading

Alper T, Cramp WA, Haig DA and Clarke MC (1967) Does the agent of scrapie replicate without nucleic acid? *Nature* 214: 764.

DeArmond SJ and Prusiner SB (1997) Prion diseases. In: Lartos P and Graham D (eds) *Greenfield's Neuropathology* 6th edn, p. 235. London: Edward Arnold.

Gajdusek DC (1977) Unconventional viruses and the origin and disappearance of kuru. *Science* 197: 943.

Prusiner SB (1998) Prions. *Proc. Natl. Acad. Sci* 95: 13363.

Prusiner SB, Scott MR, DeArmond SJ and Cohen FE (1998) Prion protein biology. *Cell* 93: 337.

Safar J, Wille H, Itri V *et al* (1998) Eight prion strains have PrP^{Sc} molecules with different conformations. *Nat. Med.* 4: 1157.

Kuru

Carlo Masullo, Institute of Neurology, Catholic University School of Medicine, Rome, Italy

Copyright © 1999 Academic Press

History

Kuru was the first naturally occurring subacute spongiform encephalopathy of humans shown to be caused by an unconventional transmissible agent. Kuru means shivering or trembling in the Fore language. It was first described by Gajdusek and Zigas in 1957 in the Fore cultural and linguistic group of isolated regions of Papua New Guinea. It was found to affect all ages, being common in male and female children and in adult females, but rare in adult males. Kuru is characterized by cerebellar ataxia and a shivering-like tremor that produces complete motor incoordination. The disease is inevitably fatal and death usually occurs in less than 1 year.

Classification

Kuru belongs to the group of subacute spongiform encephalopathies or prion diseases of humans which also include Creutzfeldt–Jakob disease (CJD), Gerstmann–Straussler syndrome (GSS) and fatal familial insomnia (FFI); related animal diseases are scrapie of sheep and goats, chronic wasting disease (CWD) of mule and deer, transmissible mink encephalopathy (TME) and bovine spongiform encephalopathy (BSE).

Geographic and Seasonal Distribution

Kuru has been found in the Eastern Highlands

Province of Papua New Guinea, which has a population of about 35 000 people living in 160 villages. These villages are located from 1000 to 2500 meters above sea level. No cases of Kuru have been found outside this geographical region. No evidence has emerged from the clinico-epidemiological studies on different seasonal trends of the disease.

Host Range and Virus Propagation

Kuru is naturally occurring only in humans and its clinical course is inevitably fatal.

Experimental transmission of Kuru has been obtained in nonhuman primates and in some small rodents, such as minks and ferrets, through intracerebral inoculation of brain material of patients who died from Kuru. Fourteen strains of Kuru have been isolated and 11 of these human strains have been inoculated into small laboratory rodents, i.e. hamsters, mice and guinea pigs. Only three of these 11 strains produced clinical disease and neuropathological lesions in an occasional mouse on primary passage, and none of these have been successfully serially transmitted from mouse to mouse. Hamsters and guinea pigs failed to develop clinical disease or evidence of brain pathology during several years of follow-up after the experimental inoculation.

A similar pattern of strain adaptation occurred in attempting the transmission of strains of Kuru adapted into nonhuman primates to small rodents. In fact, several strains of chimpanzee, capuchin, spider, rhesus and squirrel monkey-adapted Kuru virus failed to transmit the disease or induce subclinical neuropathological lesions in small rodents for their entire lifespan. On the contrary, two primate-adapted strains of Kuru have caused disease in one of several minks and one of several ferrets, respectively. Serial passage of the Kuru virus in mink has not been successful, while primary passage into ferrets required an incubation of 31 months; serial passage of this same strain in ferrets has been associated with incubation periods of 59 and 70.5 months, respectively, in the two animals which developed the disease on the first ferret-to-ferret passage, and 9 months in the one ferret which developed the disease on the second ferret-to-ferret passage. This variable behavior of a given strain of Kuru has been observed with the passage of the virus between species and, to a lesser degree, within the same species of experimental host. The time sequence of disease progression also mimics that in humans, ranging from several months to over a year until death. A single strain of Kuru virus may cause severe neuronal spongiosis in different brain areas such as the cerebral cortex in chimpanzees without any major neuropathological involvement of the brainstem or spinal cord. On the contrary, this same virus strain may produce extensive brainstem and spinal cord lesions in the squirrel monkey.

Kuru is a naturally occurring disease and its mode of dissemination and maintenance is not completely clarified. A possible explanation is the contamination of close kinsmen by opening of the skull of dead victims in a rite of cannibalism, during which all girls, women and children of the Kuru victim's family were certainly exposed to the virus. The disease is gradually disappearing with the cessation of ritualistic cannibalism.

There are several hundred Kuru orphans born since 1957 to mothers dying of Kuru and none has yet developed the disease. Thus, the many children with Kuru seen in the 1950s were not infected prenatally, perinatally or neonatally by their mothers. Kuru has progressively disappeared, first among children and thereafter among adolescents.

Genetics

Experimental studies have shown that there are several strains of the Kuru agent. In fact, at least 14 strains of Kuru have been isolated by direct inoculation of human brain into nonhuman primates.

Recent studies on the search for possible mutations of the PRNP gene found no mutations occurred in some Kuru cases. The polymorphism at the codon 129 of the PRNP (prion protein) gene has been determined in a group of 38 Kuru patients and the genotypes were M/V in 50%, M/M in 30% and V/V in 20% of the cases; in a control group of the same ethnic background, the genotypes were M/V in 48%, M/M in 30% and V/V in 22%. Therefore, no differences between Kuru patients and their controls have been found, irrespective of the codon 129 genotype.

Evolution

The origin of Kuru is not clear; it is possible that it resulted from a sporadic case of CJD, which, in that particular environment of New Guinea, produced a unique epidemic. Serial passages of brain in successive cannibalistic rituals might have changed the clinical picture of the disease. A spontaneous case of CJD in a 26-year-old native Chimbu New Guinean from the Central Highlands has been reported – the clinical diagnosis was proved only by the neuropathological study of a brain biopsy specimen; this case might represent the basis for spread of the agent, with modifications of the virulence related to serial passages through cannibalistic procedures.

Serologic Relationships and Variability

Transmission studies in experimental animals have shown that several strains of the Kuru agent do exist. Owing to the still unknown nature of the agent causing the disease and the lack of any immune-mediated response in the course of Kuru, no antigenic variations are known.

Epidemiology

The natural incubation period of Kuru can be as long as 25–30 years and it is at times identical in two or more individuals infected at the same time, even over this span of years; the natural incubation period does not seem to be determined by age at exposure.

In the Fore group, Kuru had a yearly incidence rate and prevalence ratio of 1% of the population. As mentioned earlier, there was a marked excess of deaths of adult females over males with a male:female ratio of 1:3 for the whole South Fore group. More than 2500 patients died of Kuru in the 17 year period of surveillance by year since its discovery in 1957 through 1975.

In the last 20 years, there has been a constant and progressive decline of the incidence of Kuru among Fore people. The disease has progressively disappeared from the younger age-groups up to the adult ones. No new Kuru patients have been recorded as born after 1959, and prospective evaluations estimate that Kuru will disappear by the end of the twentieth century.

Transmission and Tissue Tropism

The natural (human-to-human) mode of transmission is not totally understood, but ritual cannibalism has been the probable mode of propagation and maintenance of the disease. This is because the brain tissue, with which the officiating women contaminated both themselves and all their infants and toddlers, contained over ten infectious doses per gram, with self-inoculation occurring through the eyes, nose and skin as well as by mouth.

Experimental transmission of Kuru was first demonstrated in a chimpanzee by intracerebral inoculation of brain homogenate of a Kuru patient; since then, experimental transmission studies of Kuru were conducted in several animal species (other nonhuman primates and various small laboratory rodents).

Studies in cell cultures derived from tissues of patients and animals with Kuru have been performed, inoculating nonhuman primates by the intracerebral route. Primary cell lines that maintain the infectious Kuru agent did not largely differ in appearance from neuronal cultures derived from brains of non-Kuru cases. Some of these cell cultures became infected with Kuru and the persistence of Kuru infection was demonstrated for 170 days in human cultures and for 215 days in animal cultures. It has never been clearly proved that the Kuru agent replicates *in vitro*.

Kuru has a selective neurotropism; in fact, histological lesions are found only in the central nervous system, involving neurons as well as astrocytes. In about 10% of Kuru cases there is an accumulation and deposition of typical amyloid plaques. Lesions have never been described outside nervous tissue. It is likely that, as in other subacute spongiform encephalopathies of humans and animals, the etiological agent penetrates the lymphoreticular system, reaching the midthoracic level of the spinal cord and then spreading towards the central nervous system, resulting in the clinical appearance of the disease.

Pathogenicity

The etiological agent of Kuru has not yet been isolated; the agent produces a disease which is always fatal for the host and it is regularly detected in the brain tissue where the infectivity titer reaches 10^8 infectious doses per gram. In extraneural tissues, such as liver and spleen, Kuru agent has been found only rarely at death and with lower titers. Infectivity has never been detected in blood, urine, leukocytes, cerebrospinal fluid, placenta or embryonal membranes originating from patients with Kuru.

A pathological amyloidotic protein, PrPres (resistant), has been systematically found in the brains of patients dead from Kuru. PrPres is a distinctive pathological hallmark of Kuru and other spongiform encephalopathies of animals and humans; however, whether this pathological protein represents an important component of the infectious agent or is a by-product of the infection is still a matter of controversy.

Clinical Features of Infection

There is considerable consistency in the clinical characteristics of Kuru, suggesting genetic stability of the agent. In fact, Kuru is constantly characterized by cerebellar ataxia and a shivering-like tremor and its clinical course is remarkably uniform, with cerebellar symptomatology progressing to total inability and death, usually within 3–9 months. Generally, patients complain of joint pain, with the subsequent appearance of walking difficulties prior to clinical onset. During the clinical course of the disease, some patients develop neurological signs of cognitive impairment, mainly related to damage to the frontal lobes, but most Kuru patients show signs of dementia only in the late stages of the disease. During the progression of the disease, truncal ataxia and shivering tremor become so severe that patients are not able to walk without assistance. At least a third of Kuru patients show clinical signs of basal ganglia impairment, with rigidity and cogwheeling.

Pathology and Histopathology

Macroscopically, the cerebral hemispheres appear normal but the cerebellum regularly shows atrophy, often especially severe in the phylogenetically old paleocerebellum, i.e. the vermis and flocculonodular lobe. Microscopically, the lesions are almost homogenous and no large variations are noted that could be related to differences in age, sex or duration of the disease. The most regular and striking degeneration always occurs in the cerebellum, where there is a loss of Purkinje and granule cells. At the level of the molecular layer, masses of microglial cells are usually found. A diffuse and severe proliferation of astrocytes is observed throughout all layers of the cerebellar cortex. Amyloid plaques, a distinctive neuropathological feature of Kuru, are abundant in more than 80% of cases and are seen within the granular and molecular layers of the cerebellum. These plaques are morphologically characterized by a multicentric core with radiating filamentous deposits. The core consists of granular or homogenous substances of various sizes which are densely stained with periodic acid–Schiff reaction, birefringent with Congo red staining and fluorescent with thioflavin staining.

Immunohistochemical staining with antibodies specifically raised against the pathological protein PrPres shows an intense positive reaction in the core and the periphery of these multicentric amyloid 'Kuru' plaques. Immunocytochemistry of some Kuru brains has been recently carried out in the light of potential similarities with the amyloid plaques deposited in the brain of cases of the new variant CJD (nvCJD), recently reported in young British patients. The conclusion of these studies using antiprion protein immunocytochemistry shows that the pathology, including immunomorphology of PrP deposition, is within the lesion spectrum of CJD, although plaques are unusually prominent and the topography of PrP deposition parallels that of spongiform change and/or astrogliosis, while it seems that Kuru does not share the neuropathological hallmarks of nvCJD. The cerebellar white matter shows no signs of a primary demyelination. Spongiform changes associated with proliferation of reactive astrocytosis and some degree of neuronal loss are diffusely observed throughout the cerebral cortex. In the striatum, many large neurons show a severe and multilocular vacuolation. Other changes are variably distributed in the rest of the basal ganglia and are most frequently observed in the anterior nuclear group of the thalamus.

Immune Response

There is no recognizable inflammatory/immune-mediated response during the clinical course of Kuru, as is the case in all the other subacute spongiform encephalopathies.

Prevention and Control

The most likely mode of natural propagation and maintenance of the infection appears to be contamination during ritualistic cannibalistic ceremonies; this has been confirmed by the dramatic decrease of the number of new cases of Kuru since the cessation of cannibalistic rituals in the Fore region. This decline in Kuru incidence occurred during the period of transformation from a Stone Age cultural enviroment, in which the endocannibalistic ritual consumption of dead relatives was regularly practiced, to a modern society organized with a cash economy. The decline in the incidence of Kuru victims has therefore followed the cessation of cannibalism, and the disease has progressively disappeared from the youngest age group (4–9 years) up to the adult age groups.

The number of Kuru cases has steadily declined and each year the youngest patients have been older than those in the previous year. Now, only two or three cases are occurring annually, none younger than 40 years of age. According to prospective estimates it will probably take only a few years before the appearance of the last Kuru case.

See also: **Prions: Human and Animal.**

Further Reading

Gajdusek DC (1977) Unconventional viruses and the origin and disappearance of Kuru. *Science* 197: 943.

Gajdusek DC (1996) Infectious amyloids: spongiform subacute encephalopathies as transmissible cerebral amyloidoses. In: Fields BN, Knipe DM, Howley PM *et al.* (eds) *Fields Virology*, 3rd edn. p. 2851. Philadelphia: Lippincott-Raven.

Gajdusek DC (1996) Kuru in childhood: implications for the problem of whether bovine spongiform encephalopathy affects humans. In: Court L and Dodet B (eds) *Transmissible Subacute Spongiform Encephalopathies: Prion Diseases*, p. 15. Paris: Elsevier.

Gajdusek DC and Zigas V (1957) Degenerative disease of the central nervous system in New Guinea: the endemic occurrence of 'kuru' in the native population. *N. Engl. J. Med.* 257: 974.

Klatzo I, Gajdusek DC and Zigas V (1959) Pathology of Kuru. *Lab. Invest.* 8: 799.

Yeast and Fungi

Marie-Lise Maddelein, **Herman Edskes**, **Kim Taylor** and **Reed B Wickner**, Laboratory of Biochemistry and Genetics, National Institute of Diabetes Digestive and Kidney Diseases, National Institutes of Health, Bethesda, Maryland, USA

Copyright © 1999 Academic Press

History

The notion that a protein could be infectious without a nucleic acid as part of the infectious material arose from studies of scrapie of sheep, kuru and Creutzfeldt–Jakob disease (CJD) of man, and the equivalent diseases of other mammals. These diseases are called transmissible spongiform encephalopathies because the diseased brain has a spongy appearance due to loss of neurons and accumulation of vesicles in others. The transmissibility requires injection or feeding of the diseased tissues.

Origin of the infectious protein concept

Gajdusek showed in the 1960s that the inherited and spontaneous forms of CJD were infectious for monkeys, just like the infectious form. He believed that CJD (and scrapie) was due to a slow virus. Studies by Tikva Alper showed that the scrapie agent was remarkably UV-resistant, compared with viruses and bacteriophage. She proposed that scrapie may be infectious without a nucleic acid. Griffith proposed that an infectious protein might be an altered form of a cellular protein that had acquired the ability to change the normal form of the protein into the altered form by forming an oligomer with it. This 1967 proposal is precisely what the transmissible spongiform encephalopathies are widely believed to be today.

In 1975, Dickinson identified a critical gene involved in scrapie of mice that he named *Sinc*, for scrapie *inc*ubation period. Prusiner purified the scrapie agent and found that it contained a protease-resistant protein (named PrP). Weissmann and Chesebro cloned the PrP genes of hamster and mouse, respectively, and found they were normal cellular genes. In fact, the PrP gene was the same as Dickinson's *Sinc* gene. Weissmann showed that PrP was necessary for the propagation of scrapie, as mice deleted for the gene were immune to the disease. Prusiner showed that mice transgenic for the hamster gene had now become sensitive to the hamster scrapie agent. Although these studies have not yet proven that scrapie is due to an infectious protein, the concept was widely circulated in this connection.

The definition of 'prion'

The term 'prion' was coined by Prusiner in 1982 to mean simply the scrapie agent. In view of its unusual properties, scrapie was considered to be a new type of entity. It was suggested that if scrapie were an infectious protein, without a nucleic acid, it could be transmitted via 'reverse translation' or 'protein-dependent protein synthesis', but infectious protein was not part of the definition of the word prion. Indeed, many current authors use 'prion' as a synonym for 'scrapie agent'.

We have perhaps confused matters by using the word 'prion' to mean 'infectious protein' and have treated the question of whether there are such things as a separate issue. We continue that usage here.

Expected properties of a yeast or fungal infectious protein

If there were an infectious protein of yeast, it would be expected, like yeast viruses, to spread to other cells via the cell fusion that accompanies mating. Thus, it would appear as a nonchromosomal genetic element.

We proposed three genetic criteria that should distinguish an infectious protein (a prion) from the majority of non-chromosomal genetic elements, which are plasmids or viruses (**Fig. 1**).

1. If one can cure a prion, it should be possible for it to arise again in the cured strain (reversible curability).
2. Overproduction of the normal form of the protein should increase the frequency with which the prion form arises.
3. Recessive mutations of the chromosomal gene for the protein should produce the same phenotype as the presence of the prion, because both result in absence of the normal form of the protein. Deletion of the chromosomal gene should also result in loss of the prion.

Note that scrapie is not known to satisfy any of these criteria.

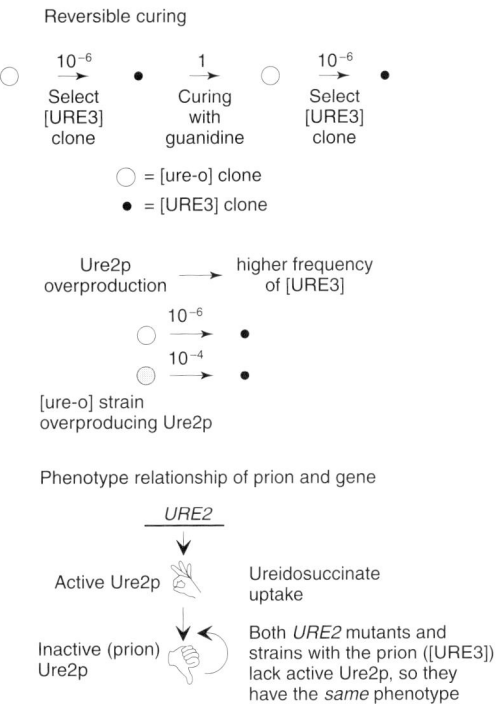

Figure 1 Genetic properties expected of a prion. We proposed that a prion should be reversibly curable, that overexpression of the normal form should increase the *de novo* appearance of the prion form and that the presence of the prion and the absence of the normal form should have similar phenotypes (if the prion phenotype comes from absence of the normal form). From Wickner RB (1994) with permission.

[URE3], an Infectious Form of Ure2p, a Regulator of Nitrogen Metabolism

[URE3] satisfies the three genetic criteria for a prion

[URE3] is a nonchromosomal genetic element identified by Lacroute in 1971 in his search for yeast mutants able to take up ureidosuccinate in the presence of a good nitrogen source, such as ammonia. Ureidosuccinate is an intermediate in uracil biosynthesis, the product of aspartate transcarbamylase (**Fig. 2**). It is taken up by Dal5p, the permease for allantoate, which is structurally similar to ureidosuccinate. Allantoate is a poor, but usable nitrogen source for yeast, but genes needed for allantoate utilization (such as *DAL5*) are repressed when a good nitrogen source is available. This 'nitrogen catabolite repression' is mediated in part by Ure2p, which blocks the positive transcription regulator, Gln3p, when a good nitrogen source is at hand. Gln3p is necessary for transcription of *DAL5* and other nitrogen-regulated genes.

Lacroute found that both the chromosomal *ure2* mutants and strains with the nonmendelian element [URE3] could take up ureidosuccinate. But Aigle and Lacroute found that *ure2* mutants could not propagate the [URE3] genetic element. This is criterion (3) above. [URE3] may be cured by growing cells in the presence of low concentrations of guanidine, but we found that from the cured strains can again be isolated strains that have spontaneously developed [URE3]. This is reversible curability (criterion (1) above). Finally, overproduction of Ure2p results in a 20–200-fold increase of the frequency with which [URE3] arises (criterion (2)).

Further evidence that [URE3] is a prion form of Ure2p

Not only can overproduction of Ure2p induce appearance of [URE3] in a normal strain, but it can do the same thing in a strain which was initially deleted for *URE2*. This argues against [URE3] being the altered form of a virus or plasmid present in the normal strains, as the putative normal replicon should depend on the same chromosomal genes (i.e. *URE2*).

If [URE3] is an infectious protein form of Ure2p, it should be possible to show some difference in Ure2p in [URE3] strains compared with normal strains. Indeed, Ure2p is more protease resistant in [URE3] strains, than in either the parent strain or in a cured strain.

One type of nonnucleic acid 'genetic element' is a sort of regulatory circuit that is self-maintaining. Since Ure2p is a transcription regulator, it is critical to show that this is not the case here. Several lines of evidence show that the regulatory capacity of Ure2p and its ability to undergo or induce the [URE3] change are distinct. Moreover, the [URE3] genetic element can be equally well propagated under conditions of nitrogen derepression or repression.

Molecular biologic proof that Ure2p is infectious

We have shown that it is actually the overproduction of the Ure2 protein, not the *URE2* mRNA or the *URE2* gene in high copy, that induces the appearance of [URE3]. This may be viewed as the molecular biological equivalent of purifying Ure2p from [URE3] strains and showing that it is infectious.

Mechanism of [URE3] generation and propagation

The Ure2 protein may be divided into an N-terminal 65-residue prion domain and a C-terminal nitrogen regulation domain. The prion domain is sufficient when overproduced to induce appearance of [URE3] at a frequency over 1000 times the spontaneous rate. It is also necessary for a Ure2p molecule to have a

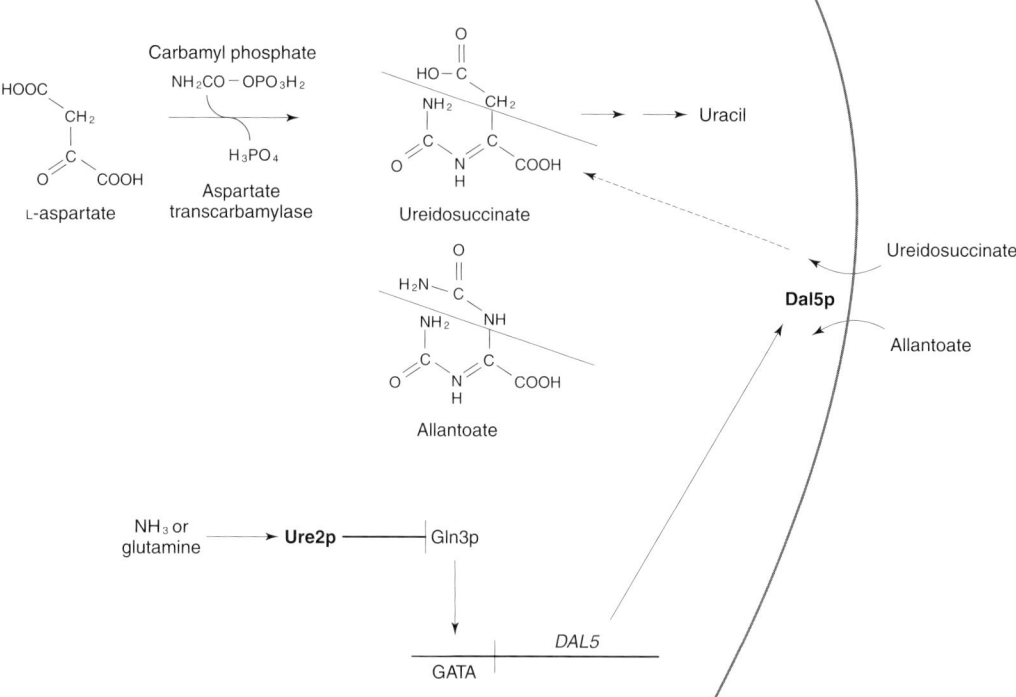

Figure 2 Nitrogen regulation affects uptake of ureidosuccinate through Ure2p. In the presence of a good nitrogen source (ammonia or glutamine) the Ure2p protein prevents the Gln3p protein from activating transcription of genes whose products are involved in utilization of poor nitrogen sources. Dal5p is such a protein, a transporter for allantoate, a poor nitrogen source structurally similar to ureidosuccinate. Ureidosuccinate is an intermediate in uracil biosynthesis.

covalently attached prion domain in order for it to be subject to the prion change as transmitted from another molecule (**Fig. 3**). Indeed, the N-terminal prion domain can transmit [URE3] in the complete absence of the C-terminal part of the Ure2 molecule. Likewise, the C-terminal part of the molecule can regulate nitrogen without the N-terminal domain.

Although the N-terminal prion domain and the C-terminal nitrogen regulatory domain of Ure2p can each act in the absence of the other, there are several lines of evidence that they have specific functional interaction: (1) the C-terminal domain must be overproduced to regulate nitrogen as well as the full-length protein, suggesting that the N-terminal domain somehow helps in this activity; (2) deletions in the C-terminal domain *increase* the frequency with which the molecule converts to the prion form, suggesting that the C-terminal domain stabilizes the N-terminal domain in the normal form; and (3) attaching the prion domain to β-galactosidase does not make that enzyme subject to inactivation by the introduction of [URE3].

The precise mechanism by which the prion domain inactivates the C-terminal nitrogen regulation domain is not yet known. It is possible that this involves a specific interaction, or that the aggregation of Ure2p in [URE3] strains prevents Ure2p from entering the nucleus, where it acts to modulate Gln3p activity.

[PSI], an Infectious Form of Sup35p, a Translation Release Factor

[PSI] as a infectious form of Sup35p

[PSI] was discovered in 1965 by Cox as a nonchromosomal genetic element that increased the strength of chromosomal suppressor mutations (suppressor tRNAs). Weak suppressors became strong and strong suppressors became lethal. Even [PSI] by itself had some weak suppressor activity. [PSI] could affect any nonsense mutation.

[PSI] can be cured by growth of strains in high osmotic strength medium, or by guanidine. But from the cured strains could again be isolated strains that had developed [PSI]. This is reversible curability. *Sup35* mutants, like [PSI], have 'omnipotent suppressor' activity, working on UAA, UGA and UAG codons. Moreover, [PSI] fails to propagate in certain *sup35* mutant strains. This is the relation expected if [PSI] is a prion form of Sup35p (**Fig. 3**). Finally, overproduction of Sup35p results in a 100-fold increase of the frequency with which [PSI] appears.

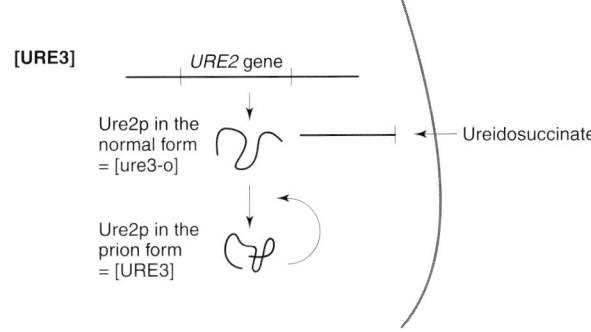

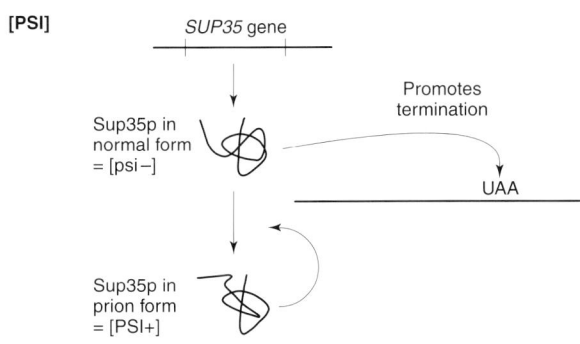

Figure 3 [URE3] and [PSI] as prion forms of Ure2p and Sup35p. If an altered protein can convert the normal form into the same altered form, this altered form can be a prion if it has a means to pass from cell to cell, or individual to individual. We proposed that [URE3] and [PSI] are altered forms of Ure2p and Sup35p, respectively.

Thus, [PSI] has the three genetic properties expected if it is an infectious protein form of Sup35p. Sup35p is a subunit of the translation release factor. It is to be expected that a change of Sup35p that partially inactivates it (or completely inactivates some proportion of the Sup35p molecules) would make translation termination less active and less able to compete with a suppressor tRNA.

Support for [PSI] being a prion

In normal strains, Sup35p is a soluble protein, complexed with the other subunit of the translation release factor, Sup45p, as a heterodimer. In extracts of [PSI] strains, most of Sup35p is present as an aggregate. The Sup35p in extracts of [PSI] strains is resistant to digestion with protease, perhaps because it is in this aggregated form.

Prion domain of [PSI]

Ter-Avanesyan and coworkers examined various deletion mutants of Sup35p and showed that the C-terminal domain is essential for cell growth, presumably the translation termination domain. They found that the N-terminal 114 residues were dispensable for cell growth, but were necessary for the propagation of [PSI]. This region has a series of repeats of an eight amino acid motif and is rich in glutamine and glycine residues. PrP also has an octapeptide repeat near its N-terminus, but transgenic mouse studies indicate that this repeat is not necessary for the propagation of scrapie.

Hsp104 is necessary for [PSI] propagation *and* can cure [PSI]

Chernoff and coworkers isolated a high-copy plasmid that cured [PSI] and found that it encoded Hsp104, a heat shock protein known to disaggregate proteins which had been denatured by heat. Overproduction of Hsp104 by other means also results in loss of [PSI]. Surprisingly, underproduction of Hsp104, for example, by deletion of the gene, also results in loss of [PSI].

The fact that a protein renaturing factor can eliminate [PSI] supports the notion that [PSI] is a conformationally altered form of a normal protein. At the same time, this important result suggests an avenue to approach the treatment of CJD and other transmissible spongiform encephalopathies. That [PSI] propagation requires Hsp104 could suggest that Hsp104 is actually involved in the conversion of Sup35p from the normal to the altered form (along with the altered form of Sup35p itself). Another possibility is that in the absence of Hsp104 there is essentially a single aggregate of Sup35p in [PSI] strains, and that when the cell divides, only one of the daughter cells will receive this aggregate (and thus receive [PSI]). Perhaps normal levels of Hsp104 breaks the aggregates into several peices, at least one of which goes to each daughter cell, insuring the stable propagation of [PSI].

In vitro propagation of [PSI]

Recently, Paushkin *et al* have reported an *in vitro* system in which soluble Sup35p, isolated from a wild-type strain, is converted to the aggregated form by addition of highly purified Sup35p aggregates from a [PSI] strain. A small aliquot of the product can prime the aggregation reaction of a new batch of soluble Sup35p. This reaction can apparently be continued as long as there is a supply of fresh normal Sup35p. The reaction requires the same N-terminal domain of Sup35p that has been shown to be critical for propagation of [PSI]. This is a remarkable confirmation of the prion model for [PSI].

[Het-s] as a Prion Form of the *het-s* Protein of *Podospora*

Heterokaryon incompatibility in fungi

A colony of the filamentous fungus, *Podospora*, is not really a collection of cells. Rather, the cells of the colony are interconnected, separated by incomplete cell walls and septae. Thus, each colony is a single multinuclear cell, a syncytium. When two colonies of a single fungal strain grow toward each other, the cellular processes (called hyphae) of the two colonies fuse, forming what is, in effect, one colony. The nuclei migrate between what was the two colonies so that a 'heterokaryon' is formed – a combination of the two colonies in which each 'cell' may have a mixture of the two kinds of nuclei, one kind from one parent colony, and one from the other. When these colonies fuse, a virus or plasmid present in one colony will spread throughout the other as well. Many fungal viruses and plasmids are quite debilitating to their hosts. For this reason, it is believed, most fungi have a system that limits with what strains it will carry out this 'hyphal fusion' (or heterokaryon formation). This system limiting heterokaryon formation is called 'heterokaryon incompatibility'.

Genetic control of heterokaryon incompatibility

Sexual mating, leading to meiosis, is a process designed to create diversity by shuffling the genetic cards. Thus, sexual mating requires *differences* between the individuals at one or more loci (the mating type loci). Heterokaryon formation, as described above, is designed to allow cooperation (e.g. sharing of nutrients) between genetically identical individuals, and so heterokaryon formation only occurs between strains identical at each of several genes, called *het* genes in the case of *Podospora*.

One of the *Podospora het* genes is called *het-s*, and it can have two alleles, *het-S* and *het-s*. Two *het-s* or two *het-S* strains readily fuse and form healthy heterokaryons with each other. But when a *het-s* strain meets a *het-S* strain, hyphal fusion is followed quickly by death of fused hyphae and the formation of a barrier to further fusion between the two colonies.

Genetic properties of *het-s* suggest a prion

The *het-s* strains can have either of two phenotypes, one showing the incompatibility described above, and another 'neutral' phenotype in which cells form heterokaryons equally well with *het-s* and *het-S* cells. This difference is controlled by a nonmendelian genetic element, called [Het-s], whose presence leads to the incompatibility phenotype, and whose absence results in the neutral phenotype (**Fig. 4**). [Het-s] can

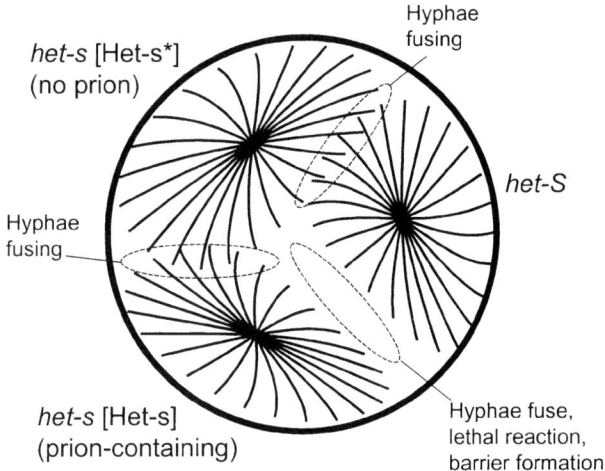

Figure 4 Heterokaryon incompatibility in *Podospora* and the [Het-s] prion. A *het-s* strain shows heterokaryon incompatibility with a *het-S* strain only if the former carries a nonmendelian genetic element, called [Het-s]. Begueret and coworkers have presented evidence that [Het-s] is a prion form of the *het-s* protein.

be cured, but then spontaneously reappears at a low frequency ('reversible curability'). Begueret and coworkers have recently found that overproduction of the *het-s* protein results in an increase of the frequency with which [Het-s] appears. Deletion of the *het-s* gene results in inability to propagate [Het-s], but the deleted strains show the same neutral phenotype as is found in the absence of [Het-s], so this does not specifically point to [Het-s] being a prion (although it is not against this conclusion). Finally, the *het-s* protein shows increased resistance to protease digestion in extracts of [Het-s] strains compared to strains lacking [Het-s].

These results all point to [Het-s] being a prion form of the *het-s* protein. This is the first case in which a prion appears to be facilitating a normal cellular function. Heterokaryon incompatibility is a phenomenon found in most filamentous fungi, and in the many other cases examined genetically, there is no evidence of any unusual genetic features suggestive of prions.

Features of the *het-s* protein

The *het-s* and *het-S* alleles differ by only 14 amino acids in a 289 amino acid open reading frame. A single difference at residue 33 is sufficient to convert *het-s* to *het-S* behavior. These proteins have no similarity to any other proteins in the databases, including the other putative prion proteins, PrP, Ure2P and Sup35p.

Table 1 Comparison of the putative prion systems

Prion	Protein	Phenotype of prion	Function of normal protein	Structure of protein
Scrapie	PrP	Ataxia, dementia, death	Unknown	Normal – α helix; prion – β sheet
[URE3]	Ure2p	Nitrogen derepression	Nitrogen repression	Asparagine-rich prion domain
[PSI]	Sup35p	Translation readthrough	Translation termination	Glutamine and asparagine rich
[Het-s]	het-s protein	Heterokaryon incompatibility	None known	??

Comparison of the Putative Prion Systems (Table 1)

Although the evidence certainly suggests that the scrapie agent is an altered form of PrP, there is other data that calls this into question. Although PrP can be made in large amounts in bacterial or yeast cells, sometimes as protease-resistant material with high β-sheet content, it has never proven infectious. Moreover, there are several reports of dissociation between the finding of abnormal PrP and appearance of infectivity. Finally, the genetic criteria proposed for fungal prions have not yet been satisfied for PrP and scrapie.

The yeast and fungal systems, because of the ease with which they may be studied genetically, have already produced some important results:

- The fungal systems have provided evidence that there can be such a thing as a prion – evidence of a type not yet available for scrapie and PrP.
- These systems show that an inherited trait can be a prion: a prion can be a 'gene'.
- The role of chaperones in prion propagation has long been speculated, but is first shown for [PSI]. It is expected that these systems will soon lead to the definition of other factors affecting prion generation and propagation.
- [Het-s] shows that a normal cellular function can be determined by a prion.
- The definition of prion domains in Ure2p and Sup35p is beginning to contribute to our understanding of how a prion arises and is propagated.
- The *in vitro* system for [PSI] is the best available for any prion to date.

We expect that many more prions will be discovered, some causing pathologic conditions of animals, plants or microorganisms, while others mediate normal cellular functions. The genetic approaches to identifying prions that have proven useful in yeast and filamentous fungi will probably continue to be valuable in identification of other prions.

See also: **Prions: Human, Human and Animal; Yeast RNA viruses (*Totiviridae*); Viroids.**

Further Reading

Chernoff YO, Lindquist SL, Ono BI, Inge-Vechtomov SG and Liebman SW (1995) Role of the chaperone protein Hsp104 in propagation of the yeast prion-like factor [psi$^+$]. *Science* 268: 880.

Coustou V, Deleu C, Saupe S and Begueret J (1997) The protein product of the *het-s* heterokaryon incompatibility gene of the fungus *Podospora anserina* behaves as a prion analog. *Proc. Natl Acad. Sci. USA* 94: 9773–9778.

Cox BS (1993) Psi phenomena in yeast. In: Hall MN and Linder P (eds) *The Early Days of Yeast Genetics*, p. 219. Cold Spring Harbor: Cold Spring Harbor Laboratory Press.

Masison DC and Wickner RB (1995) Prion-inducing domain of yeast Ure2p and protease resistance of Ure2p in prion-containing cells. *Science* 270: 93–95.

Paushkin SV, Kushnirov VV, Smirnov VN and Ter-Avanesyan MD (1997) In vitro propagation of the prion-like state of yeast Sup35 protein. *Science* 277: 381.

Wickner RB (1994) Evidence for a prion analog in S. cerevisiae: the [URE3] non-Mendelian genetic element as an altered *URE2* protein. *Science* 264: 566.

Wickner RB (1996) Prions and RNA viruses of *Saccharomyces cerevisiae*. *Annu. Rev. Genet.* 30: 109.

Wickner RB (1997) *Prion Diseases of Mammals and Yeast: Molecular Mechanisms and Genetic Features*. Austin, TX: Landes.

PROPAGATION OF VIRUSES

Contents

Animal
Bacteria
Plant

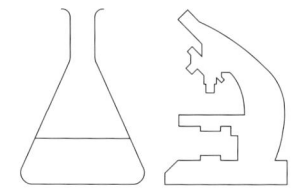

Animal

Steffen Faisst, Novo Nordisk AIS, Soeborg, Denmark

Copyright © 1999 Academic Press

Introduction

Viruses exist in two functionally distinct forms. The viral particle, referred to as virion, represents the static extracellular form without any metabolic activity, serving as a vehicle for the viral genetic material. The second, the dynamic form, consists of the viral genetic material itself once it is uncoated in a host cell. This active form of a virus uses the host cell biosynthesis machinery and energy supplies to multiply and to generate progeny virions. Hence, virus multiplication exploits host cells in a parasitic way. This results in the disturbance of normal cellular functions in many virus-infected cells, one of the basic mechanisms of viral diseases.

Virus propagation under defined laboratory conditions provides an important experimental tool in basic research in virology, allowing studies of virus multiplication, virus–host cell interactions and viral pathogenesis. Furthermore, virus propagation provides the basis for diagnoses of viral disease and vaccine production, as well as the generation of recombinant viruses for potential use in gene therapy.

Here, the mechanisms of intracellular virus multiplication are summarized, and techniques used for virus propagation, purification and titration are described.

The Virus Multiplication Cycle

To multiply, a virus has to enter a living cell. Thereafter, the viral genome is released from the capsid, and interacts with the host cell in order to replicate and to produce viral proteins. New capsids are assembled, and the newly synthesized genomes are packaged into these capsids either concomitant with or after their assembly. This results in progeny virions, which are released from the cell in order to transfer the viral genome to new host cells.

The initial step of virus–cell contact, referred to as adsorption, is mediated by the binding of a viral protein, located at the virion surface, to a receptor at the cell surface. Cellular receptors of many viruses have been identified. Most viruses adsorb to cell surface proteins that have specific metabolic functions, and that are expressed only in a subset of differentiated cells. Rabies virus, for example, binds to the acetylcholine receptor, and accordingly adsorbs to nerve cells. Human immunodeficiency virus adsorbs to CD4 molecules of T lymphocytes and macrophages, but needs co-receptors for viral entry into these cells. These co-receptors have been identified recently, and belong to the family of chemokine receptors. It should also be noted that carbohydrates have been shown to act as virus receptors. For example, polyomavirus, Sendai virus and vaccinia virus adsorb to sialyloligosaccharides of glycoproteins and glycolipids, which can be found on the surface of many cell types.

After adsorption, viruses have to cross the plasma membrane in order to enter a cell. The mechanism of penetration differs from virus to virus, depending on the respective virion structure. Adsorption to cell receptors brings viruses into intimate contact with the plasma membrane. Subsequently, viruses with a membranous envelope may directly inject the viral capsid into the cytoplasm by membrane fusion. However, the virus–receptor complex can also be internalized by coated pit-mediated endocytosis and delivered to endosomes. Subsequent fusion of viral and endosome membranes leads to the release of the viral capsid into the cytoplasm.

Viruses lacking an envelope also enter cells by coated pit-mediated endocytosis, but entry of the capsid into the cytoplasm obviously cannot occur via membrane fusion. For the non-enveloped adenovirus, evidence has been presented that capsid proteins induce the lysis of endosomes, thus releasing the capsid into the cytoplasm.

Once within the cytoplasm, the viral genome has to be liberated from the capsid and transported to the appropriate intracellular site for transcription or replication. This event is referred to as uncoating.

For RNA viruses, cellular factors like proteases are thought to dismantle the virus capsids immediately after entry, releasing the viral RNA into the cytoplasm, where it is replicated and translated. Also poxviruses, which contain a double-stranded DNA genome, replicate in the cytoplasm, using a virus-encoded DNA polymerase. Only retroviruses transcribe their RNA genome in DNA, which subsequently translocate to the nucleus and integrate into the cellular genome. The integrated retroviral genome serves as a template to synthesize new RNA genomes.

For nuclear-replicating DNA viruses, the capsid is supposed to be translocated along the cytoskeleton to the nuclear pores. At the nuclear pores, the viral DNA is released into the nucleus, where it is replicated.

When the viral genome is delivered to its appropriate intracellular site, it has to interact with the host cell biosynthesis machinery in order to get amplified and transcribed into mRNAs allowing the synthesis of viral (capsid and noncapsid) proteins. Thereafter, cellular and viral factors mediate the assembly of the capsids, and the packaging of the viral genome into these capsids. These steps are referred to as capsid maturation. The assembly of capsid proteins of nonenveloped viruses occurs either in the nucleus (e.g. parvoviruses, adenoviruses and papovaviruses) or in the cytoplasm (e.g. reoviruses). Most of the nonenveloped viruses rely on host cell lysis for their egress.

The assembly of the capsids of enveloped viruses also takes place either in the cytoplasm (most RNA viruses, poxviruses), or in the nucleus (herpesviruses), but the last step in virion assembly is linked to the release of the virions. Most RNA viruses egress by budding through the plasma membrane. Herpesviruses have been shown to leave the nucleus by budding through the inner nuclear membrane. They are then released from the cells by transport through the endoplasmic reticulum. Poxviruses may be released from the cells either by budding through the Golgi apparatus, or by cell disruption, resulting in enveloped and nonenveloped particles, respectively. Both enveloped and nonenveloped particles are infectious. Once progeny virus has been released, new cells can become infected, and further multiplication cycles are initiated.

Cytopathic Effect

Different types of interaction between viruses and host cells can be observed. Many viruses kill or morphologically modify their host cells when they multiply. This is called the cytopathic effect (CPE), and the respective virus is said to be cytopathogenic.

Generally, cytopathogenic viruses code for proteins that shut off synthesis of cellular macromolecules, or that are cytotoxic. Furthermore, the capsid proteins of nonenveloped viruses seem to be implicated in cell lysis, on which these viruses may rely for their egress. Enveloped viruses may additionally insert viral proteins into the cell membrane, which also may impair the viability of the target cells. Cell death within a few days is the result of productive infection with many types of viruses, such as togaviruses, picornaviruses or autonomous parvoviruses. Infection with poxviruses, reoviruses or adenoviruses also leads to cell death, but less rapidly.

Another type of CPE is the induction of cell fusion by viruses such as paramyxoviruses, human immunodeficiency viruses and herpesviruses. Induction of cell fusion is also due to the insertion of viral proteins into the host cell membrane, and results in the formation of syncytia (giant cells with up to several hundred nuclei).

As a result of mild CPEs, a balance between cell growth and virus production can sometimes be observed (e.g. after paramyxovirus infections). Such 'carrier cultures' may be seen as the cell culture counterparts of chronic infections in animals. Several RNA viruses that are not cytopathogenic (like arenaviruses and most retroviruses) may also provoke such steady-state infections.

Host Range, Permissiveness and Susceptibility

Any cell that can be infected by a virus is said to be susceptible. However, infection of a susceptible cell does not necessarily result in a productive infection. Productive infections occur only in cells able to support a complete viral multiplication cycle. Such cells are said to be permissive. In terms of cell cultures, the spectrum of permissive cells makes up the host range of a virus. However, the host range may also define the animal species that support a productive infection.

The host range of viruses may be wide, but it may also be very limited. For example, the host range of the parvovirus H-1 comprises humans, monkey, hamster and rat as animal species, and most cell types (fibroblasts, keratinocytes, lymphocytes) of human, monkey, hamster or rat origin. On the other hand, the host range of B19, another parvovirus, is restricted to humans and human erythroid precursor cells.

Infections of susceptible, but nonpermissive cells do not result in virus production. Three distinct types of such nonproductive infections have been described, and are referred to as abortive, latent and restrictive infections, respectively.

An abortive infection occurs in susceptible cells, which sustain some, but not all steps of the viral multiplication cycle. As stated earlier, after successful entry of a virus into a cell, the viral genome has to become uncoated, amplified and expressed. Newly synthesized genomes have to be packaged into progeny particles that need to be released from infected cells.

Virus multiplication can be blocked at all stages of this cycle in susceptible, but nonpermissive cells. For example, the polyoma virus multiplication cycle is blocked at the stage of DNA replication and transcription in embryonal carcinoma cells lacking specific DNA-binding proteins. Similarly, the multiplication of the parvoviruses H-1 and MVM is blocked at the level of DNA and RNA synthesis in some cells that are refractory to virus propagation. Furthermore, some diploid cell strains infected with parvovirus H-1 are proficient in capsid assembly, but no DNA is packaged, and no particles are released from the cells. Cellular functions implicated in these last stages of infection have not yet been identified.

It should also be stated that infection of a permissive cell with a defective virus, lacking one or several essential viral functions, results in an abortive infection. During abortive infections, the virus may exert different cytopathic effects, depending on the viral functions that the host cells allow to be expressed. Hence, an abortive infection may result in cell death, if the virus was able to express its cytotoxic proteins, but may also be inapparent.

A latent infection consists of the persistence of viral genomes in infected cells for many cell generations. The viral genomes may persist in an integrated or in an episomal state or both. For example, retroviruses have been found as 'endogenous viruses' in human cells, and have been calculated to persist in these cells since approximately 40 million years. Such latent infections do not lead to host cell killing, but may nevertheless influence biologic characteristics of the cells. As an extreme example, persistence of tumor viruses is associated with cellular transformation leading to increased growth rates, abnormal cell morphology, altered cell metabolism and chromosomal aberrations.

Most viruses establishing latent infections can be rescued from their host cells, provided they have not become defective. Latent infections that can become productive are called persistent infections. To convert a latent into a productive infection, specific treatments have to be applied. For example, superinfection with adenovirus results in a productive infection of persistent adeno-associated viruses, and treatment with phorbol esters activates the multiplication cycle of persistent human immunodeficiency virus type 1 in the human macrophage cell line U1.

Finally, a rare type of nonproductive infection is the restrictive infection, that is observed in cell cultures where only a small subset of the cell population is permissive, or where the cells are only transiently permissive.

Virus Propagation in Whole Organisms

In initial studies in virology, the experimental tools for virus propagation and purification were whole laboratory animals or embryonated hen's eggs. Laboratory animals can be infected using the natural route of virus entry. To achieve this, the virus must be brought into contact with either the skin (e.g. papillomaviruses), the digestive tract (e.g. enteroviruses), the respiratory tract (e.g. orthomyxoviruses) or the conjunctiva (e.g. herpes simplex virus). Viral replication may be confined to the site of entry, or progeny virions may spread through the body (generally via the blood or lymphatic stream) with subsequent targeting to specific organs. Laboratory animals also can be infected by injecting the virus directly into specific organs (e.g. the brain for rabies virus). Several days or weeks after infection, the animals are killed, and cell-free extracts from the organs sustaining virus multiplication are used as a source of virus.

Furthermore, fertilized hen eggs can be infected after several days of incubation (depending on the stage of embryonic development required). Most viruses can be grown in the embryonic membranes of fertilized eggs, i.e. the yolk sac (e.g. herpesviruses), the chorion (e.g. poxviruses), the allantois (e.g. influenza virus) and the amnion (e.g. mumps virus). Although laboratory animals or embryonated eggs are still the most appropriate propagation systems for some viruses (animals for arboviruses, coxsackieviruses and rabies virus; eggs for orthomyxoviruses), they tend to be replaced by cell cultures, which are much more convenient to handle. For present-day virology, the use of animals is restricted mostly to research on viral pathogenesis and for production of vaccines.

Virus Propagation in Cell Culture

Multiplicity of infection, defective-interfering particles

The term 'cell culture' refers to *in vitro* cultures derived from dispersed cells taken from original tissues by enzymatical, mechanical or chemical disaggregation. Cultured cells may serve as hosts for the propagation of a number of viruses, provided these cells express all the factors allowing a complete viral replication cycle.

The first cells to be cultured were primary cells freshly isolated from animal tissues. The growth of

Table 3 Some implications of the quasispecies structure of viral populations

- It offers a general and highly effective adaptive strategy
- In particular, it explains the pre-existence and selection in viral populations of mutants with altered phenotypic properties:
    resistant to antiviral agents
    antibody and cytotoxic T lymphocyte escape
    with altered cell receptor specificity
    with different ability to induce interferon
    with increased virulence
- It implies the existence of thresholds for phenotypic expression
- There is a possible association between the pathogenic potential of a virus and its mutant spectrum complexity

some nutritional deficiencies. Chumakov and colleagues quantitated the presence of virulent poliovirus in the mutant spectrum of attenuated poliovirus used for vaccine preparation. When the proportion of virulent poliovirus variants in the vaccine exceeded a certain value, the virulent phenotype was manifested and the vaccine failed the safety tests in monkeys. This, and additional results with other viral systems, have established that expression of a variant phenotype encoded in a subset of genomes from the mutant spectrum depends on their proportion in the mutant distribution. These results agree with theoretical predictions on the behaviour of viral quasispecies in that the fate of each individual component of the mutant spectrum is strongly dependent on the mutant cloud surrounding it.

Recent evidence suggests that the complexity of the mutant spectrum may influence the outcome of viral infections. The complexity of the coronavirus mouse hepatitis virus quasispecies may contribute to its pathogenic potential. Likewise, the nonresponse to treatment with interferon α in chronic hepatitis C virus infections may relate to the number of viral molecular species detected in the infected patients. Model experiments with the animal pathogen foot-and-mouth disease virus showed that indeed the repertoire of viral mutants that became dominant in an evolving quasispecies depended on the population size of the virus. Thus, it is not surprising that both the population size and the complexity of the mutant spectrum may be important determinants of the pathogenic potential of some viruses, although the number of well-documented cases is still limited.

Connections with Population Genetics and with Current Concepts of Complexity

The main departure of the quasispecies concept from previous models of population genetics is the emphasis on mutation (or, more generally, in genetic variation) to the point of invalidating the concept of the wild type as a defined genomic sequence. RNA viral genome sequences are statistically defined, but individually indeterminate. Recognition of such indetermination, together with the emphasis on continuous mutant generation, contributed to the success of quasispecies, rather than other quantitative models of population biology, as a descriptor of RNA viruses.

The rapid evolution of RNA viruses has been used to explore some principles and theories of population biology. A concept of increasing interest in virology is fitness (**Table 2**). This is a complex parameter which has been the object of considerable research and debate in biology. Fitness of a virus is measured as its relative ability to produce infectious progeny under a defined set of environmental conditions. Relative fitness values have been determined in tissue culture and in some cases in laboratory mice or other hosts. Cells or organisms are co-infected with the virus to be tested together with a genetically or phenotypically marked reference virus. The progeny virus is passaged for several transfers and the quantification of the proportion of the two viruses relative to the initial mixture yields a relative fitness value. Using this assay a number of observations on the dynamics of viral quasispecies have been made.

When large populations of RNA viruses are allowed to replicate in a defined environment, fitness gains are generally observed when measured in the same environment (**Fig. 1**). However, adaptation of virus to one environment (for example one cell type) may result in profound fitness losses in another environment. Two vesicular stomatitis virus clones with similar relative fitness competing in serial infections coexisted for many passages. However, in a rather unpredictable manner, one of the clones abruptly displaced the other and became dominant in the population. This observation agrees with the competitive exclusion principle of population genetics that states that unless there is a niche differentiation, one of two competing species will eventually outcompete the other. In such competitions both the

Table 4 Some practical implications of the quasispecies structure of RNA viruses

- Vaccines must be multivalent (multiple B and T epitopes)
- Antiviral agents must be used in combination (directed to independent targets; the number depends on viral population size and genome turnover)
- Completely new antiviral strategies should be explored (drugs capable of throwing viral replication into error catastrophe)
- The use of virulent RNA viruses as pest control agents should be avoided

winners and the losers gained fitness in such a manner that their relative position in the fitness landscape was similar at the end and at the start of the competition. This agrees with the Red Queen hypothesis of population biology, as, in the words of the Red Queen in Lewis Carroll's *Through the Looking Glass*, 'it takes all the running you can do, to keep in the same place'.

In contrast to large population passages, repeated bottleneck events such as those mediating serial plaque-to-plaque transfers, resulted in stochastic fitness losses (**Fig. 1**). This is known as the 'Muller's ratchet' effect, according to which asexual populations of organisms will tend to incorporate deleterious mutations in a rather irreversible fashion unless compensatory mechanisms such as recombination can restore the initial, better adapted, genomes. For well-adapted viral quasispecies, repeated plaque isolations will tend to deviate successive mutant distributions from the optimal one, resulting in average fitness losses (**Fig. 1**). The transmission population size needed to maintain viral fitness is dependent on the initial fitness of the viral clone tested. The higher the initial fitness the larger the transmission pool must be to avoid fitness losses. Studies with foot-and-mouth disease virus have documented that viral clones subjected to serial plaque-to-plaque transfers accumulate unusual mutations, providing insight into the types of low-frequency mutants that populate viral quasispecies.

RNA viruses in their evolutionary dynamics constitute attractive experimental systems of complex adaptive behaviour. They display a highly indeterminate fine structure as well as a rather unpredictable behavior. Indetermination arises from the stochastic nature of mutagenesis, in conflict with the need of the system to ensure genetic continuity. Adaptability stems from the variable degrees of success of subsets of genomes. The indetermination of mutagenesis, together with the directionality of selective forces, situate RNA viruses in a subtle border between reproducibility of some observations and unpredictability of others. Thus, RNA virus quasispecies may also become interesting model systems for studies on complexity.

Strategies for Disease Prevention and Control

The great adaptability of viral quasispecies creates difficulties for viral disease control, and may also contribute to the emergence of new viral pathogens. When quasispecies was recognized as the most adequate descriptor of pathogenic RNA viruses, the need to adjust antiviral strategies to the new findings became apparent to some scientists. These recommended strategies (**Table 4**) are not yet generally followed, probably because of an inherent tendency of thinking of RNA viruses still as genetically defined entities. If a single selective pressure is applied to limit virus replication, the highly dynamic mutant spectrum is likely to provide variants capable of overcoming the selective constraints. Research on entire new antiviral strategies, such as the possibility of displacement of virus replication into error catastrophe, seems justified in view of accumulating evidence that the copying fidelity properties of viral replicases can be modified by structural alterations of the enzymes.

See also: **Antivirals; Defective interfering viruses; Emerging and re-emerging virus diseases; Immune escape mechanisms; Persistent viral infection.**

Further Reading

Domingo E and Holland JJ (1997) RNA virus mutations and fitness for survival. *Annu. Rev. Microbiol.* 51: 151.

Domingo E, Sabo DL, Taniguchi T and Weissmann C (1978) Nucleotide sequence heterogeneity of an RNA phage population. *Cell* 13: 735.

Domingo E, Holland JJ, Biebricher C and Eigen M (1995) Quasispecies: the concept and the word. In: Gibbs AJ, Calisher CH and Garía-Arenal F et al (eds) *Molecular Basis of Virus Evolution*, p. 171. Cambridge: Cambridge University Press.

Eigen M and Schuster P (1979) *The Hypercycle – A Principle of Natural Self-Organization*. Berlin: Springer.

Holland JJ, Spindler K, Horodyski F et al (1982) Rapid evolution of RNA genomes. *Science* 214: 1577.

Nowak MA (1992) What is a quasispecies? *Trends in Ecol. Evol.* 7: 118.

| Rabbit Fibroma Virus   *see* Poxviruses |

| Rabbit Hemorrhagic Disease Virus   *see* Caliciviruses |

| Rabbitpox Virus   *see* Mousepox and Rabbitpox Viruses and Poxviruses |

RABIES VIRUS (*RHABDOVIRIDAE*)

George M Baer and **Noël Tordo**, Laboratorios Baer, Mexico City, Mexico

Copyright © 1999 Academic Press

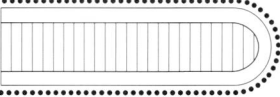

History

The dramatic clinical signs of rabies have been recorded from early times: hyperexcitability, increased tendency of animals to bite, jaw paralysis, changed facial expression, and transmission of the disease to other animals and, eventually, humans. One of the earliest references to the disease is from the third millenium BC, in the Eshnunna Code preceding the Code of Hammurabi:

> If a dog is mad and the authorities have brought it to the attention of the owner; if he does not keep it in and it bites a man and causes his death, then the owner shall pay 40 shekels of silver. If it bites a slave and causes his death he shall pay 15 shekels of silver.

Rabies in dogs and its transmission to man were well recognized by the time of Aristotle. Pliny and other writers referred to the influence of the dog-star Sirius, including the increased susceptibility of dogs to rabies during the so-called 'dog-days' of summer.

Outbreaks of rabies in dogs, foxes and wolves were reported from most European countries throughout the Middle Ages, predating the current European outbreak in foxes which began in the early 1940s. The first cases in the United States were reported in Virginia foxes in 1753. Bites by rabid wolves (animals often reported rabid in Iran, Afghanistan and the Soviet Union) still rank as the most dangerous source of the disease for humans. Mortality rates after wolf bites are well over 50%, although dogs still cause over 90% of human rabies deaths world-wide; in many developing countries the numbers of deaths still reach many thousands annually.

Rabies in vampire bats was first suggested by chronicles of Spanish conquistadores in the sixteenth and seventeenth centuries and confirmed in Brazil, Argentina and Trinidad in the early 1900s. Vampire rabies is still a major animal health problem in most Latin American countries, with hundreds of thousands of cattle deaths yearly. Insectivorous bats are a sporadic problem in North America, Latin America and Europe.

The classic studies of Pasteur beginning in 1881 showed that the central nervous system was the principal site of rabies virus replication, that the virus could be passaged in experimental animals, and that vaccines could be prepared from virus thus passaged. These studies led to his first preparing and then administering human vaccine in 1885. It is surprising that the same vaccine was not used for mass dog vaccination programs until 1921 when Umeno and Doi initiated urban control programs in Japan.

The first specific diagnostic tool, the 'Negri body', was discovered by Adelchi Negri in 1903. This rather insensitive tool was commonly used until the fluorescent antibody technique replaced it in the late 1950s.

Taxonomy and Classification

Rabies viruses belong to the family of RNA viruses *Rhabdoviridae*. These viruses have nonsegmented negative-strand RNA genomes enclosed in a lipid envelope derived from the host cell. The bullet-shaped virions are all composed of a nucleocapsid or ribonucleoprotein (RNP) core and an envelope in the form of a lipoprotein bilayer membrane closely surrounding the RNP core. The outer glycoprotein (G) coat is responsible for the induction of neutralizing (anti-G) antibodies. The virion RNP core is tightly wound into coils. Extending from the outer surface of the envelope is an array of spike-like G projections. The rabies-like viruses cross-react serologically with rabies nucleoprotein (N) antisera to varying degrees and include Lagos bat, Mokola, Duvenhage, Obodhiang and kotonkan viruses.

Geographic and Seasonal Distribution

Human rabies occurs world-wide, except in certain islands and peninsulae where the disease has never occurred (Australia and a number of small Caribbean islands) or where it has been eliminated (England, Ireland, Japan, Taiwan, Spain, Portugal). The infected countries can be divided into those that have controlled canine rabies with effective canine vaccination programs (but where wildlife rabies remains) such as all the western European countries, Canada, the US and some Latin American countries, and those countries where canine rabies is still endemic such as most of the African and Asian countries.

Genetics

Since 1981 the molecular genetics of rabies virus has followed two distinct strategies, work with viral messenger RNAs and work with the genome itself; the latter has permitted simultaneous analysis of the intergenic regions. Complete sequence is known for the PV and SAD strains of rabies and the rabies-related Mokola virus. The sequence data have helped to locate the glycosylation sites as well as the signal and transmembrane peptides on the G protein. The potential phosphorylation sites have also been characterized on the N and M1 (NS or phospho-protein). In addition, the important regions in eliciting humoral and T cell-mediated immunity were mapped along the G, M1 and N polypeptides.

Evolution

Conservation of the elements involved in transcription and replication

A comparative analysis of rabies virus strains, rabies-related viruses, rhabdoviruses in general, and paramyxoviruses indicate that strong selective pressure has stressed the following major elements controlling the gene expression: (1) the start and stop transcription signal bordering each cistron; (2) the promoters for RNA synthesis and encapsidation at the 3' and 5' genomic ends, respectively; (3) the RNA-dependent RNA polymerase (L protein), by far the most conserved polypeptide; it exhibits six highly conserved domains separated by variable areas, a distribution in agreement with the notion of independent functions (RNA synthesis, capping, polyadenylation and phosphorylation) concatenated within the polypeptide.

An intermediate place of unsegmented negative-strand RNA virus evolution

Proteins other than the L polymerase are poorly conserved. The G protein, although maintaining limited sequences around the main glycosylation site, has varied a great deal, as might be expected for the polypeptide that mediates the first contact with the host. The N protein has also retained small sequence stretches most likely involved in direct interaction with the genomic backbone. The M1 phosphoproteins and M2 matrix proteins are highly varied, as are the untranslated genomic areas.

The G–L intergene is of particular interest because of its large size and its inability to encode substantial peptides. In the same genomic location a fish rhabdovirus (infectious hematopoietic necrosis virus or IHNV) encodes an mRNA of similar size, as do the paramyxoviruses for the HN hemagglutinin protein. The rabies G–L intergene is presumed to be a remnant gene, baptized ψ for pseudogene. It places rabies virus in an intermediate position in the evolution of unsegmented negative-strand RNA viruses, between the rhabdoviruses with condensed genomes (vesicular stomatitis virus, for instance, shows the dinucleotide GA between the G and L), IHNV virus and the paramyxoviruses. The L protein homology studies independently confirm that rabies virus was closer to paramyxoviruses than to VSV.

The rabies ψ pseudogene: the best thermometer of evolution

Since it is a nonprotein coding region highly susceptible to mutation, changes in the rabies ψ pseudogene are more likely to represent the natural evolution of the virus outside any external selective pressure, and this site may therefore be a suitable target for epidemiologic studies. By use of the polymerase chain reaction (PCR) technique directly from brain samples it was shown that:

- There is up to 18% divergence in the ψ pseudogene of different vaccine strains, most of which are derived from the original Pasteur strain.
- Wild isolates from a given geographic area are clearly related, with less than 2.5% divergence.
- Wildlife isolates differ by approximately 15% from vaccine strains (but complete cross-protection by those vaccines is still achieved).
- In West Africa (Ivory Coast, Cameroon, Niger and Morocco) where vaccine failures have often been noted, there is a greater (25–40%) divergence from the vaccine strains.
- European bat isolates tend to be completely different from vaccine strains at the ψ pseudogene. At the G and N gene, those known to be important in initiating the immune response, the divergence between isolates from European bats and isolates from vaccine strains is comparable to the difference vs Mokola virus (against which rabies vaccines are ineffective).

Serologic Relationships and Variability

The lyssavirus genus includes a wide variety of rabies viruses, both laboratory-adapted and naturally occurring 'street' viruses, almost all of which can be differentiated through the use of antinucleoprotein monoclonal antibodies. Monoclonal antibody analysis of various rabies variants indicates a remarkable stability in their pattern over many years, with a bat virus from all Mexican freetail bat, for instance, giving the same pattern in the early 1980s and the early 1990s. The analysis of variants also shows that the predominant virus circulating in a given epidemiologic area or 'niche' (such as raccoon rabies in eastern US) is also found in the animals that raccoons bite such as skunks and groundhogs; bat viruses tend to give a different pattern. The common rabies vaccines prepared from 'fixed' viruses such as LEP (low egg passage Flury), HEP (high egg passage Flury), ERA, PM and PV virus strains protect against all rabies 'street' viruses.

Within the lyssavirus genus there are also 'rabies-like' viruses, originally isolated in Africa and markedly different from the rabies viruses in their NP pattern. They include a virus isolated from a bat in Nigeria (Lagos bat), from a human bitten by a bat in South Africa (Duvenhage), or from shrews in Nigeria (Mokola). Common rabies vaccines do not protect against these virus strains.

Epidemiology

Rabies is endemic world-wide, either in dogs or in wild animals, except in those limited areas of the world (mostly islands) where rabies has never existed or where it has been eliminated. Most developing countries of Asia, Africa and Latin America have many cases of rabies in dogs which result in many human antirabies vaccinations and many human deaths. In most of these countries the approximate rate of human antirabies vaccination is 1:1000 population annually.

The picture is quite different in regions where rabies in dogs has been controlled and the disease is prevalent in a variety of wild animals, such as red foxes (western and eastern Europe and Ontario, Canada), arctic foxes (all circumpolar areas), skunks (midwest US), raccoons (eastern US), mongooses (Asia, South Africa, Cuba, Puerto Rico, the Dominican Republic, Haiti and Grenada), wolves (Iran, Afghanistan and the former USSR), vampire bats (northern Mexico to northern Argentina), insectivorous bats (Latin America, the US, Canada and, rarely, western Europe), and frugivorous bats (South America and the Caribbean). In those areas rabies is mostly transmitted within one species and rarely outside, with, for instance, rabies transmitted freely within skunk populations but only occasionally to other animals they bite, such as cows. Rabies rarely 'crosses over' and begins an outbreak in a species bitten by the original species involved.

But rabies in Latin America is almost always transmitted by one species of bat, the common vampire *Desmodus rotundus*, an animal that feeds solely on blood, mostly cattle blood. Every year there are hundreds of thousands of rabies deaths in cattle bitten by vampire bats; rare human outbreaks have also been reported, mostly in Trinidad, Brazil and Peru. Rabid insectivorous bats, on the other hand, rarely infect other species such as humans, cats and wild animals.

Transmission and Tissue Tropism

Rabies is almost always transmitted by saliva via bites or scratches. In rabid animals the submaxillary salivary glands (the most commonly involved extraneural organ) are infected about 75% of the time, with levels of virus often exceeding 10^8 infectious doses (mouse or tissue culture) per ml. After its introduction by a bite the virus stays at the local site for a variable incubation period, usually several weeks, then advances up the peripheral nerves to the central nervous system; it often reaches the brain and the salivary glands before changes in the behavior of the animal occur. There is, then, a dangerous preclinical period of virus excretion in which the animal can infect other animals or humans without exhibiting any clinical abnormality such as jaw paralysis, excitation or changes in locomotion. During the terminal centrifugal spread of the disease (again by peripheral nerves) a variety of organs are commonly infected, including salivary glands, skin, lungs, kidneys and gonads.

Pathogenicity

Rabies viruses differ in their pathogenicity, but those differences have been difficult to measure. Certain laboratory adapted viruses (i.e. 'fixed' viruses) are highly invasive when injected either intracerebrally or intramuscularly. The invasiveness (as measured by the difference in mortality after intracerebral or intramuscular injection) of two 'street' isolates from one species in one geographic area can differ by as much as a thousandfold; it is not clear what factors this difference is due to, but it may include some factor in the saliva, the number of defective-interfering particles in the sample, and the particular characteristics of the virus. The pathogenicity also depends on the species of animal bitten, some species such as foxes being exquisitely susceptible to the virus, while others, such as the opossum, are much more resistant. Humans are quite resistant to rabies, with the expected mortality in persons bitten by rabid animals yet untreated being far below 50%; in observations made in the late 1800s, before rabies treatments were initiated, it was noted that 15% of persons died after severe and multiple hand bites by rabid dogs, while 85% survived without any treatment.

Clinical Features of Infection

Rabies in humans usually begins with mild and nonspecific symptoms which lead to an initial diagnosis of a common and minor bacterial or viral infection. A specific symptom often noted during the progression of the disease is pain or paresthesia at the bite site (usually the hand or foot). The acute neurological period begins with obvious nervous dysfunction, often including hyperactivity and, later, paralysis. Fever, nuchal rigidity, muscle fasciculation, convulsions, hyperventilation and excess salivation may be seen. The majority of agitated patients ('furious rabies') develop marked anxiety or agitation, sometimes accompanied by hydrophobia and aerophobia; during periods of agitation the patient's mental state fluctuates between periods of increasingly severe agitation and periods of normal behavior or depression. This acute period ends after 2–7 days. 'Paralytic rabies', with paralysis dominating the symptoms, is seen in about 20% of patients. Coma follows a transition period which begins with apneustic breathing; death is thought to be caused by respiratory arrest.

Pathology and Histopathology

There is little gross pathology in humans or animals that die of rabies; congestion of the meningeal vessels may occasionally be noted. The most common histologic change is perivascular infiltration, especially in the brainstem (the pons and medulla) as well as the spinal cord, basal ganglia and cerebral cortex. The neuronal degeneration and other inflammatory changes are variable. Negri bodies, specific (pathognomonic) cytoplasmic inclusions, are found in approximately 75% of rabid animals; these inclusions are most notable in the Purkinje cells of the cerebellum and in the hippocampal gyri (Ammon's horn). The absence of these inclusions does *not* rule out the diagnosis of rabies.

Geographic and Seasonal Distribution

The geographic distribution of the disease is summarized in the Epidemiology section. Rabies in dogs appears to have a somewhat seasonal character, with an increase in cases during the summer months; this was early attributed to the influence of the dog-star Sirius, but actually may be due to heat cycles in female dogs which lead to fighting among male dogs and an eventual increase in subsequent rabies cases. Rabies in terrestrial wild animals has not been reported to be seasonal; bat rabies, however, is distinctly seasonal in nontropical areas.

Host Range and Virus Propagation

Rabies virus infects a very broad array of animal species, perhaps the widest range of any animal virus. Commonly infected are dogs, wolves, foxes, jackals, skunks, raccoons, raccoon dogs, vampire bats, insectivorous bats and mongooses; the animals bitten by these species develop sporadic cases of rabies (these include cats, cows, horses, badgers and woodchucks) although the virus in those species rarely becomes enzootic. Humans are mostly infected after bites by rabid dogs.

Propagation is almost always by bite. Virus appears in the saliva of infected animals either when they are symptomatic, or for days or weeks before clinical signs appear. The presymptomatic excretion of virus in saliva is a very important epidemiologic characteristic for virus survival, and a crucial piece of information for physicians who judge whether an exposure has occurred in persons bitten by rabid (or possibly rabid) animals.

Experimental hosts include mice (the animal most commonly injected for confirmatory laboratory diagnosis), hamsters and rats (often used for pathogenesis studies), dogs (pathogenesis, vaccine efficacy), raccoons and skunks (oral vaccination). Suckling (1–3 day old mice) have been used for human and animal rabies vaccine production in many countries, mainly in Latin America, since their myelin content is much lower than that of adult animals, and virus titers in these young animals tend to be very high. Embryonating eggs have been used for propagation of attenuated vaccines (LEP and HEP). Street rabies viruses can be grown on mouse neuroblastoma cells with relative ease, and those cells are the most sensitive for confirming an initial diagnosis by fluorescent antibody. Tissue culture-adapted viruses grow to high titers on BHK cells. Other cells such as VERO, human diploid, chick and duck embryo cells are also commonly used for vaccine preparation.

Immune Response

Animals or humans vaccinated with classic rabies vaccines respond with a rise in neutralizing antibodies, the level reached generally being proportional to the potency of the vaccine. Neutralizing antibodies arise in direct response to the glycoprotein (G) gene; recombinant vaccines constructed with the cDNA of rabies virus glycoprotein also give rise to neutralizing (anti-G) antibodies. Animals with neutralizing antibodies, even at low levels, almost always survive subsequent challenge with 'street' rabies virus. Recently the protective role of the N gene has been recognized in experimental animals, although its significance in vaccinated animals (or humans) is not known. The cellular immune response after vaccination involves a wide array of cells. Serum neutralizing antibodies in individuals (humans or animals) that sicken with rabies are rarely noted before the eighth day of illness; antibodies appear in the cerebrospinal fluid 1 or 2 days later.

Prevention and Control of Rabies

Rabies may be controlled at three levels: human, domestic animal and wild animal. Until widespread canine vaccination programs were initiated in the late 1940s rabies was controlled only at the human level, with hundreds of thousands of persons vaccinated world-wide for exposure to rabid animals, mostly dogs. Rabies in dogs was controlled when potent animal vaccines became available (especially after the advent of proper vaccine potency tests) along with effective dog vaccination programs (those resulting in the immunization of at least 70% of community dogs) and stray dog control. This stopped dog-to-dog rabies transmission as well as serving as a barrier between infected wild animals and human populations. Recently an additional step has been taken involving the oral rabies vaccination of wild animals (foxes, raccoons) to eliminate rabies in those populations.

Future Perspectives

Many issues remain unsolved in rabies: what causes 15% of persons bitten in the hand by rabid dogs to die, while 85% survive without treatment? Where is the virus during the long incubation periods? What makes the virus break away at the end of that period? Why do some outbreaks in wild animals fade away after a few decades while others 'simmer' for much longer periods? Is there a better and less expensive treatment for exposed humans than that now administered (antiserum – or globulin – and vaccine)?

As the examination of molecular aspects of rabies permits the unravelling of the mysteries of pathogenesis we should see more investigation of antiviral substances and the development of more effective and less lengthy human treatments. Examination of viral isolates from various areas of the world will permit examination of the viral genomes of more and more rabies viruses, and clarify whether some are so far from the 'classic' strains as to require separate vaccines for the protection of humans and animals. The future should also bring a better understanding of just how effective vaccines can be delivered to unvaccinated animals such as wild animals, or, more important, community dogs in developing countries.

See also: **Epidemiology of viral diseases; Nervous system viruses; Rabies-like viruses (*Rhabdoviridae*); Vaccines and immune response; Vesicular stomatitus viruses (*Rhabdoviridae*); Zoonoses.**

Further Reading

Baer GM (ed.) (1991) *The Natural History of Rabies*, 2nd edn. Boca Raton, Florida: CRC Press.

Dietzschold B, Rupprecht CE, Zhen Fang Fu and Koprowski H (1996) Rhabdoviruses. In: Fields BN *et al.* (eds) *Fields Virology*, Third Edition, p. 1137. Philadelphia: Lippincott-Raven Publishers.

Dietzschold B *et al.* (1988) Antigenic diversity of the glycoprotein and nucleocapsid proteins of rabies and rabies-related viruses: implications for epidemiology and control of rabies. *Rev. Infect. Dis.* suppl. 4: 785.

Smith JS (1996) New aspects of rabies with emphasis on epidemiology, diagnosis, and prevention of the disease in the United States. *Clinical Microbiology* 9: 166–76.

Tordo N and Poch O (1988) Structure of rabies virus. In: Campbell JB and Charlton KM (eds) *Rabies. Developments in Veterinary Virology*, p. 25. Boston: Kluwer Academic.

[This article is reproduced from the 1st edn (1994).]

RABIES-LIKE VIRUSES (*RHABDOVIRIDAE*)

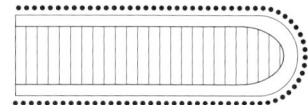

Robert E Shope, Center for Tropical Diseases, University of Texas Medical Branch, Galveston, Texas, USA

Copyright © 1999 Academic Press

History

Rabies virus was thought to be a single serotype without relatives until 1969. That year workers at Yale University and the Centers for Disease Control in Atlanta, Georgia discovered that two viruses from Africa were bullet-shaped like rabies, and were related serologically to rabies virus. One of these, Lagos bat virus had been isolated in 1956 by L.R. Boulger and James Porterfield from brains of *Eidolon helvum* fruit bats captured on Lagos Island, Nigeria. The second, Mokola virus, was isolated by Graham Kemp in 1968 from the organs of shrews of the genus *Crocidura* captured in the Mokola District of Ibadan, Nigeria. Subsequently, it was discovered that the virus Obodhiang, isolated by Jack Schmidt in 1963 from *Mansonia* mosquitoes in the Sudan, and another virus isolated in 1967 by Graham Kemp and Vernon Lee from *Culicoides* midges in Ibadan, Nigeria and named kotonkan virus, were distant serologic relatives of rabies virus. The mosquito and midge viruses have not been recovered from naturally infected vertebrate animals and may be insect viruses.

The full significance of the finding in 1969 that viruses from Africa were related to rabies virus was not realized at the time. In 1971, however, Mokola virus was isolated from a fatal human case of central nervous system disease in Ibadan, Nigeria.

In 1970, a South African farmer was bitten on the lip by a bat. He later died of what was clinically thought to be rabies. The virus isolated from his brain was recognized as a new rabies-related virus and was named Duvenhage virus.

Lagos bat virus has since been isolated from a cat and a bat in South Africa, from a bat in Central African Republic, and from a rabid dog in Ethiopia, but has not been associated with human illness. Mokola virus has been subsequently isolated from apparently rabid dogs and a cat in Zimbabwe, and from a rabid dog in Ethiopia. Both Lagos bat and Mokola viruses have thus demonstrated their potential for rabies-like pathogenicity; Mokola virus was also isolated from shrews in Cameroon and from a rodent, *Lophuromys* in the Central African Republic. The most striking finding, however, was the discovery of viruses most closely related to Duvenhage virus in bats in Germany. In 1985, a bat biologist died of this virus (since named European bat lyssavirus) infection. It is now clear that close relatives of Duvenhage virus are widely distributed in bats throughout Europe, and represent a hazard to human health.

A lyssavirus was recovered from the brains of flying foxes (fruit bats) *Pteropus alecto* and *P. scapulatus* found in New South Wales and Queensland, Australia in 1995 and 1996. These are the first reports of enzootic lyssavirus infection in Australia. A fatal human case in a woman who took care of bats occurred in 1996. Preliminary serological studies indicate that the Australian bat lyssavirus is neutralized by rabies antibody, although it is not identical to rabies in its reactivity with monoclonal antibodies. It is provisionally considered a member of the classic rabies serotype 1. A partial sequence is 92% homologous with rabies virus at the amino acid level.

Charles Calisher and his colleagues in 1989 tested 89 rhabdoviruses for antibody crossreaction by immunofluorescence and found that 19 reacted with the known rabies-related viruses or with rhabdoviruses that in turn reacted with the known rabies-related viruses. Other than rabies, Mokola, Lagos bat, Duvenhage virus and European bat lyssavirus, none of these rabies relatives has been implicated as a cause of rabies-like disease in people or domestic animals. Here, the properties of the rabies-related lyssaviruses that cause rabies in domestic animals and/or people are described, whereas kotonkan, Obodhiang, and the 19 other rhabdoviruses that have distant serological relationships to members of the genus *Lyssavirus* are not detailed.

Taxonomy and Classification

The rabies-related viruses belong to the genus *Lyssavirus* of the family *Rhabdoviridae* of RNA viruses. These viruses have nonsegmented negative-strand RNA genomes enclosed in a lipid envelope derived from the host cell. The particles are covered by glycoprotein (G), a layer of spikes contained in the envelope, which endows the particles of at least two of the viruses, Mokola and Lagos bat, with the ability to agglutinate avian red blood cells. Beneath the lipid envelope is a membrane phosphoprotein designated P associated with a helical complex containing the nucleoprotein (N) and the polymerase protein (L). A matrix (M) protein forms the inner lining of the lipid envelope. The viruses in the genus are bullet-shaped; Obodhiang and kotonkan resemble bovine ephemeral fever virus with mostly cone-shaped particles whereas the other members are indistinguishable from rabies particles. They have parallel sides, one flat end and one hemispherical end, and are approximately 180 nm in length and 65 nm in diameter.

The lyssaviruses are classified in five serotypes: serotype 1, rabies; serotype-2, Lagos bat (Lag); serotype-3, Mokola (Mok); serotype-4, Duvenhage (Duv) and serotype-5, European bat lyssavirus (EBL). These types were historically distinguished by neutralization test using polyclonal sera. Serotypes are currently typed and subtyped using a battery of anti-N monoclonal antibodies by immunofluorescence, and anti-G monoclonal antibodies by neutralization test. The serotypes correspond to genotypes except that EBL has two recognized genotypes, EBL1 and EBL2.

Geographic and Seasonal Distribution

Rabies-related viruses are geographically limited to Africa, except for European bat lyssavirus which is found in Europe. European Bat lyssaviruses are recognized throughout Europe from Spain to Russia and Ukraine. The rabies-related virus distribution is almost certainly a function of the range of reservoir hosts. There is no pattern of seasonality recognized.

Host Range and Virus Propagation

The reservoir hosts of Lagos bat, Mokola, Duvenhage, and European bat viruses are inferred from knowledge of sources of virus in nature. Lagos bat virus has been isolated at least nine times from bats. Where the bats were identified, these were fruit-eating bats: *Eidolon helvum* in Nigeria and Senegal, *Micropterus pusillus* in the Central African Republic, and *Epomophorus wahlbergi* in South Africa. The virus has presumably spilled over into domestic animals. It caused rabies in cats in South Africa and Zimbabwe, and in a dog in Ethiopia.

The reservoir of Mokola virus is believed to be the shrew, *Crocidura* spp., from which it has been isolated in Nigeria and Cameroon. A single isolation was made from a rodent, *Lophuromys sikapusi* in Central African Republic. The virus was recovered from rabid dogs in Zimbabwe and Ethiopia, and from rabid cats in Zimbabwe and South Africa indicating spillover into the domestic animal population. A fatal human case was recorded in Nigeria.

Insectivorous bats are implicated as the reservoir host of Duvenhage virus. The virus has been isolated repeatedly from *Eptisicus serotinus* throughout Europe, and once from *Nycteris thebaica* in Zimbabwe. The bat that bit the lip of the South African farmer who died of Duvenhage virus infection in 1970 was not identified.

European bat virus has been isolated repeatedly from *Eptisicus serotinus* (genotype EBL1) and *Myotis dasycneme* and *M. daubentonii* (genotype EBL2).

Lagos bat, Mokola, and Duvenhage viruses kill baby and adult mice following intracerebral inoculation. The three viruses induce plaques in Vero cells, and Duvenhage virus was readily adapted to form plaques in BHK-21 cells.

Wild-caught *Crocidura flavescens manni*, the African giant shrew, were inoculated in the laboratory with Mokola virus. Many of these became infected, including shrews exposed orally. Virus was recovered from brain, salivary glands, kidney, pancreas, lung and mouth swab. Virus was also sometimes detected in blood. Some animals became sick. They tended to save their food without eating it, to be more aggressive than uninfected animals, and to develop flaccid hind-limb paralysis. Shrews attack other animals in nature. Both sick and apparently healthy infected shrews transmitted Mokola virus to laboratory mice by bite.

Rhesus monkeys and beagle dogs were inoculated experimentally with Lagos bat and Mokola viruses. Animals inoculated intracerebrally invariably developed encephalitis indistinguishable from rabies and either died, or were killed. Dogs inoculated intramuscularly (i.m.) survived without illness as did the majority of monkeys inoculated i.m. One of five monkeys inoculated i.m. with Lagos bat virus developed unilateral paresis, but survived. One of five monkeys inoculated i.m. with Mokola virus developed tremors and died on day 19 postinoculation. Thus, Mokola and Lagos bat viruses are less pathogenic after i.m. inoculation than street rabies virus.

Mokola virus was passaged sequentially in baby mice, *Aedes albopictus* mosquito cells, and Vero cells. This passage material was found to infect *Aedes aegypti* mosquitoes by intrathoracic inoculation and was maintained by sequential passage in mosquitoes for 340 days. The virus was found in salivary glands, but in higher titer in nervous tissue of the mosquitoes. Mokola virus was transmitted transovarially in the mosquito, but infection of mice by mosquito bite was not demonstrated. Whether Mokola virus can be transmitted by arthropods in nature is still not known.

Genetics

The RNA of Mokola virus was cloned and the cDNA sequenced. The genome is very similar in length and organization to rabies virus. The length is estimated at 12 000 nucleotides. The genes, designated by the proteins they code, are arranged as follows: 3'-N-P-M-G-L-5'. The 3' and 5' end sequences of Mokola virus are highly conserved when compared to the PV strain of rabies virus, and the Mokola end sequences appear to be complementary.

Evolution

Rabies and the other lyssaviruses are postulated to have evolved initially on the African continent. This hypothesis is based on the known African distribution of nearly all lyssaviruses described. Sequence analysis of the gene coding for the N protein of the European bat lyssavirus shows that EBL1 and EBL2 have probably evolved from a progenitor on the African continent. The worldwide distribution of rabies virus can be explained by transport with people of domesticated dogs which were infected and carried extensive distances by sailing ships from Africa during the long incubation period of the virus. For this hypothesis to be credible, one also needs to postulate that rabies virus spread in the Americas, Asia, and Australia from dogs to sylvatic animals such as the skunk, fox, raccoon and bat, and that further divergent evolution occurred in these hosts.

Serologic Relationships and Variability

Serologic relationships among lyssaviruses have been measured by complement fixation, neutralization and immunization challenge tests. The N protein plays a major role in complement fixation. By this method, rabies, Mokola, Lagos bat and Duvenhage viruses differ among themselves by two- to 16-fold in each direction in reciprocal tests. This degree of closeness indicates a relative conservation of the N protein antigens.

The neutralization test measures the surface G antigen. When undiluted hyperimmune sera are tested against various dilutions of infectious virus in the baby mouse, the four lyssaviruses are very closely related. However, the same test done with constant virus dose and various dilutions of antibody shows almost no relationship among the viruses except with undiluted antibody. When the test is done in cell culture using plaque reduction and varying dilutions of antibody, Duvenhage virus is most closely related to rabies, and Mokola virus is quite distinct.

The immunization challenge test is the most likely method to indicate the utility of a rabies vaccine to protect against challenge with other lyssaviruses. Mokola and Lagos bat crossreact minimally with rabies virus; a rabies vaccine with solid homologous protection, yields only a 1.5 log protection index against Duvenhage virus challenge. If these same relationships hold in human infection, there is some rationale for use of rabies vaccines to protect against Duvenhage infection, but the efficacy would not be expected to be optimal.

Batteries of monoclonal antibodies are used to determine the variability in reactivity by immunofluorescence of the G and N antigens. The monoclonal antibodies reactive with the G antigens have also been tested for neutralization. On the basis of reactivity with these batteries, subtypes of lyssaviruses have been recognized. Lagos bat virus has three proposed subtypes (Lagos, Central African Republic and South Africa). Duvenhage and Mokola viruses have only one each, but there is some evidence that the Ethiopian Mokola virus is different from the Nigerian. European bat lyssavirus is still under study, but is considered at this time to be a single antigenic subtype (with two genotypes).

Epidemiology

Lyssaviruses related to rabies are maintained in transmission cycles of terrestrial wildlife or bats. Each serotype is found in one or a relatively limited number of related species. It is believed that transmission to humans or domestic animals represents spill-over from the wildlife cycle. These spill-over events are rare. They may occur when people intrude into wildlife habitats, such as a Finnish spelunker who was infected in 1985 with EBL, or when the wildlife enter houses such as may have happened in Ibadan, Nigeria in 1971 when a 6-year-old girl was infected fatally with Mokola virus.

There is no evidence that epidemics or epizootics occur. Animals and people may survive infection with Duvenhage, Lagos bat and Mokola viruses. Survival of experimentally infected dogs and monkeys following Lagos bat and Mokola virus infection is documented. Mokola virus was reportedly isolated from a child that recovered from poliomyelitis-like disease in Nigeria, although the patient did not develop antibody during convalescence and the validity of the isolation is in doubt. The seasonality, carrier rates, sex and age susceptibility are not known for animals or people.

Transmission and Tissue Tropism

Experimentally, Mokola virus is transmitted by bite of shrews, and there is anecdotal evidence that a bat transmitted Duvenhage virus to a person by bite. Aerosol transmission has not been eliminated as a possible mechanism of spread. Mokola virus was adapted to mosquitoes in the laboratory, but there appears to be no need to postulate mosquito transmission to explain maintenance in nature.

The limited data available from autopsy and infection of experimental animals indicate that Mokola, Lagos bat and Duvenhage viruses are neurotropic. The brain is the prominent target organ, as in rabies, and virus is also found in salivary glands late in infection.

Pathogenicity and Clinical Features of Infection

The range of pathogenicity of different strains of rabies-related viruses is not known. The clinical features of Mokola and Duvenhage virus infections are recorded in three patients; all presented with central nervous system disease. Duvenhage is associated with Guillain–Barré ascending paralysis and radiating pain in the arm and neck, followed later by agitation, increased respiration rate, muscle spasms, then coma and death. Diabetes insipidus with polyuria complicates the course. The child who died of Mokola virus infection had a prodromal illness of fever and vomiting, then flaccid paralysis of the limbs, progressing to deep coma before death.

Pathology and Histopathology

Specific lesions in the child who died of Mokola virus infection after a 9-day illness were limited to the brain. There were lymphocytic perivascular cuffing, neuronal changes of chromatolysis, eosinophilic necrosis, and nuclear pyknosis most marked in the midbrain and basal ganglia. Eosinophilic cytoplasmic inclusion bodies were found clustered in degenerating neurons. There were several lytic changes in the brain of the Finnish case of EBL. Rabies-reactive antigen was found in central nervous system neurons postmortem.

Immune Response

The very limited observations of patients infected with Mokola and Duvenhage viruses failed to show a specific serological response. The Finnish case of EBL infection was followed through 23 days of illness.

Prevention and Control of Disease Caused by Rabies-related Viruses

Prevention of human infection with rabies-related viruses is based on elimination of exposure in Europe and Africa, contact with bats should be avoided. Sick animals or those with abnormal behavior should be handled only with protective gloves. There is no vaccine available for Mokola or Lagos bat viruses. Commercial rabies vaccine and immune globulin may give limited protection against Duvenhage and EBL infection. Thus persons with bat bites and other bat exposures should receive classic rabies postexposure treatment, but should not expect complete protection. Persons whose occupations lead to exposure to bats should receive pre-exposure rabies vaccination.

Vaccines prepared from Mokola, Duvenhage and European bat lyssaviruses would be useful biologicals, but with the very low attack rates, it is not likely that such vaccines will be developed commercially.

Future Perspectives

The finding in Zimbabwe and Ethiopia of dogs and cats infected with Lagos bat and Mokola viruses is cause for concern. Human exposure and disease may be prevalent and not diagnosed. Active surveillance in Africa for Lagos bat, Mokola and Duvenhage viruses is needed.

Likewise, the threat posed by European bat lyssavirus is not yet completely appreciated. The scientific community needs to maintain vigilance for possible human cases, and needs increased research on the prevalence in bats, the possible spread to species other than serotine bats, and the extent to which terrestrial wildlife and domestic animals are exposed and infected.

See also: **Rabies virus (*Rhabdoviridae*); Rhabdoviruses (*Rhabdoviridae*): Ungrouped mammalian, bird and fish rhabdoviruses.**

Further Reading

Swanepoel R (1994) Rabies: rabies-related viruses. In: Coetzer JAW, Thomson GR and Tustin RC (eds.) *Infectious Diseases of Livestock,* vol. I, p. 520. Cape Town: Oxford University Press.

RECOMBINATION OF VIRUSES

Jozef J Bujarski, Northern Illinois University, Plant Molecular Biology Center, Montgomery Hall, DeKalb, Illinois, USA

Copyright © 1999 Academic Press

Introduction

Biochemically, recombination is a process of creating new genomic molecules by combining or substituting pieces of nucleic acids. Genetically, recombination could be defined as physical exchange of fragments among the parental genetic material. The results of recombination are progeny genomes that contain genetic information in nonparental combinations. Recombination was recognized as an important factor producing the genetic diversity upon which natural selection can operate.

Recombination events can occur in both RNA and DNA viruses. Since the molecular events behind DNA and RNA recombination differ in many aspects, they are described separately below.

Recombination in DNA Viruses

Recombination in many DNA viruses is believed to be accomplished by cellular enzymatic activities. There are two general types of genetic DNA recombination in the cell: homologous recombination (general recombination) and nonhomologous recombination. Nonhomologous or site-specific recombination occurs relatively rarely and requires special proteins that recognize specific DNA sequences to promote recombination. Homologous recombination occurs between two DNA sequences that are the same or very similar in the region of crossovers. Homologous recombination probably occurs in every DNA-based organism and it happens much more often than nonhomologous recombination.

There is plenty of information on the biochemical pathways responsible for crossovers in DNA. Besides sequence identity the requirements of general recombination include complementary base-pairing between double-stranded DNA molecules, recombination enzymes and the formation of heteroduplex within the regions of complementary base-pairing between the two recombining DNA molecules. Studies of the enzymology of DNA recombination in bacteria (and in particular of RecA, RecBCD proteins of *Escherichia coli*) have led to a large amount of literature, including many general reviews. Related recombination activities have been found and studied in eucaryotic sources, including yeast, insect, mammalian and plant cells.

Some DNA viruses encode their own proteins that function during recombination processes. In fact some DNA viruses serve as model systems for the study of recombination. For instance, certain bacteriophages encode the recombination pathways in order to avoid dependence on host systems. Such recombination can be used for repairing damaged phage DNA and for exchanging DNA between related phages to increase their diversity. High-frequency illegitimate recombination was observed at the replication origin of bacteriophage M13 in the *E. coli* host. The crossovers occurred at the nucleotide adjacent to the nick at the replication origin, by joining to a nucleotide elsewhere in the genome. This implied a breakage-and-reunion mechanism of illegitimate recombination, operating in *E. coli*.

Many of the phage recombination activities are analogous to those present in the host bacteria and studies on bacterial recombination systems were influenced by studies on phage systems. These pathways include Rec proteins of phages T4 and T7 (analogous to host RecA, RecG, RuvC or RecBCD proteins), RecE pathway in the rac prophage of *E. coli* K-12, or the phage 1 *red* system. In phage lambda there is another recombination system that can substitute for the RecF pathway components in *E. coli*. Models illustrating functions of RecA protein, RecBCD enzyme and Ruv proteins are shown in **Fig. 1**. A cartoon of the correlation of different stages of DNA recombination with transcription and DNA replication during bacteriophage T4 growth cycle is shown in **Fig. 2**.

Analogies between selected phage and *E. coli* host recombination functions are shown in **Table 1**.

Recombination between viral DNA and host genes was first observed in transducing bacteriophages in procaryotes and for retroviruses in eucaryotes. In some cases this represents a useful way for DNA viruses to acquire cellular genes. Among interesting examples of acquisition of cellular genes by DNA viruses are tRNA genes present in bacteriophage T4. These genes contain introns indicating that bacteriophage T4 must have passed through a eucaryotic host during evolution.

Genetic methods that rely on the use of mutants have been one of the most popular approaches for studying genetic recombination of DNA viruses. In viruses that have a single-component DNA genome,

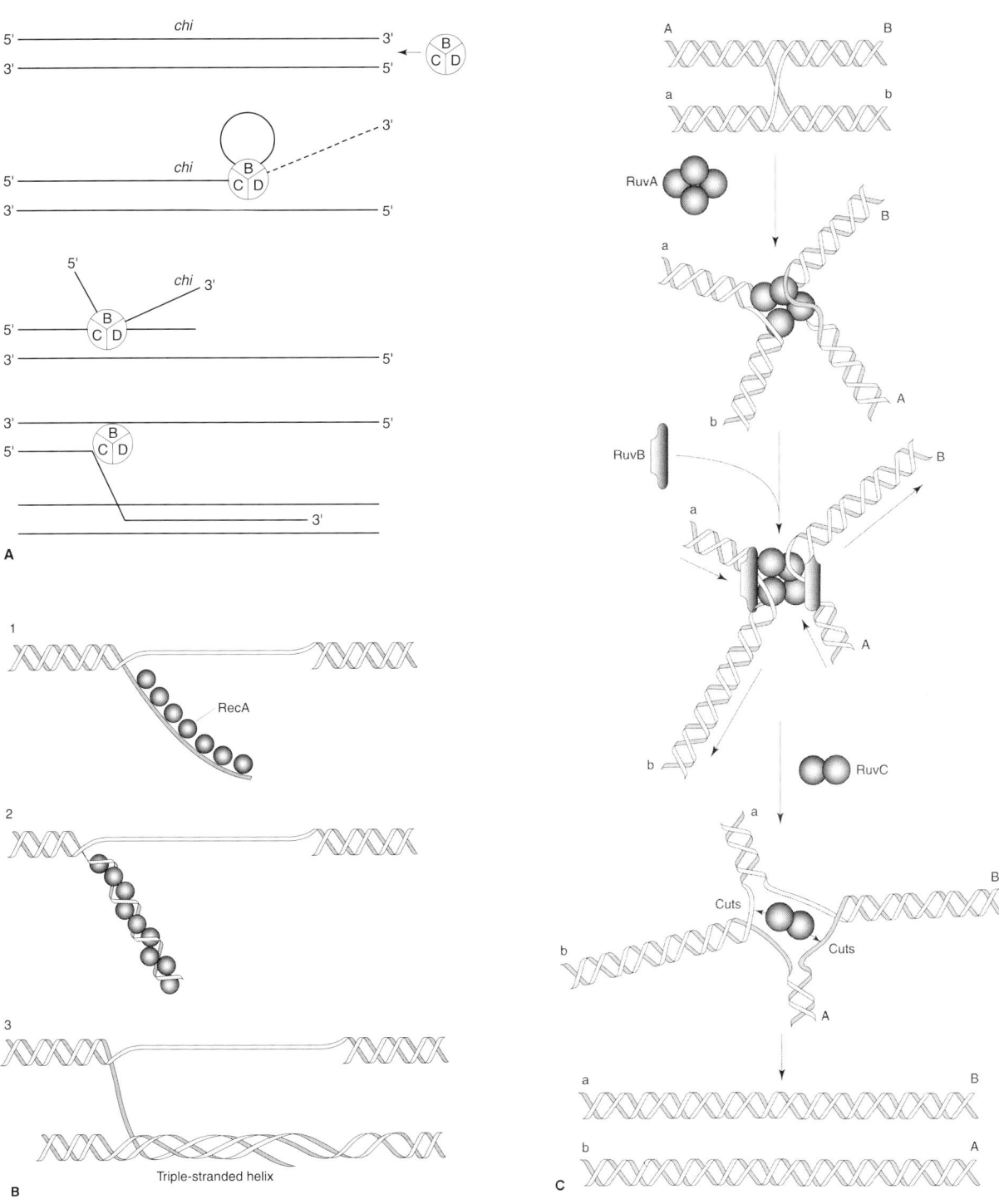

Figure 1 (**A**) Model for promotion of recombination initiation at a *chi* site by the RecBCD enzyme. The RecBCD enzyme loads on to the DNA at a free end or at a double-strand break internal to the DNA. It then moves along the DNA, displaces a loop, and the 3' end is degraded by the exonuclease activity of the RecBCD enzyme (dotted line). The exonuclease activity is inhibited at a *chi* site, the 3' end is no longer degraded and can thus invade another DNA molecule. (**B**) Synapse formation between two homologous DNAs by RecA protein. In steps 1 and 2, the RecA protein binds to the single-stranded end and forces it into an extended helical structure. In step 3, the helical single-stranded DNA can pair with a homologous double-stranded DNA in its major groove to form a stable extended triple helix. (**C**) Model for the mechanism of action of the Ruv proteins. RuvA binds to the Holliday junction. Note that the figure starts with one turn of blue-gray heteroduplex. Then RuvB binds to RuvA, and the junction migrates, deriving energy from ATP cleavage. RuvC cleaves two strands of the Holliday junction to resolve the junction into separate DNA molecules. Note the three turns of heteroduplex after junction migration. (Reproduced with permission from *Molecular Genetics of Bacteria* (1997) ASM Press.)

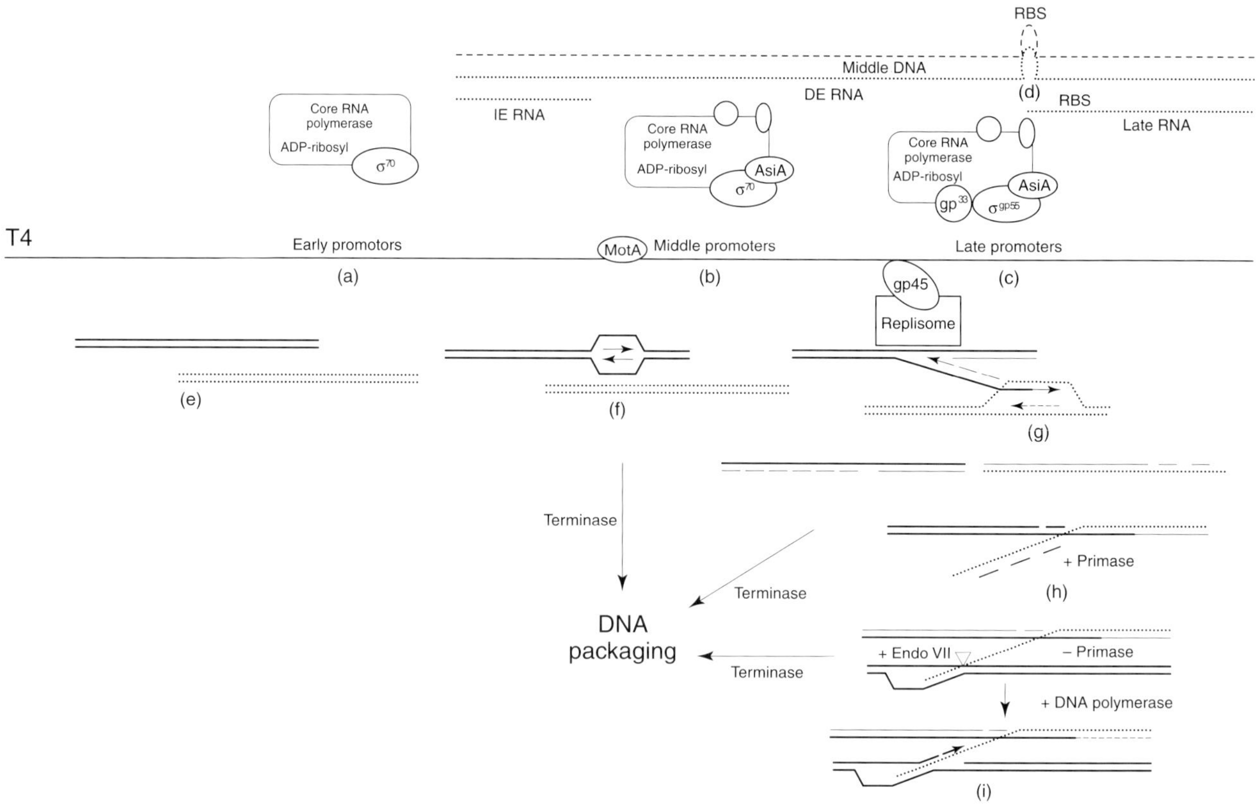

Figure 2 Cartoon showing the correlation between T4 recombination, and transcription and replication processes during bacteriophage T4 life cycle. The upper panel shows early (a), middle (b), and late (c) promoters recognized by forms of the host RNA polymerase that is modified by ADP-ribosylation of the α subunits and by T4-encoded accessory proteins. (d) shows a ribosome-binding site (RBS) of the mRNA for a late protein (Endo VII) that can be sequestered in a long early transcript but is free to initiate protein synthesis from a late transcript. The lower panel illustrates different stages of DNA replication and recombination in the context of the transcriptional program. (e) represents two T4 DNA molecules infecting a bacterium. (f) depicts bidirectional origin of replication cycle. (g) shows a replication–recombination pathway that becomes essential when the RNA polymerase modifications prevent further origin initiation. It is hypothesized that late after infection proteins required to initiate Okazaki pieces become limiting and that some join-cut-copy recombination requiring endonuclease VII occurs (h and i). Packaging proteins finally compete with replication and early recombination proteins for the recombinational intermediates, the concatamers are debranched, cut to headfull lengths, and packaged. (Reproduced with permission from *Molecular Biology of Bacteriophage T4* (1994) ASM Press.)

recombination can involve the exchange of DNA fragments. In contrast, in segmented DNA viruses, in addition to exchanges within each DNA component, the genome segments can be reassorted. This has implications for the recombination behavior observed among mutants. Recombination analyses are most easily performed using conditional-lethal type. The cells are mixedly infected with two mutants at permissive conditions and then the nonpermissive conditions are applied to select for recombinants. The so called two-factor crosses are performed through simple pairwise infections. For single-segmented DNA viruses this approach allows the mutants to be ordered into complementation groups and the relative positions of mutations to be placed on a linear map. For segmented genome DNA viruses, however, due to the reassortant factors, the data obtained in two-factor crosses do not allow mutants to be ordered on to a linear map. Three-factor crosses involve the use of three mutations, with one of them being kept unselected during selection of recombinants between the other two. These crosses are useful for determining linkage relationships between mutants and for establishing the order of marker mutations. Due to reassortment the three-factor crosses are of less use in segmented viruses.

Recombination in DNA viruses of eucaryotes was observed for both animal and plant viruses. The recombination frequencies among pairs of temperature-sensitive mutants (two-factor crossings) were studied in herpes simplex virus. A linear dependence upon the distance between mutations and the fre-

Table 1 Functional analogy between phage and *E. coli* recombination proteins.

Phage	E. coli
T7 gene 3	RuvC, RecG
T4 UvsX	RecA
T4 gene 49	RuvC, RecG
T4 genes 46 and 47	RecBCD
I ORF in nin region	RecO, RecR, RecF
Rac recE gene	RecJ, RecQ

ORF, open reading frame.

quency was observed, suggesting the lack of specific signal sequences responsible for crossover events in this virus.

Three-factor crosses were performed using herpes simplex virus. Here, a syncytial plaque morphology mutation was used as an unselected marker for ts mutations. In the case of adenoviruses the host range determined by the helper function of two mutations has been used as a third marker between ts mutants.

Epstein–Barr virus (EBV), a member of the gamma herpesvirus family, is a DNA virus with a long double-stranded DNA genome which shows a high degree of variation among strains. This variation takes the form of single base changes, restriction site polymorphism, insertions and deletions. It was found that some EBV variants arose by DNA recombination events.

Homologous genetic recombination was observed in vaccinia virus (VV) and other poxviruses. This is evident from the high frequency of intertypic crossovers, the ease of the marker rescue and the isolation of viral recombinants. Recombination of VV DNA occurs both intra- and intermolecularly, and is dependent on DNA target size. A function of the viral DNA polymerase or viral DNA replication itself has been implicated and viral proteins with DNA strand transfer activity have been identified.

Intertypic crosses between ts mutants were selected for adenoviruses. Analysis of the segregation patterns of DNA fragments and their restriction enzyme polymorphism has allowed the specific ts mutations to be mapped on adenovirus genomes.

General recombination in somatic cells was observed for SV40 (a papovavirus). The authors tested recombination events from artificially constructed recombinant circular oligomers. While this type of recombination was high, homologous recombination in this type of DNA tumor viruses was rare.

The geminiviruses are a unique group of single-stranded plant DNA viruses. Intermolecular recombination between geminivirus DNAs has frequently been observed using various combinations of mutants. Likewise, intramolecular homologous recombination between tandem repeats of a geminivirus genome was found in agro-infected tobacco plants. Both homologous recombination model and replication-based recombination model were proposed to explain the observed events. In addition, deletions, insertions and other rearrangements have frequently been detected in geminivirus infections. These illegitimate recombination processes may rely on aberrant breakage–fusion events as well as errors of DNA replication, and may be inter- or intramolecular in nature.

Cauliflower mosaic virus (CaMV) is a plant DNA virus. It belongs to the pararetroviruses, which replicate through a reverse transcription step. A high recombination rate was observed *in vivo* for CaMV. The replication cycle of CaMV offers a variety of possibilities for recombination: recombination at the DNA level, which occurs in the nucleus, and at the RNA level, which occurs during reverse transcription in the cytoplasm. In general, it is difficult to decide by which recombination route a CaMV recombinant is obtained. However, such features as recombinational hot spots and apparent mismatch repair might be indicative. Namely, the presence of hot spots reflects replicative (RNA) recombination, while mismatch repair can occur during formation of heteroduplex intermediates and is thus indicative of DNA recombination. Recombination between CaMV strains and CaMV transgene mRNA was observed. It is believed that this type of recombination represents an RNA–RNA recombination event (during reverse transcription).

Recombination in RNA Viruses

RNA viruses utilize RNA as their genetic material. The potential for variation of the RNA genome is very large owing to a high mutation rate (during copying by RNA-dependent RNA polymerase) and to recombination. The terms of classic population biology do not describe RNA viruses. Instead, a term of quasispecies was proposed to reflect the nature of RNA virus populations. The processes of genetic recombination in plus-stranded RNA viruses probably do occur at the RNA level, as these viruses most likely do not go through DNA steps in their replication cycles. RNA recombination processes are generally categorized as either homologous or nonhomologous. In 1992, Lai postulated three classes of RNA recombination: homologous, aberrant homologous and nonhomologous. Homologous recombination occurs between two related RNA molecules at corresponding sites, although homologous RNA recombination can also occur within a common region shared by otherwise unrelated RNA sequences. Aberrant homologous recombination involves crossovers between related RNAs, but does not occur at corresponding sites, leading to sequence insertions or deletions. Nonhomologous recombination occurs between unrelated RNA molecules. Slightly different definitions, based on mechanistic models and considerations, were proposed recently by several authors.

Although genetic recombination in RNA viruses such as influenza virus and poliovirus has been described, it has not been found in Newcastle disease virus. The complete nucleotide sequences of the genomic RNAs of a large number of RNA viruses belonging to different virus groups have been obtained. This revealed the relatedness of various animal, plant and other RNA viruses and allowed the definition of sequence rearrangements in the viral RNA genome.

Sequence rearrangements were found in the following animal plus-strand RNA viruses: picornaviruses: poliovirus and foot-and-mouth-disease virus (FMDV); in coronaviruses: mouse hepatitis coronavirus (MHV); Sindbis alphavirus (SIN); flock house nodavirus (FHV); and in bacteriophages Qβ, and MS-2. Recombinants were found in bunyaviruses. Genetic rearrangements were also observed in other types of RNA viruses, including influenza virus, a minus-strand RNA virus, in retroviruses, and in double-stranded Φ6 bacteriophage. The following genomes of plant RNA viruses reveal RNA rearrangements: alfalfa mosaic virus (AlMV), beet necrotic yellow vein virus (BNYVV), bromoviruses (see below), hordeiviruses, luteoviruses, nepoviruses, tobamoviruses, tobraviruses, tombusviruses and turnip crinkle carmovirus (TCV).

Recombination by reassortment was observed for multisegmented animal RNA viruses, including influenza virus and double-stranded reoviruses and orbiviruses. The reassortment mechanism functioning in reoviruses is reflected by the fact that the interpretation of two-factor crosses (using for instance temperature-sensitive mutations) appears to be difficult: the mutants cannot be ordered on to a self-consistent linear map and quite often no linkage between mutants could be detected.

The examples in which host-derived sequences have recombined with viral RNAs include an ubiquitin-coding sequence of bovine diarrhea virus, a sequence from 28S rRNA inserted in the hemagglutinin gene of an influenza virus, and a tRNA sequence in Sindbis virus RNA. For plant viruses, several potato leafroll virus isolates contain sequences homologous to an exon of tobacco chloroplast. Acquisition of chloroplast sequences during RNA recombination was observed for brome mosaic virus.

The use of transgenic plants expressing viral RNA sequences has confirmed that plant RNA viruses are able to recombine with host mRNAs. This was shown for cowpea chlorotic mottle bromovirus (CCMV), red clover necrotic mosaic virus (RCNMV), potato virus Y potexvirus (PVY) and plum pox potyvirus (PPV).

Studies on the molecular mechanism of RNA recombination have progressed when experimental systems that supported the high frequency of crossovers were established. The available data on rearrangements in picornaviruses suggest a mechanism of template switching that occurs during minus-strand RNA synthesis. These rearrangements may be facilitated by the existence of identical or completely dissimilar signal sequences between the recombining RNA substrates.

Certain RNA viruses can produce both homologous and nonhomologous RNA recombinants. The molecular mechanism involved in the formation of homologous and nonhomologous recombinants was tested using an efficient recombination system of brome mosaic virus (BMV). A partially debilitating BMV RNA3 mutant was repaired *in vivo* by exchanges with the sequences of other BMV RNA components. Low recombination frequency was overcome by construction of RNA3-based recombination vectors, where recombinationally active sequences could be inserted and analyzed. It appeared that short base-paired regions between the two BMV RNA recombination substrates can target efficient nonhomologous recombination crossovers. A model invokes the formation of local RNA–RNA heteroduplexes to be responsible for targeting the RNA crossovers as a result of: (1) bringing the RNA substrates into a close proximity; and (2) slowing down or stalling the approaching replicase enzyme complex (**Fig. 3**).

Similarly, homologous RNA recombination was studied by inserting a BMV RNA2-derived sequence into the recombination vector. Both precise and imprecise crossovers were observed. Other RNA sequences revealed that the frequency of RNA2–RNA3 homologous crossovers depends upon sequence composition and tends to occur at hot spot regions that contain stretches of GC-rich alternating with AU-rich sequences. Such nucleotide composition may act as recombination activators during switching between RNA templates by the RNA replicase enzyme (**Fig. 4**). Overall, the data on BMV RNA recombination suggest that molecular mechanisms involved in the two types of crossovers in BMV differ from each other.

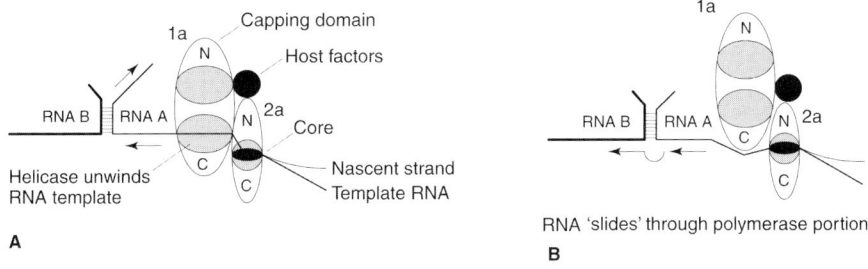

Figure 3 The model of strand switching by BMV replicase. The replicase is composed of the interacting host (smaller black circles) and viral (represented by ellipses) proteins. Functional domains of nucleotidyl transferase (capping enzyme), helicase and core RNA polymerase on proteins 1a and 2a are represented by smaller shaded ellipses. At the replication mode (**A**) the enzyme copies the original template through the double-stranded region (represented by a short 'ladder') due to the helicase action. During recombinational mode (**B**), the polymerase 'slides' under the double-stranded regions and changes the templates from RNA A to RNA B. The arrows indicate the direction of replicase migration. (Reproduced from Bujarski and Nagy (1994) Genetic RNA–RNA recombination in positive-stranded RNA viruses of plants. In: Paszkowski J (ed.) *Homologous Recombination and Gene Silencing in Plants*. Kluwer Academic.)

The term 'recombinosome' was proposed to describe a complex between the recombining RNAs, the replicase proteins and other (putative) factors involved in template switching events. The participation of replicase proteins of BMV in recombination was studied using a temperature-sensitive 1a of BMV protein mutant. This revealed a 5′ shift in crossover sites within the RNA1–RNA3 heteroduplex, suggesting that the helicase domain of 1a participates in heteroduplex-mediated crossovers. Likewise, a single amino acid mutation within the core domain of 2a protein and mutations within the N-terminal portion of 2a, the polymerase component of the replicase, inhibited the frequency of nonhomologous recombination in BMV. These studies confirm the participation of replicase proteins in recombination.

The role of replicase enzyme in RNA recombination was also studied in TCV, a small single component RNA virus that is associated with a number of subviral RNAs, such as satellite RNA D and chimeric RNA C. High frequency recombination was observed *in vivo* between RNAs C and D. A template switching model was proposed where viral replicase utilizes the nascent plus-strand of RNA D to reinitiate RNA elongation at a hairpin structure on the acceptor minus-strand RNA C template (**Fig. 5**).

The participation of TCV replicase in RNA recombination was studied *in vitro* with a TCV replicase preparation and a chimeric RNA template containing the *in vivo* hot spot region from RNA D joined to the hot spot region from RNA C. This demonstrated roles for a priming stem sequence in the RNA C portion and the TCV RNA-dependent RNA polymerase (RDRP) binding hairpin, also from the RNA3 portion. It probably reflects such late steps of the *in vivo* RNA recombination as strand transfer and primer elongation.

For coronaviruses, the animal RNA viruses containing a large RNA genome, recombination has been demonstrated between coronavirus genomes and defective-interfering RNAs, and it was postulated to account for the diversity in the genomic structure of these viruses. The mechanistic considerations suggest the nonprocessive nature of the coronavirus RNA polymerase, which might be responsible for recombination. Similarly, RNA recombination in nodaviruses, two-partite RNA viruses, occurs between RNA segments at a site, where the nascent strand could form a base-paired region with the acceptor template. Such factors as template secondary structure and the similarity of the crossover sites to an origin of replication seem to influence the choice of recombination site. A model of recombination where the polymerase interacts directly with the acceptor nodavirus RNA was postulated.

A copy-choice template switching mechanism was also suggested for recombination in a double-stranded bacteriophage Φ6. Here, the crossovers occur inside the virus capsid structure. Apparently, the crossovers can occur in regions that share little sequence similarity and the frequency of recombinants can be enhanced by conditions that prevent the minus-strand synthesis.

The bacteriophage Qβ has emerged as a unique RNA virus system for the study of RNA recombination both *in vivo* and in cell-free systems. It was demonstrated for the first time in this virus that RNA recombination can occur not by polymerase template switching events but rather via a splicing-type RNA recombination mechanism.

Genetic RNA recombination has been observed in retroviruses. Here, the efficient recombinant jumpings are secured by reverse transcriptase. In fact, the retrovirus system represents a well-established model

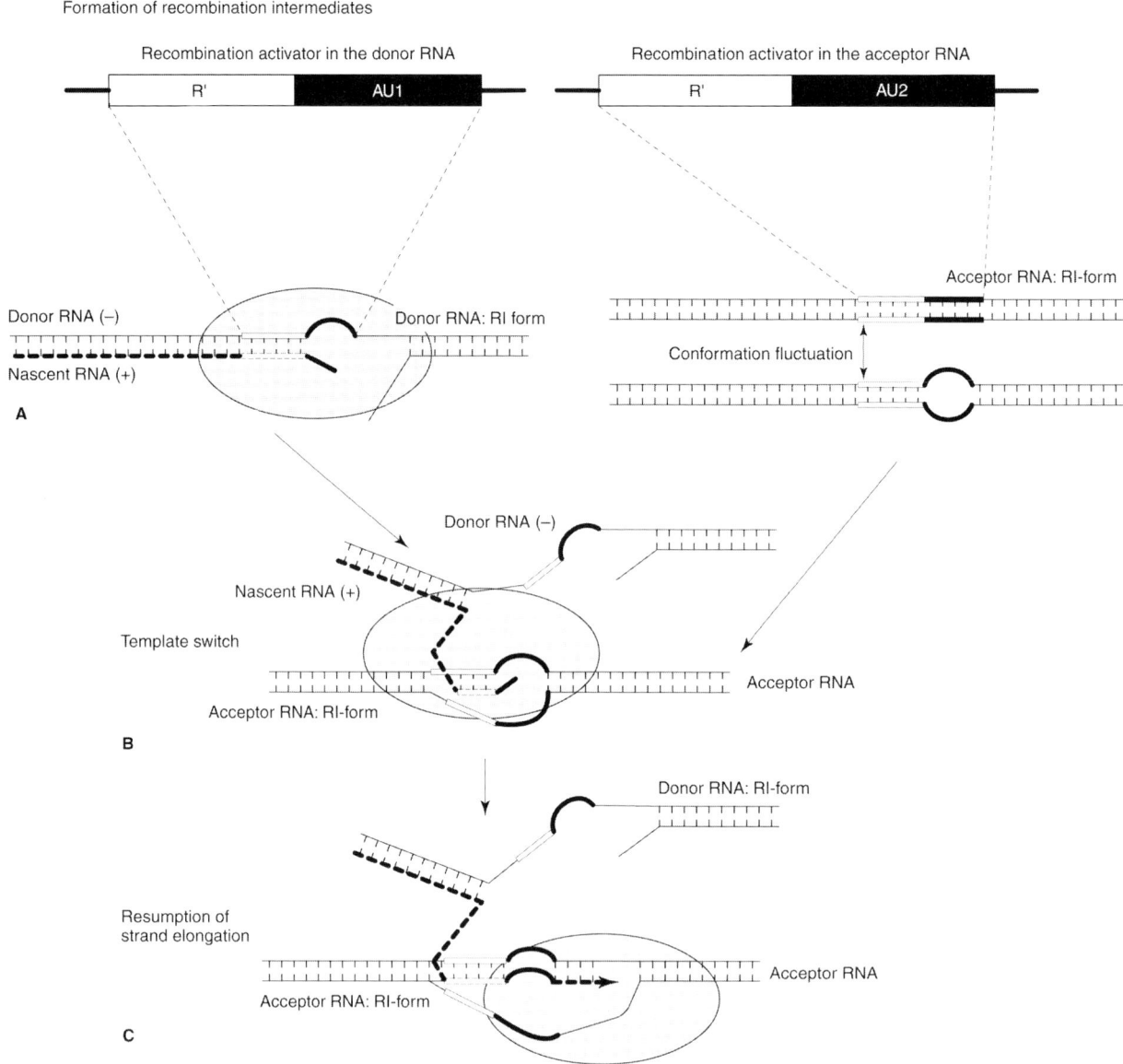

Figure 4 Processive template switching model explaining the formation of homologous recombination hot spots within the recombination activator sequences. (**A**) Template switching of the BMV replicase occurs during positive-strand synthesis. Although localized double-stranded replicative intermediates (RIs) are shown, the existence of single-stranded RNAs with negative polarity is also possible (not shown). The weak base pairing within the AU-rich region (shown on the left side of the diagram with a black line) can facilitate the release of the 3' end of the incomplete nascent RNA. The weak base pairing within the AU-rich region can also facilitate the temporary formation of a bubble structure in the RI of the acceptor strand (gray line on the right side). The replicase (large shadowed ellipse) pauses on the donor strand at the UA-rich region, and the very 3' end of the nascent strand disengages from the original template strand. (**B**) The released 3' end of the nascent strand hybridizes to the acceptor strand facilitated by the bubble structure. Hybridization of the upstream located R' (shown by empty boxes) stabilizes the recombination intermediate. (**C**) The viral replicase resumes chain elongation on the acceptor strand (shown by an arrowhead). This leads to the formation of homologous recombinant RNA3s. (Reproduced with permission from a paper by Nagy and Bujarski (1997) *J. Virol.* 71(8): 3808.)

of the polymerase/template switching reactions both *in vivo* and *in vitro*. Apparently, the virally encoded reverse transcriptases are evolutionarily selected to secure jumping during reverse transcription reactions. The recombinant jumpings are responsible for both inter- and intramolecular template switching, and for

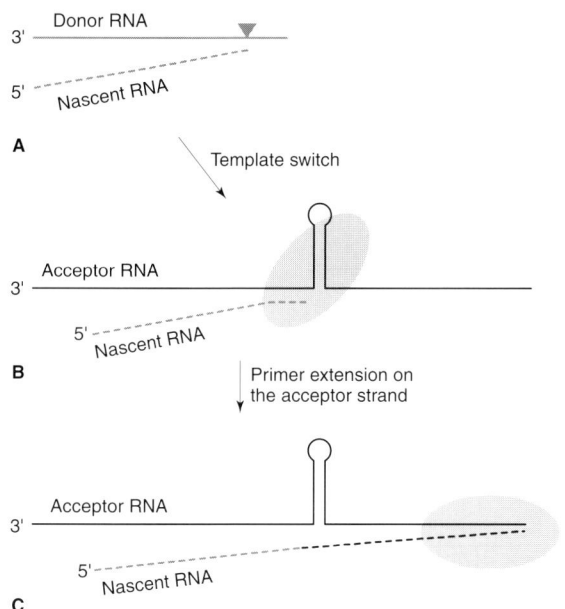

Figure 5 Model for RNA recombination in the turnip crinkle virus (TCV) system. (**A**) The TCV RDRP copying minus-strand sat-RNA D either reaches the natural 5′ end or pauses at some positions (mainly 13 nucleotides from the 5′ end, as indicated by a triangle) likely due to the presence of a protein-binding site. (**B**) The TCV RDRP, which is still associated with the nascent sat-RNA D strand, switches to the acceptor template (minus-strand sat-RNA C or TCV) facilitated by either the motif I or motif III hairpins. Hybridization between the nascent strand and the acceptor strand may stabilize the recombination intermediate. (**C**) The TCV RDRP reinitiates RNA synthesis using the 3′ end of the nascent sat-RNA D as a promoter. Further copying of the acceptor RNA by the RDRP results in a recombinant RNA molecule. (Reproduced with permission from Simon et al (1996) Semin. Virol. 7: 373.)

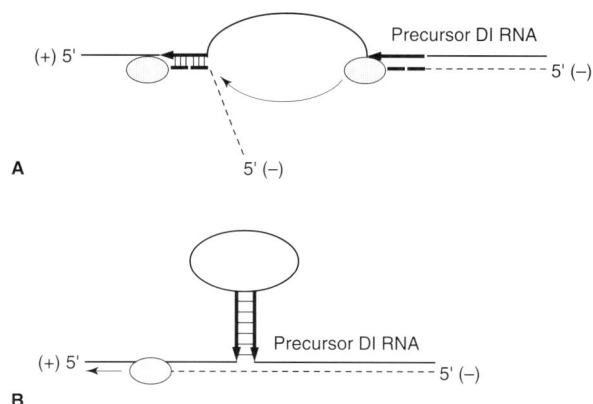

Figure 6 Proposed replicase-mediated model for deletion of segments from precursor DI RNAs. RNA templates are depicted as solid lines while nascent strands are shown as dashed lines. The viral replicase is represented by shaded ovals and its path is indicated by thin arrows. Deletion of segments from precursor DI RNA molecules may be facilitated by tracts (bold arrows) of sequence (**A**) identity or (**B**) complementarity, as discussed in the text. (Reproduced with permission from White A (1996) Formation and evolution of Tombusvirus defective interfering RNAs. Semin. Virol. 7: 409.)

the formation of defective retroviral genomes. They contribute significantly to genetic variability of retroviruses.

Defective-Interfering RNAs

Defective-interfering (DI) RNAs are subviral RNA molecules derived from the helper virus genomic RNA and typically interfere with helper virus accumulation and affect symptoms produced by the helper virus. Paul von Magnus was first (in 1954) to report DI RNAs in influenza virus. Later, DI RNAs were observed in a majority of animal and in many plant RNA virus infections. Naturally-occurring DI RNAs have been identified during infection with several coronavirus species. These molecules appear to arise by a polymerase strand-switching mechanism. In fact the DI RNAs were used in coronavirus research, to study the mechanism of high-frequency, site-specific RNA recombination events that progress through leader acquisition during RNA replication, and as vehicles for the generation of targeted recombinants of the parental virus genome.

For plant tombusviruses and carmoviruses the DI RNAs reveal a consistent pattern of rearranged mosaic-type sequences flanked by unmodified terminal regions. Analysis of these DI RNAs suggests that in some cases the base-pairing between an incomplete replicase-associated nascent strand and the acceptor template can mediate the selection of the rearrangement sites (**Fig. 6**).

Single deletion-type DI RNAs were isolated from infections with several viruses, including beet necrotic yellow vein furovirus (BNYVV), soil-borne wheat mosaic furovirus (SBWMV), peanut clump furovirus (PCV), clover yellow mosaic potexvirus (CYMV), sonchus yellow net rhabdovirus (SYNRV), and tomato spotted wilt tospovirus (TSWV). Such factors as the length of the defective RNA or its coding capacity seem to affect the selection of DI RNAs during infection.

For broad bean mottle bromovirus (BBMV) the naturally existing DI RNAs were found to be derived by single deletions in the RNA2 component. A secondary structure-mediated model for BBMV DI RNAs, where local complementary regions bring the remote parts of RNA2 together to facilitate the crossover events, has been proposed (**Fig. 5**). Similar to BBMV, single deletion-type DI RNAs have been found associated with cucumoviruses. Overall, it seems likely that the mechanisms leading to DI RNA generation are similar to those of RNA recombination.

The closteroviruses are the RNA viruses of plants that have the longest known RNA genome. Recently, multiple species of citrus tristeza closterovirus (CTV) defective RNAs, which resulted from the recombination of a subgenomic RNA with distant parts from the 5′ end of the viral genomic RNA, were identified. This suggests that closteroviruses can utilize subgenomic RNA as factors for the modular exchange and rearrangement of their genomes.

Defective-interfering particles were also found in negative-strand RNA viruses. Namely, for vesicular stomatitis virus (VSV) cis-acting terminal sequence elements play an important role during RNA replication. The formation and accumulation of certain classes of DI RNA molecules were observed: the majority of DI RNAs were of the 5′ copy-back class, reflecting the mechanisms involved in DI RNA generation.

In the case of RNA viruses both homologous and nonhomologous recombination events were observed. Various types of copy-choice mechanisms were proposed to explain the formation of RNA recombinants, and the role of special RNA signal sequences and viral proteins in recombination was observed. In some cases a mechanism of RNA breakage and religation cannot be excluded and was experimentally demonstrated for bacteriophage Qβ. Further studies are required to obtain a more general picture of genetic recombination pathways available for viruses, especially for RNA viruses.

See also: **Bromoviruses (*Bromoviridae*); Defective interfering viruses; Genetics of animal viruses; History of virology: Bacteriophages, General; Pathogenesis: Animal viruses, Plant viruses; Phage Homologous Recombination; Replication of viruses; Taxonomy and classification – general.**

Conclusions

Genetic recombination can be found in many groups of DNA and RNA viruses. Both the observed natural sequence rearrangements and the data obtained with the use of experimental systems demonstrate that recombination plays an important role in providing the genetic diversity during virus infections. The molecular mechanisms involved in genetic recombination depend on the class of viruses. DNA viruses utilize mechanisms of homologous (general) recombination available in the host cells, although some DNA viruses encode their own recombination proteins. Also, site-specific (nonhomologous) recombination events were found for certain classes of DNA viruses.

Further Reading

Bujarski J (ed.) (1996 and 1997) RNA recombination and defective RNA formation. *Semin. Virol.* 7/6 (Part I) and 8/2 (Part 2).

Gibbs AJ, Calisher CH and Garcia-Arenal F (eds) (1995) *Molecular Basis of Virus Evolution*. Cambridge: Cambridge University Press.

Holland JJ (ed.) (1992) *Genetic Diversity of RNA Viruses*. Berlin: Springer.

Karam JD (ed.) (1994) *Molecular Biology of Bacteriophage T4*. Washington: ASM Press.

Roossinck MJ (1997) Mechanisms of plant virus evolution. *Annu. Rev. Phytopathol.* 35: 191.

Snyder L and Champness W (1997) *Molecular Genetics of Bacteria*. Washington: ASM Press.

REOVIRUSES (*REOVIRIDAE*)

Contents
General features
Molecular biology

General Features

Kenneth L Tyler, Neurology Department, B-182, University of Colorado Health Sciences Center, Denver, Colorado, USA

Copyright © 1999 Academic Press

History

In 1959, AB Sabin proposed the designation reovirus (respiratory enteric orphan virus) for a subgroup of respiratory and enteric viruses not known to be associated with human disease (hence orphan) with particular distinguishing characteristics. The distinguishing features of reoviruses included: (1) their size, which at ≥75 nm was larger than other known enteric viruses; (2) their capacity to produce cytoplasmic inclusions in monkey kidney cells in tissue culture; (3) their pathogenicity for newborn but not adult mice; and (4) their capacity to hemagglutinate human type O erythrocytes. All of the viruses that would subsequently be designated the prototypes for the three reovirus serotypes (see below) were originally isolated in the 1950s from the stools of children. The first reovirus was isolated by NF Stanley and colleagues in 1951 from an aboriginal child and subsequently named hepatoencephalomyelitis virus. An enteric virus isolated by M Ramos-Alvarez and AB Sabin in 1953 from the stool of a baby named Lang initially became the prototype virus for ECHO 10, and subsequently for reovirus serotype 1 (reovirus serotype 1 strain Lang). The prototype for reovirus serotype 2 was isolated by Ramos-Alvarez and Sabin from the stool of a child named Jones with a summer diarrheal illness (reovirus serotype 2 strain Jones) in 1955. Viruses isolated by Ramos-Alvarez and Sabin in 1955 from the stool of a child named Dearing and by L Rosen in 1957 from an anal swab from a baby named Abney became the prototype strains for serotype 3 (reovirus serotype 3 strains Dearing and Abney).

Taxonomy and Classification

The genus *Orthoreovirus*, of which the mammalian reoviruses are the prototypes, is one of the nine genera belonging to the family *Reoviridae*. Viruses belonging to this family are nonenveloped spherical viruses of 60–85 nm diameter, whose genome consists of 10–12 discrete segments of double-stranded RNA (dsRNA) that is contained in two or three concentric protein capsids with icosahedral symmetry. Members of different genera can be distinguished by differences in relative size, capsid number and structure, genome segment number, nature and number of structural proteins, and patterns of reactivity with antisera. Viruses belonging to different genera also differ substantially in their host range and pathogenesis. (*See also*: **Orbiviruses and Coltiviruses, Phytoreoviruses, Rotaviruses.**) Nucleotide sequence data indicate that members of the *Orthoreovirus* genus are highly divergent from other *Reoviridae* genera (e.g. *Orbivirus, Rotavirus*) including those known to infect humans and other mammals. Members of the *Orthoreovirus* genus have 10 segments of dsRNA contained in two concentric protein capsids of approximately 85 nm diameter (**Table 1**).

The mammalian orthoreoviruses, which form the subject of this chapter (subsequently referred to as 'reoviruses'), are further classified into three serotypes (designated serotypes 1, 2, 3) on the basis of their patterns of reactivity with typing antisera and differences in their capacity to hemagglutinate human and bovine erythrocytes. Classically, serotyping was performed by hemagglutination–inhibition assay on human type O erythrocytes using serotype-specific antisera. Serotyping can also be accomplished by evaluating the capacity of serotype-specific antisera to produce neutralization as measured in plaque reduction neutralization assays. Genetic studies with reassortant viruses derived from crosses between the prototype strains for different serotypes indicate that the $\sigma 1$ protein, which is encoded by the S1 dsRNA segment, is the major serotype-specific determinant. Accurate serotyping can also be accomplished by evaluating the capacity of serotype-specific sigma 1 monoclonal antibodies to neutralize infectivity of test isolates. The most accurate information concerning the relationship between different reovirus strains can be accomplished by comparison of nucleotide and amino acid sequence variability between their cognate gene segments and encoded proteins. Detailed phylogenetic analyses of the evolutionary relationship between a number of reovirus strains based on the nucleotide sequence of their S1, S2, S3 and S4 gene segments have now been published (**Fig. 1**). Interestingly, the phylogenetic trees of individual viral strains differ depending on the dsRNA segment chosen for comparison, indicating that reassortment of reovirus gene segments occurs under natural circumstances.

Other members of the *Orthoreovirus* genus include a large group of viruses isolated from birds, the avian reoviruses, and several currently incompletely categorized viruses isolated from the flying fox (Nelson Bay virus), baboons and several species of snakes. These viruses all have basic similarities in the nature of their genomic organization (10 dsRNA segments), protein coding pattern and general virion structural organization. Reassortment between these various groups of reoviruses has not been demonstrated and their cognate gene segments and corresponding proteins are extremely divergent in their nucleotide and protein sequences. It is likely that mammalian reoviruses, avian reoviruses, and perhaps some of these other currently uncharacterized reoviruses are independent quasispecies.

Geographic and Seasonal Distribution

Reoviruses are ubiquitous in their geographic distribution. Studies of variation in the seasonal pattern of infection are extremely limited. As noted, many of the initial isolates of reoviruses from humans were made from infants and children with summer diarrheal illnesses. Studies of the prevalence of child-

Table 1 Properties of the mammalian reoviruses

Genome
    Double-stranded RNA
    10 gene segments in three size classes (L, M, S)
    Total size 23 500 bp
    Gene segments encode either one or two proteins each
    Gene segments are transcribed into full-length mRNAs
    Plus strands of gene segments have 5′ caps
    Nontranslated regions at segment termini are short
    Gene segments can undergo reassortment between virus strains

Particles
    Spherical, with icosahedral (5:3:2) symmetry
    Nonenveloped
    Total diameter 85 nm (excluding σ1 fibers)
    Two concentric protein capsids: outer capsid subunits in $T = 13$ lattice, arrangement of inner capsid subunits unknown
    8 structural proteins: 4 proteins in outer capsid (λ2, μ1 (mostly as cleavage fragments μ1N and μ1C), σ1, and σ3) and 4 proteins in inner capsid (λ1, λ3, μ2, and σ2)
    Subviral particles (ISVPs and cores) can be generated from fully intact particles (virions) by controlled proteolysis.
    Cell-attachment protein σ1 can extend from the virion and ISVP surface as a long fiber.
    Protein λ2 forms pentamers that protrude from the core surface.

Replication
    Fully cytoplasmic
    Sialic acid can serve as cell surface receptor for recognition by cell-attachment protein σ1.
    Proteolytic processing of outer capsid proteins σ3 and μ1/μ1C is essential to infection and can occur either extracellularly or in endo/lysosomes.
    Uncoating of parent particles is incomplete: genomic dsRNA does not exit particles to enter the cytoplasm.
    Transcription and capping of viral mRNAs occur within particles and are mediated by particle-associated enzymes.
    Segment assortment and packaging involves mRNAs.
    Minus-strand synthesis occurs within assembling particles.
    Mature virions are inefficiently released from infected cells by lysis.

Reproduced with permission from Nibert *et al* (1996).

---

hood illnesses associated with reovirus type 2 infection suggested an increased incidence in summer months (June–September).

Host Range and Viral Propagation

Evidence of infection as documented by virus isolation or the presence of antireovirus antibodies, has been found in an enormous variety of animal species including humans, a wide variety of nonhuman primates, swine, horses, cattle, sheep, goats, dogs, cats, rabbits, rats, mice, guinea pigs, voles, bats, a large number of marsupials and several avian species. The clinical syndrome produced by natural reovirus infection in animals includes predominantly respiratory, enteric and neurological disease. Among the more commonly described diseases are conjunctivitis, rhinitis, other upper respiratory tract infections, and pneumonia in horses, cattle, sheep and pigs. Dogs and cats can develop neurological illnesses including encephalitis and 'ataxia' in addition to respiratory and enteric illness. In birds, infection may produce arthritis, enteritis and hepatitis.

Reoviruses can be propagated in a variety of cultured cells. Cytopathic effects (CPE) can be seen in a wide variety of cell types derived from different animal species and tissues including mouse strain L clone 929 cells ('L cells' 'L929 cells', ATCC CCL1), human HeLa cells (ATCC CCL2), African green monkey kidney cells (CV-1, ATCC CCL70), and human embryonal kidney cells (HEK). Growth of virus for preparation of viral stocks, purification of virions, and quantification of viral titer by plaque assay is most commonly performed in L929 cells.

Genetics

The genome of reoviruses consists of equimolar quantities of ten discrete segments of dsRNA which can be divided into three size classes: large (dsRNA

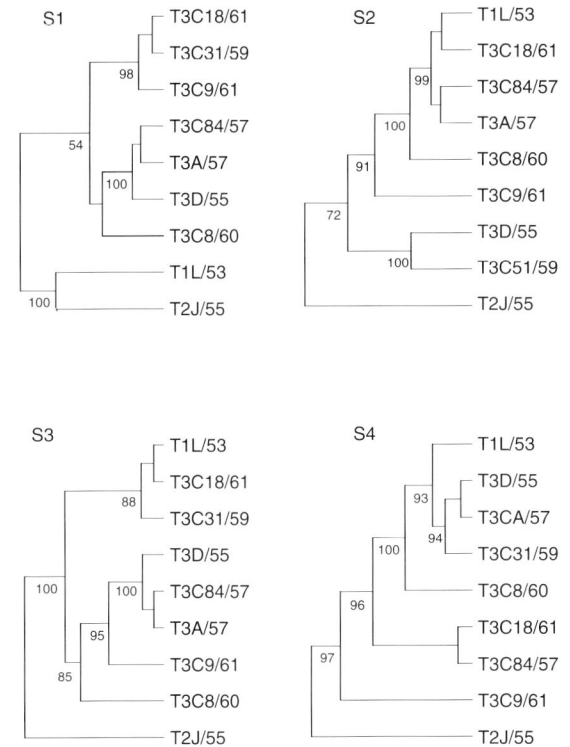

Figure 1 Phylogenetic trees indicating the potential evolutionary relationship and degree of diversity or relatedness between reovirus strains based on the nucleotide sequences of the reovirus S1, S2, S3, and S4 dsRNA segments. Each tree is rooted at the midpoint of its longest branch. (Reproduced with permission from Virgin et al (1997).)

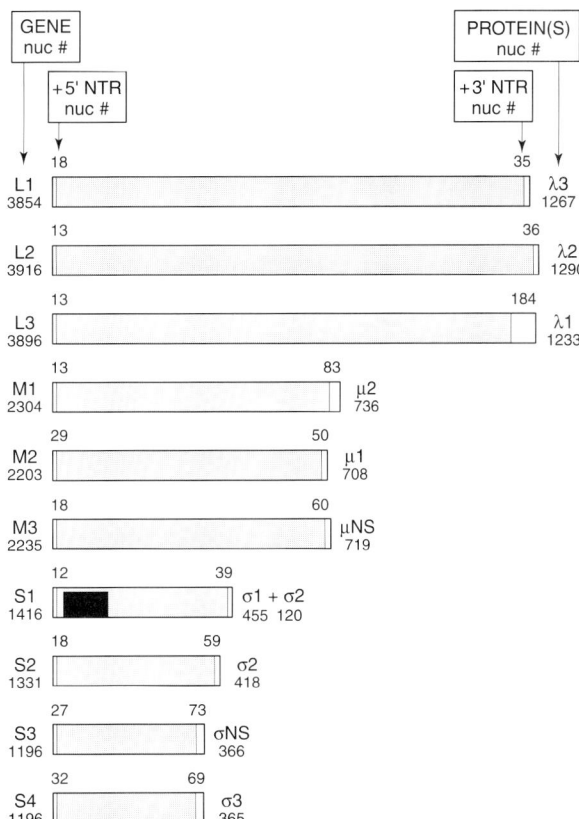

Figure 2 Coding strategies of the ten reovirus gene segments. The names of the individual reovirus dsRNA segments are shown on the left, along with their length in nucleotides. The name and size of the protein(s) encoded by each dsRNA segment are shown on the right. The lengths of the nontranslated regions (in nucleotides) are also indicated. Note that each dsRNA segment encodes a single protein with the exception of the S1 dsRNA segment. The S1 dsRNA segment encodes two proteins from different but overlapping open reading frames. (Reproduced with permission from Nibert et al (1996).)

segments L1, L2, L3), medium (M1, M2, M3) and small (S1, S2, S3, S4). dsRNA segments belonging to the three size classes can be distinguished on the basis of their different mobility patterns when subjected to polyacrylamide gel electrophoresis (PAGE). The cognate dsRNA segments of different reovirus strains often have different mobility patterns. Differences in the PAGE mobility pattern of gene segments derived from reoviruses belonging to different strains or serotypes has facilitated identification of the derivation of individual genes in reassortant viruses derived from co-infection of cells or animals with two distinct reoviruses (see below).

Nucleotide and derived amino acid sequence information is available for each of the ten dsRNA segments from at least one strain of reovirus (**Fig. 2**). The nucleotide sequence of the genome of the prototype strain T3D is 23.55 kilobase-pairs (kbp) in length. Individual dsRNA segments range in size from 1196 bp (S4) to 3916 bp (L2). The 5′-nontranslated regions (NTR) are extremely short, the largest being only 32 nucleotides. The longest 5′-NTR, that of the L3 segment, is 184 nucleotides. All other dsRNA segments have 5′-NTR of ≤83 nucleotides. The gene segments encode protein ranging in size from 365 amino acids (S4) to 1290 amino acids (L2). dsRNA segments are typically transcribed into a full-length mRNA from a single open reading frame (ORF). Each mRNA is translated into a single protein species. An exception to this scenario involves the S1 dsRNA segment which encodes two proteins ($\sigma 1$, $\sigma 1s$) from separate initiator sites in different, but overlapping, reading frames. Further details on the properties of the reovirus genome and reovirus replication are contained in the following entry on Reoviruses: Molecular Biology.

A number of mutants of reovirus have been identified or created in the laboratory. Temperature-sensitive (ts) mutants, defined by their reduced capacity to replicate at nonpermissive (39°C) compared to permissive (31°C) temperatures, have been created by chemical mutagenesis with nitrous acid, nitrosoguanidine, or proflavin. These ts mutants have been classified into ten ts groups (tsA–tsJ) representing mutations involving each of the ten reovirus dsRNA segments. Several intra- and extragenic suppressor mutants resulting in reversion of the ts− to the ts+ phenotype have also been identified. Additional reovirus mutants have been generated and selected based on their resistance to inactivation by physicochemical agents such as ethanol, or by their resistance to neutralization by monoclonal antibodies specific for the σ1 protein. Reovirus mutants, including deletion mutants, can also be identified in high passage viral stocks. These deletion mutants typically contain deletions involving the L1, L2, L3 and M1 dsRNA segments. Mutant viruses have also been selected based on their capacity to generate persistent infections (PI viruses), by selecting revertant viruses from hemagglutination-negative (HA−) T3 strains which have regained the capacity to bind to bovine erythrocytes or murine erythroleukemia (MEL) cells, and by serial passage through the brains of neonatal mice.

Evolution

Comparison between the complete nucleotide and derived amino acid sequences from the S1, S2, S3 and S4 dsRNA segments of a large number of reovirus strains has allowed the construction of phylogenetic trees indicating potential evolutionary relationships between various reovirus strains (**Fig. 2**). Of these four gene segments, the S1 dsRNA segment shows the most extreme diversity between viruses belonging to different serotypes. Within strains belonging to a particular serotype the degree of diversity in the S1 dsRNA segment is considerably less than the diversity between serotypes. It has been suggested that there were originally three 'progenitor' S1 genes representative of the current three viral serotypes, which have subsequently diverged to produce the differences seen between strains of virus belonging to the same serotype.

Comparison of the evolutionary relationships between reovirus strains differ strikingly depending on which dsRNA segment is used for analysis (**Fig. 2**). This provides strong evidence that reoviruses can and have reassorted their dsRNA segments in nature. Reovirus reassortants can be easily generated *in vitro* by co-infection of susceptible cells with two distinct strains of virus. Reassortant viruses can also be isolated from mice simultaneously co-infected with two different reovirus strains. These studies provide experimental support for the feasibility of reassortment.

In distinction to the evidence supporting reassortment of dsRNA segments between reovirus strains is the absence of evidence indicating that recombination occurs between either homologous or heterologous dsRNA segments.

Serologic Relationships and Variability

As discussed above, reoviruses are classified into three serotypes on the basis of reactivity with type-specific polyclonal or monoclonal antibodies in reactions including hemagglutination inhibition and plaque-reduction neutralization. Each serotype is represented by one or more prototype strains including reovirus serotype 1 Lang (T1L), serotype 2 Jones (T2J), and serotype 3 Dearing (T3D) and Abney (T3A). In addition to the prototype viruses, many additional strains have been isolated, characterized to varying degrees, and classified according to serotype. Variability between viruses belonging to different serotypes and/or strains has been analyzed based on variability in the nucleotide and derived amino acid sequence of their cognate dsRNA segments (see above).

Epidemiology

The majority of individuals have developed detectable serum antireovirus antibodies against all three reovirus serotypes by late childhood. Seroepidemiological studies suggest that less than 25% of children ≤1 year-old are seropositive for reovirus antibodies, but that by ≥3 years of age over 70% of individuals are seropositive. The majority of cases of reovirus infection in humans appear to be sporadic in nature, although outbreaks of infection caused by reovirus serotype 1 have been described. Age-related susceptibility to reovirus infection has also been observed in both natural and experimental infections in non-human animals. Calves, foals, piglets, and neonatal mice all appear more susceptible to reovirus infection than their adult counterparts. Experimental studies in mice indicate that the host's immune status is another important factor in determining the nature and outcome of reovirus infection. Immunocompetent adult mice develop an immune response but do not show clinical or pathological evidence of disease following reovirus infection. By contrast, after reovirus infection SCID (severe combined immunodeficient) mice develop prominent and often lethal hepatic disease. SCID mice, and mice with targeted disruptions of the transmembrane exon of IgM (i.e. antibody and B cell deficient mice), show altered

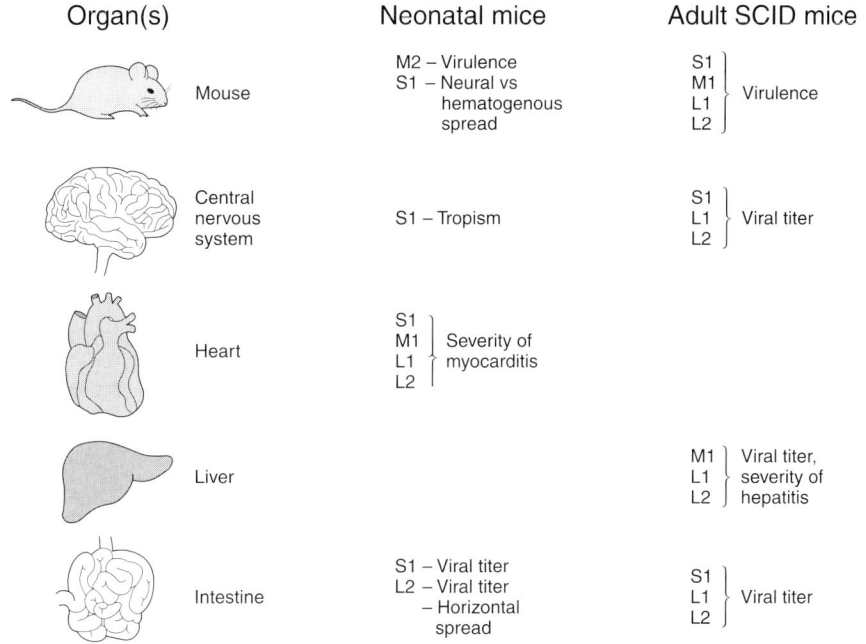

Figure 3 Reovirus dsRNA segments shown to have a role in determining organ-specific virulence in mice. (Reproduced with permission from Virgin et al (1997).)

patterns of viral clearance following peroral inoculation of reovirus.

Transmission and Tissue Tropism

Reoviruses are respiratory and enteric viruses whose transmission ('horizontal spread') under natural circumstances involves respiratory aerosols and secretions and fecal–oral transmission. Following oral inoculation in mice reovirus strains differ in their capacity to grow in intestinal tissue. There is an excellent correlation between the capacity of reoviruses to grow in the intestine, the amount of virus subsequently shed in the stool, and the efficiency with which an infected animal transmits disease to its uninfected litter mates. Genetic studies using reovirus reassortants derived from strains exhibiting high and low transmission efficiency indicate that the viral *L2* gene, which encodes the core spike protein $\lambda 2$, is the primary determinant of the efficiency of viral transmission following peroral inoculation. Both the *L2* and the *S1* genes influence growth and survival of reovirus in intestinal tissue (**Fig. 3**).

Transmission is also influenced by the capacity of the virus to survive in the environment after being shed from an infected host. Most reoviruses are generally stable at temperatures below room temperature, although at higher temperatures strain-specific differences in thermostability become apparent. One index of thermostability is the time required for a viral stock to lose 50% of its infectivity at 37°C. Reovirus T1L has $t_{1/2}$ of 19 h compared to 2.6 h for T3D. Reoviruses are also stable in aerosols, especially in the presence of high relative humidity. Studies of the genetic basis of physicochemical inactivation of reoviruses indicate that the viral outer capsid proteins are the major determinants of virion stability.

The basic steps in the pathogenesis of reovirus infection have been extensively studied in experimental animals including mice and rats. After peroral or intratracheal inoculation reoviruses adhere to the surface of epithelial M (microfold) cells. These cells overlie collections of lymphoid tissue in the small intestine and bronchi that form part of the systems of gut-associated lymphoid tissue (GALT) and bronchus-associated lymphoid tissue (BALT). In the intestinal lumen virions are partially digested by proteases into intermediate subviral particles (ISVPs). ISVPs lack the major outer capsid protein $\sigma 3$, contain a partially cleaved form of the major outer capsid protein $\mu 1C$, and contain the cell attachment protein $\sigma 1$ in an extended conformation. It appears that, at least in the intestine, ISVPs are the form of virus particles that bind to M cells. After binding to M cells ISVPs and/or virions are transported across these cells to the underlying intestinal lymphoid tissue. Studies of intestinal infection suggest that replication may occur in macrophages within mucosal lymphoid tissue.

Spread of virus from the site of primary infection to distant tissues and organs results in systemic disease. Reoviruses are capable of spreading in the host by means of the lymphatic system, through the bloodstream, or via axoplasmic transport within neurons. Reovirus strains differ both in their capacity to generate and sustain viremia and the efficiency with which they utilize neuronal transport. Following footpad or intramuscular infection in neonatal mice, reovirus T1L spreads to the central nervous system (CNS) primarily through the bloodstream, whereas T3D spreads predominantly through neural pathways. Studies of this pathway of spread using T1L × T3D derived reassortant viruses indicate that the viral S1 gene determines the pathway of spread used by reoviruses in the infected host (**Fig. 3**). Similarly, studies of the spread of reoviruses to extraintestinal organs following peroral inoculation into mice also indicate that the viral S1 gene is the major determinant of the extent of extraintestinal spread in this experimental model.

Depending on the viral strain, the route of inoculation and host factors such as the age and immune status of the host, reoviruses can produce injury in a variety of target tissues. Among the most extensively studied targets of viral infection in murine model systems are the CNS, the lung, the heart, the hepatobiliary system and the gastrointestinal tract. The specific pathology induced in these various organ systems is discussed extensively in the references included at the end of this chapter.

Reovirus strains often show striking differences in their pattern of organ and tissue tropism. These differences are particularly, but not exclusively, evident in reovirus infection of the CNS. For example, the prototype T3D strains infects neurons and retinal ganglion cells whereas the prototype T1L strain infects ependymal cells, and cells in the anterior lobe of the pituitary gland. Using T1L × T3D reassortant viruses it has been shown that differences in the tropism of reoviruses in the brain, the pituitary gland and the retina are all determined by the viral S1 gene. This gene encodes the virus cell attachment protein as well as a small nonstructural protein (σ1S). Studies with monoclonal antibody resistant σ1 variants of T3D, indicate that even single amino acid substitutions within this protein are sufficient to alter the neurovirulence, CNS growth and pattern of CNS tropism of reoviruses.

Tropism is obviously influenced by the nature and distribution of viral receptors on host cells. The nature of the reovirus receptor(s) on cells is only incompletely understood, and the nature of the reovirus receptor(s) on host cells remains controversial. Reoviruses appear to utilize different receptors on different types of cells. Sialic acid residues appear to be important for the binding of reoviruses to a variety of cultured cells and for their capacity to hemagglutinate erythrocytes. Studies with anti-idiotypic antibodies have suggested that reovirus binds to a surface receptor complex that contains components of M_r 65 kDa (p65) and 95 kDa (p95). It has been suggested that the p65 receptor component has structural similarity to the family of receptors that include the β-adrenergic receptor and that the p95 component either has or is associated with a tyrosine kinase activity. Interestingly, the state of tyrosine kinase activity in target cells has also been shown to influence the severity of reovirus-associated cytopathic effects in certain target cells. It is clear that if reoviruses bind to members of the β-adrenergic receptor family they do so without triggering any of the usual pharmacologic activities associated with β-adrenergic receptor binding (e.g. stimulation of adenylate cyclase activity). Reoviruses can also bind to the epidermal growth factor receptor (EGF-R), and the activity of this receptor may influence the efficiency of reovirus infection in certain cultured cells. Additional candidate reovirus receptor proteins that appear to be distinct from either sialic acid residues or the p65/p95 receptor complex have been identified on some cells.

Clinical Features and Infection

Reoviruses remain as much human orphan viruses as when they were first described (**Table 2**). Seroepidemiological studies indicate that human infection occurs during early childhood. The clinical correlates of this infection are difficult to determine accurately. It would appear that the overwhelming majority of human infections are either asymptomatic or produce mild symptoms of upper respiratory or intestinal infection or in some cases exanthema with fever. The predominant symptoms in children during an outbreak of T1 infection included rhinorrhea (81%), pharyngitis (56%) and diarrhea (19%), although the extent to which these were attributable exclusively to the reovirus infection itself is unclear. Over half the children shed reovirus in the stool for at least one week, and 21% shed virus for at least two weeks. The longest reported duration of stool shedding of virus was five weeks. Deliberate inoculations of adult human volunteers with reoviruses produces similar patterns of infection to those that appear to occur under natural circumstances. Reovirus seronegative volunteers nasally inoculated with T1L are typically

Table 2 Reovirus as a possible human pathogen

Probable associations
    Enteritis in infants and children
    Upper respiratory infections
Possible associations (unproven)
    Exanthema
    Neonatal biliary atresia
    Neonatal hepatitis
Isolated cases
    Meningoencephalitis
    Pneumonia
    Myocarditis
    Keratoconjunctivitis
Speculative or doubtful associations
    Chronic neuropsychiatric illnesses
    Adult cholestatic liver disease
    African Burkitt's lymphoma

From Tyler and Fields (1996), with permission.

asymptomatic. Approximately one-third of individuals develop symptomatic infection lasting 4–7 days and beginning 24–48 h after viral challenge. The predominant symptoms include fever, headache, coughing, sneezing, rhinorrhea and generalized malaise. Infection is associated with shedding of virus in the stool and seroconversion. Challenge with T2J has not been associated with clinical illness in volunteers, but is associated with seroconversion and shedding of virus in stools. Individuals challenged with T3D are also generally asymptomatic or develop mild rhinitis. Infected volunteers shed virus in the stools and show seroconversion. In general, individuals with pre-existing antireovirus antibody prior to challenge with reoviruses do not develop signs of clinical disease and do not shed significant amounts of virus in stool.

Reovirus infection of mice produces a disease whose clinical and pathological features resemble human extrahepatic biliary atresia (EHBA). Attempts to link reovirus infection to human EHBA have produced conflicting results. Some serologic studies show a higher frequency or higher titers of anti-reovirus antibodies in children with EHBA as compared to controls, whereas other studies do not. Reovirus has not been directly isolated from pathological specimens obtained at biopsy, surgery or autopsy from patients with EHBA nor has reovirus antigen been detected in liver or biliary tissues of EHBA patients by immunocytochemistry. However, reovirus nucleic acid corresponding to the L1 gene segment is detectable by polymerase chain reaction (PCR) with significantly greater frequency in liver and biliary tissues of patients with extrahepatic biliary atresia and choledochal cysts compared with liver and biliary tissues from patients with other liver diseases.

There are occasional reports of an association between reovirus infection and human diseases including meningitis, encephalitis, keratoconjunctivitis, and pneumonia. These cases are sufficiently rare and unusual as to suggest that if reovirus is involved in the production of these diseases it must be an exceedingly unusual event. It is important to recognize that currently available studies suggest that reoviruses are only responsible for a vanishingly small percentage of the total number of cases of these various illnesses.

Pathology and Histopathology

Pathological studies of material from humans infected with reovirus are exceedingly rare. Most of our current knowledge of the pathology of reovirus infection comes from studies of experimental infection in animals, notably mice. A detailed description of the pathology of reovirus infection in different organs is beyond the scope of this chapter, and interested readers should consult the references for further reading. As noted, in mice the brunt of reovirus infection and injury involves the CNS, the lungs, the heart, the liver and biliary tree, and the intestinal tract. The nature and severity of injury depends on the strain of virus, route of inoculation, and host factors include the age and immune status of the infected animals. The pattern of injury shows considerable variation. In some cases virus induces significant destruction of tissue with minimal or absent early inflammatory response. This pattern of infection can be seen in the CNS after intracerebral inoculation of T3D, and in the heart after intramuscular inoculation of reovirus 8B. Conversely, reovirus can also generate more prominent perivascular and parenchymal inflammation with less tissue injury. This pattern is often seen in skeletal muscle following intramuscular inoculation of T1L.

Recent studies indicate that reoviruses can produce apoptosis in infected L929 and MDCK cells in culture. Reovirus strains differ in this capacity with T1L strains producing less apoptosis than T3 strains. Studies using reassortant viruses derived from apoptotic-inducing (APO+) and non-inducing (APO−) strains (e.g T1L × T3D or T1L × T3A) indicate that the viral S1 gene is a major determinant of the capacity of these viruses to induce apoptosis. Recent studies indicate that apoptosis also occurs *in vivo* in the CNS following intracerebral inoculation with T3D. Virus-infected (antigen positive) and apoptotic cells (TUNEL positive) colocalize to the regions of the brain that show the brunt of neuropathological injury. At a cellular level, colocalization studies suggest that apoptotic cells may be either virus-infected or 'bystander' cells in proximity to virus-infected cells.

Immune Response

Following natural or experimental reovirus infection antibodies specific for a variety of reovirus structural and nonstructural proteins are produced. The bulk of both the immunoglobulin (Ig)A and IgG antibody response appears to be directed against viral structural proteins. There is no evidence that reovirus infection results in production of antibodies against nonprotein viral antigens (e.g. nucleic acid). The majority of the antibody response is not serotype specific, as would be expected by the high degree of homology between most reovirus proteins between viruses belonging to different serotypes. Serotype-specific immune responses are directed against the reovirus $\sigma 1$ protein, which is the least conserved of the reovirus proteins. Currently available monoclonal antibodies directed against the $\sigma 1$ protein (e.g. 9BG5, 5C6) are serotype-specific and show minimal if any crossreactivity between viruses belonging to different serotypes. Monoclonal antibodies directed against the reovirus outer capsid proteins $\sigma 3$ and $\mu 1$ are all crossreactive between reoviruses belonging to different serotypes, although in some cases they may show differing degrees of reactivity to viruses belonging to different serotypes or to individual viral strains within a serotype.

The nature of the reovirus-specific antibody response is influenced by the route of viral inoculation. Following peroral inoculation of reovirus T1L there is an increase in the number of reovirus-specific IgA-producing cells in intestinal Peyer's patches and in the spleen. Enteric infection is also associated with the induction of IgG antibody, predominantly of the IgG_{2a} and IgG_{2b} subclasses. Intradermal inoculation of reovirus does not result in significant IgA production, but instead induces predominantly reovirus-specific antibody belonging to the IgG_{2a} and IgG_{2b} subclasses. Variations in the dominant reovirus-specific IgG antibody subclass are influenced both by the route of virus inoculation and the strain of mouse: for example, IgG_1 antibodies are induced in some strains of mice following intradermal inoculation of virus.

T cell responses are induced during reovirus infection. Following peroral inoculation of reovirus, virus-specific major histocompatibility complex (MHC)-restricted cytotoxic T lymphocytes (CTLs) can be found in Peyer's patches and among the intraepithelial intestinal lymphocyte population. These cells are CD8+, bear the alpha/beta T cell receptor (TCR), and are capable of MHC-restricted lysis of reovirus-infected target cells. The number of these reovirus-specific intraepithelial CTLs increases dramatically after intestinal infection with reoviruses. Studies of Vβ TCR usage indicate that reovirus infection is associated with increases in CTLs bearing Vβ 7, 12, 14 and 17 TCRs, suggesting that reovirus infection is associated with oligoclonal expansion of specific TCR subpopulations.

Both serotype-specific and nonspecific CTL responses occur following reovirus infection. Serotype-specific CTL responses are directed against products of the S1 gene. As noted, this gene encodes the viral cell attachment protein $\sigma 1$ and a small nonstructural protein $\sigma 1S$. Nonserotype-specific CTL responses are presumably directed against epitopes on proteins other than $\sigma 1$ or on conserved epitopes within the $\sigma 1$ protein. The exact peptide epitopes recognized by MHC class I or class II restricted reovirus-specific T-cells have not yet been identified.

The role of antibody and T-cells in protection against reovirus infection has been investigated by passive transfer experiments, by selective depletion of B cells and T-cell subsets in mice, and in immunodeficient mice. Both antibody and reovirus-specific lymphocytes can protect mice against challenge with a variety of reovirus strains and from infection by a variety of different routes. Although direct comparisons are difficult, it appears that passively transferred reovirus-specific immune cells are more effective than antibody in controlling viral replication at primary sites, although systemic IgG antibody does permit viral clearance from mucosal surfaces. Conversely, antibody may be more effective than immune cells in controlling growth and spread of virus within certain tissues or organs including the CNS.

Studies with monoclonal antibodies indicate that passive protection can be conferred by antibodies specific for each of the reovirus outer capsid proteins ($\sigma 1$, $\mu 1C$, $\sigma 3$). *In vitro* studies suggest that protective antibodies may act at a variety of steps in the reovirus replication cycle including inhibition of viral binding to cell surface receptors, penetration of host cell plasma membranes, and inhibition of the intralysosomal proteolytic processing of virions to ISVPs. Similarly, *in vivo* protection can be associated with inhibition of viral replication at primary sites, spread of virus through nerves or the bloodstream to critical target tissues such as the CNS, and growth and spread of virus within these tissues.

Studies with passively transferred reovirus-specific T cells indicate that both CD4 and CD8 cells are required for optimal production and that depletion of either subset results in a significant loss of protective capacity of transferred cells. There is currently no evidence that intestinal intraepithelial γ/δ TCR+ T cells, as opposed to α/β TCR+ T cells, play a significant role in immunity to reovirus infection. As noted earlier, both SCID mice, and antibody and B cell-deficient mice show increased susceptibility to reovirus infection and diminished capacity to clear viral infection. Adult SCID mouse, unlike their congeneic immunocompetent counterparts, develop lethal hepatitis after peroral infection with reovirus T1L or T3 clone 9. Similar results have been found in immunocompetent neonatal mice depleted of CD4 and/or CD8 T cells. This suggests, that at least in certain organs, T cells play a critical role in controlling reovirus infection.

Studies of experimental reovirus-induced pulmonary infection in rats indicate that there are serotype-specific differences in the capacity of reoviruses to induce cytokine gene expression and cellular inflammatory responses. T3D is associated with significantly greater neutrophil influx into the lung than T1L. T3D-induced pulmonary neutrophilia correlates with the capacity of T3D to induce expression of tumor necrosis factor alpha (TNFα) and macrophage inhibitory protein 2 (MIP 2) mRNAs and proteins. Peroral and intradermal infection with reovirus T1L in mice is associated with the production of interferon gamma (IFN-γ), and low levels of interleukin 5, although the magnitude of these responses varies significantly among different strains of mice. Reovirus strains differ in their capacity to induce IFN-γ following infection of cultured cells, with T3D typically inducing higher levels than T1L. In mice, the level of IFN-γ induction also varies with the strain of mouse infected. Induction of IFN-γ is associated with enhanced MHC I expression.

Reovirus strains differ in their sensitivity to IFN-γ, and this effect may vary in different cell types. Reovirus T3D appears to be generally more sensitive to the effects of IFN-γ than T1L. Therefore the amounts of IFN-γ induced and the effects of this induction on reovirus replication, involve a complex interplay between the nature of the infecting viral strain, the species of animal, and the particular tissue involved. Given this complexity it is perhaps not surprising that the role of IFN-γ in the pathogenesis of reovirus infection *in vivo* remains to be established. In the case of reovirus-induced myocarditis, there is an excellent correlation between the myocarditic potential of reovirus strains and the level of viral RNA produced by these strains in infected cells. Since dsRNA is a potent inducer of IFN-γ, this raises the possibility that differences in the amount of IFN-γ induction could potentially play a role in determining the severity of reovirus-induced myocarditis.

Prevention and Control

Because reoviruses are not important human pathogens, investigations of the prevention and control of reovirus infection are limited. In experimental models of infection protection can be conferred by passive transfer of both reovirus specific antibodies and immune cells. Several reovirus vaccines have been developed for veterinary use and appear to be reasonably effective in inducing reovirus-specific antibody responses and in preventing symptomatic infection. Most veterinary vaccines against reovirus utilize either formalin or β-propiolactone-killed virus. Protease inhibitors, which can prevent the conversion of reovirus virions into ISVPs, can protect against reovirus infection after peroral inoculation. In this experimental model, ISVPs appear to be the critical form of virus responsible for initiating infection and blockage of the digestion of virions into ISVPs by intestinal proteases prevents infection. Reovirus infection *in vitro* can be inhibited by ribivarin, acivicin and cicloxolone; but none of these agents has been tested against reovirus infection *in vivo*. These agents have a variety of mechanisms of action. For example, ribivarin is a guanosine analogue, acivicin is a glutamine analogue and cicloxolone is a monesin-like Golgi apparatus inhibitor.

Future Perspectives

Future studies of reoviruses are likely to provide more detailed information at the atomic level of the structure of the reovirus particle and the mechanisms by which the various structural proteins interact. Many aspects of the reovirus replication cycle remain obscure, particularly as they relate to the methods by which equimolar quantities of the ten dsRNA segments are correctly packaged in the virion. Increased understanding of the viral replication cycle may facilitate the development of experimental systems that allow gene segments to be modified and re-inserted into virions. Many fundamental aspects of the interaction between reovirions and host cells remain to be delineated. This includes clarification of the nature of the reovirus receptor(s) on specific host cells, the nature of and mechanisms by which reovirus infection affects host cell signal transduction pathways, and the precise biochemical processes that lead to reovirus-induced inhibition of host cell macromolecular synthesis and ultimately cell death. A major theme of future reovirus research will certainly continue to be the effort to understand the molecular and genetic basis for specific steps in viral pathogenesis. Many areas of reovirus biology and pathogenesis remain to be explored. For example, the nature of the age-related susceptibility to reovirus infection remains unknown. Many aspects of the fundamental immunology of reovirus infection remain obscure, such as the exact nature of the specific peptide epitopes recognized by reovirus-specific antibodies and immune cells, and the role played by cytokines in host defense against reovirus infection. Finally, the role, if any, of reoviruses as agents of human disease remains as mysterious now as it was 40 years ago.

See also: **Immune response: Cell mediated immune response, General features; Orbiviruses and coltiviruses (*Reoviridae*): General features, Molecular biology; Phytoreoviruses (*Reoviridae*); Reoviruses (*Reoviridae*): Molecular biology; Rotaviruses (*Reoviridae*): General features, Molecular biology.**

Further Reading

Nibert ML, Schiff LA and Fields BN (1996) Reoviruses and their replication. In: Fields BN, Knipe DM, Howley PM et al (eds) *Fields Virology*, 3rd edn, p. 1557. Philadelphia: Lippincott–Raven.

Tyler KL and Fields BN (1996) Reoviruses. In: Fields BN, Knipe DM, Howley PM et al (eds) *Fields Virology*, 3rd edn, p. 1597. Philadelphia: Lippincott–Raven.

Tyler KL and Oldstone MBA (eds) (1998) *Reoviruses. Current Topics in Microbiology and Immunology*, vols 223 and 224. Heidelberg: Springer-Verlag.

Virgin HW IVth, Tyler KL and Dermody TS (1997) Reovirus. In: Nathanson N (ed.) *Viral Pathogenesis*, p. 669. Philadelphia: Lippincott–Raven.

Molecular Biology

WK Joklik, Duke University Medical Center, Durham, North Carolina, USA

Copyright © 1999 Academic Press

Introduction

Reoviruses (*R*espiratory *e*nter*o*) are members of the genus *Orthoreovirus* of the family *Reoviridae*, which also includes five other genera, namely, *Rotavirus* and *Orbivirus*, both of which are also viruses of vertebrates, *Cypovirus* of insects and *Phytovirus* and *Fijivirus*, both of which are plant viruses. The common characteristic features of all these genera are a basically similar particle morphology and size, and double-stranded RNA (dsRNA)-containing genomes that comprise 10, 11 or 12 genome segments.

Reoviruses are ubiquitous among mammals in which they usually do not cause overt disease. Mammalian reoviruses fall into three serologic subgroups or serotypes (ST1, ST2 and ST3), members of each of which are not neutralized by antisera against the other two.

Reoviruses have also been isolated from other vertebrates such as birds and reptiles, as well as from invertebrates, such as insects and molluscs. None of these viruses have been studied in biochemical or molecular terms except the avian reoviruses which fall into five serotypes. In contrast to mammalian reoviruses, they cause disease [the viral arthritis syndrome (VAS) and the stunted growth syndrome (transient digestive system disorder, TDSD)], as well as pericarditis/myocarditis, hepatitis and nephritis.

Most of our knowledge concerning the biochemistry and molecular biology/genetics of orthoreoviruses derives from studies of the mammalian reoviruses.

The Reovirus Particle

Reovirus particles consist of a core some 55 nm in diameter which is surrounded by an outer capsid shell that is about 12.5 nm thick (**Fig. 1**). Since the thickness of the core shell is about 7.5 nm, the central cavity accounts for about 12.5% of the reovirus particle volume, and the core for about 33%.

Both the outer capsid and the core shell are composed of capsomers which are arranged with icosahedral symmetry. The reovirus particle surface reveals 600 protrusions, presumably capsomers, arranged with $T = 13l$ symmetry in the form of shared hexamer rings around 120 holes. The core shell also possesses $T = 13l$ symmetry elements, but the arrangement of capsomers in them is difficult to discern (**Fig. 2**). However, cores possess 12 icosahedrally located columnar projections or spikes which are about 10 nm in diameter, possess central channels 5 nm in diameter, and project about halfway through the outer capsid shell in which they are visible as depressions or craters. The spikes, which can be removed from cores by incubating them at pH 11.4 at 4°C for 15 min, are pentamers of protein $\lambda 2$ and appear to be partially covered by 3 nm-thick 'lids' which appear to be trimers of protein $\sigma 1$ (see below).

The outer capsid shell is stable at high and physiological salt concentrations, but loses capsomers on storage at low ionic strength. It is readily digested by chymotrypsin to which the core shell is completely resistant. Virus particles and cores are readily separated by density gradient centrifugation; their sedimentation coefficients are about 630 and 470S, respectively, and their densities in cesium chloride density gradients are 1.36 and 1.43 g ml^{-1}, respectively.

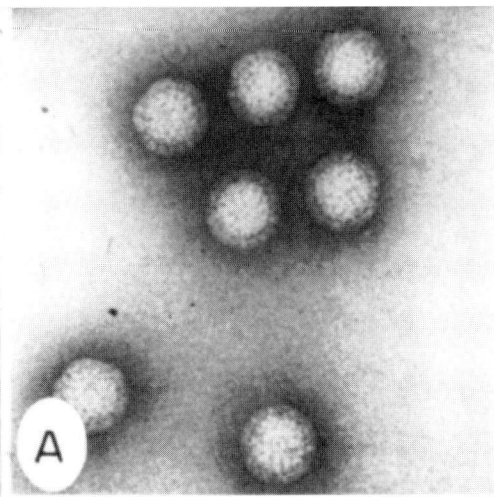
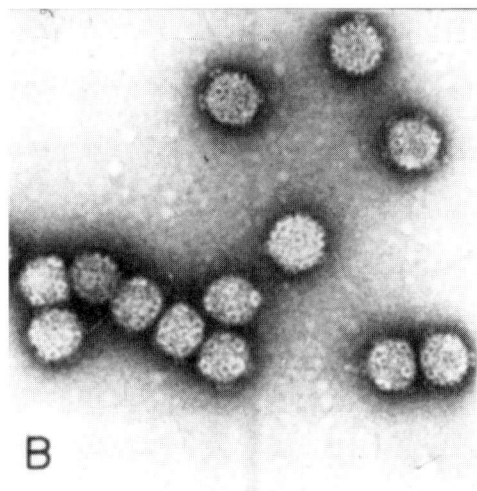

Figure 1 (A) Reovirus particles. Note double-capsid shell. The arrangement of capsomers is discernible at the periphery. (B) Reovirus cores. Note the large spikes, located as if situated at the 12 vertices of an icosahedron. Magnification for both ×120 000. (Courtesy of Dr R. B. Luftig.)

The reovirus genome

The reovirus genome consists of ten segments of dsRNA, all of which have been cloned and sequenced (Table 1). They fall into three size classes termed L, M and S, members of which are about 3900, 2250 and 1300 bp long, respectively. The total length of the reovirus genome is 23 549 bp; it is one of the largest and therefore most complex of RNA-containing genomes. Small-angle x-ray diffraction studies indicate that the RNA segments exist within the central cavity in tight well-ordered packing arrangement with adjacent helices aligned locally parallel to each other rather like the DNA in T even bacteriophages.

Each of the ten reovirus genome segments possesses a major open reading frame (ORF) which varies in length from 365 to 1289 codons. Most of them also contain short ORFs in other reading frames at least one of which, in S1, is translated in infected cells (see below). The 5′-untranslated regions are all short (12–32 nucleotides); those at the 3′-ends are longer, but still (with one exception, L3 (182 nucleotides)) less than 85 nucleotides long. The four 5′-terminal and five 3′-terminal base pairs of all ten genome segments are identical (5′-GCUA- and -UCAUC-3′ for the plus-strands).

Reovirus oligonucleotides

Reovirus particles also contain about 3200 oligonucleotides of which about 2400 are 5′-G-terminated and are the products of abortive reiterative transcription catalyzed by the reovirus transcriptase (see below), and about 800 are oligoadenylates from 2 to 20 residues long. The latter may represent either an untemplated polymerase activity of the reovirus transcriptase committed to transcribe but unable to move along its template, or slippage transcription of the three genome segments (L2, M3 and S3) the 3′

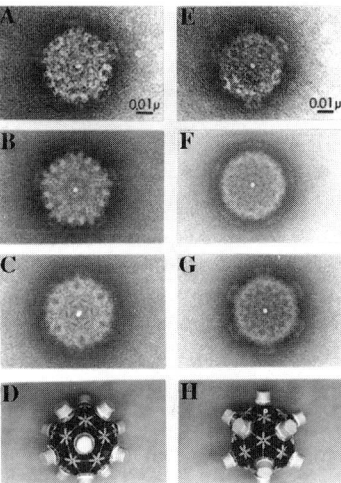

Figure 2 Two reovirus core particles the central axis of which passes through either a presumptive fivefold (A) or threefold (E) vertex. Enhancement of the five peripheral spikes of (A) was achieved by an $n = 5$ rotation (B), but not by an $n = 6$ rotation (C). (D) Model that depicts the spike orientations when the central axis is through a fivefold vertex. Enhancement of the six peripheral spikes (E) was exhibited with an $n = 6$ rotation (G), but not an $n = 5$ rotation (F). (H) Model with the central axis through a threefold vertex. The particles were stained with 2% uranyl acetate. (From Luftig RB, Kilham S, Hay AJ, Zweerink HJ and Joklik WK (1972) Virology 48: 170.)

Table 1 The reovirus serotype 3 genome segments and the proteins that they encode

Genome segment			Protein				
Segment	Length (bp)	Protein	Number of amino acids	Number of molecules/particle	Percent of viral protein	Location in particle	α-helix/β-sheet ratio
L1	3854	$\lambda 3$	1267	120	15	Core	0.9
L2	3916	$\lambda 2$	1289	60	8	Core	0.5
L3	3896	$\lambda 1$	1223	12	1.5	Core	0.9
M1	2304	$\mu 2$	687	12	1	Core	1.2
M2	2203	$\mu 1$	708	<60	1.5	OCS[a]	0.9
		$\mu 1C$	666	600	39	OCS	
		$\mu 1N$	42	?		OCS	
M3	2235	μNS	719	—	—	—	2.5
		μNSC	678	—	—	—	
S1	1416	$\sigma 1$	455	36	1.5	OCS	0.5
		$\sigma 1S$	120	—	—	—	
S2	1331	$\sigma 2$	418	120–180	10	Core	0.5
S3	1198	σNS	366	—	—	—	1.8
S4	1196	$\sigma 3$	365	600	22	OCS	0.9

[a] OCS, outer capsid shell.

ends of the minus-strands of which are CGAUUU- (see below).

Enzymes in reovirus cores

Since host cells do not contain enzymes capable of generating mRNA from dsRNA templates, reovirus particles contain the enzymes necessary for this purpose. Since reovirus mRNAs are capped at their 5′ ends, this involves possession of a transcriptase or RNA polymerase, an RNA triphosphatase to convert the 5′-terminal ppp groups generated by the transcriptase to the pp groups required by the guanylyltransferase, the guanylyltransferase itself and two methyltransferases to methylate the 7 position of the cap G and the 2′-O position of what was the 5′-terminal ribose of the uncapped RNA.

In core form the transcriptase is very stable and functions for long periods of time (more than 24 h) at elevated temperatures (up to 50°C), transcribing the genome segments many times.

The reovirus proteins

The various reovirus proteins are listed in **Table 1**. All reovirus proteins except μ1 have been isolated in native form from cells infected with recombinant vaccinia viruses with TK (thymidine kinase) genes containing reovirus genome segments inserted under the control of powerful promoters like the T7 polymerase promoter or the cowpox virus A-type inclusion body protein gene promoter.

The core shell components $\lambda 1$ and $\sigma 2$ The core shell consists of an inner layer of 120 or 180 molecules of protein $\sigma 2$ and an outer layer of 120 molecules of protein $\lambda 1$. The two proteins associate with each other *in vitro* and in cells infected with recombinant vaccinia viruses expressing them, core-like particles are formed. Protein $\lambda 1$ possesses a nucleotide-binding site –TKGKSSG– starting at residue 8; a zinc finger motif centered around residue 194 ($\lambda 1$ is a zinc-binding metalloprotein); and a weak dsRNA-binding site upstream of the zinc finger. It possesses two enzymic activities; it is a helicase and, as suggested by genome segment reassortant analysis, an RNA triphosphatase/ATPase. This enzyme activity may function in preparing transcripts for capping or to provide energy for the helicase-mediated unwinding of the dsRNA genome segments required for the transcription of their minus strands. Protein $\sigma 2$ also binds dsRNA weakly and possesses a region that bears a striking similarity to a region in the β subunit of *Escherichia coli* DNA-dependent RNA polymerase.

The spike component $\lambda 2$ Protein $\lambda 2$, in the form of pentamers, is the reovirus spike. It is also the reovirus guanylyltransferase, that is, it is the capping enzyme. Protein $\lambda 2$ exhibits strong epitopes that are exposed on the reovirus particle surface, are identical or very similar on all three (ST1, ST2 and ST3) $\lambda 2$ proteins, and elicit the formation of group-specific antibodies. It possesses strong affinity for proteins $\sigma 1$, $\lambda 1$ and $\lambda 3$. There is some evidence that is possesses SAM-utilizing methyltransferase activity, but such an activity has not yet been demonstrated for isolated protein λ2.

The minor core components λ3 and μ2 Reovirus cores contain about 12 copies of each of two proteins, λ3 and σ2, that possess no apparent structural functions, but play very important roles in two key enzymic activities. One is protein λ3 which possesses several amino acid sequences or motifs that are present, and similarly spaced, in all positive strand- and dsRNA-dependent RNA polymerases, such as DxxxxxD, GxxxTxxx(N/E)(S/T) and GDD; the genome segment that encodes it, namely L1, controls the pH optimum of the transcription of dsRNA genome segments into mRNAs by cores; and is a poly(C)-dependent poly(G) polymerase. It is very likely, therefore, that it is the catalytic component of the reovirus RNA polymerase/transcriptase, specificity being supplied by another component, most likely μ2. It should be pointed out, however, that these two proteins exhibit no affinity for each other *in vitro*. However, it is also true that the intracore concentrations of these two proteins are very high (of the order of 0.1 M), so that high affinity may not be required for them to be capable of interacting. The second enzymic activity is the nucleoside triphosphatase activity. As pointed out above, this activity has been linked to protein λ1; but genome segment reassortant analysis has also linked it to protein μ2. Either there are two such activities in cores, or protein λ1 is its catalytic subunit and protein μ2 provides specificity or some other required function.

The outer capsid shell The reovirus outer capsid shell consists of 600 μ1C–σ3 complexes, with the former -SS- bonded and internal to the latter. The cleavage of μ1, which is myristoylated at its N-terminus, to μ1C and μ1N, its 42 amino acid-long myristoylated N-terminal fragment, occurs when μ1 associates with σ3 well before the insertion of the resulting complexes into the outer capsid shell; most μ1 in cells is free, whereas most μ1C is associated with σ3. Interestingly, most μ1N remains associated with μ1C and is also present in virus particles, as is a small amount of μ1 (about one-twentieth of the amount of μ1C). The presence of myristoyl groups in the reovirus outer capsid shell raises interesting questions concerning their function in the assembly and structural stability of the outer capsid shell, as well as during the uptake and entry of reovirus particles into cells (in analogy with the presence of myristoyl groups on picornavirus and other viral proteins).

Protein μ1C accounts for almost 40% of the reovirus protein complement. Antibodies against it neither precipitate virus particles, nor neutralize infectivity. Not surprisingly, protein μ1C plays a major role in specifying how reovirus particles interact with their environment. On the one hand, it controls sensitivity to chemical reagents like ethanol and phenol; on the other, it controls some aspects of tissue tropism because susceptibility of μ1C to proteolytic cleavage controls activation of the transcription of mRNA as the first step of the reovirus replication cycle (see below). It therefore specifies the extent to which reovirus replicates in the intestine, which in turn determines the extent to which it spreads to the central nervous system; it thus controls neurovirulence. It also plays a role in inducing serotype-specific immunologic tolerance and delayed-type hypersensitivity responses. Finally, there is evidence that μ1 is cytotoxic, apparently damaging membranes; and that it is one of the two reovirus proteins, the other being σ1, that inhibits cellular DNA replication and induces apoptosis in infected cells.

The second major component of the reovirus outer capsid shell is protein σ3 which has a variety of functions. First, it possesses a Zn-binding site in a zinc finger that encompasses residues 45–72 inclusive. Interestingly, residues 45–53 inclusive are very similar to a region in picornavirus proteases. Since σ3 is strongly implicated in the cleavage of μ1 to μ1C (see above), it was at first thought that this sequence might be involved; but it turns out that μ1 is cleaved even when it complexes with σ3 variants that lack this sequence. Rather the association of σ3 with μ1, which does not proceed in the absence of the zinc finger, causes conformational changes in μ1 that cause the cleavage to be autocatalytic. Second, σ3 possesses a strong dsRNA-binding site centered around residue 265, a remarkable property for an outer capsid shell component. However, sigma 3 also binds to ssRNA transcripts in vivo very soon after they are formed (see below), which suggests that its affinity is not for dsRNA per se, but for regions of ssRNA with dsRNA character such as hairpins (stem-loops) or intermolecular complementary regions.

Protein σ1 Protein σ1 is a reovirus particle component that exists in the form of 12 trimers inserted into the spikes that are composed of pentamers of λ2 (see above). Normally σ1 appears to form a lid that covers the channel of these spikes, but mild heat causes σ1 to assume the form of 48 nm-long 4–6 nm-wide fibers topped by 9.5 nm-diameter globular heads that extend from the surface of the virus particles, the heads containing the cell attachment site. Most of the N-terminal one-third of σ1 is made up of a series of about 20 tandemly arranged heptads in which the first and fourth amino acids are hydrophobic. This type of sequence results in an alpha-helical coiled coil type structure in which the hydrophobic residues form the interfaces beween alpha-helices. It is these sequences that cause the trimerization of σ1 which in turn generates the signals for its association with insertion into the spike channels.

Although present in reovirus particles to the extent of 36 molecules (only 3 of which are essential, that is, virus particles that possess only one σ1 trimer are about one-half as infectious as virus particles that possess all twelve), protein σ1 plays an extremely important role in specifying the interactions between reovirus particles with host cells and intact hosts. Protein σ1 is the cell attachment protein (and the hemagglutinin); thus is specifies tissue tropism and is therefore the major factor in reovirus pathogenesis. It also elicits the formation of three forms of neutralizing antibodies that crossreact minimally, if at all; that is, σ1 is the reovirus type-specific antigen. Protein σ1 also induces delayed-type hypersensitivity, generates suppressor T cells and cytolytic T lymphocytes, and is recognized by cytotoxic T lymphocytes. Finally, genome segment reassortant analysis suggests that σ1 inhibits cellular DNA synthesis and induces apoptosis in infected cells, and it plays a crucial role in the maintenance of persistent infections.

The nonstructural reovirus proteins Reovirus encodes three nonstructural proteins that are not virus particle components. Two are encoded by genome segments M3 and S3 and are produced in large amounts. The former, muNS, is produced in two forms, one of which is translated from the entire M3 ORF, whereas the other, designated muNSC because it was at first thought to be a cleavage product of muNS, is translated in the same reading frame but starting at AUG at codon position 42. Protein muNS has a very high alpha-helix content and in its C-terminal region shares a periodic sequence similarity pattern with various myosins. It rapidly complexes with newly-transcribed mRNAs with which it remains associated until they are transcribed into minus-strands to form progeny genome segments (see below). It possesses affinity for elements of the cytoskeletal framework which may play an important role in morphogenesis.

Protein σNS is another ssRNA-binding protein. Like proteins muNS and σ3 it forms complexes with reovirus mRNA molecules very soon after they are transcribed. Proteins muNS and σNS possess affinity for each other as demonstrated by the fact that antibodies against either also precipitate the other.

The third nonstructural reovirus protein is the basic protein σ1S, encoded by the minor ORF in S1, which is formed in infected cells in small amounts. It

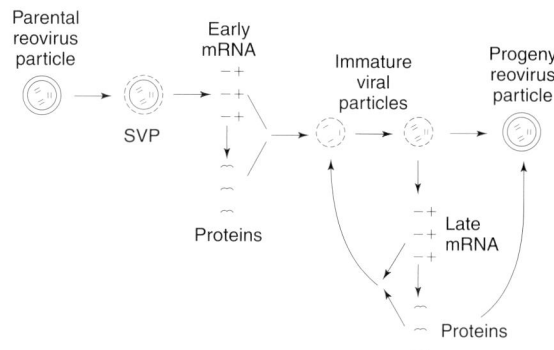

Figure 3 The reovirus multiplication cycle. SVP, subviral particle.

localizes to the cytoplasm and to nucleoli where it could interfere with both DNA and RNA synthesis and/or expression. Its actual function may only be discovered by examining the phenotypes of knock-out mutants.

Reovirus Replication

Strategy

Reovirus multiplication exhibits two unusual features, both consequences of the fact that the reovirus genome is dsRNA, which means that a virus associated polymerase is required to generate mRNA, and the fact that it is segmented. As a result, parental genomes are not uncoated to naked RNA, and a highly complex mechanism functions to assort the ten genome segments into complexes that contain one, and one only, of each (**Fig. 3**).

Reovirus particles adsorb to specific receptors (see below) and internalized in endoplasmic vesicles that fuse with lysosomes within which the reovirus capsid shell is extensively degraded: a 12 kD fragment is cleaved from the C-terminal portion of μ1C to generate the 60 kDa protein δ, and proteins σ3 and σ1 are lost. The resultant particles, which are cores covered by an outer shell that consists only of protein δ and which are known as viral particles (SVPs), are liberated into the cytoplasm. The major functional difference between reovirus particles and SVPs is that the former genome segments are not transcribed into mRNA, whereas in the latter they are transcribed. The mRNAs are then translated into the various reovirus proteins and, after a certain interval, generally at about 3 h after infection, they begin to be transcribed into minus-strands with which they remain associated, thereby generating the progeny dsRNA-containing genome segments; and at the same time equimolar amounts of them are assorted into complexes. These complexes, or particles, then transcribe the dsRNA molecules back into plus-strands, which are again either translated and/or used as templates for the generation of further ds genome segments. This cycle represents the multiplication phase of reovirus replication. As more dsRNA-containing complexes (dsRCCs) are generated and more reovirus proteins are formed, the protein complement of the dsRCCs is modified in stepwise fashion to generate first core-like particles and eventually complete, mature reovirus particles.

The nature of the reovirus receptor

There are several reovirus receptors that differ in their affinity for the cell-attachment sequences on the $\sigma 1$ proteins. Protein $\sigma 1$ itself possesses highest affinity for a 67 kDa glycoprotein and somewhat lower affinity for several other glycoproteins. The reovirus receptor on erythrocytes is glycophorin. The minimal essential receptor is the sialic acid residue at the ends of the carbohydrate prosthetic groups of glycoproteins. Presumably the remainder of the carbohydrate moiety and the protein modulate affinity and specificity.

All this evidence suggests a relatively nonstringent requirement for reovirus receptor recognition which is consistent with its very wide host range and its ability to bind to and infect a variety of cell types in the body.

The activation of the reovirus transcriptase

Reovirus particles do not transcribe mRNA; SVPs do so. This is not due to the fact that the transcriptase is inactive in virus particles; on the contrary, transcription initiation proceeds normally in virus particles, but transcription ceases before transcripts are more than four to six residues long and then reinitiates. The products of this abortive reiterative transcription are 5'-triphosphorylated – and also often capped – oligonucleotides, the sequence of most of which is $GCUA_n$ or $GCUAU_n$ where n is 1–4, and which remain associated, at least temporarily, with reovirus particles, in which they make up the bulk of the approximately 2400 5'-G-terminated oligonucleotides that they contain (see above).

SVPs, by contrast, are capable of transcribing full-length mRNA molecules, although for them also the majority (of the order of 90%) of transcripts are abortive transcripts. Clearly, what is activated is not the transcriptase, but rather the movement of template segments relative to the transcriptase catalytic site. Exactly what is involved in this release of movement is not known. Physicochemical evidence indicates that the conversion of reovirus particles to SVPs or cores triggers a conformational change in the dsRNA.

Transcription and translation of reovirus mRNA

Under optimal conditions of NTP and Mg^{2+} concentration, reovirus cores transcribe all ten genome segments at the same rate, that is, in amounts inversely proportional to their sizes. In infected cells, the relative proportions of the various species of mRNAs that are formed generally differ in two respects: there is usually a deficiency in the relative amounts of the l size class species, and during the early phase of the multiplication cycle, before progeny dsRNA genome segments have been formed, several species of mRNA ($l1$, $m3$, $s3$ and $s4$) appear to be formed in amounts larger than the rest. The basis of this effect, which is variable – often it is the $m2$, $s3$ and $s4$ species that are formed in relatively higher proportions, and often the effect is not limited to the early period – is not known.

Whereas these effects on the relative transcription frequencies are variable and quantitatively minor (that is, the excess transcription efficiencies are no more than two- to threefold), the relative translation efficiencies of the ten species of reovirus mRNAs differ enormously. The most efficiently translated mRNA species is usually species $s4$, followed by $m2$ (relative translation efficiency 0.67), $s2$ and $s3$ (slightly less than 0.5), $m3$, $l2$ and $l3$ (0.25–0.33), $s1$ (0.1) and $l1$ and $m1$ (0.01). These differences in relative translation efficiencies are due to differences in the sequences that surround and lie upstream of the initiation codons. Not only does the well-known Kozak rule apply, namely, positions -3 and $+4$ relative to the first nucleotide of the initiation codon must be G or A, but the nature of nucleotides at least as far upstream as position -8 also profoundly affects translation efficiency, depending on the nature of the nucleotides in positions -1 to -3. There is also an optimal length of the 5'-untranslated region (about 14 nucleotides), and there are also secondary structure constraints: the 5'-upstream sequence, including the initiation codon, must not be part of a stable stem-loop, and the 5'-cap must be accessible, that is, it also must not be part of or too close to, a stem-loop.

The fact that reovirus cores contain enzymes that catalyze the entire capping reaction indicates that capping is very important for reovirus mRNA translation. Some studies have suggested that late reovirus mRNAs are uncapped and that reovirus infection modifies the host cell translational machinery, so that late uncapped viral mRNAs are translated preferentially over capped cellular mRNAs, or that a factor in reovirus-infected cells stimulates translation of late uncapped reovirus mRNAs. Other studies have found that reovirus-infected cells can translate both uncapped and capped mRNAs, which confirms earlier studies that indicated that possession of a cap facilitates translation, but is not essential. It has also been suggested that the preferential translation of reovirus mRNAs in infected cells is mediated at the level of competition between mRNAs for a limited amount of a message-discriminatory factor. The resolution of all this conflicting evidence may lie in the finding that, like infection with many other viruses, infection with reovirus activates, via the generation of dsRNA or of short sequences in ssRNA with a locally dsRNA-like character, a cellular protein kinase that phosphorylates the α subunit of protein synthesis initiation factor eIF-2, thereby inactivating it and inhibiting protein synthesis, including the synthesis of reovirus proteins; and that protein $\sigma 3$, by virtue of its affinity for dsRNA (see above), prevents this activation. Thus protein $\sigma 3$ itself may be the factor that is essential for the efficient translation of late reovirus mRNAs.

The assortment of genome segments into reovirus genomes

The mechanism responsible for assorting the ten genome segments into genomes containing one of each is one of the most fascinating problems of reovirology; and very little is known about it. Since it is much easier to imagine how ssRNA molecules can be recognized by each other and by proteins than dsRNA molecules, it has always been assumed that assortment proceeds at the level of ssRNA. However, such ssRNA-containing complexes (ssRCCs) cannot be found. Rather it appears that the plus-strands associate with three viral proteins very soon after they are formed: the nonstructural protein μNS, the nonstructural protein σNS and $\sigma 3$. The resultant complexes contain one molecule of RNA and 15–30 molecules of these three proteins, depending on their length; most of them contain μNS, as well as σNS and/or $\sigma 3$. Presumably the binding is sufficiently reversible not to interfere with the RNAs being translated. The relative amounts of the various ssRNA species in the populations of these complexes reflect the relative frequencies with which they are transcribed (see above). Very significantly, however, even the first double-stranded RNA-containing complexes (dsRCCs) that can be detected (and which contain $\lambda 2$ as a major component as well as, presumably, $\lambda 3$) contain strictly equimolar amounts of all ten genome segments. This suggests that the generation of dsRNA genome segments and their assortment into genome sets are functionally linked and concomitant events; and it focuses attention on the RNA polymerase $\lambda 3$ as a key effector of assortment.

Infectious reovirus RNA

Since the only molecular links between parental and progeny virus particles are the plus-strands transcribed by SVPs, infectious reovirus should in theory be formed in cells into which the ten species of plus-stranded RNA are introduced. Conditions have indeed been found recently under which reovirus RNA is 'infectious' in this sense. The basic system consists of lipofecting into cells all ten species of ST3 ssRNA together with rabbit reticulocyte lysates in which all ten species of ST3 ssRNA have been translated for 60 min, and infecting these cells 4–8 h later with ST2 reovirus. When analyzed for their virus content 24 h later, ST3 virus is found to be present in these cells to the extent of 10^3 to 10^4 plaque-forming units (PFU)/10^6 cells. If ST3 dsRNA is also lipofected at the same time, the virus yields are 100 times higher; and most of the increased amount of virus can be shown to be the progeny of the ssRNA, not the dsRNA, the function of which is therefore to enhance the infectivity of the former.

This system is very important because it permits identification of the signals that are required for the introduction of heterologous, that is, novel, genetic information into the reovirus genome. Clearly there must be recognition signals on incoming, that is, to-be-accepted, genome segments because orbivirus or rotavirus genome segments, for example, are not accepted. What is very unexpected, however, is that there are also acceptance signals: thus the reovirus ST3 genome will not accept novel genome segments like, for example, ST2 genome segments, unless the S4 genome segment of the accepting ST3 genome is a variant of the normal wild-type S4 genome segment that contains two point mutations, one of which causes an amino acid change, whereas the other does not. The discovery of these acceptance signals permits the introduction of novel genetic information into the reovirus genome, permits identification of the nature of recognition signals, permits the construction of reovirus strains with desired properties such as, for example, highly efficient and nonpathogenic vaccine virus strains (this would be of great importance for orbiviruses and rotaviruses which, in contrast to reoviruses, include important human and domestic animal pathogens and to which this technology should be transferable), and opens the way for the development of the nonpathogenic reovirus as a highly efficient expression vector for clinical application in the fields of gene therapy, on the one hand, and cancer therapy, on the other.

Effect of reovirus infection on infected cells

There is no special mechanism for the release of reovirus progeny; reovirus particles are released when cytopathic effects have progressed sufficiently for cell necrosis to result in cell lysis. In cells infected with reovirus, masses of granular material develop in areas scattered throughout the cytoplasm which eventually move toward the nucleus and coalesce, forming characteristic inclusions or 'viral factories'. These inclusions are easily identified with fluorescein-labeled antibodies against reovirus proteins; they represent the areas where viral assembly proceeds, and quasicrystalline arrays of reovirus particles are often associated with them. Microtubules appear to extend throughout these viral factories and appear to be covered with viral protein; in particular, proteins σ1 and μNS possess affinity for elements of the cytoskeleton (CSK), which suggests that they may play a role in facilitating or mediating reovirus morphogenesis. However, microtubules *per se* are not essential, since colchicine does not inhibit reovirus multiplication or assembly. Like infection with all lytic viruses, reovirus infection causes progressive disruption of the CSK organization, but it is not known which reovirus protein(s) cause(s) this effect.

See also: **Pathogenesis: Animal viruses, Plant viruses; Reoviruses (*Reoviridae*): General features; Replication of viruses.**

Further Reading

Dryden KA, Wang G, Yeager M *et al* (1993) Early steps in reovirus infection are associated with changes in supramolecular structure and protein conformation: analysis of virions and subviral particles by cryoelectron microscopy and image reconstruction. *J. Cell Biol.* 122: 1023.

Joklik WK and Roner MR (1996) Molecular recognition in the assembly of the segmented reovirus genome. *Prog. Nucleic Acids Res. Mol. Biol.* 53: 249.

Nibert ML, Schiff LA and Fields BN (1996) Reoviruses and their replication. In: Fields BN, Knipe DM and Howley PM (eds) *Fields Virology*, 3rd edn. New York: Raven Press.

REPLICATION OF VIRUSES

V Gregory Chinchar, Department of Microbiology, University of Mississippi Medical Center, Jackson, Mississippi, USA

Copyright © 1999 Academic Press

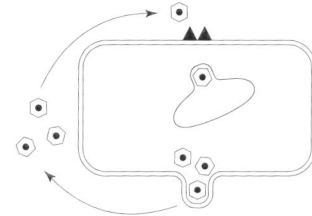

Introduction

Viruses are obligate intracellular parasites that replicate only within living animal, plant, or bacterial cells. Of the 71 taxonomically defined virus families, 24 contain members that infect vertebrates, and these families will be the focus of this overview. Among the smallest vertebrate viruses, the virion consists only of the viral genome and a closely associated protein coat (nucleocapsid), whereas larger viruses possess, in addition to the nucleocapsid, a variety of catalytic, regulatory and structural proteins, and in some cases a host-derived lipid membrane (envelope) containing one or more virus-encoded glycoproteins. In animal cells, virus replication is complete within several hours to at most a few days, and results in the synthesis of 10^3–10^5 virions per cell. Virus replication will be discussed in three stages: (1) early events (attachment to susceptible cells, penetration and uncoating), (2) viral biosynthetic events (replication of the viral genome, transcription and translation) and (3) virion assembly. However, because of space limitations, early events and mechanisms of virion assembly will be dealt with briefly so that viral biosynthetic strategies can be considered in greater detail.

Early Events

Attachment

Infection begins with the attachment of a virion, via capsid or envelope proteins, to specific cell-surface macromolecules (viral receptors). Because of the specificity of this interaction, the host range (tropism) of a given virus is determined primarily by the presence of viral receptor molecules on the cell surface. As a group, viruses utilize a variety of proteins, lipids and oligosaccharides as receptors. One class of receptors includes cellular macromolecules involved in ligand binding, endocytosis and cell recognition. For example, the receptors for poliovirus, human rhinovirus (ICAM-1), human immunodeficiency virus type 1 (CD4) and Epstein–Barr virus (CD21) are members of the immunoglobulin superfamily of proteins. In contrast, the receptor for Mahoney leukemia virus is an amino acid transporter and sialic acid-containing glycoproteins serve as receptors for paramyxo- and orthomyxoviruses.

Penetration and uncoating

Following attachment, the virion must enter the cell (penetration) and release its genome (uncoating). The process by which many viruses accomplish this dual task is termed receptor-mediated endocytosis and is the same mechanism used by the cell to import growth factors and other large molecules to which the plasma membrane is not permeable. Virions, bound to their cognate receptors, are transported laterally within the plasma membrane to clathrin-coated pits and enter the cell as the clathrin-coated pit invaginates. Subsequently, this vesicle fuses with an endosome and, within this acidic compartment, uncoating takes place. The acidic pH of the endosome is critical and agents that raise the intraendosomal pH (e.g. NH_4Cl, chloroquine, etc.) block virus uncoating. For enveloped viruses, uncoating involves fusion of the viral envelope with the endosomal membrane followed by release of the nucleocapsid into the cytoplasm. In the case of influenza virus, it is thought that low pH changes the conformation of the hemagglutinin (HA) allowing the hydrophobic fusion peptide to interact with target cell membranes. In addition, among negative-stranded viruses, the acidic environment within the endosome promotes release of the matrix (M) protein from the nucleocapsid, a step necessary for subsequent transcription. Nonenveloped viruses also appear to utilize receptor-mediated endocytosis, although here uncoating does not involve membrane–membrane fusion. For example, following attachment of poliovirus to target cells, one of the capsid proteins (VP4) is released exposing hydrophobic residues buried inside the virion. Interaction of these residues with the endosomal membrane may provide a pore through which viral RNA is extruded into the cytoplasm. In the adenovirus system, low endosomal pH induces conformational changes in the capsid which rupture the endosomal membrane at virion–membrane contact points. After its release into the cytoplasm, adenovirus is transported via microtubules to nuclear pores where viral DNA enters the nucleus. In contrast to the above mechanism, several viruses (e.g. paramyxoviruses, herpesviruses and human immunodeficiency virus type 1 [HIV]) do not require an acidic environment for uncoating and enter cells by fusion at the plasma membrane.

Although the presence of viral receptors is a primary determinant for infectivity, not all cells carrying the appropriate receptor are susceptible to infection. In several 'restrictive' systems, the synthesis of infectious progeny is blocked at a postattachment step. For example, some mammalian cell lines bind influenza virus and support the synthesis of all viral macromolecules, yet do not generate infectious virions because they lack the protease required to cleave the hemagglutinin precursor (HA_0) and generate activated (i.e. fusion-competent) HA_1 and HA_2. Conversely, some cells that lack the appropriate viral receptor can nonetheless support a productive infection if the viral genome is introduced into the cell by transfection.

Synthesis of Virus-specific Macromolecules

The 24 families of vertebrate viruses, although differing in genomic make-up, virion morphology, and their repertoire of viral-encoded enzymes, can be ordered on the basis of replicative mechanisms. However, before examination of different replication strategies, several common themes need to be addressed.

Viral transcription and genome replication

Viral nucleic acid synthesis is catalyzed by both viral and host enzymes, the relative contribution of which is determined by the type of virus and the specific molecule. Viruses with RNA genomes, except for the retroviruses, synthesize mRNA and replicate their genomes using virus-encoded RNA-dependent RNA polymerases. In contrast, retroviruses synthesize a double-stranded complementary DNA (cDNA) copy of their single-stranded RNA genome using a virion-encoded RNA-dependent DNA polymerase (reverse transcriptase). In subsequent steps, the retroviral cDNA is integrated into the host chromosome and transcribed by host-encoded DNA-dependent RNA polymerase II (pol II) to yield viral messages and genomic RNA. DNA viruses, except for poxviruses, also use host-encoded pol II to transcribe their messages. Poxviruses, because they replicate in the cytoplasm and do not have access to pol II, assemble a novel transcriptase composed of multiple poxvirus-specific (and possibly one or more host-derived) subunits. Most DNA virus families (e.g. *Poxviridae*, *Iridoviridae*, *Herpesviridae*, *Adenoviridae*) synthesize a virus-encoded DNA-dependent, DNA polymerase. However, two families (i.e. *Parvoviridae* and *Papovaviridae*) utilize host DNA polymerase, and the *Hepadnaviridae* replicate viral DNA through an RNA intermediate using a virus-encoded reverse transcriptase.

Gene regulation

Viruses have evolved a variety of mechanisms to control gene expression and maximize efficiency. In some systems, viral gene expression is divided into temporal phases in which catalytic and regulatory proteins are synthesized early in infection, whereas the synthesis of structural proteins is limited to late times. Alternatively, the expression of viral genes may be controlled by differences in the transcription rate of specific genes (e.g. rhabdoviruses and paramyxoviruses), the translational efficiency of different viral messages (e.g. reovirus) or the replication of transcriptional templates (e.g. influenza virus). Moreover, it is likely that, even within a single virus family, multiple mechanisms regulate gene expression. At the molecular level, gene expression is controlled by both *cis*- and *trans*-acting signals. In some cases, the nucleotide sequence of viral messages and transcriptional templates may be the primary factor in determining how efficiently a given sequence is translated or transcribed. For example, the differential synthesis of the various coronavirus mRNAs is thought to be controlled by interaction between *trans*-acting coronavirus leader RNA and *cis*-acting sequences located at the beginning of each gene. Furthermore, transcription and genome replication among DNA viruses (and retroviruses) is regulated by the (often) combined action of *trans*-acting viral- and host-encoded factors with *cis*-acting viral nucleotide sequences. For example, herpesvirus immediate-early gene transcription requires, aside from pol II, both host- (OTF-1) and virus-encoded (α-TIF) transcription factors. Lastly, in several families (e.g. *Orthomyxoviridae*, *Poxviridae*, *Herpesviridae* and *Iridoviridae*), there are hints that viral gene expression is also regulated at post-transcriptional and translational levels.

Viral protein synthesis

Viral protein synthesis is completely dependent on the cell's translational machinery (i.e. ribosomes, tRNAs, initiation factors, etc.). Reflecting that dependence, viral mRNAs, despite some prominent exceptions (e.g. picornaviruses), are similar in overall structure to host messages, i.e. they are capped and methylated at their 5' terminus and polyadenylated at their 3' end. Viral mRNAs are monocistronic and are translated as are other eucaryotic transcripts. However, in some systems, viral proteins are synthesized as part of a larger precursor (polyprotein) which is cleaved to generate the final products. This mechanism overcomes the inability of eucaryotic ribosomes to translate polycistronic messages and allows one viral mRNA to code for several proteins. Viruses have also developed several ways to utilize the same nucleotide sequence to encode one or more proteins:

1. HIV-1 and influenza A virus use alternative splicing to generate additional transcripts encoding novel proteins;
2. measles virus and other paramyxoviruses generate a novel P-related protein (V) by RNA editing, a process in which one or more nontemplated nucleotides are added at a site within the 3' end of some P transcripts;
3. Sendai virus synthesizes five proteins from its P transcript by using alternative translational initiation codons;
4. retroviruses use frameshifting or read-through mechanisms to circumvent a stop codon lying between the capsid and polymerase coding regions of the gag-pol transcript.

Finally, following their translation, viral proteins, like their cellular counterparts, are post-translationally modified (e.g. glycosylated, phosphorylated, etc.) using cellular enzymes.

As infection progresses, viral protein synthesis often supplants cellular translation. In some cases, this simply reflects the increased abundance of viral messages, whereas in others viral messages appear to initiate translation at a higher rate than host messages. Alternatively, virus infection may actively inhibit host translation by (1) proteolytically inactivating or covalently modifying initiation factors required solely or preferentially by cellular messages, (2) selectively degrading host messages, or (3) altering the intracellular ionic environment to favor viral over host translation. Furthermore, because infection can lead to the phosphorylation and functional inactivation of eucaryotic initiation factor 2 (eIF-2), several virus families (*Poxviridae*, *Reoviridae*, *Orthomyxoviridae*, *Adenoviridae* and *Picornaviridae*) have evolved mechanisms to block eIF-2 phosphorylation. Virus infection also blocks host cell RNA and DNA synthesis. Although transcriptional shut-off may be the direct result of inactivating specific transcription factors, the inhibition of cellular DNA synthesis is likely due to the earlier inhibition of protein synthesis.

Cytoskeleton

In addition to providing the biochemical components required for replication, the cell also supplies the virus with an intracellular highway to facilitate infection and assembly. There is growing evidence that the transport of infecting virions to the nucleus and the transport of viral proteins into assembly sites takes place along the various fibers of the cellular cytoskeleton.

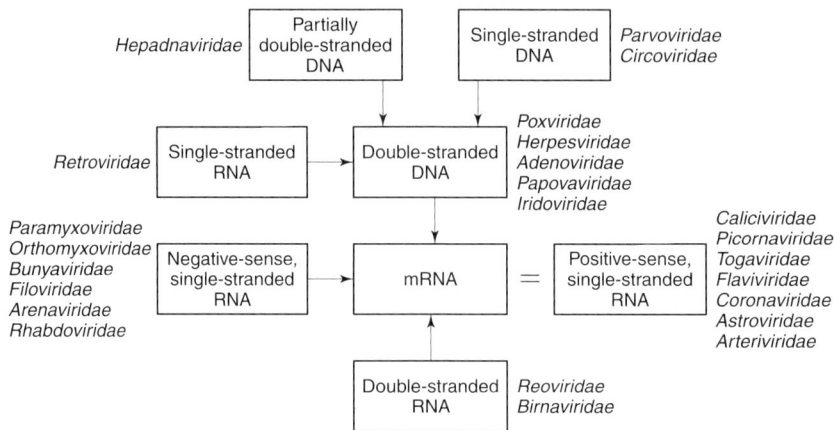

Figure 1 Strategies for the production of viral mRNA utilized by 24 families of viruses infecting humans and other animals. (Updated from Baltimore D (1971) *Bacteriol. Rev.* 35: 235.)

RNA Viruses

RNA-containing viruses are discussed in the light of four basic transcriptional strategies (**Fig. 1**). These strategies encompass viruses with message-sense (positive-strand viruses) and antisense genomes (negative-strand viruses), viruses that package their replicative form as genome (double-stranded RNA viruses) and viruses that utilize 'reverse transcription'. Although this approach is conceptually useful, not all viruses within a class conform precisely to the prototypic replication strategy. Despite this caveat, representative examples will be cited to illustrate the replication mechanism.

Positive-strand RNA viruses

Positive-strand viruses contain a single-stranded, message-sense RNA genome which is translated immediately after uncoating. To simplify this discussion, poliovirus (family *Picornaviridae*; genus *Enterovirus*) will be used as a prototype because it is the most extensively studied positive-strand virus and provides a clear view of this strategy (**Fig. 2**).

Following uncoating, the poliovirus genome is translated to yield an ~200 000 mol. wt polyprotein. Initial cleavage of the polyprotein occurs cotranslationally and is mediated by the autocatalytic activity of a virus-encoded protease, polypeptide 2A. Subsequent cleavages, catalyzed by viral protease 3C, yield structural (capsid) and catalytic (polymerase) proteins. As infection proceeds, translation of capped host mRNAs is blocked due to the virus-induced degradation of the large subunit (eIF-4G) of the mRNA cap recognition factor (eIF-4F). In contrast, viral messages, which are uncapped and possess a highly structured 5′-nontranslated region (5′-NTR), escape shut-off because the 40S ribosomal subunit binds to an internal sequence within the 5′-NTR. The ability of the 40S ribosomal subunit to bind internally, in contrast to the usual scenario in which the 40S ribosome binds at the 5′ end of the message and 'scans' until a start codon is encountered, is termed

POLIOVIRUS

Cellular receptor: A 45 kDa member of the immunoglobulin superfamily

Site of uncoating: Both the plasma membrane and endosomes have been implicated in uncoating

Translation:

1. Synthesis of viral polyprotein

2. Generation of structural (capsid) and catalytic (e.g. polymerase) proteins by proteolytic cleavage

Synthesis of antigenome

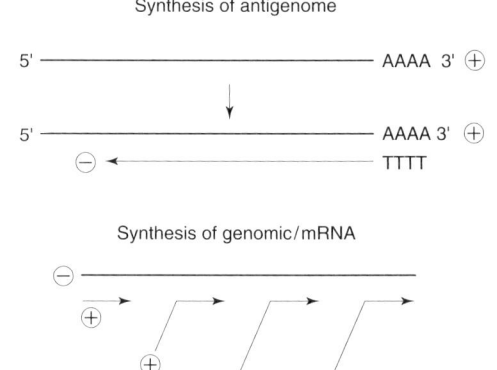

Fate of newly-synthesized genomic mRNA:

Early in infection: Additional rounds of translation and/or viral replication
Late in infection: Genomic RNA associates with viral capsid proteins and is packaged into virions

Figure 2 Replication strategy of a representative positive-stranded RNA virus.

'internal ribosome entry'. Thus cap-independent initiation and internal ribosome entry allow poliovirus messages to be selectively translated under conditions where translation of capped messages is progressively compromised.

Following its synthesis, the viral RNA-dependent RNA polymerase catalyzes the synthesis of a full-length negative-sense copy of the genome. Subsequently, the negative-strand serves as template and directs the synthesis of multiple plus-strands. Early in infection, when the concentration of viral structural proteins is low, newly synthesized positive-strands most likely are translated and serve to amplify the synthesis of viral proteins. Later when the concentration of virion precursors is high, newly synthesized plus-strands are encapsidated to generate infectious virus particles. A small virus-encoded protein (VPg) is covalently linked to the 5' end of all picornavirus RNAs except message. VPg is thought to play a role in RNA synthesis, but it is unclear whether VPg functions as a primer or in some other capacity.

Negative-strand RNA viruses

Because the genome of negative-sense RNA viruses cannot be translated, the first virus-specific biosynthetic event following uncoating is the synthesis of viral mRNA by a virion-associated RNA-dependent RNA polymerase using the viral genome as template. Negative-stranded viruses are divided into two classes: those with unsegmented (monopartite) genomes (i.e. the order *Mononegavirales* containing the families *Paramyxoviridae*, *Rhabdoviridae* and *Filoviridae*) and those with segmented (multipartite) genomes (i.e. the families *Orthomyxoviridae*, *Bunyaviridae* and *Arenaviridae*). Although each class uses the negative-strand strategy, they possess unique attributes and will be dealt with separately.

The replication of monopartite viruses is discussed using vesicular stomatitis virus (VSV), a rhabdovirus, as the prototype (**Fig. 3**). Immediately after uncoating, the VSV genome is transcribed to yield a short nontranslated 'leader' RNA followed, in decreasing molar amounts, by five capped, methylated and polyadenylated viral mRNAs. Transcription occurs within the nucleocapsid, a structure containing the viral genome and multiple copies of three virus-encoded proteins. Aside from the nucleocapsid (N) protein, which tightly encloses the genome and is present in ~2000 copies/nucleocapsid, two catalytic proteins are also present within the nucleocapsid. The polymerase, polypeptide L (mol. wt ~200 000), is present in about 50 copies per nucleocapsid and catalyzes transcriptional initiation and elongation, as well as capping, methylation and polyadenylation.

VESICULAR STOMATITIS VIRUS

Cellular receptor: phosphatidylserine

Site of uncoating: Virus enters via receptor-mediated endocytosis and uncoating occurs within acidic endosomes

Primary transcription: Synthesis of viral mRNA

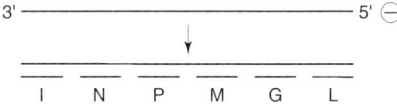

Secondary transcription: Synthesis of the viral antigenome

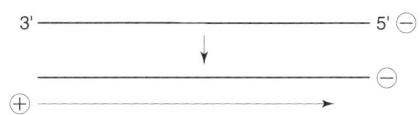

RNA replication: Synthesis of viral genomes

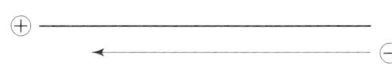

Fate of viral genomic RNA:

Early: Additional rounds of transcription and replication
Late: Virion assembly

Figure 3 Replication strategy of a representative negative-stranded RNA virus.

The phosphoprotein P, present in about 500 molecules per nucleocapsid, plays a variety of roles in RNA synthesis. It binds L to the nucleocapsid, maintains the solubility of free N and may function in chain elongation. The viral transcriptase binds genomic RNA at its 3' terminus and initiates transcription. At each intergenic junction (with the exception of the leader-N junction), a poly(A) tract is added to the newly synthesized mRNA by repetitive copying ('stuttering') of an oligo(U) sequence present at the end of the gene. After synthesis of the poly(A) tract, transcription terminates, releasing newly synthesized mRNA, but maintaining the transcriptase on its template. Re-initiation at the next gene downstream occurs via a conserved start sequence present at the beginning of each gene. However, because re-initiation does not take place every time, downstream genes (i.e. those coding for the envelope and polymerase proteins) are transcribed less frequently than upstream ones encoding the nucleocapsid, phosphoprotein and matrix proteins. Thus viral gene expression is controlled by transcriptional polarity.

Viral genome replication, i.e. the synthesis of a full-length positive-sense copy of the genome and the subsequent generation of progeny negative-strands, is catalyzed by the same polymerase that directs transcription. The switch between the transcriptive and replicative modes appears to be controlled by the concentration of the nucleocapsid protein. When N reaches a critical concentration, it binds newly synthesized RNA within the leader sequence and allows the polymerase to readthrough intergenic regions and synthesize full-size positive-strands (i.e. antigenomes) which will serve as templates for virion RNA synthesis.

Segmented viruses encode their genetic information in multiple molecules of negative-sense RNA. In the case of influenza A virus (*Orthomyxoviridae*), the genome is composed of eight unique segments of virion RNA. In contrast to most RNA virus families, orthomyxoviruses require a functional cell nucleus for replication. This requirement reflects the fact that the orthomyxovirus polymerase complex can neither initiate transcription *de novo* nor cap and methylate viral mRNAs. Instead, the complex 'pirates' the capped and methylated 5' terminus from a selected set of newly synthesized host messages and uses these to prime viral transcription. Once initiated, transcription continues until an oligo(U) tract, about 22 nucleotides from the end of virion RNA, signals addition of the 3' poly(A) tail by repetitive copying. Because of this, viral genomic and mRNAs are not completely complementary, but differ at both their 5' and 3' ends. As with unsegmented viruses, the trigger controlling the transition from transcription to replication may be the concentration of nucleocapsid protein.

Other negative-stranded viruses possess additional molecular surprises. Some bunyaviruses (tripartite genome) and all arenaviruses (bipartite genome) possess 'ambisense' genomic RNA, in which non-overlapping subgenomic messages are transcribed from the 3' ends of both virion RNA and its full-length complement. Furthermore, in what may be the prototype of a new family within the *Mononegavirales*, Borna disease virus replicates and transcribes its genome within the nucleus and utilizes RNA splicing to generate its messages.

Double-stranded RNA (dsRNA) viruses

Animal viruses with dsRNA genomes are segmented and can be viewed as a variant of the negative-sense strategy in which the virion encapsidates the replicative form of the genome. Genomic dsRNA is transcribed within partially uncoated ribonuclease-resistant viral cores by the virion-associated polymerase to yield viral mRNAs. Early in infection, some progeny plus-strands function as translational templates whereas others associate with nonstructural proteins and form complexes which are transcribed once to yield dsRNA. Newly synthesized dsRNA

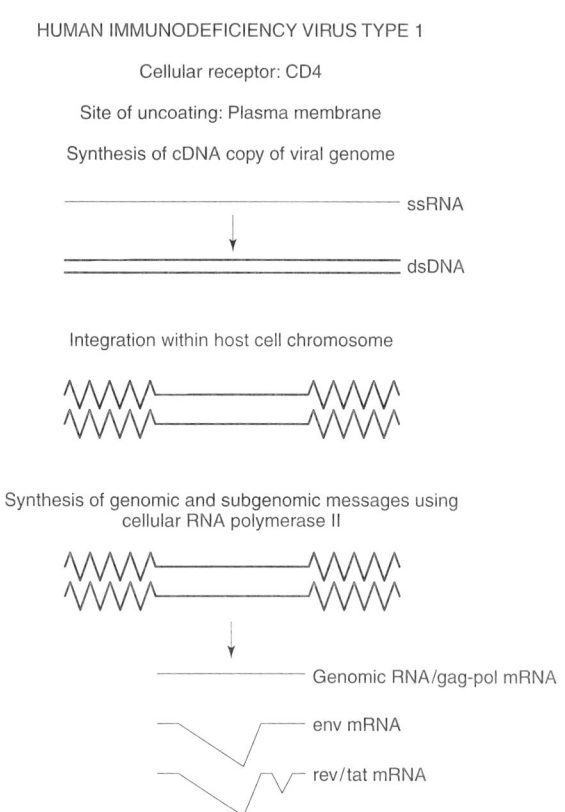

Figure 4 Replication strategy of a complex retrovirus.

serves as template for the synthesis of additional viral mRNA which amplifies the replication cycle. Later, as the concentration of core and capsid proteins increases, the dsRNA–protein complex exchanges nonstructural for structural proteins and forms mature virus particles.

RNA viruses that utilize a reverse transcription strategy

Retroviruses replicate their genome and transcribe mRNA using a dsDNA copy of viral genomic RNA as template (**Fig. 4**). This unconventional mechanism, in which single-stranded virion RNA is used as a template for dsDNA synthesis, is catalyzed by a virion-associated, RNA-dependent DNA polymerase (reverse transcriptase). After viral entry, the virion capsid is partially uncoated and a complementary DNA copy of the RNA genome is synthesized using reverse transcriptase. An endonucleolytic activity, integral to the reverse transcriptase, degrades the RNA template and second-strand DNA synthesis begins. Completion of second-strand synthesis results not only in a dsDNA copy of virion RNA, but also generates a unique structure termed the long terminal repeat (LTR). The LTR flanks the viral cDNA and is composed of unique sequences from the 5′ and 3′ ends of the genome and a repeat element common to both ends. Following cDNA synthesis retrovirus DNA is integrated into the host chromosome, and, in this form, is termed the 'provirus'. Subsequently, the provirus is transcribed by pol II to yield full-length progeny RNA and one or more subgenomic mRNAs. The upstream LTR plays a very important role in retrovirus gene expression because it contains enhancer elements which regulate pol II-catalyzed transcription. (The downstream LTR is not involved in viral gene expression, but may activate host oncogenes and play a role in cell transformation.)

Full-length genome-sized RNA can either be packaged within virions or serve as messenger for the capsid and catalytic viral proteins. Translation of retrovirus genomic RNA yields two classes of polyproteins. The majority (~95% of the total) encode the capsid, core and matrix proteins and result when translation terminates immediately after the coding region of the nucleocapsid gene. However, a minor population, encoding the aforementioned structural proteins as well as the protease, reverse transcriptase, and integrase results when the stop codon at the end of the capsid/core region is bypassed either by frameshifting or read-through. Envelope glycoproteins are translated from a singly-spliced subgenomic mRNA containing sequences primarily from the 3′ end of the genome, whereas lentiviruses, such as HIV-1, utilize doubly spliced subgenomic mRNAs to direct the synthesis of TAT, REV and several other regulatory proteins.

TAT and REV are the two best-studied of the HIV-1 regulatory proteins. TAT is a *trans*-acting protein that binds to a sequence present at the 5′ end of all HIV-1 mRNAs and enhances HIV-1 gene expression by relieving a block in transcriptional elongation or by increasing transcriptional initiation. REV mediates the switch between the synthesis of regulatory proteins (i.e. TAT and REV) and the generation of structural and catalytic proteins by binding to *cis*-acting sequences within viral mRNA and directing the transport into the cytoplasm of unspliced genomic RNA and singly-spliced envelope message.

DNA Viruses

With the exception of parvoviruses and hepadnaviruses, the genomes of which are respectively single-stranded and partially double-stranded, DNA-containing animal viruses possess a dsDNA genome. However, even in these two families, viral mRNA is ultimately transcribed from a dsDNA template using cellular DNA-dependent RNA polymerase (**Fig. 1**). In place of a detailed discussion of each family, broader issues of viral DNA replication will be discussed. To begin with, DNA viruses differ greatly in their genetic content ranging in size from 5 kbp (*Parvoviridae*) to greater than 120 kbp (*Herpesviridae*, *Poxviridae* and *Iridoviridae*). Thus the small DNA viruses are about as genetically complex as a typical RNA virus, whereas the larger DNA viruses encode 100 or more proteins. Not unexpectedly, the degree to which virus replication is dependent on cellular functions reflects the genetic complexity of the virus. Thus, parvoviruses and papovaviruses require extensive host involvement to support viral biosynthetic events (including DNA synthesis), whereas other families are progressively more independent.

Among herpes-, pox- and iridoviruses, viral genes are expressed in a coordinated temporal sequence of immediate early, early and late genes. Generally immediate early genes code for proteins required to initiate virus replication, early genes encode catalytic functions (e.g. the viral DNA polymerase), and late genes specify structural proteins. Furthermore, immediate early genes activate early and late gene transcription, whereas specific early and late genes downregulate immediate early and early gene expression respectively. Aside from specific regulatory proteins, full late gene expression also requires viral DNA synthesis, thus inhibitors of viral DNA replication block late gene expression despite the presence of functional immediate early and early activators.

Because DNA polymerase requires a primer with an available 3′-OH to initiate DNA synthesis, all viruses with a linear DNA genome have evolved specialized features that allow them to maintain intact termini during replication. For example, adenoviruses solve the 'end-problem' by using a nucleotide-linked terminal protein to initiate DNA replication, herpesviruses replicate through a rolling circle mechanism, and poxviruses and parvoviruses utilize a self-priming mechanism to ensure replication of their termini. In contrast to other DNA viruses, hepadnaviruses possess a circular, partially single-stranded DNA genome that is replicated through an RNA intermediate using virus-encoded reverse transcriptase. Upon entry into the cell the gaps are repaired and dsDNA is transcribed in the nucleus by host polymerase to yield viral mRNAs and pregenomic RNA. The latter is encapsidated and transcribed into complementary DNA using virus-encoded protein P both as the primer and the reverse transcriptase. As with retroviruses, the RNA template is degraded and second-strand DNA synthesis takes place. However, before its completion, the virion is exported from the cell leaving genomic DNA partially single-stranded.

Unlike other DNA viruses, poxviruses replicate solely within the cytoplasm in morphologically distinct viral 'factories'. Reflecting their metabolic independence from the host cell, poxviruses synthesize unique DNA and RNA polymerases, and their virions contain all the proteins needed to transcribe the earliest class of viral mRNAs. Furthermore, viral transcriptional promoters and termination sequences are unique and are regulated by virus-specific factors.

Iridoviruses, occupying a taxonomic middleground between poxviruses and the nuclear DNA viruses, possess several distinctive features. Viral DNA replication takes place in two distinct compartments (genome-length progeny DNA is synthesized in the nucleus, followed by the synthesis of concatemeric DNA in the cytoplasm), whereas virion assembly is confined to cytoplasmic viral 'assembly sites'. Viral DNA is highly methylated with nearly 25% of cytosine residues present as methylcytosine. Methylation is catalyzed by a virus-encoded enzyme and, as in some bacteriophage systems, appears to function as part of a restriction–modification system. Surprisingly, despite the high content of methylcytosine, host RNA polymerase II has been implicated in at least the early rounds of viral transcription. However, it is not known whether unmodified pol II transcribes viral DNA late in infection or whether viral-encoded proteins modify pol II and alter its specificity.

Virus Assembly

Once sufficient stores of viral nucleic acid and protein have accumulated in the infected cell, nucleocapsid formation and virion assembly begin and continue as long as the cells are metabolically competent. Despite the large number of vertebrate virus families, only three types of nucleocapsids are found: complex, helical and icosahedral (spherical). The nucleocapsids of poxviruses do not conform to the geometric symmetry found among the helical and icosahedral viruses and are considered to be 'complex'. Little is known about the molecular mechanisms controlling their assembly. Helical nucleocapsids (which, among vertebrate viruses, enclose only RNA genomes) form as viral proteins bind to nascent RNA transcripts and encapsidate them. During virus assembly, helical nucleocapsids migrate to cellular membranes where viral glycoproteins have concentrated. There, through concerted interaction between the nucleocapsid and viral glycoproteins, the nucleocapsid is enveloped by the cellular membrane in a process termed 'budding'. Host proteins are excluded from the membrane and the resulting envelope contains only virus-encoded glycoproteins. Moreover, because envelopment is not a precise process, dual infections with different strains of the same multipartite virus (e.g. influenza virus A) lead to high-frequency genetic reassortment. Although virion envelopment takes place commonly at the plasma membrane (e.g. among the *Paramyxoviridae*, *Orthomyxoviridae* and *Rhabdoviridae*), intracellular membranes (e.g. those of the Golgi, endoplasmic reticulum and, in the case of DNA viruses, the nucleus) are used by other virus families. In contrast to viruses with helical nucleocapsids, icosahedral nucleocapsids enclose both DNA and RNA genomes. It is thought that nucleocapsids form spontaneously when the concentration of capsid proteins reaches a critical level. In some families, nucleocapsids are not enveloped (i.e. virion equals nucleocapsid), whereas in others nucleocapsids are enveloped as described above. Enveloped icosahedral viruses are released from infected cells by budding, whereas non-enveloped icosahedral virions are liberated by cell lysis.

See also: **Cell structure and function in virus infections; Virus–host cell interactions.**

Further Reading

Cann AJ (1997) *Principles of Molecular Virology*, 2nd edn. San Diego: Academic Press.

Ehrenfeld E (1993) Translational regulation in virus-infected cells. *Semin. Virol.* 4: 199.

Fields BN, Knipe DM, Howley PM *et al* (eds) (1996) *Fields Virology*, 3rd edn. New York: Lippincott–Raven.

Joklik WK, Willet HP, Amos DB *et al.* (eds) (1992) *Zinsser Microbiology*, 20th edn. Norwalk, CT: Appleton and Lange.

Levy JA, Fraenkel-Conrat H and Owens RA (1994) *Virology*, 3rd edn. Englewood Cliffs, NJ: Prentice-Hall.

Wimmer E (1994). *Cellular Receptors for Animal Viruses*. Cold Spring Harbor, NY: Cold Spring Harbor Laboratory Press.

RESPIRATORY SYNCYTIAL VIRUS – HUMAN (*PARAMYXOVIRIDAE*)

Peter L Collins, Laboratory of Infectious Disease, National Institute of Allergy and Infectious Disease, National Institutes of Health, Bethesda, Maryland, USA

Copyright © 1999 Academic Press

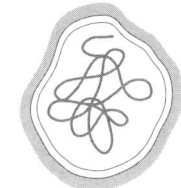

History

Human respiratory syncytial virus (RSV) was isolated in 1956 from a laboratory chimpanzee with upper respiratory tract disease. Shortly thereafter, an apparently identical virus was recovered from children ill with pneumonia or croup and was identified as a virus of humans. RSV is now recognized as the leading viral agent of pediatric respiratory tract disease worldwide. It also is gaining recognition as a significant cause of disease in the elderly and in immunocompromised individuals. Its poor growth *in vitro* and instability have impeded research. RSV lacks an approved vaccine or highly effective antiviral therapy.

Taxonomy and Classification

RSV is a member of the Order *Mononegavirales*, the nonsegmented negative-strand RNA viruses (**Table 1**). These are enveloped viruses that have as genome a single strand of protein-coated negative-sense RNA. Vesicular stomatitis and Sendai viruses are the most extensively characterized members of the group.

RSV is the type species for genus *Pneumovirus* in the subfamily *Pneumovirinae* of the family *Paramyxoviridae*. There also are bovine (BRSV), caprine (CRSV) and ovine (ORSV) versions which are related to human RSV. BRSV is one of several respiratory tract pathogens associated with shipping fever, an important disease of cattle. Pneumonia virus of mice (PVM) is a somewhat more distant relative. There is a turkey pneumovirus, formerly called turkey rhinotracheitis virus (TRTV) but now called avian pneumovirus (APV), which is sufficiently distinct (see below) so that it has been placed in a second genus, *Metapneumovirus*.

Virion Structure and Viral Proteins

RSV virions include spherical particles of 80–350 nm in diameter (**Fig. 1**) and filamentous particles of 60–100 nm in diameter and up to 10 μm in length. The nonuniform nature of the particles and the presence of large amounts of cell debris lends uncertainty as to the exact size and shape of the infectious particle. The virion contains a helical nucleocapsid (diameter 12–15 nm, compared to 18 nm for other paramyxoviruses) packaged in a lipoprotein envelope acquired from the host cell plasma membrane during budding. The genome and antigenome (positive-sense replicative intermediate) are found only in nucleocapsid form. The virion surface has spike-like glycoprotein projections of 11–20 nm spaced at intervals of 6–10 nm. RSV lacks a hemagglutinin and a neuraminidase; the former is present in all members of *Paramyxovirinae* and the latter in all but the morbilliviruses. But PVM has a hemagglutinin, and thus its absence is not a characteristic of the pneumoviruses.

RSV encodes 11 proteins (**Fig. 1, Table 2**). Four are nucleocapsid proteins, N, P, L and M2-1. The N protein binds tightly along the entire length of genomic RNA. L is the major polymerase subunit. P is thought to associate with free N and L to maintain them in soluble form and might also participate as a cofactor in RNA synthesis. N, P and L are necessary and sufficient to direct RNA replication (synthesis of antigenome and genome), whereas transcription involves in addition an elongation factor, the M2-1 protein. Although the polypeptide components of the viral polymerase are packaged in the virion, as is characteristic of the Order, virion-associated polymerase activity has not been directly demonstrated.

There are three transmembrane virion proteins, F, G and SH, which assemble separately into homooligomers that make up the membrane spikes; F and G assemble into either trimers or tetramers, and SH might be a pentamer. The F glycoprotein mediates membrane fusion, which is responsible for viral penetration and syncytium formation. It has a cleaved N-terminal signal sequence and a membrane anchor near the C-terminus. F is synthesized as a precursor, F_0, which is cleaved intracellularly by a furin-type cellular protease into the two subunits which remain disulfide-linked and constitute the biologically active form: NH_2-F_2-S-S-F_1-COOH.

The G glycoprotein mediates viral attachment. It is anchored in the membrane by a signal/anchor sequence near the N-terminus such that the large C-terminal domain is extracellular. G contains several N-linked carbohydrate side chains and approximately 24 or 25 O-linked chains (the ectodomain contains

Table 1 Order *Mononegavirales*, the nonsegmented negative-strand RNA viruses

Family	Subfamily	Genus	Example(s)
Rhabdoviridae		Vesiculovirus[a]	Vesicular stomatitis virus
Filoviridae		'Marburg-like viruses'	Marburg virus
		'Ebola-like viruses'	Ebola virus
Paramyxoviridae	Paramyxovirinae	Respirovirus	Parainfluenza virus types 1 and 3, including Sendai virus
		Rubulavirus	Mumps virus and parainfluenza virus types 2 and 4 including simian virus type 5
		Morbillivirus	Measles virus
	Pneumovirinae	Pneumovirus	RSV, animal RSVs, and pneumonia virus of mice (PVM)
		Metapneumovirus	Avian pneumovirus (APV) (formerly turkey rhinotracheitis virus)
Bornaviridae		Bornavirus	Borna disease virus

[a] Four other genera of rhabdoviruses exist which are not shown.

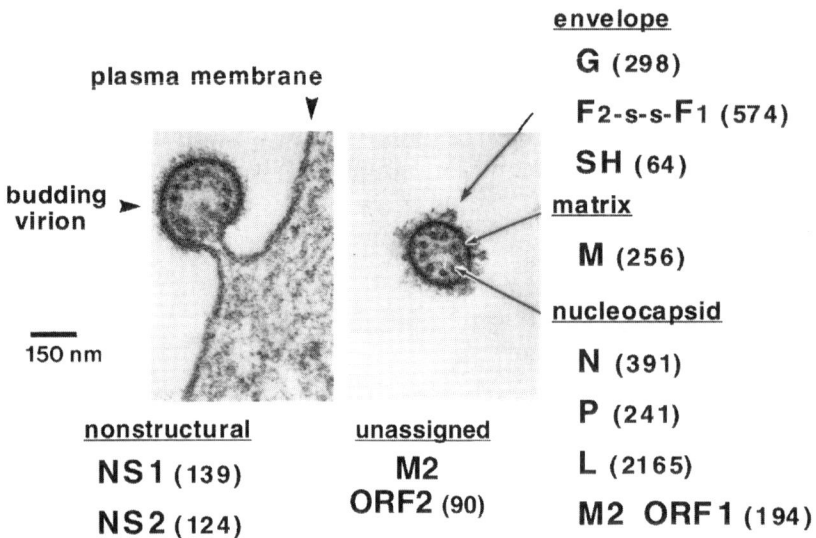

Figure 1 Locations of the RSV proteins, as illustrated on electron micrographs of thin layer sections of (left) a spherical-type RSV virion in the final stage of budding from the plasma membrane of an infected cell, and (right) a free spherical virion. Note the continuity between the envelope of the budding virus and the cell plasma membrane. Virion spikes are visible as a fringe on the exteriors of the virions, and the dense round structures in the virion interior represent cross-sections of the nucleocapsid. The amino acid lengths of the viral proteins are indicated. (The electron micrographs are adapted from Kalica *et al* (1973) *Arch. Gesamte Virusforsch.* 41: 248–258.)

more than 70 potential acceptor sites). It is speculated to have an extended, heavily glycosylated, mucin-like structure. In the middle of the ectodomain there is a predicted disulfide-linked tight turn that coincides with a conserved sequence segment presumed to be a domain important in attachment activity. Remarkably, recombinant RSV lacking the G protein gene can grow in cell culture, implying that an alternative attachment activity exists.

The function of the small SH protein is unknown. Remarkably, recombinant RSV lacking the gene in its entirety is fully viable in cell culture and chimpanzees. SH is anchored in the membrane by a centrally located signal/anchor sequence such that the C-terminal third of the molecule is extracellular. The first two methionine codons in the translational open reading frame (ORF) are alternative translational start sites, and the SH protein accumulates in a variety

Table 2 RSV proteins[a]

Protein	Function/comments	Comments on expression, post-translational modifications
Nucleocapsid-associated		
N	Binds tightly to genomic and antigenomic RNA	
P	Maintains free N and L proteins in soluble form. Polymerase cofactor	P is the most heavily phosphorylated RSV protein
L	Major polymerase subunit	
M2-1	Transcription elongation factor	Encoded by 5'-proximal ORF of M2 mRNA
Envelope-associated		
G	Transmembrane surface attachment protein. Major neutralization and protective antigen. Antigenic and sequence divergence in G defines the antigenic subgroups. Recombinant RSV lacking the G protein gene can grow in cell culture	Contains several N-linked sugar side chains and extensive O-linked glycosylation: the M_r of the unglycosylated form is 32.5 kDa and that of the fully-glycosylated form is 90 kDa. Translational initiation at the second methionine in the ORF yields an N-terminally-truncated form which, following additional N-terminal proteolytic trimming, is secreted
F	Transmembrane surface protein. Fusion activity mediates viral penetration and syncytium formation. Major neutralization and protective antigen	Synthesized as an N-glycosylated, 70 kDa precursor, F0, which is cleaved by a furin-type intracellular protease into two disulfide-linked subunits, F2 (amino acids 1–130, 19 kDa) and F1 (amino acids 137–574, 50 kDa)
SH	Transmembrane surface protein. Function unknown. Recombinant 'knock-out' virus lacking SH is fully viable	Translational initiation at first and second methionines of the ORF yields full length (SH0) and N-terminally-truncated (SHt) forms. Some of SH0 receives an N-linked sugar to form SHg, and some of the SHg is modified by the addition of polylactosaminoglycan to the N-sugar to yield SHp
M	Unglycosylated internal protein. Mediates virion assembly	
Nonstructural		
NS1[b]	Putative negative regulatory factor for replication and transcription. Recombinant 'knock-out' virus lacking NS1 is viable in cell culture but exhibits reduced synthesis of progeny virus	
NS2[b]	Recombinant 'knock-out' virus lacking NS2 is viable in cell culture but exhibits delayed synthesis of progeny virus	Unstable, with a half-life of 30 min
Newly-described, unassigned		
M2-2	Putative negative regulatory factor for replication and transcription	Encoded by the second, internal ORF of the M2 mRNA. Much less abundant than the other viral proteins

[a] Proteins known to be virion structural components: N, P, L, M2-1, SH0, SHp, G, F, M.
[b] Although the calculated molecular weight of NS1 (15 567) is greater than that of NS2 (14 674), it typically has a greater electrophoretic mobility.

of forms due to differing degrees of glycosylation. The multiplicity of forms seems to be a conserved feature, but its significance is unknown.

The nonglycosylated matrix M protein is thought to be located on the inner surface of the envelope and to have a central role in organizing the envelope and directing packaging of the nucleocapsid.

NS1 and NS2 are small proteins thought to be nonstructural. NS1 inhibits transcription and RNA replication in a minireplicon system (see below),

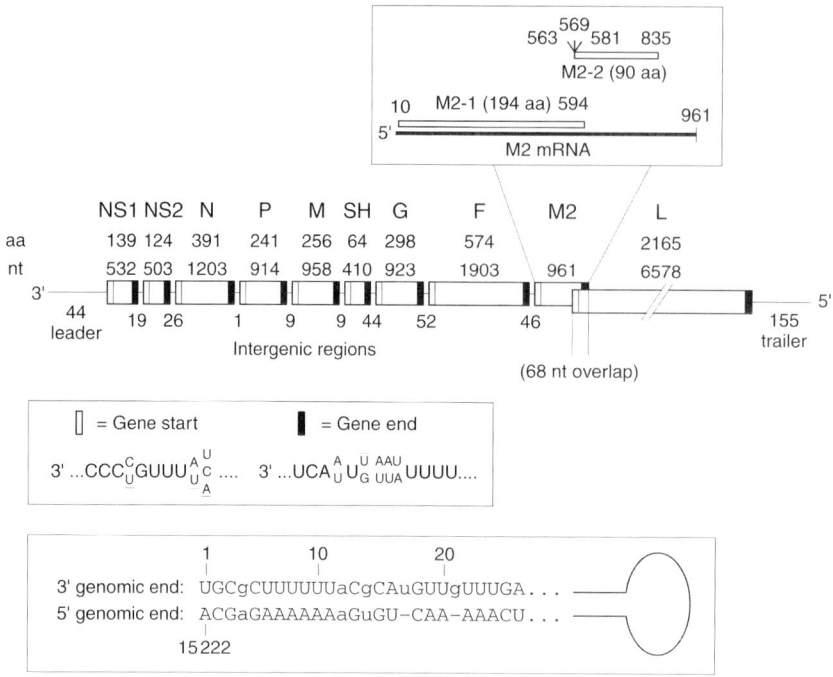

Figure 2 Gene map of RSV strain A2 (not to scale). The 15 222 nt genomic RNA is shown 3' to 5'. Each box corresponds to an encoded mRNA, with the shaded and filled regions identifying the gene-start and gene-end signals respectively. For the gene-start signal, the first nine genes are identical for the first nine nucleotides of the 10 nt signal, whereas that of the L gene has differences indicated by underlining. The gene-end signal is more variable. For both signals, variable nucleotides (or a gap representing three gene-end sequences which are each one nucleotide shorter) are listed vertically in decreasing order of prevalence. The nucleotide (nt) length of each mRNA (exclusive of nontemplated polyadenylate) is indicated immediately over its box, and the amino acid (aa) length of the encoded protein is indicated above that. An expanded drawing of the M2 mRNA illustrates the two ORFs, shown as open rectangles over the line representing the mRNA, with potential translational start and stop codons numbered according to their positions in the 961 nt M2 mRNA. The extragenic leader, intergenic and trailer regions are drawn as thin lines, with nucleotide lengths shown underneath. The complementarity between the 3' and 5' ends is illustrated at the bottom; complementary nucleotides are in capitals and the dashes indicate single-nucleotide gaps introduced to maximize the alignment. These sequences are 81% complementary, after which the degree of relatedness is insignificant.

suggesting that it is a negative regulatory factor. Recombinant RSV lacking the NS1 or NS2 gene is viable in cell culture but replicates less well than wild type. Thus, the NS1 and NS2 genes encode nonessential accessory proteins. The M2 mRNA has a second ORF (**Fig. 2**), encoding the M2-2 protein, a nonabundant species which has been detected in preliminary experiments. Expression of the M2-2 ORF inhibited transcription and RNA replication by an RSV minireplicon, suggesting that M2-2 is a negative regulatory factor.

Genome Organization, Transcription and Replication

The RSV genome is a single, negative strand of RNA that encodes ten mRNAs (**Fig. 2**). Nucleotide lengths for three different RSV genomes sequenced to date are: 15 222 (strain A2 of antigenic subgroup A; see below for a description of the antigenic subgroups), 15 225 (strain B1 of antigenic subgroup B) and 15 133 (BRSV strain A51908). The RSV gene order is conserved within genus *Pneumovirus* but, interestingly, that of APV has two differences: it lacks the NS1 and NS2 genes, and part of its gene order has a different arrangement: 3'-F-M2-SH-G-5' (**Fig. 3**).

As is the case with the Order in general, RNA replication involves the synthesis of a complete positive-sense replicative intermediate that is called the antigenome and serves as the template for the synthesis of progeny genomic RNA. Genomic RNA contains extragenic 3' 'leader' and 5' 'trailer' regions of 44 and 155 nt, respectively (**Fig. 2**). The first 26 nucleotides at the 3' end of genomic RNA have 81% complementarity with the last 24 nucleotides at the 5' end (**Fig. 2**). One possibility is that this complementarity allows the two ends to interact. However, an alternative and more likely possibility is that the complementarity reflects sequence conservation at the 3' ends of the genome and antigenome due to the

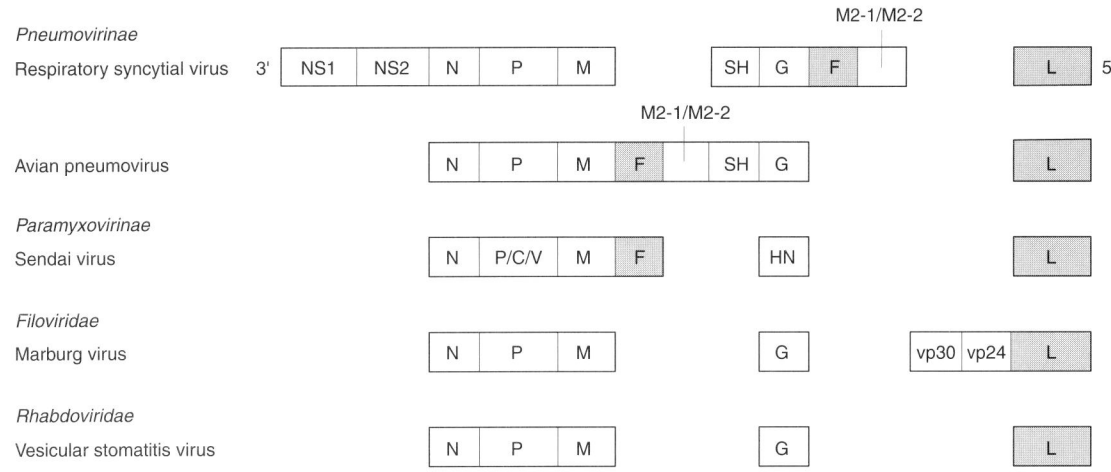

Figure 3 Comparison of the gene maps (not to scale) of the two paramyxovirus subfamilies, *Pneumovirinae* and *Paramyxovirinae*, with those of the filovirus and rhabdovirus families. Each box represents a separate mRNA, with the encoded protein(s) indicated; for mRNAs which contain more than one ORF, the encoded proteins are separated by slashes. The maps were drawn to align analogous proteins vertically when possible. The F and L proteins are shaded to indicate that each exhibits sequence relatedness among the different families. RSV and APV also share sequence relatedness for other proteins, but only F and L have unambiguous relatedness extending beyond the pneumoviruses. The identification of the filovirus P and M proteins is preliminary.

presence of a conserved promoter in each. Also, the conserved 5' ends might each contain a conserved signal for initiating encapsidation of the nascent RNA. Studies with minireplicons indicate that the RNA signals required for replication are contained in their entirety within the 33–40 nucleotides at the 3' and 5' ends of genomic and antigenomic RNA. While certain viruses like Sendai and measles viruses have the remarkable requirement that the genome length be an even multiple of six for efficient replication, there is no such requirement for RSV.

As is characteristic of the Order, RSV transcription initiates at the 3' genomic promoter and copies the genes by a sequential stop–start mechanism that yields subgenomic mRNAs. Each gene begins with a conserved 10 nt gene-start motif that directs initiation of transcription and encodes the 5' end of the mRNA, and ends with a 12–13 nt gene-end motif that directs polyadenylation and release of the mRNA (**Fig. 2**). These motifs are self-contained signals that switch the polymerase between transcribing and nontranscribing modes. The first nine RSV genes are separated by intergenic regions, which are of various lengths (1–52 nt for strain A2) and lack apparent conserved sequences. The intergenic regions do not appear to have a significant role in gene expression. In human and animal RSVs, but not in PVM or APV, the last two genes (M2 and L) overlap by 67 (BSRV) or 68 (RSV) nucleotides (**Fig. 2**) and are expressed as separate mRNAs which each contain the overlap sequence. The mechanism for transcribing overlapped genes is not known but does not appear to involve independent internal polymerase entry.

As is typical of this Order, transcription is polar: promoter-proximal genes are transcribed more frequently than downstream ones due to polymerase fall-off. This provides a gradient of transcription thought to be the major factor determining the relative amounts of expression of the various genes. There is no evidence of temporal regulation of gene expression. During transcription, there is a low frequency of readthrough of the gene-end signals, such that 5–10% of the total mRNA consists of readthrough transcripts each representing two or more adjacent genes.

The RSV mRNAs contain a virally-encoded methylated 5' cap [$m^7G(5')ppp(5')Gp$] and 3' polyadenylate typical of eucaryotic mRNA, the latter produced by reiterative copying by the viral polymerase on a tract of 4–7 U residues at the downstream side of each gene-end signal. Each mRNA encodes a single major viral protein except for the M2 mRNA, which contains two overlapping ORFs (**Fig. 2**) present in all pneumoviruses. The two ORFs are expressed as separate proteins, although the mechanism for translation of the internal ORF is unknown.

The synthesis of mRNA and antigenome ostensibly occur on the same template, and the factors which regulate the two processes are unknown. The M2-1 elongation factor does not appear to regulate transcription and RNA replication, nor does encapsidation of the nascent RNA by the N protein shift synthesis from that of mRNA to antigenome.

Genetics

Nonsegmented negative-strand viruses in general do not undergo recombination, apart from the polymerase jumping which is involved in the production of short helper-dependent defective-interfering RNA. The differences in the gene orders of RSV and APV (**Fig. 3**) suggest that recombination to yield nondefective infectious genomes can occur, but presumably is very rare.

Negative-sense genomic RNA is not directly infectious alone. However, infectious recombinant RSV can be produced in cultured cells by expression from transfected plasmids of a complete antigenomic RNA and the N, P, L and M2-1 proteins. These components presumably assemble into a nucleocapsid that initiates a productive infection. This method can be used to introduce predetermined changes into infectious virus through the cDNA intermediate.

An alternative genetic system that is very useful for basic studies involves short, internally-truncated, cDNA-encoded genome or antigenome analogues, or minireplicons, in which the viral genes have been replaced with one or more reporter genes under the control of RSV transcription signals. When complemented in *trans* by the appropriate mix of plasmid-encoded RSV proteins, the minireplicons are transcribed, replicated and packaged into virus-like particles which can be passaged to fresh cells. Identification and analysis of the functions of *cis*-acting RNA signals and *trans*-acting proteins using these systems is an active area of research.

Antigens and Antigenic Subgroups

Postinfection human or animal serum contains antibodies to various viral proteins, notably the F, G and N proteins. The F and G proteins are by far the major antigens for neutralizing antibodies, but have markedly different antigenic properties. Many of the available F-specific monoclonal antibodies (MAbs) efficiently neutralize RSV *in vitro*, whereas those for the G protein neutralize weakly or not at all. However, polyclonal antibodies to G neutralize efficiently. The high content of O-linked carbohydrate in the G protein is likely to be a factor in its antigenic properties, and indeed the sugars have been shown to be important, directly or indirectly, for the binding of many, but not all, MAbs. Since the sugar side chains are host-specific, they might mask the virus-specified polypeptide chain. Microheterogeneity in the placement of side chains among the many potentially available acceptor sites might result in subpopulations of molecules among which epitopes are variably altered or masked.

RSV is monotypic serologically, with up to fourfold differences between disparate strains in cross-neutralization *in vitro* by postinfection serum. However, binding studies with MAbs showed that RSV isolates can be segregated into two distinct antigenic subgroups designated A and B. Epitopes for F MAbs tend to be conserved, whereas those for G are not, such that antigenic relatedness between the two subgroups is greater than 50% for the F protein, compared with only 5% for the G protein. Comparably distinct antigenic subgroups also have been described for BRSV and APV.

The amino acid sequences of the various RSV proteins are 87% or more identical between the two subgroups, except for the extracellular domains of the SH and G proteins which are only 50% and 43% conserved, respectively. Potential acceptor sites in the G protein for N- and O-linked sugars also are poorly conserved. These sequence differences provide a structural basis for the observed antigenic dimorphism. The amount of sequence variation between strains within a given subgroup is considerably less, although the G protein is more variable than the others, with as much as 12% amino acid difference. While the presence of antigenic dimorphism in circulating virus is thought to be one mechanism for mitigating host immunity, RSV has not been observed to undergo significant antigenic divergence on the time scale of months or a few years.

RSV infection also generates virus-specific CD4+ helper T cells (Th) and CD8+ cytotoxic T cells (CTLs). Depending on the host and genetic background, various viral proteins have been shown to be T cell antigens. The G protein seems to be a relatively poor antigen for CTLs, perhaps a consequence of its high content of sugar side chains.

Antigenic and Sequence Relatedness of RSV to Other Viruses

Antigenic crossreactivity has been observed between RSV and BRSV for most of the proteins, and between RSV and PVM for the N and P proteins. The amount of sequence divergence between BRSV and RSV is approximately two times greater than between the two RSV subgroups. (For example, the N and F proteins are, respectively, 7% and 19% divergent between RSV and BRSV, compared with 4% and 9% divergence between the RSV subgroups.) As would be expected, the BRSV G protein is the most divergent relative to RSV, being 70% divergent with RSV, compared with 47% divergence between the G proteins of the RSV subgroups. As an example of the divergence of PVM and APV relative to RSV, the PVM or APV N protein is 40% or 59% divergent, respectively, from its RSV counterpart.

RSV lacks antigenic relatedness with paramyxoviruses outside of its subfamily. The F protein has low but significant sequence relatedness with the F proteins of the other paramyxoviruses. The L protein has low but significant relatedness with L proteins within the Order and contains sequence motifs conserved among a wide range of polymerases and thought to represent catalytic domains. Although the other RSV proteins lack obvious, unambiguous sequence relatedness with their nonpneumovirus counterparts, it is likely that functional similarity (and evolutionary relatedness) exists between these viruses for proteins such as N, P and M (**Fig. 3**).

Virus Infection in Cell Culture and Animals

RSV initiates infection by binding to a cellular receptor(s) which remains to be identified, and the viral envelope fuses with the plasma membrane. Genome expression and replication are entirely cytoplasmic. Progeny virus buds at the plasma membrane in areas of coalesced viral envelope proteins.

RSV can be grown in a variety of cultured cells of human, simian or bovine origin, and can also be adapted to grow in chick cells. The human epidermal HEp-2 or the African green monkey kidney Vero cell lines are the most commonly used. During infection with strain A2 at an input multiplicity of 5, the intracellular production of viral proteins and nucleic acids can be detected by 6–10 h postinfection and reaches maximum at 15–24 h. Virus release begins by 10–16 h and is maximal by 29 h; syncytia become evident by 20–30 h, and extensive cytopathology and destruction of the monolayer occurs at 30–48 h. Host cell macromolecular synthesis does not appear to be inhibited except by the indirect effects of cytopathology. Although most cells infected in culture are killed, persistent infection *in vitro* can be readily established. Much of the progeny virions remain cell-associated and are released by freeze–thawing or sonication. RSV is very labile to inactivation during unfrozen storage or freeze–thawing, although stability can be greatly improved if the harvested culture supernatants are adjusted to pH 7.5 and to contain 0.1 M magnesium sulfate. Virus yield is 10^5 to 5×10^8 PFU ml^{-1} depending on the cell, strain and growth conditions. A yield of 10 PFU per cell is typical, indicating that the production of infectious virus is inefficient indeed. The instability and size heterogeneity of the virion reduces the efficiency of purification and concentration.

The only hosts that are fully permissive for RSV are the human and the chimpanzee. RSV also can replicate in the respiratory tract of several species of monkey as well as in hamsters, guinea pigs, ferrets, mice, and cotton rats. But in these animals the infection is semipermissive: the titer of recoverable virus is 100–1000-fold lower than in the fully-permissive chimpanzee, and disease either does not occur or is greatly reduced in severity.

RSV buds from the apical surface of polarized cultured cells. *In vivo*, RSV infection is generally restricted to the superficial layers of the respiratory tract epithelium; however, it can spread to secondary organs under conditions of immunosuppression or immunodeficiency, indicating that systemic spread is normally restricted by host immunity rather than a viral factor. Infection of monocytes and macrophages has been reported but is of unknown significance. While individuals can shed virus for sustained periods, there is no evidence of persistent infection *in vivo*. RSV inoculated intramuscularly undergoes a single cycle of replication without the production of infectious virus.

Epidemiology and Clinical Factors

RSV is worldwide. It causes yearly epidemics centered in the winter months in temperate climates or in the rainy season in the tropics. It is highly contagious. It is an important cause of nosocomial infection. Spread involves inoculation of conjunctival or mucosal surfaces by hand or aerosolized particles containing respiratory secretions. Essentially everyone is infected by 1–2 years of age, with the greatest incidence of serious disease occurring between 6 weeks and 6 months of age. The relative sparing of newborns is thought to be due to the transient protective effects of maternally-derived serum IgG. The higher incidence of serious disease in young infants probably reflects in part the greater susceptibility of smaller airways to obstruction by edema and secretions. RSV regularly accounts for more than 20% of pediatric hospitalizations due to respiratory tract disease. In developed countries, mortality is very low for normal children. However, infants and children with bronchopulmonary dysplasia, congenital heart disease or immunodeficiency are at special risk for serious, life-threatening RSV disease. In these cases, mortality can be as high as 30%. In the USA, RSV causes an estimated 91 000 hospitalizations and 4500 deaths annually. In developing countries the infant death rate from respiratory disease can exceed 2000 per 100 000 births, and it is estimated that 20–25% of these would be due to RSV, which can be extrapolated to one million deaths per year worldwide.

During natural infection, RSV has an incubation period of 4–5 days. It causes upper respiratory tract disease, with symptoms of a common cold. Between 25 and 40% of primary infections progress to the lower respiratory tract and cause bronchitis, bronchiolitis or pneumonia. Symptoms include rhinorrhea, middle-ear disease, fever, coughing and wheezing. Seriously ill infants have increased coughing and wheezing, rapid respiration and hypoxemia, requiring the administration of humidified oxygen. The duration of illness is 7–12 days. Virus is shed in large amounts (10^4–10^6 PFU ml^{-1} nasal wash) throughout infection and sometimes during recovery.

RSV infection can be diagnosed rapidly and efficiently by the detection of viral antigens by immunofluorescence of exfoliated cells or enzyme-linked immunosorbent assay (ELISA) of respiratory secretions. Other methods in common use include isolation of the virus in cell culture or detection of an increase in RSV-specific antibodies during convalescence.

RSV is unusual in that it can infect young infants despite the presence of maternally-derived virus-neutralizing serum IgG. This reflects the inefficiency with which serum IgG moves by transudation on to the respiratory tract mucosa and indicates the importance of local immunity in restricting virus replication in the upper respiratory tract. It is not clear why RSV is more infectious under these conditions than are other viruses of the respiratory tract. Another striking feature of RSV is its ability to reinfect repeatedly during childhood and throughout life. Certainly the transient nature of local secretory immunity and the relative ineffectiveness of serum antibodies in accessing the luminal surface of respiratory mucosa are factors in frequent reinfections. But it is not clear why reinfections are so much more frequent with RSV than with other viruses of the respiratory tract. The two antigenic subgroups have been described as alternating in local prevalence from year to year, supporting the idea that the degree of antigenic variation can contribute to reinfection. That the G protein, one of the two protective antigens, might be sheathed in sugar, might exhibit microheterogeneity in side-chain location and structure, and is produced in part as a secreted form, presents other possible mechanisms for mitigating the effectiveness of host immunity. Although the virus can reinfect, serious disease is associated mostly with first or second infection. Sparing during subsequent infections is due to immunological restriction of virus replication in the lower respiratory tract, and indicates that immunoprophylaxis is feasible.

Much of the pathogenesis of RSV is the direct result of destruction of epithelial cells by virus replication and the concomitant edema, mucus secretion and influx of lymphocytes and macrophages. Pathogenesis can probably also be influenced by additional immune factors, such as antibody-mediated or cell-mediated hypersensitivity, which remain to be elucidated. In some individuals, airway reactivity in RSV disease might involve an allergic-type reaction mediated by IgE. The ability of immune factors to profoundly influence RSV pathogenesis is illustrated by the enhancement of RSV disease associated with immunization with a formalin-inactivated RSV vaccine (see below). A long-term reduction in pulmonary function is a common sequel to serious RSV disease, but it is not clear whether this is due to the infection or whether such individuals already had underlying pulmonary deficiencies which predisposed them to serious RSV infection.

Immunity

The major mechanisms for resolving primary infection appear to be innate immune mechanisms, CTLs and antibodies. In naive mice, the reduction in pulmonary RSV replication coincided with the appearance of RSV-specific CD8+ CTLs and was inhibited by prior depletion of that subset. Children deficient in cell-mediated immunity experience more serious disease and have difficulty resolving infection. Studies in calves and humans indicated that the appearance of secretory antibodies is coincident with viral clearance. The late appearance of serum antibodies suggests that they are less important in resolving the primary infection.

In experimental animals immunized with individual RSV proteins, antigens which elicited predominantly either (1) neutralizing antibodies or (2) RSV-specific CTLs could induce resistance to subsequently challenge virus replication. However, the resistance induced by CTL antigens was short-lived compared with that afforded by neutralizing antibodies. This suggests that, while CTL clearly have an important role in resolving infection, the long-term resistance to virus replication that develops from prior infection or immunization is more likely to be mediated by antibodies. The F and G proteins are the major RSV antigens which induce virus-neutralizing antibodies and protection. Secretory IgA antibodies are important mediators of resistance in the upper respiratory tract but are relatively short-lived. Virus-neutralizing serum antibodies alone can restrict virus replication in the lower respiratory tract, an effect due to their transudation, albeit inefficient, on to the respiratory epithelium.

Immunoprophylaxis and Treatment

Because natural RSV infection does not provide complete, long-lasting resistance to reinfection, it seems unlikely that a vaccine will do so. None the less, early immunization could reduce the incidence of serious disease associated with the first one or two infections of life. It is likely that natural infections would not be prevented, but their consequences would be reduced in severity and would have the desirable effect of boosting immunity. Very young infants, who would be the targets for immunization, have been shown to have reduced immune responses to RSV infection owing to immunologic immaturity. Also, maternally-derived serum antibodies can suppress the induction of antibodies and CTLs, although this effect can be abrogated to a considerable extent by direct immunization of the respiratory tract. Recent vaccine trials suggest that very young infants can mount a satisfactory immune response against live attenuated RSV administered intranasally.

Vaccine safety is a major consideration. A vaccine made from formalin-inactivated, concentrated RSV and tested in 1966 failed to prevent natural infection and, paradoxically, primed the vaccinees for an increased frequency and severity of disease upon subsequent natural infection. The lack of protective efficacy was probably due to denaturation of neutralization epitopes, and the disease enhancement appears to be due to an exaggerated Th response, perhaps one imbalanced in favor of a Th2-type response instead of the Th1-biased response typical of natural infection. The elucidation of this phenomenon, and the testing of RSV vaccines in general, is complicated by the semipermissive nature of RSV infection in convenient experimental animals like the mouse.

Live attenuated RSV strains for immunization by intranasal infection are under development and might represent the safest, most effective vaccine. Recombinant vaccinia and adenoviruses which express the F or G glycoproteins have been tested in experimental animals as prototype vaccines but, to date, have not been sufficiently immunogenic. Purified F and G glycoproteins for intramuscular immunization have been produced from cultured mammalian cells infected with RSV or from cultured insect cells infected with recombinant baculoviruses. The noninfectious nature of a subunit vaccine might be especially appropriate for immunization of the very young. But these purified antigens appear to induce antibodies with low neutralizing activity, perhaps due to denaturation during preparation, and there are indications that they, like the formalin-inactivated vaccine, prime for immune-mediated pathology upon subsequent infection.

Ribavirin treatment of hospitalized normal or high-risk infected children is well established, although debate as to its level of efficacy has continued. The administration of aerosolized ribavirin to children who were seriously ill and supported by mechanical respirators is associated with improvement and reduced hospital stay. As another approach, the systemic or topical application of RSV-neutralizing antibodies (either polyclonal serum antibodies or murine MAbs) to infected experimental animals was shown to be efficacious both in immunoprophylaxis and therapy. This concept led to the recent development of a strategy in which a pooled human serum antibody preparation with high RSV-neutralizing activity (RespiGam^{TM}) is administered intravenously to high-risk children as a method of passive immunoprophylaxis. A further improvement will be to increase the specific antiviral activity by replacing the preparation of serum antibodies, of which only a small component is RSV-specific, with humanized or human RSV-specific MAbs. Also, application of antibodies directly to the respiratory tract of infected individuals might be effective in curtailing infection and disease.

See also: **Parainfluenza viruses (*Paramyxoviridae*) – Human; Respiratory viruses; Sendai virus (*Paramyxoviridae*); Defective interfering viruses; Vesicular stomatitis viruses (*Rhabdoviridae*).**

Further Reading

Collins PL, Hill MG, Cristina J and Grosfeld H (1996) Transcription elongation factor of respiratory syncytial virus, a nonsegmented negative strand RNA virus. *Proc. Natl. Acad. Sci. USA* 93:81.

Collins PL, McIntosh KM and Chanock RM (1996) Respiratory syncytial virus. In: Fields BN, Knipe DM, Howley PM et al (eds) *Fields Virology* 3rd edn, p. 1313. New York: Lippincott-Raven.

Hall CB (1994) Prospects for a respiratory syncytial virus vaccine. *Science* 265: 1393.

Murphy BR, Hall SL, Kulkarni AB (1994) An update on approaches to the development of respiratory syncytial virus (RSV) and parainfluenza virus type 3 (PIV3) vaccines. *Virus Res.* 32: 13.

Pringle CR and Easton AJ (1997) Monopartite negative strand RNA genome. *Semin. Virol.* 8: 49.

Wright PF (1997) Respiratory diseases. In: Nathanson N, Ahmed R, Gonzalez-Scarano F et al (eds) *Viral Pathogenesis,* p. 703. New York: Raven Press.

RESPIRATORY VIRUSES

David O White and **Lorena E Brown**, Department of Microbiology and Immunology, The University of Melbourne, Parkville, Victoria, Australia

Copyright © 1999 Academic Press

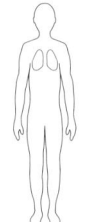

Introduction

The respiratory tract is a major portal of entry for pathogenic organisms; infections at this site are the most common afflictions of humans. Children contract up to half a dozen respiratory illnesses each year, adults perhaps two or three, and most of these are caused by viruses. Though trivial colds and sore throats account for the majority of respiratory disease, their impact on communities is significant; millions of lost working hours and a considerable proportion of all visits to family physicians can be attributed to this type of infection. More serious lower respiratory tract infections tend to occur at the extremes of life, and in those with pre-existing pulmonary conditions. The most important human respiratory viruses are influenza and respiratory syncytial viruses (RSV), the former killing mainly the aged and the latter the very young. Of the estimated 5 million deaths from respiratory infections in children annually worldwide, at least one million are viral in origin.

Altogether, there are over 200 human respiratory viruses, falling mainly within six families: orthomyxoviruses, paramyxoviruses, picornaviruses, coronaviruses, adenoviruses and herpesviruses (see corresponding entries elsewhere in this text). Here we shall confine ourselves to those that enter the body via the respiratory route and cause disease confined largely to the respiratory tract. Many other 'respiratory' viruses become disseminated via the bloodstream to produce a more generalized disease, as is the case with most of the human childhood exanthems such as measles, rubella and varicella, or rinderpest and foot-and-mouth disease in cattle. Yet other viruses, entering by nonrespiratory routes, can reach the lungs via systemic spread, and pneumonia may represent the final lethal event, e.g. in overwhelming infections with herpesviruses or adenoviruses in immunocompromised neonates or patients with the acquired immune deficiency syndrome (AIDS).

Epidemiology

By definition, respiratory viruses are transmitted via the respiratory route. Virions are shed from the respiratory tract of an infected human or animal, particularly during sneezing, coughing, talking or barking. A sneeze generates an aerosol comprising up to a million tiny droplets less than 10 μm in diameter that quickly evaporate to yield droplet nuclei which remain suspended in the air for several minutes. This particulate material containing virions transmits infection following inhalation by someone nearby. Larger droplets (up to 100 μm) contain more virions but fall to ground within seconds. They are a danger to anyone directly in the line of fire. Alternatively, respiratory infections can spread by direct contact, e.g. kissing, or by transfer of nasal or oral secretions via hands to nose or mouth. At the height of a common cold such secretions are particularly copious and readily find their way on to handkerchiefs, towels, toothbrushes, eating utensils, doorknobs and so on, as well as hands.

Enveloped viruses such as orthomyxoviruses, paramyxoviruses and coronaviruses tend to be rather susceptible to inactivation by desiccation or by summer temperatures, but icosahedral viruses such as adenoviruses and picornaviruses are more stable; for example, certain outbreaks of foot-and-mouth disease have been attributed to virus carried in the wind for 100 km.

We associate respiratory infections with cold, wet weather but there is no evidence that the winter incidence of the common cold, or indeed any other respiratory disease, is attributable to cold or wet *per se*. Colds are not common in Arctic or Antarctic explorers, for example. It seems more likely that the striking winter peaks of respiratory disease caused by influenza and RSV (**Fig. 1**) are a reflection of our predilection during that season for avoiding the invigorating outdoor climate and shutting ourselves away in ill-ventilated centrally-heated buildings and vehicles, in close apposition to others of like mind. This hypothesis is supported by the observation that in the tropics, where summer and winter are replaced by 'wet' and 'dry' seasons, respiratory infections are more prevalent during the monsoonal rains when people spend more time indoors, exchanging parasites in crowded, often squalid conditions. An additional factor in the less developed world is the domestic air pollution (smoke) generated by the ever-present fire, lit for cooking and warmth inside poorly ventilated huts. Outbreaks of influenza often occur in boarding

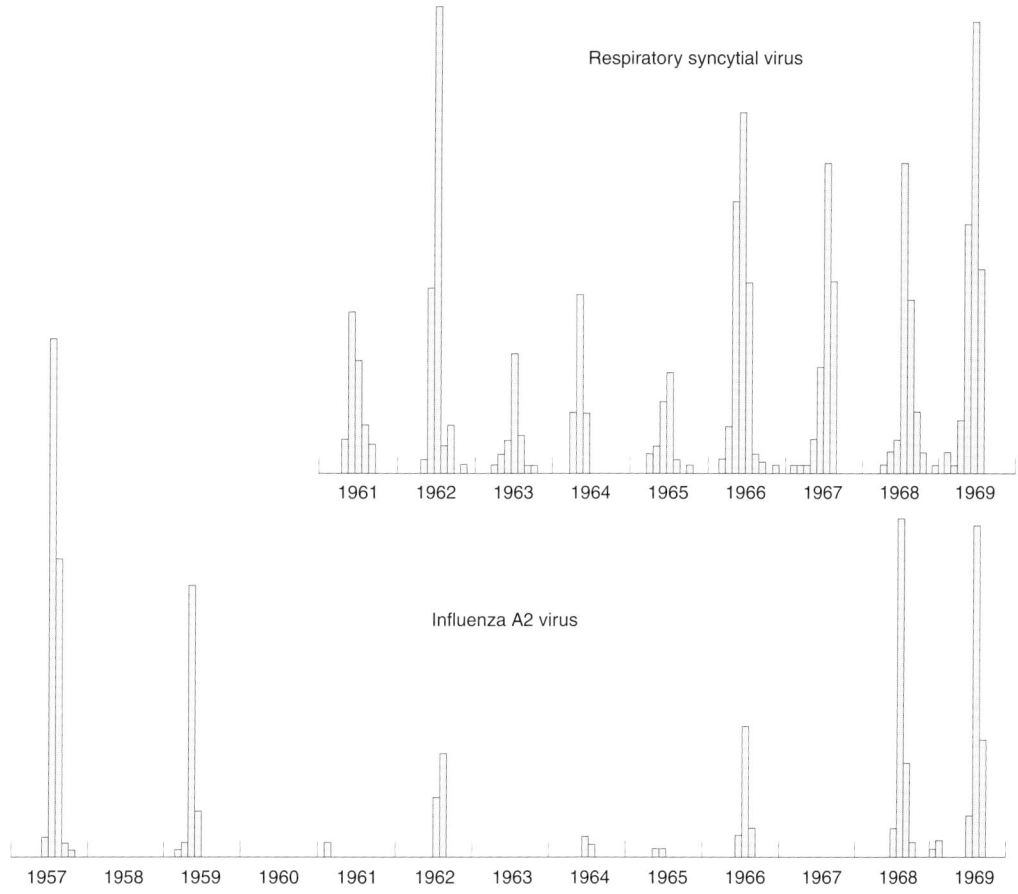

Figure 1 Epidemic occurrence of influenza A and respiratory syncytial viruses. The histograms show the monthly isolations of these two viruses from patients admitted to the Fairfield Hospital for Infectious Diseases, Melbourne, over the periods indicated. Compare the regular winter epidemics of RSV (causing significant disease mainly in infants) with the less regular winter epidemics of influenza. There were major peaks of influenza in 1957 (first appearance of the new human influenza subtype H2N2, known as 'Asian flu') and then again in 1968 (marking the emergence of the novel subtype H3N2, known as 'Hong Kong flu'). (Data courtesy of Drs A. A. Ferris, F. Lewis and I. D. Gust. From Fenner F and White DO (1976) *Medical Virology* 2nd edn. New York: Academic Press.)

schools, army camps, nursing homes, etc.; similarly, nosocomial spread of RSV is common in hospital nurseries. Livestock such as cattle are particularly vulnerable when crowded together in feed-lots or transport vehicles, e.g. shipping fever.

Respiratory viruses spread with great facility and speed, albeit not with the explosive onset that characterizes certain 'common source' outbreaks of enteric viruses when feces contaminate food or water supplies. First, respiratory diseases have a very short incubation period, usually 2–7 days. Second, very large numbers of virions (10^3–10^9 per ml of respiratory secretions) are shed, commencing even before symptoms develop, and peaking around the time the patient is coughing or sneezing with greatest abandon. A single infectious particle may infect a susceptible contact. Typically, a young child picks up the latest virus at school, brings it home and passes it on to the rest of the family and perhaps to the neighbours' children. Within 2 or 3 months up to half the population of a city may have contracted the infection and developed immunity to the virus. As the proportion of uninfected susceptibles in the community falls, the epidemic burns itself out (**Fig. 1**).

Respiratory viruses may evolve quite rapidly in the field. RNA viruses in particular display a very high rate of mutation, because their RNA polymerase is error prone and lacks the error-correcting capability that accompanies DNA replication. Any spontaneously arising mutant that is capable of replicating in the presence of antibody against the wild-type virus will have a growth advantage. Eventually mutants emerge that contain amino acid substitutions in most or all of the immunodominant antigenic domains on the critical surface protein of the virion. Such multiple mutants, no longer neutralizable by wild-type antibody, are designated a new strain and may initiate another epidemic. This phenomenon is known as

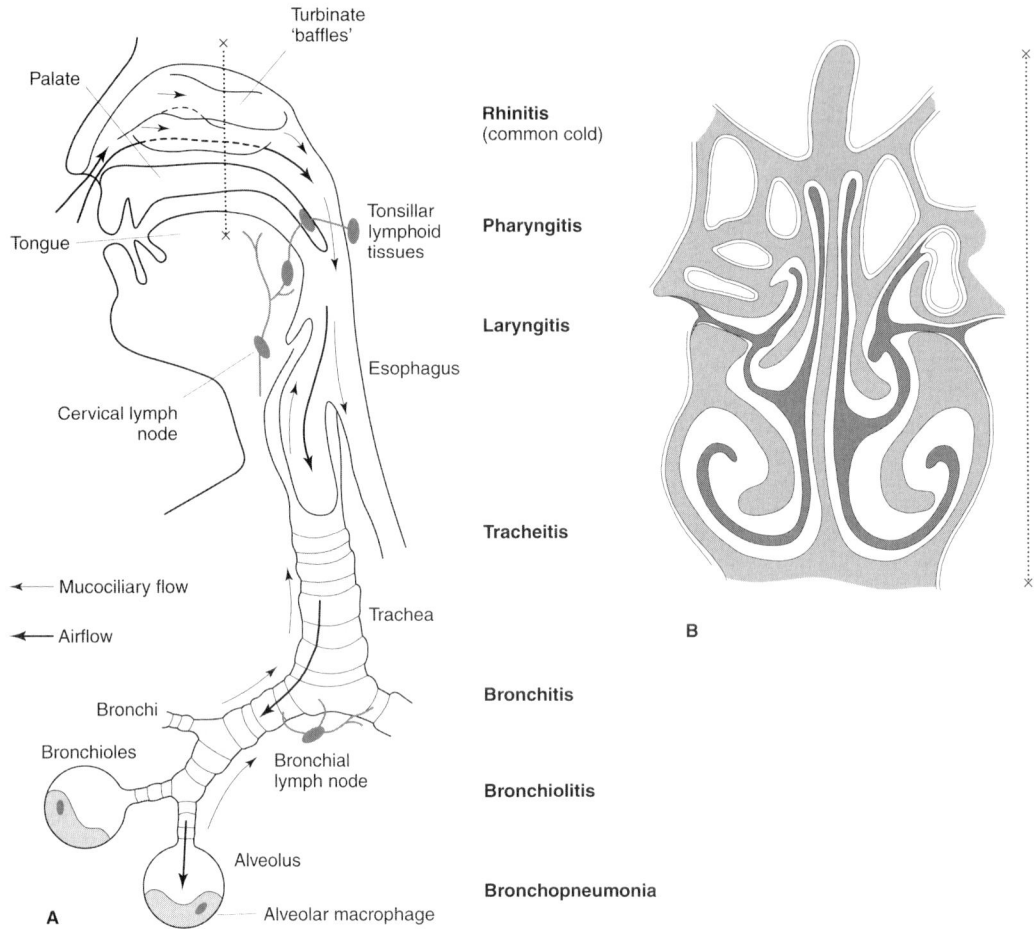

Figure 2 (**A**) Pathways of infection and mechanical protective mechanisms in the respiratory tract. On the right, clinical syndromes produced by infection at various levels of the respiratory tract. (**B**) Section of the turbinates (X—X) magnified 2.5 times, showing the narrow and complicated pathway of inspired air, and thus the ease with which slight swelling 'blocks the nose'. (From White and Fenner (1994), as modified from Mims CA and White DO (1984) *Viral Pathogenesis and Immunology.* Oxford: Blackwell Scientific.)

antigenic drift. While best characterized for influenza, it is presumably the mechanism that has also given rise to the dozens of known serotypes of rhinoviruses, enteroviruses, adenoviruses, and so on. A second, more dramatic type of change, known as antigenic shift, is observed in RNA viruses with segmented genomes that can undergo genetic reassortment. Novel subtypes of human influenza A viruses, capable of initiating pandemics that can infect the majority of the world's population within a year, arise every generation or so as a result of reassortment following co-infection of, say, a pig with a human and an avian influenza virus simultaneously.

Pathogenesis and Immunity

Inhaled droplets of more than 10 µm in diameter are trapped in the turbinates of the nose (**Fig. 2**), whereas those measuring 5–10 µm often reach the trachea and bronchioles. Many of these particles become trapped in the layer of mucus that blankets the ciliated epithelium and are carried by ciliary action to the pharynx, where they are swallowed or coughed out. Smaller particles still can be inhaled directly into the lung and some may reach the alveoli. Here, virus may be phagocytosed and destroyed by alveolar macrophages (although some viral species undergo an abortive cycle of replication and others have developed the capacity to replicate in macrophages). A few virions will succeed in attaching to susceptible epithelial cells via the appropriate ligand–receptor pairing and thereby initiate infection. Progeny virions will be released a few hours later, often by budding from the apical surface of the cell into the lumen of the respiratory tract, and then initiate a second cycle of infection in adjacent or more distant cells. Some of the enveloped species of respiratory viruses are dependent upon a particular cellular protease to cleave the appropriate viral envelope glycoprotein, e.g. influenza HA, or RSV F protein, otherwise the progeny are noninfectious. Moreover, mucus contains glycoprotein inhibitors which can neutralize the infectivity of certain viruses, e.g. influenza. Mannose-binding lectins such as those in lung surfactant can also neutralize virus. Interferon, synthesized by and secreted from virus-infected cells, binds to interferon receptors on nearby uninfected cells and protects them by inhibiting viral replication.

If specific neutralizing antibodies of the IgA class are already present in the mucus coating the respiratory tract as a result of previous infection or vaccination, they will bind to the corresponding epitopes on the surface of the virion and neutralize its infectivity by blocking attachment or fusion of viral envelope with plasma membrane or endocytic vesicle, thus preventing uncoating of the viral genome. In the absence of pre-existing antibody, however, infection can progress because primary antibody synthesis does not become significant for several days. Additional mechanisms are brought into play to control viral replication during this early period, with the first cells to be mobilized being the natural killer (NK) cells from bone marrow, which become activated by interferon (IFN) to lyse virus-infected cells. Shortly thereafter, the relevant clones of T lymphocytes are activated. Helper T (Th) cells (CD4+) recognize peptides generated from endocytosed virions by proteolysis and presented in the peptide-binding groove of the class II major histocompatability complex (MHC) molecules on the surface of antigen-presenting cells (dendritic cells and macrophages) and are triggered to proliferate and to secrete a range of lymphokines that mediate inflammation by attracting macrophages and other leukocytes to the site, and by upregulating macrophages, B cells and T cells. Cytotoxic T cells (CD8+), on the other hand, see endogenous viral peptides generated by proteolysis of newly synthesized viral proteins and bound to class I molecules on the surface of infected cells.

A major mechanism of recovery from viral infection is lysis of infected cells by activated CD8+ T lymphocytes, preferentially but not exclusively by a perforin/granzyme-mediated process. Children with a congenital T cell deficiency may die from measles or RSV infection; conversely, influenza virus-infected athymic mice may be saved by adoptive transfer of virus-specific CD8+ T cells. CD4+ T cells also contribute to the process of recovery by secretion of cytokines such as IFN-γ and through provision of help to B cells in the developing humoral response. Specific antibodies may act by (1) neutralizing virus, (2) complement-mediated lysis of infected cells, or (3) antibody-dependent cell-mediated cytolysis (ADCC). In addition, IgA, during its active passage through respiratory epithelial cells, may combine with viral proteins produced within these cells, resulting in reduced output of infectious progeny.

Whereas the immune response to respiratory infection is instrumental in recovery, it can also, paradoxically, exacerbate the disease itself. CD4+ Th1 cells may induce such a strong inflammatory response (delayed-type hypersensitivity or DTH) as to cause lethal consolidation of the lung (pneumonia). Furthermore, responses orchestrated by the type 2 cytokines IL-4 and IL-5, namely IgE production and eosinophil degranulation, can precipitate a life-threatening attack of asthma in a young infant infected with RSV. Other factors may also contribute to RSV bronchiolitis: virus infection not only enhances bronchial reactivity to antigen but also destroys the ciliated epithelial cells responsible for mucociliary clearance, thus allowing the infant's narrow bronchioles to become plugged with mucus, inflammatory cells and necrotic cell debris, while bronchoconstriction may also be triggered by vagal nerve reflexes or by release of mediators by inflammatory cells. Blockage of airways causes hypoxia and a pathophysiologic cascade that leads to acidosis and uncontrollable fluid exudation into airways.

Superinfection with bacteria, typically *Streptococcus pneumoniae*, *Haemophilus influenzae* or *Staphylococcus aureus*, often complicates viral pneumonitis, and without chemotherapy can lead to a fatal outcome. The very young and very old are particularly at risk, as are the immunocompromised, and premature or malnourished infants.

Systemic viral infections such as measles generate a strong memory response and prolonged production of IgG antibodies, which protect against reinfections for life. In contrast, viruses that cause infection localized to the respiratory tract, with little or no viremia, e.g. RSV or rhinoviruses, induce only a relatively short-lived mucosal IgA antibody response, and reinfections with the same or a somewhat different strain can recur repeatedly throughout life. In addition, numerous strains arising by antigenic drift may cause sequential episodes of the same disease in a single individual.

Viral Diseases of the Human Respiratory Tract

While some viruses have a predilection for one particular part of the respiratory tract, most are capable of causing disease at any level and the syndromes to be described below overlap somewhat (**Fig. 3**). Nevertheless, for ease of description we will

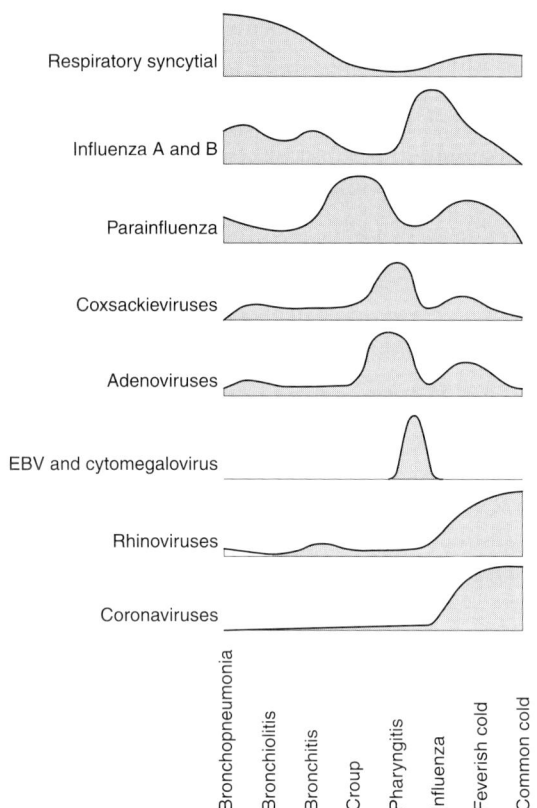

Figure 3 Frequency with which particular viruses produce disease at various levels of the human respiratory tract. (Data courtesy of Dr D. A. J. Tyrrell. From White and Fenner (1994).)

designate six basic diseases of increasing severity as we descend the respiratory tract: rhinitis, pharyngitis, croup, bronchitis, bronchiolitis and pneumonia (Table 1).

Rhinitis (common cold)

The classical common cold (coryza) is marked by copious watery nasal discharge and congestion, sneezing, and perhaps a mild sore throat or cough, but little or no fever. Rhinoviruses are the major cause, several serotypes being prevalent all year round and accounting for about half of all colds. Coronaviruses are responsible for about another 15%, mainly those occurring in the winter months. Certain enteroviruses, particularly coxsackieviruses A21 and A24, and echoviruses 11 and 20 cause febrile colds and sore throats in the summer. In children, RSV, parainfluenza viruses and the lower-numbered adenoviruses are between them responsible for up to half of all upper respiratory tract infections (URTI or URI).

Otitis media or sinusitis sometimes complicate URI. Bacterial superinfection is generally involved, but viruses have also been recovered from the effusion. Respiratory infections with RSV, influenza, parainfluenza, adenovirus or measles viruses predispose to otitis media. Indeed, repeated viral infections can precipitate recurrent middle ear infections, leading to progressive hearing loss.

Pharyngitis

Most pharyngitis is of viral etiology. URI with any of the viruses just described can present as a sore throat, with or without cough, malaise, fever and/or cervical lymphadenopathy. Influenza, parainfluenza and rhinoviruses are common causes throughout life, but other agents are prominent in particular age groups: RSV and adenoviruses in young children; herpesviruses in adolescents and young adults. Adenoviruses, though not major pathogens overall, are estimated to be responsible for about 5% of all respiratory illnesses in young children, often presenting as pharyngoconjunctival fever. Primary infection with herpes simplex virus (HSV), if delayed until adolescence, presents as a pharyngitis and/or tonsillitis rather than as the gingivostomatitis seen principally in younger children; the characteristic vesicles, rupturing to form ulcers, can be confused only with herpangina, a common type of vesicular pharyngitis caused by coxsackie A viruses. Infectious mononucleosis (glandular fever) is usually marked by a very severe pharyngitis, often with a membranous exudate, together with cervical lymphadenopathy and fever; this syndrome is generally caused by Epstein–Barr (EB) virus in 15–25-year-olds, and less commonly by cytomegalovirus.

Laryngotracheobronchitis (croup)

Croup is one of the serious manifestations of parainfluenza and influenza virus infections. A young child presents with fever, cough, inspiratory stridor and respiratory distress, sometimes progressing to complete laryngeal obstruction and cyanosis. Parainfluenza viruses are responsible for about half of all cases, type 1 being more common than type 2. Influenza and RSV are important causes during winter epidemics.

Bronchitis

Influenza, parainfluenza and RSV are the main viral causes of acute bronchitis. There is also evidence that chronic bronchitis, which is particularly common in smokers, may be exacerbated by acute episodes of infection with influenza viruses, rhinoviruses or coronaviruses.

Table 1 Human respiratory viral diseases

Disease	Virus Common	Less common
Rhinitis (common cold)	Rhinoviruses	RSV, parainfluenza, influenza
	Coronaviruses	Adenoviruses
		Coxsackie A21, 24; echo 11, 20
Pharyngitis	Parainfluenza 1–3	Rhinoviruses
	Influenza	Adenoviruses 1–7
	Herpes simplex	RSV
	EB virus	Cytomegalovirus
	Coxsackie A	
Laryngotracheobronchitis (croup)	Parainfluenza	RSV
	Influenza	
Bronchiolitis	RSV	Influenza
	Parainfluenza 3	
Pneumonia	RSV	Adenoviruses 3, 7
	Parainfluenza 3	Cytomegalovirus
	Influenza	Measles
		Varicella

Bronchiolitis

RSV is the most important respiratory pathogen during the first year or two of life, being responsible, during winter epidemics, for about half of all bronchiolitis in infants. Parainfluenza viruses (especially type 3) and influenza viruses are the other major causes of this syndrome. Breathing becomes rapid and labored, and is accompanied by a persistent cough, expiratory wheezing, cyanosis, a variable amount of atelectasis, and marked emphysema visible by x-ray. The disease can develop with remarkable speed and is one of the causes of sudden infant death syndrome (SIDS), where an infant may die overnight.

Pneumonia

Whereas viruses are relatively uncommon causes of pneumonia in adults, they are very important in young children. RSV and parainfluenza (mainly type 3) are between them responsible for 25% of all pneumonitis in infants in the first year of life. Influenza also causes a considerable number of deaths during epidemic years. Adenoviruses 3 and 7 are less common but can be severe; long-term sequelae such as obliterative bronchiolitis or bronchiectasis may permanently impair lung function. Up to 20% of pneumonitis in infants has been ascribed to perinatal infection with cytomegalovirus (CMV). CMV may also cause potentially lethal pneumonia in immunocompromised patients, as may measles, varicella and adenoviruses. Moreover, viral pneumonia not uncommonly develops in adults with varicella, and in military recruits involved in outbreaks of adenovirus 4 or 7, while measles is often complicated by bacterial pneumonia, especially in malnourished children in Africa and South America. In the elderly, and particularly in those with underlying pulmonary or cardiac conditions, influenza is a major cause of death, either via influenza pneumonitis or more commonly via secondary bacterial pneumonia.

Viral pneumonitis often develops insidiously following URI and the clinical picture may be atypical. The patient is generally febrile, with a cough and a degree of dyspnea, and auscultation may reveal some wheezing or moist rales. Unlike typical bacterial lobar pneumonia with its uniform consolidation, or bronchopneumonia with its streaky consolidation, viral pneumonitis is usually confined to diffuse interstitial lesions. The radiological findings are not striking; they often show little more than an increase in hilar shadows or, at most, scattered areas of consolidation.

Space does not permit a discussion of veterinary diseases, but **Table 2** lists some of the most important respiratory viral diseases of farm and companion animals. Most of these agents are relatively specific to a single animal species, or to closely related species, and do not infect humans. Influenza is occasionally transmitted to humans following close contact with

Table 2 Major respiratory viral diseases of animals

Host	Disease (virus)	Virus family
Cattle	Infectious bovine rhinotracheitis	Herpesviridae
Cattle	Respiratory syncytial virus	Paramyxoviridae
Cattle, swine	Foot-and-mouth disease	Picornaviridae
Horse	Equine rhinopneumonitis	Herpesviridae
Cat	Feline calicivirus	Caliciviridae
Cat	Feline rhinotracheitis	Herpesviridae
Dog	Canine laryngotracheitis	Adenoviridae
Dog	Canine distemper	Paramyxoviridae
Chicken	Infectious laryngotracheitis	Herpesviridae
Chicken	Avian infectious bronchitis	Coronaviridae
Birds	Newcastle disease	Paramyxoviridae
Birds, horses, swine	Influenza	Orthomyxoviridae

pigs or birds infected with a swine or avian influenza virus respectively, but generally fails to spread beyond the first human case. At the time of writing an avian influenza strain has caused a small number of deaths in Hong Kong residents recently in contact with infected chickens. The greater danger in such a situation is the possibility of genetic reassortment occurring between the avian strain and a human strain already well adapted to human–human transmission. A recently discovered paramyxovirus, known as equine morbillivirus because it was responsible for the death from pneumonia of several racehorses as well as their well-known trainer, now appears to be native to Australian fruit-eating bats.

Laboratory Diagnosis

The etiology of respiratory viral infection can be established in the laboratory by identifying the virus itself, viral antigen or the viral genome. The most appropriate specimen is generally a throat swab or, better still, mucus aspirated from the nasopharynx, taken early in the disease. Because enveloped respiratory viruses with helical nucleocapsids are notoriously labile, the specimen is kept cold and moist, transported promptly to the laboratory and processed as soon as practicable.

Enzyme immunoassay (EIA) is the method of choice for the rapid detection of antigen in respiratory secretions. Diagnostic kits, based on appropriate monoclonal antibodies for antigen-capture and detection respectively, and often incorporating a biotin–avidin readout system, are now available for all common human respiratory viruses and many of the important animal pathogens. EIA is replacing immunofluorescence (application of fluorescein-labeled monoclonal antiviral antibody to infected cells aspirated from the throat). Multiple target (multiplex) polymerase chain reaction (PCR) for the amplification of the viral genome, followed by its identification using an appropriate nucleic acid probe, is fast becoming popular as a diagnostic technique for respiratory infections and in epidemiologic investigations.

Most of the known respiratory viruses can quite readily be cultivated in appropriate cell lines from the corresponding host species, e.g. diploid lung fibroblasts or HUT-292 cells for human viruses. Growth of the virus is detected by cytopathic effects and/or hemadsorption or immunofluorescence, and the virus recovered from the supernatant is then typed using any of a variety of serological techniques. However, this sequence is so time consuming and expensive that isolation and identification of virus is today undertaken mainly by reference laboratories requiring a large supply of the virus for further characterization, for research, or for antigen or vaccine production. Viral culture nevertheless remains a vital first step in the identification of agents responsible for newly emerging diseases.

'Serology', i.e. identification and quantification of antibody in the patient's serum, is also far too slow to be of value in influencing the management of the patient, hence it is used principally in seroepidemiological surveys to assess the immune status of populations. IgM-capture EIA does provide a rapid diagnosis but fills only a limited role in the routine diagnostic laboratory.

Vaccines and Chemotherapy

Very successful live attenuated vaccines are in general use against certain 'respiratory' viruses like measles, mumps and rubella, which, though naturally transmitted via the respiratory route, are absolutely dependent upon viremic spread to their target organs elsewhere in the body. In contrast, it is a much more challenging assignment to develop effective vaccines against viruses whose pathogenicity is essentially confined to the respiratory tract. The major reasons for this are that (1) secretory IgA memory is relatively short-lived, and (2) numerous antigenically distinct strains or serotypes are capable of causing the same clinical syndrome. Thus, a common cold vaccine might need to contain dozens of different serotypes of rhinoviruses (± coronaviruses). An inactivated vaccine is used to protect the aged and other risk groups against the currently prevalent strains of influenza, but its composition must be updated regularly to keep abreast of antigenic drift and shift and, even so, its efficacy in the aged is only of the order of 50–80%. The incorporation into vaccines of mucosal adjuvants, e.g. low-toxicity mutants or individual subunits of cholera toxin and *Escherichia coli* heat-labile toxin, is being examined in the hope of stimulating potent antiviral mucosal IgA responses. Improved antigen-delivery strategies, many of which utilize the size and multivalent antigen presentation properties of the viruses themselves, are also being investigated. Immunostimulatory complexes or 'ISCOMs', which are small adjuvant- and lipid-containing particles into which viral proteins can be inserted, already form the basis for an equine influenza vaccine. Live 'cold-adapted' mutants, for many years licensed as influenza vaccines in Russia, replicate only at the low temperature of the nose and are generally avirulent. Although it has proven difficult to walk the tightrope between genetic stability of avirulence on the one side, and adequate replication (hence immunogenicity) on the other, there is currently considerable interest in re-exploring the potential of such viral mutants for intranasal vaccination in other parts of the world. Another potentially exciting vaccine strategy is the use of recombinant DNA encoding the vaccine antigen, delivered in the form of a plasmid by syringe or 'gene gun'. Such vaccines, encoding the nucleoprotein and hemagglutinin of influenza A virus, have successfully elicited protective responses in animals. Subsequent efforts in this area include methods for enhancing the efficiency of transfection of host cells to increase the feasibility of application in humans.

In the long term another source of hope may lie with antiviral chemotherapeutic agents (see Antivirals), although significant barriers still remaining are (1) the multiplicity of viruses involved and the specific antiviral spectrum of available agents; (2) difficulties with drug delivery, efficacy and toxicity; (3) the fact that high titers of virus may be produced even before the onset of symptoms; and (4) emergence of drug-resistant mutants. Since the discovery of interferon in 1957, the field of antiviral chemotherapy has moved slowly. Although IFN-α is effective when given intranasally shortly before or after virus exposure, its use is not practical because of cost of production, frequency of doses required and problems with local bleeding and discharge. The only agents currently in use against respiratory viruses are (1) amantadine and its methylated derivative rimantadine, which display activity against influenza A if given prophylactically and act by interfering with the ion flux mediated by the M2 channel-forming protein of the virus, thereby inhibiting its uncoating; and (2) ribavirin, a nucleoside analogue, which may be of value in severely ill infants with RSV bronchiolitis/pneumonia when administered as a small-particle aerosol. More recently, thanks to x-ray diffraction and cryoelectron microscopy techniques, sites on viral proteins essential for interaction with the host cell receptor or otherwise critical to the infectious process can be visualized. From this has blossomed the age of computer-aided drug design for the development of antivirals. Among the compounds already in clinical trial are those that block the enzyme active site of influenza neuraminidase, a glycoprotein whose role is to facilitate the release of progeny virions from infected cells and prevent self-aggregation of the virus. Others target a small hydrophobic pocket within the canyon region of the coat proteins of rhinoviruses; these drugs stabilize the coat proteins, thereby preventing uncoating and release of viral RNA for replication. Viral mutants resistant to these drugs can be derived in the laboratory but their significance *in vivo* remains to be established.

See also: **Adenoviruses (*Adenoviridae*): Animal viruses, General features, Malignant transformation and oncology, Molecular biology; Coronaviruses (*Coronaviridae*); Diagnostic techniques: Detection of viral antigens, nucleic acids and specific antibodies, Isolation and identification by culture and microscopy; Influenza viruses (*Orthomyxoviridae*): General features, Molecular biology, Structure of antigens; Parainfluenza viruses (*Paramyxoviridae*) – Human; Rhinoviruses (*Picornaviridae*); Vaccines and immune response; Interferons: General features, Therapy of aids and cancer; Immune response: Cell mediated immune response, General features; Antivirals.**

Further Reading

Brown LE, Hampson AW and Webster RG (eds) (1996) *Options for the Control of Influenza III.* Elsevier: Amsterdam.

Fenner F, Gibbs EPJ, Murphy FA et al (1993). *Veterinary Virology*, 2nd edn. San Diego: Academic Press.

Fields BN, Knipe DM, Howley PM et al (eds) (1996) *Fields Virology*, 3rd edn. Philadelphia: Lippincott-Raven.

Mims CA and White DO (1984) *Viral Pathogenesis and Immunology*. Oxford: Blackwell.

White DO and Fenner FJ (1994). *Medical Virology*, 4th edn. San Diego: Academic Press.

RETICULOENDOTHELIOSIS VIRUSES (*RETROVIRIDAE*)

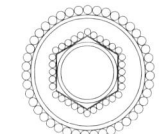

Radmila Hrdlickova, **Jiri Nehyba** and **HR Bose**, Department of Microbiology and Institute for Cellular and Molecular Biology, University of Texas, Austin, Texas, USA

Copyright © 1999 Academic Press

Introduction

The reticuloendotheliosis (RE) viruses constitute a small group of avian retroviruses which are genetically and immunologically unrelated to the avian leukosis-sarcoma viruses (ALSV) complex. Interesting aspects of RE viruses include their evolution, tumorigenicity, and the immunosuppression they induce.

Taxonomy, Classification and Evolution

RE viruses belong to the *Retroviridae*, a large family of RNA viruses that replicate through a DNA intermediate. Seven genera of retroviruses are recognized and the RE viruses belong to the same genus (*Betaretrovirus*) as the murine leukemia viruses (MLV). The RE group includes the acutely transforming reticuloendoeneliosis virus, strain T (REV-T), its helper virus, reticuloendotheliosis associated virus (REV-A), spleen necrosis virus (SNV), chicken syncytial virus (CSV), duck infectious anemia virus (DIAV), and other isolates from chickens, ducks, geese, pheasants and turkeys. A total of 26 replication-competent RE virus isolates have been biologically cloned. Only one acutely transforming replication-defective member (REV-T) has been identified. Three antigenic subtypes of RE viruses are distinguished on the basis of their reactivity with monoclonal antibodies, but all RE viruses belong to a single interference group. No endogenous RE viruses have been recognized.

Nucleotide sequence analysis has demonstrated that the RE viruses are more related to mammalian retroviruses than to the other avian retroviruses. The *gag* and *pol* sequences of RE viruses are closely related to gibbon ape leukemia virus (GALV), a primate type C retrovirus, whereas, the nucleotide sequences of *env* gene are approximately 50% identical at the amino acid level to those of simian type D retroviruses and two type C retroviruses – feline endogenous virus (RD114) and baboon endogenous virus (BAEV). All of these viruses share a common receptor. However, the *env* sequence of RE viruses also shares 30% identity at the amino acid level with the *env* sequence of GALV. The receptor of GALV appears to be a ubiquitous permease protein. It is likely, therefore, that the receptor for RE and primate type D oncoviruses is also a permease.

It has been proposed that a common ancestor of BAEV and RE viruses existed and was related to GALV (**Fig. 1**). This ancestor evolved an envelope protein which recognizes a new cellular receptor. From this retrovirus arose the RE virus group as a result of adaptation to avian species. The subgroup D primate viruses evolved by a recombination event between the proposed common ancestor of BAEV and the RE virus which provided the *env* gene and a subgroup B retrovirus. This recombination explains why the subgroup D primate viruses and RE viruses have a similar *env* sequence and share a common receptor.

Virion Structure, Genome and Proteins

RE virus particles have C-type particle morphology resembling MLV more closely than ALV virions. The viral particles are about 100 nm in diameter and are covered with surface projections approximately 6 nm long and 10 nm in diameter. The density of RE virions in sucrose is 1.16–1.18 g ml^{-1}, and RE viruses can be distinguished from those of the ALSV complex by morphology and by density gradient centrifugation. Cell-free stocks of RE viruses may be stored for long periods at −70°C. These viruses are relatively stable

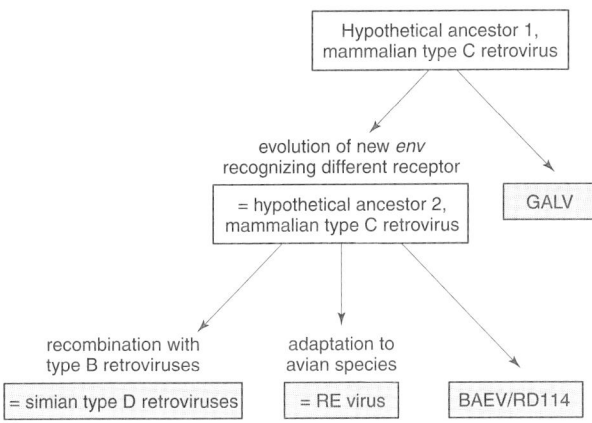

Figure 1 The suggested evolutionary relationship of RE viruses with GALV, BAEV/RD114 and simian type D retroviruses. The shaded boxes indicate currently existing retroviruses. The white boxes indicate hypothetical viral ancestors.

at 4°C but 50% of the infectivity is lost within 20 min when incubated at 37°C.

The genomic RNA of RE viruses consists of a 60–70S complex composed of two identical single-stranded (ss) RNA subunits about 3.9×10^6 Da. The genome of replication-competent RE viruses is approximately 8–9 kilobases (kb) and consists of *gag*, *pol* and *env* genes. The *gag* gene of RE viruses encodes five structural proteins, p10, p12, pp18/pp20 and p30. The *pol* gene encodes a protease (p15), a reverse transcriptase (p84) which is related to the Mn^{2+}-dependent group C mammalian retroviruses and an integrase which facilitates proviral integration (p44). The *env* gene encodes two glycoproteins – a gp90 surface unit and a gp20 transmembrane peptide. REV-T, which is replication-defective, has a genome about 5.7 kb since it contains extensive deletions in the *gag*, *pol* and *env* genes. The transforming gene of REV-T, *v-rel*, has been inserted into *env* sequences.

Replication

Entry of RE viruses is mediated by the envelope glycoproteins which bind to specific receptors on the cell surface. Entry of SNV is pH independent and may involve the direct fusion between the viral envelope and the cell membrane. Shortly after attachment and penetration of the virions, viral DNA is synthesized in the cytoplasm of the infected cell by the reverse transcriptase in uncoated viral cores. Linear as well as circular DNA copies of the retroviral RNA genome are found in the infected cells and the linear DNA serves as the immediate precursor for proviral integration. Two size classes of RNA – genomic-length and spliced subgenomic – are transcribed from the integrated provirus. Translation of genomic-length viral RNA results in the synthesis of two polyprotein precursors: the *gag* and *gag-pol* polyproteins (**Fig. 2**). The *gag* and *pol* genes are in the same reading frame and separated by a stop codon. Expression of the *gag-pol* polyprotein is dependent on stop codon suppression. The *gag* and the *gag-pol* polyproteins are proteolytically cleaved into mature *gag* and *pol* proteins by the virally encoded p15 protease. *Env* proteins are expressed from spliced viral RNA. The primary polyprotein precursor $gPr77^{env}$ is glycosylated and myristoylated and is converted into a second polyprotein precursor $gPr115^{env}$, which is rapidly proteolytically processed by a cellular protease to form gp90 and gPr22(E). A final modification of gp22(E), the transmembrane glycoprotein precursor, to mature gp20 occurs after its incorporation into the virion. The nucleocapsid is assembled in the cytoplasm as a ribonucleoprotein complex and acquires an envelope by budding through the plasma membrane. Release of virus particles begins approximately 24 h after infection.

Hosts and Tissue Tropism

RE viruses have been isolated from chickens, ducks, geese, Japanese quail and turkeys. They can replicate in a wide range of avian cells but specific species or a tissue tropism has not been described. RE viruses are also able to infect certain mammalian cells, including primate cells (HeLa and COS-7). Human cells transfected by SNV produce low levels of infectious virus. Although antibodies against p30 have been detected in human tissue, the health significance of these findings remains to be evaluated.

Immune Response

RE viruses are generally strongly immunosuppressive and the immunosuppression they induce may contribute to their virulence (see below, *Nonneoplastic diseases*). However, most birds are able to develop a strong immune response which efficiently controls the infection.

Humoral immunity

Birds infected at hatching or later develop a 'nontolerant' infection characterized by a transient viremia and antibody synthesis. Some birds develop a persistent virus infection which can be detected in peripheral blood lymphocytes in the absence of a viremia. Infection of embryos with RE viruses results in a 'tolerant' infection characterized by the lack of antibody production and by a viremia that can persist for 2 years. Also, neonatal bursectomy leads to the

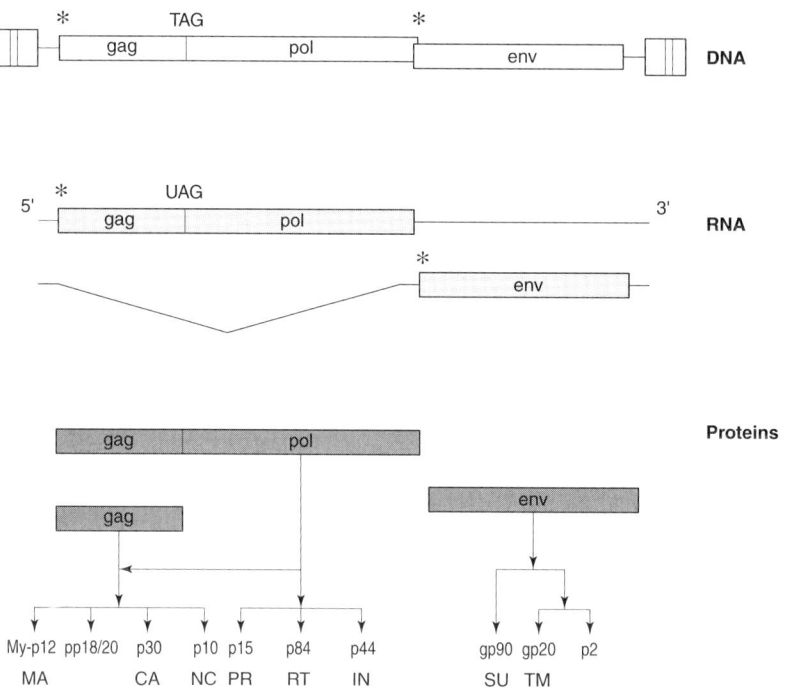

Figure 2 Genome structure, RNA splicing pattern and polyprotein processing pattern of RE viruses. White boxes indicate the genomic regions encoding proteins. Lightly colored boxes represent coding regions in genomic and spliced RNA and dark boxes represent translated proteins. Asterisks indicate the ATG/AUG codons known to be used in initiation of translation. The *gag* stop codon TAG/UAG is shown. The polyproteins and mature processed proteins derived from the *gag*, *pol* and *env* genes of RE viruses are shown. Proteins are designated according to molecular weight (kDa). The following designations are used: My-p, myristoylated protein; p, protein; pp, phosphoprotein; gp, glycoprotein; MA, *gag* matrix protein; CA, *gag* capsid protein; NC, *gag* nucleocapsid protein; PR, protease; RT, reverse transcriptase; IN, integrase; SU, *env* surface unit; TM, *env*, transmembrane protein. pp18/20 proteins are two differentially post-translation modified proteins encoded by the same *gag* sequence.

establishment of a tolerant infection, which suggests that B lymphocytes are involved in the elimination of the viremia. Tolerance to RE viruses does not depend on immunodepression. In contrast to nontolerantly infected chicken, tolerantly infected dams transmit the virus to their progeny but at low efficiency.

Cell-mediated immunity

Thymectomy increases the mortality of REV-T-infected birds suggesting the involvement of cell-mediated immunity in the elimination of RE virus-infected cells. Cytotoxic T lymphocytes (CTL) lyse virus-infected cells which present viral antigens in conjunction with the major histocompatibility complex (MHC) class I molecules. CTL are induced 7 days after infection with RE viruses and may persist at least 21 days. The CTL response against RE viruses is mediated by $\gamma\delta$ T CD8+, CD4− cells which express MHC class I and II molecules. RE viruses do not appear to activate natural killer cells.

Transmission, Diagnosis, Prevention and Control

Despite the fact that RE viruses are widespread in commercial poultry flocks, they do not create a real economical problem. However, the contamination of vaccines against Marek's disease virus (MDV) by RE viruses has been associated with a runting disease and chronic neoplasia. In addition, occasional outbreaks of neoplastic diseases in turkeys have also been described.

Both vertical and horizontal routes of transmission have been observed but at low levels in the viremic birds. Vertical infections may occur when viruses released from the mother contaminate the egg resulting in the infection of the embryo. Alternatively, infectious virus may be transmitted to the offspring from the semen of a viremic male. RE viruses are transmitted horizontally by contact and may also be transmitted by insects.

RE virus epidemics are prevented by testing commercial vaccines for contamination by these viruses. RE viruses can be detected by the presence of the viral genome, viral antigens, reverse transcriptase or the induction of a cytopathic effect by some strains. The sensitive polymerase chain reaction (PCR) and reverse transcriptase PCR can be used for detection of viral genomes. RE viruses specific antigens may be detected by immunofluorescence, complement fixation assays or enzyme immunoassays. Antibodies to RE viruses may be monitored by immunofluorescence, virus neutralization, agar-precipitation, Western blot analysis, enzyme immunoassays and pseudotype neutralization tests.

A commercial vaccine is not available since RE viruses do not create a significant economic impact. It is, however, feasible to develop an effective vaccine against RE viruses. Fowlpox virus recombinants expressing the *env* gene of SNV induce neutralizing antibodies and reduce the viremia and runting disease in infected chickens.

Pathogenesis

Nonneoplastic diseases

All replication-competent RE viruses induce to some degree a rapid and severe immunosuppression, in which T cells fail to undergo a blastogenic response to antigens or mitogens. This immunosuppression probably facilitates expression of the oncogenic potential of the virus and is responsible for the increased susceptibility of RE virus-infected birds to other pathogens. Other nonneoplastic disease syndromes include a runting disease syndrome, enlarged peripheral nerves, abnormal feather development, bursal and thymic atrophy and anemia. Several of these syndromes may be the direct or indirect consequence of the immunosuppression. These syndromes develop during the first month after infection and may either be transient or result in death.

The induction of nonneoplastic diseases by RE viruses correlates with their ability to induce a cytopathic response in cultured cells. The replication-competent RE viruses induce an acute infection characterized by an extensive cytopathic effect and cell killing. Large amounts of unintegrated and integrated proviral DNA accumulate in the infected cell during this acute phase. Surviving cells which replicate and become persistently infected contain much lower levels of both unintegrated and integrated proviral DNA. The correlation between the transient accumulation of large numbers of proviral DNA and the transient development of a cytopathic effect suggests that cell death results from the toxic effect of this DNA or proteins coded by this DNA.

The primary determinants of the runting disease syndrome have been mapped to distinct regions in the structural genes of RE viruses by comparing highly pathogenic REV-A with the less pathogenic CSV. Both *env* and *gag* sequences were necessary for the full expression of the pathogenic effect of REV-A. The *env* genes of REV-A and CSV encode the immunosuppressive peptide (ISP) which is conserved in a number of mammalian retroviruses including human T-cell leukemia virus (HTLV) I and II, feline leukemia virus, MLV and GALV. The murine env protein which contains the ISP, suppresses the proliferation of an interleukin-2-dependent cytotoxic T lymphocytes cell line, the mixed lymphocyte response of T and B cells, the respiratory burst of monocytes, immunoglobulin production, the cytolytic activity of natural killer cells, monocyte-mediated tumor cell killing and the production of γ-interferon by peripheral blood lymphocytes. Interestingly, ISP is an inhibitor of protein kinase C and this may explain its profound suppressive effect on immune cells. However, the sequence of ISP is conserved in both CSV and REV-A and, therefore, the other regions of the *env* genes of REV-A and CSV must be responsible for the difference in pathogenicity of these viruses. These *env* sequences may influence how the ISP immunosuppressive region is exposed on the virion surface accounting for the difference in pathogenicity between REV-A and CSV. The *gag* sequences may directly influence the replication efficiency of the virus. The matrix region of *gag* is responsible for the increased replication efficiency of REV-A in some cell types relative to other replication-competent RE viruses. Therefore, the cytopathogenicity and immunosuppressive ability of RE virus is most likely determined by *env*. By increasing replication ability, the *gag* sequence of REV-A also enhances the virulence of the virus.

Syncytia formation has also been observed in certain cell lines infected by RE viruses. The viral envelope glycoproteins expressed on the surface of the infected cell may interact with cellular receptors of neighboring cells, resulting in fusion and syncytia formation. This phenomenon may contribute to the pathology induced by RE viruses.

Chronic neoplasia

Two types of chronic neoplasia induced by replication-competent RE viruses have been described. In the first type, RE viruses induce B cell lymphomas after a relatively long latent period (17–35 weeks). Tumor induction may be prevented by surgical or chemical bursectomy. This type of disease is indistinguishable from lymphoid leukosis induced by ALV. As is the case with ALVs, RE proviruses are integrated upstream from the second exon (the first exon is a noncoding exon) of the c-*myc* locus in the same transcriptional orientation in these tumor cells. Invariably these RE proviruses have deleted the 5' LTR and/or large parts of the viral genome. When the 5' LTR is lacking, the 3' LTR becomes transcriptionally active leading to constitutive expression of c-*myc* RNA.

The second type of neoplasia induced by replication-competent RE viruses is a T cell lymphoma which develops after a shorter latent period (6 weeks) and does not involve the bursa. This lymphoma involves the thymus, but also the liver, spleen, heart and peripheral nerves. Induction of this T cell lymphoma is also associated with insertional activation of c-*myc*, but one half of the proviruses are oriented in the opposite transcriptional direction from the c-*myc* gene. Whereas some of the proviruses in these T cell lymphomas use the 3' LTR promoter to transcribe the downstream c-*myc* gene, others apparently activated a cryptic promoter located in the first intron of c-*myc*. This insertion pattern contrasts with that observed in B cell lymphomas induced by the same virus. The proviral integration pattern in these T cell lymphomas induce lower levels of c-*myc* and it has been suggested that T cell lymphomas can be induced at lower levels of c-*myc* than the B cell lymphomas.

Interaction with herpesvirus

Recently, the recombination of RE viruses with Marek's disease virus (MDV) an avian herpesvirus, has been described. This interaction represents the first example of genetic recombination between an RNA and a DNA virus. This phenomenon has important biological consequences for the transmission of RE viruses into cells which would otherwise not be susceptible to RE virus infection. The presence of RE viral sequences in MDV also alters MDV gene expression and pathogenesis. Co-infection of avian cells with MDV and RE viruses frequently leads to the integration of RE proviral sequences within the MDV genome. Although usually only the LTR sequences become stably integrated into the MDV genome, a complete infectious RE provirus has been detected in one case.

REV-T induced neoplasia

REV-T was initially isolated from a lymphoma of a turkey in 1958. Subsequently, it was discovered that the original isolate contains both REV-T which is a replication-defective virus encoding the v-*rel* oncogene and a replication-competent helper virus REV-A. In experimentally infected avian species REV-T induces tumors in the liver, spleen and other visceral organs and causes death within 2 weeks. REV-T transforms a number of cell types at different stages of differentiation including B and T cells, macrophage-like cells and dendritic cells and birds die from a lymphoproliferative disease. REV-T can transform these cell types *in vitro* and also morphologically transforms avian fibroblasts. REV-T-transformed fibroblasts have a distinct morphology, prolonged life-span and induce sarcomas in susceptible birds. REV-T(REV-A) can infect mammalian cells but fails to transform them. Transgenic mice which constitutively express the v-*rel* gene under the control of the *lck* promoter in T cells develop thymic lymphomas in approximately 10 months. However, these murine T cell tumors grow poorly in culture and they do not induce tumors in syngenic mice.

The role of v-*rel* mutations in transformation REV-T induces an acute neoplastic disease due to the expression of the v-*rel* oncogene. v-*rel* arose as a result of the transduction of the c-*rel* proto-oncogene into envelope sequences of REV-A. c-Rel is a member of the Rel/NF-κB family of transcription factors, a ubiquitously expressed group of proteins which participate in the control of cell proliferation, differentiation and apoptosis. The transduction of c-*rel* resulted in the deletion of 2 N-terminal and 118 C-terminal amino acids. Since c-*rel* was transduced into envelope sequences, translation of the v-*rel* subgenomic RNA results in the formation of an oncogene fusion protein with 11 amino acids of envelope protein at the N-terminus and 18 out-of-frame envelope sequences at the C-terminus. Two critical functions of c-Rel were lost or modified during the initial transduction event. The loss of the C-terminal amino acids of c-Rel removed sequences responsible for cytoplasmic anchoring allowing v-Rel increased nuclear access. The C-terminal deletion also removed a significant portion of the sequences involved in transactivation. v-Rel, therefore, activates transcription of some genes less efficiently than c-Rel. One of the genes immediately activated when Rel/NF-κB complexes translocate to the nucleus is IκB-α. IκB-α inhibits the ability of Rel/NF-κB complexes to regulate target genes through cytoplasmic retention and displacement of Rel/NF-κB complexes from DNA. v-Rel, because it has deleted a portion of its transactivation domain induces the transcription of IκB-α much more weakly and with reduced kinetics relative to c-Rel. Decreased IκB-α synthesis may lead to the constitutive activation of v-Rel in transformed cells.

Following the initial transduction event, v-*rel* sustained multiple mutations many of which altered the amino acid sequence of v-Rel and contribute directly to its oncogenicity. These mutations are

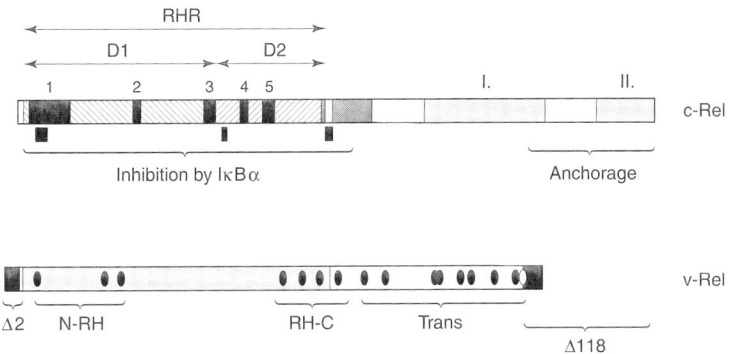

Figure 3 The functional domains of c-Rel and the position of mutations in v-Rel. The Rel homology region (RHR) consists of two domains D1 and D2. The five loops in the RHR that contact DNA directly are indicated by black boxes and numbered above. Loop 1 contains the major DNA recognition motif RxxRxRxxC. A hinge-like loop 3 connects domains D1 and D2. The region flanking D2 on the C-terminal side (white diagonals on black background) contains the nuclear localization signal indicated by the white box. The region of c-Rel that is both necessary and sufficient for inhibition of DNA binding of c-Rel by IκB-α is shown (Inhibition by IκBα). Small black boxes identify the amino acids believed to be in contact with IκB-α. Two transactivation domains (light gray boxes) and a cytoplasmic anchorage region (Anchorage) are present in the C-terminus. The RHR of v-Rel is represented by an intermediate color pattern. Mutated amino acids in v-Rel are indicated. Deletions of 2 N-terminal and 118 C-terminal amino acids resulting from the transduction of c-rel into REV-A are indicated below (Δ2, Δ118). The black boxes represent amino acids encoded by env-derived sequences which are fused to the truncated N- or C-termini. Internal mutations are identified by black or white ellipses. These mutated amino acids can be divided into three groups: N-RH, RH-C and Trans mutation clusters. The groups contain mutations that may affect a similar structural/functional domain. The N-RH and RH-C mutation clusters are situated at N- and C-termini of the RHR and contain, respectively, three and four single amino acid substitutions. A group of mutations designated Trans contains six single amino acid substitutions and three internal deletions of one or two amino acids. The majority of the Trans mutations are situated in the transactivation domain. (Adapted from Nehyba J, Hrdlickova R and Bose HR, Jr (1997) Differences in κB DNA-binding properties of v-Rel and c-Rel are the result of oncogenic mutations in three distinct functional regions of the Rel protein. *Oncogene* 14, 2881.)

located in several functional regions of v-Rel (**Fig. 3**). Two clusters of mutations are located in the N-terminus (N-RH) and C-terminus (RH-C) of the Rel homology region (RHR). The RHR is conserved among all members of the Rel/NF-κB family of transcription factors. This region contains the sequence responsible for DNA binding, dimerization, nuclear localization and IκB-α association. A third cluster of mutations (Trans) maps to the sequences in the C-terminus of v-Rel with the majority of them present in the transactivation region. The mutated amino acids in v-Rel are located in regions normally involved in the regulation of c-Rel. The functions of c-Rel including DNA-binding activity, the ability to form dimeric complexes as well as transcriptional activity are required for v-Rel to be transforming. The conversion of c-Rel into a highly oncogenic protein is due, therefore, to alterations which modify rather than eliminate the functional domains of c-Rel which are responsible for interacting with other proteins and/or DNA. The amino acid substitutions in the N-terminal part of RHR inside of or near the DNA contact motif are responsible for the altered DNA-binding specificity of v-Rel. Amino acid changes in the C-terminal portion of RHR, in the region responsible for dimerization, enables v-Rel to escape IκB-α-mediated inhibition of DNA binding. Finally, alteration in the amino acid sequence in the extreme C-terminal region of v-Rel may be responsible for altered transcriptional activity or may modulate the DNA-binding activity of v-Rel. These changes created an oncogenic protein which is no longer responsive to normal cellular regulatory constraints.

Altered gene expression in v-*rel* transformed cells Disruption of the ability of v-Rel to bind DNA abolishes its oncogenicity indicating that v-Rel must bind κB sites and directly alter gene expression in order to induce transformation. Although the role of some v-Rel mutations in the activation of the transformation potential of c-*rel* are known, how altered regulation of gene expression by v-Rel results in transformation remains largely unknown. Numerous genes have been identified in which the expression pattern is altered in cells transformed by REV-T. To date, all the genes which display an altered pattern of transcription in REV-T transformed cells are regulated by the Rel/NF-κB family members. These genes are listed in **Table 1**.

A few of the genes altered by v-*rel* expression are known to contribute to the transformed phenotype of v-Rel infected cells. The expression of the gene

Table 1 Genes induced by v-Rel. The genes are grouped into classes with similar function of their protein products. All genes were detected in avian cells unless indicated otherwise

Functional groups	Genes induced by v-Rel
Rel/NF-κB family	nfkb1, nfkb2, Ikba
Cell surface receptors	The MHC genes class I and II, DM-GRASP[a], the interleukin-2 receptor, p75 membrane protein, sca-2
Cytokines	mip-1β, ctca, CEF-4 (avian homologue of interleukin-8), interleukin-6[b], tumor necrosis factor-α[b]
Transcription factors	c-fos, c-jun, fra-2, interferon response factor 1 and 3, interferon consensus sequence-binding protein, the high-mobility-group protein 14b
Inhibitors of apoptosis	ch-IAP1
Structural proteins	δ-crystallin, vimentin, type I collagen α, β-tubulin
Proteins of oxidative metabolism	Mitochondrial cytochrome b
Chaperons	GRP-78

[a] Upregulated in T cell lymphomas in transgenic mice expressing v-Rel under the control of the lck promoter and in avian v-Rel transformed cells.
[b] Upregulated in T cell lymphomas in transgenic mice expressing v-Rel under the control of the lck promoter, not tested in avian v-Rel transformed cells.

encoding the cell surface receptor DM-GRASP and the cytokine *mip-1β* are altered in v-Rel transformed cells. Antibody against the DM-GRASP inhibits the *in vitro* proliferation of v-*rel*-transformed cells. The overexpression of *mip-1β* induces limited colony formation in soft agar and prolongs the life span of avian fibroblasts. Activation of an inhibitor of apoptosis, ch-IAP1, contributes to the immortalization of lymphocytes transformed by v-Rel. Expression of exogenous ch-IAP1 in temperature-sensitive v-Rel mutant transformed lymphocytes inhibits apoptosis of these cells at nonpermissive temperature. The fos/jun family of transcription factors also plays an important role in the Rel transformation pathway. v-Rel binds to the c-*jun* promoter inducing the constitutive expression of c-*jun* in transformed cells. Sup*jun*, a dominant inhibitor of c-*jun* significantly reduces the transformation efficiency by oncogenic Rel proteins.

v-Rel directly up- or downregulates genes which are normally under the control of c-Rel, but with different efficiencies. For example, the c-*jun* promoter is transactivated by v-Rel more efficiently than by c-Rel. The *Ikba* promoter is transcriptionally upregulated by both v-Rel and c-Rel, however, v-Rel is a much weaker inducer than c-Rel. To date, no genes have been identified which are activated by c-Rel but inhibited by v-Rel or the reverse. v-Rel, therefore, functions as constitutively activated c-Rel but modulates gene expression in a qualitatively different way than c-Rel. The differences in the DNA-binding specificity of v-Rel versus c-Rel may be partly responsible for this behavior. This suggestion is in agreement with the fact that v-Rel binds to the c-*jun* κB site with a higher affinity than c-Rel.

Retroviral Vectors

REV-A and SNV-based retroviral vectors have been successfully used to study retrovirus replication, recombination, cell transformation and to establish transgenic chickens. Moreover, several properties of RE viruses make them candidates for human gene therapy. The use of retroviral vectors for human therapy must address potential safety concerns. It is desirable to avoid homologous recombination which could reconstitute a replication-competent virus. Therefore, RE viruses are produced from packaging cell lines which express genes encoding structural retroviral proteins under the control of nonretroviral promoters. After transfection by the plasmid form of the retroviral vector which encodes only the desired therapeutic protein controlled by its own promoter, the viral RNA is packaged into virions. Unlike other retroviral vectors, RE vectors have no homology with structural genes coded by the packaging cell lines, therefore, replication-competent viruses are not produced. Also, it is essential that the retroviral vectors used in gene therapy are unable to undergo homologous recombination with endogenous viruses in target cells. Human cells do not contain endogenous RE virus sequences. The integration of the strong retrovirus LTR promoter/enhancer element into the DNA of target cells which could influence the transcription of neighboring genes must also be avoided. The construction of SNV-derived self-inactivating vectors which produce proviruses lacking LTRs addresses this safety concern.

The delivery of retrovirus vectors into specific cell types is also required for human therapy. The envelope protein of RE viruses contains multiple binding domains and, therefore, can tolerate the extensive modification associated with the introduction of cell specific targeting sequences. Retroviruses that recognize specific target cells have been generated by the incorporation of sequences encoding antigen binding sites into the *env* gene of SNV. These targeted SNV-derived vectors are very efficient at infecting specific human cell types.

See also: **Avian type C retroviruses (*Retroviridae*); Gibbon ape leukemia virus (*Retroviridae*); Murine leukemia viruses (*Retroviridae*); Retroviral Oncogenes; Recombination of viruses; Retroviruses – type D (*Retroviridae*); Vectors: Animal viruses.**

Further Reading

Coffin JM (1996) Retroviridae and their replication. In: Fields BN, Knipe DM, Howley PM *et al* (eds) *Fields Virology*, 3nd edn, p. 1767. New York: Lippincott-Raven.

Dornburg R (1995) Reticuloendotheliosis viruses and derived vectors. *Gene Ther.* 2: 301.

Gilmore TD (1995) Malignant transformation of cells by the v-Rel oncoprotein. In: Cooper GM, Temin RG and Sugden B (eds) *The DNA Provirus: Howard Temin's Scientific Legacy*, p. 105. Washington, DC: American Society for Microbiology.

Johnson ES (1994) Poultry oncogenic retroviruses and humans. *Cancer Detect. Prev.* 18: 9.

Payne LN (1992) Biology of avian retroviruses. In: Levy JA (ed.) *The Retroviridae*, vol. 1, p. 299. New York: Plenum.

Witter RL (1991) Neoplastic diseases/reticuloendotheliosis. In: Calnek BW, Barnes HJ, Beard CW, Reid WM and Joder HW, Jr (eds) *Diseases of Poultry*, 9th edn, p. 439. Ames: Iowa State University Press.

RETROTRANSPOSONS OF FUNGI

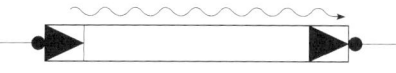

Jef D Boeke, Department of Molecular Biology and Genetics, Johns Hopkins University, Baltimore, Maryland, USA

Copyright © 1999 Academic Press

History

Transposable elements in eucaryotes can nearly all be classified into three basic types. The first type, typified by the Ac elements of plants and the P elements of *Drosophila*, resemble bacterial transposons in that they bear short inverted repeat termini; the available evidence strongly suggests that this type of element transposes directly via a DNA intermediate. However, most eucaryotic transposons differ from the bacterial elements in that they encode a reverse transcriptase (RT) or RT-like protein. Two basic types of these 'retrotransposons' are known – the LTR (long terminal repeat)-containing type, which are structurally highly reminiscent of retroviruses, and the poly(A)-type, which lack LTRs and usually (but not always) contain an oligo(A), poly(A) or similar sequence tract at their extreme 3′ end. These two types of retrotransposon are shown in **Fig. 1**. Both classes of retrotransposons are now known from organisms as phylogenetically distinct as fungi, trypanosomes, insects and mammals. Hence this brief review will focus on what is currently known about fungal retrotransposons, principally the retrotransposons that are more retroviral-like and are distinguished by the presence of LTRs. Thus, only a small and highly selective glimpse of the total picture of retrotransposons is provided.

Structural Features

The structural features of the known fungal retrotransposons are summarized in **Table 1**. LTR-containing retrotransposons isolated from fungi resemble retroviral proviruses in structure. They contain LTR sequences of a few hundred base pairs long flanking a central coding region that contains one or two open reading frames (ORFs), called *gag* and *pol* by analogy to the retroviral counterparts. As is the case with proviruses and DNA-based transposons, target site duplications of a fixed length flank the elements. These vary greatly in sequence and are presumably generated during the integration process

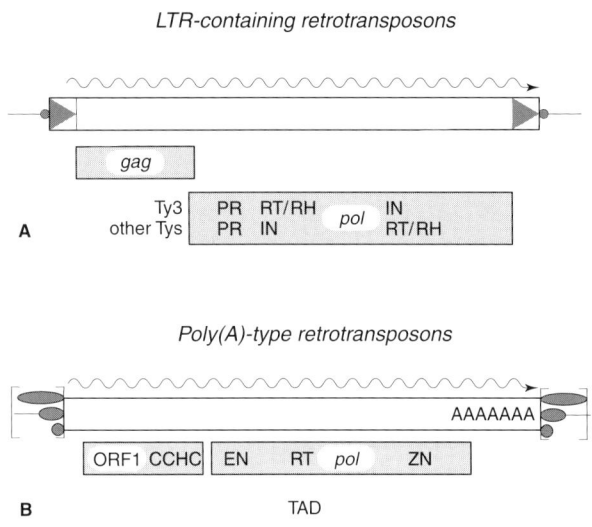

Figure 1 Retrotransposon types in fungi. All elements found to date in the yeasts, *Saccharomyces cerevisiae* and *Schizosaccharomyces pombe* are LTR-containing transposons (**A**). PR, protease; IN, integrase; RT, reverse transcriptase; RH, RNase H. Boxed triangles represent the LTRs; wavy line represents the transcript; shaded circles represent fixed-length target site duplications. Note that the order of functional domains differs between Ty3 (*Metaviridae*) and the other yeast elements (*Pseudoviridae*). (**B**) Two elements of the 'poly(A)' type have been found in the filamentous fungi (see **Table 1**). Note that unlike almost all members of this class of elements, TAD does not contain the 3′ poly(A) tract, but instead contains an AT-rich sequence. Abbreviations and symbols as above except: CCHC, retroviral Gag Zn-finger-like sequence; EN, endonuclease domain; FZN, zinc-finger-like domain found in *pol* genes of this class of elements; bracketed shaded ovals represent variable-length target site duplications.

by a transposon-encoded integrase function. In the cases where the RNA has been examined, it resembles retroviral genomic RNA in that it extends from LTR to LTR and is terminally repetitious, allowing definition of U3, R and U5 regions of the LTR sequence in a manner formally analogous to that used by retrovirologists. The elements with two ORFs clearly contain the equivalents of *gag* and *pol*, but no analogue of retroviral *env*. The elements with single ORFs, Tf1 and Tf2, (and possibly also Ty5) apparently translate a Gag/Pol fusion protein only. In all cases, the primary translation products are then cleaved into smaller final products by the element encoded aspartyl protease.

The elements with LTRs fall into two basic classes, distinguishable by the order of the functional domains in pol (see **Fig. 1**). In the class typified by Ty3, the RT domain precedes the IN domain, as it does in retroviruses. This family of elements has recently been classified as the *Metaviridae*. In the other type, typified by Ty1 and the other yeast elements except Ty3, the order of these domains is reversed. This family of elements has recently been classified as the *Pseudoviridae*.

Thus far there is only one report in the literature of a fungal retrotransposon that lacks LTRs, the TAD element from the filamentous fungus *Neurospora crassa* Adiopodoume strain, although structurally similar elements have now been isolated from other filamentous fungi. As these elements are much less retroviral-like, they are not reviewed here.

Transposition Mechanism

There is probably more known about the LTR-containing retrotransposons of fungi than about those of any other species. By far the most heavily studied elements are the Ty1 and Ty3 elements of *Saccharomyces cerevisiae*, and the Ty5 elements of the related species *Sac. paradoxus*, and the Tf1 elements of *Schizosaccharomyces pombe*. The life cycles of these

Table 1 Fungal retrotransposons

Host[a]	Element name	Type	ORFs	Target site duplication (bp)	LTR length (bp)	Primer (−) strand
Sac. cerevisiae	Ty1	LTR	2	5	334	tRNA$^{Met}_i$
Sac. cerevisiae	Ty2	LTR	2	5	334	tRNA$^{Met}_i$
Sac. cerevisiae	Ty3	LTR	2	5	340	tRNA$^{Met}_i$
Sac. cerevisiae	Ty4	LTR	2	5	371	tRNA^{Asn}
Sac. paradoxus	Ty5	LTR	1	5	250	tRNA$^{Met}_i$
Sch. pombe	Tf1,2	LTR	1	5	358	self-priming
N. crassa	TAD	polyA	2	14, 17	N.A.	?
M. grisea	MAGGY	LTR	2		253	
A. fumigatus	Afut	LTR	2	5	282	

[a] Generic abbreviations: *M.*, Magnaporthe; *Sac.*, Saccharomyces; *Sch.*, Schizosaccharomyces; *N.*, Neurospora; *A.*, Aspergillus.

are quite similar. In contrast, except for the presence of a cytoplasmic transposition intermediate, and evidence for reverse transcription during its transposition, relatively little is yet known about TAD transposition. This is because these poly(A)-type elements are generally less well known (and retroviral analogies are uncertain at best). Thus the discussion below applies to yeast Ty elements specifically, and to LTR retrotransposons generally.

A transposon copy (usually studied in the laboratory in the form of a *GAL* promoter/Ty element fusion) produces a transcript that extends from a point in the 5′ LTR to a different, downstream point in the 3′ LTR. Thus, a terminally redundant RNA is generated. This RNA is polyadenylated and exported to the cytoplasm, where it can have two different fates; it can serve (1) as an mRNA for Gag and Gag-Pol protein products and/or (2) as genetic material for transposition.

Translation of Ty elements is somewhat unconventional. Gag is produced directly by conventional translation of this mRNA, whereas Pol is expressed as a Gag-Pol fusion protein (readthrough protein); this 'frameshifting' process is mediated at a special sequence within the region of overlap of *gag* and *pol*. Both the Ty1 and Ty3 frameshifts differ from those of more conventional retroviruses in that they are +1 frameshifts rather than −1 frameshifts, and the intrinsic mechanism used to effect the frameshift is different. In the −1 frameshifts used by retroviruses, coronaviruses, and the yeast killer double-stranded RNA virus, a 'slippery site' allows for a simultaneous slip of the ribosome during the translational step in which the ribosomal P and A sites are simultaneously occupied. Stem–loop structures or pseudoknots that are often found just downstream of the slippery site are thought to cause ribosomal pausing and perhaps even to induce the ribosome to slip backwards. In contrast, the Ty1 element appears to utilize a completely different mechanism. There appears to be no requirement for any special RNA secondary structure; rather the frameshifting appears to be sequence-mediated, because a seven nucleotide sequence from the overlap region readily confers frameshifting on a heterologous reporter gene. Ribosomal pausing, thought to be required for frameshifting, is apparently caused by limiting amounts of a rare tRNA, $tRNA^{Arg}_{CCU}$. The stalled ribosome, which unlike the retroviral case, has an empty A site, has the P site occupied by a specific $tRNA^{Leu}$ that recognizes all six Leu codons. The stall caused by low $tRNA^{Arg}$ levels allows time for the slippage event to occur; the $tRNA^{Leu}$ slips to an overlapping Leu codon in the +1 (*pol*) frame. This then exposes a Gly codon recognized by an apparently abundant tRNA in the A site, allowing translation to continue in the *pol* frame. This mechanism results in an efficiency of frameshifting that varies somewhat with context, but on average is about 10–20%.

Once sufficient Ty protein products, in the form of intact Gag and Gag-Pol readthrough proteins, are produced, an assembly process that is not yet well understood begins. What follows is a working model for this assembly process, although this is based largely on interpretations of the limited experiments that have been done on Ty assembly and by analogy with retroviral systems and models. Ty RNA is apparently selectively packaged, together with at least one specific tRNA, the primer tRNA, into a capsid initially consisting of a coassemblage of unprocessed Gag and Gag-Pol proteins. Presumably, these coassemble via Gag-Gag interactions, and these are made in such a way that the C-termini of the proteins, and the RNA, reside in the internal cavity of the virus-like particle (VLP). The aspartyl protease encoded within *pol*, presumably activated by a dimerization process facilitated by the high protein concentration involved in the assembly process, then cleaves the precursor Gag proteins and Gag-Pol proteins to their mature, presumably physiologically relevant forms. This results in a change in the morphology of the VLPs, as well as an apparent activation of the endogenous reverse transcriptase activity.

Once reverse transcriptase is activated, the initial DNA products, corresponding to the left end of the transposon are synthesized, using a cellular tRNA as primer. This primer was recently shown to be $tRNA^{Met}_i$ for Ty1. Eventually, a full-length double-stranded (ds) DNA is made through a series of priming and DNA strand transfer events. In the Ty5 element, the same tRNA is apparently cleaved to form a half-molecule; the 5′ half-molecule is then used to prime reverse transcription. The identity of the enzyme that effects this cleavage is unknown.

In the Tf elements of *Sch. pombe*, a different type of reverse transcriptase priming occurs – self priming. In these unusual elements, the primer for reverse transcription is a piece of the retrotransposon RNA itself. The 5′ end of the RNA folds into a complex secondary structure, and an 11 nucleotide (nt) fragment is then released, apparently by the RNase H activity associated by the reverse transcriptase. A number of other retroelements from fungi and other organisms are thought to use a similar mechanism.

The dsDNA remains associated with Gag and Pol proteins such as reverse transcriptase inside the cell. These DNA-containing VLPs (isolated as a mixture of RNA-containing and DNA-containing VLPs) have been shown to contain all the macromolecular factors needed to carry out an *in vitro* transposition (integration) reaction. Like retroviral core particles, which have this same activity, these VLPs require only a divalent cation for activity. The Ty DNA is apparently synthesized inside VLPs inside the cytoplasm. It is interesting to consider how and in what form this DNA is delivered to the nucleus. This is a particularly interesting question to ask in yeast, because fungi, unlike mammalian cells, undergo a 'closed mitosis' in which the nuclear membrane does not break down and reform during each mitosis, but apparently remains intact. Recent experiments implicate a small basic amino acid sequence at the C-terminus of the integrase in this process. This 'nuclear localization signal' may be responsible for delivering not only the integrase but also the DNA to the nucleus.

Once the Ty DNA and Ty integrase enter the nucleus, a concomitant cleavage of host DNA and joining to transposon ends similar to that occurring during retroviral integration occurs. Ty3 is extremely selective for its integration, and apparently inserts only at the transcription initiation sites for RNA polymerase III. Ty1 also targets tRNA genes, but probably by recognizing a unique chromatin structure associated with their 5' ends. Ty5 elements appear to target 'silenced' chromatin. All of these mechanisms tend to ensure that these Ty elements will not destroy host genes, as most of the Ty targets do not encode genes, or at least not essential ones.

Virus-like Particles: Evolutionary Vestige or Transposition Intermediates?

The presence of VLPS in Ty elements has often raised the question of the evolutionary relationship between retroviruses and LTR-containing retrotransposons. Is the VLP a degenerate leftover of some decaying retrovirus? Or are LTR-containing retrotransposons a family of modern-day descendants of the precursor of the retroviruses? Presumably all retroelements descended ultimately from a 'cellular reverse transcriptase gene' as originally proposed by Temin. This gene may be ancient, and its original product may have been the molecule that archived the genetic information of the RNA world into DNA. Examination of the spectrum of modern-day retroelements from this perspective, reveals a natural progression from the simple to the very complex, as follows: starting with a simple RT gene (perhaps represented by modern-day telomerase?), to the poly(A)-type retrotransposons, which contain a second ORF in addition to RT, to the LTR-containing retrotransposons, which have the above plus LTRs, to the simple retroviruses, which have acquired a third ORF, *env*, and on to the most elaborate of all, the lentiviruses, with multiple additional regulatory reading frames in addition to the basic three. Since all LTR-containing retrotransposons studied appear to involve a VLP intermediate (that is, all examined to date have many properties of a transposition intermediate), the implication is that, as is the case in all complex biological reactions, a structure is built to ensure (1) high local concentration of numerous macromolecules required for the reaction and (2) appropriate orientations/conformations of these macromolecules to allow the reactions to proceed appropriately. The strongest support for this idea comes from studies on Ty1, which suggest that the VLP is a direct, functional transposition intermediate. Thus, if LTR-containing retrotransposons predated retroviruses, and their VLP structure evolved in response to selection for this organizing function, it does not stretch the imagination too far to suggest that these elements were 'preadapted' for subsequent selection for infectivity. In fact, one may see such transitional forms within the *gypsy* family of LTR-containing retrotransposons, in which some family members resemble the Tys in having two ORFs, but a few elements have

Table 2 Host genes affecting Ty1

Gene name	Normal function/product	Function for Ty1	Found by
Transcriptional effect genes			
SPT3, 7, 8	Transcription factor	Transcription initiation	Suppression of Ty- or LTR-induced mutation
SPT4, 5, 6	Chromatin factors	Transcription initiation	Suppression of Ty- or LTR-induced mutation
SPT10, 21	Repressor and activator	Repress 3' LTR	Suppression of Ty- or LTR-induced mutation
Post transcriptional effect genes			
IMT1-4	Translation initiation, tRNA$^{Met}_i$	Prime reverse transcription	Intentional mutagenesis of genes to reveal interaction
(none)	tRNA$^{Arg}_{CCU}$	Low level causes ribosome stalling, frameshifting	Search for genes which interfere with transposition when overexpressed
DBR1	Debranch intron lariats (2'-5' phosphodiesterase)	Unknown	Search for chromosomal mutations that interfere with transposition

a third *env*-like ORF in the appropriate genomic position.

Host Functions in Retrotransposition

The Ty1 system has provided some insights into the roles of host-encoded proteins and RNAs on the retrotransposition process, and it is anticipated that many more remain to be discovered. A large number of host genes that play roles in Ty and host gene transcription have been uncovered genetically; these are called *SPT* genes because they were originally identified by mutations that *su*ppressed the effect of Ty or LTR insertions. Although some of these affect Ty transcription, they do not affect the production of GAL/Ty mRNA. The development of sensitive assays for transposition of GAL/Tys *in vivo* has led to the identification of a number of host factors that are important for transposition at a post-transcriptional level; these are reviewed in **Table 2**.

See also: **Coronaviruses (*Coronaviridae*); Retroviruses – type D (*Retroviridae*); Yeast RNA viruses (*Totiviridae*).**

Further Reading

Boeke JD and Sandmeyer SB (1991) Yeast transposable elements. In: Broach J, Jones E and Pringle J (eds) *The Molecular and Cellular Biology of the Yeast Saccharomyces*. Cold Spring Harbor, NY: Cold Spring Harbor Laboratory.

Devine SE and Boeke JD (1996) Integration of the yeast retrotransposon Ty1 is targeted to regions upstream of genes transcribed by RNA polymerase III. *Genes Dev.* 10: 620.

Eichinger DJ and Boeke JD (1988) The DNA intermediate in yeast Ty1 element transposition copurifies with virus-like particles: cell-free Ty1 transposition. *Cell* 54: 955.

Kinsey JA (1990) *Tad*, a LINE-like element of *Neurospora*, can transpose between nuclei in heterokaryons. *Genetics* 126: 317.

Levin HL, Weaver DC and Boeke JD (1990) Two related families of retrotransposons from *Schizosaccharomyces pombe*. *Mol. Cell. Biol.* 10: 6791.

Levin HL (1995) A novel mechanism of self-primed reverse transcription defines a new family of retroelements. *Mol. Cell. Biol.* 15: 3310.

RETROVIRAL ONCOGENES

Paula J Enrietto and **Gabriela Maldonado-Codina**, Genomica Corporation, Boulder, Colorado, USA

Michael J. Hayman, Department of Molecular Microbiology and Genetics, SUNY at Stony Brook, Stony Brook, New York, USA

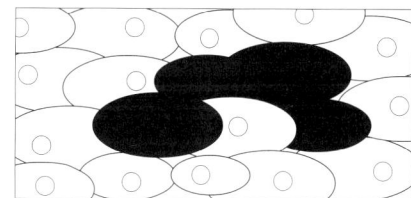

Copyright © 1999 Academic Press

Introduction

The role of viruses in the etiology of cancer was suggested by the work of Peyton Rous who isolated the first acutely transforming retrovirus, Rous sarcoma virus (RSV), from a chicken sarcoma. These viruses are highly oncogenic and induce malignant transformation of cells because of the presence of cellular sequences, oncogenes (v-*onc*) within the viral genome. The cellular sequences from which viral oncogenes are derived, proto-oncogenes, are cellular genes converted into oncogenes by mutation, rearrangement or deletion. Retroviral oncogenes are generally mutated versions of their respective proto-oncogene. These changes result from the transduction process and additional changes are acquired during viral replication. Consequently, the oncogenic potential of the viral oncogene is significantly enhanced when compared to the cellular oncogene.

In this entry we will focus on retroviral oncogenes, which will be discussed in functional groups. The description of oncogenes within each group is meant to be broad. Specific details have been excluded but can be found in the references listed at the end.

Nuclear Oncogenes

ErbA

V-*erbA* is found in the avian erythroblastosis virus, AEV-ES4 and -R strains, isolated in 1934 by Englebreth-Holm. AEV transduced two different oncogenes, v-*erbA* and v-*erbB*. V-*erbB* is a homologue of the epidermal growth factor receptor tyrosine kinase (see below).

The two *erb* genes are inserted between *gag* and *env* and are separated by an *erbB* intron sequence, which encodes the C-terminal four amino acids and termination codon of v-*erbA*. The 11 preceding Erb-A amino acids are encoded by *env* sequence. At the N-terminus a substitution of 254 amino acids encoded by the viral *gag* gene is also apparent. Giving rise to the protein product of v-ErbA, p75$^{gag\text{-}erbA}$, v-ErbA is derived from c-ErbA, the thyroid hormone receptor α (THRA1). V-ErbA is a mutated form of chicken THRA1. In addition to deletions resulting from transduction (nine amino acid N-terminal deletion and a 13 amino acid C-terminal deletion), V-ErbA has two point mutations in the DNA-binding domain and 11 in the hormone-binding domain. These changes result in the loss of hormone-binding capacity but do not abrogate sequence-specific DNA binding. The p75$^{gag\text{-}erbA}$ protein is localized to the nucleus. P75$^{gag\text{-}erbA}$ is phosphorylated on Ser16/17 by protein kinase A or protein kinase C. Mutation of the Ser16/17 phosphorylation site releases the block of erythroid differentiation exerted by v-ErbA.

THRA1 is a zinc-finger transcription factor, which binds to the response element TCAGGTCAT-GACCTGA, repressing its promoter activity. V-ErbA suppresses transcription of several genes, including avian erythrocyte anion transporter (band III), carbonic anhydrase II and β-globin genes. Transcriptional repression of erythrocyte-specific genes correlates with the biological properties of v-Erb-A and requires formation of heterodimeric complexes with retinoid X receptor (RXR).

V-ErbA is not tumorigenic but cooperates with v-Erb-B to cause avian erythroleukemia and fibrosarcomas. *In vitro*, v-ErbA blocks erythroid differentiation in cooperation with v-ErbB and other sarcoma-inducing oncogenes in transformation. V-ErbA stimulates chicken embryo fibroblast (CEF) growth and enhances the tumorigenicity of v-ErbB transformed fibroblasts.

Ets

The avian retrovirus E26, which carries the *ets* oncogene, was isolated in 1962 at the Bulgarian Academy of Sciences from a case of avian erythroblastosis. The E26 genome consists of deleted viral *gag* and *env* genes, a truncated version of *myb*, and *ets* (δgag-v-myb-v-ets-δenv). The *myb-ets* junction was created by an aberrant splice between a cryptic donor in *myb* and the normal splice acceptor in *ets* exonα. The result is the generation of five additional amino acids at this junction (HGTSE). Comparison of c-Ets (ETS-1) with v-Ets reveals amino acid substitutions at Ala285 and Ile445, which are replaced by Val in v-Ets. The 13 C-terminal residues of c-Ets have been replaced by 16 amino acid residues in v-Ets, 13 of which are derived from an inverted Ets-1 sequence. This results in a contiguous Gag-Myb-Ets open reading frame encoding a protein of 135 kDa, p135$^{gag\text{-}myb\text{-}ets}$ that is in the nucleus.

V-Ets is a member of a family of transcription factors that bind to DNA motifs containing (C/A)GGA (A/T) through a conserved 85 amino acid region called the Ets domain. V-Ets has less stringent target sequence requirements than c-Ets and binds to a broad spectrum of DNA sequence motifs, suggesting that v-Ets transforms cells by altering expression of tightly regulated genes with nonconsensus Ets binding sites.

The predominant disease induced by E26 in chickens is erythroblastosis. *In vitro*, both myeloid and erythroid cells can be transformed by E26, reflecting the fact that E26 also contains the myeloid-specific oncogene, v-Myb (see below). E26 transforms quail fibroblasts, NIH-3T3 cells, immature erythroid cells, and stimulates proliferation of CEF.

Fos

The *fos* oncogene is carried by the Finkel–Biskis–Jinkins (FBJ-MSV) and Finkel–Biskis–Reilly (FBR-MSV) murine osteogenic sarcoma viruses. Dr Miriam Finkel isolated both viruses from mice with ^{90}Sr-induced osteosarcomas. A virus isolated from an avian nephroblastoma, NK24, also contains the *fos* gene. The genome structures of FBJ and FBR-MSV differ significantly. FBJ-MSV contains v-*fos* and has no additional viral structural gene information, whereas FBR-MSV v-*fos* is fused to *gag* and non-*fos* sequences from the *fox* gene.

FBJ-MSV has five amino acid changes compared to c-Fos. A 104 bp deletion shifts the reading frame resulting in a C-terminus with 49 novel amino acids. Comparison with c-Fos reveals that FBJ-MSV v-Fos has lost 24 amino acids at the N-terminus (replaced with 310 gag amino acids) and 98 C-terminal amino acids (replaced with eight amino acids from fox). There are two C-terminal in frame deletions of 13 and 9 amino acids. The NK24 virus expresses an unaltered Fos protein linked to the gag encoded sequence.

The FBJ-MSV Fos protein product is 39 kDa, whereas the FBR-MSV fusion protein is p75$^{gag\text{-}fos\text{-}fox}$. Fos is a member of the helix–loop–helix/leucine zipper transcription factor superfamily. Each member of the family contains a basic domain, a leucine zipper, two homology boxes (HOB1 and HOB2) within a transactivation domain, and a *trans*-repression domain. FBJ-MSV and FBR-MSV both lack the *trans*-repression domain at the C-terminus. Both FBJ and FBR-MSV v-Fos proteins are localized in the nucleus.

FBR-MSV v-Fos, but not FBJ v-Fos, is myristylated at the N-terminus. Both proteins are phosphorylated on serine and threonine residues but not to the same extent as c-Fos, as the predominant phosphorylation sites on c-Fos are within the C-terminal sequences deleted from v-Fos. A basic motif, KCR, is conserved in the Fos family and redox-regulation of the cysteine residue mediates DNA binding. All Fos proteins display DNA binding activity at a site (TGAc/GTCA) termed either activating protein-1 site (AP-1) or TPA response element (TRE) and form heterodimers with Jun proteins. These function as positive or negative transcription regulators binding to DNA via the basic domain.

FBJ, NK24 and FBR-MSV transform fibroblasts *in vitro*. FBR immortalizes murine cells in culture, while FBJ does not. Transforming ability appears to correlate with the presence of a C-terminal transactivation domain.

Jun

Avian sarcoma virus 17 (ASV17), which contains V-Jun, was isolated from a chicken sarcoma in 1987; 220 viral Gag residues (p19 and δp10) are joined in frame to 296 Jun-encoded amino acids. Comparison to c-Jun reveals a 27 amino acid deletion in the N-terminus of v-Jun and three nonconservative substitutions in the C-terminal half; two of which are in the DNA binding domain. The v-Jun protein product p65$^{gag-jun}$ is localized in the nucleus and has several domains: the A1 activator domain, two homology box regions, HOB1 and HOB2, the ε region and δ region (the region of 27 amino acids deleted in v-Jun), A2 activation domain, and a Pro/Gln-rich ancillary DNA-binding domain. The primary DNA-binding domain, a basic region and leucine zipper, are in the C-terminal 110 residues. This region and the activation domain are necessary for transformation by Jun. V-Jun forms heterodimers with members of the Fos family and Fos-related antigens (FRA1 and FRA2) and binds with high affinity to a TPA response element (TGAc/gTCA), TRE.

Oncogenic activation of c-Jun results from 27 amino acid deletion in the N-terminus. This region contains a MAP kinase site allowing for control of c-Jun activity by phosphorylation. V-Jun is not subject to control by phosphorylation. Two of the three nonconservative amino acid substitutions may be important functionally. A Ser222 to Phe mutation prevents the glycogen synthase kinase-3 phosphorylation of a negative regulatory site. Mutation of Cys248 to Ser disrupts the oxidation of Cys248, inactivating DNA binding.

V-Jun induces tumors when injected into the wing web of young chicks. *In vitro*, v-Jun transforms chicken embryo fibroblasts.

Maf

The v-*maf* oncogene was identified in an avian retrovirus, AS42, isolated from a spontaneous musculoaponeurotic fibrosarcoma of chicken. The v-*maf* gene is inserted into the viral genome in the *gag* gene and v-*maf* encodes a 42 kDa basic region/leucine zipper protein, which is localized in the nucleus. The coding region of v-*maf* has only two structural changes when compared to c-*maf*.

V-Maf and other Maf family members form homodimers and heterodimers with each other and Fos and Jun. The DNA target sequence to which Maf binds is termed the Maf response element (MARE). It is a 13 or 14 bp element that contains a core TRE or CRE palindrome.

In vitro v-Maf transforms avian fibroblasts. *In vivo* the virus induces musculoaponeurotic fibrosarcomas.

Myb

The v-*myb* oncogene is found in two acutely transforming avian retroviruses, avian myeloblastosis virus (AMV) and E26. AMV v-*myb* replaces 26 codons at the 3′ end of *pol* and most of *env*. There are 6 *gag*-coded amino acids at the N-terminus and 11 *env* amino acids at the C-terminus. E26 v-*myb* is fused in frame with v-*ets*, see above. Comparison of AMV v-*myb* with c-*myb* revealed extensive 5′ (71 N-terminal amino acids) and 3′ (198 C-terminal amino acids) deletions and 11 point mutations. E26 v-Myb lacks 80 N-terminal and 278 C-terminal amino acids of c-Myb and has one point mutation.

The AMV v-Myb protein product is p45^{v-myb}. The E26 v-Myb protein product is p135$^{gag-myb-ets}$. Both proteins are nuclear. C-Myb contains a DNA-binding domain with three repeat regions, R1, R2, R3, transactivation domain, leucine zipper, *trans*-repression domain and a conserved domain in the C-terminus. N-terminal deletions in AMV v-Myb remove most of the R1. The C-terminal conserved region is also deleted. E26 v-Myb lacks almost all of R1, the leucine zipper region, the MAPK/CDC2 site, and the conserved domain. All Myb related genes contain a Cys residue at position 65.

Phosphorylation of a casein kinase II site at the N-terminus decreases c-Myb DNA binding. This site is absent in both E26 and AMV v-Myb. A MAPK/CDC2 site in the C-terminus of c-Myb is not phosphorylated in AMV v-Myb. V-Myb binds directly to double stranded DNA and regulates transcription through a consensus site YAACT/(C)/GGYCA. V-Myb regulates the expression of mim-1 and c-Myb.

AMV induces myeloid leukemia in chickens. *In vitro*, AMV transforms macrophage precursors (monoblasts). E26 transforms fibroblasts, myeloid and, as a result of the presence of ets, erythroid cells.

Myc

The v-*myc* gene was first identified in avian myelocytomatosis virus, MC29, but was subsequently found in four other virus isolates, CMII, OK10, MH2 and FH3. All the v-*myc* genes are highly homologous and contain only eight single nucleotide changes when compared with c-*myc*. MC29 contains deleted *gag*, 422 v-*myc* amino acids, no *pol* and a complete *env* gene. CMII contains deleted *gag*, 421 v-*myc* amino acids, and complete *pol* and *env* genes. OK10 contains all of *gag*, 426 v-*myc* amino acids, deleted *pol* and *env* genes. P58$^{\delta gag\text{-}myc}$ is a second Myc protein product translated from a subgenomic RNA, which contains a small piece of *gag* sequence at the N-terminal end. MH2 contains deleted *gag* and *env* genes and 417 v-*myc* amino acids and a second oncogene, *mil*, which is homologous to v-*raf*. FH3 contains deleted *gag* gene and 421 *myc* amino acids.

All v-*myc* genes are expressed as fusion proteins with viral structural information. MC29: P110$^{\delta gag\text{-}myc}$; CMII: P90$^{\delta gag\text{-}myc}$; OK10: P200-gag$^{\delta pol\text{-}myc}$, P58$^{\delta gag\text{-}myc}$; MH2: P57$^{\delta gag\text{-}myc}$; FH3: P145$^{\delta gag\text{-}myc}$. Several functional domains have been defined in the Myc family. A central acidic region influences the transforming host range of v-Myc proteins. Two nuclear localization signals have been defined. The C-terminus contains elements essential for DNA binding, a basic region, a helix–loop–helix motif and a leucine zipper. All v-Myc proteins are localized to the nucleus except P200$^{gag\text{-}\delta pol\text{-}myc}$, which is found in the cytoplasm and the nucleus. The Ser62 is phosphorylated by MAP kinases, lies in a highly-conserved proline-rich region and carries transcriptional activation capacity.

Myc forms a sequence specific (CACGTG) DNA binding heterodimer with a helix–loop–helix protein, Max. The leucine zipper and the helix–loop–helix region are required for heterodimer formation. Both positive and negative regulation of gene expression has been associated with Myc family members.

In vivo, MC29, CMII or FH3 cause myelocytomatosis. MC29, MH2 or OK10 cause liver and kidney carcinomas. *In vitro*, MC29, CMII, OK10, MH2 or FH3 transform immature macrophages or fibroblasts. Primary fibroblasts are immortalized by v-Myc but are rendered tumorigenic only when an activated Ras is also expressed.

Rel

V-*rel*, the oncogene in avian reticuloendotheliosis virus strain T (REV-T), was isolated from a turkey with lymphoid leukosis. V-Rel is a member of the NF-κB family of transcription factors. Incorporation of c-*rel* into the viral genome resulted in truncation of *gag*, *pol* and *env*. Using the *env* initiation codon, v-*rel* begins with 12 *env* amino acids and ends with 18 amino acids which are out of frame with respect to *env*. Comparison of v-Rel and turkey c-Rel revealed that v-Rel has lost two N-terminal amino acids and 118 amino acids at the C-terminus. V-Rel has 14 amino acids changes, ten of which are nonconservative, and three sites of deletion where a total of five amino acids are deleted.

The protein product of v-*rel* is p59$^{v\text{-}rel}$, which is localized to both the cytoplasm and nucleus of infected cells. At the N-terminal end of v-Rel is the Rel homology domain, a DNA-binding domain conserved in all members of the NF-κB family. This region also specifies nuclear localization and protein–protein interaction. C-Rel contains sequences in the C-terminus important for cytoplasmic retention and transcriptional activation which are deleted from v-Rel. In the cytoplasm, v-Rel exists in a complex with several other cellular proteins, including the inhibitor IκB. Dissociation of IκB from this complex allows translocation of v-Rel to the nucleus. V-Rel forms heterodimers with other members of the NF-κB family and binds to NF-κB motifs (NGGNN^A/TTTCC). In most cells, v-Rel represses gene expression; however, in transformed avian cells v-Rel activates transcription of MHC class I, HMG 14b, NF-κB, macrophage inflammatory protein-1 and an interleukin (IL)-8 related gene.

In vivo, REV-T causes acute reticuloendotheliosis. *In vitro*, v-Rel transforms a bone marrow-derived dendritic cell precursor, spleen-derived lymphoid cells, and fibroblasts.

Qin

The *qin* oncogene is the cell-derived insert in the genome of the avian sarcoma virus, ASV31. V-Qin is fused to Gag sequences at the N-terminus and eight cell coded amino acids link the cellular *qin* coding domain with the viral *gag* domain. Comparison of v-Qin with chicken c-Qin demonstrated several differences between the two. There are two non-conservative amino acid substitutions in the Qin coding region, a truncation in the C-terminus of the viral protein due to a premature stop codon. V-Qin is a nuclear protein.

V-Qin contains two domains: a winged helix domain and a repression domain. Regions between residues 74–141 and 383–395 are required for transformation. Qin is a member of the winged helix transcription factor family which function as important regulators of embryonal development and tissue differentiation in vertebrates and invertebrates, regulating expression of a number of genes. It is most closely related to brain factor-1. Qin also functions as a transcriptional repressor.

In vivo ASV31 induces fibrosarcomas in chickens. *In vitro*, the virus transforms avian fibroblasts.

Ski

V-ski is the oncogene found in the Sloan–Kettering viruses, SKV. Inially two molecular weight forms of v-Ski proteins were described. A 125 kDa form, in which the *ski* sequence was inserted into the *gag* gene, and a 110 kDa form, which was derived from the former via deletion of *gag* sequence 3′ to the *ski* gene resulting in a Gag-Ski-Pol fusion protein. Both proteins are located in the nucleus of infected cells. By comparison to the c-Ski protein, v-Ski is truncated at both the N- and C-terminus. Both v-Ski and c-Ski can transform fibroblasts and so these truncations do not seem to be essential for oncogenic activity.

Ski has several protein motifs, including two amphipathic helices which are required for transforming activity. Ski can both transform cells and induce differentiation of muscle cells. The exact function of ski is unknown. However it appears to be capable of acting as a repressor of retinoic acid-induced transcription and this may be important for hematopoietic cell transformation. It can also activate transcription and this may be important for its effects on differentiation.

In vivo ski can effect the differentiation of muscle cells. It can also cause fibrosarcomas and stem cell leukemia when coexpressed with the v-*sea* oncogene. *In vitro* it can transform fibroblasts and hematopoietic cells.

Growth Factors

Sis

The v-*sis* oncogene is the transforming oncogene of the simian sarcoma virus. The oncogenic sequences of the Parodi–Irgens (PI) FSV are homologous with the v-*sis* sequences of the simian sarcoma virus but very little is known about this feline virus-encoded protein. The v-*sis* oncogene product is a protein of 28 kDa, which shares 92% homology with the platelet-derived growth factor (PDGF) B chain. *V-sis* is presumed to transform cells via autocrine activation of the endogenous PDGF receptor. The location of these autocrine interactions between the v-Sis protein and PDGF receptors remains somewhat controversial; however, it is thought that internal autoactivation of PDGF receptors may be essential for transformation by v-Sis. V-Sis can transform fibroblasts in culture and causes fibrosarcomas *in vivo*.

Protein Tyrosine Kinases

Abl

The v-*abl* oncogene was originally found in the Abelson murine leukemia virus. Subsequently the Hardy–Zuckerman 2, HZ2, feline sarcoma virus was also found to have transduced the feline *abl* gene. The protein encoded by the murine v-*abl* oncogene is a 160 kDa fusion protein, p160, which contains N-terminal gag sequences and is a truncated version of the cellular *c-abl* gene. A 120 kDa protein encoded by a variant Abelson MuLV has been described, in which 263 codons have been deleted from the middle of the p160 sequence. The feline v-Abl protein is a fusion protein of 110 kDa, which is comprised of N-terminal Gag sequences followed by Abl sequences and then sequences from the viral *pol* gene. The c-Abl protein is composed of several structural motifs. An SH3 domain is located close to the N-terminus, followed by an SH2 domain, then the tyrosine kinase domain, and a DNA-binding domain followed by an F-actin-binding domain has been located at the C-terminus. The murine p160 v-Abl protein contains all of these domains, apart from the N-terminal SH3 domain. In contrast, the feline v-Abl protein contains the SH3, SH2 and kinase domains, but lacks the C-terminal DNA-binding and actin-binding domains. A model has been proposed in which association of the N-terminal SH3 domain with C-terminal sequences keeps the tyrosine kinase activity of the c-Abl protein in an inactive state. This model would predict that the murine v-Abl protein would be an active kinase due to the loss of the SH3 domain, and the feline v-Abl protein would also be active owing to the loss of the C-terminal sequences. Consistent with this model, both v-Abl proteins are constitutively active tyrosine kinases and this activity is essential for their transforming abilities.

The v-Abl protein is located at the plasma membrane of the cell by virtue of the myristylated N-terminus provided by the Gag sequences. This is in contrast to the cellular Abl protein, which is primarily found in the nucleus of the cell. These myristylation sequences not only direct membrane localization but also activate tyrosine phosphorylation and are necessary for cell transformation. *In vivo* the murine Abelson MuLV causes lymphocytic leukemias, whereas the feline HZ2 virus causes multicentric sarcomas. *In vitro* v-Abl can transform fibroblast cell lines and also transforms hematopoietic cells of the myeloid and lymphoid lineages. The transformation of these hematopoietic cells is of particular interest as the *c-abl* gene is rearranged by a balanced translocation between chromosomes 9 and 22, (t9;22)[q34;q11], in over 95% of the human malignancy chronic myelogenous leukemia (CML). This translocation forms a fusion protein between Bcr and Abl that gives rise to a constitutively active tyrosine kinase similar to the v-Abl proteins.

ErbB

The v-*erbB* oncogene was originally identified in the replication-defective avian erythroblastosis virus AEV-ES4. This retrovirus also contains the *erbA* oncogene (see above, Nuclear Oncogenes). The AEV-H strain of avian erythroblastosis virus also contained the *erbB* oncogene but did not contain any other oncogenes. This identified *erbB* as the oncogene that was primarily responsible for the induction of disease. In addition to erythroblastosis, AEV-ES4 and AEV-H also caused fibrosarcomas. A specific strain of chickens, L15, is very susceptible to erythroblastosis induced by avian leukosis virus, and analysis of these diseased birds demonstrated that the *erbB* oncogene was activated by retroviral insertions into the *c-erbB* gene. Furthermore the *erbB* sequences were frequently transduced into the retroviral genomes, giving rise to new strains of avian erythroblastosis viruses that encoded v-ErbB proteins. These proteins have sustained the N-terminal truncations but not the C-terminal truncations. Upon further passage, AEVs acquire the ability to cause other tumors in addition to erythroblastosis, for example fibrosarcomas and angiosarcomas. This increase in oncogenic potential is associated with point mutations and deletions within the cytoplasmic region of the ErbB protein.

The *erbB* oncogene is a truncated version of the epidermal growth factor receptor (EGFR). The EGFR is a member of the tyrosine kinase family of growth factor receptors. In comparison to the EGFR, the different forms of ErbB have been truncated at the N-terminus and frequently they are also truncated at the C-terminus. The N-terminal truncations all involve deletion of the ligand-binding domain of the EGFR and this results in constitutive activation of tyrosine kinase activity. The v-ErbB proteins of AEV-ES4 and AEV-H are glycoproteins of approximate molecular mass 74 kDa, which are located at the plasma membrane. Kinase activity and membrane localization are necessary for full oncogenic potential. The EGFR can induce mitogenic signals, which are accompanied by tyrosine phosphorylation of several cellular substrates. Presumably the constitutive activation of v-ErbB leads to the activation of similar substrates. V-ErbB is a much more powerful oncogene than the EGFR, thus the possibility exists that the mutations have somehow altered the specificity of v-ErbB for some substrates. To date no novel substrates for v-ErbB have been identified. Potential substrates identified in v-ErbB transformed include caldesmon, the catenin-like protein p120cas, Shc and Stat5b. In addition, the Grb2 adapter protein binds to v-ErbB and the mitogen-activated protein kinase pathway is constitutively active.

Eyk (ryk)

The v-*eyk* oncogene was found in the avian retrovirus RPL30. It was originally termed v-*ryk*, but the name was changed to avoid confusion with another gene that had been previously termed *ryk*. The v-*eyk* sequences are 1.39 kb in length and code for a tyrosine kinase domain that is fused in frame to the gp37 Env sequences. Unlike other acute transforming retroviruses, the transduction of the v-*ryk* gene did not result in the loss of viral sequences. The v-Eyk protein is first synthesized as a 150 kDa precursor Env-Eyk fusion protein. This protein undergoes the normal proteolytic processing of the *env* gene product to release the Env protein gp85 and a gp69 fusion protein containing gp37 and Eyk sequences. The gp69 protein is located in the membrane of transformed cells and possesses tyrosine kinase activity. C-Eyk encodes a receptor-type tyrosine kinase of 974 amino acids, which is a member of the UFO/Axl/Ark subfamily of receptors. The v-Eyk sequences are truncated by comparison to c-Eyk and have lost the regions that encode the extracellular and transmembrane domains; in addition there are two amino acid changes. RPL30 causes fibrosarcomas when injected into chickens and the cloned *eyk* gene can transform chicken embryo fibroblasts *in vitro*.

Fes/fps

The *fes/fps* oncogene has been isolated from both avian and feline sarcoma viruses. It was identified in the avian viruses: Fujinami sarcoma virus, Poultry Research Center viruses II and IV, PRCII, PRCIV, University of Rochester virus 1, UR1 and 16L. The name *fps* was derived from Fujinami-PRCII Sarcoma, as these were the first two viruses described to contain this gene. The cognate oncogene *fes* was found in the Snyder–Theilen, Gardner–Arnstein and Hardy–

Zuckerman 1 strains of feline sarcoma viruses and the name is derived from *feline sarcoma*. The c-*fps/fes* oncogene encodes a cytoplasmically located 98 kDa protein tyrosine kinase that contains an SH2 domain. All of the viral Fps/Fes forms are fusion proteins between N-terminal Gag sequences and fps sequences. The v-Fps/Fes sequences have lost the N-terminus of Fps/Fes but retain the SH2 domain and the tyrosine kinase domain. The v-Fps/Fes proteins are of varying sizes: Fujinami sarcoma virus v-Fps is 140 kDa; PRCII v-Fps is 105 kDa; PRCIV v-Fps is 150 kDa; 16L v-Fps is 142 kDa; UR1 v-Fps is 150 kDa; ST-FSV v-Fes is 85 kDa; GA-FSV v-Fes is 95 kDa; and HZ1-FSV v-Fes is 100 kDa.

The fusion of the Fps/Fes sequences to Gag is sufficient to activate the transforming potential. This fusion seems to be important for the activation of the tyrosine kinase and membrane location of the virally-encoded proteins. Although the feline proteins have lipid modification, there is no evidence of myristylation for any of the avian proteins. *In vitro* the v-Fps proteins can transform fibroblasts and *in vivo* these viruses cause fibrosarcomas and/or myxosarcomas. The tyrosine kinase activity of the Gag-fusion proteins is essential for transformation, and the identity of several cellular substrates is known. These include the GTPase-activating protein, the Shc adapter protein and fibronectin receptor proteins. A key pathway involved in transformation appears to be the Ras pathway, as microinjection of anti-Ras antibody blocks Fps-induced transformation. Interestingly the Bcr protein, which is fused to the Abl oncoprotein in CML, has recently been identified as a substrate of the Fps/Fes kinase. Phosphorylation of BCR provides a docking site for Grb-2 and in this way links Fps/Fes to Ras activation.

Fgr

The v-*fgr* oncogene was first identified in the Gardner–Rasheed feline sarcoma virus, GR-FSV and was subsequently found in the Theilen–Petersen feline sarcoma virus, TP1-FSV. Fgr encodes a cytoplasmic tyrosine kinase activity and is a member of the Src family. In the GR-FSV virus the *fgr* sequences are expressed as a fusion between Gag, followed by γ-actin and then the Fgr sequences to generate a 70 kDa protein. In the TP1-FSV the Gag sequences are fused to the Fgr sequence to generate an 83 kDa protein. The Gag sequences are myristylated and this explains the plasma membrane location of the v-Fgr protein. There is no actin domain in the TP1 v-Fgr protein, and in fact deletion of this region from the GR-FSV v-Fgr protein actually increases both tyrosine kinase activity and transformation.

In vitro Fgr has been shown to transform most mammalian fibroblasts. *In vivo* the GR-FSV causes fibrosarcomas and rhabdosarcomas upon infection of kittens. The c-Fgr protein is a 55 kDa protein tyrosine kinase that is most abundantly expressed in hematopoietic cells. c-*fgr* mRNA levels are increased up to 50-fold in Epstein–Barr virus-associated lymphoproliferative disease; however, viral infection does not readily lead to tumors of hematopoietic cells.

Fms

The *fms* oncogene is the transforming oncogene of the Susan McDonough (SM-FSV) and Hardy–Zuckerman 5 strains of feline sarcoma virus. C-Fms is a growth factor receptor tyrosine kinase that is activated by the ligand, macrophage colony-stimulating factor, CSF-1. V-Fms protein is initially synthesized as a Gag-Fms fusion protein in which the Gag sequences are rapidly removed upon cleavage at the Fms-signal peptide sequence. V-*fms* and c-*fms* encode mature glycoproteins of approximately 140 kDa in size that differ in a few scattered amino acids and at the C-terminus, where in the SM-FSV encoded protein the last 50 amino acids of c-Fms have been replaced by 14 residues that come from c-*fms* 3′ untranslated sequences. This substitution has removed a C-terminally-located tyrosine residue, which plays a role in activating the oncogenic potential of v-Fms. V-Fms is a constitutively activate tyrosine kinase and, of the scattered amino acid changes, the substitution of two serine residues in the extracellular domain seems to be particularly important in activating the tyrosine kinase. Membrane localization and tyrosine kinase activity are necessary for transformation. V-Fms-transformed cells contain similar tyrosine phosphorylated substrates to those seen following c-Fms activation, for example PI3-kinase. Interestingly, tyrosine residue 809 is involved in Myc gene expression and this seems to be key for mitogenesis induced by Fms.

In vivo SM-FSV causes fibrosarcomas and does not normally induce hematopoietic malignancies in spite of the fact that v-Fms is derived from the receptor for CSF-1; however *in vitro* v-*fms* can induce the growth factor-independent growth of CSF-1 dependent cell lines in addition to transforming fibroblast cell lines.

Kit

V-*kit* is the oncogene found in Hardy–Zuckerman 4 feline sarcoma virus, HZ4-FSV. V-Kit is derived from the tyrosine kinase growth factor receptor for stem cell factor, c-Kit. V-*kit* is expressed as a Gag-Kit fusion protein of 80 kDa. V-*kit* contains sequences encoding the tyrosine kinase domain from c-*kit* (residues 558–925). The N-terminal sequences, which include the extracellular domain and the transmembrane domain, are deleted, and 50 amino acids from the C-terminus of c-Kit are replaced by five unrelated residues. Thus the v-Kit protein is not a transmembrane glycoprotein like its cellular homologue. However the P80$^{gag\text{-}kit}$ protein is myristylated, which suggest that it is membrane associated and it was shown to display a tyrosine-specific autophosphorylation activity.

Comparison of the v-Kit and c-Kit sequences revealed, in addition to the deletions mentioned above, three additional v-Kit mutations: deletion of Tyr569 and Val570, and the exchange of Asp at position 761 to Gly. Examinations of the consequences of the deletion of Tyr569 and Val570 revealed significant enhancement of transformation. Tyr568 and Tyr571 in c-Kit are a potential binding site for Src family members. Thus the repositioning of Y571 by this two-codon deletion has been postulated to play a role in the enhancement of v-Kit oncogenic activity.

In vitro v-Kit can transform the murine NIH3T3 fibroblast cell line. *In vivo* HZ4-FSV has been reported to cause fibrosarcomas in cats.

Ros

Ros is the transforming oncogene of the University of Rochester UR2, replication-defective avian sarcoma virus. It is derived from c-Ros, which is an orphan growth factor receptor that has similarity in overall structure to the drosophila sevenless protein. C-Ros is a large glycoprotein of 260 kDa. In contrast v-Ros is a 68 kDa protein that is expressed as a Gag-fusion protein. V-Ros contains the transmembrane and the tyrosine kinase domain of c-Ros, and has lost C-terminal sequences that have been replaced by 12 amino acids. In addition the transmembrane sequence in v-Ros contains a three amino acid insertion compared to c-Ros which seems to increase the transforming ability of v-Ros. This Gag-Ros fusion protein is a transmembrane protein in which the Gag moiety protrudes extracellularly. This Gag-Ros fusion protein is an active tyrosine kinase, is autophosphorylated and is found in a complex with phospholipase Cγ. In addition the mitogen-activated protein kinase pathway is activated in v-Ros transformed cells.

In vitro the UR2 virus can transform fibroblasts and *in vivo* cause fibrosarcomas.

Src

V-*src* is the transforming oncogene of the avian Rous Sarcoma virus, RSV. RSV is unique amongst acutely transforming retroviruses in being a replication competent virus in which the v-*src* sequence is located between the *env* gene and the 3' end of the viral genome.

C-Src is a cytoplasmic protein tyrosine kinase and is the founding member of the Src superfamily of kinases, which includes Blk, Fgr, Fyn, Hck, Lck, Lyn, Src and Yes. All of these kinases have been implicated to some extent in oncogenesis and Src, Fgr and Yes have viral homologues. The cellular proteins are N-terminally myristylated and are membrane located. They contain a tyrosine kinase domain and Src-homology 2 and 3 domains (SH2 and SH3). In addition the cellular proteins have a C-terminal Tyr, which is important for regulation of the tyrosine kinase activity. In c-Src this tyrosine is Tyr527 and its phosphorylation *in vivo* inhibits the tyrosine kinase activity. In v-Src this tyrosine is deleted and thus v-Src has a constitutive tyrosine kinase activity which is essential for its transforming ability.

In vivo Src causes fibrosarcomas that are rapid and fatal in young birds. *In vitro* v-Src is capable of transforming several different cell types including fibroblasts, chondrocytes and hematopoietic cells. V-Src transformed cells have very high levels of tyrosine phosphorylation and over 30 different proteins are reported to be phosphorylated on tyrosine. The contributions to the transformed phenotype by these proteins are not always clear. However the activation of proteins in the MAP kinase pathway and cytoskeletal proteins clearly have roles in the uncontrolled growth and morphological changes associated with v-Src transformation.

Sea

V-*sea* is the transforming oncogene of the S13 avian erythroblastosis virus. The cellular c-Sea protein is a member of the hepatocyte growth factor (HGF) receptor family, which is comprised of Met, Ron and Sea. V-Sea is expressed as a fusion protein between the viral *env* gene and the cytoplasmic sequences from the c-*sea* gene. The Env-Sea fusion protein is initially synthesized as a precursor molecular weight of 155 kDa, which is then subject to proteolytic cleavage at the normal site in Env to give rise to a disulfide-linked complex comprising the Env protein gp85 and a gp37-Sea fusion protein called gp70. The Env protein sequences provide the extracellular domain and transmembrane domain and serve to oligomerize this complex. Oligomerization activates the tyrosine kinase activity. Oligomerization, plasma membrane localization and tyrosine kinase activity are all necessary for transformation by v-Sea.

The HGF family of receptors all have two tyrosine located near to the C-terminus of the receptor which are autophosphorylated and serve as a multifunctional binding site for SH2-domain signaling proteins. The v-Sea protein has retained this site and it has been shown to be essential for transformation. *In vitro* v-Sea can transform chicken and rat fibroblasts and also chicken erythroid progenitor cells. *In vivo* infection of young chicks by the S13 virus causes sarcomas, erythroblastosis and anemia.

Yes

V-*yes* is the transforming oncogene of the avian sarcoma viruses Y73 and Esh. The name derives from these two strains, Y73 and Esh. C-Yes is a member of the Src family of protein tyrosine kinases and encodes a 61 kDa protein. V-*yes* is expressed as Gag-Yes fusion proteins in both Y73 and Esh of molecular weights 90 kDa and 80 kDa respectively. In the Yes sequences in the Y73 virus the C-terminal eight amino acids of c-Yes are replaced by three amino acids, which are encoded by the avian leukemia virus *env* gene. This alteration changes the position and context of a tyrosine residue in $p61^{c-yes}$. In addition, there are the six amino differences between v-Yes and c-Yes sequences. Based on the importance of the C-terminal sequences in regulating Src protein kinase family members, it is thought that the differences at the C-terminus of v-Yes are important for the activation of the tyrosine kinase. The c-Yes protein is found associated with the plasma membrane and also with the cell cytoskeleton. V-Yes is more diffusely distributed and, in a similar manner to v-Src, is also found associated with adhesion plaques.

Analysis of proteins phosphorylated on tyrosine in v-Yes transformed cells has identified multiple substrates as in Src transformed cells. These substrates include proteins associated with the cytoskeleton proteins and those involved in adhesion, such as integrins, $p130^{cas}$, and focal adhesion kinase as well as PI3 kinase.

In vitro the Y73 and Esh viruses can transform chicken embryo fibroblasts and *in vivo* they cause fibrosarcomas.

Cytokine Receptors

Cytokine receptors do not possess intrinsic tyrosine kinase activity; however, upon ligand activation cytoplasmic tyrosine kinases are activated. Although this is a very large gene family, to date only one member has been found as a retrovirally encoded oncogene, and this is v-*mpl*.

Mpl

V-*mpl* is the transforming oncogene of the murine myeloproliferative virus, MPLV. C-Mpl has been recently identified as being the receptor for the cytokine, thrombopoietin, and plays a role in the growth and differentiation of cells into megakaryocytes. V-*mpl* encodes a transmembrane protein that is expressed as an Env-Mpl fusion gene and is a truncated form of the c-Mpl receptor. The v-Mpl protein contains 100 amino acids of Env followed by 184 amino acids derived from c-Mpl, which contains the transmembrane and cytoplasmic sequences.

In vivo MPLV causes an acute hematological disorder characterized by the rapid growth of cells from several lineages. In contrast to most acutely transforming retroviruses, MPLV does not transform fibroblasts but *in vitro* infection of bone marrow cells will lead to the rapid outgrowth of immortalized cells from several lineages.

Adapter Proteins

Recently a class of proteins has been identified that has no intrinsic biochemical activity but they serve as linker molecules to connect proteins in key signaling pathways. These proteins are known as adapter molecules and they possess structural motifs that allow for protein–protein interaction. They also frequently serve as targets for tyrosine protein kinases, and upon phosphorylation can act as scaffolding molecules that bind to several downstream effector molecules. Two such molecules have been identified in acute transforming retroviruses; these are the *cbl* and *crk* oncogenes.

Cbl

Cbl is the transforming oncogene of the murine Cas NS-1 virus. The c-Cbl protein is a cytoplasmic protein of approximately 120 kDa. V-Cbl is a Gag-fusion protein of 100 kDa, which contains only 355 amino acids from the N-terminus of c-Cbl. V-Cbl is found in the nucleus of transformed cells. C-Cbl is associated with the Grb2 adapter protein and is phosphorylated upon tyrosine residues following growth factor stimulation. C-Cbl is related to the *Caenorhabditis elegans* gene Sli-1, which is a negative regulator of growth factor signaling. The N-terminal region of c-Cbl contains a putative phosphotyrosine binding domain and a ring-finger motif. Cbl is thought to function as a scaffold protein and associates with several SH2 and SH3 domain-containing molecules, including the Crk adaptor family and Vav. The deletion of C-terminal sequences up to the ring-finger motif, as found in v-Cbl, causes Cbl to become oncogenic. This deletion is suggested to generate a structural alteration, allowing the oncogenic forms of v-Cbl to displace wild-type c-Cbl from the receptor complex and in doing so to abrogate c-Cbl's negative regulatory function.

The Cas NS-1 murine retrovirus induces lymphomas and leukemias *in vivo*.

Crk

V-*crk* is the transforming oncogene of the avian sarcoma viruses, CT10 and ASV-1. C-Crk is an adapter protein of molecular weight 28 kDa that contains both an SH2 and two SH3 domains. Although the CT10 virus was isolated in the 1920s and the ASV-1 virus in 1983, the v-crk sequence in these viruses is virtually identical and is a Gag-fusion protein of 47 kDa. Although v-Crk does not possess a tyrosine kinase domain, fibroblasts transformed by v-Crk have greatly elevated levels of tyrosine phosphorylated proteins. This is thought to be due to the activation of a cellular tyrosine kinase by v-Crk and potentially also the stabilization of tyrosine phosphorylation upon association of tyrosine phosphorylated proteins with v-Crk. Abl is a candidate for a tyrosine kinase that may be regulated by v-Crk, as it forms a stable complex with v-Crk via the SH3 domain of v-Crk. Src-family members have also been implicated as being regulated by v-Crk. V-Crk is associated with several proteins in transformed cells. These include the proteins paxillin and p130Cas, which bind to Crk SH2 domain, and are thought to play roles in adhesion. The C3G protein, a guanine nucleotide exchange protein for Rap1, was shown to be bound to Crk SH3 domains. The SH3 domain of Crk also binds to Sos, and Eps15. The nature of the proteins bound to Crk implies that Crk influences the activities of effector proteins that are included in pathways involving cell morphology and growth.

V-Crk transforms fibroblasts *in vitro* and infection of birds with the AVS-1 and CT10 viruses causes fibrosarcomas.

Serine/Threonine Kinases

Akt

V-*akt* is the transforming oncogene of the acute transforming retrovirus AKT8 which was isolated from a spontaneous mouse T-cell lymphoma. V-*akt* has two human cellular homologues, AKT1 and AKT2, also known as protein kinase B. These genes encode protein kinase C-related serine/threonine kinases.

V-*akt* arose by recombination between MuLV and c-*akt*, 785 nucleotides downstream of the Gag ATG codon and 60 nucleotides upstream of the ATG codon in the 5′ untranslated region of the c-*akt* protooncogene. The 60 base pairs of 5′ c-*akt* noncoding sequence and the entire coding and 3′ untranslated regions are fused to viral Gag giving a 763 amino acid, 105 kDa fusion phosphoprotein of structure (p12, p15, Δp30)-X-c-*akt*, where X is 21 amino acids that result from the translation of the 60 c-*akt* 5′ noncoding nucleotides plus three additional nucleotides inserted at the junction between *Gag* and c-*akt*. The Akt protein sequence of v-Akt is identical to c-Akt. V-Akt and c-Akt contain a pleckstrin homology domain and a serine/threonine homology domain.

C-Akt kinase activity is positively regulated by phosphorylation at a Thr residue in the T-loop and Ser473 in the C-terminal regulatory domain. The PIP3-dependent kinase 1 (PDK1) is responsible for phosphorylation at Thr308. Currently the kinase that phosphorylates the Ser473 residue is unknown. C-Akt is activated by growth factors, including platelet-derived growth factor. Akt interacts directly, via its pleckstrin homology domain, with PI(3,4)P2 and PIP3, promoting a conformational change, a change in localization from the cytoplasm to the plasma membrane, as well as an increase in kinase activity. Although Akt is a serine/threonine kinase, part of its regulatory region is similar to the Src homology domain (SH2), a characteristic of cytoplasmic tyrosine kinases that function in protein–protein interactions. Possible c-Akt targets include glycogen synthase kinase 3 (GSK3), ribosomal protein S6 kinase p70^{S6K} and the Bcl-2 family member BAD, phosphorylation of which makes it unable to inhibit the survival activity of proteins like Bcl-2.

Fusion of Gag sequences to Akt provides a myristylation site at the N-terminus of the v-Akt protein that mimics the pleckstrin homology domain, anchoring the protein to the membrane. Localization of v-Akt is unregulated as dependence on PIP3 formation is lost. As a result of its permanent presence at the plasma membrane, v-Akt kinase activity is unregulated.

Raf

V-*raf* is the transforming oncogene of the murine retrovirus 3611-MSV derived from the mouse *Raf-1* proto-oncogene. The avian homologue of *Raf-1*, v-*mil* (originally termed v-*mht*), occurs in the Mill Hill 2 (MH2) virus isolated from a spontaneous ovarian tumor in chickens.

The 3611-MSV genome structure is 5' gag(Δp15, p12, Δp30)-v-raf-Δpol-env-3'. The 5' v-raf junction has 12 nucleotides identical to the 3' end of mouse Raf-1 exon 9 and differs from MuLV p30^{gag} by only one nucleotide. At the 3' end, eight nucleotides of v-raf, MuLV and mouse Raf-1 exon 17 are identical. V-raf is a truncated version of Raf-1 starting with a few nucleotides of exon 9 and ending with part of exon 17 coding for amino acids 326–648 from full length Raf-1. The N-terminal regulatory conserved regions 1 and 2 (CR1 and CR2) are deleted in v-raf. Therefore, the kinase domain (CR3) is joined to viral gag sequences. The resulting protein is cytosolic like its cellular counterpart, and is phosphorylated and myristylated. The v-mil oncogene of the MH2 virus begins in exon 7 and encodes the last 380 amino acids of chicken Mil (Raf) with 19 amino acid substitutions and one deletion. None of these mutations appear critical for transformation.

C-Raf is positively regulated by serine/tyrosine phosphorylation, which occurs mainly in response to mitogenic signals. Serine phosphorylation may also exert a negative effect, as phosphorylation of Ser357 and Ser359 in the ATP-binding domain of Raf-1 may inhibit Raf-1 activity. C-Raf is a serine/threonine kinase, which activates MAP kinase-kinase (MAPK-K), which in turn stimulates the mitogen-activated protein kinases ERK1 and ERK2. V-Raf has constitutive kinase activity and consequently MAPK-K, ERK1 and ERK2 are constitutively active in v-raf transformed cells. The ΔGag-v-Raf and ΔGag-v-Mil proteins have autophosphorylating protein kinase activity, which is essential for transforming activity. These oncoproteins trans-activate expression of genes driven by AP-1, ETS and NFκB binding motifs.

V-raf induces fibrosarcomas, erythroblastosis and occasionally erythroleukemia in vivo. Raf-induced tumors are more frequent in the hematopoeitic cell lineages, followed by pancreatic epithelium and connective tissues. Raf and Myc act synergistically to transform cells of all hematopoeitic lineages.

Ras

The v-H-ras and v-K-ras oncogenes, found in Harvey and Kirsten murine sarcoma virus (Ha-MuSV and Ki-MuSV), are derived from H-ras and K-ras cellular oncogenes, members of the Ras superfamily of transforming small G proteins. These viruses were isolated from rats infected with mouse leukemia viruses, Mo-MuLV and Ki-MuLV. Following the induction of leukemia, plasma from these animals was injected into BALB/c mice, which rapidly developed solid tumors. BALB-MuSV, AF-1 and Rasheed-MuSV viruses have also acquired Ras genes.

The viral genomes of Ha-MuSV (5.5 kb) and Ki-MuSV (6.5 kb) are composed of three types of nucleotide sequences: sequences homologous to MuLV (0.2 kb at the 5' end and 1 kb at the 3' end), sequence homologous to rat retrovirus-like 30S RNA, and the oncogene sequences which are 1.5 kb in Ha-MuSV and 1.75 kb in Ki-MuSV inserted towards the 5' end of the 30S RNA.

V-H-ras and v-K-ras both encode full-length proteins with two and four point mutations, respectively. The v-H-Ras point mutations are Lys12 to Gly and Lys143 to Gln. The v-K-Ras point mutations are Gly12 to Ser, Glu37 to Gln, Ala59 to Thr, Ile100 to Leu. The v-H-ras and v-K-ras oncogenes encode a 189 amino acid protein, p21^{ras}. Ras proteins are modified by polyisoprenylation and palmitoylation, and as a consequence bind tightly to the inner surface of the plasma membrane. Ras-encoded proteins are GTPases that are activated by a variety of growth factors. Normal p21^{ras} molecules hydrolyze GTP and exist in an equilibrium between active (GTP bound state) and inactive states (GDP bound). Two other proteins are involved in determining the state of the Ras proteins: GAPs (GTPase activating proteins), which catalyze the GDP bound state; and GEFs (guanine nucleotide exchange factor), which catalyze the release of bound GDP, thereby activating the protein. Three residues are critical for activating oncogenic potential: Gly12, Ala59 and Gln61. Gly12 and Ala59 are assumed to interfere with the action of the Gln61 side chain that forms a complex with the γ-phosphate in GTP. All inhibit GTP hydrolysis by diminishing GTPase activity or modulating the rate of nucleotide exchange (Ala59). Oncogenic mutations allow the GTP.p21^{ras} complex to remain active, thereby stimulating cell growth. Ras activates a cascade of serine/threonine protein kinases that include c-Raf, MAP kinase kinase (MAPK-K) and extracellular signal-regulated kinases (ERKs or MAP kinases). Via this cascade v-Ras activates FOS, JUN and other AP1 components and therefore modulates transcription, which eventually results in DNA synthesis.

Injection of mice with Ha-MuSV and Ki-MuSV gave rise to sarcomas. It is important to note that activating mutations of Ras have been detected in a wide variety of human tumors. Normal fibroblasts are not transformed by v-Ras unless coinfected with viruses containing immortalizing oncogenes such as Myc. However, cell lines such as NIH3T3 can be transformed by v-Ras. Ras oncogenes can efficiently transform murine erythroid, myeloid and mast cells in vitro.

See also: **Transformation: Animal viruses.**

Further Reading

Glover D, Hall A and Hastie N (1994) *Cell Biology of Cancer*. Cambridge: Company of Biologists.

Hesketh R (1994) *The Oncogene Handbook*. London: Academic Press.

Hesketh R (1995) *The Oncogene Facts Book*. London: Academic Press.

Macdonald F and Ford CHJ (1997) *Molecular Biology of Cancer*. Oxford: BIOS Scientific.

Weinberg RA (1989) *Oncogenes and the Molecular Origins of Cancer*. New York: Cold Spring Harbor Laboratory Press.

RETROVIRUSES – TYPE D (*RETROVIRIDAE*)

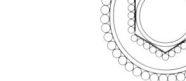

Maja A Sommerfelt, Department of Microbiology and Immunology, Gades Institute, University of Bergen, Bergen, Norway

Eric Hunter, Department of Microbiology, University of Alabama at Birmingham, Birmingham, Alabama, USA

Copyright © 1999 Academic Press

History

The first type D retrovirus described was isolated in 1970 from a spontaneous mammary carcinoma of an 8-year-old rhesus macaque. This virus, named Mason Pfizer monkey virus (M-PMV), has since become the prototype for an enlarging family of both endogenous and exogenous viruses (**Table 1**). Although isolated from a mammary carcinoma, M-PMV is not oncogenic; instead, infected primates succumb to a severe and often fatal immunosuppressive disease, which is distinct from that caused by the simian immunodeficiency viruses (SIVs) that are lentiviruses. Simian acquired immune deficiency disease (SAIDS-D) was first defined in 1983 as a disease entity caused by type D viruses. The precise mechanism of type D virus-induced immune suppression is not known, but the syndrome is currently restricted to the genus *Macaca* (subfamily Cercopithecinae) of old world monkey.

Approximately 12 years after the discovery of M-PMV, several additional horizontally transmitted type D viruses were isolated. They were called simian AIDS D-type (SAIDS-D) viruses together with the primate center of origin (for example, the virus from the New England Primate Center was named SAIDS-D/NE; **Table 1**). Based on the observation that the type D viruses could be divided into distinct neutralization groups, a new nomenclature was devised to distinguish these viruses from each other and to differentiate them from the HIV-like AIDS-inducing SIV. Members of the group are now named simian retrovirus (SRV) followed by the serological type. Serotypes 1–3 have all been molecularly cloned and sequenced. SRV-2, isolated at the Washington and Oregon primate centers, in addition to causing immune suppression, is directly associated with a severe retroperitoneal fibromatosis (RF). SRV-1–5 correspond to the exogenous type D viruses. It is presently unclear whether SRVPc isolated from an Ethiopian baboon at the Washington primate center represents an accidental laboratory infection or a new serotype. Two endogenous viruses have been isolated, one endogenous to the New World squirrel monkey *Saimiri sciureus* (squirrel monkey retrovirus SMRV) and the other to the Old World spectacled langur *Presbytis obscurus* (PO-1-Lu). An endogenous virus considered to be ancestral to the exogenous type D retroviruses has been recently identified in baboon genomic DNA. There have been reports of type D viruses isolated from human permanent cells lines: Hep-2V and PMFV, but these appear to be contaminants as only certain cell stocks carried the virus. The host species of origin for the exogenous type D viruses has not yet been defined.

Taxonomy and Classification

Type D retroviruses, classified in the family *Retroviridae*, are members of the *Betaretrovirus* genus. These are positive-strand RNA viruses that replicate by reverse transcription to form a proviral DNA intermediate which can integrate covalently into the host chromosomal DNA. M-PMV has a morphogenesis similar to that of the type B mouse mammary tumor virus (MMTV), in that it preassembles immature capsids (referred to as intracytoplasmic A-type particles (ICAPs)) within the infected cell cytoplasm.

Table 1 Type D retroviruses

Virus	Full name	Previous nomenclature	Accession number[a]	Exo/Endo	Initially isolated from
SRV-1	Simian retrovirus type 1	SAIDS-D/CA, SAIDS-D/NE	M11841	Exo	*Macaca mulatta*
SRV-2C	Simian retrovirus type 2	SAIDS-D/OR	M16605	Exo	*Macaca nigra*
SRV-2R	Simian retrovirus type 2	SAIDS-D/OR		Exo	*Macaca mulatta*
SRV-2W	Simian retrovirus type 2	SAIDS-D/WA	L38695 (env)	Exo	*Macaca nemestrina*
SRV-3	Simian retrovirus type 3	Mason Pfizer monkey virus	M12349	Exo	*Macaca mulatta*
SRV-4	Simian retrovirus type 4	None		Exo	*Macaca fascicularis*
SRV-5	Simian retrovirus type 5	None		Exo	*Macaca mulatta*
SRVPc	Simian retrovirus Pc	None	U16843 (p27) U16844 (gp20)	Exo	*Papio cynocephalus*
PO-1-Lu	Endogenous langur virus	None	None	Endo	*Presbytis obscurus*
SMRV	Squirrel monkey retrovirus	None	M23385[b]	Endo	*Saimiri sciureus*
SERV	Simian endogenous retrovirus	None	U85505/U85506	Endo	*Papio cynocephalus*

Exo, exogenous; endo, endogenous; SAIDS-D, simian acquired immunodeficiency syndrome D; RF, retroperitoneal fibromatosis; CA, California; NE, New England; W, Washington; OR, Oregon regional primate centers.
[a] DNA sequences are stored at the EMBL Nucleotide Sequence Database, GenBank. Three subtypes of SRV-2 are shown. Accession numbers for two SERV clones are shown.
[b] The accession number for SMRV-H isolated from human cells is shown.

The morphology of the mature extracellular virion is different, in that it has a centrally located nucleoid similar to type C retroviruses and a much less dense fringe of glycoprotein than MMTV. Being of primate origin with these differences, a new morphological class of retrovirus was designated type D.

Properties of the Virion

Type D viruses assemble an immature capsid in the cytoplasm. These intracellular spherical particles, 60–95 nm in diameter, migrate to the plasma membrane, where they acquire, during release by budding, an envelope containing virus-encoded glycoproteins (**Fig. 1A, 1B**). These particles have a diameter of 100–120 nm. Following release, a proteolytic event termed 'maturation' results in a morphological change in the virion from an electron-lucent core to an electron-dense core (**Fig. 1C**). Surface projections corresponding to the viral glycoproteins can be seen in negatively stained preparations (**Fig. 1D, 1E, 1F**). Type D viruses exhibit a buoyant density of $1.17\,\text{g ml}^{-1}$ in sucrose, and $1.21\,\text{g ml}^{-1}$ in cesium chloride. The three-dimensional structure of the virion remains to be determined.

Properties of the Genome

The genome of type D retroviruses that have been sequenced to date is composed of two identical positive-sense, single-stranded RNAs of approximately 8 kb in length (7943 nt for M-PMV). The RNA molecules are proposed to be hydrogen-bonded to each other and to a host tRNA^{lys}. This diploid structure of about 5.3×10^6 Da (70 S) is denatured by heat (80°C for 2.5 min) or 40% formamide to 2.65×10^6 Da (35 S). Like eucaryotic mRNA, the retroviral RNA genome is capped at the 5′ end with a 7-methyl GTP, polyadenylated at the 3′ end and internally methylated on scattered adenosine residues.

As with any replication-competent retrovirus genome, coding regions of type D viruses are flanked at both ends by 5′- and 3′-terminal sequences that are important for virus replication and regulation of gene expression. The 5′ sequences include a binding site for a host tRNA^{lys} which serves as a primer for the synthesis of negative-strand DNA by the viral reverse transcriptase enzyme, and an untranslated region preceding the coding regions. The RNA splice donor-site (AAGUAAGU) for subgenomic mRNAs is located 21 nucleotides upstream of the *gag* AUG for M-PMV. A packaging signal sequence for encapsidation of genomic RNAs into virions is also present. The 3′-terminal sequences contain at least two transcriptional elements: the AUUAAA signal sequence for poly(A) addition, and the UAUAUAAG sequence corresponding to the TATA box as promoter for viral RNA synthesis.

Properties of the Proteins

Four genes, arranged as 5′-*gag-pro-pol-env*-3′, encode type D virus proteins. The most detailed information is available for the prototype virus M-PMV. Viral

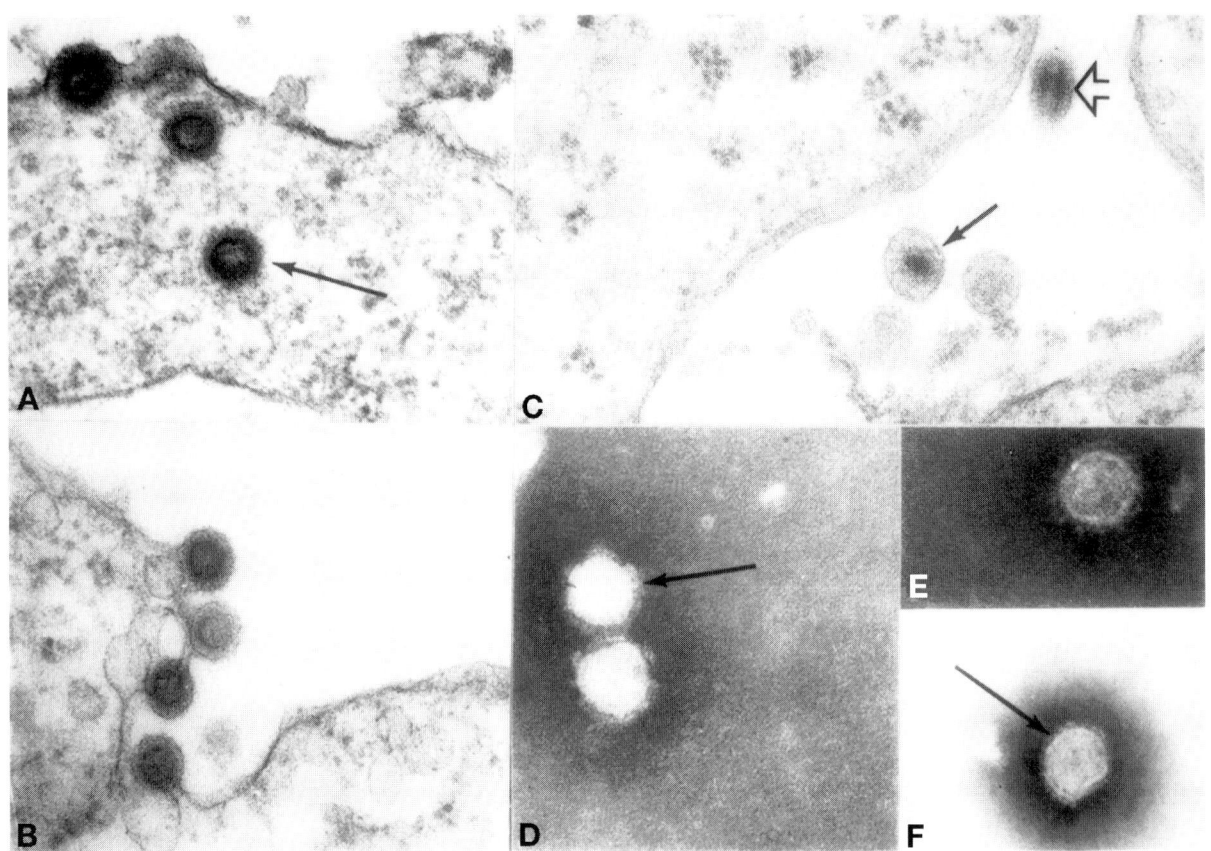

Figure 1 Electron micrographs of M-PMV-infected cells and M-PMV virions. (**A**) Thin section of an M-PMV-infected cell showing immature capsids deep in the cytoplasm (arrow) and in process of budding. (**B**) Immature capsids at a late stage of budding. (**C**) Mature virions showing electron-dense core (arrow) and section through cylindrical core (open arrow). (**D–F**) Negatively-stained virions showing glycoprotein surface projections (arrows).

genes are expressed as polyprotein precursors: Pr78 is encoded by *gag*, and Pr95 by *gag-pro* through a −1 frameshift event at the end of *gag*. The *pol* gene is similarly expressed as a Pr180 *gag-pro-pol* product that is generated from two −1 frameshifts, one at the end of *gag* and a second at the end of *pro*. The envelope glycoprotein is translated from a spliced mRNA as a Pr86 precursor. This polyprotein is comprised of the surface (SU) glycoprotein gp70 that interacts with receptors on susceptible cells, and the transmembrane (TM) glycoprotein gp22, which spans the viral membrane and catalyzes the process of membrane fusion. During virus maturation the gp22 is cleaved to gp20 by the viral protease, a process which appears to activate the fusogenic potential of the glycoprotein complex.

Immature intracytoplasmic A-type particles are composed of Pr78, Pr95 and Pr180 in an approximate 80:15:5% ratio. Expression of the precursor proteins in an *in vitro* translation system results in assembly of these immature capsids in a process that is dependent on ATP hydrolysis. During maturation, the Pr78 precursor is cleaved, by the virus-encoded protease, to yield six internal structural proteins in the order NH_2-p10(MA)-pp24/16-p12-p27(CA)-p14(NC)-p4-COOH (**Fig. 2**). The 10 kDa matrix protein (MA) forms the envelope-associated outer shell of the mature particle and is modified with myristic acid. The 27 kDa polypeptide capsid protein (CA) is the major structural component of the mature capsid, while the 14 kDa nucleic acid binding protein (NC) presumably functions in genomic RNA packaging and dimer formation. The exact functions of the 12 kDa (p12), 4 kDa (p4) proteins and the phosphorylated 24/16 protein remain to be determined. However, the p12 domain of Pr78 is critical for immature capsid assembly both in infected cells and *in vitro*, and a proline-proline-proline-tyrosine (PPPY) motif in pp16/24 is critical for the final stage of virus budding from the cell. SMRV particles contain a major capsid protein p35, which is likely to represent a fusion protein of p12 and p27.

The protease gene of M-PMV could potentially encode a protein of 314 amino acids, fused to the Gag

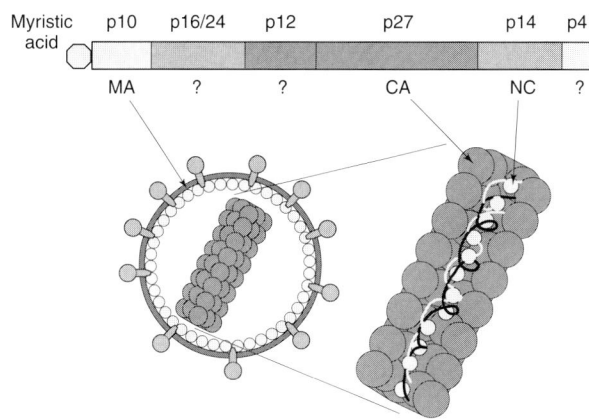

Figure 2 M-PMV *gag* gene-encoded precursor showing the organization of the mature products and their location within the mature virion. A section through the core shows the association of the NC protein with the diploid RNA genome.

precursor that is truncated at the frameshifting site. This *pro*-encoded region is cleaved by the viral protease to two proteins of 17 kDa; the N-terminal protein has dUTPase activity, while the C-terminal portion has protease activity and can be further cleaved to a 12 kDa protein with protease activity. The protease is an aspartyl protease, which remains inert while it is part of the Pr95 and Pr180 precursors within the cell. It is activated by an unknown mechanism following virus release. The importance of dUTPase activity in the virus life cycle is unknown.

The reverse transcriptase enzyme (80–90 kDa) for all the type D retroviruses has a divalent cation preference for magnesium in contrast to manganese, which is utilized by many of the nonhuman mammalian type C viruses. This enzyme also has RNase H and integrase activity.

Physical Properties of the Virion

Type D virions are rapidly inactivated when exposed to high temperature (56°C for 30 min) and are also sensitive to lipid solvents and detergents. The mature virions of M-PMV are easily disrupted in mild detergent concentration (0.5% Triton X-100), whereas immature intracytoplasmic capsid particles remain stable under these conditions. Recent evidence from cryoelectron microscopy indicates that the immature capsids, despite their assembly in the absence of membranes, are not icosahedral and exhibit a broad distribution of sizes.

Although retroviruses are quite resistant to UV light or gamma irradiation, UV irradiation of M-PMV results in inhibition of virus-induced syncytial formation in rhesus monkey embryonic lung cells.

Type D viruses are composed of approximately 60–70% protein, 30–40% lipid, 2–4% carbohydrate and 1% nucleic acid by weight.

Strategy of replication of the nucleic acid

In common with other retroviruses, the type D retroviral RNA genome is reverse transcribed within the infected cytoplasm to form a double-stranded DNA intermediate. The nascent DNA migrates to the nucleus and integrates covalently into the host chromosomal DNA, where it exists as a provirus. Transcription of the provirus results in messenger RNA that will function to produce virus-specific polyprotein precursors, and also genomic RNA that will be packaged into assembling virions.

Characterization of Transcription

Cellular RNA polymerase II transcribes the integrated type D provirus genome into RNA. In the cytoplasm of infected cells, two classes of viral RNA transcripts are detected. A genomic-sized mRNA (8 kb), which is either translated into polyprotein precursors or encapsidated into progeny virus particles, and a 3 kb mRNA representing subgenomic-spliced mRNA which is translated into Env polyproteins. Transport of the unspliced genomic RNA from the nucleus to the cytoplasm is dependent on the presence of a short (~ 200 nucleotide) element called the constitutive transport element (CTE) that is located between the *env*-gene and the 3′ long terminal repeat (LTR). This element forms a hairpin structure that is presumably recognized by a host protein(s) capable of diverting the genome-length RNA from the splicing machinery and out of the nucleus.

Characterization of Translation

Genome-length RNAs are translated on free polysomes into the Gag polyprotein and, as a result of ribosomal frameshifting, into the Gag-Pro and Gag-Pro-Pol polyproteins. The heptanucleotide sequence motifs for the -1 frameshift have been localized in both M-PMV and SRV-1 genomes: GGGAAAC for Gag-Pro fusion and AAAUUUU for Pro-Pol fusion. Due to the frequency of frameshifting, the majority of precursor proteins are Gag polyproteins, approximately 15% are Gag-Pro polyproteins and around 5% are Gag-Pro-Pol polyproteins.

The spliced subgenomic *env* mRNA is translated on polysomes associated with the endoplasmic reticulum. The cotranslationally glycosylated product is transported via the secretory pathway of the cell to the plasma membrane, where it is anchored and oriented as a type I glycoprotein.

Post-translational Processing

Cellular enzymes post-translationally modify the Gag-containing polyproteins. The N-terminal methionine residue is cotranslationally removed and myristic acid is added to the new N-terminal glycine residue. The polyproteins are also phosphorylated following translation, but the significance of this modification is not clear.

Following entry into the endoplasmic reticulum of the cell, Env polyproteins form an oligomeric structure (estimated to be a trimer), which is the transport-competent form of the precursor. During transport to the cell surface through the secretory pathway, core oligosaccharide side chains on the SU domain of M-PMV Env polyproteins are processed to complex oligosaccharide chains. The single high-mannose oligosaccharide chain added to the TM domain during translation is maintained in an unmodified form. In a late Golgi compartment the Pr86 polyprotein is cleaved into the two mature glycoproteins, gp70(SU) and gp22(TM), by a furin-like cellular endopeptidase. The gp22 is further processed, by a C-terminal cleavage event, to gp20 during virus maturation by the viral aspartyl protease.

Assembly Site, Release and Cytopathology

Type D viruses are characterized by the assembly of immature intracytoplasmic A type particles (ICAPs). These are assembled from uncleaved precursor proteins and migrate to the plasma membrane, where they are released by budding. They acquire an outer membrane, which is derived from the host cell plasma membrane and contains virus-specific envelope glycoproteins, during this process. The assembly of immature capsids appears to occur at a site in the cytoplasm where precursors congregate in sufficient quantities to allow self-assembly. A signal, which directs the proteins to the intracytoplasmic assembly site, has been identified in the MA protein of M-PMV. Immature capsids appear to contain a full complement of genomic RNA. As with other retroviruses, RNA packaging requires a sequence (psi) found within the 5′ end of genomic RNA. This region has been shown to fold into a specific secondary structure that is presumably recognized by the Gag precursor protein during capsid assembly.

Although the pathway of intracytoplasmic transport has not been defined, the transport of immature capsids to the membrane requires a specific protein-mediated targeting process, in addition to the presence of myristic acid, which is also required for intracellular transport. During the budding process, immature capsids associate with the plasma membrane, presumably via the MA protein, and are extruded from the cell. It has been postulated for M-PMV that there is an interaction between the cytoplasmic domain of the TM glycoprotein, gp22, and the matrix protein, which directs incorporation of envelope glycoproteins into the virion. As with other retroviruses, the viral glycoproteins are not essential for virion release but are required for virus infectivity.

Other Subjects Relevant to Virus Group

Type D viruses are capable of inducing cell fusion *in vitro*. This is mediated by the interaction of virus envelope glycoproteins expressed at the cell surface with available receptors present on adjacent uninfected cells and has provided a method for titrating the virus in culture.

Geographic Distribution

The primates that are infected with exogenous type D viruses primarily comprise the *Macaca* (Cercopithecinae) genus of Old World monkey which naturally inhabit India and Southeast Asia (**Table 2**). Studies of seropositivity to type D retroviruses in feral macaques is limited. At present the disease spectrum of this virus group has mainly been associated with primate research centers in the USA, although seropositivity to type D infection in imported or wild caught monkeys has been noted in primate centers in Europe and China. The spectacled langur, which harbors the endogenous virus PO-1-Lu, inhabits India and Southeast Asia and the squirrel monkey, harboring SMRV, inhabits central and southern America.

Host Range and Virus Propagation

Viruses enter cells following attachment to specific cell surface receptors. These viruses enter cells by a pH-independent pathway, suggesting that they penetrate cells at the plasma membrane. Type D virus receptors appear to be constitutively expressed on human cells. The same receptor moiety appears to be used by all the type D viruses, as well as two related mammalian type C viruses, RD114 (an endogenous virus of cats) and baboon endogenous virus (BaEV), as well as the type C avian reticuloendotheliosis viruses (REV). Viruses within this group exhibit receptor interference where cells chronically infected with one virus will be resistant to superinfection by a second in the group. The receptor gene has been

Table 2 Primates from which exogenous SRVs have been isolated

Genus and species	Common name	Primate center
Macaca mulatta	Rhesus macaque	California, New England
Macaca arctoides	Stumptail macaque	California
Macaca cyclopsis	Formosan/Taiwanese rock macaque	New England
Macaca fascicularis	Crab-eating macaque	New England, Washington
Macaca nemestrina	Pigtail macaque	Washington
Macaca fuscata	Japanese macaque	Washington
Macaca radiata	Bonnet macaque	New England, California
Macaca nigra	Celebese macaque	Oregon
Macaca assamensis[a]	Assamese macaque	China
Papio cunocephales	Ethiopian baboon	Washington

[a] Seropositivity confirmed by western blotting, no reported virus isolation.

assigned to human chromosome 19q13.1–13.3. The distinct neutralization specificities suggest that the type D retroviruses utilize distinct epitopes of the same cell surface receptor. Exploiting the neutralization epitope of SRV-2, a molecule of 60 kDa has been identified as a putative receptor on Raji cells. Further work is required to confirm a receptor function for this molecule. Type D viruses are not considered to be cytopathic; instead, they integrate into the cell genome and persist as a chronic infection where the cells do not die but continuously shed virus.

The *in vivo* host range of SRV-1–5 is broad, infecting many tissue types, including lymph nodes, salivary gland, spleen, thymus and brain. There have been reports that the SRVs may remain latent in the brain.

The *in vitro* host range of SRV-1–5 is extensive and includes a variety of human lymphoblastoid (H9, Raji) and nonlymphoblastoid cell lines (HeLa and HOS). Mink, chimp lung, African green monkey (COS), horse epithelial and dog thymus cells are also susceptible. Cells that appear to be resistant to productive infection include hamster, rat and mouse.

The endogenous viruses have a more restricted *in vitro* host range. PO-1-Lu infects only human and bat lung cells. It cannot infect langur cells, indicating that it has a xenotropic host range typical of endogenous viruses. SMRV has a broader xenotropic host range infecting cells of dog, chimp, mink, rhesus, human, marmoset, owl monkey and howler monkey, but not baboon. Simian endogenous retrovirus (SERV) has only been studied as cloned DNA. It is present in all *Papio* and *Cercopithec* species, but genomic DNA from African or Asian members of the Colobinae has not yet been analyzed. As no infectious SERV has been isolated, the *in vitro* and *in vivo* host range of this member remains to be determined.

Genetics

The type D retroviruses, in common with other retroviruses, contain two identical RNA genomes; this diploidy allows for genetic recombination.

SRV-1, -2 and -3 have been fully sequenced and show a high degree of both nucleotide and amino acid identity. They have slightly different restriction endonuclease patterns but are uniform within each group. The difference between the SRV genomes probably results from basepair mutations over time rather than large recombinational events. The exogenous SRVs have been described as variants of M-PMV. The major differences are found in regions encompassing the Gag phosphoproteins, the p12 proteins and the envelope glycoproteins. SRV-1 and SRV-3 (M-PMV) appear to be more related than SRV-2, which is also associated with RF.

The viral genome is comprised of four genes in the order 5'-*gag-pro-pol-env*-3', where *gag* encodes the structural components of the capsid, *pro* encodes the viral aspartyl protease, *pol* encodes the polymerase enzyme (reverse transcriptase) and integrase and *env* encodes the surface envelope glycoproteins. The type D retroviruses have neither regulatory genes, found in the immunosuppressive primate lentiviruses, nor oncogenes, found in members of the avian and mammalian type C retroviruses.

Evolution

The type D viruses such as M-PMV exhibit immunological crossreactivity in their envelope glycoproteins to two related endogenous type C retroviruses, namely baboon endogenous retrovirus (BaEV) and RD114. In contrast, the Gag and Pol proteins of the type D viruses are unrelated to these type C viruses.

The genomic organization, reverse transcriptase and Gag proteins of type D viruses are related to those of the B-type MMTV and the intracisternal A-type particles (IAPs). The type D viruses may therefore have arisen as a recombinational event in which the *env* gene was acquired from a virus ancestral to the C-type BaEV, and the capsid and reverse transcriptase genes were derived from a retrovirus ancestral to MMTV or the IAPs.

Early hybridization studies with tissues of different monkey species showed that M-PMV and SRV-1 DNA hybridized more readily to langur DNA (in the subfamily Colobinae) than to rhesus DNA, suggesting that M-PMV may have been derived from a virus similar to that endogenous in the langur monkey. Recently an endogenous type D retrovirus (SERV) genome was isolated from a baboon (*Papio cynocephalus*) genomic library. DNA sequence analysis showed that the *gag, pro, pol* and *env* (gp20 region) genes were similar to SRV-1, -2 and -3, whereas the gp70-encoding region was more closely related to that of BaEV. No analysis of langur DNA for SERV sequences has yet been undertaken.

The Jaagsiekte sheep retrovirus (JSRV) associated with ovine pulmonary carcinoma (OPC) of sheep, shows both antigenic and proviral DNA sequence similarity to M-PMV in the *gag-pro-pol* genes, while the *env* gene is similar to the prototype type B retrovirus MMTV and may represent a novel recombinant.

The presence of type D retroviral sequences in both Old and New World primates clearly shows that these viruses are ancient. Tracing their evolution is complicated by their potential for extensive recombination and zoonoses.

Serologic Relationships and Variability

There are five different serotypes, each with distinct neutralization epitopes, among the exogenous SRVs. These neutralization epitopes lie in the external envelope glycoproteins, which may show variability because of adaptation to different macaque species. The viruses can also be distinguished using antibodies to the smaller Gag proteins, p10 and p12. In addition to these type-specific determinants, the type D retroviruses demonstrate a high level of antigenic cross-reactivity within the major capsid protein. The type D envelope glycoproteins appear conserved for each serotype and do not show the same degree or kinetics of variation as the human and simian immunodeficiency viruses (HIV/SIV) and SIV. Minor variations are present in each serotype depending on the host species of isolation. Studies addressing sequence variability following infection have not been undertaken.

Epidemiology

Type D retroviruses have been targeted in the development and maintenance of specific-pathogen-free (SPF) colonies of rhesus macaques. Seroepidemiological surveys have shown that up to 20% of captive macaques at US primate centers and commercial suppliers are infected with SRV. Seropositivity to type D retroviruses has also been reported in China in wild-caught macaques (**Table 2**). Since certain infected macaques fail to make detectable antibody, or exhibit a long interval between infection and seroconversion, serologic testing alone is not sufficient for epidemiological studies. The polymerase chain reaction (PCR) provides a rapid means of detecting type D proviral DNA. However, PCR is limited to the detection of viruses for which DNA sequence information is available. Type D retrovirus infection is undoubtedly widespread, although its distribution in primate holding facilities worldwide, in zoos or in the wild has not been fully investigated.

Transmission and Tissue Tropism

Transmission of the exogenous SRVs requires close physical contact and is probably spread by saliva and blood through biting, grooming and fighting – the way such primates establish a social hierarchy. Unlike HIV, SRV transmission does not appear to be via sexual contact. High titers of virus can be found in infected macaque saliva, allowing entry to the bloodstream of a recipient individual following trauma.

The virus can be experimentally transmitted by inoculation of primates, as was done to prove the disease association of these viruses. The *in vivo* tissue tropism shows a broad host range for both lymphoid and nonlymphoid organs. Perinatal transmission and *in utero* transmission of the exogenous type D viruses appears to be infrequent. SRV can be recovered from peripheral blood lymphocytes, saliva, urine, feces and breast milk of viremic animals.

Transmission of the endogenous viruses occurs vertically as inherited genetic elements.

Pathogenicity

SAIDS-D is a naturally occurring, experimentally reproducible infection, where infected rhesus monkeys show a broad spectrum of clinical and pathological abnormalities (**Table 3**). Following infection of juvenile rhesus macaques, the animals may die within 1 year. The course of infection can result in fulminating viremia and death, a relatively mild acute

Table 3 Clinical features of SAIDS-D infection

Immune deficiency
Chronic wasting/ weight loss (>10%)
Persistent diarrhea unresponsive to appropriate therapy
Splenomegaly
Neutropenia
Lymphopenia or histologic lymphoid depletion
Abnormal peripheral blood lymphocytes
Mesenchymal proliferative disorders
Noma
Increased incidence of tumours
Opportunistic infections including:
    Disseminated cytomegalovirus infection
    Bacterial pneumonia
Progressive generalized lymphadenopathy (PGL)
Anemia
Bone marrow hyperplasia

phase of disease resulting in a chronic carrier state, or recovery from both viremia and latent infection.

The endogenous viruses are not associated with any pathogenic effects in their hosts.

Clinical Features of Infection

Infection of macaques with all of the SRVs isolated to date is associated with a severe and often fatal immune suppression (**Table 3**.) There is a decrease in both T and B cell populations and a low response of peripheral blood lymphocytes to mitogens, together with an increased incidence of tumors. Virus can be isolated from persistently infected animals from saliva, peripheral lymph nodes, plasma, peripheral blood leukocytes and exfoliated cells in milk.

One feature unique to SRV-2 is that this virus is also associated with retroperitoneal fibromatosis, which has been compared to Kaposi's sarcoma in humans. However, RF tissue is infected with SRV-2, unlike Kaposi's sarcoma and HIV. Particularly prevalent in Celebes and pigtailed macaques, RF is a highly vascular mesenchymal proliferative lesion that commonly originates in the subserosa of the intestine at the ileocecal junction and which can aggressively spread throughout the abdominal and thoracic cavity. A cutaneous form of RF has also been recognized in a small number of animals; immunohistochemical studies show a factor VIII-related antigen in endothelial cells and scattered fibroblast-like cells throughout the RF lesions, similar to those described for human Kaposi's sarcoma. RF is restricted to the Oregon and Washington regional primate centers.

Pathology and Histopathology

Typical type D virus particles can be found in the salivary gland acinar cells (secretory cells), mucosal epithelial cells, macrophages, lymph nodes, Langerhans cells, peripheral blood lymphocytes, thymus and spleen, but not in muscle or brain. Viral nucleic acid can be found in brain parenchyma, suggesting that the virus may remain latent in this organ. Neuropathy, however, is not a characteristic of SAIDS-D. Brain cells may thus present a post-transcriptional block to SRV replication. The tissue localization of SRV-1 is also dependent on the severity of the disease. In severe SAIDS-D, virus is present in a higher percentage of cells of the salivary gland, as well as in the sinusoidal cells lining the spleen, and the stellate cells of the thymus. If the primate presents with persistent generalized lymphadenopathy or splenomegaly, virus antigen is not as prevalent, being limited to germinal centers of lymphoid organs and scattered salivary gland acinar cells. There have been reports that some virus may also be found in other secretory cells, e.g. sweat glands, mammary glands and pancreatic acinar cells.

The histology of RF associated with SRV-2 infection reveals thymic atrophy and follicular and paracortical atrophy of the lymph nodes, as well as variable myeloid and lymphoid hyperplasia in the bone marrow.

Immune Response

Infection usually results in an overall decline in both B and T lymphocytes. Unlike in human AIDS, hypergammaglobulinemia is not a feature of SAIDS-D. Impairment of B cell function has been demonstrated by a diminished antibody response to antigenic stimulation, *in vivo* and *in vitro*, and progressively decreasing levels in the serum of all immunoglobulin subclasses. Secondary immune responses may be impaired with no switch from IgM to IgG. Complement C3 and C4 levels remain intact or are slightly elevated through the course of the disease. Antibodies are mounted predominantly to the Gag antigens. Resistance to type D infection corresponds to the presence of high levels of neutralizing antibodies directed against the envelope glycoproteins.

Prevention and Control

Effective vaccines have been generated against SRV-1, SRV-2 and SRV-3. Juvenile macaques inoculated with formalin-inactivated SRV-1 generate neutralizing antibodies that are protective upon challenge. Recombinant vaccinia virus expressing the envelope glycoproteins of SRV-1, SRV-2 and SRV-3 protect against the respective virus challenge, even years later, demonstrating that the envelope glycoproteins alone are sufficient to elicit a protective immune response. These vaccines have limited crossprotection: SRV-3 vaccinated animals were protected from SRV-1 challenge but no crossimmunity has been observed between the SRV-1 and SRV-2 serotypes. Vaccines are useful for limiting the spread of SRV infection. Control of infection *in vitro* has also been successful using zidovudine (AZT) or 9-(2-phosphonylmethoxy-ethyl)adenine (PMEA), which inhibit the reverse transcriptase, as well as inhibitors of the HIV proteinase.

Future Perspectives

Although type D virus-induced immunosuppression has been a problem at primate centers in the USA, effective screening measures are possible to identify infected primates. Polyvalent vaccines may eventually be generated to protect primates from all the different serotypes identified to date. A report of the isolation of a type D virus, highly related to M-PMV, from an AIDS patient suffering from lymphoma raised the possibility of human infections by type D viruses; however, human seropositivity to type D antigens remains controversial. Recently, a DNA sequence of 932 bp with similarity to type B/D retroviruses was identified in patients with Sjögren's syndrome. This sequence appears to represent an acquired genome that has been provisionally called human retrovirus 5. Further research is required to establish the significance of this finding.

See also: **Feline immunodeficiency virus (*Retroviridae*); Human immunodeficiency viruses (*Retroviridae*): Molecular biology, Anti-retroviral agents, General features; Mouse mammary tumor virus (*Retroviridae*); Simian immunodeficiency viruses (*Retroviridae*).**

Further Reading

Coffin JM, Hughes SH and Varmus HE (1997) *Retroviruses*. Cold Spring Harbor, NY: Cold Spring Harbor Laboratory Press.

Fine D and Schochetman G (1978) Type D primate retroviruses: a review. *Cancer Res.* 38: 3123.

Hunter E (1994) Macromolecular interactions in the assembly of HIV and other retroviruses. *Semin. Virol.* 5: 71.

Weldon R Jr and Hunter E (1997) Molecular requirements for retrovirus assembly. In: Chiu W, Burnett RM and Garcea R (eds) *Structural Biology of Viruses*, p. 381. New York: Oxford University Press.

RETROVIRUSES OF DROSOPHILA: THE GYPSY PARADIGM

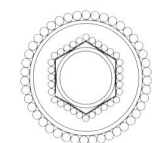

Alain Bucheton, Alain Pélisson and **Christophe Terzian**, Institut de Génétique Humaine, CNRS, Gif-sur-Yvette, Montpellier Cedex 5, France

Copyright © 1999 Academic Press

History, Taxonomy and Classification

The *Drosophila melanogaster gypsy virus* has been recently classified in the family *Metaviridae* of the genus *Errantivirus*. However, in context of the earlier classification, this virus is referred to as a retrovirus. Gypsy was first described as a transposable element present in the genome of *Drosophila melanogaster*. Although its structure is very much similar to that of vertebrate retroviruses (see below and **Fig. 1**), it was considered as a long terminal repeat (LTR)-containing retrotransposon. Infectious properties were demonstrated in 1994.

Control of Gypsy by the Host Genome

The transposition and infective properties of Gypsy are controlled by a host gene called *flamenco*. This gene is located on the X chromosome. Restrictive *flamenco* alleles repress Gypsy transposition and infectivity; permissive alleles allow high rates of

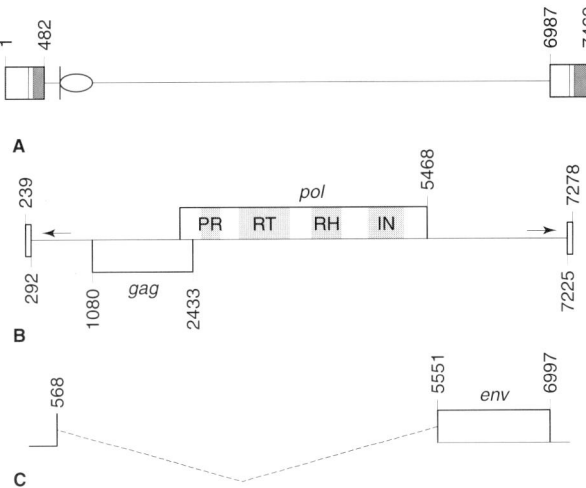

Figure 1 Gypsy proviral structure and transcription (**A**) Structure of a *D. melanogaster* Gypsy provirus. Numerical designations refer to coordinates (in nucleotides) from the first sequence deposited in the databank. Boxes represent the proviral long terminal repeats (LTRs), including U3, R and U5 (light shading, open box and dark shading, respectively). The oval and the vertical bar represent two DNA-binding regions, the SU(HW)-binding site and the downregulating palindrome, respectively. (**B**) Structure of the full-length transcript and its coding potential. The viral RNA is bounded at either end by the short direct repeat R. The U5 and U3 LTR sequences are unique in the transcript. The leftwards and rightwards arrows indicate respectively the positions of the primer binding site (PBS), including nucleotides 482–492, and of the polypurine tract (PPT), including nucleotides 6977–6986. The coordinates of the *gag* first AUG codon and of the *gag* and *pol* stop codons are given. The *pol* open reading frame begins at nucleotide 2363. Position of *pol* domains is as follows: PR, protease; RT, reverse transcriptase; RH, RNAse H; IN, integrase. (**C**) Structure of the *env* subgenomic RNA. The splicing event is figured by the broken line. The vertical bar at position 568 corresponds to the two first nucleotides of the AUG initiator codon which are spliced to a G at position 5551. The 5′ end of this RNA has not been precisely mapped.

transposition and the expression of its infective properties. Transposition only occurs in the progeny of females homozygous for the permissive *flamenco* alleles, indicating that this gene has a maternal effect on Gypsy activity.

Overview of the Strategy of Replication

The typical retroviral replication cycle mainly consists of the following sequence of events: (1) transcription of the provirus; (2) translation; (3) RNA packaging; (4) reverse transcription; and (5) integration as a proviral DNA into the chromosome of the infected host. There is already a wealth of evidence showing that most, if not all, of these steps are involved in the biology of Gypsy. Moreover, like a typical endogenous retrovirus, Gypsy is a germline parasite which can therefore just rely on the chromosome DNA replication machinery for its proviruses to be passively transmitted from generation to generation. Unlike endogenous retroviruses in vertebrates, however, the proviral copy number can dramatically increase in permissive *Drosophila* genotypes. This results from very efficient transfer from the soma towards the germen. Requirement of the infectious potential of Gypsy for this transfer has yet to be demonstrated.

Sequence of the Proviral Genome

Three Gypsy proviruses have been thoroughly sequenced to date in *D. melanogaster*. Despite some differences, these sequences all display the same three open reading frames (ORFs), each of which show at least some similarities to either of the main three genes, *gag*, *pol* and *env*, shared by all retroviruses (**Fig. 1**). Near the C-terminus of the *gag* homologue gene, an arginine-rich region, conserved in proviruses isolated from two other *Drosophila* species (*D. virilis* and *D. subobscura*), was described as a putative ARM RNA binding motif. The protein putatively encoded by the second ORF is highly homologous to the enzymatic activities, protease, reverse transcriptase, RNAse H and integrase, encoded by other retroviruses. Translation of the third ORF produces a *bona fide* retroviral envelope with a 32 amino acid intracellular domain.

Cis sequences involved in the retroviral replication cycle can also be found: (1) there are two LTRs; (2) adjacent to 5′ LTR, complementarity to $tRNA_1^{Lys}$ discloses a minus-strand primer binding site (PBS); (3) an oligopurine stretch just upstream of 3′ LTR, assumed to be resistant to RNAse H, should be able to prime synthesis of the plus-strand DNA.

Gypsy is not framed by the typical TG...CA nucleotides. Instead, the inverted repeats AGTTA... TAA^T/$_C$T are found at the LTR ends.

Transcription

Basal transcriptional activity requires a TATA-less upstream element, located between nucleotides −38 and −24, the TCAGTT Inr sequence at the start site and a downstream sequence between +13 and +60. Polyadenylation of the viral RNA occurs in the 3′ LTR downstream of the Inr sequence, thus leaving short direct repeats (R) which flank unique LTR regions at the 5′ (U5) and 3′ (U3) ends (**Fig. 1B**). A subgenomic RNA (**Fig. 1C**) has been partially characterized in adult females and in Schneider-2 tissue cell cultures; it only seems to differ from the full-length transcript by the splicing of a 5 kb sequence removing the end of the leader and the *gag* and *pol* ORFs. This splicing event generates a putative initiator codon for ORF 3.

No transcription initiation has ever been described from the 3′ LTR. By contrast, insertion of Gypsy in direct orientation into introns of the *forked* gene may result in mutant phenotypes when polyadenylation of the readthrough transcript occurs in the 5′ LTR before the intron plus the insertion have been spliced.

In addition to the two major transcripts, a rather abundant population of transcripts of various sizes is assumed to originate from the subfamily of defective proviruses, in particular as a result of readthrough transcription in either orientation.

Transcriptional Regulation

The molecular basis of the precise patterns of developmentally regulated Gypsy expression is not yet known. The two following transregulators are currently being studied:

- The product of the *flamenco* gene reduces the accumulation of Gypsy transcripts, especially that of the subgenomic transcript (see below, Transmission and Tissue Specificity). As judged from the ability of a transcriptional fusion to be repressed by *flamenco*, all the relevant *cis*-regulatory sequences must be located within a region encompassing the 5′ LTR and the leader sequence.
- The Gypsy leader region (**Fig. 1A**) contains two elements which bind proteins from nuclear extracts. One is an imperfect palindrome having some homology with the *lac*-operator of *Escherichia coli*. The other contains 12 copies of the binding site (5′PyPu$^T/_C$TGCATA$^C/_T$PyPu) for the *Drosophila* zinc-finger protein SU(HW). When binding of the ubiquitous SU(HW) factor is prevented, Gypsy transcription is uniformly reduced in every tissue. It can act both as an insulator and as a tissue-specific enhancer. This insulating ability is responsible for the SU(HW)-dependent mutant phenotypes induced by Gypsy insertions in the regulatory regions of various genes.

Translation and Post-translational Processing

Very little is known about the ORF 1 and ORF 2 products. From sequence analogy with retroviruses, ORF 2 is assumed to be translated by a -1 frameshifting process. An anti-IN monoclonal antibody failed to detect the GAG-POL fusion protein. Only a 50 kDa polypeptide was lighted up, whereas a 40 kDa IN subunit is expected. In preparations containing extracellular Gypsy particles from the supernatant of *Drosophila* cell cultures (see below, Characteristics of the Viral Particles), a 37 kDa polypeptide was shown to have some specific affinity to Gypsy nucleic acids.

Products of the *env* gene can be detected in ovary extracts of permissive *flamenco* females (see below, Transmission and Tissue Specificity). Treatment by endoglycosidase F reduces the apparent molecular mass of the 66 kDa ENV precursor such that it comigrates with the product of ORF 3 translated *in vitro*. This glycosylated precursor is cleaved into a 34 kDa surface polypeptide (SU) and a 28 kDa transmembrane subunit (TM). Transfection of *Drosophila* cell cultures by the *env* gene under control of the *actin* promoter results in accumulation of the ENV products in the cell membranes.

Characteristics of the Viral Particles

Particles containing Gypsy RNA were first described in the supernatant of *Drosophila* cell cultures (*D. melanogaster* 67j25D and *D. virilis* 79f9 cell lines). Later, fractionation by sucrose density gradients of permissive *flamenco* female extracts produced low-density fractions characterized by the co-occurrence of the ENV product and an endogenous reverse transcriptase activity able to synthetize Gypsy DNA without addition of any Gypsy template. On immunoelectron microscopic and negative staining pictures of these fractions, one can surmise particle-like structures about 100 nm in diameter, the outside of which tends to be decorated by the anti-ENV monoclonal antibodies. In the follicle cells of the same females, much smaller intracytoplasmic particles (40–45 nm in diameter, see **Fig. 2**), lighted up by a Gypsy DNA probe, were found to accumulate close to the membrane domains where ENV is targeted. Neither budding nor enveloped extracellular virions could be observed, as if the replication cycle of this type D-like retrovirus was somewhat abortive in this tissue.

Reverse Transcription

The sophisticated process of reverse transcription of LTR retroelements results in production of DNA with LTRs starting from an RNA template flanked with short terminal repeats. Reconstruction of the complete Gypsy LTR DNA was actually documented in *Drosophila* cultured cells transfected with Gypsy constructs missing the 5′ U3 sequence.

This process is due to the ability of reverse transcriptase to switch templates several times, involving formation of several distinct molecular

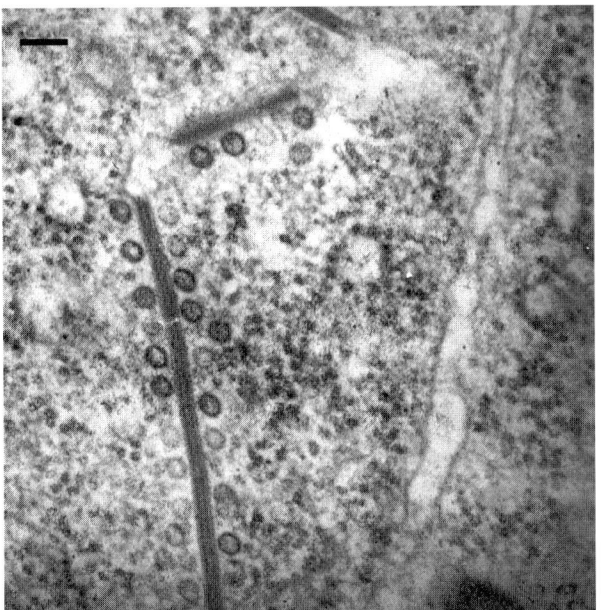

Figure 2 Localization and ultrastructure of Gypsy particles inside *flamenco* permissive follicle cells. In transverse sections, the cellular membranes appear connected together, from place to place, by some junction-like dense material. In immunoelectron microscopic experiments, not shown here, these particular membrane domains were specifically decorated by the anti-ENV antibodies. The picture also shows that these specific membrane domains are covered internally by numerous 40–45 nm particles which, in another experiment, were shown to hybridize with a Gypsy probe. Bar = 100 nm.

forms composed of the template RNA and the nascent DNA strands, organized in a highly specific fashion. Such RNA–DNA hybrids (including the 'minus strong-stop DNA', associated to an RNA primer, the 'plus strong-stop DNA' and full-length minus-strand cDNAs with one or two LTRs), could be actually identified, after oligo(dT) chromatography of nucleic acids extracted from the cell line 67j25d, as permanent cellular ingredients in the absence of exogenous retroviral infection. Similarly, Gypsy strong-stop DNAs are to be found even in females where neither particles nor insertions can be detected, suggesting that they result from the incomplete reverse transcription cycle of the endogenous Gypsy transcripts.

Integration and Excision

In the absence of any external infection, the insertion frequency of germinal proviruses ranges from 10^{-4} to 10^{-1} per haploid genome per active provirus, depending on the host genetic background. In the few insertional mutations analyzed so far, the PyPuPyPu*PyPu consensus sequence – (Py) pyrimidine; (Pu) purine; (*) insertion site – was used as a target, the first four nucleotides being duplicated at both ends of the insertion.

Three different insertional mutations were reported to revert at a frequency of 5×10^{-4} as a result of precise Gypsy excision. The mechanism of this amazing phenomenon is not yet understood.

Transmission and Tissue Specificity

Gypsy is generally transmitted vertically through the germline as a provirus and is not contagious in normal breeding conditions. However, infectious properties of Gypsy were demonstrated by experiments in which crude extracts of pupae issued from a *flamenco* permissive strain containing a high copy number of active Gypsy were put in contact with permissive larvae lacking active Gypsy. Using a genetic assay (based on the screening of mutations due to *de novo* insertion of Gypsy), new sites of Gypsy insertion were observed in the progeny of the flies subjected to the extracts. These results suggest that Gypsy can be efficiently transmitted to the germline of permissive individuals.

The regulation of Gypsy by the *flamenco* gene is tissue-specific. The Gypsy RNAs and ENV proteins accumulate in the ovaries of *flamenco* permissive females. This accumulation takes place near the apical membrane of the somatic follicle cells that surround the oocyte, whereas no derepression occurs in the germline which gives rise to the progeny where integration occurs. This pattern of accumulation is reminiscent of the targeting of enveloped viruses to membrane domains of epithelial cells.

Gypsy ORF 3 is expressed from a spliced messenger RNA that encodes a membrane glycoprotein containing a signal peptide and an endopeptidase cleavage site characteristic of retroviral ENV protein. Direct evidence of Gypsy ENV infectious properties was obtained using a Moloney murine leukemia virus-based retroviral vector pseudotyped by the Gypsy ENV protein. Such particles, produced in the 293GP human cell line, can infect *Drosophila* cells. *Drosophila* cell receptors for Gypsy entry remain to be determined.

Distribution

Southern blot experiments using the Gypsy sequence as a probe have shown that Gypsy-related sequences are widespread in the *Drosophila* genus.

Sequences homologous to Gypsy from *D. subobscura* (GypsyDs) and *D. virilis* (GypsyDv) were cloned and entirely sequenced. The sequenced GypsyDs and GypsyDv ORF 3s do not have the coding capacity for

Table 1 Insect endogenous retroviruses containing an *env*-like gene.

Element	Host species	env-like spliced RNA	ENV protein	Infectivity
Gypsy	D. melanogaster	Yes	Yes	Yes
ZAM	D. melanogaster	Yes	Yes	?
tom	D. ananassae	Yes	Yes	?
TED	Trichoplusia ni	?	Yes	?
roo/B104	D. melanogaster	Yes	?	?
Tirant	D. melanogaster	?	?	?
297	D. melanogaster	?	?	?
17.6	D. melanogaster	?	?	?
Idefix	D. melanogaster	?	?	?
Osvaldo	D. buzzatii	?	?	?

functional envelopes because they contain several stop codons generating truncated proteins. The phylogenetic relationship of these three elements is not consistent with the phylogeny of the three host species, suggesting horizontal transfer(s) of the Gypsy elements across species.

All *D. melanogaster* strains contain defective Gypsy proviruses located in pericentromeric heterochromatin. The strains caught in the wild studied so far contain a few additional putatively active Gypsy proviruses (fewer than five) located in euchromatin.

Putative endogenous retroviruses are common in insects. Gypsy is not the only endogenous retrovirus found in insects. Many other envelope-containing insect elements have a similar ORF 3 (**Table 1**) but Gypsy is the only invertebrate retroelement for which infectivity has been shown.

See also: **Endogenous viruses; Host genetic resistance; Replication of viruses; Retroviruses – type D (*Retroviridae*).**

Further Reading

Arhipova IR, Lyubomirskaya NV and Ilyin YV (1995) *Drosophila* retrotransposons. New York: RG Landes, Springer.

Bucheton A (1995) The relationship between the *flamenco* gene and Gypsy in *Drosophila:* how to tame a retrovirus. *Trends Genet.* 11: 349.

Kim A, Terzian C, Santamaria P *et al* (1994) Retroviruses in invertebrates: the Gypsy retrotransposon is apparently an infectious retrovirus of *Drosophila melanogaster. Proc. Natl Acad. Sci. USA* 91: 1285.

Pélisson A, Song SU, Prud'homme N *et al* (1994) Gypsy transposition correlates with the production of a retroviral envelope-like protein under the tissue-specific control of the *Drosophila flamenco* gene. *EMBO J.* 13: 4401.

Pélisson A, Teysset L, Chalvet F *et al* (1997) About the origin of retroviruses and the co-evolution of the Gypsy retrovirus with the *Drosophila flamenco* gene. *Genetica* 100: 29–37.

RHABDOVIRUSES (*RHABDOVIRIDAE*)

Contents

Plant Rhabdoviruses

Ungrouped Mammalian, Bird and Fish Rhabdoviruses

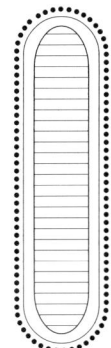

Plant Rhabdoviruses

Andrew O Jackson, **Michael Goodin**, **Ignacio Moreno**, **Jennifer Johnson** and **Diane M Lawrence**, Department of Plant and Microbial Biology, University of California, Berkeley, California, USA

Copyright © 1999 Academic Press

Introduction

Plant viruses have traditionally been included in the Rhabdovirus family based on their distinctive enveloped bacilliform or bullet-shaped particles. These large complex particles can be distinguished readily from the constituents present in uninfected tissue by electron microscopy of extracts or thin sections of infected tissue. Therefore, numerous putative rhabdoviruses have been described in many different plant families. Microscopy of infected cells reveals that plant rhabdoviruses can be distinguished depending on whether the viruses elicit inclusions in the nucleus, bud from the inner nuclear envelope, and accumulate in the perinuclear spaces, or whether they undergo morphogenesis from cytoplasmic membranes and accumulate in the cytoplasm. Thus, the cytopathology of most plant rhabdoviruses differs in several respects from that of the prototype animal rhabdovirus, vesicular stomatitis virus (VSV), which replicates in the cytoplasm and undergoes morphogenesis at the plasma membrane.

Plant rhabdoviruses infect a large number of monocot and dicot plant species (**Table 1**). In some instances, serious disease outbreaks occur on economically important crop plants, some of which result in substantial losses on a recurring basis. The most serious pathogens include maize mosaic virus (MMV), lettuce necrotic yellows virus (LNYV), rice transitory yellowing virus (RTYV) which may be identical to rice yellow stunt virus (RYSV), strawberry crinkle virus (SCV), potato yellow dwarf virus (PYDV), and barley yellow striate mosaic virus (BYSMV). A number of other rhabdoviruses also have considerable disease potential that can be affected by agronomic practices and biological variables of the insect vectors that facilitate their transmission.

Most plant rhabdoviruses are highly dependent on transmission by phytophagous insects, so their prevalence and distribution is influenced to a large extent by the ecology and host preferences of their vectors. Virus–vector interactions are highly specific, and in all cases where known vectors have been carefully examined, they have been shown to support the replication of the plant rhabdoviruses they transmit. Although some rhabdoviruses can be transmitted mechanically by abrasion of leaves, this mode of transmission does not contribute significantly to natural spread in nature due to the labile nature of the virion. Moreover, seed or pollen transmission of plant rhabdoviruses has not been described; thus, aside from vegetative propagation, direct plant to plant transmission is unlikely to be a major factor in the ecology or epidemiology of these pathogens.

Taxonomy and Classification

The International Committee on Taxonomy of Viruses used subcellular distribution patterns to assign plant rhabdoviruses into the *Cytorhabdovirus* and the *Nucleorhabdovirus* genera (**Table 1**). Individual members within these groups have also been shown to be distinct based on host range, vector transmission, serology and nucleic acid hybridization analyses. Presently, eight viruses (BYSMV, broccoli necrotic yellows virus (BNYV), festuca leaf streak virus (FLSV), LNYV, northern cereal mosaic virus (NCMV), sonchus virus (SV), SCV, and wheat American striate mosaic virus (WASMV)) are assigned to the *Cytorhabdovirus* genus. The *Nucleorhabdovirus* genus has seven members (Datura yellow vein virus (DYVV), eggplant mottled dwarf virus (EMDV), MMV, PYDV, RTYV, sonchus yellow net virus (SYNV), and sowthistle yellow vein virus (SYVV)). Of these viruses, SYNV and LNYV have been the most extensively characterized in terms of sequence analysis.

Table 1 List of plant rhabdoviruses and their host and insect specificity

Virus	Host	Vector	Virus	Host	Vector
Cytorhabdovirus			*Unassigned Plant Rhabdoviruses* (cont.)		
Barley yellow striate mosaic virus (BYSMV)	M	L	Finger millet mosaic virus (FMMV)	M	L
Broccoli necrotic yellows virus (BNYV)	D*	A	Gerbera symptomless virus (GRBSV)	D	
Festuca leaf streak virus (FLSV)	M		Gomphrena virus (GoV)	D*	
Lettuce necrotic yellows virus (LNYV)	D*	A	Holcus lanatus yellowing virus (HLYV)	M	
Northern cereal mosaic virus (NCMV)	M	L	Iris germanica leaf stripe virus (IGLSV)	M	
Sonchus virus (SonV)	D*		Ivy vein clearing virus (IVCV)	D*	
Strawberry crinkle virus (SCV)	D*	A	Laelia red leafspot virus (LRLV)	D*	
Wheat American striate mosaic virus (WASV)	M	L	*Launea arborescens* stunt virus (LASV)	D	
			Lemon scented thyme leaf chlorosis virus (LSCTV)	D	
Nucleorhabdovirus			Lolium ryegrass virus (LoRV)	M	
Datura yellow vein virus (DYVV)	D		Lucerne enation virus (LEV)	D	A
Eggplant mottled dwarf virus (EMDV)	D*		Lupine yellow vein virus (LYVV)	D	
[Pittosporium vein yellowing virus]			*Malva sylvestris* virus (MaSV)	D	
[Tomato vein yellowing virus]			Maize sterile stunt virus (MSSV)	M	L
Maize mosaic virus (MMV)	M	L	Meliotus latent virus (MeLV)	D*	
Potato yellow dwarf virus (PYDV)	D*	L	Melon variegation virus (MVV)	D	
Rice yellow stunt virus (RYSV)	M	L	Oat striate mosaic virus (OSMV)	M	L
[Rice transitory yellowing virus (RTYV)]			Orchid fleck virus (OFV)	D*	
Sonchus yellow net virus (SYNV)	D*	A	Parsley virus (PaV)	D*	
Sowthistle yellow vein virus (SYVV)	D	A	Pelargonium vein clearing virus (PVCV)	D*	
			Pigeon pea proliferation virus (PPPV)	D	
Unassigned Plant Rhabdoviruses			Pineapple chlorotic leaf streak virus (PCLSV)	M	
Atropa belladonna virus (AtBV)	D		Pisum virus (PiV)	D*	
Beet leaf curl virus (BLCV)	D	LW	Plantain mottle virus (PIMV)	D	
Callistephus chinensis chlorosis virus (CCCV)	D		*Ranunculus repens* symptomless virus (RsRSV)	D	
Carnation bacilliform virus (CBV)	D		Raphanus virus (RaV)	D*	
Carrot latent virus (CLV)	D	A	Raspberry vein chlorosis virus (RVCV)	D	A
Cassava symptomless virus (CasSV)	D		Red clover mosaic virus (RCIMV)	D	
Cereal chlorotic mottle virus (CCMV)	M		Sainpaulia leaf necrosis virus (SLNV)	D	
Chrysanthemum frutescens virus (CFV)	D		Sambucus vein clearing virus (SVCV)	D	
Chrysanthemum vein chlorosis virus (CVCV)	D		*Sarracenia purpurea* virus (SPV)	D	
Clover enation virus (ClOEV)	D		Sorghum virus (SV)	M	L
Coffee ringspot virus (CoRSV)	D*	M	Soursop yellow blotch virus (SYBV)	D	
Colocasia bobone disease virus (CBDV)	D	P	*Triticum aestivum* chlorotic spot virus (TaCSV)	M	
Coriander feathery red vein virus (CFRVV)	D*	A	*Vigna sinensis* mosaic virus (VSMV)	D	
Cow parsnip mosaic virus (CPMV)	D*		Winter wheat Russian mosaic virus (WWMV)	M	L
Cynara virus (CyV)	D*		Wheat chlorotic streak virus (WCSV)	M	L
Digitaria striate virus (DSV)	M	L	Wheat rosette stunt virus (WRSV)	M	L
Euonymus fasciation virus (EFV)	D		*Zea mays* virus (ZMV)	M	

Names in brackets are synonomous to those immediately above. Host: D = Dicot, M = Monocot. (*) indicates ability to be mechanically transmitted. Vectors: A = Aphid, L = Leafhopper, LW = Lacewing, M = Mite, P = Planthopper. Blank spaces indicate that no insect vector has been defined.

Most other plant rhabdoviruses have not been investigated in much detail beyond cursory infectivity studies, crude physicochemical analyses of virus particles, and electron microscopic observations of morphogenesis. Consequently, nearly sixty rhabdoviruses await assignment to a genus (**Table 1**). Moreover, sufficient comparative information to determine whether individual descriptions from disparate hosts are due to distant, closely related, or identical viruses is not available from many preliminary descriptions. Hence, more definitive morphological, serological and molecular studies need to

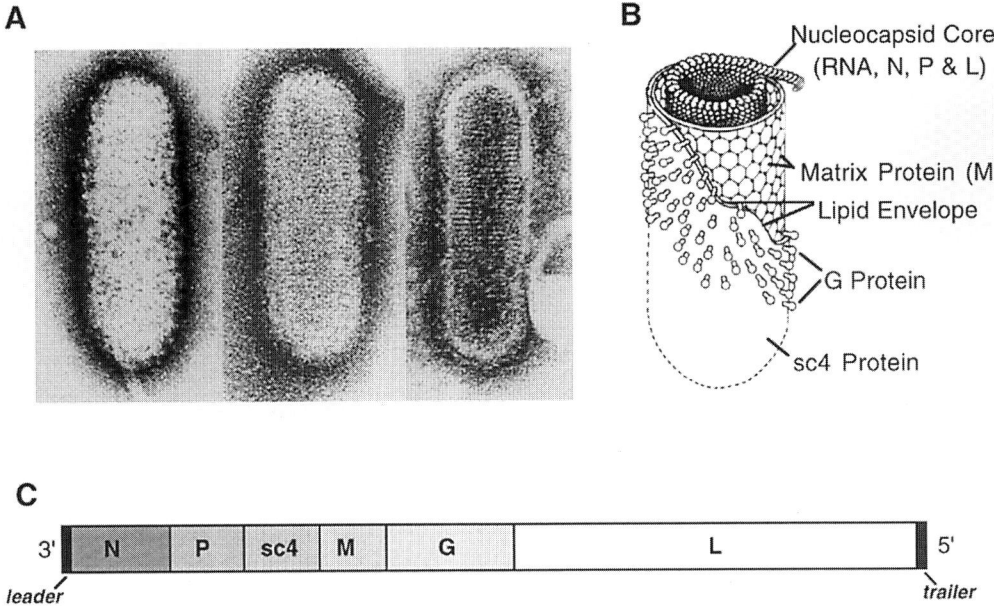

Figure 1 Plant rhabdovirus morphology and depiction of the sonchus yellow net virus genome. (**A**) Electron micrographs of negatively stained particles of SYNV. The panel on the left shows a lightly stained particle illustrating the hexagonal subunit associations at the surface of the virion. The slightly more intense negative stain in the center highlights the surface glycoprotein spikes surrounding the particle. The right panel illustrates a particle with deeper penetration revealing the internal striated nucleocapsid core. (**B**) Depiction of the architecture of the virus particle. The nucleocapsid core is composed of the minus-sense genomic RNA, the nucleocapsid protein (N), the phosphoprotein (P), and the polymerase protein (L). The matrix protein (M) is involved in the attachment of the nucleocapsid core to the envelope. The membrane lipids are host-derived and are interspersed with an orderly array of the glycoprotein (G) spikes. The location of the sc4 protein has not been precisely defined, but it is solubilized by nonionic detergent treatment of virions. (**C**) Depiction of the genome organization of SYNV. The 13 720 nucleotide minus-strand genomic RNA from 3′ to 5′ consists of the leader sequence, the N, P, sc4, M, G and L protein genes and the trailer sequence. The relative sizes of the genes are proportional to the size of the viral RNA. Adapted from Jackson and Wagner (1998).

be carried out to establish reliable criteria for the taxonomic grouping of plant rhabdoviruses, and to more readily verify their roles as causal agents of specific diseases. Additional biological data also need to be acquired with numerous poorly characterized rhabdoviruses whose host range, vector relations and distribution have received only cursory attention. Nevertheless, even though taxonomy assignments and our understanding of the relatedness of the rhabdoviruses are presently rudimentary, modern molecular and cell biological methodology provides great potential for identifying and characterizing unassigned plant rhabdoviruses, and developing additional criteria to better appreciate stages in their evolution.

Virion Morphology and Composition

Plant rhabdoviruses are normally bacilliform after careful fixation, but are bullet-shaped in unfixed preparations (**Fig. 1A**). Estimates of the sizes of virus particles range from 45 to 100 nm in width and 130 to 350 nm in length; however it is very difficult to determine accurately the sizes of the virus particles due to swelling of the fragile virions, shrinking of the nucleocapsid core, and other artifacts. Electron microscopy of particles reveals three distinct layers of varying electron density whose composition has been determined for several viruses by particle disruption, gel electrophoresis and RNA analyses. The outer layer containing 5–10 nm spike-like surface projections is composed of the G protein (**Fig. 1B**). The spikes appear to be arranged as hexamers on the surface and, by analogy with animal rhabdoviruses, G protein trimers may participate in forming the surface lattice. The middle layer consists of a host-derived membrane penetrated by the G protein. The striated inner core, with a periodicity of 4–5 nm, is composed of a helical ribonucleoprotein consisting of the genomic RNA, the nucleocapsid protein (N), the phosphoprotein (P), and the L polymerase protein (**Fig. 1 A, B**). The exact location of the matrix protein (M), has not yet been clearly determined, but it probably participates in coiling of the nucleocapsid and interacts with the G protein to stabilize the particle. A sixth protein (sc4) found in SYNV particles has no known function, but it can be solubilized from membrane components on treatment with nonionic detergents.

The overall chemical composition (~70% protein, 2% RNA, 20–25% lipid, and a small amount of carbohydrate associated with the G protein) of the plant and animal rhabdoviruses is similar. The minus-sense RNA genomes of plant rhabdoviruses range in size from ~11 to 14 kb based on sedimentation and gel electrophoretic analyses, and are slightly larger than those of most described animal rhabdoviruses. The lipids of plant and animal rhabdoviruses have differences in fatty acid and sterol composition that are related to their respective hosts and sites of morphogenesis. Two nucleorhabdoviruses, SYNV and PYDV, have been examined in the most detail, and the results indicate that a variety of fatty acids, free and esterified sterols are present in purified virus particles. Four sterols predominating in SYNV closely approximate the sterols of the nuclear envelope, whereas those of NCMV, a cytorhabdovirus, are more typical of cytoplasmic membranes.

	I	II	III
Consensus	AP_yUP_yUUUU	^G_CN	P_yUNNN
SYNV	AUUCUUUUU	GG	UUG^{AA}_{UC}
LNYV	AUUCUUUU	$G(N)_x$	CU^{AAG}_{UUU}
VSV	ACUUUUUU	^G_CU	UUGUC
RV	ACUUUUUU	$C(N)_x$	$UUGU^A_G$

Figure 2 Alignment of the intergenic regions of selected plant and animal rhabdoviruses. The rhabdovirus consensus sequence is shown at the top followed by the sequences of sonchus yellow net virus (SYNV), lettuce necrotic yellows virus (LNYV), vesicular stomatitis virus (VSV) and rabies virus (RV). The intergenic sequences ('gene-junction' sequences) are separated into three elements: element I constitutes the poly(U) tract at the 3' end of each gene on the genomic RNA; element II is a short sequence that is not transcribed during mRNA synthesis; element III constitutes the start site for transcription of each mRNA. The bold type in the viral sequences indicates the consensus nucleotides, P_y indicates pyrimidine, $(N)_x$ corresponds to a variable number of nucleotides.

Genomic Structure and Organization

The nucleotide sequence of SYNV RNA and genome mapping studies of LNYV show that both viruses encode six proteins, but otherwise, their genome organization is similar to those of VSV, which encodes five genes. The gene order for SYNV is 3'-leader-N-P-sc4-M-G-L-trailer-5' (**Fig. 1C**), and the order for LNYV is 3'-leader-N-4a-4b-M-G-L-trailer-5' (where 4a is thought to represent a phosphoprotein derivative and 4b an undefined extra gene). The coding regions of SYNV and LNYV are flanked by leader sequences at the 3' end of the minus-sense genomes, and by a noncoding trailer sequence at the 5' end of the genomes. The leader and trailer sequences of the plant rhabdoviruses have complementary regions, as is the case with other minus-strand viruses, and both sequences are considerably longer than those of animal rhabdoviruses. Another difference is that the transcribed leader RNA of SYNV is polyadenylated, which may represent an adaptation to facilitate its nuclear mode of replication.

The leader and trailer genes of SYNV have little obvious sequence relatedness to those of LNYV or other animal rhabdoviruses. In contrast, the intergenic 'gene-junction' sequences of SYNV and the animal rhabdoviruses are generally highly conserved (**Fig. 2**). These intergenic regions can be grouped into three components constituting a poly(U) tract at the 3' end of each gene on the genomic template (element I), a short nontranscribed element which separates each gene (element II), and a conserved element located at the beginning of each subsequent gene (element III). The SYNV 'gene junctions' are very similar to the intergenic region following the N gene of the nucleorhabdovirus, RYSV. LNYV also has some similarity to other rhabdoviruses in element I, but elements II and III diverge substantially. Element 1 (AUUCUUUUU) of SYNV is also nearly identical to the analogous regions (AUUCUUUUU) of Ebola virus, suggesting that some conservation of regulatory regions may extend to the *Filoviridae*. Sequence similarities in this region are also found in paramyxoviruses and in borna disease virus. Thus, intergenic regions of the genome that play an important role in regulating mRNA transcription and replication appear to have been stringently conserved. However, the leader and trailer genes and the genes encoding the proteins appear to have undergone extensive evolution to accommodate diverse host requirements.

Properties of the Encoded Proteins

The structural properties of plant rhabdovirus proteins deduced from nucleotide sequence analyses are presented below in the order of their appearance from the 3' end of the genome (**Fig. 1C**). Only rudimentary biochemical analyses have been conducted on the proteins and these are mostly confined to SYNV and LNYV. Overall, the plant rhabdovirus proteins appear to have very little sequence relatedness to analogous proteins of animal rhabdoviruses, with the exception of the L protein which has conserved motifs common to those of most rhabdoviruses. A description of these proteins and their probable functions is outlined below.

The nucleocapsid protein (N)

The N protein functions to encapsidate the genomic and antigenomic RNAs and it is a component of the viroplasms and of the polymerase complex that can be isolated from nuclei of SYNV-infected plants. The N protein genes of the nucleorhabdoviruses, SYNV and RYSV, and the cytorhabdovirus, LNYV, have been sequenced. The deduced proteins of these viruses have no extensive sequence relatedness to animal rhabdovirus proteins, although their hydropathy patterns have some similarity. However, the SYNV and RYSV N proteins have limited regions of weak homology that are more closely related to each other than to analogous regions of the N protein of LNYV. The 475 amino acid SYNV N protein contains a nucleoplasmin-like nuclear localization signal close to the carboxy terminus that has some involvement in mediating the nuclear localization of the N protein. A related consensus element is also present in the RYSV N protein, but this element is lacking in the cytorhabdovirus, LNYV. The SYNV, LNYV and RYSV N proteins all contain regions located approximately two-thirds of the way towards the carboxy termini that appear to be weakly conserved with that of VSV.

The phosphoprotein (P)

Sequence information for the P protein and the remaining encoded genes are available only for SYNV. The P gene encodes a 362 amino acid protein with no direct amino acid sequence relatedness to the P proteins of other rhabdoviruses. However, the SYNV P protein appears to have functions similar to those of other rhabdoviruses because it is a component of the viral nucleocapsid core and the nuclear associated replicase complex. The P protein is also capable of forming complexes *in vivo* with the N and L proteins that are analogous to N:P and P:L complexes found in VSV-infected cells that may function in transcription and replicase recycling. The amino terminal half of the SYNV P protein is negatively charged, as is the case with the other rhabdoviruses, but little charge similarity or sequence resemblance is present at the carboxy terminus. The SYNV P protein is phosphorylated *in vivo* at threonine residues and hence differs from the VSV P protein, which is phosphorylated at serine residues. The SYNV P protein accumulates in the nucleus and a basic region approximately 150 amino acids from the amino terminus may have some karyophilic properties.

The sc4 protein

The sc4 protein appears to be associated with the SYNV envelope because nonionic detergent treatments can facilitate its release from virus particles. sc4 does not contain an obvious transmembrane domain or a nuclear localization signal. However, it could be associated with membranes by acylation through attachment of palmitic acid residues found in the viral envelope and thioester (cysteine) or ester (serine or threonine) linkages. Recent studies suggest that sc4 may be phosphorylated *in vivo*. Analysis of the sequence reveals that 16% of the amino acids are serine or threonine residues and that four potential consensus casein kinase II phosphorylation sites are present. The sc4 protein also contains a motif related to an aspartic protease site found in α-amylases and cellular and acid proteases. The function of sc4 has not been elucidated, but it may play a role in aphid transmission or in cell to cell movement. However, irrespective of its function, sc4 appears to be unique to plant rhabdoviruses because its predicted sequence has no similarity to sixth genes encoded by infectious hematopoietic necrosis virus, Sigma virus, Flanders virus, or bovine ephemeral fever virus.

The matrix protein (M)

The 286 amino acid M protein is basic and is thought to function in nucleocapsid coiling and interactions with the G protein, as is the case with other rhabdovirus M proteins. Multiple alignments of the M protein fail to reveal conserved consensus motifs, but short stretches of amino acids display some similarities in composition to the M proteins of other rhabdoviruses. A hydrophobic region of 67 amino acids extending almost to the middle of the protein could be involved in membrane–lipid interactions with the G protein. Recent studies suggest that the SYNV M protein is phosphorylated *in vivo* at both threonine and serine residues.

The glycoprotein (G)

The G protein forms the glycoprotein virion spike. The 632 amino acid sequence deduced for the G protein has no significant homology to G proteins of other rhabdoviruses, but it does contain putative signal sequences, a transmembrane anchor domain, and glycosylation signals. In addition, the SYNV G protein contains a putative nuclear targeting signal near the carboxy-terminus which could be involved in transit to the inner nuclear membrane prior to morphogenesis. Glycosylation inhibitors interfere with G protein N-glycosylation and the protein is stable in tunicamycin-treated cells. This treatment blocks SYNV morphogenesis and results in striking arrays of condensed nucleocapsid cores that fail to bud and accumulate in the nuclei.

The polymerase protein (L)

The SYNV L gene encodes a 2116 amino acid protein that is present in low abundance within the nucleocapsid. The L protein is required for polymerase activity, because antibodies raised against a fragment containing the GDNQ (polymerase) motif inhibit transcription. As is the case with other rhabdoviruses, the L protein is positively charged and contains polymerase and RNA binding domains. Alignment of the L protein sequence with polymerases of several other nonsegmented negative-strand RNA viruses reveals conservation within 12 motifs that appear sequentially in the protein. A cluster dendrogram derived from the L protein alignments suggests that SYNV is more closely related to animal rhabdoviruses than to paramyxoviruses, and that animal rhabdoviruses have diverged less from each other than from SYNV.

Polymerase Activity

A viral RNA-dependent RNA polymerase is activated after treatment of LNYV and BNYV cytorhabdovirus virions with mild nonionic detergents. This activity cosediments with the 40–45S loosely coiled nucleocapsid filaments that are released from virions by detergent treatment. The transcribed products are complementary to the genome, as expected of mRNAs. Thus, the described polymerases of these plant rhabdoviruses appear to be similar to the extensively studied polymerase of the animal rhabdovirus prototype, VSV.

In contrast, no appreciable polymerase activity is evident in dissociated preparations of SYNV and other nucleorhabdovirus members. In this regard, the negligible levels of activity are similar to those obtained from rabies virus preparations. However, an active polymerase can be recovered from the nuclei of plants infected with SYNV. The polymerase activity is associated with a nucleoprotein complex consisting of the N, P, and L proteins, and it cosediments with SYNV nucleocapsid cores. The complex can be precipitated in an active form by P protein antibodies, and L protein antibody inhibition experiments show that the L protein is a functional component of the polymerase. Kinetic analysis of transcription products also reveals that the complex is capable of sequentially transcribing a polyadenylated plus-sense leader RNA, and polyadenylated mRNAs corresponding to each of the six SYNV-encoded proteins. Potential replication intermediates consisting of short incomplete minus-strand products homologous to the genomic RNA are also transcribed. These results thus support the hypothesis that polymerases of cytorhabdoviruses are present in an active form in virions and that released cores are capable of initiating primary transcription immediately upon uncoating. Nucleorhabdovirus particles differ by containing an inactive polymerase that appears to require activation by host components early in infection.

Defective Interfering RNAs

Animal rhabdoviruses passaged at high multiplicities of infection commonly accumulate defective-interfering (DI) particles. These DIs are dependent on the wild-type virus for their replication, and their presence results in a substantial decrease in the titer of the helper virus. The RNA molecules associated with DIs are typically internally deleted forms of the wild-type viral genomic RNA that retain the complementary 3′ and 5′ terminal sequences.

Formation of plant rhabdovirus DIs has been observed with PYDV and SYNV. PYDV passaged at high multiplicities of infection developed DIs after 30 successive mechanical transfers. The slowly sedimenting particles appeared not to be infectious in local lesion assays, but their protein composition was similar to those of the parental virus. In addition, the presence of the DIs decreased the amount of PYDV that could be isolated from infected plants. In the case of SYNV DIs, calyx tissues of *Nicotiana edwardsonii* examined 5 months after inoculation were shown to contain a high proportion of particles approximately three quarters as long as those of wild-type SYNV. Purified short particles were not infectious when inoculated alone, but when coinoculated with wild-type virions, short particles predominated upon reisolation. RNA isolated from these short particles was approximately 25% shorter than RNA from complete virions. The DI RNAs were able to hybridize to SYNV cDNA probes, but additional information about their structure has not been reported. From these results, the appearance of plant rhabdovirus DIs appears to be an uncommon occurrence that contrasts with the high frequency of animal rhabdovirus DIs.

Cytopathology and Replication

Unlike the animal rhabdoviruses which replicate and assemble in the cytoplasm, the plant rhabdoviruses vary profoundly in their sites of replication and morphogenesis (**Fig. 3**). The nucleorhabdoviruses, typified by SYNV, replicate in the nucleus, bud in

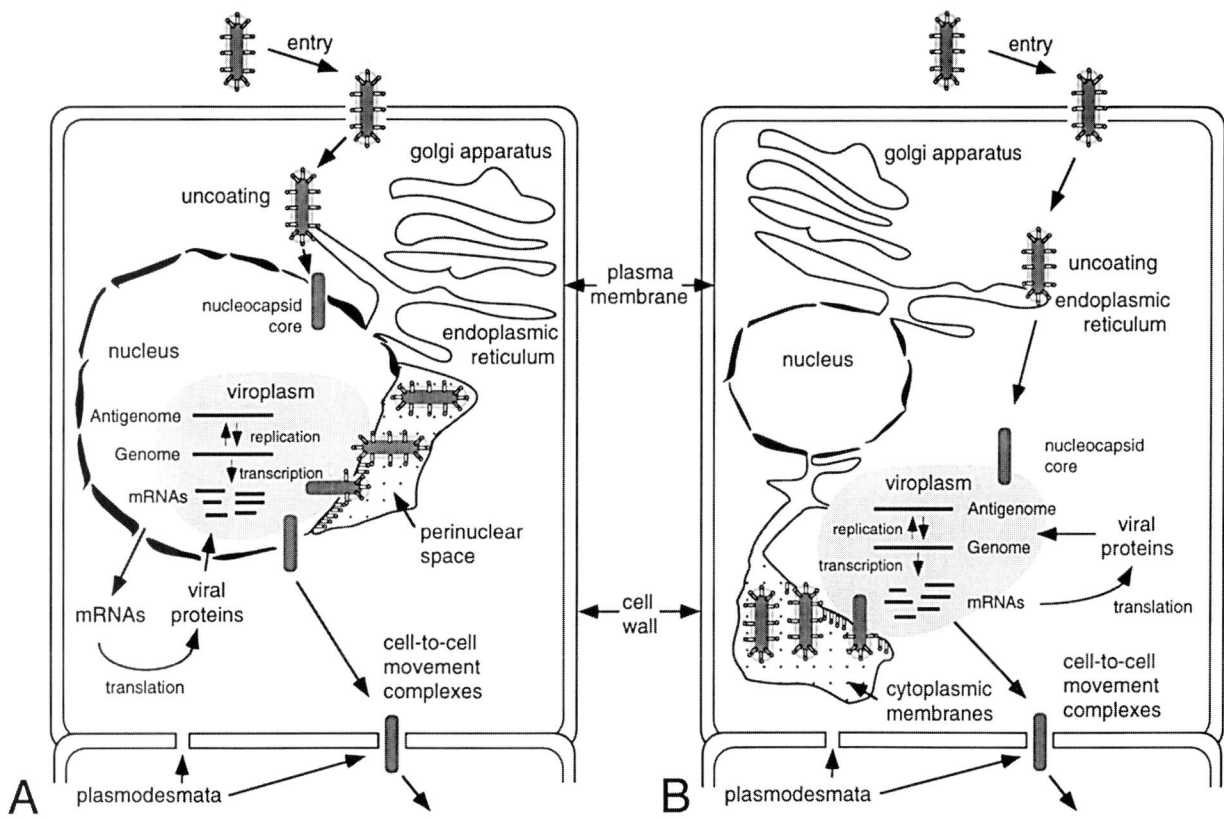

Figure 3 Model for the replication cycle of plant nucleorhabdoviruses (**A**) and cytorhabdoviruses (**B**). See text for details.

association with the inner nuclear envelope, and accumulate in enlarged perinuclear spaces formed between the inner and outer envelopes. Considerable attention has been focused on SYNV, and these studies support the model illustrated in **Fig. 3A**. The early entry and uncoating events are obscure, but based on observations with SYNV-infected protoplasts, it has been hypothesized that during entry into the cell, virus particles associate with the endoplasmic reticulum to release the nucleocapsid cores into the cytoplasm. It is thought that the cores utilize the host nucleocytoplasmic transport machinery to facilitate movement and entry into the nucleus via the nuclear pore complex. During the early stages of infection the virion-associated polymerase probably is activated by host components to produce an active transcriptase that participates in primary transcription. The transcribed mRNAs are transported to the cytoplasm and translated. The newly translated N, P and L polymerase core proteins are transported to the nucleus where they participate in multiple rounds of replication of antigenomic and genomic RNAs and secondary rounds of mRNA transcription. As replication proceeds, the nuclei increase dramatically in volume, and granular electron-dense viroplasms form discrete foci that appear near the periphery of the nuclei.

Several recent lines of evidence show that SYNV viroplasms contain the N, P and L proteins, suggesting that the viroplasms are the source of the polymerase activity that can be recovered from nuclei. During the late stages of replication, the matrix protein is thought to participate in coiling of nucleocapsid cores containing the minus-sense RNA genome. These cores then associate with G protein concentrated at sites on the inner nuclear envelope that are in close proximity to the viroplasms. Virus budding apparently requires G protein glycosylation because tunicamycin interrupts budding and causes the appearance of large numbers of the nucleocapsid cores around the periphery of the nucleus. During normal budding, numerous enveloped particles accumulate in perinuclear spaces between the inner and outer nuclear envelope, but in some instances, a few virus particles are present in cytoplasmic vesicles. Since the outer nuclear envelope is continuous with the endoplasmic reticulum and is part of the endomembrane system, this observation is not surprising. However, it does indicate that assignments to the nucleorhabdovirus group need to be based on several different types of ultrastructural evidence. Such evidence should include use of virus specific probes for *in situ* hybridization, immunochemical localization of nucleocapsid proteins, and high resolution immunoelectron microscopy to probe virus morphogenesis at different stages of infection.

The cytorhabdoviruses appear to replicate in the cytoplasm, bud in association with the endoplasmic reticulum, and accumulate in endoplasmic reticulum-derived vesicles (**Fig. 3B**). Two variations have been proposed based on extensive electron microscopic observations of LNYV and BYSMV cells. During the early stages of LNYV infection, indirect evidence suggests that LNYV may undergo a nuclear phase because the outer nuclear membrane blisters and develops small vesicles that contain some virus particles. However, later in the life cycle masses of thread-like viroplasms appear in the cytoplasm and these are in close proximity to dense networks of the endoplasmic reticulum. These membranes serve as sites for morphogenesis of the majority of virus particles which bud into vesicles that appear to be derived from the proliferated host membranes. A slightly different scenario lacking a nuclear phase has been outlined for BYSMV. In this case, membrane-bound viroplasms appear in the cytoplasm and virus particles are found exclusively in association with cytoplasmic membranes that proliferate in close proximity to the viroplasms. Unfortunately, both of the cytorhabdovirus models have been derived solely from ultrastructural observations, and none of these studies have utilized specific antibodies to individual virus proteins or viral-specific probes for *in situ* hybridization. Clearly more direct cell biological studies must be conducted with such reagents before detailed models of the replication cycles of these viruses can be proposed.

Vector Relationships, Distribution and Evolution

Many members of the rhabdoviruses are transmitted by insects and other arthropods in which they also multiply, so it is possible that members of the rhabdovirus family radiated from a primitive arthropod. This mode of transmission more than any other property, may have been responsible for the widespread occurrence of the rhabdoviruses within the plant and animal kingdoms. Although some plant rhabdoviruses have no known vector, most are transmitted by aphids (*Aphidae*), leafhoppers (*Jassidae*), or planthoppers (*Delphicidae*). Two poorly characterized putative rhabdoviruses, beet leaf curl virus and coffee ringspot virus, have lacebug and mite vectors, respectively, but these viruses need to be examined more rigorously before they can be unambiguously accepted as members of the *Rhabdoviridae*.

Several general patterns indicate that host–vector relationships have profoundly affected plant rhabdovirus distribution. For example, leafhoppers, planthoppers and aphids are prevalent on both monocots and dicots, but rhabdoviruses causing diseases of the *Gramineae* are all transmitted by leafhoppers or planthoppers. Except for PYDV and CBDV, which have leafhopper and planthopper vectors, respectively, the rhabdoviruses infecting dicots are commonly transmitted by aphids. The available evidence indicates that rhabdovirus–vector interactions are highly specific and that generally, a single rhabdovirus is transmitted by closely related species of the same genus. In all cases of insect transmission that have been carefully examined, the rhabdovirus is persistently transmitted in a propagative fashion. Comprehensive transmission trials conducted with PYDV in leafhoppers and SYVV in aphids, as well as less extensive studies with several other leafhopper and aphid transmitted rhabdoviruses, are all consistent with replication in the vector. Indirect evidence for replication is that long latent periods are required before transmission occurs, that virus is often retained throughout the life of the insect, and that transovarial passage can be observed through eggs and nymphs. More persuasive results have been obtained by continued transmission after repeated serial dilution passages from insect to insect. Strain specific infection of tissue culture lines and explants and serological detection of virus in vectors provides additional proof that rhabdoviruses replicate with high specificity in leafhopper and aphid vector cells.

Genetic experiments with PYDV have shown that highly efficient and inefficient leafhopper vectors can be selected. Continuous passage of PYDV by serial injection of insects can also result in isolates that are unable to infect plants. Additional studies have shown that strains that have lost their capacity to be insect transmitted can be recovered after protracted passage in plants. This phenomenon could provide a mechanism for evolution of vectorless rhabdoviruses particularly in cases where infections were established in vegetatively propagated hosts. Rhabdoviruses normally have the capacity to infect a greater range of hosts than the narrow range of species colonized by their vectors, because experimental host ranges usually can be extended considerably by mechanical transmission. One appropriate example is transmission of SCV, which is restricted in nature to cultivated and native strawberry due to feeding preferences of its aphid vector. SCV is very difficult to transmit mechanically from strawberry (**Table 1**). However, alternate solanaceous hosts can be infected by surrogate nonvector aphids injected with extracts from the strawberry aphid, and the virus can then be mechanically transmitted from these plants. In addition, cowpea protoplast infectivity experiments with the grass rhabdovirus FLSV and with SYNV show that both viruses are able to infect legume protoplasts, but they are unable to infect cowpea plants. These results indicate that plant rhabdoviruses have the ability to infect cells of hosts that are quite distantly related to their native hosts, but that vector feeding and requirements for systemic movement constrain their host specificity.

Plant rhabdoviruses are faced with two major evolutionary challenges of a fundamentally different nature brought about by the necessity to alternately infect plants and insects. In each host, the virus must utilize different entry methods and accommodate distinct cellular and defense mechanisms. Establishment of effective vector relations requires nonpathogenic infections of the insect without substantial interference with longevity, fecundity or normal feeding activities necessary for efficient virus dispersal. Rhabdovirus acquisition by the vector probably necessitates attachment to specific receptors at the surface of cells in the digestive system and active invasion of the reproductive organs, fat bodies and salivary glands. It is highly likely that vector specificity is regulated at the entry stages of infection via receptors on the surface of the host alimentary system. This hypothesis is supported by experiments showing that aphid vector specificity can be extended if the gut barrier is avoided by direct injection of virus. Very different barriers must be circumvented to establish systemic infections of plants. In order to establish a primary infection focus, the cell wall must first be breached by mouthparts of the insect, the virus must be regurgitated into the cell, uncoated and replicated. Then, to establish systemic invasions, the virus must move from cell to cell through very small plasmodesmatal connections, into the phloem cells of the vascular system and throughout the plant. Because the plasmodesmata normally restrict movement of macromolecules, viruses generally move to adjacent cells via mechanisms that increase the permeability of the plasmodesmatal openings. Many plus-strand RNA viruses encode specific nucleic acid binding proteins that function to enlarge plasmodesmata, bind viral RNA and shuttle the genome through the plasmodesmata to neighboring cells. Plant rhabdoviruses face a special challenge at this stage of infection because the approximately 3 nm plasmodesmata are at least an order of magnitude smaller in diameter than virus particles. Therefore, transit of intact viruses would require enormous plasmodesmatal alterations that ought to be easily visible by electron microscopy. Moreover, since the naked genomic RNA of minus-strand viruses is not infectious, the polymerase proteins must accompany the infectious derivative. These constraints probably mandate that rhabdovirus-encoded gene products facilitate enlargement of the plasmodesmata, and that nucleocapsid cores function in cell to cell and vascular movement. These movement activities may well require functions of the sixth genes that have been identified by mapping of SYNV and LNYV.

Epidemiology and Disease Control

Plant rhabdoviruses have been identified in most major crops throughout the world. Although the factors affecting their dispersal have not been investigated extensively, several studies suggest that transmission depends on a delicate balance of interactions involving vector–host plant associations. These include the specificity of the virus–vector relationship, the dependence on insect vectors for local and long distance spread, and possible pathological effects of rhabdovirus infections on the insects. The ecology of host plant and insect vector interactions also has a major role in distribution and spread of plant rhabdoviruses. Therefore, a number of interacting factors, including changes in vector species and weed host populations could affect rhabdovirus ecology and disease cycles. In Berkeley, California, an interesting example resulting in a marked decline of SYVV in natural sowthistle populations has been attributed to the displacement of the aphid vector (*Hyperomyzus lactucae*) with an aggressive invader aphid (*Uroleucon sonchi*) that is not a vector for SYVV. Other obvious components affecting the biology of plant rhabdoviruses and their capacity to cause disease are virus reservoirs in weed hosts or volunteer crop plants that bridge the season between crops, and vectors that survive from one crop generation to the next. An additional element that often is not considered is that synergistic or antagonistic interactions with other viruses may affect viral ecology. One possibility of such interactions comes from a correlation of the presence of bidens mottle virus (BMoV), a potyvirus, in all beggarticks (*Bidens* sp.) harboring SYNV. Potyviruses often act synergistically with a number of viruses, including SYNV; thus it is likely that BMoV may serve to facilitate high levels of SYNV that aid in aphid acquisition.

Several additional interactions also contribute to disease outbreaks. These include populations of viruliferous aphids early in the growing season that can establish infection foci when crops are most susceptible to invasion. After initial infections have been established, rapid distribution of the virus probably is most dependent on a sufficient density of host plants capable of supporting the vector and transmission of virus to juvenile insects. Concurrently, environmental conditions conducive to short incubation periods after acquisition feeding by vectors, and optimal for rapid disease development in plants after virus transmission will facilitate efficient dissemination of the virus. Consequently, seemingly minor changes in climate, agronomic practices, crop varieties or vector populations may alter virus spread and disease development profoundly, and manipulation of these factors can lead to reductions in yield losses.

For these reasons, rhabdovirus disease control has emphasized a broad range of different strategies. Agronomic or cultural controls applied with some success include elimination of natural weed reservoirs, spraying to reduce vector populations, and production of virus-free vegetative stocks. However, the efficacy of these measures relies on the particular host/virus/vector relationships, and no common method suitable for rhabdovirus disease control has yet been described. In particular, the reported successes indicate that development of effective control measures requires a detailed knowledge of the ecology of the particular virus under consideration, the biology of the host plant and the natural vector reservoirs.

Major factors that can affect rhabdovirus disease incidence are external agents that alter the ecology of host/vector interactions. An interesting anecdotal description of such a situation relates to the epidemiology of LNYV outbreaks in lettuce that occurred in Australia in the early 1960s. These epidemics have been speculated to coincide with the introduction of myxomatosis in Australia to control rabbit populations. The reduced rabbit populations permitted increases in sowthistle plants that constitute a natural reservoir for LNYV and its aphid vector, *Hyperomyzus lactucae*. This combination resulted in disease epidemics due to invasion of newly planted lettuce by large numbers of viruliferous aphids that had increased on viruliferous sowthistle. Fortunately, elimination of weeds for a short distance around fields reduced the entry of vectors into the lettuce crops and provided acceptable disease control. Elimination of rhabdoviruses from vegetatively propagated crops also has considerable potential for disease control. Certification strategies to produce disease-free stock by selection of strawberry propagules free of SCV are proving to be beneficial in California. In other cases, production of virus-free stock, combined with insecticide applications, can provide disease control. Infections of PYDV, which caused serious yield losses before the 1940s in the northeastern United States, appear to have been reduced to a very low frequency as a serendipitous consequence of combinations of insecticides and elimination of the virus from seed potatoes.

Incorporation of disease resistance into crop plants normally provides more effective, durable and economical control than any other measure. Two notable examples of the employment of this strategy exist in rhabdoviruses. The first relates to MMV in Hawaii, where up to 100% losses have been observed in maize lacking disease resistance genes. Useful control is obtained by incorporation of a single gene for tolerance into cultivars, which ameliorates the disease. Another example exists for infections with raspberry veinal chlorosis virus, an unassigned plant rhabdovirus. Raspberries possessing this form of resistance appear to be immune because resistant scions can not be infected by graft inoculation.

The major problem with application of disease resistance is identification of useful genes. Traditionally, such genes have been isolated by screening wild species found near centers of origin of crop plants. However, two major advances in biotechnology provide optimism that resistance can be more widely applied for disease control. Disease resistance genes with specificity to viruses, bacteria and fungi have been cloned from several crops, and some of these genes retain their function when transferred to distantly related species. The evidence also suggests that the recognition motifs of these genes can be engineered to produce novel sources of resistance. A second approach involves engineering synthetic sources of pathogen-mediated resistance by producing transgenic plants expressing portions of the viral genome. Although both strategies have enormous potential for disease control, neither has yet been applied to plant rhabdoviruses. Thus, these approaches represent an important challenge for the future.

See also: **Defective interfering viruses; Fish viruses; Parainfluenza viruses (*Paramyxoviridae*): Animal, Human; Plant virus disease – economic aspects; Rabies virus (*Rhabdoviridae*); Rhabdoviruses (*Rhabdoviridae*): Ungrouped mammalian, bird and fish rhabdoviruses; Vectors: Animal viruses, Plant viruses; Vesicular stomatitus viruses (*Rhabdoviridae*).**

Further Reading

Black LM (1979) Vector cell monolayers and plant viruses. *Adv. Virus Res.* 25: 192.

Francki RIB, Kitajima EW and Peters D (1981) Rhabdoviruses. In: Kurstak E (ed.) *Handbook of Plant Virus*

Infections – Comparative Diagnosis, p. 455. Amsterdam: Elsevier/North Holland.

Jackson AO, Francki RIB and Zuidema D (1987) Biology, structure and replication of plant rhabdoviruses. In: Wagner RR (ed.) The Rhabdoviruses, p. 427. New York: Plenum Press.

Jackson AO and Wagner JDO (1998) Procedures for plant rhabdovirus purification, polyribosome isolation, and replicase extraction. In: Foster G and Taylor S (eds) Plant Virology Protocols: From Virus Isolation to Transgenic Resistance, vol. 81, p. 77. Totowa, NJ: Humana Press.

Sylvester ES and Richardson J (1989) Aphid-borne rhabdoviruses – relationships with their vectors. Adv. Vector Dis. Res. 9: 313.

Ungrouped Mammalian, Bird and Fish Rhabdoviruses

Bishnu P De and **Amiya K Banerjee**, Department of Molecular Biology, The Lerner Research Institute, The Cleveland Clinic Foundation, Cleveland, USA

Copyright © 1999 Academic Press

Introduction

The family *Rhabdoviridae* comprises a diverse collection of viruses linked by a common bullet-shaped or bacilliform morphology. They are among the most widely distributed viruses in nature, infecting vertebrates, invertebrates and many plants. A large number are included so far in five genera: *Vesiculovirus, Lyssavirus, Ephemerovirus, Cytorhabdovirus* and *Nucleorhabdovirus*. Many others are virtually uncharacterized and, because of the lack of any serological relatedness to other viruses, they remain ungrouped. This entry deals with those ungrouped rhabdoviruses, including Gossas virus, Klamath virus, Navarro virus, and fish rhabdoviruses. Except for the fish rhabdoviruses, very little is known about these ungrouped viruses. The mammalian and bird rhabdoviruses are grown in most common laboratory cell lines, e.g. BHK-21, Vero, etc., while fish rhabdoviruses are grown in some special cell types such as epithelioma papulosum cyprini (EPC) cells. In common with other rhabdoviruses, mammalian and bird rhabdoviruses readily infect newborn or weanling mice when injected intracerebrally. No human disease is known for any of these viruses.

Gossas Virus

The Gossas virus was originally isolated in 1984 by Bres from the salivary glands of an adult bat (*Tadarida* sp.) caught in Dakar, Senegal. Neither the pathology of infection nor the neutralizing antibody was detected in the bat at that time. However, in laboratory infections antibody can be detected in mice as well as rabbits. The virus did not crossreact antigenically with many other viruses, including Sindbis, Semliki Forest, West Nile or blue tongue virus. Like vesicular stomatitis virus (VSV), the virus grows in BHK-21 and also in Vero cells. Oita rhabdovirus, another ungrouped virus, was isolated from bat by Oya in Japan. No other information is available on this virus.

Klamath Virus

Klamath virus was originally isolated in 1965 by Johnson from a 3-month-old (immature) meadow vole (*Microtus montanus*) collected at Klamath Falls, Oregon. The virus was subsequently detected in Alaska at Dot Lake (red-backed mice, *Clathrionomys rutilus*) and at the University of Alaska (meadow vole, *Microtuseconomus*). The virus is bullet-shaped (167×80 nm) in morphology, typical of a rhabdovirus. When inoculated intracerebrally into newborn mice, infectious virus was detected in the lung and brain. The virus grows in chicken embryonated eggs as well as laboratory cell lines. In infected cells, cytoplasm contains the nucleocapsids and matured virions found around the cisternae of endoplasmic reticulum. Antigenic crossreactivity tests using 154 different viruses indicate that Klamath virus is antigenically distinct.

Navarro Virus

The Navarro virus was isolated in 1984 by the Cali Virus Laboratory (Cali, Colombia) from the spleen of an adult wild turkey vulture (*Cathartes aura*) shot in Navarro, Colombia. The known properties of the virus are very similar to the Klamath virus.

Fish Rhabdoviruses

The rhabdoviruses that infect fish are particularly interesting because their hosts live in a wide variety of habitats and include such diverse fish as salmon, trout, cod, carp, pike, perch, etc. These viruses were initially designated as members of either the *Lyssavirus* or *Vesiculovirus* genera on the basis of electrophoretic migration of their proteins. Recently, it has been recognized that these classifications require modification, and the fish rhabdoviruses are now classified as 'unassigned' (formerly known as *Lyssavirus*) and 'vesiculo-like' (formerly known as *Vesiculovirus*) in accordance with the sixth report (1995) of the International Committee on Taxonomy of Viruses (ICTV). The members of the 'unassigned' subgroup include infectious hematopoietic necrosis virus (IHNV), viral hemorrhagic septicemia virus (VHSV) and hirame rhabdovirus (HIRRV). The members in the 'vesiculo-like' subgroup include spring viremia of carp virus (SVCV) and pike fry virus (PFV). These viruses may also be classified into two divisions reflecting their host: salmonoid and nonsalmonoid. The IHNV and VHSV are examples of salmonoid fish rhabdovirus, whereas SVCV and PFV belong to the nonsalmonoid group. Because of rapid progression of infection and high mortality, these viruses represent a major threat to aquaculture. Unlike other rhabdoviruses, the fish rhabdoviruses infect and cause disease at characteristically low temperatures (12–15°C), probably due to adaptation to colder aquatic habitats. In the laboratory, these viruses grow in standard cell lines such as BHK-21 and WI-38 and also some poikilothermic cell lines such as FHM, RTG-2 and STE-137. In all cases, the optimum temperature for growth and virus stability is 15–18°C. Like other rhabdoviruses, ultrastructurally they display a bullet-shaped morphology with glycoprotein spikes projecting from the viral envelope. Like VSV, the SVCV and PFV virions have been shown to contain protein kinase activity. Specific characteristics of individual fish rhabdoviruses are described below.

Infectious Hematopoietic Necrosis Virus

The IHNV is enzootic in the sockeye salmon population on the west coast of North America. In recent years, another major host for IHNV was found to be rainbow trout. The infectious hematopoietic necrosis disease was introduced into Japan in 1977 and it appeared in Europe in 1987. The IHNV-infected disease now represents a major threat to aquaculture all over Europe. The virus infection and the disease appear to be cold-dependent, with the characteristic of epizootics at 13°C which disappears at a higher temperature (above 15°C). Two other viruses, namely Oregon sockeye salmon disease virus (OSDV) and Sacramento River Chinook disease virus (SRCDV), are antigenically similar to IHNV and produce diseases with nearly identical symptoms.

Clinical features and pathology

An epizootic of IHNV usually begins with a sudden rise in mortality. Clinical signs are the appearance of dark color, loss of appetite, anemia, exophthalmia, distension of the abdomen with ascites, general viremia and fecal casts. Petechial hemorrhages occur near the base of the fins and on the mesenteries surrounding the viscera. Necrosis of the hematopoietic tissues in the anterior kidney and spleen can be detected by histological examination. With increasing severity of the disease, necrosis is also detected in liver, pancreas, and granular cells in the wall of the alimentary tract.

Fish infected with SRCDV and OSDV do not feed and have symptoms similar to those produced by IHNV. Extensive subcutaneous hemorrhaging occurs, accompanied by the appearance of red blotches on the skin and the gills turning pale. Like IHNV, infection with these viruses also causes necrotic lesions in kidney, pancreas, spleen and adrenal cortex. Virus particles are detected in the interstitial spaces of the infected organs and in some cases in the cytoplasmic vacuoles.

Transmission

The IHNV is transmitted through water, either by feeding on infected carcasses or by exposure to eggs from infected fish. Gills and gastrointestinal tracts are the most probable route of entry of the virus. Transmission also occurs from adult carriers to fry. The virus is readily detected in ovarian or seminal fluid of the infected fish. In the laboratory, defective interfering (DI)-like particles are produced when the cells are infected at higher multiplicity of infection (m.o.i).

Molecular aspects

The morphology and genome size (11 kb) of IHNV is identical to VSV. However, several differences are observed among IHNV and other rhabdoviruses. IHNV specifies six mRNAs rather than five mRNAs as is found in VSV. The five mRNAs encode the viral structural proteins RNA polymerase (L, 225 kDa), envelope glycoprotein (G, 59 kDa), nucleocapsid protein (N, 42 kDa) and two matrix proteins (M1, 26 kDa and M2, 22 kDa. Like P protein of VSV, the M1 protein is phosphorylated and believed to function in transcription, similar to other rhabdoviruses. The sixth mRNA encodes a unique nonstructural protein (NV) that is expressed in infected cells but is not present in purified virions. Recently, the complete nucleotide sequence of the genome of IHNV has been determined. This represents the first complete nucleotide sequence of a fish rhabdovirus genome. The genome organization is 3′-N-M1-M2-G-NV-L-5′. The intergenic region contains the conserved sequence 5′-AGAYAG/C-3′ (antigenomic polarity) which is followed by a stretch of seven adenosine residues. This sequence is present at the end of every sizeable open reading frame found in the IHNV genome and is similar to that found in the intergenic region of VSV.

Viral Hemorrhagic Septicemia Virus

History

VHSV was initially isolated from the rainbow trout (*Oncorhynchus mykis*) in the Egtved region of Jutland (Denmark) in 1950. It represents a major threat to the fish farming industry in continental Europe, causing devastating viral disease in fish. Brown trout (*Salmo trutta*) and brook trout (*Salvelinus fontinalis*) were found to be immune to the disease; however, they could be infected experimentally. Recently, both the geographical distribution and host range of the virus were shown to be wider, as VHSV was isolated in routine control of other species of fish in the USA. The antigenic crossreactivity and the electrophoretic pattern of the viral structural proteins indicate that these viruses are similar to those originating in Europe. The North American isolates, however, were not associated with any specific clinical condition, and no experimental overt infection could be obtained with these strains.

Clinical features and pathology

Infected trout appear black, especially on the head and abdomen, and show exophthalmia of the eyes (sometimes with protruding eyeballs giving a popeye effect due to the hemorrhages in the connective tissues of the eye pit), distended abdomen and severe anemia. The gills appear pale pink or greyish white. Acute hemorrhages are seen at the base of the pectoral fins. At the lateral line they are less frequent or may be entirely absent. In some cases the fish also show neurological and motor disorders, such as spiral swimming at the bottom of the pond, tilted swimming and darting through and out of water. Death occurs within several days.

The most prominent pathological changes are the scattered hemorrhages in skeletal muscles, mouth cavities and sex organs. Histology of the liver and kidney shows necrotic foci with hepatocytes including cytoplasmic vacuoles, karyolysis and pyknosis. Lymphoid and spleen tissues show accumulation of mononucleated and immune erythrocytes.

Immunology and interferon production

Neutralization studies of 76 natural isolates of VHSV from Danish, Norwegian and Swedish rainbow trout showed that 72 of them were essentially identical to the F1 strain, suggesting that the four others may represent different serotypes. However, in cell cultures all were recognized by fluorescein isothiocyanate-conjugated anti-F1 antibody. Diagnosis of the disease is made by immunofluorescent staining of tissue or by direct isolation of the virus from tissue homogenates.

Experimental infection of rainbow trouts with VHSV has been shown to produce interferon that reaches a maximal level (about 2800 units ml^{-1}) at 3 days postinfection. Physicochemical properties of fish interferon have been determined as the molecular mass of about 26 kDa, sedimentation coefficient of 2.5 S and isoelectric point of 4.5–6.2. It has been suggested that the production of interferon may play a role in the antiviral response of the fish at temperatures above 15°C.

Molecular aspects

The VHSV genome, like IHNV, encodes five structural proteins: the nucleocapsid protein N (41 kDa), the polymerase-associated protein M1 (28 kDa) similar to the P protein of VSV, the matrix protein M2 (24 kDa) similar to the M protein in VSV, the glycoprotein G (74 kDa), the polymerase protein L ($\sim$150 kDa) and a nonstructural protein NV (14 kDa). By direct sequencing VHSV genome organization was confirmed to be 3′-N-M1(P)-M2(M)-G-NV-L-5′. The NV protein has no significant sequence similarity to the NV protein of IHNV or any other known protein. The predicted sequence of the M1 and M2 proteins are rich in Ser and Thr residues and both are phosphorylated. The RNA polymerase activity of all fish rhabdoviruses, including VHSV, have a lower optimum temperature (15–20°C), as opposed to 30–32°C in VSV. Also, unlike other rhabdoviruses, the RNA polymerase activity of VHSV is stimulated by Mn^{2+} rather than Mg^{2+}.

Spring Viremia of Carp Virus

SVCV belongs to the vesiculo-like genus of the family *Rhabdoviridae*. The infectious dropsy of carp (*Cyprinus carpio*) was originally reported in Europe as early as 1930, but the origin of the disease remained unknown until 1950. Now it is clearly established that SVCV is the causative agent of hemorrhagic swimbladder inflamation and infectious dropsy in common carp. Clinical signs of the virus infection are external and internal hemorrhages, peritonitis and ascites. The symptoms of the disease, however, vary depending on the form of the disease: acute, chronic, asymptomatic or latent. In an overt disease, the central nervous system and peripheral nerves are affected. The fish becomes hyperactive, with the appearance of ulcerative dermal vesicles (carp erythrodermatitis). The kidneys and spleen become enlarged and contain the highest titer of the virus. Peak viremia appears on the 6th day postinfection and again on the 9th and 10th days. Excretion of the virus in feces and mucus occurs on the 11th day, and finally the fish dies around the 20th day. Since the first isolation of the virus several other fish hosts have been reported, suggesting that SVCV has a wider host range than the carp family. The virus causes significant mortality in both juvenile and adult fish, and therefore it has a large economic impact on the fish farming industry in Europe. In experimental infections, fingerling carp, pike fry and the larvae and carp fry are also susceptible.

Pike Fry (Rhabdo) Virus

The PFV belongs to the vesiculo-like genus of the *Rhabdoviridae* family. It is involved in two diseases of fry of the northern pike (*Esox lucius* L.): a 'head disease' identified by swelling or lumps on the body, or a 'red disease' identified by swelling and reddish color of large areas of the body. These diseases were first seen in the Nieuw-Vennep hatchery in The Netherlands around 1959. Both diseases have a high mortality rate. The hydrocephalus associated with the 'head disease' makes the fish lose equilibrium and swim erratically near the surface of the water. Clinical symptoms are poor growth, hemorrhages in the brain, spinal cord, spleen and pancreas, and degenerative necrotic changes in kidney tubules. The 'red disease' is characterized by pale gills, hemorrhages in trunk and muscle connective tissue, and red swollen areas above the pelvic fins. The virus is detected in the hematopoietic tissues of the kidney. At the molecular level, the PFV is similar to VSV, encoding the structural proteins, N, P, M, G and L.

Hirame Rhabdovirus

The HIRRV is a member of the 'unassigned' genus of the *Rhabdoviridae* family. It was first isolated from Japanese flounder (*Paralichthys olivaceus*) and from ayu fish (*Plecoglossus altivelis*), both of which are valuable cultured fish species in Japan. The clinical signs of HIRRV infection are similar to those caused by SVCV. Crossreactions in serological studies have suggested that HIRRV is related to the well-characterized North American fish pathogen IHNV. The genes of the two matrix proteins (M1 and M2) and the glycoprotein (G) of HIRRV have been sequenced. Sequences of all of the internal gene junctions have also been determined. The matrix protein genes have been shown to share a high amino acid similarity (81.5% for M1 and 86.0% for M2) with the respective genes of IHNV. The G protein shared the highest sequence identity (74.3%) and similarity (83.3%) with the G protein of IHNV.

See also: **Fish viruses; Defective interfering viruses; Rabies virus (*Rhabdoviridae*); Interferons: General features, Therapy of aids and cancer; Vesicular stomatitis viruses (*Rhabdoviridae*).**

Further Reading

Basurco B and Benmansour A (1995) Distant strains of the fish rhabdovirus VHSV maintain a sixth functional cistron which codes for a nonstructural protein of unknown function. *Virology* 212: 741.

Benmansour A, Paubert G, Bernard J and DeKinkelin P (1994) The polymerase-associated protein (M1) and the matrix protein (M2) from a virulent and an avirulent strain of viral hemorrhagic septicemia virus (VHSV), a fish rhabdovirus. *Virology* 198: 602.

Bjorklund HV, Higman KH and Kurath G (1996) The glycoprotein genes and gene junctions of the fish rhabdoviruses spring viremia of carp virus and hirame rhabdovirus: analysis of relationships with other rhabdoviruses. *Virus Res.* 42: 65.

Kurath G, Higman KH and Bjorklund HV (1997) Distribution and variation of NV genes in fish rhabdoviruses. *J. Gen. Virol.* 78: 113.

Pilcher KS and Fryer JL (1980) The viral diseases of fish: a review through 1978. Part I: Diseases of proven viral etiology. *Crit. Rev. Microbiol.* 7: 287.

Schutze H, Enzmann PJ, Kuchling R, Mudt E, Niemann H and Mettenleiter TC (1995) Complete genomic sequence of the fish rhabdovirus infectious hematopoietic necrosis virus. *J. Gen. Virol.* 76: 2519.

Schutze H, Enzmann PJ, Mudt E and Mettenleiter TC (1996) Identification of the non-virion (NV) protein of fish rhabdoviruses viral haemorrhagic septicaemia virus and infectious haematopoietic necrosis virus. *J. Gen. Virol.* 77: 1259.

Wolf KE (1988) Fish viruses and fish viral diseases. Ithaca, NY: Cornell University Press.

Thus, many serotypes seem to coexist within the human population. The multiplicity of serotypes is in contrast to two other medically important picornaviruses, the polioviruses (three serotypes) and hepatitis A virus (a single serotype). Several serotypes fall into groups on the basis of low-level immunological crossreactivity with hyperimmune serum (HRV-36, HRV-58 and HRV-89; HRV-2 and HRV-49 for example), but it is not known whether this plays any role in protection from heterologous serotypes. These antigenic groups seem to correlate with close molecular relationships (**Fig. 3**).

Epidemiology

Rhinoviruses are a major cause of morbidity and economic loss. They have been implicated in 10–40% of cases of acute respiratory disease, a category accounting for around half of all acute illnesses in the developed world. Thus, although the common cold is less severe than some respiratory diseases, rhinoviruses are responsible for a significant proportion of working days lost in industry, commerce and education.

Rhinovirus infections are most common in young children and babies and the infection rate decreases with age, possibly due to prior exposure to a growing number of serotypes. Estimates of the average incidence of rhinovirus colds have varied, but it is probably at least 0.5 per adult per year. It is agreed that the rate in babies and infants is approximately three times that in adults. Once an individual is infected, the virus often spreads to other members of the family, the home being a major site of transmission. Young children are frequently causes of introduction into the family unit and other young children and the mother the most frequent recipients. The infection rate in mothers possibly reflects greater exposure to infected individuals, although other factors may be involved as it has been shown that the susceptibility to colds varies with the stage of the menstrual cycle. Schools and preschool groups also facilitate rhinovirus transmission.

Transmission and Tissue Tropism

Two routes may be important in rhinovirus spread: direct contact and airborne transmission. People with colds contaminate their hands and environmental surfaces with virus from nasal secretions. The hands of uninfected individuals can then become contaminated by direct contact with the person with a cold or by touching the contaminated surface. The virus can enter the body when the hand is used to rub an eye or pick the nose, common features of human behavior. In experiments which exclude this route, some transmission still occurred, suggesting that contaminated airborne particles or aerosols may also be important. Transmission in the family context correlates with time of exposure to the infected individual, severity of their symptoms and titer of rhinovirus in nasal secretions.

Once introduced into the body, the primary and major site of infection is the epithelial surface of the nasal mucosa. Rhinoviruses thus show a restricted tissue tropism, which may be correlated, among other factors, with their optimum growth temperature (33°C). Clinical manifestations are therefore largely limited to common-cold-like symptoms. Sometimes though, rhinoviruses infect other tissue, particularly the lower respiratory tract, the maxilliary sinus and the middle ear.

Pathogenicity and Clinical Features of Infection

Rhinovirus infections are usually relatively trivial and not life-threatening. Extensive work has been performed on their etiology and pathogenesis using human volunteers. These studies show that a rhinovirus infection can be initiated by less than one $TCID_{50}$ (50% tissue culture infectious dose) of virus, if it is administered to the nasopharynx. Virus shedding can be detected within 24 h and reaches a maximum after 2–3 days, coinciding with the onset of symptoms. Virus titers thereafter fall rapidly but may remain detectable for 3 weeks.

Rhinovirus infection is accompanied typically by the symptoms of a common cold. These vary with the individual and possibly the particular rhinovirus, but usually include nasal discharge and obstruction, often with sneezing, coughing and sore throat. Fever and malaise are less commonly seen than in infections with other respiratory viruses, but gastrointestinal disorders are not uncommon, particularly in children.

Although limited largely to the upper respiratory tract, rhinovirus infections are believed to predispose some individuals to bacterial sinusitis and otitis media. In addition, rhinoviruses can produce serious and debilitating lower respiratory infections, particularly in the elderly, young children and patients with existing disorders, such as cystic fibrosis and bronchopulmonary dysplasia. Up to 40% of exacerbations of chronic bronchitis may be due to rhinovirus infections. Respiratory infections are known to increase the severity and frequency of asthma attacks in susceptible individuals and rhinoviruses are the most important pathogens associated with increased asthma.

Pathology and Histopathology

Physical examination of patients with a rhinovirus infection usually reveals nasal obstruction and discharge, the nasal mucosa being pale and edematous. Elevated levels of bradykinin found locally, possibly contribute to this edema. Neutrophil infiltration is observed in the common cold and this may be caused by rhinoviruses inducing the expression of interleukin 8 (IL-8), a neutrophil chemoattractant. IL-8 may also be involved in asthma exacerbation, which is characterized by rhinovirus-induced enhancement of allergic inflammation and responsiveness to histamine.

The detailed histopathology of rhinovirus infections is not well documented. Nasal mucosa biopsies reveal few histological abnormalities, although shed, virus-containing, columnar epithelial cells can be detected in nasal secretions, suggesting that the epithelial surface of the nasal mucosa is primarily involved. Infection of bovine tracheal organ cultures with bovine rhinovirus leads to the shedding of large numbers of ciliated epithelial cells, leaving a smooth epithelial surface.

Immune Response

Rhinovirus infection stimulates the production of type-specific IgA, IgG and IgM antibodies in up to 90% of individuals. These are detectable within 2–3 weeks in serum and nasal secretions and their levels rise for 5–6 weeks. Most immunoglobulin in nasal secretions is IgA and this is probably a major factor in protection against re-infection (or at least reduction of disease symptoms) by the homotypic rhinovirus. Serum and secretory antibody persist for several years after infection, although their levels decline. As antibody appears late in the infection, it probably plays little part in recovery but it may be involved in final virus clearance. Other mechanisms, including interferon involvement, may therefore be involved in the recovery process. T cell responses which are serotype-crossreactive have been observed, but their contribution to subsequent protection is not known.

Prevention and Control

At present, there is no generally available means of protecting against or treating common colds produced by rhinoviruses. The large number of serotypes apparently precludes conventional vaccines and few attempts have been made to pursue this approach. Most effort has been expended on the development of chemical antivirus agents, but of the many shown to have antirhinovirus activity *in vitro*, none has yet proved clinically useful, although some are currently at the clinical trials stage. An alternative approach is interferon, produced in large amounts by recombinant DNA means. High, intranasal doses, initiated several days before virus challenge, have proved to be effective in preventing illness. However, side effects limit long-term use and as symptoms are only reduced if treatment is commenced before virus infection, interferon has limited applicability. It may prove useful in the family context when it is important to prevent virus spread to specific individuals, e.g. asthmatics and bronchitics. In these cases, it may also be possible to use what we know about the properties of rhinoviruses and their mode of transmission to limit spread. Interrupting transmission by avoiding direct contact with the infected person and by frequent hand-washing is sensible. Furthermore, experiments have been performed in which paper tissues impregnated with virucidal agents (mild acid to exploit rhinovirus lability at low pH) were used for frequent nose-blowing and hand-wiping by infected and uninfected individuals kept together under confined conditions for prolonged periods. The tissues were effective in preventing infection. One semi-empirical approach is the regular topical application of warm, moist air to the upper respiratory tract. Its beneficial effect may be due to the temperature increase in the nose, making it less conductive to rhinovirus replication, although the stimulation of host mechanisms may also be involved. In the absence of specific antivirus agents, proprietary treatments which reduce symptoms are widely used. In addition, both large amounts of vitamin C and zinc acetate tablets have been reported to reduce the severity and duration of colds, although their efficacy have been frequently questioned.

Future Perspectives

The past few years have seen major advances in the study of rhinoviruses, particularly the determination of three-dimensional structures and the identification of receptors. Several nucleotide sequences have been determined, revealing conserved regions which have been exploited by PCR-based systems for rapid detection. These are an improvement on virus isolation procedures for detection and are giving a more complete picture of the role of rhinoviruses in human disease, for instance the recognition of their importance in asthma exacerbation. Rhinovirus serotype diversity means that broadly reactive prophylactic or therapeutic approaches must be devised. The economic and social significance of the common cold continues to stimulate research and our knowledge of the structure of the virus particle, the determinants of antigenicity and cellular receptors, together with

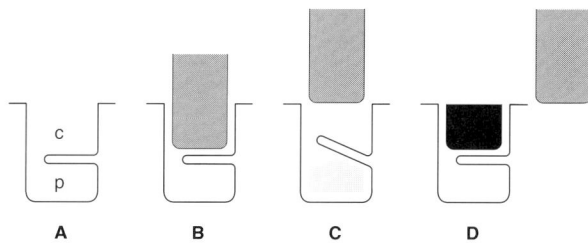

Figure 4 Targets for antirhinovirus therapeutic agents. (**A**) Underneath the canyon (c), which is the site for receptor binding, there is a hydrophobic pocket (p). (**B**) The receptor (gray) docks with the canyon. (**C**) A class of effective antirhinovirus compounds binds strongly to the pocket. This distorts the canyon floor, preventing receptor binding and/or uncoating. (**D**) An alternative approach is to saturate the receptor binding domains with a soluble form of the receptor, thus preventing receptor binding.

other advances, will contribute greatly to the development of rational approaches. It still seems unlikely that a vaccine can be produced, although the ability to pin-point areas of antigenic importance means that it may become possible to construct molecules which can mimic the antigenicity of several serotypes and thus reduce the complexity of the antigenic diversity problem. Even so, several components to the vaccine would be necessary and there may be a reluctance to use such a vaccine, with possible side effects, against what is usually a mild pathogen.

The antirhinovirus drug route may prove more feasible and there are at least three potential targets. Best studied are agents which bind within a hydrophobic pocket located underneath the canyon, blocking virus attachment to cells and/or uncoating (**Fig. 4**). They have high specificity and efficacy against rhinoviruses *in vitro* and seem to lack toxicity. As the pocket is well conserved, the drugs are potentially broadly reactive and it is possible that one, or a small number, of agents would be effective against all rhinovirus serotypes. Following success with inhibitors of the HIV-1 protease, agents (e.g. peptidylaldehydes) which specifically interfere with processing by inhibiting the rhinovirus 3C^{pro} are being widely studied. A third approach is to use soluble ICAM-1 to block early virus/cell interactions. However, even such highly specific reagents are likely to suffer from problems which may limit their usefulness. For example, in common with other RNA viruses, rhinoviruses have a high mutation rate and drug-resistant mutants can appear rapidly *in vitro*. Furthermore, maximal benefit from most agents tested is possible only if they are administered before infection. Thus, despite improvements in understanding, rhinovirus infections may continue to be a familiar feature of our lives.

See also: **Antivirals; Interferons: General features, Therapy of aids and cancer; Pathogenesis: Animal viruses; Respiratory viruses; Vaccines and immune response; Viral receptors; Virus structure: Atomic structure, Principles of virus structure; Virus–host cell interactions.**

Further Reading

Couch RB (1996) Rhinoviruses. In: Fields BN, Knipe DM, Howley PM *et al* (eds) *Fields Virology*, 3rd edn, p. 713. Philadelphia: Lippincott-Raven.

Johnson SL (1997) Problems and prospects of developing effective therapy for common cold viruses. *Trends Microbiol.* 5: 58.

Racaniello VR (ed.) (1990) Picornaviruses. *Current Topics in Microbiology and Immunology*, vol. 161. Berlin: Springer-Verlag.

Stott EJ and Garwes DJ (1990) Rhinoviruses, adenoviruses and coronaviruses: their role in repiratory disease. In: Collier LH and Timbury MC (eds) *Topley and Wilson's Principles of Bacteriology, Virology and Immunology*, 8th edn, p. 243. London: Edward Arnold.

RIBOZYMES

Robert H Symons, Department of Plant Science, University of Adelaide, Glen Osmond, South Australia, Australia

Copyright © 1999 Academic Press

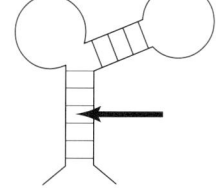

History

Ribozymes are catalytic RNA molecules, first identified in the early 1980s. They have the intrinsic ability to break and form covalent bonds in RNA molecules. In many ways they can be compared to the protein enzymes which catalyze cleavage of peptide bonds in other proteins or peptides. However, ribozymes can

Table 1 RNAs involved in RNA-catalyzed splicing/cleavage reactions

RNA present in	Reaction in vivoz	End groups on cleaved RNAs	Nucleotide cofactor	Mechanism
Ribonuclease P	Processing tRNA precursors	5'-P,3'-OH	No	Hydrolysis
Group I introns	Self-splicing of ribosomal introns	5'-P,3'-OH	Yes	Transesterification
Group II introns	Self-splicing of organelle introns	5'-P,3'-OH	No	Transesterification
Three plant viroids, four circular (virusoids) and four linear satellite RNAs	Cleavage of oligomeric precursors	5'-OH,2',3'-cyclic phosphate	No	Transesterification
Hepatitis delta virus (HDV) RNA	Cleavage of oligomeric precursors	5'-OH,2',3'-cyclic phosphate	No	Transesterification
Newt satellite II RNA transcript	Unknown	5'-OH,2',3'-cyclic phosphate	No	Transesterification
Neurospora mitochondrial plasmid transcript VS RNA	Unknown	5'-OH,2',3'-cyclic phosphate	No	Transesterification

also be *cis*-acting since the ribozyme component of an RNA molecule can cleave at a specific site in another part of the same molecule. All except one of the naturally occurring ribozymes (**Table 1**) are of the latter type.

In 1983, Altman and his colleagues described the first, and so far the only, truly naturally occurring catalytic ribozyme. The bacterial ribonuclease P is involved in the processing of precursor transfer RNA (tRNA) by specific cleavage of a 5'-terminal sequence (**Fig. 1A**). The enzyme consists of one molecule of protein and one molecule of single-strandard RNA; the isolated RNA can carry out the same processing reaction in *trans* as in the holoenzyme with multiple turnover and without being changed in the reaction.

The term ribozyme was first used by Cech and his colleagues in 1982 to describe the self-splicing activities of an intervening sequence (IVS) of ribosomal RNA precursor sequences in the protozoan *Tetrahymena* (**Fig. 1B**). This is an intramolecular reaction and the ribozyme component only catalyzes a single turnover and is modified during the reaction. It can, therefore, be considered to be acting in a quasicatalytic manner. All introns which self-splice as in **Fig. 1B** are called Group I introns. The molecular aspects of this self-splicing reaction continue to be extensively investigated.

In 1986, three groups reported a new type of intron self-splicing as in **Fig. 1C** and such introns are called Group II introns. They are less common than Group I introns and are found in organellar and bacterial genomes. They exist in fungal mitochondria, plant mitochondria and chloroplasts, algae and bacteria.

Also in 1986 two new ribozymes were identified in small circular plant pathogenic RNAs which were subsequently called the hammerhead and hairpin ribozymes. They both carry out the reaction summarized in **Fig. 1D**. A total of 14 plant pathogenic RNAs have so far been identified which can carry out either the hammerhead or hairpin ribozyme reaction or both the reactions (**Table 1**). Interestingly, only one nonpathogenic RNA has been reported to carry out the hammerhead reaction, the RNA transcripts from satellite DNA of the newt, and none have been reported for the hairpin ribozyme.

The only animal RNA pathogenic RNA known so far to undergo self-cleavage was reported in 1988 for hepatitis delta RNA which is essentially a satellite RNA dependent on hepatitis B virus for its replication. Both plus and minus forms of the approximately 1700 nt circular RNA self-cleave via a pseudoknot structure.

And, finally, a second nonpathogenic RNA was reported in 1990 to undergo the self-cleavage reaction of **Fig. 1D**; this was an 881 nt transcript of a circular mitochondrial DNA plasmid of *Neurospora*. Two-dimensional structural models around the self-cleavage site are different from other known self-cleavage structures.

It is perhaps surprising that all currently known types of self-processing or self-cleaving naturally occurring RNAs in **Table 1** were identified between 1982 and 1990. It remains to be seen whether any new types of reactions will be found from 1998 onwards.

Ribozymes of Non-viral Origin

Since the emphasis in this encyclopedia is on Virology, the nonviral ribozyme systems are only considered briefly here; the newt hammerhead ribozyme system is considered in the following section.

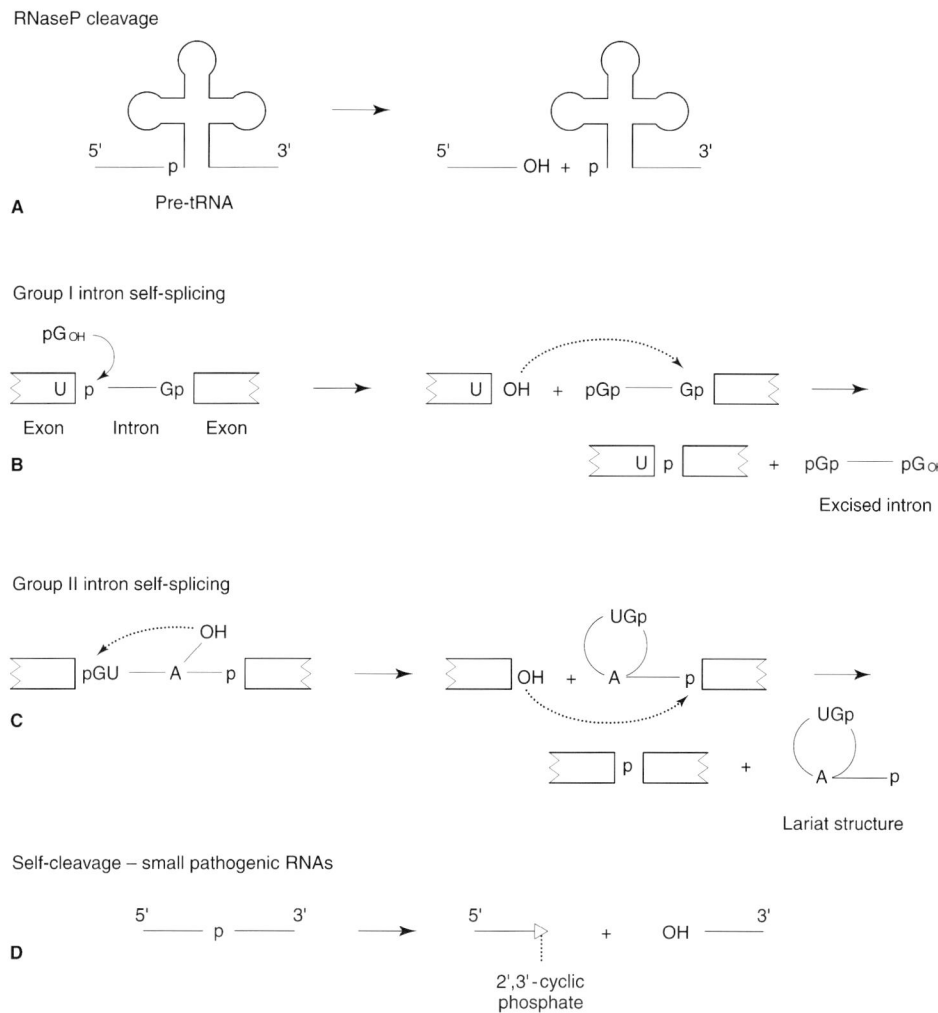

Figure 1 RNA processing reactions that are naturally RNA catalysed. See text and Tables 1 and 2 for further details.

Ribonuclease P (RNase P)

The reaction carried out by this ribozyme is summarized in **Fig. 1A**. RNase P is an endoribonuclease which cleaves precursor tRNAs at their 5' ends to give the mature 5' termini of tRNAs (**Fig. 1A**). The best characterized enzymes are those from the eubacteria *Escherichia coli* and *Bacillus subtilis*. The RNase P holoenzyme is composed of one basic protein subunit of approx. M_r 14000 (119 amino acids) and one single-stranded RNA molecule of 377 nucleotides (*E. coli*) or 401 nucleotides (*B. subtilis*). The RNAs make up 90% by weight of these enzymes and are not covalently coupled to the protein component.

The purified RNAs of bacterial RNase P can carry out the same reaction as the holoenzyme but high ionic strength is required in the reaction mixture. This result indicates that, *in vivo*, the catalytic component of RNase P is the RNA moiety.

The nucleotide sequences of the substrate tRNAs are not conserved around the cleavage sites for RNase P; hence there must be common structural features which allow specific recognition. The basic substrate requirements for RNase P activity are shown in **Fig. 2**; a base paired stem, one strand of which contains the eventual 3' terminal–NCCA of the tRNA and the other strand the cleavage site. Hence, the RNA component of RNase P can act as a true ribozyme in *trans* to specifically cleave pre-tRNAs as well as unrelated RNAs which contain the basic sequence and structural requirements of **Fig. 2**.

Group I introns as ribozymes

The best characterized Group I system is that of the 413 nucleotide intervening sequence (IVS) in the nuclear rRNA precursor from *Tetrahymena thermophila*. The intron can be excised and the two exons

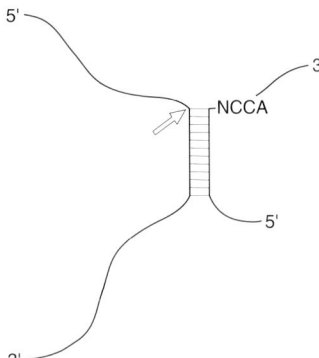

Figure 2 Basic structural and sequence requirements of a substrate for specific cleavage (site indicated by arrow) by RNase P or its RNA.

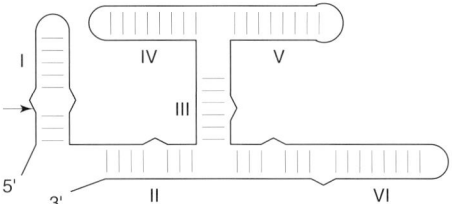

Figure 3 Secondary structure model of part of the 881 nt *Neurospora* VS RNA required for self-cleavage. The minimal sequence required contains 154 nt with only 1 nt 5′ to the self-cleavage site indicated by an arrow.

ligated in the complete absence of protein but there is a requirement for guanosine or a guanosine nucleotide as a cofactor as indicated in **Fig. 1B**. Hence, the IVS catalyzes only its own excision and is modified during the process. The released intron can then undergo further RNA-catalyzed cyclization and cleavage reactions that remove a total of 19 nucleotides from the 5′ end to produce an intron core (L-19 IVS) of 395 nucleotides.

The L-19 IVS RNA can be used *in vitro* in a classical enzymatic fashion in several in *trans* reactions, catalyzing the turnover of more than one substrate molecule and remaining unchanged. One of these reactions is a sequence-specific endonuclease.

Group II introns as ribozymes

Group II introns are found in eubacteria and eubacterial-derived organellar genomes of plants, mitochondria and chloroplasts. They have never been reported in the nucleus of eukaryotes. The overall self-splicing of Group II introns (**Fig. 1C**) involves the initial nucleophilic attack by a 2′-hydroxyl near the 3′

Table 2 Plant and animal pathogenic RNAs with *cis*-ribozyme activity

	Viroid or satellite abbreviation	Size (nt)	Catalytic motif Plus RNA	Minus RNA
A. Viroids				
Avocado sunblotch viroid	ASBV	246–251	Hammerhead	Hammerhead
Chrysanthemum chlorotic mottle viroid	CChMV	398–399	Hammerhead	Hammerhead
Peach latent mosaic viroid	PLMV	337–338	Hammerhead	Hammerhead
B. Satellite RNAs				
Sobemoviruses (Virusoids)				
Lucerne transient streak virus	vLTSV	322–324	Hammerhead	Hammerhead
Solanum nodiflorum mottle virus	vSNMV	377	Hammerhead	—
Subterraneum clover mottle virus	vSLMoV	322–388	Hammerhead	—
Velvet tobacco mottle virus	vVTMoV	365–366	Hammerhead	—
Nepoviruses				
Arabis mosaic virus	sARMV	300	Hammerhead	Hairpin
Chicory yellow mottle virus	sCYMV	457	Hammerhead	Hairpin
Tobacco ringspot virus	sTRSV	359–360	Hammerhead	Hairpin
Luteovirus				
Barley yellow dwarf virus	sBYDV	322	Hammerhead	Hammerhead
Hepatitis delta virus				
Hepatitis delta virus RNA	HDV RNA	1860	Pseudoknot	Pseudoknot
Uncharacterized				
Carnation stunt associated viroid-like RNA	CarSV RNA	275	Hammerhead	Hammerhead
Cherry small circular RNA	CSC RNAs	451	Hammerhead	Hammerhead

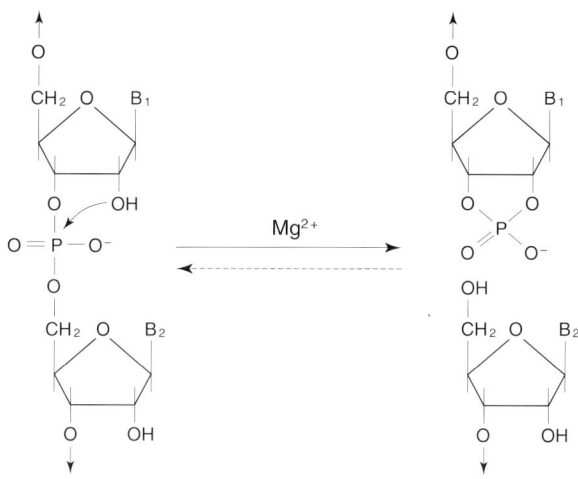

Figure 4 The self-cleavage reaction of RNA catalysed by Mg^{2+} or other divalent cations. This nonhydrolytic, transesterification reaction is theoretically reversible.

end of the intron on the 5'-terminal phosphate of the intron followed by the two steps of **Fig. 1C** to give the ligated exons and the released intron as a lariat structure. The splicing of intron-containing pre-mRNAs follows the same route but it occurs in the nucleus and requires the assistance of the spliceosome complex.

Demonstration of self-splicing of Group II introns *in vitro* requires very unphysiological conditions of high concentrations of salt and of Mg^{2+} and higher than normal temperatures. Only a minority of Group II introns have been shown to have ribozyme activity *in vitro*. Hence, progress in characterizing this ribozyme activity has lagged behind that of the Group I introns.

Neurospora VS RNA can self-cleave

VS RNA is a self-cleaving 881 nt RNA transcript of a mitochondrial DNA plasmid of *Neurospora*. Only 154 nt is required for self-cleavage and a potential two-dimensional structure is shown in **Fig. 3**. As for the hepatitis delta ribozyme (see below), only a single nucleotide 5' to the cleavage site is required for activity. The RNA can be divided into a two-component in *trans* ribozyme system. Even though VS RNA is present at high concentrations in mitochondria, its function is unknown.

Ribozymes of Viral Origin

The plant and animal pathogenic RNAs which have been shown so far to undergo self-cleavage *in vitro* are listed in **Table 2**. In all cases, this self-cleavage activity involves the divalent metal ion-catalyzed nucleophilic attack of the oxygen of the 2'-hydroxyl group at the cleavage site on the phosphate of the internucleotide linkage (**Fig. 4**). The cleavage products contain a 3' end terminal 2',3'-cyclic phosphate and a 5'-hydroxyl. The reaction is theoretically reversible.

Experimental evidence, at least for some of the RNAs of **Table 2**, indicates that this self-cleavage reaction is an essential step in their rolling circle replication (**Fig. 5**). Where both the plus RNAs (the dominant form *in vivo*) and the minus RNAs (the minor form) self-cleave, replication follows (**Fig. 5A**). The circular plus strand is copied by a host or viral-coded RNA-dependent RNA polymerase to produce a multimeric minus strand which is processed into unit length minus monomers. These are circularized by a host RNA ligase and the circular molecules copied by the RNA polymerase to give a multimeric plus strand which is cleaved specifically to monomers. These are then circularized to give the progeny circular RNAs, the dominant form found *in vivo*.

Of the RNAs in **Table 1**, only three plant satellite RNAs follow the replication cycle of **Fig. 5B** where the dominant plus form undergoes self-cleavage and the multimeric minus strand is copied directly to give

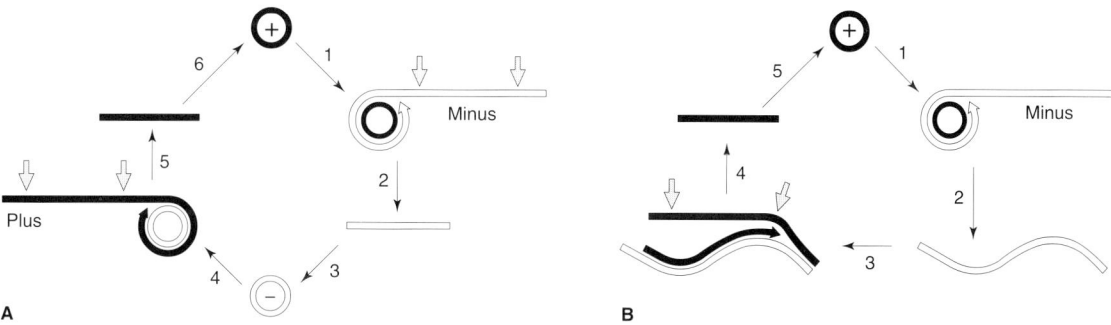

Figure 5 Two routes for the rolling circle replication of small, circular pathogenic RNAs, by an RNA polymerase. (**A**) Six-step pathway where both the multimeric minus and plus linear RNAs self-cleave (open arrows) to give monomers which are ligated *in vivo* to the circular forms. (**B**) Five-step pathway where only the multimeric plus RNA self-cleaves.

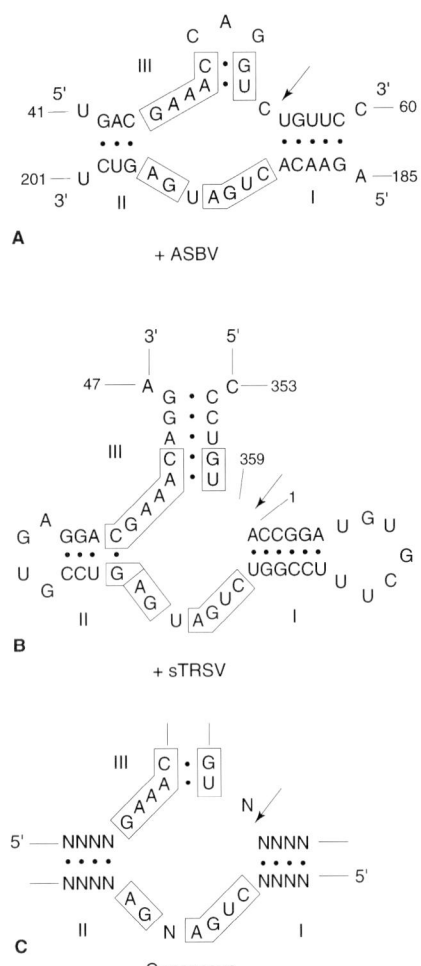

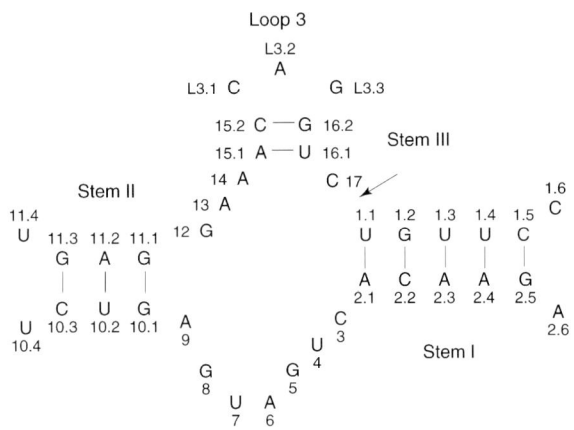

Figure 6 Two-dimensional hammerhead structures in self-cleaving RNAs. (**A**) Hammerhead structure that can form from opposite strands in the 247 nt rod-like structure of plus ASBV. (**B**) Hammerhead structure in the plus strand of the 359 nt satellite RNA of tobacco ringspot virus. (**C**) Consensus hammerhead structure for RNAs in Table 2. Self-cleavage site indicated by arrow. The 13 nucleotides that are highly conserved in all RNAs which cleave by the hammerhead structure are boxed.

the plus strand which self-cleaves to monomers which are then circularized.

Only the three viroids listed in **Table 2**, out of 27 so far identified, undergo self-cleavage *in vitro*. Viroids are single-stranded circular RNAs which vary in size from 246 to 463 nucleotides and infect a wide range of plant species. Many are of agricultural importance. Most of the remaining self-cleaving RNAs in **Table 2** are satellite RNAs in that they are dependent on a helper virus for their replication, including the only animal virus member, the hepatitis delta virus RNA which depends on hepatitis B virus. Two other self-cleaving plant pathogenic RNAs have yet to be characterized at the biological level.

Figure 7 Standard convention for numbering the residues in a hammerhead structure.

So far only three types of two-dimensional structural motifs have been identified at the self-cleavage sites of the 14 pathogenic RNAs of **Table 2**. These are the hammerhead, hairpin and pseudoknot structures.

Hammerhead ribozyme

The hammerhead self-cleavage motif was first recognized in the plus and minus self-cleaving RNAs of avocado sunblotch viroid (ASBV) and of the satellite RNA of lucerne transient streak virus (sLTSV) and the plus form of the satellite RNA of tobacco ringspot virus (sTRSV). The original hammerhead structures predicted around the self-cleavage sites of (+)ASBV and (+)sTRSV together with the highly conserved nucleotides (boxed) in all hammerhead structures are given in **Fig. 6** together with the consensus hammerhead structure for all naturally occurring RNAs. *In vitro*, the RNA sequences in **Fig. 6** are all that are required to ensure efficient self-cleavage in the presence of Mg^{2+}. Hence, such RNAs can be considered as ribozymes since they catalyze a single turnover, intramolecular (*cis*) cleavage reaction.

In addition to the well-studied plant viroids and satellite RNAs in **Table 2**, there are two other naturally occurring circular RNAs where both plus and minus strands self-cleave via the hammerhead structure but which have yet to be characterized in detail at the biological level. One of these is the 275-nt circular RNA from carnation and named carnation small viroid-like RNA (CarSV RNA) which has a dsDNA counterpart in the form of head-to-tail monomers. The other self-cleaving viroid-like RNA is the 451 nt cherry small circular RNA which is associated with a series of double-stranded RNAs of putative viral origin in cherry trees showing the cherry chlorotic rusty spot disease.

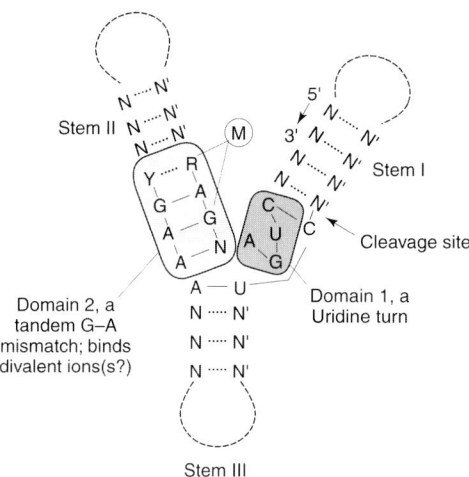

Figure 8 Schematic drawing of the structure of the hammerhead as determined by x-ray crystallography. (Reproduced with permission from McKay (1996).)

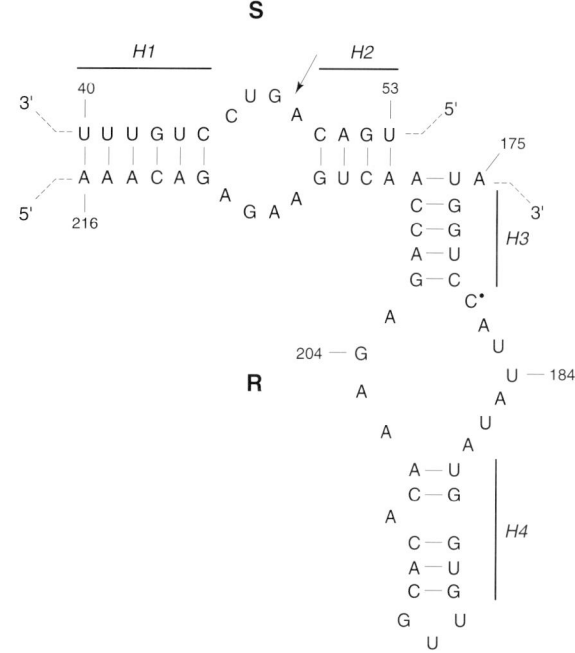

Figure 9 Secondary structure model of the hairpin ribozyme of the minus strand of the satellite RNA of tobacco ringspot virus ((−)sTRSV). The model is divided into a ribozyme component R and a substrate component S which form part of the 359 nt sTRSV. The self-cleavage site between G48 and A49 is indicated by an arrow; note that the residue numbering is of the plus strand so that the numbering increases in the 3' to the 5' direction. Helices are numbered H1 to H4. UV irradiation of the ribozyme leads to cross-linking between G204 and U184.

In 1987, Epstein and Gall reported that *in vitro*-produced transcripts of tandemly repeated 330 bp satellite II DNA of the newt self-cleaved by a hammerhead structure. This is the only non-viral RNA identified so far which self-cleaves via the hammerhead structure; the role of this reaction *in vivo* is unknown.

The small size of the hammerhead structure has led to its extensive characterization and manipulation. To aid in the description of various hammerhead constructs, a standard numbering system was introduced in 1992 (**Fig. 7**) and is now widely used.

Hammerhead reaction in *trans*

The plus and minus hammerhead structures of ASBV as identified in the native rod-like molecules are constituted from sections of the top and bottom RNA strands in the 247 nucleotides viroid. This led Uhlenbeck in 1987 to demonstrate hammerhead self-cleavage in *trans* using a 19 nt ribozyme to catalyze cleavage with multiple turnover of a 24 nt substrate as well as to cleave sequences embedded in a number of different RNAs. Haseloff and Gerlach in 1988 extended this approach by the design of small riboyzmes for the cleavage of specific sites in native RNA molecules *in vitro*, an approach which is now extensively used *in vitro* and *in vivo*.

Crystal structure of the hammerhead

The first crystal hammerhead structure was reported by McKay in 1994; it consisted of a 34-ribozyme and a 13-mer deoxynucleotide substrate. This was soon followed by Klug in 1995 and 1996 with crystal structures of an all RNA hammerhead. The three-dimensional structures developed from the three approaches are essentially the same (**Fig. 8**). Stem III of the hammerhead forms the stem of a Y-shaped structure where the arms are formed by stems I and II. Stems II and III are nearly collinear.

The hairpin ribozyme

This ribozyme (**Fig. 9**) has it origins in a 359 nt linear satellite RNA of tobacco ringspot virus (sTRSV) which is encapsidated within viroids of the helper virus. Circular forms of sTRSV are found *in vivo* in infected plants but these are not encapsidated, in contrast to the encapsidation of the circular viroid-like satellite RNAs or virusoids associated with the Sobemoviruses (**Table 2**). The dominant plus form of sTRSV self-cleaves via the hammerhead structure and the minus form via the hairpin structure. Only three satellite RNA examples of the hairpin ribozyme have been identified, all within the Nepovirus group and having hammerhead self-cleavage in the plus strand.

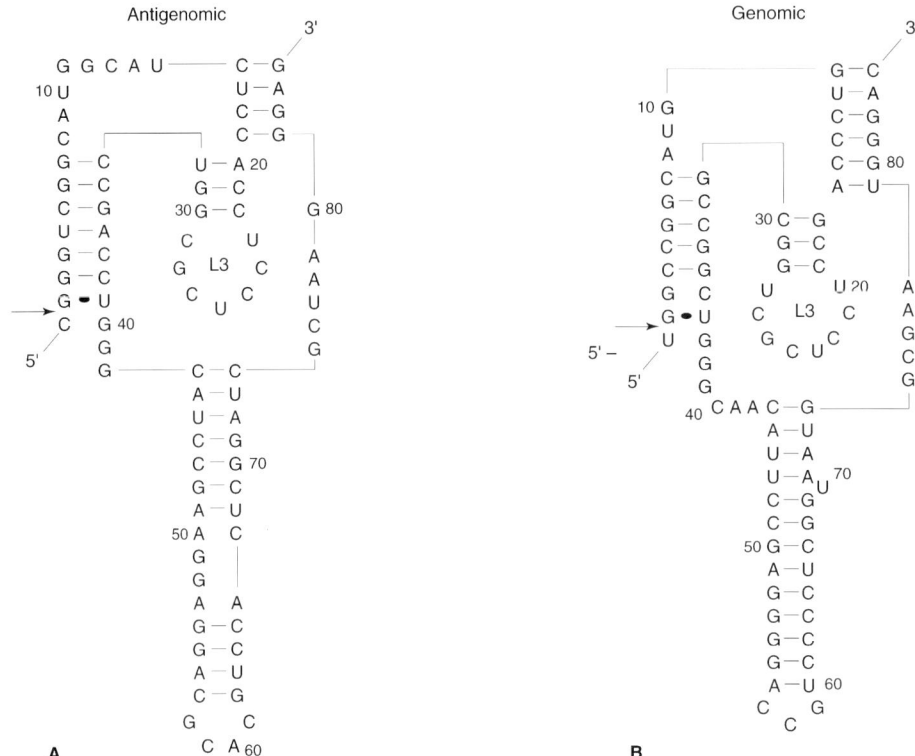

Figure 10 Secondary pseudoknot structures of the (**B**) genomic and (**A**) antigenomic ribozymes of hepatitis delta virus. The self-cleavage site in each ribozyme is indicated by an arrow. Only one nucleotide is needed 5' to the self-cleavage site for cleavage to occur *in vitro*.

As for the hammerhead sequences in plus and minus ASBV, the nucleotide sequences required for self-cleavage of minus sTRSV are from two well-separated regions of the RNA molecule (**Fig. 9**). This allowed the demonstration of self-cleavage in *trans in vitro* and the manipulation of the hairpin ribozyme to target unrelated RNAs *in vitro* and *in vivo*. This work is at an early stage as compared to the application of the hammerhead ribozyme.

The pseudoknot riboyzme of hepatitis delta virus RNA

Hepatitis delta virus (HDV) is a subviral satellite virus of hepatitis B virus (HBV). The approx. 1680 nt circular genomic RNA is encapsidated in HBV-coded proteins and can fold into an unbranched rod-like structure as can the nonencapsidated complementary antigenomic RNA found *in vivo*. The antigenomic RNA contains an open reading frame coding for a 195 amino acid protein called the delta antigen which is essential for HDV RNA replication. At one end of these molecules there is a viroid-like domain containing the ribozyme domains required for the processing of multimeric intermediates during the rolling circle replication of HDV RNA. There are no known coding regions on the genomic RNA.

The two-dimensional structures of genomic and antigenomic riboyzmes are given in **Fig. 10** and each contain approx. 85 nt. By common usage they are referred to as pseudoknot structures. There is a high conservation of sequence between the two structures. The naturally occurring *cis* ribozyme activity can be converted into in *trans* ribozyme activity by splitting the structures in **Fig. 10** in at least two single-stranded regions to give ribozyme and substrate fragments.

See also: **Hepatitis Delta virus; Luteovirus; Nepoviruses (*Comoviridae*); Satellite RNAs and Satellite viruses; Sobemoviruses; Viroids.**

Further Reading

Been MD and Wickham GS (1997) Self-cleaving ribozymes of hepatitis delta virus RNA. *Eur J Biochem* 247: 741.

Birikh KR, Heaton PA and Eckstein F (1997) The structure, function and application of the hammerhead ribozyme. *Eur J Biochem* 241: 1.

Cech TR and Herschlag D (1996) Group I ribozymes:

substrate recognition, catalytic strategies, and comparative mechanistic analysis. *Nucleic Acids Mol. Biol.* 10: 1.

Hampel A (1998) The hairpin ribozyme: discovery, two-dimensional model, and development of gene therapy. *Prog. Nucleic Acid Res. Mol. Biol.* 58: 1–39.

McKay DB (1996) Three-dimensional structure of the hammerhead ribozyme. *Nucleic Acids Mol. Biol.* 10: 161.

Nolan JM and Pace NR (1996) Structural analysis of the bacterial RNase P. *Nucleic Acids Mol. Biol.* 10: 109.

Pyle AM (1996) Catalytic reaction mechanisms and structural features of Group II intron ribozymes. *Nucleic Acids Mol. Biol.* 10: 75.

Scott WG and Klug A (1996) Ribozymes: structure and mechanism in RNA catalysis. *Trends Biochem. Sci.* 21: 220.

RINDERPEST AND DISTEMPER VIRUSES (*PARAMYXOVIRIDAE*)

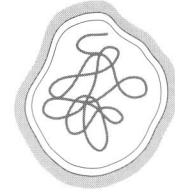

Tom Barrett, Institute for Animal Health, Pirbright Laboratory, Pirbright, Surrey, UK

Copyright © 1999 Academic Press

History

Rinderpest virus

Rinderpest (or cattle plague) is one of the oldest known plagues of domestic livestock, with recognizable descriptions dating back to the fourth century AD. It is of ancient Asiatic origin but in more recent times devastating plagues of rinderpest swept across Europe in the eighteenth and nineteenth centuries. In 1711 the disease entered Europe through Venice and had spread as far as Britain by 1714. The economic effect of the subsequent European plagues was so drastic that it led to the establishment of veterinary schools to deal specifically with the problems of animal health, the first being the veterinary school at Lyon in France in 1762. A vigorous slaughter and quarantine policy succeeded in controlling the disease and by the beginning of the twentieth century Europe was free of rinderpest. Subsequently there have been periodic introductions through importation of live infected animals; the last serious outbreak in domestic cattle occurred in Belgium in 1920 and was caused by infected zebu cattle in transit from India to Brazil mixing with local cattle at the docks. Following the 1920 outbreak in Europe, the Office International des Epizooties (OIE) was set up in Paris to deal with matters concerning animal health in relation to international trade. The last known case reported in Europe was in an imported zoo animal in Rome in 1949. Isolated cases of rinderpest have occurred in Brazil (1920) and Australia (1924), again in association with importation of live infected cattle.

In 1889 a catastrophic outbreak of rinderpest occurred in Africa and was caused by the importation of infected cattle from India to feed Italian soldiers engaged in a military campaign in Abyssinia (Ethiopia). The subsequent panzootic spread to nearly all parts of the continent, reaching South Africa by 1897. Over 90% of domestic cattle, along with other highly susceptible wild animals such as buffalo (*Syncerus caffer*), eland (*Taurotragus* spp.), kudu (*Tragelaphus imberbis*), giraffe (*Giraffa* spp.) and wildebeest (*Connochaetes* spp.), were wiped out (**Table 1**). At the time most transport relied on oxen and, as the South African railway system had not been fully established, the economic consequences were devastating. In Kenya the Masai tribe suffered greatly and many people starved. Descriptions at the time stated that the East African Plains were so littered with dead carcasses that the vultures were unable to clear the carrion. Previously rinderpest was only seen in Africa in Egypt and parts of Senegal, where it was periodically introduced from Europe or the Middle East.

A similar plague in small ruminants, peste des petits ruminants, was first described in West Africa in 1942 by Gargadennec and Lalanne. This disease is

Table 1 Susceptibility of wildlife to rinderpest

Susceptibility	Animals
Very high	Buffalo, eland, kudu, warthog
High	Giraffe, bushbuck, bushpig, sitatunga, Uganda cob, bongo, wildebeest
Moderate	Reedbuck, topi, gemsbok, blesbok, bontbok, oribi, impala, springbok
Low	Waterbuck, dukier, orynx, Grant's gazelle, dikdik, hartebeest
Very low	Thomson's gazelle, hippopotamus, gerenuk

also caused by a virus and is known as kata in West Africa. At first it was thought to be a variant of rinderpest virus adapted to grow in sheep and goats; however, it was subsequently shown to be an immunologically distinct virus with a separate epizootiology in areas where both viruses were enzootic. A disease of small ruminants, which was almost certainly caused by peste des petits ruminants virus, was first described in Senegal in 1871.

Canine distemper virus

Canine distemper virus is also a disease with a long history. Edward Jenner studied its neurological symptoms but it was Carré in 1906 who first showed that it was caused by a virus. In French the virus is known as 'la maladie de Carré'. In the summer of 1988 a large number of harbour seals (*Phoca vitulina*) died in the Baltic Sea and on the North Sea coasts of Northern Europe with clinical signs very similar to canine distemper in dogs. The epizootic was eventually shown to have been caused by a virus, at first thought to be canine distemper. Monoclonal antibody analyses and nucleic acid hybridization showed that it was a new virus distinct from canine distemper and it is now named phocid distemper virus. A disease with similar clinical signs caused mass mortality in Siberian seals (*Phoca sibirica*) in Lake Baikal in the winter of 1987. There was no obvious link between the virus outbreaks in the two seal populations and subsequent work showed that, in contrast to the European situation, the Russian epizootic was caused by a virus indistinguishable from canine distemper. The source of virus in this outbreak is thought to have been lakeside dogs which were suffering from canine distemper at that time. So, in addition to a wide range of land mammals, canine distemper virus can also infect aquatic carnivores.

In 1990 large numbers of striped dolphins (*Stenella coeruleoalba*) in the Mediterranean Sea were found dying from a virus infection which was referred to as the dolphin morbillivirus. Two years previously a virus had been isolated from porpoises (*Phocoena phocoena*) which was then found to be very closely related to the new dolphin virus. They were shown to be genetically distinct from other morbilliviruses, including phocid distemper virus. Serological evidence of infection with this virus was subsequently found in many other cetacean species in the Atlantic Ocean and the term cetacean morbillivirus has been suggested as a suitable name.

Taxonomy and Classification

Rinderpest was first shown to be a filtrable agent in 1902 and, along with the other viruses described above, is classified in the *Morbillivirus* genus (from the latin *morbus* meaning disease) within the *Paramyxoviridae* family. Antigenically the animal morbilliviruses are closely related to human measles virus, the type virus of the genus. Morbilliviruses are large enveloped viruses with a negative-strand RNA genome of about 16 kb. The virus particles are pleomorphic with an average diameter of around 200–300 nm. Measles virus is the only member of the group which has been shown to haemagglutinate red blood cells reproducibly. Unlike other members of the *Paramyxoviridae*, neuraminidase activity is generally not found in morbilliviruses; however, a highly substrate-specific neuraminidase activity has recently been demonstrated in rinderpest and peste des petits ruminants viruses.

Geographic Distribution

Rinderpest is enzootic on the Indian subcontinent and in parts of the Middle East and Eastern Africa. Sporadic outbreaks occur in countries bordering the enzootic regions. Peste des petits ruminants is enzootic in parts of West Africa but in the past few years it has spread across a broad belt of sub-Saharan Africa and eastwards through the Middle East and to southern Asia as far as Bangladesh (**Fig. 1**). It was thought until recently that India was free from peste des petits ruminants virus and that the morbillivirus-like disease prevalent in small ruminants was caused by rinderpest virus. However, in 1988 its presence in southern India was confirmed using specific cDNA hybridization probes.

Canine distemper has a worldwide distribution but is not found in very hot, arid regions. The development of an attenuated vaccine for canine distemper virus in the 1950s greatly reduced the incidence of disease in domestic dogs. However, many wild-life species are susceptible to the disease and can act as reservoirs of infection.

The origin of the European seal morbillivirus is unknown but it appears to be enzootic in Arctic waters, as sera collected from Greenland seals dating back to the early 1980s have been shown to be positive for morbillivirus antibodies. Arctic harp seals (*Phoca groenlandica*) show a high seropositivity and, unlike seals in European waters, are present in sufficient numbers to maintain the disease. The morbilliviruses isolated from porpoises and dolphins were probably transmitted by contact with another cetacean species in which the virus is enzootic. The most likely candidate in this case is the pilot whale (*Globicephalus melas*), which is gregarious and present in sufficient numbers to maintain the virus.

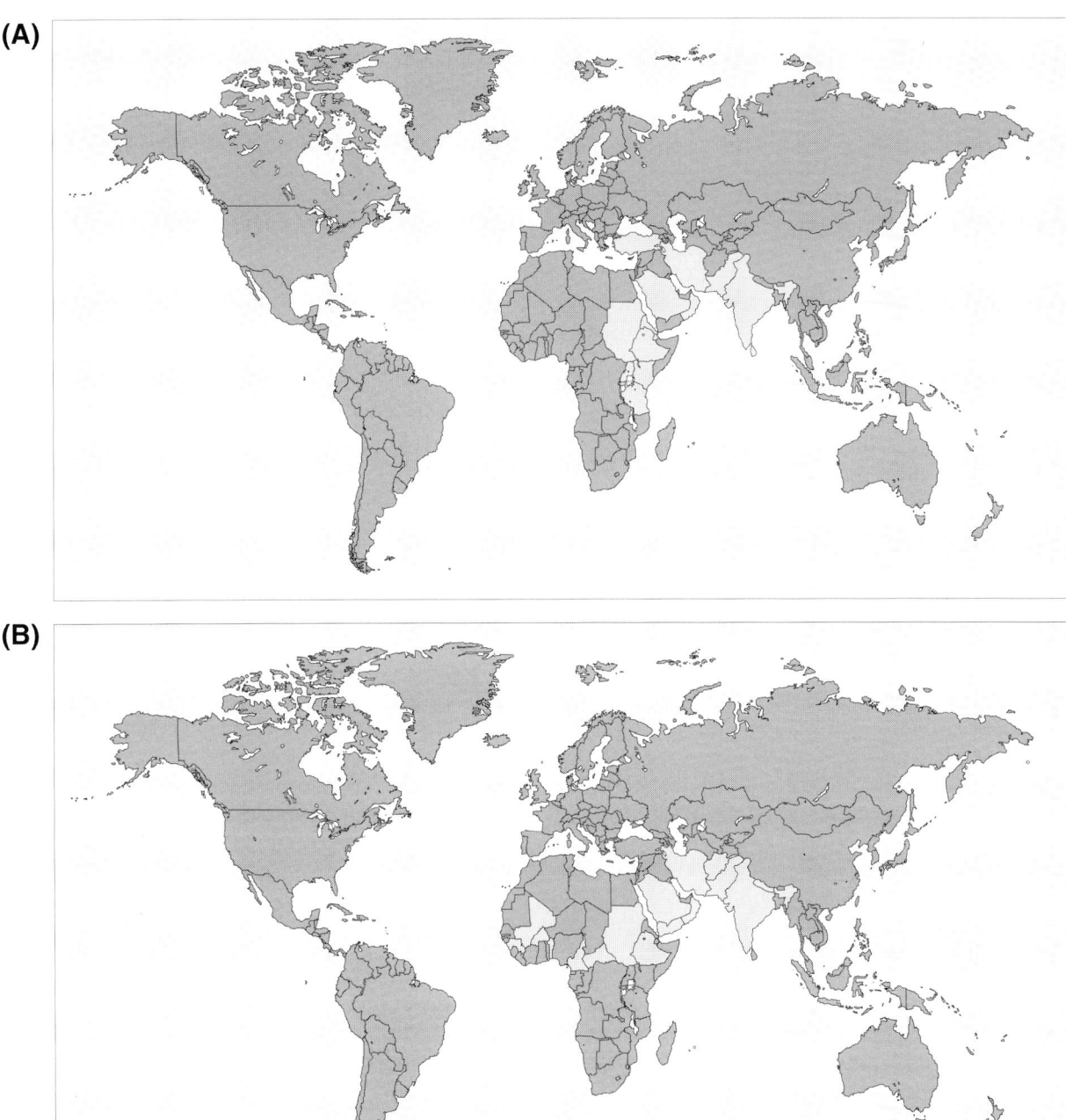

Figure 1 The present (1999) distribution of **(A)** rinderpest and **(B)** peste des petits ruminants viruses. Countries reporting disease since 1990 are in lighter shading.

Host Range and Virus Propagation

All species of the order *Artiodactyla* can be infected with rinderpest virus but some species are more susceptible to disease than others. In the case of cattle, Asian breeds are more resistant than European, while the opposite is the case in pigs. In the case of domestic ruminants, peste des petits ruminants virus only causes clinical disease in sheep and goats – goats being particularly susceptible. Peste des petits ruminants virus can also infect wild ruminants, as was illustrated by an outbreak of peste des petits ruminants virus in a zoo in the United Arab Emirates, but its full host range is unknown. In that outbreak gazelle (*Gazella dama*), ibex (*Capra ibex nubiana*) and gemsbok (*Oryx gazella*) were involved. Some large ruminants and pigs can be infected subclinically but they are dead-end hosts and do not transmit the disease.

Canine distemper causes disease in all *Canidae* (dog, wolf, fox), *Mustelidae* (ferret, weasle, mink), *Procyonidae* (racoon, panda) and collared peccaries (*Tayassu tajacu*). Canine distemper can probably infect all carnivore species but in certain cases, e.g. some *Felidae* (cats), the infection may be subclinical. Until recently it was thought that canine distemper could not cause disease in large cats such as tigers, lions and panthers; however, in 1991–1992 canine distemper was found to have been responsible for the deaths of large cats in several zoos in the USA. Shortly afterwards a distemper outbreak had a devastating effect on the population of lions in the Serengeti in Africa. The virus responsible for infection in large cats was most closely related to that circulating in local wild carnivores, e.g. racoons in the USA and hyaenas (*Hyaena crocuta*) in Africa, and not a new strain adapted specifically to felids. The outbreak of canine distemper virus in Siberian seals has extended its range to aquatic carnivores.

Phocid distemper virus is known to infect several species of seal, ranging from the harp seals and ringed seals (*Phoca hispida*) of the North Atlantic to the grey (*Halichoerus grypus*) and harbor seals which have a more southerly distribution. During the 1988 European epizootic, although few grey seals succumbed to the infection, many were found to have developed morbillivirus-specific antibodies. This indicated a difference in susceptibility to disease as harbor seals died in large numbers. Phocid distemper virus accidentally infected mink in Denmark during the 1988 epizootic and so it can also cause disease in terrestrial carnivores.

The morbilliviruses can be isolated in a variety of cell types. Primary bovine kidney cells are usually used to isolate field strains of rinderpest virus and primary lamb kidney cells for peste des petits ruminants virus. More recently a marmoset lymphoblastoid cell line (B95a) and a *Theileria parva*-transformed bovine lymphocyte cell line have been reported to be suitable for rinderpest virus isolation. Virus can be best isolated from tissues such as mucosal lesions, lymph nodes or by cocultivation of washed buffy coat with susceptible cells such as bovine kidney or B95a cells. Cytopathic effects are usually evident between 3 and 12 days after infection, whereas control cells treated with antirinderpest antiserum should remain healthy.

Canine distemper virus is usually isolated by cocultivation of lymphocytes from infected animals with mitogen-stimulated canine or ferret lymphocytes and can then be adapted to grow in MDCK or Vero cells. Lung tissue is also a good source of virus for canine distemper and phocid distemper virus isolation. Primary seal kidney cells were used initially to isolate phocid distemper virus but the virus can also be adapted to grow in Vero cells. Typical cytopathic effects such as cell elongation, cell rounding, the formation of stellate cells and syncytia can be observed between 3 and 12 days postinfection. Several blind passages may be necessary before cytopathic changes are observed in the cells.

Properties of the Virion and Genome

The rinderpest virus particle is made up of a lipid envelope derived from the host cell, six virus structural proteins and a genome consisting of a single strand of negative-sense RNA. Two other virus-specific proteins (C and V) found in infected cells, but not so far in virus particles, are termed nonstructural proteins. All morbilliviruses are identical in genetic configuration. In the case of rinderpest, the virion RNA consists of a short 3' leader RNA (55 nucleotides) followed by the coding regions of the six structural protein genes and ending in a short 5' trailer RNA (37 nucleotides). There are semiconserved start–stop sequence motifs at the start and end of each gene, and between these is a trinucleotide untranscribed intergenic sequence (usually GAA). Measles, rinderpest and canine distemper viruses have been completely sequenced; measles virion RNA is 15 894 nucleotides long, rinderpest 15 882 nucleotides long and and canine distemper virion RNA slightly shorter, at 15 690 nucleotides.

The two virus encoded glycoproteins, the haemagglutinin (H protein) and fusion proteins (F protein), are embedded in a lipid membrane which is derived from the host cell during budding and this forms the virus envelope. A nonglycosylated matrix protein (M protein) interacts both with the cytoplasmic domains of the envelope glycoproteins and with the nucleocapsids formed within the host cell during genome replication. The M protein is thought to be essential for virus morphogenesis and budding. The newly synthesized virion RNA is surrounded and protected in the cytoplasm by the nucleocapsid (N protein) protein which, in association with the virus polymerase (L protein) and phosphoprotein (P protein), forms the ribonucleoprotein complex (**Fig. 2**).

Replication

The two nonstructural proteins found in infected cells are derived from messenger RNAs transcribed from

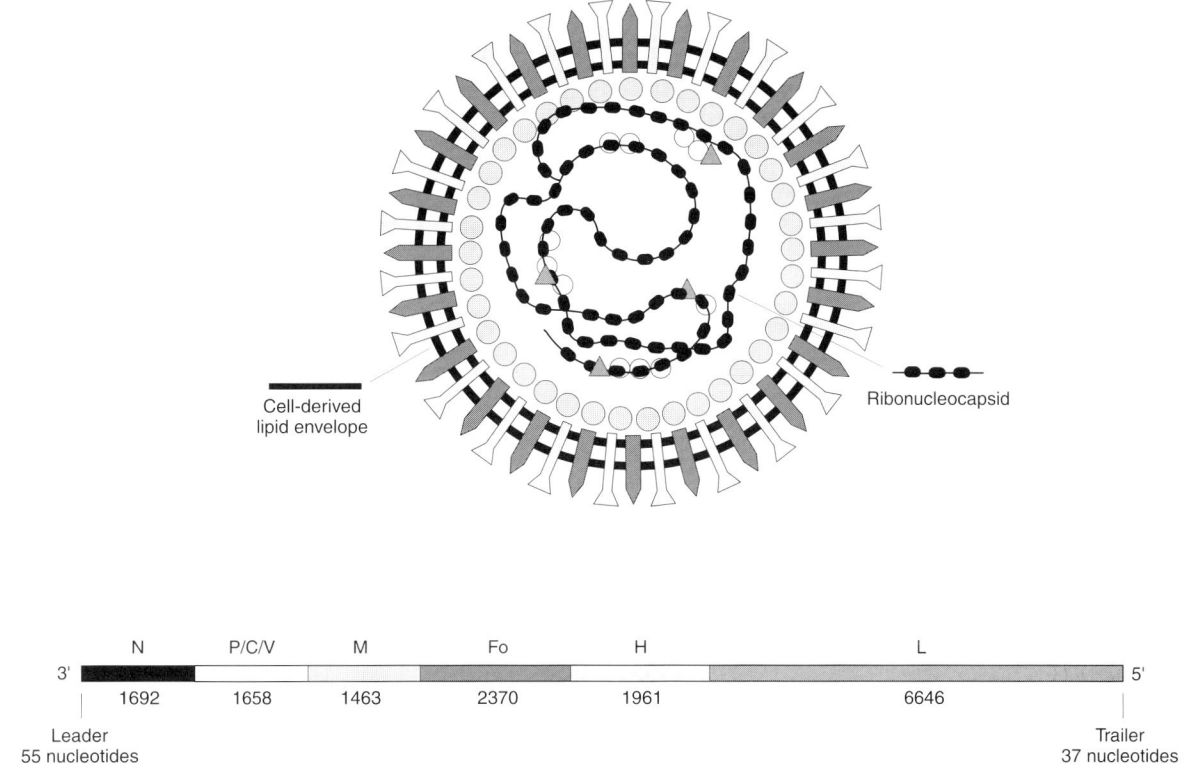

Figure 2 A typical morbillivirus showing the outer envelope with the two projecting surface glycoproteins and the inner helical nucleocapsid containing the virion RNA. The matrix protein is shown underneath the virus envelope. The arrangement of the genes along the virion RNA is shown below.

the P gene. The C nonstructural protein is translated from an alternate reading frame in the phosphoprotein mRNA beginning at the second AUG codon. The V protein is translated from an mRNA which is not an exact copy of the P gene sequence but from one which has an extra G residue inserted about halfway along the gene. This process is often referred to as 'editing' but is more correctly called alternative transcription and is a property of the virus polymerase, as it does not occur in other artificial systems. A conserved sequence motif is found in the region where the insertion occurs. Addition of an extra G occurs in about 50% of the mRNAs transcribed from the P gene in the case of measles and rinderpest viruses and there is evidence that it occurs in all other morbilliviruses. Translation of this mRNA produces a chimeric protein consisting of the N-terminus of the P protein with a new C-terminus, rich in cysteine residues, derived from RNA sequence in the third reading frame. This mRNA is also capable of translating the C protein as its coding region is located in front of the editing sequence position. The functions of these proteins are unknown but they most likely play a part in the control of transcription and replication of the genome RNA.

Evolution

Rinderpest virus

Monoclonal antibody and sequence analyses indicate that rinderpest virus is most closely related to measles virus, and phocid distemper virus to canine distemper virus. The nucleic acid homology between the N genes of phocid and canine distemper viruses is only about 77%. The two viruses are, therefore, almost as different as rinderpest and measles (70% homology) and must have had a long period during which they diverged from a common ancestor. The new dolphin and porpoise morbilliviruses are very closely related to each other, being different strains of the same virus, and are now often referred to as the cetacean morbillivirus. They are antigenically more related to rinderpest and peste des petits ruminants viruses than to phocid and canine distemper viruses but they fall into a distinct lineage group when their sequences are compared with other morbilliviruses (**Fig. 3**).

The exact evolutionary relationship between the different morbilliviruses is unknown but rinderpest has been proposed as the 'archevirus' of the group. Monoclonal antibody reactivities support this conclusion as rinderpest reacts with a broader range of

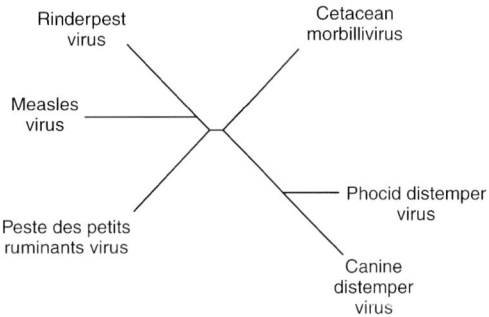

Figure 3 A computer-generated tree showing the phylogenetic relationships between the different morbilliviruses. The tree was generated using the PHYLIP programs to analyze the complete N gene coding region.

monoclonals produced against other morbilliviruses. The fragility of the virus particle and the lifelong immunity following infection (see Prevention and Control) dictate that morbilliviruses have a constant supply of susceptible hosts for their survival. Populations of 300 000 or more are required to maintain measles virus. Animal populations of the required size would most likely have been large herds of ruminants before humans formed sufficiently large settled groups. When cattle were domesticated they could have passed a morbillivirus infection to humans which eventually evolved into measles virus.

Canine distemper virus

Canine distemper virus infects a wide range of carnivores and is maintained by a virus reservoir in a large variety of wild carnivore species. This virus, unlike rinderpest virus, can in rare cases maintain a persistent infection from which the disease can reactivate as old dog distemper. It is conceivable, though less likely, that canine distemper is the progenitor of the group and that predators passed the disease to other nonpredator species, which then evolved into the distinct morbilliviruses. Little is known about the evolution of the morbilliviruses isolated from aquatic mammals. It is possible that seals contracted canine distemper from dogs or other carnivores with which they came into contact while hauling up on land or ice flows to breed. Their relatively close genetic relationship supports this suggestion. In the case of cetaceans the situation is much less clear. They do not come on land to breed and there are not many opportunities for contact with terrestrial mammals. This, and the great genetic distance between the cetacean and other morbilliviruses, indicates that the virus must have been present in cetaceans for a very long time. Pilot whales have been suggested as the most likely species in which the virus is naturally enzootic, as they are present in relatively large numbers and serological studies have shown a high prevalence of morbillivirus-specific antibodies in this species.

Serologic Relationships and Variability

All viruses in the group are antigenically related – the matrix, fusion and nucleocapsid proteins being the most highly conserved across the group. In fact, immunity induced to the F protein may be responsible for the strong crossprotection seen after vaccination with heterologous virus. Rinderpest vaccine is routinely used to vaccinate against peste des petits ruminants virus, and inactivated canine distemper virus vaccine has been shown to protect seals against infection with phocid distemper virus. It has also been shown experimentally that measles virus can protect dogs against distemper and cattle against rinderpest, and that distemper virus can protect humans against measles. This has no epidemiological significance as the viruses do not naturally crossinfect. The H protein, responsible for attachment to the host cell receptor, is the least conserved and least crossreactive morbillivirus protein. In immunoprecipitation reactions only the H protein fails to crossprecipitate with heterologous antisera, although some one-way precipitations are seen, e.g. measles antiserum will precipitate canine distemper H but not vice versa. Strain variations within each virus group can be readily demonstrated using monoclonal antibodies but these variations do not result in different serotypes for each virus.

Epizootiology

Rinderpest virus

Traditionally, rinderpest outbreaks follow wars and civil disturbance where there is unrestricted movement of people and troops with live food animals which can carry the virus. Recent outbreaks in Lebanon, the Middle East and Sri Lanka follow this pattern. The outbreak in Sri Lanka in 1987 was seen after a 40 year span free from the disease and the likely source was live goats brought from India with the troops and traded locally. More recently rinderpest reappeared in Turkey as a consequence of the Gulf war.

Rinderpest and peste des petits ruminants viruses are normally introduced into an area by importation of live infected animals from an enzootic area. Transmission by infected meat is very rare and considered to be a low risk. The most dangerous sources of virus are subclinically infected animals. Subclinically infected pigs act as a source of virus for cattle. Sheep, goats and possibly other small ruminants can be infected with rinderpest virus and pass the infection to cattle. Experimentally this has been shown to occur with Asian strains of rinderpest virus which readily infect small ruminants. In contrast, African strains of rinderpest do not appear to productively infect sheep and goats. Another factor which may be important in the maintenance of rinderpest is the presence of strains which cause mild or subclinical infections in some enzootic areas. The incubation period for these viruses can be up to 15 days and this, along with their low transmission rates, means that they can persist unnoticed for many years in cattle populations. It is possible that the disease may flare up clinically when animals are put under stress, such as when they are moved to markets. In Africa the situation is also complicated by the presence of large numbers of susceptible wildlife species which can help spread the virus in an uncontrolled manner. Wild ruminants vary greatly in their response to rinderpest infection with species such as buffalo, kudu, eland and warthog (*Phacochoerus aethiopicus*) being highly susceptible, and others such as the hippopotamus (*Hippopotamus amphibius*) and Thompson's gazelle (*Gazella thomsoni*) highly resistant. The epizootiology of rinderpest virus on the two continents is therefore quite different. In Asia there is one known lineage of the virus, while in Africa two distinct virus lineages coexist (**Fig. 4**).

The role of wildlife species in maintaining the disease is unclear. There is no good evidence that wild ruminants act as a reservoir of infection for domestic animals but they may be important in helping to spread disease once an outbreak occurs. To date the evidence suggests that domestic animals are generally the source of infection for wildlife species. The virus was successfully eradicated from South Africa and Tanzania, despite the presence of considerable numbers of wild animals. In fact some highly susceptible wild animals may act as sentinels for the disease, as illustrated by the recent severe outbreak of rinderpest virus in lesser kudu, eland and buffalo in Kenya. The epizootiology of peste des petits ruminants virus and the role wildlife plays in its maintenance has not been studied in any detail.

Canine distemper virus

Canine distemper virus is enzootic in wild carnivores and it remains a problem in poor urban areas where there are many stray dogs and vaccination is not carried out rigorously. The virus is also an important factor in the ecology of wild animal populations. The last free-living population of black-footed ferrets in

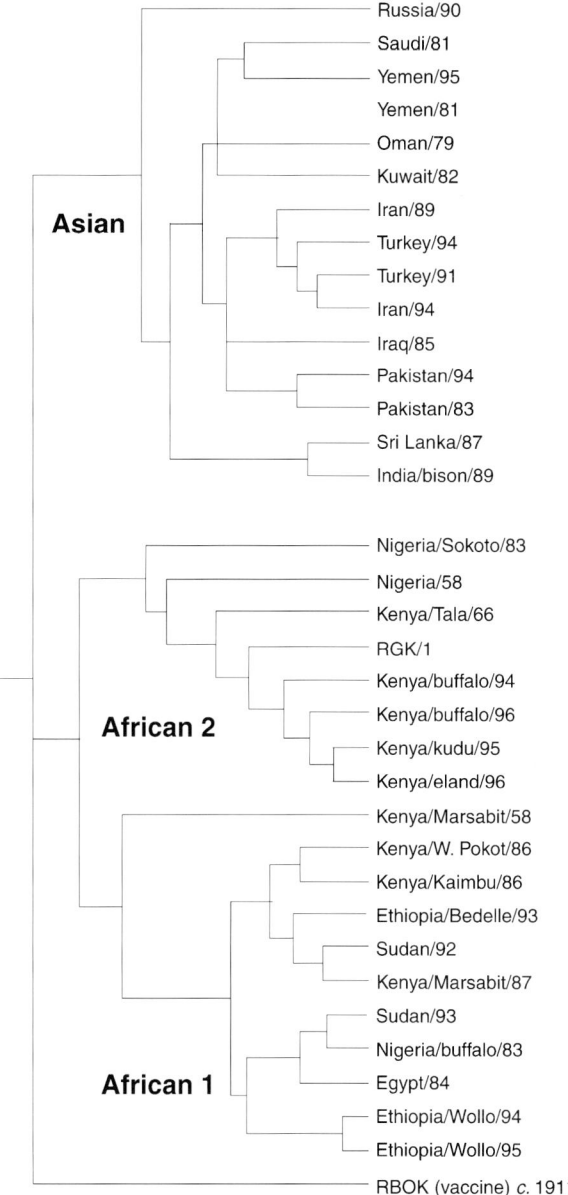

Figure 4 A computer-generated tree showing the relationship between African and Asian lineages of rinderpest virus. The tree was generated with the PHYLIP programs using partial sequence data from the F protein gene.

Wyoming was almost wiped out by a canine distemper infection. The recent canine distemper outbreak in free-living lions in the Serengeti and in captive lions, tigers and panthers in zoos in the USA indicate that it must now be considered a threat to these species. As noted previously, canine distemper and a closely related phocid distemper virus have recently been isolated from several species of pinniped. Such a serious disease could have a devastating effect on small populations of rare sea mammals, such as that of the monk seals (*Monachus monachus*) in the Mediterranean Sea and the Atlantic Ocean or in the Siberian seals in Lake Baikal. It is important to monitor these species for signs of infection and possibly vaccinate those taken into seal sanctuaries with safe subunit vaccines. The epizootiology of phocid distemper virus is poorly understood. Analysis of historic sera from Canadian harp seals and arctic ringed seals indicated that they were infected with a morbillivirus several years before the appearance of phocid distemper along the coasts of northern Europe. It has been suggested that climatic changes caused the harp seals to migrate further south, so passing the infection to other seal species which lacked herd immunity to the virus and as a result suffered a severe epizootic.

Transmission and Tissue Tropism

Morbillivirus transmission is by direct contact with secretions or excretions of infected animals. The morbilliviruses are highly contagious: all discharges can carry the virus. However, since the virus is extremely sensitive to environmental factors, such as heat, sunlight and chemical inactivation, it requires close contact with an infected animal for successful transmission. It is therefore relatively easy to control by regulating animal movements, in conjunction with a strict quarantine and slaughter policy where necessary. Even without the availability of vaccines rinderpest was successfully controlled and eliminated from Europe by these means.

The morbilliviruses are highly lymphotropic and cause a transient immunosuppression in infected animals. The more virulent strains of the virus also have a strong tropism for epithelial tissues and this helps the spread of the disease by contact, as high titres of virus are then excreted. Mild strains do not replicate so readily in epithelial surfaces and so are more difficult to transmit by contact. With the exception of rinderpest and peste des petits ruminants, morbilliviruses are known to infect brain cells, where they can set up persistent, eventually fatal, infections.

Pathogenicity

Although there is only one serotype of each virus, differences between isolates can be shown using monoclonal antibodies, and strains also vary in their ability to cause disease in infected animals. In the case of rinderpest, extreme variation in pathogenicity has been reported, ranging from the mild strains currently circulating in eastern Africa to highly virulent strains, such as those found in the Middle East, which can cause 90–100% mortality in susceptible hosts.

Variation in the severity of clinical disease and neurotropism have also been reported with different strains of canine distemper, which are known as 'biotypes'. Very little is known about the pathogenicity of the marine morbilliviruses. Different hosts are known to have different susceptibilities, as evidenced by the greater number of deaths in harbor seals relative to gray seals during the European seal epizootic in 1988. Likewise, pilot whales show a high level of seropositivity to cetacean morbillivirus but only dolphins and porpoises were severely affected during the epizootic in the Mediterranean Sea in 1990–1991. However, because of the immunosuppressive nature of morbilliviruses, secondary bacterial and concurrent parasitic infections can greatly influence the outcome of the disease and it is sometimes difficult to assess the contribution of virus infection. Nothing is yet known concerning the molecular basis of pathogenicity in morbilliviruses.

Clinical Features of Infection

Rinderpest virus

Typical rinderpest is an acute febrile disease, with mortality reaching close to 100% with some of the most virulent strains of rinderpest virus, such as the Saudi/81 strain. The course of the disease is divided into five stages: after a short (1) incubation period of 3–5 days, the (2) prodromal phase is seen in which there is a rapid rise in temperature. This is followed by the (3) mucosal phase in which severe mouth lesions are seen and there is a copious nasal and ocular mucopurulent discharge. The affected animals become depressed and anorexic and on postmortem examination many lesions are seen throughout the digestive and lymphatic system. This is followed by the (4) diarrheal phase where there is severe bloody diarrhea, the animal is prostrated and dies from dehydration and weakness. In nonfatal cases there follows the (5) convalescent phase which may take many weeks and during which pregnant animals may abort. Some strains, such as those prevalent in Eastern Africa, are generally mild and there may be no clinical signs in many cases, even though the animals seroconvert. With the mild strains the incubation period can extend up to 15 days.

Clinically peste des petits ruminants virus infection closely resembles rinderpest. There is an incubation period of 4–5 days, then a rise in temperature followed by nasal and ocular discharges, which can be very severe. Mucosal lesions and severe diarrhea then appear and the animals, in fatal cases, die of dehydration within 6 days of the onset of fever. Bronchopneumonia is a frequent complication.

Canine distemper virus

The incubation period for canine distemper virus is usually about 1 week. There are often two temperature peaks, the second corresponding with other signs such as nasal discharge, conjunctivitis and anorexia. As in the case of rinderpest, respiratory and gastrointestinal lesions follow and severe leukopenia is also seen. In some cases central nervous system (CNS) signs, such as convulsions and seizures, are seen as part of the clinical disease, or they may follow a subclinical infection. Recovered dogs frequently show persistent nervous 'ticks' or involuntary movements of one or more legs. Old dog encephalitis is a rare disease thought to be caused by canine distemper virus persistence in the brain and nervous tissue. Seals infected with phocid distemper virus show clinical signs, including CNS lesions, reminiscent of canine distemper infection in dogs, and this gave the first clue to the nature of the etiological agent.

Pathology and Histopathology

Severe morbillivirus infections are accompanied by a marked leukopenia, leading to a deficiency in the immune system. This often results in the activation of latent or other concurrent infections. In addition, secondary bacterial infections are common. These factors may complicate both the clinical and pathomorphological findings. In the case of rinderpest, leukopenia is most marked during the erosive mucosal phase. Histologically the virus shows a tropism for lymphoid and epithelial cells. All lymphoid organs are affected, with the greatest damage occurring in the mesenteric lymph nodes and gut-associated lymphoid tissue; severe destruction of the B and T cell areas is seen. Intracytoplasmic and intranuclear eosinophilic inclusion bodies are commonly found in the cells of morbillivirus infected animals.

Epithelial tissues of the upper respiratory, urogenital and alimentary tracts are also infected by the highly pathogenic, and highly contagious, strains of the virus. In acute rinderpest and peste des petits ruminants infections there is extensive erosive inflammation of mucosal surfaces of the digestive and upper respiratory tracts, with cellular necrosis and the formation of syncytia. Mild strains induce less extensive mucosal lesions and this may account for the reduced ability of these strains to transmit by contact. In the cecum, colon and rectum of animals infected with rinderpest and peste des petits ruminants viruses, so-called zebra or tiger stripes are commonly found. The stripes are caused by greatly distended capillaries packed with erythrocytes. Similar pathological changes are seen in infections with the other animal morbilliviruses. Dehydration in acute morbillivirus infections, the result of profuse diarrhea, causes changes in hematology and blood chemistry. There is an apparent increase in erythrocyte count and the packed cell volume increases by 40–65%. At death the blood is dark, thick and slow to coagulate. In acute canine distemper, phocid distemper and peste des petits ruminants virus infections a serous inflammation of intestinal and respiratory surfaces, associated with interstitial pneumonia, occurs. A nonsuppurative encephalitis is also seen.

Immune Response

There is a strong cell-mediated component in the response to morbillivirus infection. In the case of measles virus, individuals with a genetic defect leading to agammaglobulinemia can quite easily overcome measles infection but immunosuppressed individuals are at extreme risk from the disease. Animals with any detectable neutralizing antibody are considered immune to rinderpest and immunity following morbillivirus infection is lifelong. Either the F or H surface glycoprotein can confer immunity to disease, as poxvirus recombinant vaccines, expressing either the H or F proteins of rinderpest virus, are protective. Similar observations were made in animal model systems in the case of measles virus. In addition, it was found that vaccinia recombinants expressing the N protein could protect mice from lethal intracerebral challenge with measles virus, whereas a similar recombinant expressing the N gene of rinderpest virus gave no protection. In contrast, purified H and F antigens are not protective unless presented as immune stimulating complexes in association with Quil A (ISCOM vaccines). ISCOM vaccines are known to stimulate cytotoxic T cell responses in animals.

Prevention and Control

Morbilliviruses are extremely fragile; they are sensitive to sunlight, high temperature, low and high pH and chemicals which can destroy their outer lipid-containing envelope. Outbreaks of these viruses are therefore easily controlled by proper quarantine and hygienic measures. There is only one serotype of each virus and, once recovered from the infection, the animal is immune for life. As there is no evidence for a persistent or carrier state in the recovered animals, vaccination is a very effective means of controlling these diseases.

Diagnosis

Rapid and accurate differential diagnosis is the key to success in controlling a morbillivirus outbreak. Identification of the morbilliviruses is generally based on the species in which the disease is seen, e.g. measles in humans, rinderpest in cattle, canine distemper in dogs, etc. However, this is not always accurate as the viruses can sometimes infect unusual hosts and the diseases share clinical signs with other virus infections, so diagnosis can not be based solely on the host and clinical signs. For example, rinderpest and bovine virus diarrhea are often confused, and peste des petits ruminants virus can be mistaken for pasteurellosis or other microbial pleuropneumonias. Laboratory diagnosis, based on either virus isolation or specific antigen detection, is essential to confirm the presence of these diseases. A general morbillivirus-specific antigen detection test, the agar gel immunodiffusion (AGID) test, is currently used in field situations in Africa and Asia but it cannot distinguish between the viruses of rinderpest and peste des petits ruminants. Differential neutralization tests can be used to classify virus isolates but these are time consuming. However, rapid competitive ELISA systems using morbillivirus species-specific monoclonal antibodies, which can distinguish rinderpest and peste des petits ruminants viruses, have been developed for virus antigen and antibody detection. Rapid penside tests for the detection of rinderpest and peste des petits ruminants viruses have been developed based on latex bead technology and specific monoclonal antibodies. These new techniques are now being introduced into countries where these diseases are endemic. The most recent advance has been the introduction of the polymerase chain reaction for specific morbillivirus diagnosis (**Fig. 5**). This technique, in combination with sequence analysis of the DNA produce, has enabled a much more precise analysis of the epidemiology of these viruses in the field.

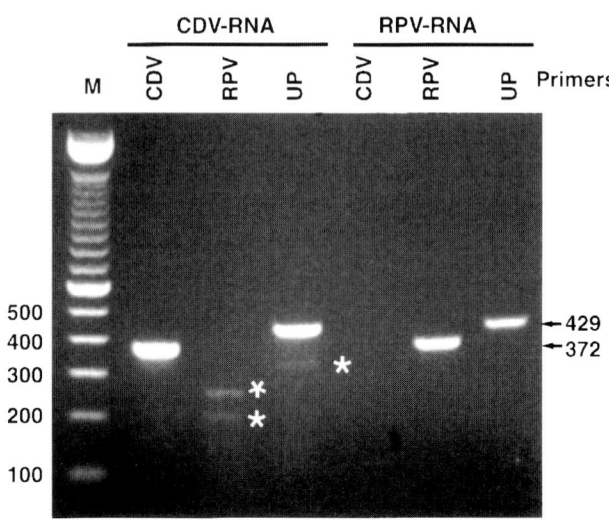

Figure 5 Example of a differential RT/PCR test to distinguish rinderpest (RPV) and canine distemper virus (CDV). Both a universal primer set (based on P gene sequences) and specific primer sets (based on F gene sequences) were used. Nonspecific amplification products are indicated by asterisks.

Vaccination

During the 1930s attenuated rinderpest vaccines were developed by passage of the virus in nonnatural hosts, e.g. rabbit and embryonated eggs (lapinized/avianized) or goats (caprinized). The Japanese lapinized/avianized vaccine was used extensively to control the disease in Asia. In India and Africa the caprinized virus was used; however, this virus was not completely attenuated and it may have been responsible for the circulation of rinderpest in small ruminants in India. In the early 1960s the Plowright tissue culture attenuated vaccine was introduced; it is safe and relatively easy to produce, with no clinical signs following vaccination in domestic animals. In addition, the virus does not replicate at epithelial surfaces and cannot be transmitted by contact. Immunity following vaccination is complete and lifelong. The vaccine is, however, very heat labile and establishment of an effective cold-chain and follow-up seromonitoring to determine the level of herd immunity are essential prerequisites for a successful vaccination campaign. Improvements in freeze-drying techniques have greatly increased the stability of the vaccine in the dry form but it is still very labile when reconstituted and must be used within a very short period.

In the 1960s an internationally funded rinderpest eradication campaign (Joint Programme 15 or JP 15) was carried out in Africa, using the tissue culture attenuated vaccine, and almost succeeded in clearing the disease from Africa. However, political instability, lack of funds to continue vaccination and disease surveillance and the existence of mild strains of the disease resulted in a resurgence in the 1980s. Quite often countries are reluctant to report cases of rinderpest or peste des petits ruminants virus infection because of the repercussions for trade in live animals and this makes the task of controlling outbreaks more difficult. An internationally funded vaccination campaign has been underway in Africa, the Pan African Rinderpest Campaign (PARC), since the mid-1980s and has successfully contained rinderpest virus to eastern Africa. Currently a Global Rinderpest Eradication Programme (GREP) has been established by the United Nations Food and Agricultural Organization in an attempt to eradicate the disease early in the twenty-first century.

Generally rinderpest vaccine is used to control the spread of peste des petits ruminants virus but a homologous vaccine has now been developed and is being field tested in West Africa. The role that wildlife species play in maintaining rinderpest and peste des petits ruminants viruses needs to be more clearly understood before it will be possible to be certain that vaccination of domestic animals alone can eliminate these diseases.

Canine distemper vaccines are not attenuated for all species, and in some, such as the lesser panda (*Ailurus fulgens*), they cause quite severe disease. There are two widely used vaccines for canine distemper virus: the Onderstepoort strain was attenuated by growth in avian cells and the Rockborn strain in canine tissue culture cells. Immunity lasts for several years following vaccination with either vaccine. A less effective ISCOM subunit vaccine (see Immune Response) must be used for nondomestic species, particularly in the case of valuable zoo animals. Since there is a large wildlife reservoir of canine distemper virus and the vaccines are not attenuated for many wild animal species, it may be impossible to eradicate this virus disease.

Future Perspectives

Much research has gone into the development of poxvirus recombinants expressing morbillivirus antigens in an effort to obtain more heat-stable vaccines, which would make them easier to use in hot climates. They have proved to be effective vaccines in short-term protection studies; however, the duration of immunity and the level of protection these vaccines give in comparison with the conventional tissue culture vaccines needs to be established. The most exciting new development in the field of morbillivirus research has been the ability to rescue live virus from DNA copies of their genomes. This technology will enable us to study the molecular mechanisms that underlie pathogenic variation in the morbilliviruses. Identification of attenuating mutations will help in the design and production of safer vaccines. Another great advance will be the ability to introduce genetic markers into the viruses, which will enable vaccinated animals to be distinguished serologically from animals which have been naturally infected. A genetically marked vaccine will be a very valuable tool for GREP in its aim to eradicate rinderpest virus by the end of the first decade of the twenty-first century.

See also: **Parainfluenza viruses (*Paramyxoviridae*): Animal; Measles virus (*Paramyxoviridae*); Bovine diarrhea virus and Border disease virus (*Flaviviridae*); Immune response: Cell mediated immune response, General features; Pathogenesis: Animal viruses.**

Further Reading

Anderson J, Barrett T and Scott GR (1996) *Manual on the Diagnosis of Rinderpest*, 2nd edn. Rome: Food and Agriculture Organization.

Appel M (1987) Canine distemper virus. In: Appel MJ (ed.) *Virus Infections of Carnivores*, p. 133. Amsterdam: Elsevier.

Barrett T, Blixenkrone-Moller M, DiGuardo G et al (1995) Morbilliviruses in aquatic mammals: report on round table discussion. *Vet. Microbiol.* 44: 261.

Losos G (1986) Peste des petits ruminants. In: *Infectious Tropical Diseases of Domestic Animals*, p. 549. Harlow: Longman.

Plowright W (1982) The effects of rinderpest and rinderpest control on wildlife in Africa. In: Edwards MA and McDonnell U (eds) *Animal Disease in Relation to Animal Conservation*, p. 1. Symposia of the Zoological Society of London, no. 50. London: Academic Press.

Scott GR (1985) Rinderpest in the 1980s. In: Pandey R (ed.) *Infections and Immunity in Farm Animals*, p. 145. Progress in Veterinary Microbiology and Immunology, no 1. Basel: Karger.

ROSS RIVER VIRUS AND BARMAH FOREST VIRUS (*TOGAVIRIDAE*)

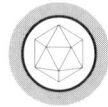

Lynn Dalgarno and **Ian D Marshall**, Division of Biochemistry and Molecular Biology, School of Life Sciences, The Australian National University, Canberra, Australia

Copyright © 1999 Academic Press

History

The first reports of a disease probably caused by Ross River virus (RRV) appeared in 1928, describing epidemics of transient arthritis and rash in two Murrumbidgee River towns on the semiarid inland plains of New South Wales (NSW), south-eastern Australia. During World War II, epidemics of arthritis with rash were described in troops serving in the tropical regions of Australia and on islands to the immediate north. Most of these outbreaks were differentially diagnosed against a background of endemic dengue fever, and published reports allowed the description of a syndrome adequate for clinical diagnosis of the disease, at least during epidemics. Several attempts failed to isolate or define the nature of the causative agent. These wartime reports provided the terms 'epidemic polyarthritis' and 'epidemic polyarthritis with rash' to characterize the disease; although these are still widely used, the noncommittal 'Ross River virus disease' is gaining currency. As fever is usually absent or unremarkable, 'Ross River fever' is inappropriate.

The first large, adequately documented community epidemic occurred in the Murray Valley of south-eastern Australia in 1956, but again two groups of investigators failed to isolate the causative agent. However, following consideration of the epidemiology and nature of the disease, and subsequent serological testing of convalescent sera, it was concluded that a mosquito-borne Group A arbovirus was the most likely candidate, and for several years the Malaysian alphavirus Bebaru was used as a surrogate diagnostic and survey antigen. Eventually, in 1963, the specific alphavirus was isolated from a pool of *Aedes vigilax* mosquitoes collected during dengue investigations near the Ross River at Townsville, coastal north Queensland. The first human isolate was in 1971 from the serum of a mildly febrile 7-year-old aboriginal boy, but, as is usual before puberty, characteristic signs and symptoms did not develop. The final incrimination of RRV did not occur until 1979, when the virus was introduced to Fiji, presumably by a viremic tourist from Australia; RRV was isolated in newborn mice inoculated with the acute stage serum of the indicator case. Numerous isolations were subsequently made during the ensuing series of virgin soil epidemics which, over the next 2 years, extended across the south Pacific from New Caledonia to the Cook Islands. RRV has since been isolated from patients in Australia but only from sera incidentally taken before onset of symptoms (see below).

Over recent years it has become apparent that a significant number of clinically well-defined cases of viral polyarthritis with rash are due to Barmah Forest virus (BFV), which was first isolated from mosquitoes in 1974 (see below). In 1988 BFV was shown to be the causative agent of a disease that is currently regarded as being clinically indistinguishable from that due to RRV infection. Although RRV and BFV are both alphaviruses, BFV has a number of features which are atypical. RRV and BFV are antigenically quite distinct. There have been several epidemics where both viruses circulated concurrently and the causative virus of individual cases was distinguished serologically.

Taxonomy and Classification

RRV and BFV are mosquito-borne arboviruses belonging to the genus *Alphavirus* of the *Togaviridae* family. RRV is a subtype of Getah virus in the Semliki Forest virus (SFV) serological complex. BFV is the sole member of a seventh alphavirus complex.

Properties of the Virion

Purified RRV virions have two glycosylated envelope proteins: E1, the hemagglutinin (molecular mass, 52 kDa) and E2, the neutralizing antigen (49 kDa). The nucleocapsid protein, C, is 32 kDa. RRV is sensitive to chloroform, ether, detergents, ultraviolet irradiation and low pH. The infectivity titre of wild-type RRV is virtually unaffected by incubation in cell growth medium at 50°C for 45 min. Under the same conditions, a mutant of RRV T48 with a deletion of seven amino acids (residues 55–61) in the E2 glycoprotein is thermolabile, showing a three log unit loss of infectivity.

Cryoelectron microscopy and image reconstruction have provided a detailed structural picture of RRV, the first for an alphavirus. The nucleocapsid (approximately 40 nm in diameter) possesses icosahedral symmetry with a triangulation number (T) of 4 and is surrounded by a lipid bilayer (4.8 nm thick). The core structure, at a radius below 17 nm, is composed of both the genomic RNA and the basic, N-terminal domain of the nucleocapsid protein. The surface of the virion is largely protein. There are 240 heterodimers of E1 and E2 assembled into 80 trimeric spikes on the surface. The E1 protein forms the core of the trimeric spike and E2 is found largely on the outer surface. The trimers separate immediately above the lipid bilayer to form a propeller-like, tripartite head; at the end of each heterodimer E1 and E2 appear to separate. Fab fragments from neutralizing monoclonal antibodies directed against E2 determinants bind to one tip of the heterodimer. The spike has a hollow base which may have a role in fusion mediated by an E1 homotrimer. The heterodimers form one-to-one associations with nucleocapsid monomers across the lipid bilayer; this contact is due to the association of the 'cytoplasmic domain' of E2 and the ordered, C-terminal domain of the nucleocapsid protein.

Properties of Genome

The prototype RRV (T48) genome is a single-stranded, positive-sense RNA molecule of 11 851 nucleotides excluding the poly(A) tail. The 5′ two-thirds of the RNA encodes the nonstructural proteins (NSPs); the 3′ one-third is expressed as a subgenomic (26S) mRNA which is transcribed from full length negative strands. In the genome, a 5′ noncoding region of 78 nucleotides is followed by an open reading frame (ORF) of 7440 nucleotides which is interrupted after 5586 nucleotides by a UGA termination codon. By analogy with Sindbis virus (SIN), the 5′ two-thirds of the genome encodes two polyproteins. One is NSP1-2-3 (1862 amino acids), and the second is produced by read-through of the 'leaky' UGA codon to generate NSP1-2-3-4. Four in-phase stop codons, three of which are in a region corresponding to the 5′ noncoding sequence of the 26S subgenomic RNA, ensure termination of NSP translation. The 3′ one-third of the genomic RNA has an ORF of 3762 nucleotides which encodes the polyprotein C-E3-E2-6K-E1. The length of the 3′ noncoding region can vary between isolates. For the prototype the length is 524 nucleotides; four closely related sequence blocks, 48–58 nucleotides in length, are found in the 3′ noncoding region of RRV (T48). Deletions, insertions, sequence rearrangements and single nucleotide substitutions are commonly observed in the 3′ noncoding region of different isolates of RRV.

The RRV genome has three regions which are strongly conserved between alphaviruses, including BFV. These are (1) a tract of 23 nucleotides next to the 3′ poly(A) tail; (2) 21 nucleotides at the 3′ terminus of the *NSP4* gene; and (3) 50 nucleotides near the 5′ end of the *NSP1* gene. The genome also contains a moderately conserved sequence element close to its 5′ end. All four sequence elements appear to have roles in the regulation of viral RNA replication. The 23 nucleotide tract is believed to be a promoter for negative strand synthesis; the complement of the 21 nucleotide element may be recognized, in the negative strand, by the 26S RNA transcriptase.

The prototype BFV (BH2193) genome is 11 488 nucleotides long, excluding the poly(A) tail. The 5′ and 3′ noncoding regions are 62 and 445 nucleotides in length respectively. The genome encodes an NSP of 2411 amino acids and a structural polyprotein of 1239 amino acids. The 3′ noncoding region has two unrelated sequence blocks of around 50 nucleotides which are each repeated once. One of these is unrelated to sequences in other sequenced alphaviruses; the other is closely similar to a repeat in the 3′ noncoding region of RRV and Getah RNAs. Thus recombination in the 3′ noncoding region of the RNA of common ancestor viruses may be part of the evolutionary history of these three alphaviruses. SIN, the fourth Australian alphavirus, shows no homology in its 3′ noncoding region with those of RRV/BFV/Getah.

Virus Proteins

Sequence data predict that for RRV, C, E3, E2, the '6K' protein and E1 are 270, 64, 422, 60 and 438 amino acid residues in length respectively, assuming no post-translational trimming. The RRV polyprotein is 75 and 48% homologous with the SFV and SIN polyproteins respectively. The capsid protein is highly basic in its N-terminal half, consistent with a role in interacting with genomic RNA. The N-terminal ten amino acids of E3 are hydrophobic and presumably form part of a signal sequence for the insertion of p61, the E2 precursor, into the host endoplasmic reticulum. Three neutralization epitopes on RRV E2, which together make up a significant antigenic site, have been mapped to residues 216 (epitope *a*), 232 and 234 (epitope *b1*) and 246, 248 and 251 (epitope *b2*). These epitopes are flanked in the primary sequence by asparagine-linked glycosylation sites at residues 200 and 262. This site is important in early virus-cell interactions and in virulence, as judged by biological studies on RRV mutants selected during epidemics (see below), selected during passage in cell culture or mice, or generated using infectious RNA derived from cDNA clones. The existence of a '6K' protein has not been reported in RRV-infected cells. The hemagglutinin, E1, has an uncharged tract (residues 80–96) which is highly conserved between alphaviruses and may be involved in fusion with cell membranes during virus entry. Comparative sequence data predict that the genomic RNA encodes two polyproteins (NSP1-2-3, the major species; NSP1-2-3-4, a minor species) which are processed to four NSPs of 533, 798, 531 and 611 residues respectively.

Sequence data predict that for BFV (BH2193), C, E3, E2, 6K and E1 are 253, 68, 421, 58 and 439 residues in length. For the NSPs the corresponding figures are 533, 798, 470 and 610. BFV E2 appears to be unique among alphavirus proteins in its relatively low observed molecular mass (43 kDa) and in the absence of N-linked glycosylation sites; the molecular mass of BFV E1, which has two glycosylation sites, is high (56 kDa) relative to other alphaviruses.

Replication and Virus Assembly

In cultured vertebrate cells RRV infection is cytopathic. The latent period is 3–5 h; maximum extracellular virus titers (10^8 Vero PFU ml^{-1}) and levels of viral RNA synthesis are at 8–10 h, at which time the shutdown of host cell protein synthesis is virtually complete. Virus-specific RNAs formed in BHK and Ae. albopictus cells include RF, RI, 45S, 26S and small amounts of 38S and 33S RNA (conformational variants of 45S and 26S RNAs respectively). Seven major virus-specific polypeptides are detected in vertebrate cells: p127, p95, p61 (E2 precursor), p52 (E1), p49 (E2), p32 (capsid protein) and E3. In Vero cells RRV is commonly found in small cytoplasmic vesicles; 'type 1 cytopathic vacuoles' are observed. There is a pronounced accumulation of nucleocapsids, particularly late in infection. In vertebrate cells BFV replication appears to involve analogous steps to those seen for RRV and other alphaviruses.

In cultured Ae. albopictus cells at 28°C RRV generates a non-cytopathic, persistent infection with peak titers (2×10^7 Vero PFU ml^{-1}) at 2–3 days. At 12 and 48 h after infection, 85 and 5% of cells respectively assay as 'infective centres'. Viral protein synthesis is sustained over the period 10–24 h after infection but is quantitatively less than in vertebrate cells; no p95 is observed. There is no shutdown of host protein synthesis, and cell division rate is unaffected by infection. Virus matures within large electron-dense, cytoplasmic inclusions and at the cell membrane. Free nucleocapsids are infrequent. When titers decrease during the later stages of infection, inclusions are transformed into microvesiculated vacuoles which may result from fusion with lysosomal vesicles.

Geographic and Seasonal Distribution

An extensive serological survey of neutralizing antibodies in humans has established that before 1979 RRV occurred only in Australia, the islands of New Guinea, New Britain and the Solomons, with activity in these islands decreasing from west to east. Chikungunya virus was the predominant alphavirus west and north of New Guinea through to south-east Asia. No alphavirus activity was detected in island groups further to the east. Unfortunately the pathogenicity of BFV was not appreciated at that time, and evidence for BFV activity outside Australia has not been sought.

RRV and epidemic polyarthritis occur in every state of Australia. Limited surveys in New Guinea indicate that activity is confined to the lowlands and deep valleys of the central mountain ranges. The south Pacific island epidemics which started in 1979 petered out early in 1981, and there is no evidence that the virus has become enzootic in the region.

RRV infection occurs throughout the year in tropical and subtropical northern regions of Australia, with the highest incidence during the wet season, December to April. In temperate southern regions outbreaks occur mainly in late summer and autumn. Major RRV epidemics occasionally occur in years of flood in the Murray-Darling basin and persist from spring through to the fall. The epidemics are particularly severe in irrigation districts. Frequent localized outbreaks occur in coastal regions of eastern and southern Australia, including Tasmania. Cases have occurred on the fringes of most major cities during periods of increased coastal activity. Brisbane and Perth have experienced infrequent but significant suburban outbreaks.

The prototype BFV strain was isolated from Cx annulirostris mosquitoes trapped in February 1974 at Barmah Forest on the Murray River, north-eastern Victoria. It was independently isolated from mosquitoes collected at about the same time near Charleville, southern Queensland. In 1975 it was isolated from Culicoides spp collected near Darwin in the Northern Territory. BFV continued to be isolated sporadically in the eastern States, both inland and in coastal regions, but it was not until 1989 that it was recorded in Western Australia (in the far north). BFV distribution appears to coincide with that of RRV at least in eastern and northern Australia. In Western Australia more than 85% of the population is concentrated in the coastal districts of the south-west corner of the state. In and to the south of Perth, RRV is endemic in the area, with an average of 154 cases annually. In the early spring and through the summer of 1992–1993 RRV appeared to be completely replaced by BFV; 18 BFV isolates were obtained from mosquito pools and there were 22 serologically confirmed BFV polyarthritis cases, the first indication of the virus in the region. The explanation for the apparent replacement of RRV by BFV during this episode is not known. No RRV was isolated from >70 000 mosquitoes tested during 1993, but since then, as in other States, both viruses have been active.

Host Range and Virus Propagation

In the primary cycle the vertebrate host range of RRV is effectively limited to placental and marsupial mammals. There is a lack of specificity in mosquito vector species; the virus has been recovered from 11 species encompassing five genera. Horses are commonly infected, sometimes resulting in lameness and constitutional or nervous disturbances of varying severity; RRV is suspected as a cause of equine death, but proof is lacking. No other domestic or native animal is known to show signs, but naturally acquired antibodies are found in most mammals, and virus has been recovered from macropods and from a horse. Antibodies are rarely found in birds, and, in the laboratory, viremia has been demonstrated only in recently-hatched chickens. It has been concluded that birds are not involved in the primary or amplification cycles for RRV. Viremia has been readily produced in a range of small and large adult marsupial species and in the small native rodent, *Pseudomys novaehollandiae*.

The host range of BFV is not known but limited serological investigations indicate that marsupials are more likely to be the primary hosts than are birds.

Newborn and weanling outbred mice have been the most commonly used experimental host. Many cell lines are susceptible to RRV and are used to prepare stocks, and in virus assay by plaque formation or induction of cytopathic effects. The C6/36 line of *Ae. albopictus* mosquito cells is the most sensitive available cell line, and is now the most common means of recovering RRV from patients and field material. Infection of mosquito cell monolayers cannot usually be visualized by cytopathic effect so they are commonly used together with immunofluorescent detection methods or in conjunction with Vero or BHK cells.

Genetics and Evolution

RRV genetic types and subtypes have been demonstrated from *Hae*III restriction digest profiles of cDNA to virion RNA and by sequencing genomic RNA. The examination of 14 isolates of RRV led to the identification of three genetic types with an estimated 1.5–5% nucleotide sequence divergence between types. RRV is not a bird virus and the relative immobility of mammalian hosts may allow the emergence of geographic variants adapted to local hosts. Based on pathogenicity for outbred infant mice there are a number of variants of RRV with degrees of mouse virulence. The prototype T48, from north Queensland, kills all infant mice in 5–6 days; a Nelson Bay (central coastal NSW) isolate kills 0–25% of infant mice in 10–12 days. There is no evidence for an association between a particular RRV genetic type and vector species.

Sequence studies on the genomes of RRV (T48) (genetic type I), and a strain from Nelson Bay (type III), showed 284 nucleotide differences, equivalent to 2.4% nucleotide sequence divergence. Most of the differences are 'silent'. There are 36 amino acid differences in the NSPs and 12 in the structural proteins, five of which are in E2. The distribution of these differences correlates with the location of nonconserved regions in the proteins of alphaviruses more generally.

Under conditions of natural selection in 'virgin soil' outbreaks the RRV genome is remarkably stable. During the first 10 months of the RRV epidemic in Pacific island communities (1979–1981), involving thousands of infections of humans, domestic animals and mosquitoes, changes in the E2 gene from the sequence seen in the earliest isolate obtained during the outbreak (the April 1979 Fijian strain) were confined to a single nucleotide which altered residue 219 (in the region of an antigenic site; see above). This mutation was first detected in a strain from an American Samoan patient infected in August 1979; there was no further change in the E2 gene in a strain from a Cook Islands patient infected in February 1980. No changes were observed in the 3′ noncoding region of the genome during the entire outbreak.

For BFV, the nucleotide sequence of the E2 gene from 12 isolates (1974–1995) differed by up to 1.7% in pairwise comparisons. The 3′ noncoding region can vary markedly between isolates, as is seen with RRV. BFV (BH2193) pathogenesis in infant mice is inconsistent even within a litter of day-old outbred mice; some will die within 24 h of peripheral inoculation, with high concentrations of virus generated in brain and muscle. Other mice will gradually develop signs and die 6–7 days after inoculation. No evidence has been obtained for differences in pathogenicity for infant mice between isolates.

In comparisons between the sequences of the BFV, RRV and SFV structural and nonstructural polyproteins, the percentage amino acid identity is relatively uniform along their lengths. There is therefore no evidence that BFV results from recombination between ancestral viruses in the coding region of the genome. Phylogenetic trees derived from sequence comparisons show that BFV, RRV and SFV arise from a separate evolutionary branch to that giving rise to SIN and the equine encephalitis viruses. RRV and SFV are more closely related to each other than either is to BFV.

Serological Relationships and Variability

RRV shares group- and genus-specific antigens with other alphaviruses. Based on antigenic relationships determined by hemagglutination inhibition (HAI), complement fixation tests and plaque reduction neutralization tests, RRV is in the SFV complex, and is a subtype of Getah virus. BFV shows little crossreaction in complement fixation tests or neutralization tests with RRV, SFV and other alphaviruses, although BFV is clearly related to RRV and SFV at the nucleotide and amino acid sequence levels.

Differences between the surface antigens of RRV geographic variants have been demonstrated with kinetic HAI and kinetic complement fixation tests. Homologous and heterologous virus/polyclonal antibody kinetic tests with RRV strains collected over a period of 13 years in north Queensland indicated antigenic identity. Similarly, strains collected over 3 years at Nelson Bay, NSW were antigenically identical by kinetic tests. However, heterologous kinetic tests between Queensland and Nelson Bay viruses and antibodies gave no crossreaction in HAI and significantly reduced crossreaction in complement fixation tests. The control crossreaction tests using standard incubation times suggested that all virus strains were antigenically identical.

Epidemiology

In Australia, the most important RRV vectors in coastal regions are brackish-water mosquitoes breeding in mangrove or melaleuca swamps. In these habitats *Ae. vigiliax* is the dominant vector in tropical and subtropical coastal regions, but in cooler southerly coastal regions such habitats are shared with or dominated by *Ae. camptorhynchus*. In the inland regions of Australia the major vector is the summer-breeding *Cx. annulirostris*. BFV has been isolated from a range of mosquito species similar to that for RRV in tropical and temperate ecosystems on the Australian mainland.

In Australia, RRV persists in a mammalian wildlife–mosquito primary cycle, probably augmented by a low-level transovarial cycle in *Aedes* mosquitoes. Year-round sporadic cases and the initiation of epidemics are presumably due to mosquitoes that have been infected in the primary cycle. It has now been demonstrated that there is a symptomless prelude of viremia prior to the onset of disease manifestations in Australian patients so that, as in the Pacific islands, a direct man–mosquito–man cycle can develop and accelerate into an epidemic.

Clinical Features and Infection

There are three major manifestations of RRV disease: rheumatic, rash and constitutional. Arthralgia usually develops very rapidly; the most common signs are pain on movement, tenderness and slight swelling. Wrists are most frequently involved, followed closely by knees, ankles and fingers. Elbows, toes and tarsal joints are also commonly affected. Pain is often more intense than indicated by observed signs. Rash occurs in about two-thirds of patients, but is rarely the sole manifestation of the disease. Most commonly it appears as erythematous macules and papules 1–5 mm across, distributed sparsely to thickly on trunk and limbs, and less frequently on face and scalp. Appearance on palms, soles and digital webs is characteristic, particularly when there is no rash elsewhere. Scattered purpura may be found, usually on the feet and lower legs. Except for hyperesthesia of the palms there is usually no discomfort due to the rash, and it resolves within 7–10 days. Pyrexia, one of the most common of the constitutional effects of other virus infections, is usually absent or slight. Myalgia is common, and carpal tunnel syndrome can be induced or exacerbated. Fatigue is the most consistently apparent constitutional effect and seems to be independent of other manifestations. Clinical signs and symptoms of RRV are rarely detected in infected prepubertal children but there is a normal antibody response.

Although diagnostic criteria of 'chronic fatigue syndrome' are difficult to define it seems that, in Australia, RRV infection might now be the most common precursor of the syndrome. In these cases fatigue is usually accompanied by persistent intermittent arthralgia. Such complications are uncommon in patients under the age of 30 years.

Although BFV causes disease in humans with a similar set of signs and symptoms to that caused by RRV, the possibility that BFV is responsible for milder symptoms than RRV has been suggested. Chronic fatigue has not been reported following BFV infections.

Pathogenicity

Differences in the pathogenicity of RRV strains involved in various outbreaks can be inferred from differences in the duration and severity of signs and symptoms, which can range from subclinical to a so-called chronic form. In reports of discrete epidemics there are differences in the incidence, severity and persistence of rash; in the presence or absence of muscle pain; in the average duration of incapacity; in the occurrence of relatively rare signs such as buccal and palatal enanthems; and in the correspondence of disease onset with viremia or antibody production.

By comparison with earlier unsuccessful attempts at virus isolation during outbreaks in Australia, virus isolation from humans was readily accomplished during the Pacific island outbreaks. In successfully isolating virus, investigators used mice, Vero or mosquito cell monolayers or *Toxorhynchites amboinensis* mosquitoes. Differences in the disease profile were also apparent. The incubation period (days from infection to onset of symptoms) was 2–3 days in the Pacific islands, compared with 9–11 days in Australia. The Pacific island patients were viremic for up to 7 days and HAI antibodies were usually detected by day 10; in some cases a brief remission of symptoms occurred after viremia, followed by relapse as antibodies developed. The onset of symptoms in Australian patients usually coincides with antibody production, so the level and duration of the symptomless viremia has not been determined.

Considering the apparent dearth of potential primary cycle mammals on these Pacific islands, it is probable that only an RRV strain which induces a relatively prolonged high level viremia in humans could sustain a 'virgin soil' epidemic for 2 years.

Studies on the molecular basis of RRV virulence for mice have demonstrated the involvement in virulence of a number of genetic determinants including E2, the NSPs and E1. The introduction of the E2 gene from the mouse-attenuated Nelson Bay RRV strain into a cDNA clone of RRV (T48) attenuates mouse virulence. Chimeric viruses have been constructed in which the 5' and 3' noncoding regions of the RRV and SIN genomes have been exchanged. Virus containing heterologous 5' noncoding regions show host-dependent defects in replication; exchange of the 3' noncoding regions gives rise to virus that grows surprisingly well.

Pathology and Histopathology

In the early stages of RRV infection in humans, cells in the synovial fluid and joint effusions are predominantly mononuclear and remarkable for the proportion of mitotic figures and highly vacuolated and phagocytic macrophages. In later effusions macrophages appear less activated and small lymphocytes predominate. RRV antigen has been detected by immunofluorescence on the surface of 20–30% of the larger cells in synovial fluid during the first few days after onset of symptoms, but attempts to isolate virus have failed. There is no erosion nor permanent damage to joints. In a minority of cases relapses occur over a year or more; these gradually decline in incidence and intensity.

The histology of the rash is variable. The dermis shows a chiefly perivascular mononuclear cell infiltrate, vasodilatation and varying degrees of edema. Diffuse to dense erythrocyte extravasation is quite common. Histologically detectable changes in the epidermis are present in about half the cases, although rarely recognized macroscopically. It is not clear whether rash is due to the direct action of virus or is the result of immunological processes.

Signs and symptoms of epidemic polyarthritis can be confused with those of rubella infection. There is no evidence that RRV is teratogenic, so, if termination is being considered in first trimester pregnant women, it is important to differentially diagnose cases of polyarthritis with rash.

The pathology and histopathology of BFV infection has not been explored.

Immune Response

The detection of RRV and BFV antibodies is now routinely performed by ELISA, although their first appearance can usually be detected several days earlier by standard alphavirus HAI tests. ELISA can also be used in antibody class capture assays to detect IgM, but precautions must be taken to avoid false positives due to the presence of rheumatoid factor, which is not causally present in epidemic polyarthritis. Specific IgM often persists for many months in RRV infection so is not a reliable indicator of recent infection; as with many other arbovirus infections, a rising titer of IgG antibodies from acute to convalescent stages is a more reliable diagnostic tool. Signs and symptoms can persist in the presence of antibodies. It is likely that infection bestows immunity to all genetic types of RRV.

In the laboratory, RRV titers in mice and in macrophage cultures are readily enhanced by low levels of specific antibody. Whether waning levels of antibody can exacerbate a second infection in humans is unknown but should be explored when considering the development of vaccines.

Prevention and Control

As with other zoonoses involving wildlife as vertebrate hosts, particularly those that are vectored by insects, there can be no prospect of eradicating RRV or BFV. A degree of control can be achieved by reducing the interaction of vectors and humans through education, and at the community level by carrying out mosquito abatement programmes appropriate to the district. At the personal level the avoidance of mosquito attack can be achieved by screening windows and doors, remaining indoors during periods of maximum vector mosquito activity, and by the use of efficient repellents.

Vaccination against a disease which is not life-threatening and is without permanent sequelae can only be administered on a request basis. RRV-infected children rarely express signs and symptoms, which, superficially, augurs well for the development of a live virus childhood vaccine. However, little is known about persistence or the nature of immunity after subclinical or frank RRV infection, nor whether the wide range of individual responses to infection, including long-term relapses, is related in any way to the prior immune status of the patient. Before developing candidate vaccines, prospective studies should be carried out to assess the duration of effective immunity following natural infection.

See also: **Chikungunya, O'nyong nyong and Mayaro viruses (*Togaviridae*); Epidemiology of viral diseases; Equine encephalitis viruses (*Togaviridae*); Immune response: General features, Cell mediated immune response; Pathogenesis: Animal viruses; Replication of viruses; Sindbis and Semliki Forest viruses (*Togaviridae*); Vectors: Animal viruses; Zoonoses.**

Further Reading

Faragher SG, Meek ADJ, Rice CM and Dalgarno L (1988) Genome sequences of a mouse-avirulent and a mouse-virulent strain of Ross River virus. *Virology* 163: 509.

Fraser JRE (1986) Epidemic polyarthritis and Ross River virus disease. *Clin. Rheum Dis* 12: 369.

Lee E, Stocks C, Lobigs P *et al* (1997) Nucleotide sequence of the Barmah Forest virus genome. *Virology* 227: 509.

Marshall ID and Miles JAR (1984) Ross River virus and epidemic polyarthritis. In: Harris KF (ed.) *Current Topics in Vector Research*, p. 31. New York: Praeger.

Strauss JH and Strauss EG (1994) The alphaviruses: gene expression, replication, and evolution. *Microbiol. Rev.* 58: 491.

ROTAVIRUSES (*REOVIRIDAE*)

Contents
General features
Molecular biology

General Features

Robert D Shaw, State University of New York at Stony Brook, Northport VA Medical Center, Northport, New York, USA

Harry B Greenberg, Division of Gastroenterology, Stanford University Medical School, Stanford, California, USA

Copyright © 1999 Academic Press

History

Diarrhea was long recognized worldwide as a leading cause of morbidity and mortality, but the search for important etiologic agents of human disease was not fruitful until the early 1970s. Rotavirus was known as a mouse diarrheal pathogen in the 1950s and as a simian and bovine pathogen in the 1960s, but it was not until 1972 that a virus was positively implicated as a cause of human gastroenteritis when Kapikian and coworkers used immune electron microscopy to identify Norwalk virus in diarrheal stools. The following year, investigators in several locations identified rotaviruses in intestinal biopsies and diarrheal stools of children. Rotaviruses are now identified as the leading cause of severe dehydrating gastroenteritis in infants and children. Efficient *in vitro* cultivation of many human rotavirus strains in the early 1980s, followed by the successful cloning of the rotavirus genome and expression of individual rotavirus proteins in recombinant systems, has provided a detailed knowledge of rotavirus structure and function, as well as many aspects of rotavirus serology, immunity and pathogenesis.

Classification

The family *Reoviridae* contains the *Rotavirus* genus and eight other genera. Rotaviruses share several common features that form the basis of the classification. Viral particles are approximately 102 nm in diameter (including surface spikes) and consist of two protein capsids surrounding a central protein core that contains the genome (designated as a 'triple-layered' particle). The extracellular icosahedral particles are not enveloped by a lipid membrane. Ten monocistronic and one bicistronic genomic segments form the organization of double-stranded RNA. The negatively stained electron microscopic appearance of the complete rotavirus particle is responsible for the name *rotavirus*, which derives from the Latin word *rota*, meaning wheel. The outer capsid appears as a sharply defined rim, to which spokes appear to radiate from a large central hub. Recent advance in cryo-electron microscopy with computer-enhanced reconstructed images has provided a more detailed view of rotavirus structure (**Fig. 1**). Notable features include the presence of spikes on the outer capsid that extend over 10 nm and pores that penetrate from the virion surface into the viral genome. These channels may permit importation of metabolites required for viral RNA transcription and export of the nascent RNA transcripts for subsequent viral replication processes.

Geographic and Seasonal Distribution

Rotaviruses are ubiquitous among humans and many animal species throughout the world, and are usually important causes of gastroenteritis wherever they occur. Human rotavirus illness predominantly occurs in the cooler months in developed countries, peaking in January and February, while it is an unusual cause of gastroenteritis in the summer months. Rotavirus infections in the USA occur in a wave, starting in the Southwest in November and spreading on to New England and the Canadian Maritime provinces in March. This seasonality does not occur in tropical climates (10° latitude from the equator) where rotavirus infections occur throughout the year.

Host Range and Virus Propagation

Rotaviruses are recovered from diarrheal stools shed by a multitude of animal species. As an indication of the breadth of the host range of group A rotaviruses, infection in species other than human occurs in simian, equine, porcine, canine, feline, lapine, murine, bovine, ovine and avian, although rotavirus is not an important cause of disease in all of these species. Among laboratory animals, group A rotaviruses do not infect guinea pigs or rats, although group B rotaviruses infect the latter. Animal strains, even those with serotypes indistinguishable from human strains, rarely infect humans. Recently, a few human rotavirus isolates have been described that are probably derived from feline, canine, bovine or porcine rotaviruses. The potential of animal rotavirus reservoirs as a source of genetic diversity for the evolution of new human strains is unknown.

Rotaviruses were first propagated *in vitro* in 1963, when Mahlerbe and coworkers reported the isolation of simian SA11 from a vervet monkey kidney cell culture. Cultivation of human rotaviruses was not successful until the discovery that trypsin exposure, which cleaves amino acid bonds at three closely spaced sites of the VP4 protein, dramatically enhances virus infectivity in culture. Group B and C viruses are not generally cultivatable, with the exception of several porcine and bovine group C strains. Group A rotaviruses are usually cultivatable in simian kidney cell lines in the presence of trypsin. The most efficiently cultured animal rotaviruses typically yield 10^7–$10^{8.5}$ plaque-forming units (PFU) per milliliter in tissue culture systems. Human viruses tend to produce one to two orders of magnitude fewer PFU in tissue culture, although they are often shed in diarrheic stools in quantities of 10^9–10^{10} particles per milliliter.

Genetics

The double-stranded RNA (dsRNA) segments of the rotavirus genome have masses between 2×10^5 and 2.2×10^6 Da. The genes distribute by size into four classes that produce a characteristic pattern (the 'electropherotype') when separated by polyacrylamide gel electrophoresis. Electropherotype classification of rotaviruses was particularly important before *in vitro* cultivation of human rotaviruses. The wide variability of electropherotypes and the observation that serotypes and electropherotypes do not correlate well has decreased the importance of this technique in classification. However, some epidemiologic studies continue to use electropherotypes for detection and characterization of rotavirus, and it is still a useful technique for detection of non-group A rotaviruses.

Rotavirus RNA lacks 3′-terminal polyadenylated sequences and contains 5′-capped structures. Both ends of each segment contain short highly conserved regions of approximately eight nucleotides. These highly conserved sequences may be of importance in transcription, replication and assortment of the virus genome. These features are also characteristic of other *Reoviridae*.

The RNA itself is not infectious; rotaviruses contain within the double-layered particle an endogenous RNA-dependent RNA polymerase that tran-

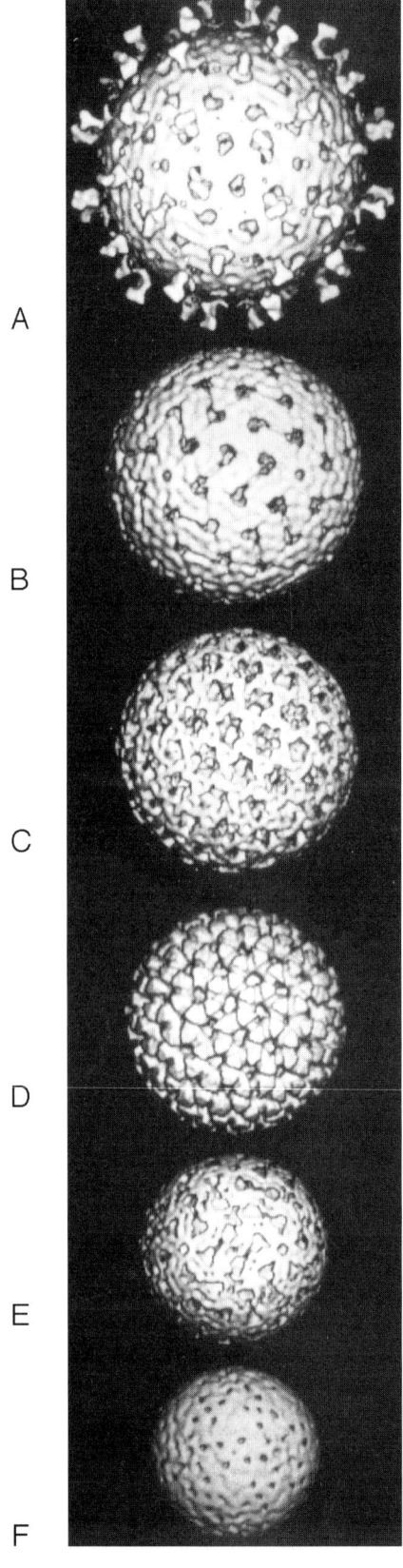

scribes the gene segments into mRNA. Transcripts are full-length positive strands from which negative-strand synthesis occurs following the formation of replicase particles in the cytoplasm. RNA transcripts can be identified 3 h postinfection. The proteins and structural requirements of RNA replication are not fully understood. Reassortment of gene segments occurs at high frequency during mixed infection with two or more rotavirus strains, although, unlike influenza, there is no evidence that this is a mechanism for generation of serotypic diversity in nature.

Gene-coding assignments for group A rotavirus genes have been clearly established as follows. Genes 5, 7, 8, 10 and 11 code for nonstructural proteins, which were originally designated by the prefix 'NS' followed by the molecular mass, but are presently known as 'NSP' 1–5. The gene product of genes 5 (nonstructural protein NSP1) seems to have a role in the early stages of virus assembly. The gene 7 product (NSP3) has been detected in infected cells in association with complexes containing replicase activity and has specific RNA-binding function, but little else is known. The gene 8 product (NSP2) is associated with replicase activity but has a poorly defined function. NSP4, coded by gene segment 10, is a membrane-associated glycoprotein which plays an important role in viral assembly, in which the protein serves as a receptor for VP6 in the endoplasmic reticulum. In addition, NSP4 has been implicated in diarrheal pathogenesis (see below). NSP5, coded by gene segment 11 is a phosphoprotein of unknown function coded by gene segment 11. Genes 1–4, 6 and 9 code for structural proteins VP1–4, 6 and 7, respectively (in most group A viruses). VP4 and VP7 are the two

Figure 1 Three-dimensional structure of rhesus rotavirus by cryoelectron microscopy and icosahedral image reconstructure (Yeager et al (1990) J. Cell Biol. 110: 2133). The surface-shaped representations were obtained by truncating the three-dimensional maps with spherical envelopes to reveal the internal structure. The six structures from top to bottom with their corresponding diameters (in parenthesis) are as follows: (**A**) The virion outer capsid surface displays 60 spikes attributed to the VP4 hemagglutinin (102 nm). (**B**) The smoothly-rippled outer capsid surface attributed primarily to VP7, is perforated by 132 aqueous holes (79 nm). (**C**) The space between the outer and inner capsids forms an open aqueous network that may provide pathways for the diffusion of ions and small regulatory molecules as well as the extrusion of RNA (72 nm). (**D**) The inner capsid has a 'bristled' outer surface composed of 260 trimeric columns, attributed to VP6 trimers (66 nm). (**E**) The VP6 trimers merge with a smooth, inner capsid shell which is perforated by holes in register with those in the outer capsid (58 nm). (**F**) A third protein shell (referred to as the 'core') is thought to be formed by VP1, VP2 and VP3 and encapsidates the dsRNA segmented genome (53 nm).

surface proteins of the virion while VP6 is the major constituent of the double-layered particle.

The electropherotypes of non-group A rotaviruses differ from group A viruses primarily in gene segments 7, 8 and 9. The organization of the non-group A 7–9 genome segments lacks the tight triplet formation in polyacrylamide gel electrophoresis that characterizes the group A electropherotype. Non-group A rotaviruses are morphologically identical to group A strains but they are antigenically distinct and they do not crosshybridize in Northern blot analyses, even under conditions of low stringency. There appear to be at least five (B–F) non-group A rotavirus types. Groups B and C have been identified in humans as well as in animals. Sequence data are now available for several non-group A rotaviruses and this has allowed some gene coding assignments to be made. The development of serologic reagents from expressed viral proteins will extend the understanding of the epidemiology and importance of non-group A viruses.

Evolution

Little is known about the evolution of rotaviruses. While strong similarities in genomic sequences exist among some human and animal strains, there remains little evidence as to the origin of any particular strain. High rates of mutation exist in RNA genomes, and the capacity of the segmented genome to reassort during mixed infections provides theoretical opportunities for rotaviruses to mutate and evolve rapidly. However, during multiple passages in cell culture without the presence of obvious selection pressure, rotaviruses do not appear to change appreciably.

Serologic Relationships and Variability

Six of the viral proteins are structural, but only three have played important roles in the classification of group A rotaviruses by virtue of antigenic or functional properties. Non-group A rotaviruses have not been widely cultivated *in vitro* and far less is presently known about the structure and serologic classification of these viruses. VP6, the major structural protein of the group A secondary capsid, bears most of the common group antigens as well as the subgroup antigens. Rotaviruses that cause most human disease are classified as group A strains but occasionally group B and C also infect humans (see below, Epidemiology). Animal viruses have been classified into groups A–F. Human and animal group A rotaviruses are subdivided into subgroups (I and II) on the basis of serologic reactivity with subgroup-specific monoclonal antibodies directed at VP6. All group A rotaviruses share antigenic determinants on VP6, and some shared epitopes appear to be present on group C rotaviruses as well.

The glycoprotein VP7, the major neutralization protein of the outer capsid constituting 20% of the viral mass, induces serotype-specific neutralizing antibodies. VP4 is the other outer capsid protein, which is only 2% of the viral mass. It is the viral hemagglutinin, an important determinant of virulence, and is the cell attachment protein. VP4 is also responsible for inducing neutralizing antibodies. The contribution of VP4-specific neutralizing antibodies seems to be less important than VP7-specific neutralizing antibodies in hyperimmune sera used in determination of viral serotypes, but evidence delineating the relative roles of these antibodies in natural infections and following vaccination in many species is conflicting. A combined role of VP7- and VP4-specific immunity in the serologic classification of rotaviruses (such as the influenza binary system using hemagglutinin and neuraminidase antigens) has been adopted. In this system the VP7 serotype is classified as a G (glycoprotein) type and the VP4 type as a P (protease) type.

At least 14 group A G types have been identified, 10 of which have been isolated from humans (G1–4 are the major human pathogens worldwide; 8, 9 and 12 have been occasionally recovered from humans; and porcine G5 and bovine G6 and 10 have been recovered from children with diarrhea). Initially, serotyping required tissue culture growth of the viruses in the presence of defined serotype-specific sera, but serotype-specific monoclonal antibodies as well as serotype-specific nucleic acid probes are now readily available and have dramatically reduced the time and expense of the serotyping procedure. A total of 18 P types have been defined by amino acid sequence homologies, including seven in humans (P4, 6, 8, 9, 10, 11 and HCR3). The number of serotypes is steadily increasing as larger numbers of isolates are tested. In some studies, 70–80% of human isolates are either G1P8 or G2P4. Although it is assumed that the serotype classification of rotavirus strains is important in determining immunity to these viruses, the relationship of serotype to protective immunity is not entirely clear. For instance, VP6, the subgroup determinant, has recently been shown to elicit antibodies that mediate intracellular viral neutralization. A VP6 DNA vaccine has also resulted in protection from infection in a murine model, and particles containing only VP2 and VP6 have induced protective immunity in mice and rabbits.

Epidemiology

Group A rotaviruses are the principal cause of severe gastroenteritis in infants and young children throughout the world, accounting for 12–71% (median 34%) of all diarrheal episodes requiring hospitalization in children under the age of 2 years. In developing countries, the annual toll includes roughly 18 million cases of severe diarrhea and nearly a million deaths. In the USA, over 60 000 children are hospitalized, and about 50 deaths are annually attributed to rotavirus infection.

Infants in the first 2–3 months of life seem to be relatively protected from severe rotavirus disease, probably because of residual maternal immunity mediated by transplacental antibodies. Severe disease is most common among children of 6 months to 2 years of age. Rotavirus infections occur beyond 3 years of age and into adult life but they are typically mild or asymptomatic. However, group A rotavirus may occasionally cause severe diarrhea in immunologically competent adults. Epidemics are known to occur in institutional settings, especially among the elderly in nursing homes, and occasional cases may be fatal.

The epidemiology of rotavirus infections and viral shedding can be monitored by serologic assays or by electrophoretic patterns of viral RNA (electropherotype) obtained from fecal specimens. Electropherotype studies have demonstrated that several genomic patterns may coexist within a community, but these patterns do not necessarily correlate with serotypic classifications. Several serotypes may also coexist within a community, but each season is usually dominated by a single serotype that may vary from year to year. Group A serotypes G1–4 cause most human disease and appear to be equally virulent. These serotypes have been identified in developed and underdeveloped settings and have been in circulation for at least 30 years.

Transmission and Tissue Tropism

Rotaviruses are transmitted by the fecal–oral route, as has been conclusively demonstrated by transmission of illness in human volunteers by oral inoculation of fecal filtrates. Transmission by the respiratory route has been considered but the evidence to support this route is weak. Rapid appearance of antibodies to rotaviruses is noted by 3 years of age in all areas of the world regardless of hygiene. Viral shedding is not always associated with symptoms, and asymptomatic infection occurs frequently in newborn nurseries and daycare centers. The virus is quite stable on environmental surfaces for prolonged periods. These factors complicate efforts to control hospital outbreaks, which are not always successful even if patients are carefully monitored for virus excretion and appropriate control measures are followed.

Rotaviruses replicate within and are primarily shed from mature small intestine epithelial cells located at the villous tips. Recent evidence of rotavirus infection of the liver in a small number of immunocompromised children has demonstrated that infection of other tissues is possible in some rare cases.

Pathogenicity

The genetic correlates of rotavirus pathogenicity have not yet been completely determined. Host range restrictions limit crossinfection between species in most cases. Animal strains have been used as human vaccine candidates as they possess antigenic similarity with human viruses but do not cause disease, except when given in very large doses. Animal rotavirus vaccine candidates appear to replicate in humans at a low level and stimulate local and systemic immunity. All serotypes of rotavirus seem to be equally virulent, although some neonatal strains have been associated with asymptomatic infection. Other studies, however, have indicated that it is the newborn host rather than the rotavirus strain that determines the avirulent phenotype in the newborn.

Clinical Features of Infection

Rotavirus gastroenteritis is seen most commonly in children between the ages of 3 months and 2 years. Asymptomatic infection is common in infants less than 2 months old or individuals older than 2 years, although episodic severe disease in adults may result from group A rotavirus infection. Group B rotavirus infection causes epidemics in older children and adults in China.

In some animal species, illness is strictly limited to the very young. Age-related restriction of rotavirus illness appears to be due, at least in part, to nonimmune mechanisms. The incubation period in humans and most animals appears to be 24–72 h. Malnutrition may increase the severity of the symptoms. In addition to the symptoms listed in **Table 1,** those related to severe volume depletion, such as lethargy, irritability, confusion, and eventually vascular collapse and death, can be seen.

Pathology and Histopathology

The pathologic lesion resulting from rotavirus infection varies somewhat depending on the species and age in question. For instance, porcine rotavirus causes a particularly large amount of cellular damage, whereas murine infection may be characterized by much more selective destruction. Infection of the very young of most species will characteristically produce more cell destruction than infection in adults. Blunt-

Table 1 Clinical features of rotavirus gastroenteritis

Symptom	Frequency (%)
Diarrhea	98
Diarrhea >10 times daily	28
Vomiting	87
Vomiting >5 times daily	51
Fever	84
Abdominal pain	18
Blood in stool	1
Hospitalization	39

Adapted from Uhnoo et al (1986) Arch. Dis. Child. 61: 732–738. British Medical Association, Tavistock Square, London, WC1H 9JR, with permission.

ing of intestinal villi and vacuolation of enterocytes may be seen within hours after infection, prior to the presence of detectable viral antigen. Also seen are mononuclear cell infiltration of the lamina propria, distended endoplasmic reticulum, mitochondrial swelling and denuded microvilli. Viral particles may be seen within columnar epithelial cells, goblet cells, phagocytic cells and M cells in the small intestinal mucosa (the colon is generally spared). Production of viral antigen in the intestine peaks around 48–72 h postinfection in most species. Large amounts of viral proteins accumulate in the cytoplasm (viroplasm), which may appear swollen and vacuolated. However, some damaged cells may be seen without detectable viral antigen present. Intestinal cellular morphology returns to normal in about 7 days, although much of the damage is repaired as quickly as 3 days after infection.

The mechanism of virus-induced diarrhea is not clear. Lytic infection is not prominent in intestinal cell lines, nor is the histologic damage in the host clearly related to diarrhea. Toxin-like effects have been suggested, as exogenous administration of the rotavirus NSP4 protein has been reported to induce diarrhea in mice, and inactivated rotaviruses that do not cause tissue damage have also been demonstrated to cause diarrhea in mice. NSP4 has been reported to stimulate chloride secretion, but the role of this effect in disease is as yet unclear. Water absorption by the small intestine is impaired, but can be corrected by the administration of glucose–salt solutions. Abnormal motility may contribute to rotavirus-induced diarrhea. Also, carbohydrate malabsorption and secondary osmotic diarrhea may occur. An integrated understanding of the roles of these many factors in the pathogenesis of diarrhea has not yet been achieved.

Group B and C rotaviruses also cause small intestinal lesions in several animal species as well as in humans. Villous blunting is seen in various small intestinal regions. Syncytia including up to 20 enterocytes are seen during group B infection, a finding not observed in group A infections.

Immune Response

The antibody-based immune response to rotavirus infection has been studied in many animals as well as in humans. Serum and mucosal antibodies are detected, beginning several days after primary infection. Cytotoxic T cells have been identified in the intestinal mucosa of mice undergoing experimental rotavirus infection. The rapid resolution of rotavirus diarrhea during an acute infection occurs somewhat before the immune response is fully developed, so at least some of the factors responsible for resolution of the illness may be nonimmune. Immune factors are most likely to have substantial roles in the prevention of subsequent infections, although it is still unclear precisely which factors determine susceptibility to rotavirus infection.

Genetic studies using specific viral reassortants and passive transfer studies using monoclonal antibodies directed at specific rotavirus proteins have demonstrated that antibodies directed at either VP4 or VP7 (but not other rotavirus proteins) can neutralize virus and protect susceptible hosts. However, the bulk of antibodies elicited by rotavirus infection are directed at the major structural protein of the inner capsid VP6 (which constitutes 51% of the viral mass). While antibodies to VP6 may not neutralize virus in the intestinal lumen or in tissue cultures, VP6-specific IgA antibodies may prevent viral replication intracellularly during the process of transcytosis through intestinal epithelial cells. Protective efficacy against infection of IgG antibodies raised in mice following systemic vaccination (including adjuvant) with recombinant proteins assembled into virus-like particles has also been recently shown, despite the absence in the particle of VP4 or VP7. In addition, murine protection appears to be conferred by DNA vaccination with the gene that codes for VP6. Thus, several mechanisms and antigens appear to be capable of mediating protection from infection in animal models. The utility of these mechanisms in vaccine strategies or their role in response to natural infection remains to be determined.

The locations of the amino acid-defined regions of VP4 and VP7 that elicit neutralizing antibodies have been mapped. One large and complex conformationally determined neutralization domain exists on VP7, and at least two domains are found on VP4 (one on each of the two fragments resulting from trypsin cleavage of VP4, which are referred to as VP5* and VP8*). Most neutralizing antibodies elicited by VP7 are serotype-specific, although at least one epitope is heterotypic and binds antibodies that are broadly crossreactive. VP4 serotypic diversity is still not well understood. There are at least two important neutralization regions on VP4, one on either side of the site of trypsin cleavage (cleavage of this site enhances growth in tissue culture; see above, Host Range and Virus Propagation). The N-terminal fragment, VP8*, contains neutralization sites that are limited to particular strains. The C-terminal fragment VP5* has a domain that is crossreactive among several human strains, and a similarly crossreactive region is shared among several animal strains.

Primary rotavirus infection induces neutralizing antibodies to VP7 and VP4. There is conflicting evidence, in various animal models and in humans, concerning the relative importance of these two groups of antibodies in the establishment of protection against subsequent infections. Prevailing opinion at the present time could be simplified to state that a primary human infection results in predominantly serotype-specific immunity, although heterotypic immunity is frequently detected at lower levels. Individuals gradually establish broader immunity with reinfections, although whether this is due to accumulated diversity of homotypic responses to serial VP7 exposures or a gradual increase in the immune response to the major heterotypic regions on VP4 or VP7, or even VP6, remains unknown.

The complexities of the intestinal immune environment have impaired the development of a complete understanding of the immune response to rotavirus infection and vaccination. The immunological environment of the intestinal mucosa is relatively difficult to monitor, either by serum or intestinal fluid measurements. Animal studies have confirmed that most of the specific antirotavirus antibodies generated in response to infection are IgA, which is secreted predominantly by lymphocytes in the small intestinal lamina propria. It has long been inferred from animal studies that replication of the virus in the intestinal tract was a prerequisite for the development of substantial local immunity. While infectious rotavirus administered directly into the intestinal tract has been demonstrated to be a powerful mucosal antigenic stimulus to specific antibody formation, it is not yet clear that replication is vital; or, if it is, the mechanism by which replication enhances the response is not determined. Furthermore, rotavirus-specific cytotoxic lymphocytes have been identified in the intestinal mucosa following parenteral administration of killed rotavirus. In immunodeficient murine model studies, passive transfer of immune cytotoxic T cells has been shown to prevent acute rotavirus infection and resolve ongoing rotavirus infection.

The mechanisms of rotavirus antigen processing and presentation in the mucosal immune compartment are largely unexplored. Rotaviruses, like many other particulate antigens, including reoviruses, are known to bind to and be internalized by M cells overlying intestinal lymphoid aggregates, at least in a porcine model. The importance of this route of contact with immune cells, as opposed to penetration of virus directly into the lamina propria or presentation of viral antigens by major histocompatibility complex (MHC) class I- or II-bearing enterocytes, is unknown.

Prevention and Control of Rotavirus

Two avenues leading to prevention and control of rotavirus disease are vaccination and oral rehydration therapy. Treatment with oral rehydration solutions containing glucose and electrolytes is highly effective for ameliorating the consequences of rotavirus infection, but there are serious logistical, cultural and educational difficulties limiting the distribution of this treatment resource into underdeveloped areas. Recent evaluations of this approach in the USA suggest that it is underutilized even in a developed setting.

Breast feeding has been advocated as an inexpensive and effective means of rotavirus disease suppression, as breast milk is effective in the reduction of morbidity and mortality caused by bacterial gastroenteritis. However, despite the presence of antirotavirus antibodies in breast milk, there is little evidence that breast feeding can protect against rotavirus infection or serious rotavirus disease.

Vaccination strategies that have been tested have utilized the host range restrictions of animal rotaviruses in a 'Jennerian' approach to disease prevention. For example, simian and bovine rotaviruses have been used as naturally attenuated vaccine strains in children. Field trials demonstrated these vaccines to be safe and immunogenic, and efficacy against severe disease was high in developed countries. Efficacy in underdeveloped countries has been more difficult to demonstrate, although at least one large study showed substantial efficacy. Animal rotaviruses have induced both homotypic and heterotypic protection in some studies, but in other circumstances these vaccines have failed to protect in both developed and less-developed settings. Overall, these findings have been considered encouraging by most authorities, and live attenuated 'Jennerian' vaccines with significant protection against severe disease may soon be commercially available. However, further investigation may reveal an optimal vaccine strategy that will routinely provide reproducible protective efficacy in all parts of the world.

Future Perspectives

Vaccine strategies currently under consideration are varied. Both nonpathogenic neonatal rotavirus strains and multivalent collections of reassortant rotaviruses that contain human gene 4 segments are presently undergoing intensive testing. One example of the latter has now been approved by the FDA for use in the USA. Vaccines made from synthetic viral proteins or particles administered systemically or enterally are planned or under investigation, but the ability of these constructs to stimulate protective immunity in humans is unknown.

A better understanding of the mechanisms of viral antigen processing and presentation, the determinants of the magnitude and specificity of the antibody and cytotoxic T cell responses and a more precise determination of the mechanisms of naturally-occurring protective immunity may permit a more efficient and effective design for synthetic vaccine products that will elicit sufficiently broad protective immunity.

See also: **Enteric viruses; Norwalk and related viruses (*Caliciviridae*); Pathogenesis: Animal viruses, Plant viruses; Rotaviruses (*Reoviridae*): Molecular biology; Vaccines and immune response.**

Further Reading

Ball JM, Tian P, Zeng CQ, Morris AP and Estes MK (1996) Age-dependent diarrhea induced by a rotaviral nonstructural glycoprotein [see comments]. *Science* 272 (5258): 101.

Blacklow N and Greenberg H (1991) Viral gastroenteritis. *N. Engl. J. Med.* 325: 252.

Burke B and Desselberger U (1996) Rotavirus pathogenicity. *Virology* 218: 299.

Iqbal N and Shaw R (1997) Rotaviruses. In: D. Richman, R. Whitley and F. Hayden (eds) *Clinical Virology*, p. 765. New York: Churchill Livingstone.

Midthun K and Kapikian AZ (1996) Rotavirus vaccines: an overview. *Clin. Microbiol. Rev.* 9: 423.

Offit PA (1996) Host factors associated with protection against rotavirus disease: the skies are clearing. *J. Infect. Dis.* 174: S59.

Patton JT (1994) Rotavirus replication. [Review]. *Curr. Top. Microbiol. Immunol.* 185: 107.

Perez-Schael I, Guntinas MJ, Perez M *et al* (1997) Efficacy of the rhesus rotavirus-based quadrivalent vaccine in infants and young children in Venezuela [see comments]. *N. Engl. J. Med.* 337: 1181.

Ramig RF (1997) Genetics of the rotaviruses. *Annu. Rev. Microbiol.* 51: 225.

Molecular Biology

Mary K Estes, Division of Molecular Virology, Baylor College of Medicine, Houston, USA

Copyright © 1999 Academic Press

Properties of the Virion

Rotaviruses are members of the *Reoviridae* and are characterized by a genome of double-stranded (ds) RNA and a nonenveloped icosahedral structure (**Figure 1** also see Plate 31 for color). The rotaviruses were named (from the Latin *rota*, meaning wheel) based on the distinctive morphologic appearance of particles visualized by negative-stain electron microscopy. Virus particles resemble a wheel, with short spokes and a well-defined rim. The virion contains six structural proteins (VP1, VP2, VP3, VP4, VP6 and VP7) that make up a triple-layered protein shell. In the interior of particles, the genomic dsRNA is highly ordered, with about 25% of the genome making up a dodecahedral structure (**Figure 2**). Surrounding the genome is the innermost shell that is composed of VP2. VP2 shells also are called single-layered particles, and two internal proteins, VP1 and VP3, interact with the inner surface of VP2 at the fivefold axes where they are visualized as flower-shaped structures in three-dimensional reconstructions of virus-like particles containing proteins 1/2/3/6. VP1 is the viral transcriptase and VP3 is the guanylyltransferase. The addition of VP6 to single-layered particles results in structures called double-layered particles. These particles possess an active transcriptase activity and mRNAs are extruded from particles at the fivefold axes. The outer protein shell has a rippled surface composed of trimers of a glycoprotein, VP7; dimeric spikes composed of VP4 emanate through the VP7 surface and the base of the VP4 spikes interacts with the inner capsid protein VP6.

Three-dimensional reconstructions of rotavirus particles using images of particles embedded in vitreous ice have provided the most detailed description of particle structure (**Figures 1** and **2** see Plates 31 and 32 for color). The outer shell has a diameter of 76.5 nm, the second shell is 70.5 nm and the inner core shell is 50 nm in diameter. The two outer icosahedral layers have a $T = 13\, l$ symmetry, and the inner shell is composed of 120 molecules of VP2 arranged with a $T = 1$ symmetry. The most distinctive feature of the outer shell is the presence of 60 spikes, at least 10 nm

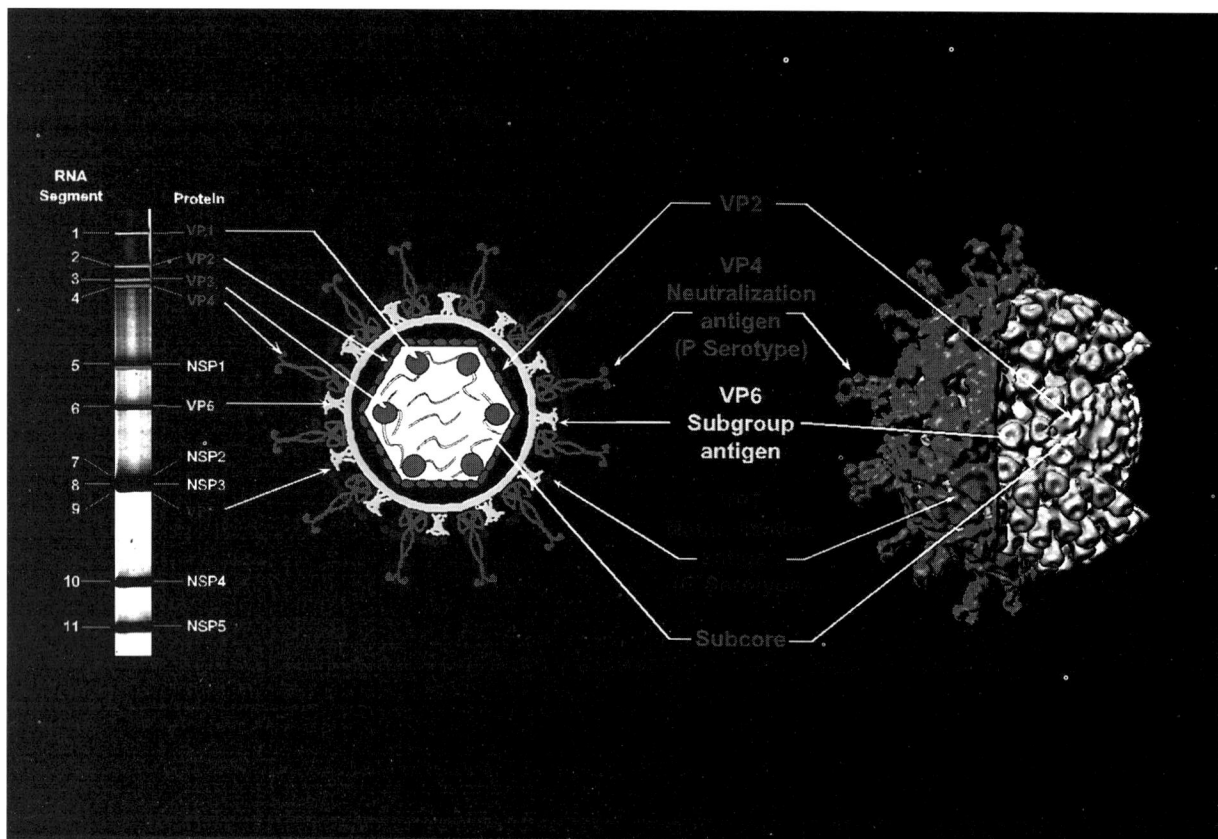

Figure 1 Rotavirus genes, proteins and structure. The left panel shows the RNA segments and the gene coding assignments for the simian rotavirus SA11. See **Table 1** for details on the genes and proteins. The location of the viral structural proteins in the different shells of the virus particles is shown in the schematic in the center. The major structural proteins that make up the outer shell of particles (VP4 and VP7), the intermediate shell (VP6), the inner shell (VP2) and the subcore region composed of ordered viral RNA are illustrated in the ~25 Å three-dimensional structure of particles shown in the right panel. (This reconstruction was kindly provided by B.V.V. Prasad.) (**For color references see Color Plate 28.**)

(100 Å) in length, that extend from the surface of particles. These spikes are made up of dimers of VP4, the protein product of genome segment 4. The spikes are situated at the edge of a subset of three types of 132 channels that lead from the viral surface to the center of the virion. The channels are involved in importing the metabolites for RNA transcription and exporting nascent RNA transcripts for subsequent virus replication processes. The channels at the fivefold axes are the conduits for the export of mRNA that first interacts with the enzyme complexes at the inner surface of these axes. Cleavage of VP4 is associated with enhanced viral infectivity. This proteolytic cleavage results in the appearance of two products, VP5* and VP8*, that both remain associated with virions. Cleavage of VP4 is thought to be important in viral penetration into cells. The VP6 shell has a bristle-like structure composed of trimers of VP6. These trimers have a central indentation and 132 channels lie in register with the channels in the outer capsid.

Properties of the Genome

The sequences of the genome of several rotaviruses (the simian rotavirus SA11, bovine rotavirus RF, and human rotavirus K8 strains) have been determined completely. The following summary of information about the genome is based on data known primarily for the group A rotaviruses, of which SA11 is the prototype strain. The viral genome consists of 11 RNA segments that range in size from 667 (segment 11) to 3302 (segment 1) base pairs, with the total genome containing 18 556 base pairs (**Table 1**). The RNA segments are thought to be encapsidated in association with protein molecules. Each RNA segment encodes one protein, with the exception of gene 11 which codes for two proteins.

Each genomic RNA segment contains a methylated cap 5′ sequence $m^7GpppG^{(m)}GPy$ followed by a 5′ nontranslated sequence, an open reading frame coding for the protein product, another set of noncoding sequences, and ending with a 3′-terminal

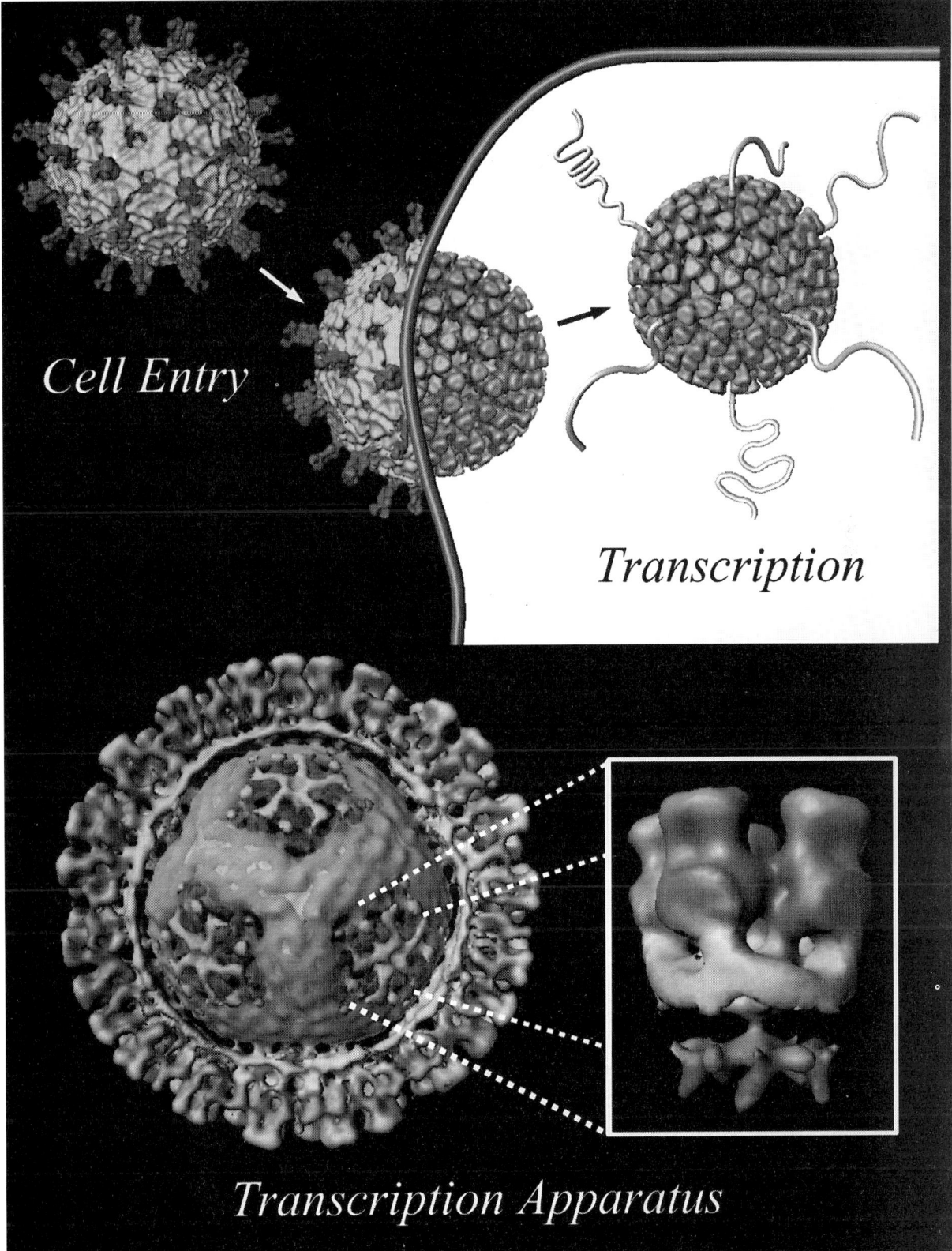

Figure 2 Rotavirus transcription. The top panel illustrates the early changes in rotavirus structure that lead to transcription and release of the mRNA molecules from the double-layered particles. The bottom panel shows the internal structure of rotavirus double-layered particles that are surrounded by trimers of the intermediate shell protein VP6 (blue). The double-stranded RNA genome is organized as a dodecahedral shell inside the particles and the minor internal proteins VP1 and VP3 are organized in a flower-shaped structure at the fivefold axes. The right-hand insert shows a side view of this structure highlighting VP6 (blue), VP2 (green) and the complex of VP1 and VP3 (orange). The newly made transcripts are extruded from these complexes at the fivefold axes (see top panel). (Figure kindly provided by J. Lawton.) (**For color references see Color Plate 29.**)

Table 1 Rotavirus genome RNA segments and protein products[a]

Segment	Number of base pairs	Number of noncoding sequences[b] 5'	Number of noncoding sequences[b] 3'	Protein product[c]	Nascent polypeptide mol.wt (no. of amino acids)[d]	Mature protein modified	No. molecules per virion[e]	ts mutant group[f]	Remarks
1	3302	18	17	VP1	125 005 (1088)		12	C	Core protein, slightly basic, polymerase
2	2690	16	28	VP2	102 431 (880)	Cleaved	120	F	Single-layered particle RNA binding, leucine zipper
3	2591	49	34	VP3	98 120 (835)		12	B	Core protein, basic, guanylyltransferase
4	2362	9	22	VP4	86 782 (776)	Cleaved VP5*(529)[g] VP8*(247)[g]	120	A	Surface spike protein, dimer, hemagglutinin, protease-enhanced infectivity, neutralization antigen, cell attachment protein, virulence, putative fusion region
5	1611	30	93	NSP1	58 654 (491)			NA	Slightly basic, zinc fingers
6	1356	23	139	VP6	44 816 (397)	Myristilated	780	G	Inner capsid protein, trimer, hydrophobic subgroup antigen
7	1104	25	131	NSP3	34 600 (315)			NA	Slightly acidic, RNA binding, oligomer
8	1059	46	59	NSP2	36 700 (317)			E	Basic, role in RNA replication?
9	1062	48 135	33 33	VP7(1) VP7(2)	37 368 (326) 33 919 (297)	Cleaved signal sequence, N-linked high mannose glycosylation and trimming[h]	780	NA	Surface glycoprotein, rough ER integral membrane glycoprotein, neutralization antigen, 2 hydrophobic NH$_2$-terminal regions, Ca^{2+}-binding
10	751	41	182	NSP4	20 290 (175)	Uncleaved signal sequence N-linked high mannose glycosylation and trimming		NA	Nonstructural rough ER transmembrane glycoprotein, 2 hydrophobic NH$_2$-terminal regions, role in morphogenesis, putative Ca^{2+}-binding site, enterotoxin
11	667	20	49	NSP5	21 725 (198)	Phosphorylated, O-linked glycosylation		NA	Nonstructural, slightly basic; serine–threonine-rich, RNA binding, protein kinase
				NSP6	21 000	Phosphorylated		NA	Nonstructural phosphoprotein

[a] For the Group A/Si/SA11 strain. Modified from Estes (1996) and Mattion et al. (1994). [b] Number of 5' noncoding sequences does not include the termination codon. [c] Determined by biochemical and genetic approaches. The size (in thousands) of the primary translation product is given for the nonstructural (NSP) proteins. [d] Molecular weights are calculated from the deduced amino acid sequences from nucleotide sequence data. The molecular weights are calculated from the largest potential open reading frame. [e] The calculated numbers of molecules of VP2, VP4, VP6 and VP7 are made from predicted structural analyses of individual particles using electron cryomicroscopy. [f] NA indicates none assigned. [g] There are two trypsin cleavage sites in SA11 4fM VP4 at amino acid 241 and 247. The indicated mature products are those based on use of only the preferred second cleavage site. [h] Mature cleaved VP7 contains 276 amino acids.

cytidine. A poly(A) tract is not found in the genomic RNAs and viral RNA transcripts are not polyadenylated. The 5′- and 3′ ends of each genome segment contain terminal consensus sequences of 7–10 nucleotides (nt). These consensus sequences are present in each RNA segment as part of the noncoding sequences. The 5′- and 3′-terminal consensus sequences are unrelated, implying they have functional differences. The terminal consensus sequences are assumed to be important *cis*-acting signals, which presumably include, at the 3′ ends, the viral promoters. The termini are also thought to contain sequences important in packaging and in the regulation of rotavirus gene expression at the levels of transcription, replication and translation. Both the 5′ and 3′ termini have been shown to be important for *in vitro* replication of the genome and they likely interact during translation of the viral mRNAs.

Properties of the Proteins

Descriptive properties of the six structural and six nonstructural proteins are quite well characterized (**Table 1**). Biochemical and antigenic information about the structural proteins is quite extensive, but molecular mechanisms of how these proteins function remain unknown. The two outer capsid proteins (VP4 and VP7) are the proteins studied in most detail because of their expected important roles in virus replication and in the induction of protective immunity. Indeed, VP4 and VP7 each have been shown to induce antibodies with neutralizing activity, and they function to mediate early events (attachment and penetration) in the replication cycle. Virus serotypes are defined based on antigenic properties of VP4 and VP7. VP7 serotypes (also called G for glycoprotein types) now are easily characterized and classified using monoclonal antibodies (MAbs). VP4 types (also called P for protease types) are still being characterized and VP4 typing MAbs are not yet available. VP4 and VP7 also interact with one another in still undefined ways, and these interactions can affect specific biologic and antigenic properties of virions. VP6 is the most immunogenic protein based on the ease of detection of antibodies to this protein following infection, and the most sensitive diagnostic assays are based on detection of this protein or antibodies to it. The minor subcore proteins, VP1 and VP3, are part of the RNA-dependent RNA polymerase activity associated with double-shelled particles. VP1 functions as the polymerase in association with VP3, which is the guanylyltransferase responsible for capping the newly made transcripts. VP2 is an RNA-binding protein that can self-assemble into single-layered particles. It is unclear if VP2 has an active role in the transcription process. VP2 is needed for replication of genomic RNA, and it may be one of the key proteins responsible for the packaging of the nascent RNA segments into newly forming particles in infected cells. VP6 is needed for transcriptase activity. However, it is not known whether VP6 simply functions as a structural component required to keep VP1, VP2, VP3 and the RNA segments in the proper conformation to permit transcription or if VP6 participates actively in the transcription process. Based on electron cryomicrograph studies, it is estimated that particles contain 120 molecules of VP2, 120 molecules of VP4, and 780 molecules of each VP6 and VP7.

The nonstructural proteins, found only in infected cells and not in mature virions, function in the steps of genome replication, mRNA translation and virion assembly. However, the precise role of only two of the nonstructural proteins (NSP3 and NSP4) in these processes is currently clear. Several of the nonstructural proteins involved in RNA replication may function as complexes. The nonstructural protein NSP3 binds specifically to four nucleotides at the 3′ end of viral RNAs and initially was suggested to be involved in RNA encapsidation. While this remains a possibility, recently NSP3 was found to interact with eIF4GI, a human eukaryotic initiation factor, and this interaction has been confirmed in rotavirus-infected cells by coimmunoprecipitation. In addition, the amount of poly(A) binding protein (PABP) present in eIF4F complexes decreases during rotavirus infection, and PABP is removed from eIF4F complexes after incubation with NSP3. These results indicate a physical link between the 5′ and the 3′ ends of mRNA is necessary for efficient translation of viral mRNAs and strongly support a closed loop model for the initiation of translation. These results also suggest that NSP3, by taking the place of PABP on EIF4GI, is responsible for the shut-off of cellular protein synthesis. Thus, NSP3 is involved in a new kind of viral mRNA translational regulation.

The nonstructural glycoprotein NSP4 is a unique protein that functions in the unusual rotavirus morphogenesis pathway that includes the transport of subviral particles across the membrane of the endoplasmic reticulum membrane, and acquisition and subsequent loss of a transient envelope on particles. This process culminates in the assembly of the outer capsid glycoprotein on to particles in the lumen of the ER. NSP4 has been found to have other properties including modulating intracellular calcium levels and chloride secretion. These activities relate to NSP4 functioning as an enterotoxin; NSP4 represents the first viral enterotoxin to be described.

Physical Properties of the Virions

The three forms of particles (triple-layered, double-layered and single-layered) are easily distinguished by electron microscopy and these also can be separated easily by centrifugation in gradients of cesium chloride (CsCl). The physical property of virions used most often to purify virus particles is virion density. In CsCl gradients, virions are relatively stable and viral infectivity is stable to extremes of pH (3.5–9.0). Virion stability is strain-dependent and some strains, particularly human virus strains, may be much less stable than viruses isolated from animals. Studies with reassortants suggest that virion stability during purification and storage at 4°C is determined by a particular gene 4 or its encoded protein VP4, and by specific interactions of VP4 with VP7. The outer capsid proteins can be removed by treatment of virions with chelating agents, such as 10 mM EDTA, or with ethanol, and this results in inactivation of infectivity. VP7 is a calcium-binding protein. In some cases, virus infectivity is less stable when virions contain cleaved VP4. In addition, the VP4 spikes can be removed by treatment of virions at pH 11.2 with ammonium hydroxide; removal of VP4 also may occur during other physical or chemical manipulations such as treatment with organic solvents. The ease of removing the VP4 spikes suggests that most virus preparations are quite heterogeneous and they probably contain many noninfectious particles (that lack a full complement of VP4 spikes). This heterogeneity of virus preparations may explain why early estimates of the approximate percent of each protein in particles determined by biochemical methods did not agree with the calculations made from electron cryomicrographs.

Replication

General features of the replication of rotaviruses are that infectious triple-shelled rotavirions bind to a host cell receptor and virions enter cells by still poorly characterized mechanisms. The outer shell of the virion apparently is disrupted or removed as part of the virus entry process and this allows activation of the RNA-dependent RNA polymerase (transcriptase) activity that is associated with the particles that contain VP1, VP2, VP3 and VP6. The virion-associated transcriptase synthesizes viral messenger RNAs (mRNAs) that are end-to-end transcripts of each of the 11 genome segments. These mRNAs are capped by the virion-associated capping enzyme. The mRNAs subsequently are translated, giving rise to all the viral proteins. The accumulation of viral proteins in the cytoplasm results in the formation of large perinuclear electron dense inclusions, termed viroplasms, that are thought to be the sites of genome replication and the assembly of progeny subviral particles. Subviral particles that contain a subset of newly made structural proteins (VP1, VP2, VP3, VP6) and of nonstructural proteins and mRNAs are apparently formed. Some subviral particles contain an associated RNA polymerase (replicase) activity that uses the mRNAs as templates for the synthesis of minus-strand RNA resulting in the formation of dsRNA. It has been proposed that the replicase particles mature into double-layered particles, and some of these nascent double-layered particles will function as transcriptase particles and synthesize additional mRNAs, thus leading to an amplification of the level of RNA replication in the cell. Other newly-formed double-layered particles associate with regions of the endoplasmic reticulum (ER) containing the nonstructural protein NSP4 and bud into the endoplasmic reticulum. During this process, the particles acquire a membrane that is subsequently lost, while VP4 and VP7 condense around the particles producing the outer shell of protein found on mature virus particles. VP4 probably associates with NSP4 and VP6 prior to the budding of particles into the ER.

Stages of the Replication Cycle

Adsorption, penetration and uncoating

The initial stages of virus replication have been examined by biochemical and morphologic (electron microscopic) procedures and they are not yet completely understood. Only triple-layered particles attach to cells when monitored by electron microscopy or by infectivity assays. Virus attachment is thought to occur via VP4 but VP7 may be involved in this process as well. Binding to cells does not require cleaved VP4 or glycosylated VP7.

The identity of the cellular receptor for rotaviruses appears to be different for different virus strains and cells. Some virus strains bind to cells in a sialic acid (SA)-dependent fashion. A study of the binding of radiolabeled simian rotavirus SA11 (a SA-dependent virus) to monkey kidney (MA104) cells found approximately 13 000 receptor units per cell. Binding is sodium-dependent, pH-insensitive between 5.5 and 8, and is dependent on sialic acid residues in the membrane. Virus binds but is not internalized at 4°C. The SA-dependent porcine rotavirus OSU has been shown to bind to ganglioside receptors NeuGcGM3 and NeuAcGM3 on porcine enterocytes. The SA-independent receptor has not yet been identified.

Many rotavirus strains contain a hemagglutinin, as demonstrated by their ability to bind to red blood cells. The hemagglutination activity has been mapped to VP8*, the N-terminal cleavage fragment of VP4. Studies of virus binding to red blood cells were the first to show that neuraminidase treatment reduces virus binding, indicating a role of SA in virus attachment. SA-containing compounds such as fetuin and mucin also inhibit virus binding to cells. These results add rotaviruses to an increasing number of viruses (such as reoviruses and influenza) that require SA for binding to cells. However, these studies have not determined whether virus binds directly to SA or whether SA maintains the configuration of the binding site without directly interacting with the virus. Binding to SA is not essential for rotavirus infectivity, as most human and animal rotaviruses infect cells in a SA-independent manner.

After binding to susceptible cells occurs, virus is internalized. Rotavirus infectivity is enhanced by proteolysis and this effect is not due to increased efficiency of virus attachment to host cells, but to facilitation of the virus internalization (penetration) step. Internalization will not take place at 0–4°C, indicating that this step requires active cellular processes. All virus is internalized by 60–90 min after binding. The mechanism of internalization (penetration) into cells remains unclear and controversial.

Both morphologic and biochemical approaches have been used to investigate the mode of entry of rotaviruses into cells. Current data indicate that trypsin-treated and nontrypsin-treated virus enter cells by different mechanisms. Nontrypsin-treated virus is thought to enter cells by receptor-mediated endocytosis, while trypsin-activated rotavirus is thought to enter cells more quickly by inducing permeability alterations in the plasma membrane which result in direct penetration of the cell membrane. Either pathway is essential for initiating penetration of the cell membrane but not for further steps in virus infectivity, as double-layered particles that lack the outer capsid proteins are infectious if they are delivered into the cytoplasm of cells by using a facilitator such as lipofectamine.

Other viruses that initiate infection by mechanisms involving receptor-mediated endocytosis often depend on the acidification of endosomes for partial uncoating or entry into the cell. The acidification of endosomes is not important for the entry of rotaviruses into cells. Unlike other viral systems, including reoviruses, lysosomotropic agents (ammonium chloride, chloroquine, methylamine, amantadine) or endocytosis inhibitors (dansylcadaverine and cytochalasin D or the vacuolar proton-ATPase inhibitor bafilomycin A1) have little inhibitory effect on rota virus replication as measured by RNA synthesis, polypeptide synthesis or virus yields. Energy inhibitors (sodium azide and dinitrophenol) have a minimal effect on rotavirus infection suggesting that rotaviruses do not use endocytosis to enter cells. However, it remains possible that these inhibitors (and the conditions tested) specifically affect the cell processes (if any) required for rotaviruses to enter cells.

It seems clear that the passage of rotaviruses from endocytic vesicles to the cytoplasm does not occur by a pH-dependent fusion mechanism, but this does not prove that rotaviruses are not taken up by endocytosis. The most direct support for the idea that rotaviruses enter the cell through direct penetration of the plasma membrane is the demonstration that trypsin-treated triple-layered rotavirus (but not non-trypsinized virus or double-layered particles) causes release of a fluorophore encapsulated within liposomes. A putative fusion region in VP5* has been identified that has sequence homology with Sindbis virus, and it has been suggested that this region might mediate virus penetration into cells. This remains to be demonstrated. It also remains to be determined if the interaction of cleaved VP4 with lipids occurs only at the plasma membrane or if this might occur in the endosome, or during virus morphogenesis (see below). It is possible that more than one mechanism, including endocytosis and direct passage, is operative for rotaviruses, as has been proposed for poliovirus and reoviruses. Recently, internalization of rotavirus or virus-like particles composed of proteins 2/4/6/7, but not of proteins 2/6/7 or 2/6, were shown to be able to induce a rapid and transient coentry of α-sarcin, a toxin that inhibits translation. Studies of the entry of this toxin may be useful to reveal the route used by rotaviruses to traverse the cell membrane and initiate productive infection.

Transcription and replication

The synthesis of viral transcripts is mediated by a viral RNA-dependent RNA polymerase (transcriptase) which has a number of enzymatic activities. The transcriptase is a component of the virion and properties of this enzyme (or enzyme complex) have been inferred by studying the characteristics of products from *in vitro* transcription reactions. Rotavirus particles presumably contain the same enzymatic activities found in reoviruses, including transcriptase, nucleotide phosphohydrolase, guanyltransferase and two methylases. These activities are inferred because rotavirus transcripts made *in vitro* in the presence of S-adenosyl methionine possess a methylated 5′-terminal cap structure, m^{7}GpppGm, and transcription is inhibited by pyrophosphate. Particles also contain a poly(A) polymerase activity whose precise function remains unknown; it has been postulated to be responsible for the synthesis of oligo(A) molecules.

The virus-associated transcriptase is latent in triple-layered particles and can be activated *in vitro* by treatment with a chelating agent or by heat shock treatment. Such treatments result in removal of the outer capsid proteins with conversion of triple-layered particles to double-layered particles. In infected cells, triple-layered particles have been shown to be uncoated to double-layered particles, and transcription in cells occurs from such particles (**Figure 2**). Transcription is asymmetric and all transcripts are full-length (+) strands made off the (−) dsRNA strand. The intracellular site of transcription is unknown.

Activation of transcriptase activity is a process that is not well understood. 'Activation' may be a misnomer, since in reoviruses it has been suggested this process does not actually modify the enzyme complex but instead releases the templates from structural constraints, allowing them to move past the transcriptase catalytic site. Rotavirus transcription requires a hydrolyzable form of ATP and studies with analogues that inhibit transcription suggest that ATP is required in reactions other than polymerization. ATP may be used for initiation or elongation of RNA molecules, as has been described for vesicular stomatitis virus or vaccinia virus RNA polymerases. It remains unclear if distinct polypeptides in the transcriptively active particles perform distinct functions or if the inner core polypeptides function as an enzymatic complex, but the location of VP1 and VP3 as a structural complex at the fivefold axes favor the latter hypothesis. VP1 has been crosslinked with a photoreactable nucleotide analogue, indicating that VP1 is a component of the transcriptase. VP3 in virus particles and expressed alone in insect cells can bind GTP, suggesting this protein is the guanyltransferase. Whether VP3 also possesses transcriptase activity alone or in association with VP1 remains unclear. Similarly, the role of VP2 in the transcription process is unclear.

The synthesis of plus- and minus-strand RNA has been studied in SA11-infected cells and in a cell-free system. Optimization of an electrophoretic system that allows separation of the plus and minus strands of rotavirus RNAs based on the complementary strands migrating at different rates in acid urea agarose gels facilitated these studies. Analysis of the kinetics of RNA synthesis in infected cells showed that plus- and minus-strand RNAs are detected initially at 3 hours postinfection, in agreement with other studies that looked at the time of incorporation of [^{3}H]uridine into rotavirus RNA. After 3 hours, the level of transcription increases until 9–12 hours, at which time the levels of plus-strand RNAs are maximal. The ratio of plus- to minus-strand RNA synthesis changes during infection and the maximal level of minus-strand RNA synthesis is seen several hours prior to the peak of plus-strand RNA synthesis.

The delay in obtaining maximal plus-strand RNA synthesis has been hypothesized to be due to a requirement for the accumulation of stoichiometric amounts of a protein (e.g. VP6) necessary for the assembly of transcriptase particles. Both newly synthesized and pre-existing plus-strand RNA can act as templates for minus-strand RNA synthesis throughout infection, an unexpected result based on earlier studies with reoviruses. The observation that the level of RNA replication does not increase continually in conjunction with the increasing levels of plus-strand RNA suggests that RNA replication is regulated by factors other than the level of plus-strand RNAs in the infected cell.

The synthesis of dsRNA also has been analyzed using a cell-free system to study the replication of rotavirus RNA. The components of this system include: (1) open core particles prepared from purified double-layered particles or virus-like particles composed of VP1/2/3/6; (2) exogenously added viral mRNA or a synthetic transcript; and (3) salts and nucleoside triphosphates. The *in vitro* replication system does not require the nonstructural proteins and specifically replicates rotavirus templates. The synthesis of dsRNA *in vitro* is an asymmetrical process in which a nuclease-sensitive positive-strand RNA acts as template for the synthesis of negative-strand RNA. After its synthesis, dsRNA remains associated with subviral particles, suggesting free dsRNA is not found in cells.

This *in vitro* system supports the initiation of negative-strand RNA using exogenous viral positive-strand RNA as template. The conversion of exogenous mRNA to dsRNA by subviral particles provides a method of studying (1) the specificity of viral proteins in recognition and replication of rotavirus mRNAs, and (2) the effect of adding exogenous synthetic RNAs containing specific mutations on replication. Finally, the possibility exists that nascent replicated dsRNA can be assembled into these viral particles in this *in vitro* replication system. Unfortunately to date, the efficiency of the system has not been adequate to achieve this goal. Together these results suggest that a cell-free system to support rotavirus RNA replication, transcription and the assembly of subviral particles can be established. This system should be useful to help define the defects in rotavirus mutants and to study the RNA sequences and proteins involved in virus replication and assembly. The role of individual proteins and specific protein complexes in RNA replication and viral morphogenesis will probably not be solved until they are studied *in vitro* with pure species of native rotavirus proteins and viral RNAs.

The sites and precise details of RNA replication remain unclear. However, electron-dense viroplasms are probably the sites of synthesis of the single-shelled particles that contain RNA. This conclusion is based on the localization of several of the viral proteins (VP2, NSP2, NSP5) to viroplasms and of VP4 and VP6 to the space between the periphery of the viroplasm and the outside of the ER, and on the observation that particles emerging from these viroplasms often seem to directly bud into the ER that contains VP7 and NSP4.

Assembly

The distinctive feature of rotavirus morphogenesis is that subviral particles, which assemble in cytoplasmic viroplasms, bud through the membrane of the ER and maturing particles are transiently enveloped. This is one of the more interesting aspects of rotavirus replication differing from virus members of other genera in the *Reoviridae* family. The envelope acquired in this process appears to be lost as particles move toward the interior of the ER, and it is replaced by a thin layer of protein which ultimately comprises the outer capsid of mature virions.

The sites of synthesis or localization of the viral proteins have been examined by ultrastructural immunocytochemistry using polyclonal monospecific or monoclonal antibodies and by studying the distribution of proteins by immunofluorescence or by subcellular fractionation. Taken together, the morphologic and biochemical data are consistent with rapidly assembling double-layered particles serving as an intermediate stage in the formation of triple-layered virions. Most of the rotavirus structural proteins and all of the nonstructural proteins are synthesized on the free ribosomes, although the nascent proteins on free ribosomes have not been analyzed. Instead, this conclusion has been drawn based on the absence of signal sequences that would indicate targeting to the ER and lack of protection to digestion in *in vitro* protease protection studies. In contrast, the glycoproteins VP7 and NSP4 are synthesized on ribosomes associated with the membrane of the ER and they are cotranslationally inserted into the ER membrane due to signal sequences at their N-termini. The glycoprotein NSP4 is a homotetramer oriented with the C-terminus on the cytoplasmic side of the ER membrane. This cytoplasmic domain of NSP4 acts as a receptor to bind to VP6 on the outer surface of nascent double-layered particles. This binding is thought to be the first step that initiates the membrane budding event.

VP7 is detected in the ER of SA11-infected cells in two pools. One pool is found only on intact particles and is detected only by a neutralizing monoclonal antibody. The second pool of VP7 is unassembled, it remains associated with the ER membrane, and it is detected by a polyclonal antibody made to denatured VP7. A kinetic study of the assembly of VP7 and of other structural proteins into particles has shown the incorporation of the inner capsid proteins into double-layered particles occurs rapidly, while VP4 and VP7 appear in mature triple-layered particles with a lag time of 10–15 minutes. Kinetic analyses of the processing of the oligosaccharides on the two pools of VP7 have shown the virus-associated VP7 oligosaccharides have a 15 minute lag compared with that of the membrane-associated form, suggesting that the latter is the precursor to virion VP7. This lag appears to represent the time required for virus budding and outer capsid assembly. NSP4, VP7 and VP4 also can form hetero-oligomers that are not associated with any known subviral particle; these hetero-oligomers are thought to be present at sites on the ER membrane where maturation to triple-layered particles begins. The proteins of the outer shell apparently are assembled on to the double-layered particles either during the budding process or once the particles reach the ER lumen.

Rotavirus maturation is a calcium-dependent process, based on the observation that virus yields are decreased when produced in cells maintained in calcium-depleted medium. Viruses produced in the absence of calcium were found to be exclusively double-layered, and budding of virus particles into the ER was not observed. Among the viral proteins, reduced levels of VP7 were observed, and subsequent studies showed that such reduced levels were due to the preferential degradation, and not to the impaired synthesis, of VP7. An interesting finding of these studies is that unglycosylated (but not mature) VP7 made in the presence of tunicamycin is relatively stable in a calcium-free environment. It is possible calcium stabilizes or modulates folding or compartmentalization of the newly glycosylated VP7 for subsequent assembly into particles. Alternatively, calcium deprivation may destabilize the ER or ER proteins required for the stable association of glycosylated VP7 with the membrane.

Virus release

Electron microscopy studies of infected tissue culture cells have shown the infectious cycle ends when progeny virus is released by host cell lysis. Extensive cytolysis during infection and drastic alterations in the permeability of the plasma membrane of infected cells resulting in the release of cellular and viral proteins have been demonstrated. In spite of cell lysis, most double-layered and many triple-layered particles remain associated with the cellular debris, suggesting these particles interact with structures within cells. Interactions with cell membranes and the cell cytoskeleton have been suggested to occur and these may play a role in movement of the viral proteins or particles within the cell. Whether the cytoskeleton provides a means of transport of viral proteins and particles to discrete sites in the cell for assembly or acts as a stabilizing element at the assembly site and in the newly budded virions or if particles are simply trapped by the cytoskeleton remains to be determined. It also is possible that virus may not be released from infected enterocytes because of cytopathic effect and cell lysis. Instead, virus-infected enterocytes may merely be sloughed intact into the intestinal lumen. This possibility has been suggested by studies of rotavirus replication in polarized human intestinal epithelial cells. These cells are infected in a symmetric manner and cell functions are shut off before the development of cytopathic effect and extensive virus release. Recent studies in polarized epithelial cells have suggested that rotaviruses are released from cells by a novel vesicular transport that does not result in extensive cytopathic effects.

Future Perspectives

Future basic research is expected to define the functions of each of the nonstructural proteins in the replication cycle and to understand the mechanisms of RNA replication and genome packaging. This may lead to the ability to use reverse genetics to probe in great detail the functions of any gene and to construct virions with desired properties. Knowledge of the three-dimensional structure of these complex virions is awaited for further understanding of the interactions between the outer capsid proteins and between the proteins in each of the capsid shells.

See also: **Rotaviruses (*Reoviridae*): General features; Reoviruses (*Reoviridae*): Molecular biology; Influenza viruses (*Orthomyxoviridae*): General features.**

Further Reading

Chen D, Zeng Q-Y, Wentz M et al (1994) Template-dependent *in vitro* replication of rotavirus RNA. *J. Virol.* 68, 7030.

Estes MK (1996) Rotaviruses and their replication. In: Fields BN, Knipe DM, Howley PM et al (eds) *Fields Virology*, 3rd edn. Philadelphia: Lippincott-Raven.

Lawton JA, Estes MK and Prasad BVV (1997) Three-dimensional visualization of mRNA release from actively transcribing rotavirus particles. *Nat. Struct. Biol.* 4: 118.

Mattion NM, Cohen J and Estes MK (1994) The rotavirus proteins. In: Kapikian AZ (ed.) *Virus Infections of the Gastrointestinal Tract*, 2nd edn, p. 169. New York: Dekker.

Patton JT (1995) Structure and function of the rotavirus RNA-binding proteins. *J. Gen. Virol.* 76: 2633.

Prasad BVV and Estes MK (1997) Molecular basis of rotavirus replication: structure–function correlations. In: Chiu W, Burnett RM and Garcea R (eds) *Structural Biology of Viruses*, p. 239. Oxford: Oxford University Press.

Prasad BVV, Rothnagel R, Zeng CQ-Y et al (1996) Visualization of the ordered genomic RNA and the transcription complex in rotavirus by three-dimensional electron cryomicroscopy. *Nature* 382: 471.

RUBELLA VIRUS (*TOGAVIRIDAE*)

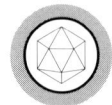

Teryl K Frey, Department of Biology, Georgia State University, Atlanta, Georgia, USA

Jerry S Wolinsky, Department of Neurology, The University of Texas Health Science, Center at Houston, Houston, Texas, USA

Copyright © 1999 Academic Press

History

Acute rubella virus infection causes a generally benign disease known as rubella or German measles that is usually acquired during childhood. The virus is endemic worldwide and causes epidemics at irregular intervals. First described by German physicians in the eighteenth century as distinct from scarlet fever and proteins indicates that rubella virus is more closely related to HEV and beet necrotic yellow vein virus than to the alphaviruses. This dissimilarity is borne out by differences in order of motifs in the NS-ORF. Thus, it is hypothesized that the evolution of the genera of the *Togavirus* family may have been more complicated than simple divergence from a common ancestor and probably involved recombination between progenitors of the current alphaviruses, rubella virus, HEV and possibly plant viruses.

Serologic Relationships and Variability

Rubella virus is monotypic and immunological characterization of diverse strains has only revealed subtle antigenic differences. These reside on C and E2 as E1 has been found to be antigenically identical using a variety of assays. The recent discovery of the second Asian genotype raised the possibility of greater antigenic variation, however the two genotypes only vary by 1–3% in predicted amino acid sequence of E1 and none of the recognized monoclonal epitopes contain major changes. Additionally, immune human serum neutralizes viruses from both genotypes with similar kinetics. As might be anticipated by the lack of serologic crossreaction with the alphaviruses, there is no important homology between rubella virus and sequenced alphaviruses in the subgenomic region that specifies the structural polypeptides of the virion.

Epidemiology

Rubella virus is endemic worldwide. In temperate zones, seasonal peaks occur in the spring and before widespread vaccine use, rubella epidemics occurred at 5–9-year intervals. There is considerable geographic variation in rubella attack rates in different age groups. In developed, temperate zone countries, peak infection rates occur in 5–9-year-old children. However, in much of Africa, the highest infection rates occur in children under 5, and 80% of all children are immune by 10 years of age. In contrast, in island and rural tropical populations the incidence of rubella is low, with high percentages of susceptible women of childbearing age. Much of this regional variation is explained by population densities, socioeconomic factors, and levels of medical sophistication. An additional factor in rubella epidemiology is that rubella virus is not as transmissible as is measles virus and thus even during epidemics, susceptibles are missed. Thus, infection of adolescents and young adults in any population is not uncommon.

Needless to say, vaccination programs have considerably altered the epidemiology of rubella in countries in which they are employed. Vaccination strategies and their effect on the incidence of rubella are discussed below.

Transmission and Tissue Tropism

Rubella virus is transmitted between individuals by aerosolation. Congenitally infected infants shed virus for three to six months following birth and are a source of transmission. Although vaccine virus can be recovered from vaccinees, transmission of vaccine virus to susceptible individuals has not been observed.

The epithelium of the buccal mucosa provides the initial site for rubella virus replication after infection and the mucosa of the upper respiratory tract and nasopharyngeal lymphoid tissue serve as portals of virus entry. The virus is then spread by local lymphatics which seed regional lymph nodes where further virus replication occurs. After an incubation period of 7–9 days, virus appears in the blood. The secondary sites of replication which account for the maintenance of viremia have not been identified, however infection of mononuclear cells contributes. Viremia ceases with the onset of detectable rubella-specific antibody shortly after the rash appears 2–3 weeks postinfection. Through the viremia, virus is seeded into the nasopharynx where it is shed by aerosolation. Patients are most infectious immediately preceding and during the rash; virus generally disappears from nasopharyngeal secretions within four days of appearance of the rash.

Reinfection with rubella virus does occur and is more frequent among vaccinees than naturally infected individuals due to lower antibody levels. Reinfection usually proceeds without viremia, clinical illness or virus shedding, however, reinfection with clinical illness has been reported. There are a small number of cases in which rubella virus reinfection of pregnant women with well-documented immunity has resulted in CRS.

During pregnancy, placental tissues are very susceptible to infection. Placental infection results in scattered foci of necrotic syncytiotrophoblast and cytotrophoblast cells and damage to vascular endothelium. Following placental infection, virus can spread to the fetus but this does not always occur and rubella virus is more often recovered from placental tissue than from fetal products of conception. Once fetal infection occurs, virus spreads throughout the fetus and almost any organ may be infected. *In vitro* cell cultures derived from infected fetuses are persistently infected with rubella virus. Severe fetal damage is only associated with infection during the first trimester of pregnancy. This is due to a combination of an apparent decline in the efficiency of placental transfer after the first trimester and a reduction in the ability of the virus to inflict fetal damage after this time of gestational development.

Clinical Features of Infection

Rubella acquired in childhood or early adulthood is usually mild, however symptoms in adults tend to be more severe than in children. It is estimated that up to 50% of rubella infections are clinically inapparent. Symptomatic rubella encompasses combinations of maculopapular rash, lymphadenopathy, low-grade fever, conjunctivitis, sore throat and arthralgia. The rash is the most prominent and earliest feature and appears following an incubation period of 16–20 days. The rash begins as distinct pink maculopapules on the face that then spread over the trunk and distally onto the extremities. The maculopapules coalesce and the rash rapidly fades over several days. An associated posterior cervical and suboccipital lymphadenopathy is also characteristic. Fever is typically low grade. The entire clinical syndrome usually resolves in a few days. Infrequently occurring complications include thrombocytopenia and post-infectious encephalitis. Acute polyarthralgia and arthritis following natural rubella virus infections of adults are common and occur more frequently and with greater severity in women than in men. Joint involvement is usually transient, resolving within one to several weeks, however chronic arthritis persisting or recurring over several years has been reported. The most common symptoms of rubella, lymphadenopathy, erythematous rash, and low-grade fever, are nonspecific and easily confused with similar illnesses caused by other common viral and nonviral pathogens or drug-induced eruptions. Therefore, a definitive diagnosis of rubella requires confirmation by virus isolation or, more commonly, by serology.

Fetal infection with rubella virus has dire consequences for fetal development. The rate of CRS following maternal infection is highest early in pregnancy; 50%, 25% and 10% during the first, second, and third months, respectively. CRS is rare following maternal infection after week 16 of gestation. The clinical manifestations of CRS apparent at birth vary widely, most frequently including thrombocytopenia purpura ('blueberry muffin syndrome'), intrauterine growth retardation, congenital heart disease (patent ductus arteriosus or pulmonary artery or valvular stenosis), psychomotor retardation, eye defects (cataract, glaucoma, retinopathy), suspected or confirmed hearing loss and hepatomegaly and/or splenomegaly. Less frequent features include adenopathy, bony radiolucencies, hepatitis usually with jaundice, and hemolytic anemia. Nearly 80% of CRS children show some type of neural involvement, particularly neurosensory hearing loss.

Most clinical manifestations of congenital rubella are evident at or shortly following birth and some are transient. However, recognition of retinopathy, hearing loss and mental retardation may be delayed for several years in some cases. Progressive consequences of congenital rubella have become increasingly appreciated as CRS children from the 1964 epidemic have been followed longitudinally. These predominantly involve endocrine dysfunction (diabetes mellitus, which ultimately affects 40% of CRS patients, and thyroid dysfunction). A rare, fatal neurodegenerative disease, progressive rubella panencephalitis (PRP), was also described in CRS patients that bears superficial resemblance to subacute sclerosing panencephalitis associated with measles virus. Subsequently, PRP cases were also reported in individuals who were infected postnatally.

Pathogenesis, Pathology and Histopathology

There is limited information on the pathogenesis of uncomplicated rubella because of the benign nature of the illness. With respect to the complications that can accompany acute rubella, the postinfectious encephalitis is thought to be autoimmune in nature since rubella virus cannot be isolated from cerebrospinal fluid or the brain at autopsy. Interestingly, however, extensive inflammation and demyelination are not observed. In a few cases of rubella arthritis, the presence of rubella virus in synovial fluid and/or cells has been demonstrated and therefore it is assumed that virus persistence is involved. However, considering the age and sex factors in the incidence of arthritis, it seems likely that immunopathological mechanisms also play a role. No predisposition for development of arthritis following rubella, immunological or otherwise, has been identified.

Following fetal infection, virus can be isolated from practically every organ of abortuses or infants who die soon after birth. However, only 1 in 10^3 to 1 in 10^5 cells are infected and it is not known how such a low infection rate leads to the profound birth defects exhibited in CRS. Affected organs are routinely small for gestational age and contain reduced numbers of cells. Considering the inhibitory effect of rubella virus on primary cells, it is thought that virus infection early in organogenesis inhibits cell division leading to both retardation and alteration in organ development. Virus persistence continues after birth as evidenced by shedding which generally ceases within six months of age. Whether virus persistence continues beyond cessation of shedding and plays a role in the delayed and progressive manifestations of CRS is not known.

Histologically, affected organs from CRS show a limited number of well-recognized malformations with noninflammatory histopathology predominating. Particularly apparent are vascular lesions and focal destruction in tissue bordering these lesions. These lesions are likely to be due to virus replication in the vascular endothelium and the damage to neighboring tissue may play a role in the pathogenesis of CRS. The neuropathology of CRS is of interest not only because of the defects manifest shortly after birth, but also because some CRS patients develop schizophrenia-like symptoms later in life. CRS brains are generally free of gross morphological malformations with a common tendency towards microcephaly. Vascular damage, leptomeningitis, decreased numbers of oligodendroglial cells, and alteration of white matter are observed. Recently, magnetic resonance imaging of a group of CRS adults with schizophrenia-like symptoms revealed specifically reduced cortical gray matter and enlargement of the ventricles, which were not previously observed aspects of CRS-induced neuropathology. Interestingly, the comparative finding that non-CRS schizophrenia patients exhibit a pattern of brain dysmorphy similar to CRS patients with schizophrenia-like symptoms supports the hypothesis that the pathogenesis of schizophrenia is developmental in nature (there is some evidence for a viral trigger to schizophrenia).

Immune Response

The earliest detectable serological response to rubella virus infection is the presence of immunoglobulin (Ig)M antibodies at the time of onset of the rash. Since these antibodies generally wane within a month or two, serodiagnostic testing for the presence of IgM is the primary means for diagnosis of acute rubella virus infection currently employed. In the succeeding weeks, antirubella virus antibodies appear in all immunoglobulin classes. The dominant early and persistent IgG response is in the IgG_1 subclass and antibodies of this class persist indefinitely after natural infection in healthy individuals. Immunoprecipitation studies disclose that the majority of the antibody response is directed to the E1 glycoprotein, with proportionally lesser amounts of the response directed at E2 or C. Although neutralizing and complement fixing antibodies are induced as well, the classical assay for the presence of antirubella virus antibodies was hemagglutination inhibition (HAI) and the current standard titer recognized for immunity of $10\ IU\ ml^{-1}$ is based on a reciprocal HAI titer of roughly 1:8. Because of the importance of serodiagnostic testing for rubella, a worldwide commercial market for rubella tests exists and a number of companies offer such kits, most of which are based on latex agglutination or enyzme immunoassay.

Rubella virus-specific cellular immune responses are measurable within one to two weeks of onset of rubella. These decline over several years but persist at low levels indefinitely following natural rubella. MHC-restricted CD4+ epitopes have been mapped to all three of the virus structural proteins, however CD8+ epitopes have thus far only been mapped to the C protein.

Following fetal infection, the fetus produces IgM antibody, detectable at 18–20 weeks of gestation, and maternal IgG antibody crosses the placenta. Both types of antibody exhibit virus neutralizing activity *in vitro*, however neither is sufficient to resolve virus infection during gestation. As discussed above, the intracellular maturation of virus probably shields it from antibody. After birth, the presence of IgM or a lack of decline of IgG titer are both considered diagnostic of fetal infection. CRS infants exhibit impairment in the cellular immune response to rubella virus to varying degrees and it is thus a deficiency in this arm of the immune response that allows the virus to persist. Considering this deficiency in CRS infants, it is curious that detectable virus persistence ends relatively shortly after birth. The means by which virus persistence is cleared under these conditions is not understood.

Prevention and Control of Rubella

As discussed above, live attenuated vaccines were developed and placed in use by 1970. The vaccine used in most countries, with two exceptions, is the RA 27/3 vaccine. This vaccine was developed by multiple passaging of a virus isolate from an explant culture of a fetal human kidney in WI-38 human fetal diploid lung cells. Several of the passages were done at 30°C and limiting dilutions were used at some of the passages. Production of the vaccine is done in both WI-38 and MRC-5 diploid human cell cultures. In Japan, five attenuated vaccine strains were developed and are currently in use. Additionally, at least one Chinese vaccine strain is currently in use in China.

Rubella attenuated vaccines cause subclinical infection with transient viremia in susceptible recipients. However, transmission of vaccine virus has not been reported. The RA27/3 vaccine strain produces seroconversion in greater than 95% of recipients. Vaccine-induced titers are lower than those induced by natural infection but appear to last indefinitely. The rubella vaccine is generally administered to children in trivalent form with the measles and mumps attenuated vaccines. Additional testing has shown that the recently licensed varicella vaccine can be combined with these vaccines in a tetravalent vaccines with no detectable interference between the component vaccine viruses.

In general, the rubella vaccines have been among the most successful in terms of induction of immunity with an absence of side effects. However, two issues have arisen concerning rubella vaccination. The first is that the vaccine virus can cross the placenta and infect the fetus. However, in a registry kept in the US between 1971 and 1988 of over 300 deliveries to women inadvertently vaccinated within three months of conception or during the first trimester of pregnancy, no congenital abnormalities were reported. Nevertheless, vaccination during pregnancy is contraindicated and is deferred until post-partum. Second, is the occurrence of arthralgia and arthritis following vaccination. Joint complications are nonexistent in children with the currently used rubella vaccines, however transient arthralgia and arthritis is reasonably common among adult female vaccinees. There have also been reports of chronic arthritis and related neurological involvement following vaccination of adult women. Although these complications are consistent with complications that can accompany natural rubella in adult females, recent studies have shown that the incidence of such vaccine-related complications is rare and cannot be statistically differentiated from the incidence of similar symptoms in control, unvaccinated populations.

Since the inception of rubella vaccination, the US has employed a strategy of universal vaccination at 15 months of age augmented with vaccination of seronegative 'at-risk' individuals (women planning pregnancy, health care workers) which was successful in bringing the incidence of rubella and CRS to record low levels by 1988. However, a resurgence occurred between 1989 and 1991 among foci of unvaccinated individuals concentrated primarily on college campuses, among Amish communities in the Northeast, and among the Hispanic population in the Southwest. Since most of the infected individuals were of adolescent age or older, the ratio CRS to rubella cases was higher than in unvaccinated populations and over 50 CRS cases occurred despite the fact that only 3000 rubella cases were reported. Since the resurgence, a second vaccine at age 5–10 has been included in the vaccination program as well as more strict enforcement of vaccine requirements for school admission. The incidence of rubella and CRS has subsequently dropped to minuscule levels. Most of these cases are thought to be imported and no rubella was reported during a two month period in 1996, possibly indicating a break in endemic transmission.

In Japan and Europe, a strategy of vaccination of adolescent girls was initially adopted since it was felt that natural immunity was more robust than vaccine-induced immunity and thus it was considered desirable that as many individuals as possible should contract natural rubella. Predictably, rubella virus continued to circulate and thus postadolescent women who managed to break through without a rubella titer were infected and CRS was not eliminated. Therefore, most of these countries adopted the universal strategy in the late 1980s. Aggressive implementation of the universal policy in the UK and Scandinavia has brought rubella down to very low levels; however, in many countries with rubella vaccination programs, vaccination is not comprehensively pursued and thus both rubella and CRS still occur.

Rubella vaccination is practiced in only a few countries outside of the US, Canada, Europe and Japan. In underdeveloped countries, this is primarily because of the expense of the vaccine, the nature of national public health infrastructures, and the general mildness of the disease in comparison to those caused by life-threatening pathogens. However, rubella exacts a societal load in every country in which it is endemic. Because rubella virus is exclusively a human virus and excellent vaccines for use against it exist, it is potentially eradicable and recently attention has been focused on the possibility of elimination or eradication efforts for two major reasons. First, because the rubella and measles vaccines are administered together in most childhood vaccination programs, it would be efficient to include the rubella vaccine in currently ongoing worldwide measles elimination efforts. In addition to controlling two diseases with one effort, measles surveillance requires diagnosis of rubella because of the similarity of symptomology and thus inclusion of rubella vaccine would also concomitantly reduce surveillance costs by reducing rubella cases. Secondly, rubella elimination is potentially of great benefit to the countries which maintain expensive comprehensive vaccination and control programs. In these countries, most rubella outbreaks are due to importation and thus a substantial reduction or elimination of rubella would allow easing of control efforts as well as eventual discontinuation of vaccination. Therefore, a concerted worldwide effort on rubella control appears to be forthcoming.

Future

Because of its association with a diverse group of clinical diseases, rubella virus will remain a fascinating pathogen. As an example, the incidence of diabetes in CRS patients is the best statistically direct association between a specific human virus and a specific autoimmune disease. The mechanism of viral involvement in each of these diseases is not fully understood. Unfortunately, our present understanding of disease mechanisms in the rubella virus-related syndromes is hindered by the current lack of a suitable animal model system that fully mimics the infection seen in humans and development of an animal model is a research priority. Virologically, rubella virus is taxonomically unique and appears to have evolved as a recombinational hybrid of other distantly related viruses. Thus, investigation of its molecular biology will likely reveal novel replication strategies and yield insight into virus evolution. The biggest challenge concerning rubella virus, however, will be potential forthcoming elimination efforts which could well consume the next quarter to half century.

See also: **Defective interfering viruses; Diagnostic techniques: Detection of viral antigens, nucleic acids and specific antibodies; Sindbis and Semliki Forest viruses (*Togaviridae*); Nervous system viruses; Epidemiology of viral diseases; Immune response: Cell mediated immune response, General features; Persistent viral infection; Vaccines and immune response.**

Further Reading

Frey TK (1994) Molecular biology of rubella virus. *Adv. Virus Res.* 44: 69.

Frey TK (1997) Neurological aspects of rubella virus infection. *Intervirology* 40: 167.

Gillam S (1994) The Jeanne Mannery Fisher memorial lecture 1994: Molecular biology of rubella virus structural proteins. *Biochem. Cell. Biol.* 72: 349.

Plotkin SA (1994) Rubella vaccine. In: Plotkin SA and Mortimer Jr EA (eds) *Vaccines*, 2nd Edn, p. 303. Philadelphia: WB Saunders.

Pugachev KV, Abernathy ES and Frey TK (1997) Improvement of the specific infectivity of the rubella virus infectious clone: determinants of cytopathogenicity induced by RUB map to the nonstructural proteins. *J. Virol.* 71: 562.

Wolinsky JS (1996) Rubella virus. In: Fields BN, Knipe DM, Howley PM *et al.* (eds) *Virology* 3rd edn., p. 899. Philadelphia: Lippincott-Raven Publishers.

Russian Spring Summer Encephalitis   *see* Encephalitis Viruses

SALMONELLA PHAGE P22 (*PODOVIRIDAE*)

Anthony R Poteete, Department of Molecular Genetics and Microbiology, University of Massachusetts Medical Center, Worcester, Massachusetts, USA

Copyright © 1999 Academic Press

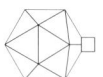

Introduction

P22 is a temperate bacteriophage that mediates generalized transduction of its host, *Salmonella typhimurium*. This capability forms the basis of the first claim of P22 to distinction: the discovery of transduction described by Zinder and Lederberg in 1952 involved the transfer of *Salmonella* genes by P22. P22 continues to the present day to be an indispensable tool of *Salmonella* genetics. It is an unassigned species in the family *Podoviridae*.

The molecular genetics of P22 itself have been studied intensively. Research with P22 has contributed to our understanding of a number of biological processes, including replication, recombination, and regulation; protein folding and assembly; and viral morphogenesis and evolution.

Virion Structure

The P22 virion can be described as an icosahedral head, with a diameter of approximately 570 Å, attached at one vertex to a short tail/baseplate structure, from which a single, slender fiber extends (radially with respect to the head) (**Fig. 1**). The virion is roughly half protein and half DNA by weight.

P22 virions contain nine protein species. The major one is the coat protein, which is present in about 400 copies arranged in an icosahedral ($T = 7$ laevo) shell. One minor structural polypeptide, the portal protein, forms a ring-shaped dodecamer around the place in the head where the tail/baseplate attaches. Another, described as the tailspike protein, forms trimers (**Fig. 2**); six trimers attach to the tail to form the baseplate. The remaining six proteins of the capsid have structurally undefined roles in forming the tail and in DNA injection.

The single P22 chromosome is a linear double-stranded DNA molecule of approximately 43 400 bp. Its precise structure varies from one virion to another, due to the nature of the viral assembly process. P22 DNA is packaged from a large DNA molecule, called a concatemer, consisting of multiple tandem repetitions of the phage genome. Packaging into a preformed head structure, called a prohead, starts at a specific sequence, *pac*, and proceeds unidirectionally until a headful of DNA has been taken up. At that point, wherever it occurs in the phage DNA sequence, packaging into the first prohead terminates, and packaging into a second prohead initiates. This sequential packaging can continue for many headfuls. The process, in the case of wild-type P22, results in

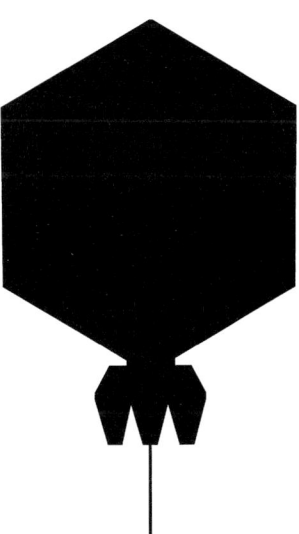

Figure 1 Schematic drawing representing the appearance of P22 virions in electron micrographs of negatively stained preparations. The capsid is icosahedral, but can appear hexagonal in outline. The baseplate is hexagonally symmetric. Adapted from Casjens S and Hendrix R (1988) Control Mechanisms is dsDNA backeriophage assembly. In: Calendar R (ed.) *The Bacteriophages,* vol. 2. New York: Plenum

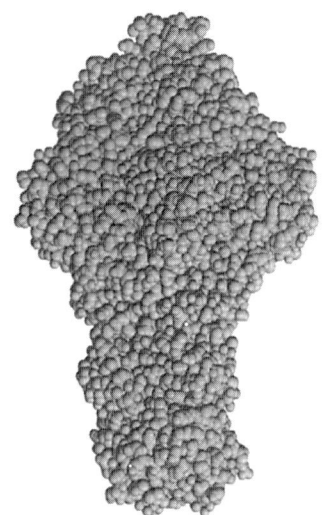

Figure 2 Tailspike trimer. Six of these trimers constitute the baseplate. The drawing is based on the crystal structure of a truncated version of the molecule, lacking only a small domain that attaches it to the head (on top, as oriented here). Steinbacher S, Baxa U, Miller S *et al.* (1996) Crystal structure of phage P22 tailspike protein complexed with *Salmonella* sp. O-antigen receptors. *Proc. Natl. Acad. Sci. USA* 93: 10584; coordinates from the Protein Data Bank.

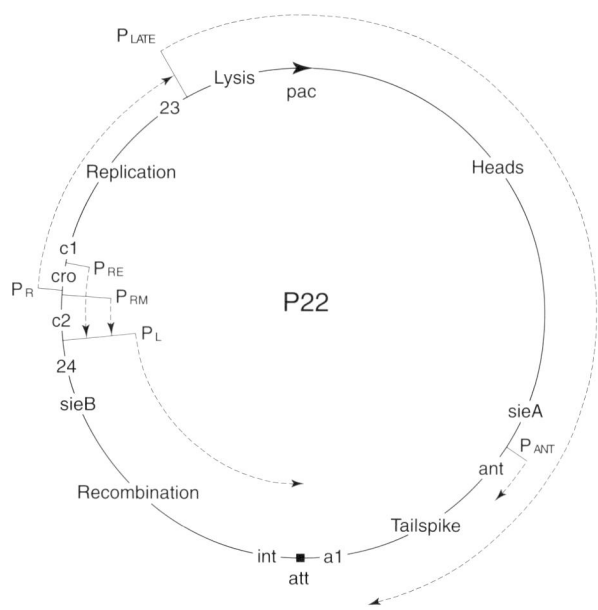

Figure 3 Map of the circular P22 chromosome, roughly to scale, showing the origins and extents of most of the major known transcripts, as well as some sites and structural genes.

the packaging of one complete genome, plus a variable amount of DNA, averaging 1600 bp, that constitutes a repetition, at one end, of the sequences present at the other end. The repetitious ends of the P22 chromosomes are cyclically permuted over much of the phage genome. This 'headful' DNA packaging process, first established in studies of P22, is thought to be characteristic of generalized transducing phages; generalized transduction can be viewed as a consequence of headful packaging of the bacterial chromosome, starting at spurious *pac*-like sites.

Genetic Structure

The genome of P22 consists of 41 725 bp. Genetic maps, based on recombination frequencies observed in phage crosses, or on sequences of DNA extracted from the phage, are circular. The map determined by recombination frequencies is distorted relative to that determined by physical methods, as a consequence of a gradient of recombination frequencies that peaks in the vicinity of the *pac* site (**Fig. 3**).

P22 genes are clustered by function. Thus, genes involved in recombination, early transcriptional regulation, DNA replication, lysis, DNA packaging and head assembly are located in discrete blocks.

P22 is a relative of coliphage λ, with which it can exchange blocks of genes by recombination *in vivo*. These two phages, and other members of the family, exhibit a remarkable conservation of genetic organization, far in excess of their limited sequence homology. Some P22 genes are related by partial sequence identity to their λ counterparts; most are not. Sequences shared by P22 and λ are scattered over the genomes of the two phages.

Lytic Cycle

The P22 tailspike protein is an enzyme that binds and hydrolyzes the *S. typhimurium* O-antigen (the outer polysaccharide component of the outer membrane lipopolysaccharide), which serves as the initial receptor for the phage. Following attachment of the virion to a secondary receptor, phage DNA is piloted into the cell by three capsid proteins.

In the cytoplasm of the infected cell, phage DNA is transcribed (throughout the lytic cycle) by the host-encoded RNA polymerase. Three key transcripts are produced in the 'immediate early' phase of transcription, from the promoters P_L, P_R and P_{ant}. The P_L transcript encodes the gene *24* protein, which induces RNA polymerase to transcribe past terminators at the ends of the short P_L and P_R RNAs. This antitermination activity is needed for expression of the rest of the genes in the P_L and P_R operons. The P_R transcript encodes Cro protein, a transcriptional repressor, which binds to operators that overlap P_L and P_R, turning down transcription from these two promoters. This action of Cro protein is essential for the shift from early to late transcriptional patterns, and, consequently, for lytic growth. The third transcript, from P_{ant}, encodes antirepressor, which induces lytic growth of any P22-related prophage that happens to be resident in the infected cell.

The P22 genes that are expressed as a result of gene 24 protein action include ones that promote homologous recombination, DNA replication, and late transcriptional regulation. The late transcriptional regulatory gene, 23, encodes a protein that antiterminates transcription from the promoter P_{LATE}. The late transcript thus extended is over 20 000 bp in length, and includes all of the genes required for phage assembly and host cell lysis.

Replication of P22 DNA requires the action of two phage-encoded proteins, whose function is to recruit host replisomes to the phage replication origin. The key product of replication is the linear concatemer that serves as a substrate for sequential headful DNA packaging. This concatemer is generated from a circular P22 chromosome by a rolling circle mechanism. The circular form of the P22 chromosome is formed by homologous recombination between the repetitious ends of the linear DNA molecule injected by the phage.

Assembly of P22 virions proceeds by an ordered pathway that starts with the formation of proheads. Coat protein aggregates into a roughly spherical shell around a core of scaffolding protein. Four minor proteins, including the portal protein, also participate in this process. Proheads of normal appearance in electron micrographs can assemble in the absence of any of these minor proteins; however, they cannot mature into infectious phage. During the DNA packaging process, the scaffolding protein is ejected intact; it subsequently participates, catalytically, in the formation of new proheads. The coat protein shell also expands and rearranges. Addition of three minor proteins is required for the formation of a stable head with a short tail, to which trimers of the tailspike protein attach as a final step.

Packaging of DNA by the prohead requires the action of two proteins which are not incorporated into the final structure, one to bring the prohead to the pac site, and the other to pump DNA inside. P22 mutants, called HT, direct the synthesis of altered versions of the first of these, and reduce the specificity of *pac* recognition. HT mutants exhibit elevated frequencies of transduction of bacterial genes, and are especially useful for *Salmonella* genetics.

Lysis of the infected cell results from the action of two proteins. One of the proteins, called a holin, inserts into the cytoplasmic membrane, creating channels that permit the passage of small proteins. The second protein, a lysozyme, thereby gains access to the cell wall peptidoglycan, which it hydrolyzes to effect disruption of the host cell.

Lysogeny

Like other temperate phages, P22 can follow either of two pathways following infection of a sensitive host cell: it can grow lytically, or form a lysogen. Which of these pathways is favored depends on a variety of factors, including the multiplicity of infection and the nutritional status of the cell. The key element in the choice between pathways is a transcriptional regulatory protein, the product of gene *c1*, which is transcribed as a result of antitermination by gene 24 protein. Regulation of c1 protein synthesis and stability is complex and only partially understood. When present at sufficient levels, c1 protein stimulates transcription from the promoter P_{RE}. The c2 protein, encoded in the P_{RE} transcript, is then synthesized, and acts by binding to operators overlapping P_L and P_R, repressing transcription; at the same time, it turns on its own transcription from the otherwise silent promoter P_{RM}. An additional transcriptional repressor, the product of the *mnt* gene, is required for maintenance of the lysogenic state; the function of this protein is to turn off transcription of antirepressor.

Establishment of stable lysogeny requires, in addition to transcriptional repression, integration of the phage DNA into the bacterial chromosome to form a prophage. This function is carried out by integrase, a protein that promotes reciprocal recombination between specific sequences called attachment sites in the circular phage and bacterial chromosomes.

In the lysogenic state, a number of P22 genes are expressed. In addition to the c2 and Mnt repressors, these include *sieA*, *sieB* and *a1*. The functions of the latter genes all involve keeping out infecting phages: the product of *sieA* interferes with DNA injection by P22 and related phages; *sieB* causes the lytic cycle of certain other *Salmonella* phages (not P22 itself) to abort at an early stage; and *a1* alters the structure of the lysogen's O-antigen, interfering with adsorption by P22 and related phages.

The lysogenic state is homeostatic. The c2 protein turns on its own gene, and turns off most of the other phage genes; spontaneous induction is a rare event. On the other hand, treatment of lysogens with agents that damage DNA results in efficient induction. The mechanism of this induction is based on the host cell's normal reaction to such agents. A signal, perhaps single-stranded DNA, generated as a consequence of DNA damage, activates RecA protein, which in turn promotes proteolysis of LexA protein, a cellular repressor that controls transcription of the global SOS regulon. Some phage repressors, including c2 protein, are homologues of LexA protein; they are similarly cleaved in response to activated RecA protein. With repressor thus rendered inactive, transcription from P_L and P_R initiates. The resulting lytic growth requires the reversal of integration–excision, promoted by the combined action of the phage-encoded integrase and excisionase, but is otherwise similar to lytic growth following infection.

Research Directions

Current research with P22 is focused on the molecular mechanisms of selected aspects of the phage's biology. Some of this research is comparative. For example, P22 frequently serves as a system in which particular mechanisms of λ gene regulation can be tested for generality. P22 has also found use as a component of certain specialized cloning systems. In addition, a few P22-encoded proteins serve as model systems for the study of protein folding and stability, of DNA binding, and of transcriptional regulation.

Antirepressor

P22 departs from the familiar pattern of lambdoid phage transcriptional regulation by possession of an antirepressor (the protein product of gene *ant*). Embedded in the late operon of P22, *ant* is subject to regulation by its own set of three repressors: two proteins, the products of genes *arc* and *mnt*, and one antisense RNA, the *sar* transcript. All of these have been extensively characterized.

The *ant* operon has been employed in the construction of a specialized cloning system. In it, a DNA sequence thought to function in gene regulation is installed in P22 in place of the operator that normally controls *ant* expression. The resulting hybrid phage will invariably kill a bacterium that can not control its synthesis of antirepressor; it can be used to select among bacterial clones for those which express a protein that can bind specifically to the DNA site in question. A closely related P22 strain provides a direct selection for bacteria expressing a protein that can bind specifically to a site in RNA. The phage is constructed so that the RNA site question overlaps the *ant* ribosome binding site.

DNA packaging

The molecular basis of the limited sequence specificity of one of the DNA packaging proteins (the product of gene *3*) has been the subject of recent investigation. This research has led to understanding of the sequence determinants of *pac* activity, as well as a picture of what constitutes a *pac*-like site. The DNA packaging apparatus of P22 has been used in a cloning system in which it is combined with the ends of the transposon-phage Mu. The resulting replicon, when inserted into the host cell's chromosome (essentially anywhere), becomes a locked-in prophage, unable to excise. However, upon induction, it packages the host chromosome, one headful at a time; sequences located near and to one side of the insertion are packaged with particularly high efficiency.

Homologous recombination

P22 depends on genetic recombination to circularize its chromosome following infection. This recombination must take place at high efficiency within the 1600 bp sequence repeated at the ends of the linear DNA injected by the phage. The recombination system of the bacterial host is inefficient in this process. P22 encodes proteins that work in conjunction with the host system to increase its efficiency. One of these proteins, Abc, binds to the host cell's RecBCD nuclease/helicase and modulates its nuclease activity. Another, Erf, is a single-stranded DNA-binding protein that accelerates association of complementary strands. A third protein, Arf, is a general recombination enhancer of unknown mechanism. Though the phage and host proteins work together, the combined system contains functional redundancies, and can operate at nearly normal efficiency in the absence of any of the known host functions.

Like P22, phage λ encodes a homologous recombination system, called Red, that can function in the absence of the known host recombination proteins, but that works most efficiently in their presence. Both phages encode strand exchange-promoting proteins (Erf and Redβ, respectively) analogous to RecA. However, the two phages use different strategies for interactions with RecBCD. Whereas P22 modifies RecBCD and uses it in promoting phage recombination, λ completely nullifies RecBCD and elaborates its own exonuclease. The two phage recombination systems share no apparent sequence homology, but are functionally interchangeable. The functional significance of such an efficient recombination system for λ is not obvious, as it is in the case of P22, as the λ chromosome circularizes by an entirely different mechanism. The explanation may reside in the idea of the lambdoid phages as mosaics of interchangeable genetic modules; efficient recombination systems are required to retain the capability of headful packaging in the group.

Tailspike

The P22 tailspike protein has proven to be an interesting object for studies of protein structure, folding and assembly, and aggregation. The mature form of the protein is a trimer of identical 666 amino acid residue subunits. The most prominent feature of the monomer is a large β-helix, consisting of 13 helical turns of parallel β strands. In the trimer, the helical coils pack into a parallel bundle. Distally, the three polypeptides intertwine to create an extremely stable bundle of β sheets.

Folding and assembly of the tailspike occur in concert: monomers partially fold, assemble into a structure called a protrimer, then complete folding together. Folding and trimerization of the tailspike polypeptide are slow *in vivo* under certain physiological conditions, and the various forms of the tailspike exhibit different solubilities and electrophoretic mobilities. It has thus been possible to dissect the tailspike folding and assembly pathway *in vivo* as well as *in vitro*.

The mature tailspike trimer is an unusually stable protein. However, its folding/assembly process is unusually temperature sensitive. At 40°C, most of the subunits fail to fold correctly, and end up in insoluble aggregates. Investigators have characterized mutant proteins that exhibit increased and decreased tendencies to aggregate.

P22 in novel settings

P22 does not form plaques on *Escherichia coli*, but only because it cannot adsorb. If *E. coli* is given the capability of synthesizing the *S. typhimurium* O-antigen, it will support lytic growth, lysogeny and generalized transduction by P22. Plasmid-borne *rfb* and *rfc* genes from *S. typhimurium* are sufficient for this purpose. This observation suggests the possibility of using P22 as a generalized transducing phage in other, less genetically characterized Gram-negative bacteria.

Early in this century, a key aim of bacteriophage researchers was to use these viruses as antibacterial therapeutic agents. This line of investigation was discontinued due to technical difficulties and the advent of antibiotics. However, the recent proliferation of antibiotic resistant strains has revived interest in this area. Recently, investigators have described the isolation of mutants of phages λ and P22 that have extended lifetimes in the murine circulatory system, and can abort experimental infections.

See also: **Coliphage lambda (*Siphoviridae*); Lysogeny and prophage; Phage Homologous Recombination.**

Further Reading

Campbell A and Botstein D (1983) Evolution of the lambdoid phages. In: Hendrix RW, Roberts JW, Stahl FW and Weisberg RA (eds) *Lambda II*. New York: Cold Spring Harbor Laboratory.

Casjens S and Hendrix R (1988) Control mechanisms in dsDNA bacteriophage assembly. In: Calendar R (ed.) *The Bacteriophages*, vol. 2, New York: Plenum.

King J, Haase-Pettingell C, Robinson AS, Speed M and Mitraki A (1996) Thermolabile folding intermediates: inclusion body precursors and chaperonin substrates. *FASEB J* 10: 57.

Poteete AR (1988) Bacteriophage P22. In: Calendar R (ed.) *The Bacteriophages*. vol. 2, New York: Plenum Press.

Susskind MM and Botstein D (1978) Molecular genetics of bacteriophage P22. *Microbiol. Rev.* 42: 385.

SATELLITE RNAs AND SATELLITE VIRUSES

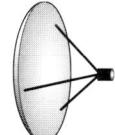

ME Taliansky and **PF Palukaitis**, Virology Department, Scottish Crop Research Institute, Invergowrie, Dundee, UK

Copyright © 1999 Academic Press

Introduction

Satellites are a heterologous collection of subviral agents which comprise nucleic acid molecules that depend for their productive multiplication (replication) on a helper virus, but which contain sequences substantially distinct from those of the genomes of either their helper virus or their hosts. Satellites are thus distinct from either defective (D) or defective interfering (DI) RNAs, because the latter are wholly derived from their helper virus genomes. However, there are some hybrid RNAs between satellites and parts of the viral genome, such as the chimeric molecules formed from part of a satellite RNA associated with turnip crinkle virus (TCV) and part of a DI RNA formed from the virus genome. Satellites may encode their own coat protein (CP) (satellite viruses), or they may rely on the helper virus for encapsidation as well as replication (the satellite RNAs or satellite DNA). Satellites are not needed

Table 1 Satellite viruses

Helper virus/satellite virus	Particle size (nm)	CP (NW)	Size of satellite RNA (nt)
Subgroup 1			
Tobacco necrosis necrovirus (TNV)/Satellite TNV (STNV)	17	~21 600	1239 620[a]
Panicum mosaic sobemovirus (PMV)/Satellite PMV (SPMV)	17	~17 000	826
St. Augustine decline sobemovirus (SADV)/Satellite SADV (SSADV)	17	~17 000	24
Tobacco mosaic tobamovirus (TMV)/Satellite TMV (STMV)	17	~17 500	1059
Maize white line mosaic virus (MWLMV)/Satellite MWLMV (SMWLMV)	17	23 961	1168
Subgroup 2			
Chronic bee-paralysis virus (CPV)/CPV associated satellite virus (CPVA)	17	NR[b]	~1100 (three species)

[a] Satellite RNA of STNV.
[b] NR, not reported.

by helper viruses for their accumulation. However, some RNA molecules which are not required by the helper virus for experimental infection, appear to be essential for the natural life cycle of the virus, by contributing to vector transmissibility. Such examples are the RNAs associated with groundnut rosette virus (GRV) and beet necrotic yellow vein virus (BNYVV), which have been described and are referred to as satellite-like RNAs. A related group of subviral agents is that containing RNAs that resemble satellites but which depend on a helper virus only for encapsidation rather than for replication [e.g. hepatitis delta virus (HDV) and beet western yellows virus (BWYV) ST9-associated RNA].

History

The term satellite virus was adopted by Kassanis to describe the small 17 nm diameter particles associated with tobacco necrosis virus (TNV), in 1962. It was serologically unrelated to TNV and hence encoded its own CP. In 1969, a satellite was found associated with tobacco ringspot virus (TRSV), which was encapsidated by the helper virus, and the term 'satellite' was broadened to include satellite RNAs. In recent years, a large number of other satellite viruses and satellite nucleic acids associated with different groups of viruses have been described. Most known satellites consist of single-stranded (ss) RNA, with ssRNA plant viruses as helpers. However, satellite ssDNAs and double-stranded (ds) RNAs have also been described.

Classification

Satellites do not constitute a homogeneous taxonomic group. They represent quite different disparate groups of subviral agents associated with plant, animal, protozoan and fungal viruses containing different types of genetic material such as ssRNA, dsRNA or ssDNA. It seems very unlikely that such different groups of satellites might be evolutionarily related. There are also no taxonomic correlations between the viruses that support satellites. Satellitism would appear to have arisen independently a number of times during the evolution of viruses. Thus, classification of satellites is based largely on features of the genetic material of the satellites. The nature of the helper virus and helper virus host range are important secondary characters. All known satellites appear to be included into the following categories.

Satellite viruses

   Subgroup I. Satellite tobacco necrosis virus (STNV)
   Subgroup II. Chronic bee paralysis associated satellite virus (CPVA)

Satellite nucleic acids

ss satellite DNA
ds satellite RNA
ss satellite RNA
   Subgroup I. Large ss satellite RNA with messenger properties
   Subgroup II. Small linear ss satellite RNA
   Subgroup III. Circular ss satellite RNA

As mentioned above, satellite-like RNAs and subviral agents dependent on a helper virus only for encapsidation may also be regarded as satellite-related agents. A complete list of satellites and satellite-related agents is presented in **Tables 1–3**.

Table 2 Satellite nucleic acids

Helper virus/satellite nucleic acid	Size of satellite nucleic acid (encoded protein MW)
ss sat-DNA (circular)	
Tomato leaf curl virus (TLCV)/TLCV sat-DNA	682 nt (NR)[a]
ds sat-RNAs (linear)	
L-A ds RNA virus of *Saccharomyces cerevisiae*/M sat-RNA	~1000–1800 nt (NR)
Trichomonas vaginalis virus (TVV)/TVV sat-RNA	~500 nt, ~700 nt, ~1700 nt (NR)
ss sat-RNAs	
Large sat-RNAs with messenger properties	
Nepovirus	
Arabis mosaic virus (ArMV)/ArMV large sat-RNA	1104 nt (~39 kDa)
Chicory yellow mottle virus (CYMV)/CYMV large sat-RNA	1145 nt (~39 kDa)
Grapevine Bulgarian latent virus (GBLV)/GBLV sat-RNA	~1500 nt (NR)
Grapevine fanleaf virus (GFLV)/GFLV sat-RNA	1114 nt (~37 kDa)
Myrobalan latent ringspot virus (MLRV)/MLRV sat-RNA	~1400 nt (~45 kDa)
Strawberry latent ringspot virus (SLRV)/SLRV sat-RNA	1118 nt (~36 kDa)
Tomato black ring virus (TBRV)/TBRV sat-RNA	1372–1375 nt (~48 kDa)
Potexvirus	
Bamboo mosaic virus (BaMV)/BaMV sat-RNA	836 nt (~20 kDa)
Small linear ss sat-RNAs	
Carmovirus	
Turnip crinkle virus (TCV)/TCV sat-RNA	194 nt, 230 nt, 356 nt
Cucumovirus	
Cucumber mosaic virus (CMV)/CMV sat-RNA	333–405 nt
Peanut stunt virus (PSV)/PSV sat-RNA	393 nt
Robinia mosaic virus (RbMV)/RbMV sat-RNA	~390 nt
Umbravirus	
Pea enation mosaic virus (PEMV)/PEMV sat-RNA	717 nt
Necrovirus	
Tobacco necrosis virus (TNV)/TNV small sat-RNA	620 nt
Nepovirus	
Chicory yellow mottle virus (CYMV)/CYMV small sat-RNA	457 nt
Tombusvirus	
Artichoke mottled crinkle virus (AMCV)/AMCV sat-RNA	~700 nt
Cymbidium ringspot virus (CymRSV)/CymRSV sat-RNA	621 nt
Carnation Italian ringspot virus (CIRV)/CIRV sat-RNA	~700 nt
Pelargonium leaf curl virus (PLCV)/PLCV sat-RNA	~700 nt
Petunia asteroid mosaic virus (PAMV)/PAMV sat-RNA	~700 nt
Tomato bushy stunt virus (TBSV)/TBSV sat-RNA	612 nt, 822 nt
Circular ss sat-RNAs	
Polerovirus	
Barley yellow dwarf virus (BYDV-RPV)/BYDV-RPV sat-RNA	322 nt
Nepovirus	
Arabis mosaic virus (ArMV)/ArMV small sat-RNA	~300 nt
Tobacco ringspot virus (TRSV)/TRSV sat-RNA	359 nt
Sobemovirus	
Lucerne transient streak virus (LTSV)/LTSV sat-RNA	324 nt
Rice yellow mottle virus (RYMV)/RYMV sat-RNA	~210 nt
Solanum nodiflorum mottle virus (SNMV)/SNMV sat-RNA	377 nt
Subterranean clover mottle virus (SCMV)/SCMV sat-RNA	332 nt, 388 nt
Velvet tobacco mottle virus (VTMoV)/VTMoV sat-RNA	365 nt–366 nt

[a] NR, not reported.

Table 3 Related subviral agents

Helper virus/satellite-like RNA/subviral agent	Size of satellite-like RNA/subviral agent (MW of encoded protein)
Satellite-like ssRNAs (dependent on a helper virus for replication and encapsidation, but essential for vector transmission of a helper)	
Umbravirus	
Groundnut rosette virus (GRV)/GRV sat-RNA	895–903 nt
Benyvirus	
Beet necrotic yellow vein virus (BNYVV)/	
BNYVV RNA3	1774 nt ($\sim$25 kDa)
BNYVV RNA4	1467 nt ($\sim$31 kDa)
BNYVV RNA5	1342–1347 nt ($\sim$26 kDa)
Agents dependent on a helper virus for encapsidation but not for replication	
Hepadnavirus	
Hepatitis B virus (HBV)/	
Hepatitis delta virus (HDV)	1679 nt ($\sim$22 kDa; δAg-S) (δAgS+19 aa; δAg-L)
Luteovirus	
Beet western yellows virus (BWYV)/BWYV-associated RNA ST9	2843 nt ($\sim$85 kDa) + several others

General Properties of Satellites and their Effects on Helper Virus and Host Plants

The satellite viruses

Satellite viruses occur as nucleoprotein particles that are morphologically and serologically distinct from their helper viruses. No serological relationships were found between different satellite viruses except between satellite panicum mosaic virus (SPMV) and satellite St Augustine decline virus (SSADV), the helper viruses of which, PMV and SADV, respectively, are closely related. All known satellite viruses including CPVA contain ssRNAs between 800 and 1200 nucleotides (nt). Particles of all known satellite viruses are isometric and are 17 nm in diameter. Whereas helper viruses of most satellite viruses also have isometric particles, the helper virus of satellite tobacco mosaic virus (STMV) has rod-shaped particles.

Subgroup I The most studied of satellite viruses are plant virus satellites belonging to subgroup I. The three-dimensional structures of STNV, STMV and SPMV have been determined at high resolution by x-ray crystallography. The shell of all these satellite viruses is composed of 60 protein subunits. Most satellite virus RNAs are presumably monocistronic. The CP is the sole product of *in vitro* translation of the STNV, satellite maize white line mosaic virus (SMWLMV) and SPMV RNAs, although the last contains several additional open reading frames (ORFs) which are untranslatable *in vitro*. However, in the case of STMV, in addition to the CP, another product of about 6.8 kDa is produced during *in vitro* translation, although it remains unclear if this product is functionally active.

Although the STNV CP is not related to that of the helper virus, TNV, both particles bind specifically to the surface of zoospores of the fungal vector *Olpidium brassicae*. The replication of STNV inhibits that of TNV and the extent of the inhibition depends on the particular combination of strains of STNV and TNV. A second satellite RNA of about 620 nt has been detected in STNV particles. It is distinct from STNV RNA, in that it has no messenger RNA activity, but still depends on TNV for replication. Therefore this RNA may be considered as a satellite of TNV for replication, and a satellite of STNV for encapsidation (**Table 1**).

The effect of the multiplication of SPMV on the accumulation of its helper, PMV, is unknown, but it is known that the presence of SPMV alters the mild mosaic symptoms induced by PMV in maize to severe mosaic and necrosis. On the other hand, no differences in symptomatology have been observed between isolates of MWLMV or TMV containing or lacking satellite viruses.

Subgroup II Less is known about satellite viruses belonging to the subgroup II (**Table 1**). RNA of CPVA satellite virus consists of three species, each about 1.1 kb, which are distinct from CPV helper RNA, although some T1 oligonucleotides appear in common between CPV and CPVA RNA. The satellite virus interferes with CPV replication.

Satellite nucleic acids

ss Satellite DNAs This category comprises tomato leaf curl virus (TLCV) satellite DNA with a circular ssDNA genome, which does not encode a satellite CP (**Table 2**). The 682 nt DNA contains no ORFs and shows little sequence similarity to the helper virus genome, limited to two short motifs present in two separate stem–loop structures. One of these motifs is universal for all geminiviruses, and the other motif is identical to a replication-associated protein binding site in TLCV. The satellite DNA is strictly dependent on the helper virus replication-associated protein and is encapsidated by TLCV CP. Replication of TLCV satellite DNA is also supported by other taxonomically distinct geminiviruses, including African cassava mosaic virus and beet curly top virus.

ds Satellite RNAs These RNAs have been found in association with viruses of the family *Totiviridae*. The dsRNA range from 0.5 kb to 1.8 kb and are encapsidated by the helper virus CP. These particles often also contain a positive-sense ssRNA copy of the dsRNA. The presence of satellites in helper virus cultures can affect markedly the virulence of the helper virus infection. This category comprises the M satellites of L-A dsRNA virus of *Saccharomyces cerevisiae* and satellites of *Trichomonas vaginalis* virus (TVV) (**Table 2**).

Some strains of *S. cerevisiae* secrete a protein toxin that is lethal to other strains, but not to the toxin-secreting strain, which is said to be immune or resistant. The protein responsible both for the killer phenotype and for immunity to the toxin (in the form of the prototoxin) is encoded by M_1, a dsRNA satellite of the major yeast dsRNA virus L-A. Several other satellite dsRNAs of L-A, each encoding a toxin-immunity system, have been described and are called M_2, M_3, M_{28}, etc. The family of these satellites comprises dsRNAs, varying from ca. 1.0 kb to 1.8 kb. These RNAs completely depend on the helper virus (L-A) encoded proteins Gag and Gag-Pol for encapsidation and replication. In addition, a strict dependence of M_1 satellite multiplication on host chromosomal genes has also been described. M_1 needs 30 so-called *MAK* (maintenance of killer) genes, of which only three are required by the helper virus L-A. The M_1 satellite represses the copy number of the L-A helper virus.

Another series of dsRNA satellites is associated with a virus infected with a sexually transmitted protozoan, *T. vaginalis* (TVV). Three different dsRNA satellites of TVV have been found, containing approximately 500 bp, 700 bp and 1700 bp. All these RNAs are synthesized conditionally and are present in only some *T. vaginalis* isolates harboring the virus, which seems to replicate and encapsidate them.

ss Satellite RNAs This is the most numerous group of known satellites. The ss satellite RNAs range in size from just under 200 nt to approximately 1500 nt. The larger satellite RNAs appear to contain functional ORFs, although as yet no precise function has been assigned to any of their gene products. Small ss satellite RNAs do not appear to encode any functional ORFs, but tend to be highly structured. Small ss satellite RNAs may be either linear or circular. Despite their small size and the usual absence of any potential products, these ss satellite RNAs may have a dramatic effect on the symptoms induced by their helper virus, ranging from amelioration to severe exacerbation. These symptom effects vary with the helper virus, host plant, and satellite.

Subgroup I: Large ss Satellite RNAs with Messenger RNA Properties The most studied of this type of satellite RNAs is that of the nepoviruses (**Table 2**). These satellite RNAs, ranging in size from approximately 1100 to 1500 nt, resemble the genomic RNA of their helper viruses in that they have a 3′-terminal poly(A) sequence and a 5′-terminal genome-linked protein (VPg). The VPgs of satellite RNAs of tomato black ring virus (TBRV), arabis mosaic virus (ArMV) and grapevine fanleaf virus (GFLV) are indistinguishable from those attached to the helper virus genome RNA and therefore must be encoded by the helper virus genome. These satellites encode a nonstructural protein with M_r ranging from 36 to 48 kDa, which at least in some cases, such as in TBRV, GFLV and ArMV satellites, has been shown to be essential for satellite RNA replication. Comparison of amino acid sequences of proteins encoded by different satellite RNAs of nepoviruses revealed several domains: the terminal regions are strongly basic, most notably the N-terminal region, and the central region contains both basic and acidic residues. The satellite-encoded proteins are also relatively rich in cysteine and histidine residues, mostly in the 3′-terminal halves. It has been suggested that these proteins may be involved in adapting the helper virus replicase to the satellite RNA. The most characteristic biological property of these RNAs is that the symptoms induced by infection with the helper virus are only slightly or not at all affected by the presence of the satellite RNA. TBRV, strawberry latent ringspot virus (SLRV), chicory yellow mottle virus (CYMV) and GFLV satellite RNAs induce no changes in the symptoms induced by the helper virus. However, in the case of the large ArMV satellite RNA, the satellite RNA was found to exacerbate symptoms in three species and ameliorate symptoms in ten species out of 42 plant species tested. The large satellite RNAs of nepoviruses have little or no effect on the accumulation of their helper viruses, even in plants in which satellite RNA enhanced or ameliorated the symptoms of ArMV infection.

Another large ssRNA satellite which may be included in this category is associated with the potexvirus bamboo mosaic virus (BaMV). This RNA is a linear molecule of 836 nt [excluding the poly(A) tail] and like other satellite RNAs is encapsidated by the CP of its helper virus. However, it differs from all other known satellites in that the RNA is encapsidated into rod-shaped particles. The BaMV satellite RNA contains an ORF for a protein of 183 amino acids (20 kDa). This protein shares 46% sequence identity with the CP amino acid sequence of SPMV (see above). The ORF for the BaMV satellite RNA appears to be translated *in vitro* and *in vivo*. However, the encoded protein is not essential for satellite RNA replication. The presence of the BaMV satellite RNA caused a reduction of BaMV genomic RNA accumulation, in the range 65–85%.

Subgroup II: small linear ssRNAs This subgroup comprises the satellites with genomes less than 0.8 kb (**Table 2**). No circular molecules are present in infected cells. Some of these satellites contain potential ORFs, but the evidence indicates that there are no *in vivo* functions for these ORFs. Although small satellite RNAs of some cucumber mosaic virus (CMV) strains have been shown to direct the synthesis of protein products *in vitro*, these ORFs are not conserved among different isolates. Moreover, neither mutagenesis of the 5′-proximal initiation codon in a biologically active cDNA clone nor a frameshift mutation of the ORFs altered the biological activity of CMV satellite RNAs. Other small, linear, ssRNA satellites also do not appear to encode functional proteins, and hence the biological functions of these satellite RNAs must rely on the nucleotide sequence and the corresponding secondary structure. The small satellite RNAs have highly ordered secondary structures. The small size and high degree of secondary structure are probably responsible for the high stability and survivability of satellites both *in vitro* and *in vivo*. The latter may in turn account for the highly infectious nature of many satellite RNAs.

Small RNA satellites can dramatically alter the symptoms induced by the helper virus. The alterations can be either an attenuation or an exacerbation of the virus-induced symptoms. Some satellite RNAs of CMV can ameliorate the symptoms induced by the helper virus on one host and intensify them on another host. The symptom modulation can also be affected by the particular strain of helper virus. Thus, a three-factor interaction involving the particular satellite, the strain of helper virus, and the species of host determines the type of host response. In most cases, satellites attenuate the symptoms. Exacerbation of symptoms is much rarer. Attenuation of symptoms is usually accompanied by a reduction in the virus titer. This has led to the suggestion that the competition for the replicase between the satellite and helper virus genomes results in a reduction in the concentration of the helper virus elicitor of host pathogenesis. However, it has also been shown that the chimeric satellite RNA of TCV may inhibit movement of the virus helper (rather than replication), thus reducing its accumulation and symptom expression; the CP of TCV is involved in this type of interaction. However, in some other satellite virus: helper combinations [for example CMV satellite RNA and the helper tomato aspermy virus (TAV)], a reduction in pathogenicity was not accompanied by a reduction in the titer of the helper virus. Thus, more than one mechanism may be responsible for satellite RNA-mediated symptom attenuation.

A few satellites exacerbate the symptoms induced by the helper virus. Of these, the best characterized are the satellite RNAs of CMV. Examples of symptom intensification include chlorosis on tobacco (and pepper), chlorosis on tomato, and necrosis on tomato. As in the case of satellite-mediated symptom attenuation, there might be different mechanisms for symptom intensification. One of them may be based on the interaction of the satellite RNA with a helper virus-encoded product. Chlorosis and some forms of necrosis involve interaction between specific regions (pathogenicity domains) of CMV satellite RNA and a factor(s) derived from CMV RNA 2, i.e. either the encoded 2a or 2b proteins or RNA 2 itself. In addition, whereas interactions between certain satellite RNAs and either RNA 2 or the 2a protein induce severe pathogenic responses in some host species, on other plant species the same combinations attenuate symptoms. The host component(s) involved in the above interactions is (are) clearly a crucial factor. Another possible mechanism of symptom exacerbation seems to involve direct interaction between the pathogenicity domain in the negative strand of the CMV satellite RNA with some helper component(s) without essential contribution from a helper virus.

Subgroup III: small circular ss satellite RNAs This subgroup comprises satellites with genomes that contain about 350 nt and occur as circular as well as linear molecules (**Table 2**). Replication of some has been shown to involve self-cleavage of linear, multimeric, progeny molecules by an RNA-catalyzed reaction. The helper viruses of these satellite RNAs come from three different genera. The sobemoviruses specifically encapsidate the circular satellites (these satellites have been referred to as virusoids in some of the literature because of their structural resemblance to viroids and the erroneous, premature conclusion that they were essential for the replication of the helper virus). Members of the other two virus genera (*Nepovirus* and *Polerovirus*) encapsidate the linear form of the satellite RNA. However, the circular forms, which are essential for rolling circle replication (see below), can be found in infected tissues. As with small, linear satellite RNAs, circular satellites do not display messenger RNA activity, although some short ORFs are detected in the genomes of some of these circular satellites. The effect on symptoms induced by helper viruses may vary from attenuation to exacerbation, as in the case of small, linear, satellite RNAs. Satellite RNAs of TRSV generally reduce the titer of the helper virus as well as the severity of TRSV-induced symptoms. The satellite RNA of barley yellow dwarf virus (BYDV)-RPV (Rho-palosiphum padi virus) also reduces the accumulation of the helper virus and attenuates symptoms. By contrast, circular satellite RNAs of sobemoviruses, such as velvet tobacco mottle virus (VTMoV) sat-RNA, greatly enhance the severity of symptoms induced by the helper virus.

Satellite related agents

Satellite-like ssRNAs Two examples have been reported of RNA molecules which have many similarities to satellites and are not required for mechanical transmission/infection of the helper virus; however, in contrast to the true satellites these RNAs are required for the natural infection of the helper virus (**Table 3**). One of these, GRV (an umbravirus) ss satellite-like RNA, contains 895–903 nt. This RNA relies on GRV for its replication, but it is needed in addition to groundnut rosette assistor virus (a luteovirus) for aphid transmission of GRV. Therefore, it is essential for the survival of GRV in nature and is thus regarded as a satellite-like RNA. This RNA shares no significant sequence similarity with the GRV genomic RNA and does not code any functional proteins. It is the satellite-like RNA that is largely responsible for the symptoms of groundnut rosette. The GRV satellite contains two nontranslatable elements involved in symptom induction. Symptoms produced by different GRV satellites are independent of the helper GRV isolate, and indeed indistinguishable symptoms are produced when a different virus, pea enation mosaic virus (PEMV) is substituted for GRV as a helper virus. Thus it seems that this RNA may induce symptoms itself without an essential contribution from the GRV helper. Normally, satellite-like RNA isolates of GRV do not affect the accumulation of GRV genomic and subgenomic RNAs in infected plants, but a few, so-called mild GRV satellites have been identified that drastically diminish the replication of the helper GRV in infected or transgenic plants. Sequence alignment revealed striking similarities between GRV satellite-like RNAs and a true satellite RNA of PEMV, belonging to the subgroup II of small, ss, linear, satellite RNAs.

Although beet necrotic yellow vein virus (BNYVV) (a benyvirus) has a bipartite RNA genome, field isolates of BNYVV have two or three additional satellite-like RNAs of which RNA 3 (1774 nt) and RNA 4 (1467 nt) are essential for spread in root tissues and transmission by the fungal vector of the virus, respectively (**Table 3**). However RNA 5 (1342–1347 nt) of BNYVV may be a true satellite RNA, since it is not essential for spread of the virus in nature. The satellite-like RNA 3 has been also implicated in symptom expression (rhizomania). The 25 kDa protein encoded by the longest ORF of the RNA 3 is probably needed for symptom production. Another ORF, ORF N, which is translationally silent on full-length RNA 3 but is translationally activated by a long, internal deletion, may also contribute to symptom production in some hosts. RNA 4 also contains a long ORF encoding a potential 31 kDa protein, although it is not clear if it is essential for the functional activity of RNA 4. RNA 5 can intensify the severity of symptoms induced by BNYVV, and a 26 kDa protein encoded by this RNA may be important for the expression of symptoms.

Other satellite related agents *Hepatitis Delta Virus (HDV)* HDV is a subviral, human pathogen that propagates only in the presence of its helper. With this helper, HDV can replicate most efficiently in hepatocytes and can greatly increase the severity of liver damage caused by a hepatitis B virus (HBV) infection. The replication of HDV genome takes place in the nuclei of infected cells. The host RNA polymerase II (that usually directs DNA-dependent RNA synthesis) is probably responsible for this RNA-directed transcriptional event in infected cells, which is independent of the hepadnavirus helper. Therefore, by definition, HDV is not a satellite. However, HDV is dependent on the envelope proteins of the helper virus required for the assembly and release of infectious virions. The HDV genome is a single-stranded, circular, 1679 nt RNA that folds into an unbranched rod-like structure in which 70% of its nucleotides are paired. This genomic RNA exists both within virions and in infected nuclei as a ribonucleoprotein (RNP), which contains the only protein encoded by HDV, the delta antigen. Two forms of this antigen are observed during infection. The small delta antigen (δAg-S), a 22 kDa nuclear phosphoprotein, is synthesized early and is required for replication to occur. Later in infection, a specific RNA-editing event leads to the mutation of the δAg-S termination codon and the synthesis of the large antigen, δAg-L, which contains an additional 19 amino acids at its C-terminus. δAg-L acts as a potent inhibitor of HDV genome replication and in combination with δAg-S promotes the assembly of the HDV RNP into HBV envelope particles.

Beet western yellows virus (BWYV)-associated RNA The ST9 strain of BWYV encapsidates not only the 5.6 kb genomic RNA that is typical of luteoviruses, but also a ss, linear 2843 nt-associated RNA (ST9aRNA), which has a distinct nucleotide sequence. The ST9aRNA was postulated to be a satellite RNA. However, this RNA has been shown to be able to replicate without a helper virus. Thus, ST9aRNA is an infectious, subviral agent of plants which depends on its associated virus, BWYV (ST9 strain), for encapsidation but not for replication. Plants infected with BWYV containing the ST9aRNA exhibit a more severe symptom phenotype and contain ~10-fold more virions than do plants infected with BWYV containing no ST9aRNA. The ST9aRNA contains three large ORFs, which, at least *in vitro*, can be translated to yield several products, the largest of which is ~85 kDa, derived from various combinations of readthrough of the three ORFs. The deduced amino acid sequence of two regions of an 85 kDa protein contain significant homology with the RNA-dependent RNA polymerase of carmoviruses.

Structure and Replication of Satellite RNA

Information on secondary structure and replication mechanisms has been obtained mostly for ss satellite RNAs. These small satellite RNAs have highly ordered secondary structures with base pairing up to 73%. The small size and high degree of secondary structure are probably responsible for the high stability, survivability and infectivity of many satellites. As mentioned above, small satellite RNAs may strongly modify symptoms induced by their helper viruses. The sequences involved in pathogenicity are located in discrete small domains. For example, in the case of the CMV satellite RNAs, distinct RNA elements, present in the positive or negative strands, may program chlorosis induction in tobacco and tomato or necrosis in tomato.

RNAs of some satellites can form a tRNA-like domain similar to some plant virus RNAs. For example, the 3' end of the STMV RNA folds into a tRNA-like structure similar to that in TMV RNA. Accordingly, functional assays have shown that STMV RNA can be aminoacylated *in vitro* with histidine as is the case for TMV. The biological implications of these observations remains unknown.

Satellites are dependent on their helper viruses for replication. The helper virus in turn is dependent on the host plant to supply some components necessary for replication, and thus a complex three-way interaction between satellite, helper virus and plant host is required for satellite replication. The specificity of satellite replication occurs at the level of both the helper virus and the host plant species. With the satellite RNAs of TRSV and CMV, the apparent level of satellite replication varies widely with the strain of helper virus. In addition, related viruses may or may not replicate the same satellite RNAs. For example, most satellite RNA isolates of CMV are replicated efficiently by the related cucumovirus, TAV, but not by another cucumovirus, peanut stunt virus (PSV). Moreover, PSV satellite RNA replication is not supported by CMV. In addition to the helper virus specificity, the host plant often plays a significant role in the efficiency of satellite replication. The small satellite RNA of ArMV replicates very efficiently in *Chenopodium quinoa*. By contrast, the large satellite RNA of another nepovirus, TBRV, replicates poorly in *C. quinoa*, but replicates very efficiently in *Nicotiana clevelandii*. Replication of satellite RNAs has been presumed to occur using the replicase of the helper virus. However, satellite RNA replication does not always involve the same mechanism as replication of the viral RNAs, and it seems likely that other factors which are specific for satellite replication are involved. For large satellite RNAs associated with nepoviruses, the satellite RNA-encoded proteins may function as such factors interacting and modifying the helper virus replication complex. In the case of noncoding, linear, satellite RNAs like the CMV or TRSV satellites, such factor(s) might be host component(s).

Circular, ss, RNA satellites are replicated by a rolling circle mechanism. The replication cycle involves the copying of the encapsidated circular plus (+) strand by an RNA-dependent RNA polymerase to yield a longer than unit length minus (−) strand, which in most cases can self-cleave to yield monomeric products. (For satellite RNAs present in virions as linear molecules this stage is preceded by a ligation of (+) linear molecules to yield a circular (+) strand.) Then, these (−) RNA monomers are circularized and copied to produce a multimeric, linear (+) strand, which self-cleaves to form linear (+) monomers, which then self-ligate to form circular satellite RNAs. For those multimeric (−) RNAs which are not processed (e.g. satellites of some sobemoviruses), the multimeric (−) RNA is copied to give a multimeric (+) strand which then undergoes cleavage to monomers. The (+) RNA monomers are either circularized and then encapsidated in the circular form (as in the case of sobemovirus satellite RNAs), or packaged as a linear form [as in the case of the BYDV-RPV satellite RNA (a luteovirus), and the small nepovirus satellite RNAs]. Replication of HDV RNA also occurs via a rolling circle mechanism and self-cleaving reactions. HDV is the only animal pathogenic RNA which replicates via a rolling circle mechanism.

There are two types of ribozyme structure found in satellite RNAs possessing self-cleavage activity: the hammerhead and the hairpin ribozymes. Hammerhead structures have been identified in both (+) and (−) RNA strands of lucerne transient streak virus (LTSV) (a sobemovirus) and BYDV-RPV (a luteovirus), as well as in the (+) strands of small satellite RNAs of nepoviruses. Hairpin structures have been found in (−) strands of small nepoviruses. The HDV RNA also contains self-cleaving sequences. However, these appear different from hammerhead and hairpin ribozymes.

Sequence Variation, Evolution, Origins

Some sequence variants of plant satellite viruses (in particular STMV, STNV and SSADV) as well as plant satellite RNAs (predominantly satellite RNAs of CMV and TRSV) have been described. The STNV and CMV satellite RNAs exhibit differences in biological properties, often in a particular host. The large number of CMV satellite RNA isolates sequenced has been used to establish the evolutionary relationships between different groups of CMV satellite RNAs and to demonstrate the presence of structural constraints on satellite RNA evolution. In the case of CMV satellite RNAs, the actual evolution of satellite RNAs in the greenhouse as well as in the field has been observed, as a function of passage with different helper virus strain.

Nothing is known about the origin of satellite RNAs. Limited sequence similarity was observed between one satellite RNA of CMV and chloroplast RNA sequences, and between a satellite RNA of CMV and the potato spindle tuber viroid.

Strategies for Virus Control

The ability of satellite to attenuate the disease symptoms induced by their helper viruses has led to the suggestion that satellite may be useful as biological control agents of pathogenic molecules. Two approaches to test the viral control potential of satellite have been used. In the first approach, the application of mild strains of CMV containing satellite RNA to greenhouse and field crops has been evaluated. In several cases, CMV containing satellite RNA are able to protect plants to various extents against infection by more virulent strains. In the second approach, transgenic plants expressing CMV satellite RNA, TRSV satellite RNA, or GRV satellite-like RNA sequences were found to be either resistant or tolerant to virus infection. Moreover, plants expressing CMV satellite RNA sequences are also resistant to potato spindle tuber viroid, with which CMV satellite RNA shares some similarity.

Further Reading

Colmer CW and Howel SH (1992) Role of satellite RNA in the expression of symptoms caused by plant viruses. *Annu. Rev. Phytopathol.* 30: 419.

Roossinck MJ, Sleat D and Palukaitis P (1992) Satellite RNAs of plant viruses: structures and biological effects. *Microbiol. Rev.* 56: 265.

Symons RH (1997) Plant pathogenic RNAs and RNA catalysis. *Nucleic Acids Res.* 25: 2683.

S13m Bacteriophage see Coliphage ϕX174 and Related Phages (*Microviridae*)

San Miguel Sea Lion Virus see Caliciviruses

Scrapie see Prions

Semliki Forest Virus see Sindbis and Semliki Forest Viruses

SENDAI VIRUS (*PARAMYXOVIRIDAE*)

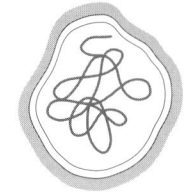

Morio Homma, Department of Home Economics, Kobe Women's University, Kobe, Japan

Masato Tashiro, Department of Viral Diseases and Vaccine Control, National Institute of Infectious Diseases, Tokyo, Japan

Copyright © 1999 Academic Press

History

Sendai virus was first discovered in 1952 by Kuroya, Ishida and Shiratori at Tohoku University Hospital, Sendai, Japan, during an epidemic of fatal pneumonitis among newborn babies. A new virus with hemagglutinating activity antigenically different from known influenza viruses was recovered from mice inoculated with the autopsied lung tissues. The virus was originally named newborn pneumonitis virus, type Sendai. However, the question soon arose as to the causative agent of human disease because this virus was reported to be widely spread among laboratory rodents and pigs in Japan at that time. Since then, Sendai virus has been shown to prevail worldwide and to cause enzootic or epizootic infections in mice and rats. Sendai virus was designated hemagglutinating virus of Japan (HVJ) in 1955 by the Society of Japanese Virologists. Later, Sendai virus was shown to be related to human parainfluenza virus type 1, isolated by Chanock in 1955 and named hemadsorption virus type 2 (HA2). As Sendai virus causes a respiratory infection in mice, this virus–animal system has been widely investigated in pathogenesis and immunology as a suitable model of respiratory viral infections. Okada's finding of cell fusion by Sendai virus in 1958 has developed a new field of cell biology, e.g. the production of hybrid cells such as heterokaryons and hybridomas. Proteolytic activation of the fusion glycoprotein was first described for Sendai virus by Homma and Ohuchi in 1973. Additionally, most of the information on the molecular biology of paramyxoviruses has been obtained from studies on Sendai virus, the prototype of the family *Paramyxoviridae*. Recently, a reverse genetics technology to recover infectious viral particles from a cDNA copy of the Sendai virus genome was developed by Kato, by which any mutant viruses could be obtained.

Taxonomy and Classification

Sendai virus belongs to the genus *Respirovirus* in the subfamily *Paramyxovirinae* of the family *Paramyxoviridae* of RNA viruses. Based on serological relationships, Sendai virus is assigned to a murine subtype of human parainfluenza virus type 1, the classification being supported by phylogenetic analyses of the genome nucleotide sequences among paramyxoviruses.

Properties of Virion and Genome

The virions are pleomorphic in size and shape. They are roughly spherical and 150–250 nm in diameter but larger particles are common. The particles consist of a nucleocapsid with helical symmetry (18 nm in width, 1 μm in length), which is enclosed by a lipid envelope derived from host cell plasma membrane. The nucleocapsid is composed of a nonsegmented, linear, negative-stranded genomic RNA (15 384 nucleotides) containing six genes, covalently linked in tandem, and associated proteins NP, P and L (**Fig. 1**). The envelope contains protein M beneath the inner layer, and two spike-like projections, composed of tetramers of glycoprotein HN and trimers of glycoprotein F, respectively. They penetrate the lipid bilayer beyond the outer surface to make the fuzzy appearance of the envelope surface when viewed by electron microscopy. The NP protein (58 kDa), bound directly to the genomic RNA, is the major structural component of the nucleocapsid. Proteins P (72 kDa) and L (255 kDa) act in concert as RNA polymerase complexes with transcriptase and replicase activities. The P–NP complex functions to encapsidate the RNA genome. The C and V proteins, nonstructural proteins and possible minor virion components encoded by overlapping reading frames within the P gene region, are not essential for viral replication but

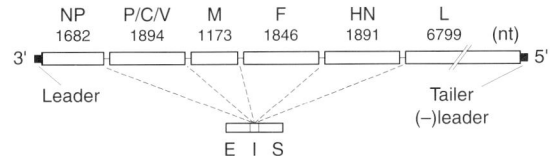

Figure 1 Sendai virus genome RNA. The extragenetic 3'-terminal leader and the complementary 5'-tailer regions are shown by bold lines. The conserved transcription regulatory sequences (E, end; I, intergenic; S, start) are located at the gene boundaries.

appear to regulate mRNA transcription and genome replication. The M protein (40 kDa) has a dual affinity for the NP protein and the cytoplasmic domain of the glycoproteins and plays an important role in the virus assembly process. The larger glycoprotein HN (68 kDa) has receptor binding, hemagglutinating and neuraminidase activities, while the smaller glycoprotein F (63 kDa), when proteolytically cleaved into disulfide-linked F_1 and F_2 subunits, has membrane fusing and hemolytic activities and mediates virus entry through envelope fusion.

Replication

In common with other paramyxoviruses, virus replication takes place exclusively in the cytoplasm and does not require DNA synthesis of host cells. A one-step replication cycle takes about 12–15 h and one infected cell usually yields thousands of progeny viral particles.

Virus Entry

The HN glycoprotein mediates attachment of viral particle to the sialic acid-containing receptors on the carbohydrate side chains of the glycoproteins or glycolipids of host cell surface. After adsorption, the F ($F_1 + F_2$) glycoprotein mediates, at neutral pH, an envelope fusion between the viral envelope and the plasma membrane, by which the nucleocapsid is introduced into the cytoplasm to initiate the primary transcription catalyzed by the virion-associated RNA polymerase complexes.

Characterization of Transcription

Transcription of the genome RNA to synthesize mRNA occurs in the cytoplasm, for which host factors, e.g. tubulin, are required. The genomic RNA consists of the leader sequence at the 3' end and the related tailer sequence at the 5' end. There is a tandem set of six genes ordered NP, P/C/V, M, F, HN and L, and bound by the consensus transcriptional regulatory sequences for the poly(A) initiation site (E), intergenic (I) and a gene start sequence (S). The P–L polymerase complexes associated with the nucleocapsid catalyze the primary transcription to synthesize monocistronic mRNA species, with adding poly(A) tail at the 3' end, corresponding to each polypeptide. Several polycistronic mRNAs may also be synthesized by reading through the stop signals at the intergenic sequence. The P/C/V gene encodes the P mRNA of the complementary copy of the genomic RNA, from which the P protein is translated. The C protein, a small basic protein, is also translated from a (+1) open reading frame in the 5' end region of the P mRNA by internal translational initiation at another site. In addition to the P gene transcript, a second mRNA species is synthesized by RNA editing, with insertion of an additional G residue not coded by the genome at the specific editing site, resulting in a frameshift downwards. The second mRNA encodes the V protein, a hybrid protein with the N-terminus half of the P protein and a new reading frame downwards for a cysteine-rich C-terminus region. The secondary transcription is catalyzed by the RNA polymerase complexes of the viral proteins newly synthesized in infected cells.

Characterization of Translation

Each monocystronic mRNA translates a corresponding polypeptide. With the P mRNA, however, four nonstructural proteins (C, C', Y_1, and Y_2) are synthesized from reading frames overlapping the P gene using different initiation codons by ribosomal scanning. The glycoproteins HN and F are synthesized on membrane-bound polysomes and subjected to post-translational processing.

Post-translational Processing

The F protein, a type I membrane protein, is translated and inserted into the membrane of the rough endoplasmic reticulum by the signal peptide at the N-terminus, which is removed after insertion. On the other hand, the HN is a type II membrane protein anchored to the lipid bilayer at a hydrophobic region in the N-terminus. Both proteins are glycosylated and during transport to the smooth endoplasmic reticulum the carbohydrate side-chains are processed to mature forms. The HN polypeptide forms homotetramers, a pair of disulfide-linked dimers, while the F polypeptide forms homotrimers by noncovalent bonds.

This precursor form of F glycoprotein is biologically inactive, and gains the fusion activity by proteolytic cleavage into the disulfide-linked subunits, F_1 and F_2 (**Fig. 2**). The cleavage site of the F protein,

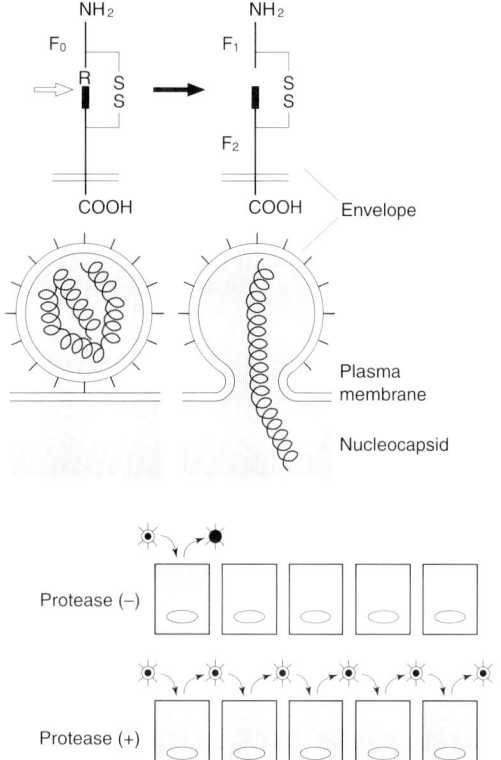

Figure 2 Proteolytic activation of Sendai virus F glycoprotein and infectivity. Upper panel: Sendai virus infects target cells through envelope fusion between viral envelope and plasma membrane. Sendai virus possessing the precursor F_0 is noninfectious. Proteolytic cleavage of F_0 by an activating protease at residue 116-arginine (indicated by open arrow) into disulfide-linked subunits, F_1 and F_2, results in the exposure of hydrophobic fusion-inducing domain (shown by bold lines), which is required for membrane fusion activity and infectivity. Lower panel: Sendai virus can undergo multiple cycles of replication and show pathogenicity in tissues where suitable activating protease(s) is present. Open circles indicate activated (infectious) virus particles and closed circle indicates nonactive (noninfectious) particle.

consisting of a single arginine residue, is not cleavable by ubiquitous cellular proteases present in the trans-Golgi region that cleave preferentially dibasic or multibasic motifs. Accordingly, Sendai virus produced in most tissue culture cells possesses uncleaved F protein and remains nonactive, lacking cell fusion and hemolytic activities and infectivity. These activities are restored by *in vitro* treatment of the virus with trypsin, blood clotting factor Xa in the chorioallantoic fluid of chicken eggs, and tryptase Clara, a serine protease secreted by Clara cells of rat bronchial epithelia. By contrast, progeny virus is recovered in the activated form in several host cells or tissues, such as the chorioallantoic membrane of chick embryos, primary monkey kidney cells and mouse lungs. In these cases, the cleavage of F protein takes place extracellularly by secreted host proteases which cleave the single arginine residue of the F protein.

Strategy of RNA Replication

Replication of the genome RNA is mediated by polymerase complexes composed of the gene products of the primary transcripts, P, L and probably some of the nonstructural proteins. The NP proteins assembled with the genomic RNA also interact with the replication complexes. The leader sequence at the 3' end and the tailer sequence at the 5' end of the genomic RNA are required for genome replication. The C protein appears to regulate the switch between mRNA transcription and genome replication. Genome replication provides templates for secondary transcription and for further amplification of the genome, and finally supplies the mature progeny genome for incorporation into virus particles. The entire nucleotide sequence of the negative-stranded genomic RNA is copied complementarily to the antigenomic positive-stranded RNA that serves as an intermediate template for the synthesis of progeny genome RNA. Subgenomic RNA species are frequently synthesized and incorporated into viral particles producing defective-interfering (DI) particles.

Assembly and Release

The progeny genome RNA is combined with the NP protein to form a helical structure to which the P and L proteins are incorporated to form the assembled nucleocapsid. The glycoproteins F and HN are transported through the Golgi apparatus to the cytoplasmic membrane, where they replace host membrane proteins. In polarized epithelial cells, the glycoproteins are transported to the apical membrane domain, where virus assembly occurs. The M protein accumulates beneath the cytoplasmic domain of the glycoproteins and binds the glycoprotein tails with the nucleocapsid. Viral particles are then assembled by budding with incorporation of the lipid bilayer of the host plasma membrane to form the viral envelope. Cellular actin, which is incorporated into the envelope, plays a role in the budding process. The neuraminidase residing on the HN glycoprotein facilitates the release of viral particles from infected cells by destroying cellular receptors.

Cytopathology

Sendai virus usually produces a lytic-type cytopathic effect, which is associated with disruption of the cytoskeletal systems likely caused by the M protein. Apoptotic cytolysis is also reported with Sendai virus-infected cells. Since the F protein is not activated in ordinary tissue culture cells, syncytial formation mediated by 'fusion from within' is not observed, unless trypsin is added to the culture medium. Inhibition of cellular RNA or protein synthesis is not remarkable. Sendai virus can set up a variety of persistent infections in tissue culture cells without killing infected cells.

Cell Fusion

Sendai virus causes cell fusion and produces multinuclear giant cells. The F protein is directly responsible for the fusion activity for which proteolytic activation is required. Coincidence of the HN glycoprotein is specifically required for inducing cell fusion. Cell fusion falls into two categories: 'fusion from without (FFWO)' and 'fusion from within (FFWI)'. FFWO occurs in cells within a few hours after infection at high multiplicity of virus infection and does not require virus replication. FFWO has been used for producing hybrid cells, such as heterokaryons and hybridomas, and for introducing macromolecules into cells. On the other hand, FFWI occurs late in the replication cycle and is mediated by, in concert with the HN glycoprotein, the F protein synthesized in infected cells and expressed at the cell surface in the activated form.

Geographic Distribution

Retrospective serological surveillance revealed that Sendai virus initially appeared in Japan in the early 1950s and became prevalent worldwide by 1970 as a most common contaminant in laboratory rodent colonies under conventional conditions.

Host Range and Virus Propagation

Mice and rats are natural hosts of Sendai virus, while other rodents, including hamsters, guinea pigs and rabbits, and also pigs can be infected. Suckling and weanling mice are highly susceptible to the respiratory infections. Susceptibility to experimental infections varies considerably among mouse strains, probably due to differences in immunological responses. Sendai virus can grow efficiently in the chorioallantoic cavity of embryonated chicken eggs and replicates productively in a broad spectrum of tissue culture cell lines as well. However, exogenous trypsin is usually needed for proteolytic activation of the F glycoprotein to support multiple cycles of replication in tissue culture cells. Primary monkey kidney cells support multiplication of the virus without exogenous proteases. Sendai virus isolated from mice and passaged only in mouse lungs or monkey kidney cells retains original pathogenicity in mice, whereas it becomes less pathogenic, due to a mutation in the C gene, when passaged in chick embryos. Sendai virus replication is detected by hemagglutination of chicken erythrocytes and the virus is identified by the hemagglutination inhibition test.

Serological Relationship and Variability

The Sendai virus core soluble (S) antigen, mainly composed of the NP protein, exhibits a serological relationship to, but distinguishable from, human parainfluenza virus type 1. Envelope components, HN, F and M proteins, share antigenicity with their human counterparts among the members of the *Paramyxoviridae*, as determined by analyses of the genome nucleotide sequences. Sendai virus is antigenically homogeneous, i.e. there are no subtypes.

Epidemiology

Sendai virus is a most frequent contaminant maintained persistently in conventional colonies of laboratory mice and rats, while no evidence for the infection in wild rodents has been obtained. Both acute enzootic and epizootic infections occur in laboratory rodents.

Curiously, in the 1950s, Sendai virus was prevalent nationwide among pigs in Japan, but by 1961 the virus had disappeared from pigs. Infection of Sendai virus in pigs has not been reported in other countries.

Transmission and Tissue Tropism

Virus replication in the respiratory tract of mice reaches a peak 4–6 days after infection, declines gradually, and virus shedding terminates within 2 weeks. However, the virus may be recovered for up to 6 weeks after infection. In suckling mice, the virus persists longer. Virus transmission occurs either by direct contact with infected mice or by airborne route. Vertical transmission is suggested to occur from pregnant mice to fetus, resulting in stillbirths or a variety of malformations in offspring.

Sendai virus is exclusively pneumotropic in weanling and adult mice, the target tissues being restricted to the epithelial cells of the upper respiratory tract, trachea, bronchi and bronchioles. Neither subepithelial invasion from the surface mucosa nor spread to systemic organs via viremia occurs. Alveolar cells are not infected under usual conditions. Infection of alveolar and peritoneal macrophages results in abortive infections. In newborn and suckling mice, the virus may spread from the nasal epithelium to the brain via the olfactory route. Intracranial inoculation of the mice causes infections in the ependyma and meninges.

Pathogenicity

Pneumotropism of Sendai virus in mice cannot be explained by cellular receptors in the lungs, as receptors for the virus are also present in other organs not permissive for Sendai virus infection. Instead, pneumotropism has been shown to be primarily determined by host protease-mediated activation of the F glycoprotein. Activated virus with the cleaved F ($F_1 + F_2$) protein will infect the respiratory mucosa and replicate in multiple cycles, as the F protein of progeny virus undergoes cleavage activation in the bronchial lumen by tryptase Clara, an arginine-specific serine protease secreted by Clara cells of the bronchial epithelium. Upon Sendai virus infection, secretion of tryptase Clara is stimulated, whereas that of pulmonary surfactant, an inhibitor of the protease also secreted by Clara cells, is reduced, thereby producing a condition in the bronchial lumen preferable for activation of progeny virus. As a result, infected cells are increased in number and lung lesions are extended. In contrast, infection by a protease-activation mutant, whose F protein is not cleavable by trypsin and tryptase Clara but by chymotrypsin, terminates after a single cycle of replication in the lung, because the progeny virus remains noninfectious. Various organs of mice other than lungs, which lack the protease(s) required for the activation of wild-type F protein, have a potential capacity to support replication of wild-type virus but only for a single cycle. On the other hand, a pantropic mutant, whose F protein is cleavable by ubiquitous host proteases distributed in various organs, causes a systemic infection in mice. These results, together with similar observations on the virulence of Newcastle disease virus and avian influenza viruses, indicate that organ tropism and pathogenicity of Sendai virus are primarily determined by the presence of activating proteases for the F protein in target tissues.

The mode of virus budding at the primary target of infection is considered an additional determinant for organ tropism. The budding site of wild-type Sendai virus in the bronchial epithelial cells is restricted to the apical membrane domain, whereas the pantropic mutant buds bidirectionally at the apical and basolateral domains, due to amino acid exchanges in the M protein. This may explain why infection by wild-type virus remains localized in the surface epithelium of the respiratory tract, whereas the pantropic mutant readily invades subepithelial tissues to gain access to the spread to distant organs via viremia.

A deletion mutant in the V protein replicates less efficiently in mouse lungs, causing a slighter lung lesion, although it is highly cytopathic in tissue culture cells. The results suggest a regulatory role of the V protein in the pulmonary pathogenicity.

Clinical Features of Infection

With enzootic infections the virus usually produces a subclinical infection in mice and rats. Experimental infections as well as epizootic infections cause symptoms characteristic of acute respiratory infection. Moderate fever, ruffled furs and nasal discharge are common signs of the upper respiratory infection, appearing 2–3 days after exposure. Dyspnea, cough, anorexia and loss of body weight, which usually appear on the sixth or seventh day after infection, will indicate progression to bronchopneumonia. With weanling mice, retardation of body weight gain reflects the severity of the disease. In the second week of infection, infected animals die of bronchopneumonia or begin to recover from the infection. In newborn or 1- to 2-day-old suckling mice, intracranial inoculation causes meningitis and ependymitis, resulting in hydrocephalus.

Pathology and Histopathology

Major pathology of Sendai virus infection in mice is mild rhinitis, moderate tracheitis and severe bronchopneumonia. Immunohistological studies reveal that target tissue of the virus is confined to the epithelial mucosa of the upper respiratory tract, trachea, bronchi and bronchioles. Subepithelial tissues, alveolar epithelium and infiltrating cells are not usually involved. Macroscopically the lungs become swollen and hyperemic in a few days after intranasal infection, and lung consolidation, looking like the liver or spleen, begins to appear around day 7. Light microscopic studies reveal infected epithelial cells to be swollen and pyknotic with destruction of cilia within day 1. Submucosal edema and hyperemia occur with a peribronchial infiltration by neutrophils and mononuclear cells. For several days such infected cells increase progressively in number, meanwhile becoming necrotic and desquamated. The cellular infiltration progresses for 2 weeks, with massive edema and bleeding in the interstitium and alveolar spaces. Resolution of the lesion, if it occurs, begins about day 10 and proceeds rapidly, but complete resolution takes more than a month. When 1- to 2-day-old mice are infected intracranially, meninges, ependyma, choroid plexus and labyrinth are involved with respective inflammations.

Immune Response

Recovery from Sendai virus infections involves both humoral and cellular immunities. Envelope glycoproteins, HN and F, are mainly responsible for the humoral response and internal proteins, NP and M, are also of importance as target antigens for the cellular responses. Virus is cleared mainly by CD8+ cytotoxic T lymphocytes (CTLs) in a class I-restricted manner, and therefore, in nude mice, virus infection persists for more than 2 months. CTL response in mice depends on the H-2 haplotype. Macrophages, natural killer cells and interferons contribute to the virus clearance in concert with the T lymphocytes. Lung consolidation is mainly caused by CD4+ T cells primed by the internal proteins.

Mucosal IgA antibodies to the HN are primarily responsible for resistance to infection. Serum IgG antibodies are less effective for preventing replication of initially infecting virus, but can minimize further replications and lung lesions. The role of cellular immunity in protection is controversial.

The HN molecule contains at least four antigenic epitopes. Antibodies against HN inhibit hemagglutinating and neuraminidase activities, and neutralize infectivity. Antibodies to the F protein, with at least four antigenic sites, inhibit fusion and hemolytic activities, and can also prevent infection, specifically cell-to-cell infection. When mice are infected, considerable titers of serum antibodies become detectable. Since the HN, F, NP and M proteins share antigenic determinants with other members of paramyxoviruses, most closely to human parainfluenza virus type 1, heterotypic antibody responses may occur when Sendai virus-primed animals are immunized or boosted with a related virus, or vice versa.

Sendai virus is a strong inducer of interferons in tissue culture cells and in mice.

Prevention and Control

Control of Sendai virus infection is practically important for breeding and maintenance of laboratory animals and for the performance of animal experiments. Contamination with the virus will interfere with experimental data, specifically in immune responses and lung histology, and often interrupts animal experimentation by causing epizootic acute infections, with or without devastating animal death. A drop in breeding efficiency as a result of infection can be critical for maintenance of animal strains.

Virus-free animals are produced by cesarean birth and can be maintained under specific pathogen-free conditions isolated from conventional colonies. Once Sendai virus-free colonies are established, frequent serological surveillance and quarantine of contaminated colonies are needed for maintenance of laboratory animals.

Inactive vaccines prepared from egg-grown virus are commercially available, but are presently far from being in general use. Experimental live vaccines of protease-activation mutants, temperature-sensitive mutants or defective-interfering particles with considerable efficacy have been developed. Recombinant vaccinia viruses with genes encoding Sendai virus proteins or oligopeptides corresponding to the epitopes responsible for immune protection have been shown to induce protection in mice.

See also: **Defective interfering viruses; Genetics of animal viruses; Parainfluenza viruses (*Paramyxoviridae*): Animal, Human; Immune response: Cell mediated immune response, General features.**

Further Reading

Brownstein DG (1986) Sendai virus. In: Bhatt PN, Jacoby RO, Morse HC III and New A (eds) *Viral and Mycoplasmal Infections of Laboratory Rodents*, p. 37. New York: Academic Press.

Collins PL, Chanoock RM and McIntosh K (1996) Parainfluenza viruses. In: Fields BN, Knipe DM and Howley PM (eds) *Fields Virology*, 3rd edn, p. 1205. Philadelphia: Lippincott-Raven.

Ishida N and Homma M (1978) Sendai virus. *Adv. Virus Res.* 23: 349.

Lamb A and Kolakofsky D (1996) Paramyxoviridae: the viruses and their replication. In: Fields BN, Knipe DM and Howley PM (eds) *Fields Virology*, 3rd edn, p. 1177. Philadelphia: Lippincott-Raven.

Okada Y (1988) Sendai virus-mediated cell fusion. *Curr. Top. Memb. Trans.* 32: 297.

Tashiro M and Rott R (1996) The role of proteolytic cleavage of viral glycoproteins in the pathogenesis of influenza virus infections. *Semin. Virol.* 7: 237.

SEQUIVIRUSES (*SEQUIVIRIDAE*)

MA Mayo and AF Murant, Scottish Crop Research Institute, Invergowrie, Dundee, UK

Copyright © 1999 Academic Press

History

The genus name *Sequivirus* was adopted in 1995 for the former 'parsnip yellow fleck virus group'. The eponymous member (PYFV) was first described in 1968 and two serotypes have been recognized, both infecting plants in the family Umbelliferae: parsnip serotype, found in parsnip, celery and *Heracleum sphondylium*; and anthriscus serotype, found in carrot and *Anthriscus sylvestris*. Both serotypes depend on a helper virus, anthriscus yellows virus (a tentative member of the genus *Waikavirus* of the family *Sequiviridae*) for transmission by aphids in a semipersistent manner. The only other species in the genus *Sequivirus* is dandelion yellow mosaic virus (DYMV) which was first isolated from diseased *Taraxacum officinale* (Compositae), but causes a severe necrotic disease in lettuce (*Lactuca sativa*: Compositae). DYMV has been relatively little studied but it is aphid-transmitted and the limited data available suggest a semipersistent mode of transmission. There is no evidence to show if a helper virus is involved.

Taxonomy and Classification

Viruses in the genus *Sequivirus* have isometric particles of c. 30 nm diameter and monopartite, positive-sense, single-stranded (ss) RNA genomes of about 10 kb. The RNA-dependent RNA polymerase encoded by PYFV RNA is 'picorna-like'. The genus is classified, together with the genus *Waikavirus* (type member, rice tungro spherical virus), in the family *Sequiviridae*. Viruses in both genera have genomes that encode a large polyprotein from which the mature virus proteins are cleaved by protease action. The viruses possess three coat proteins whose genes are located near the 5′ ends of the genomes, properties which are shared with picornaviruses. Sequiviruses have sometimes been referred to as 'plant picornaviruses'.

Properties of the Virion

Although PYFV may have an infectivity dilution end-point of up to 10^{-5} in sap of *Spinacia oleracea* (spinach), the virus concentration is often very low in extracts of glasshouse-grown plants. Best virus yields have been obtained by growing infected *S. oleracea* plants at 15°C with light at 10 000 lux for 8 h per day, and collecting systemically infected leaves 19 days after inoculation of the plants. Yields of about 5–20 mg of viral nucleoprotein per kilogram of leaf material are obtained by clarifying leaf extracts with diethyl ether or butan-1-ol followed by differential centrifugation.

Particle preparations of PYFV contain 30 nm diameter isometric particles which sediment either as 'top component' (apparently empty protein shells) or 'bottom component' (infective nucleoprotein particles). The top component particles are relatively fragile. Top and bottom components of an isolate of the parsnip serotype, separated by sedimentation in sucrose density gradients or by isopyknic banding in CsCl or Cs$_2$SO$_4$ solutions, respectively had sedimentation coefficients ($s_{20,w}$) of 60 S and 152 S, buoyant densities in CsCl of 1.29 and 1.49 g ml^{-1}, and $A_{260}:A_{280}$ ratios of 0.8 and 1.7. Top and bottom component particles of PYFV contain three major protein species of M_r ($\times 10^{-3}$) 31, 26 and 22.5 (parsnip serotype) or 31, 26 and 24 (anthriscus serotype). Bottom component particles of PYFV each contain one ssRNA molecule of c. 10 kb.

The infectivity dilution end-point of DYMV in sap of *Chenopodium amaranticolor* or *C. quinoa* may be up to 10^{-5}. Purification involves clarification of phosphate-buffered extracts of leaf by adding butan-1-ol to a concentration of 8% (v/v), followed by differential centrifugation; however, the yields are low. The nucleoprotein particles are isometric, c. 30 nm in diameter, and have an $s_{20,w}$ of 159 S, $A_{260}:A_{280}$ of 1.67 and a buoyant density in Cs$_2$SO$_4$ of 1.42 g ml^{-1}. DYMV particles have three protein species, of M_r ($\times 10^{-3}$) 32, 29.5 and 27, and one ssRNA molecule of c. 10 kb.

Properties of the Genome

Most of the 9871 nucleotide ssRNA genome of PYFV comprises one large open reading frame that encodes a polyprotein of 3027 amino acids. Mature coat proteins, such as the virion proteins, are produced from the primary polyprotein translation product by proteolysis. **Figure 1** illustrates the position of this open reading frame in PYFV RNA. The genome RNA does not have a 3′-terminal poly(A) sequence and is thought to have a 5′-terminal genome-linked protein.

Figure 1 also shows the polyprotein translation product of the PYFV genome RNA and indicates

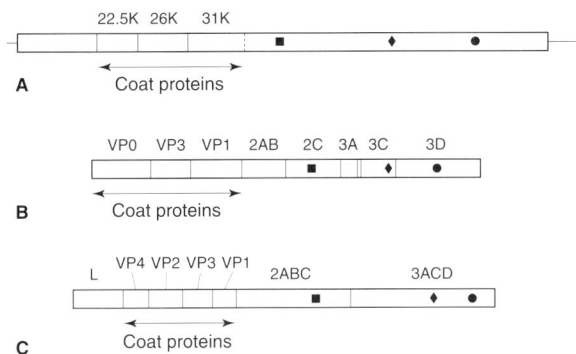

Figure 1 Genome organization of (**A**) PYFV, and comparison of the PYFV polyprotein with those of (**B**) poliovirus 1 and (**C**) foot-and-mouth disease virus. The locations of conserved domains are shown as filled squares (NTP-binding), filled diamonds (protease) or filled circles (polymerase).

where coat proteins have been mapped in the polyprotein. Other cleavage sites are unknown. However, some sequences in the polyprotein have striking similarities to those of domains in other virus proteins that are thought to have NTP-binding, protease or RNA-dependent RNA polymerase functions. The positions are shown on the diagram. Viruses in several families of plant viruses have genomes that are expressed by the cleavage of a large polyprotein. However, the genomes most resembling those of sequiviruses (and of waikaviruses which form the other genus in the family *Sequiviridae*) are those of viruses in the family *Picornaviridae*. Two examples of the polyproteins of such viruses are shown for comparison in **Fig. 1**. In some, the coat proteins are N-terminal; in others there is a protein to the N-terminal side of the coat proteins. The relative positions of the three domains with putative functions in the PYFV polyprotein are the same as in the picornavirus polyproteins (**Fig. 1**).

Sequence Comparisons

Some small regions of the structural and nonstructural proteins of PYFV seem to resemble sequences in picornaviral structural proteins. But there is little overall percent identity much in excess of that between unrelated proteins. This is also true in comparisons between PYFV nonstructural proteins and corresponding proteins of viruses in the genus *Waikavirus*, or of viruses such as comoviruses and nepoviruses (family *Comoviridae*). **Table 1** shows the only values of percent identity between pairs of proteins that were above the background level in comparisons of PYFV proteins and corresponding proteins of other 'plant picornaviruses' (family *Comoviridae*) and viruses in the genera *Enterovirus* and *Hepatovirus* (family *Picornaviridae*).

Evolution

The similarity between the genome expression strategies of sequiviruses and picornaviruses has prompted speculation about common ancestry of these groups. Some picornaviruses have insect hosts, and sequiviruses and waikaviruses are transmitted by insects (see below), albeit in a nonpropagative fashion. This has prompted further speculation about a common origin from an insect virus ancestor. As in most such speculation, there is no evidence to support or to counter these ideas.

Serology

PYFV and DYMV are moderately to highly immunogenic. The virus concentrations in plant extracts are usually too low for reactions to be obtained in gel diffusion tests but satisfactory results can be obtained in other kinds of test, including ELISA and immunosorbent electron microscopy (ISEM). The parsnip and anthriscus serotypes differ by a serological differentiation index of 4–5. Results of ISEM tests suggest the possibility of an extremely distant serological relationship between PYFV and DYMV.

Geographic Distribution

PYFV is reported only from the UK, The Netherlands

Table 1 Comparison of parsnip yellow fleck virus proteins with those of other viruses

Virus	% identity with corresponding polypeptides of PYFV		Classification
	NTP-binding	Polymerase	
Rice tungro spherical	41	49	*Sequiviridae*
Tomato black ring	29	33	*Comoviridae*
Cowpea mosaic	30	40	*Comoviridae*
Poliovirus 1	33	31	*Picornaviridae*
Hepatitis A	30	30	*Picornaviridae*

and Germany. DYMV is reported from these countries and also from Czechoslovakia, Scandinavia and China.

Host Range and Virus Propagation

Both PYFV and DYMV have restricted natural and experimental host ranges. In nature, PYFV is reported only from a few species of Umbelliferae: the parsnip serotype from parsnip (*Pastinaca sativa*), celery (*Apium graveolens*) and hogweed (*Heracleum sphondylium*); the anthriscus serotype from cow parsley (*Anthriscus sylvestris*), carrot (*Daucus carota*) and dill (*Anethum graveolens*). Experimentally, isolates of both PYFV serotypes can infect a few other species of Umbelliferae, notably chervil (*Anthriscus cerefolium*) and coriander (*Coriandrum sativum*), and a few plants in the families Amaranthaceae, Chenopodiaceae, Portulacaceae and Solanaceae. *Chenopodium amaranticolor* and *C. quinoa* are good local lesion assay hosts. *Spinacia oleracea* (spinach) and *Nicotiana clevelandii* (for the parsnip serotype only) are good systemic hosts for maintenance and propagation. *N. benthamiana* is a very sensitive indicator host, developing a lethal systemic wilt and necrosis in 4–7 days.

DYMV has been found naturally only in two species of Compositae (dandelion and lettuce). Experimentally, it has been transmitted to a few species in each of the families Amaranthaceae, Chenopodiaceae, Compositae and Solanaceae. *Chenopodium amaranticolor* and *C. quinoa* are useful both for local lesion assay and as systemic hosts for propagating the virus for purification.

Transmission and Tissue Tropism

Sequiviruses are mechanically transmissible, although mechanical transmission of DYMV to lettuce or dandelion is difficult. The natural vectors of sequiviruses are aphids: *Cavariella aegopodii* for PYFV and *Aulacorthum solani*, *Myzus ascalonicus*, *M. ornatus* and *M. persicae* for DYMV. Detailed information on aphid transmission of DYMV is lacking, but PYFV is transmitted only by aphids that also transmit a so-called helper virus (anthriscus yellows virus; AYV). The helper virus must be acquired either before or at the same time as PYFV. The AYV–PYFV complex is transmitted in a semipersistent manner. The minimum acquisition access time (AAT) is about 10–15 min and the minimum inoculation access time (IAT) is 2 min. The transmission efficacy of aphids increased with increasing AAT and IAT of up to 24 h. Adult aphids retain the ability to transmit for up to 4 days after the end of the AAT, but nymphs cease to transmit after molting. Aphids did not transmit virus after injection into the hemocele with purified preparations of PYFV or with extracts of aphids carrying PYFV and AYV. Electron microscopic examination of viruliferous aphids suggested that the virus is carried in the aphid foregut.

Sequiviruses are thought to infect cells in all host tissues. Virus can be acquired by aphids when they feed on mesophyll cells. Sequiviruses are not seed-transmitted.

Pathogenicity

The symptoms in parsnip plants of infection with the parsnip serotype range from yellow flecking to yellow and green mosaic with some stunting. Symptoms can be more severe in infected celery plants. The symptoms of infection of carrot plants with the anthriscus serotype range from mild mottling to severe necrosis, wilting and death.

Available evidence indicates that *Anthriscus sylvestris* is the main wild host of the anthriscus serotype, which infects carrot, and that *Heracleum sphondylium* is the main wild host of the parsnip serotype, which also infects celery. Both these wild hosts are infected symptomlessly. Carrot, celery and parsnip are immune to the helper virus, AYV, so that all the infections observed in these crops are primary and there is no secondary spread within the crop. Nevertheless, PYFV is common in parsnips in the UK. In celery, plants infected with PYFV are usually confined to the edges of fields. In The Netherlands, infection by the anthriscus serotype is uncommon in ware crops of carrot but common in carrot seed crops, in which infection results in 'early-season dieback', which in some years causes severe losses in seed production.

DYMV was so called because it was isolated from dandelion plants showing a bright yellow mosaic with rings and oak leaf patterns. It has also been isolated from lettuce showing a severe necrotic disease: veinal chlorosis and necrosis, thickening and curling of the leaves, severe stunting and prevention of heading. The virus was transmissible from diseased dandelion and lettuce plants to lettuce both by aphids and by manual inoculation. However, evidence that the virus that causes the necrosis in lettuce is the cause of the yellow mosaic in dandelion is either lacking or negative; the appropriateness of the name dandelion yellow mosaic virus for this virus is therefore in some doubt.

Prevention and Control

The diseases caused by PYFV in celery and parsnip, and in ware crops of carrot, do not seem to be sufficiently serious to warrant specific control measures, although insecticides applied for the control of aphids or carrot fly (*Psila rosae*) may serve to decrease the incidence of PYFV. The disease caused by PYFV in carrot seed crops in The Netherlands is economically important but spraying with systemic biological control insecticide seems of only limited usefulness in preventing infection.

The restricted host range of the AYV helper virus suggests possible control measures by eliminating overwintering weed hosts in the vicinity of susceptible crops.

Little is known about the epidemiology or importance of DYMV. Most outbreaks of necrosis disease in field crops of lettuce occurred in the vicinity of yellow mosaic-diseased dandelion, which suggested that dandelion is an important overwintering host. There is no information about resistance genes.

See also: **Polioviruses (*Picornaviridae*): General features, Molecular biology; Waikaviruses (*Sequiviridae*); Picornaviruses – insect (*Picornaviridae*).**

Further Reading

Elnagar S and Murant AF (1976) The role of the helper virus, anthriscus yellows, in the transmission of parsnip yellow fleck virus by the aphid *Cavariella aegopodii*. *Ann. Appl. Biol.* 84: 169.

Mayo MA, Murant AF, Turnbull-Ross AD *et al* (1995) Family *Sequiviridae*. In: Murphy FA, Fauquet CM, Bishop DHL *et al* (eds) *Virus Taxonomy*. Sixth Report of the International Committee on Taxonomy of Viruses, p. 337. Wien: Springer.

Murant AF (1988) Parsnip yellow fleck virus, type member of a proposed new plant virus group, and a possible second member, dandelion yellow mosaic virus. In: Koenig R (ed.) *The Plant Viruses*. Vol. 3: *Polyhedral Virions with Monopartite RNA Genomes*, p. 273. New York: Plenum Press.

Turnbull-Ross AD, Mayo MA, Reavy B & Murant AF (1993) Sequence analysis of the parsnip yellow fleck virus polyprotein: evidence of affinities with picornaviruses. *J. Gen. Virol.* 74: 555.

Sheep Poxvirus   *see* **Poxviruses**

SHRIMP VIRUSES

Philip C Loh, Department of Microbiology, University of Hawaii, Honolulu, Hawaii, USA

Copyright © 1999 Academic Press

Introduction

Since the first shrimp virus *Baculovirus penaei* (BP) was isolated from wild penaeid shrimp (*Penaeus duorarum*) in the early 1970s, a number of penaeid shrimp viruses have assumed great importance because of the severe effect on the growth and sustenance of the penaeid shrimp aquaculture industry. Several of these viruses have been associated with large epizootics and massive mortalities in shrimp farms and hatcheries. The number of penaeid shrimp viruses reported at present belong to six families (**Table 1**). This number, however, is expected to increase and additional studies of viral diseases of penaeid shrimp result in more being isolated and characterized. Many of the penaeid shrimp viruses have only been observed through electron microscopy and have not been extensively characterized in regard to their biological, immunological, biochemical and physical properties.

The Host Animal

Depending on the geographic location, the following penaeid shrimp species have been commercialized on a large scale: *Penaeus monodon* (giant tiger shrimp); *P. vannamei* (whiteleg shrimp); *P. stylirostris* (blue shrimp); *P. japonicus* (kuruma shrimp); *P. chinensis* (orientalis) (fleshy prawn); *P. duorarum* (northern pink shrimp); *P. merguiensis* (banana shrimp); *P. indicus* (Indian white prawn); and *P. setiferus* (northern white shrimp).

The Virus: General Features

Host range

The penaeid shrimp viruses implicated in epizootics and associated with massive mortality in cultured shrimp belong to four groups: *Baculoviridae*, *Rhabdoviridae*, *Parvoviridae*, *Picornaviridae* (**Table 1**).

Table 1 Penaeid shrimp viruses

Family	Name/acronym	Shape/size (nm)	Nucleic acid/sense	Envelope	Growth in cell culture
Rhabdoviridae	Rhabdovirus of penaeid shrimp/RPS	Bullet, 70 × 125	ssRNA (−)	+	+
	Yellowhead virus/YHV	Bacilliform, 45 × 160	ssRNA (−)	+	+
Picornaviridae	Taura syndrome virus/TSV	Icosahedron, 31–32	ssRNA (+)	−	−
Reoviridae	Type III reolike virus/REO-III	Icosahedron, 50–70	dsRNA (segmented)	−	−
	Type IV reolike virus/REO-IV				
Togaviridae	Lymphoid organ vacuolization virus/LOVV	?, 55	?	+	−
Parvoviridae	Infectious hypodermal and hematopoietic necrosis virus/IHHNV	Icosahedron, 22–25	ssDNA	−	−
	Hepatopancreatic parvovirus/HPV	Icosahedron, 22–24	ssDNA	−	−
	Lymphoidal parvo-like virus/LPV	Icosahedron, 25–30	?	−	−
Baculoviridae					
Occluded Type A					
	Baculovirus penaei/BP	Rod, 75 × 228	dsDNA	+	−
	Monodon baculovirus/MBV	Rod, 69 × 275	dsDNA	+	+
Nonoccluded Type C					
	Baculoviral midgut necrosis/BMN	Rod, 72 × 310	dsDNA	+	−
	Bacilliform virus/BV	Rod, 83 × 275	dsDNA	+	−
	Chinese baculovirus/CBV	Rod, 120 × 265	dsDNA	+	+
	Systemic ectodermal mesodermal baculovirus/SEMBV	Rod, 121 × 276	dsDNA	+	+
	Whitespot baculovirus/WSBV	Rod, 87 × 330	dsDNA	+	+
	penaeid rod-shaped DNA virus/PRDV	Ovoid, 84 × 226	dsDNA	+	+

The susceptibility of the different species of cultured penaeid shrimp to these viruses varies from infection of only a few to infection of a large number of species. Although the range of these viruses in feral or wild shrimp has not been fully documented, a member of the non-occluded group of baculoviruses, the white spot baculovirus (WSBV), has not only been detected in several species of wild penaeid shrimp but also in other wild decapods. Wild shrimp populations have also been reported to carry the parvovirus, infectious hypodermal and hematopoietic necrosis virus (IHHNV).

Infection and severity

The mortality and morbidity of the penaeid shrimp to several of these pathogenic viruses are affected by age. The older shrimp are generally less susceptible to infection than younger ones. The viruses can infect the penaeid shrimp at various stages of its development, from protozoea to adult, with the highest mortality occurring at the early postlarval stage. Depending on the virus and the species of penaeid shrimp, infected animals exhibit gross physical changes and histopathological aberrations of their organs and tissues. Primary organ and tissue targets may vary with the viral pathogen.

Transmission

There is very little information available on the natural routes of transmission of these viruses. Transmission via the oral route has been demonstrated through feeding of either contaminated foods or infected carcasses and appears to be a dominant route of natural infections. Transmission by way of the gills is another possible route. Although asymptomatic infections have been reported, little is known concerning the mechanism of latent or persistent viral infections in the penaeid host.

Control and prevention

Currently the most effective means of controlling the viral disease problem is to destroy the infected animals, decontaminate the ponds, and start again with virus-free stocks. Although specific-pathogen-free (SPF) shrimp has been developed as a way to control the disease problem, it represents a partial solution since the animals were tested for only a limited number of viral pathogens. Such SPF animals have been found to be equally susceptible as wild stock to other shrimp viral pathogens.

Growth and assay

Until recently penaeid shrimp viruses were grown only in a sensitive indicator shrimp bioassay system. Primary shrimp cell cultures such as primary lymphoid cell lines are currently used to isolate, grow and assay some of the shrimp viruses. Such primary cell lines have been used in limited studies on the synthesis of viral proteins, viral pathogenesis, of antiviral chemicals, and the development of virus detection/diagnosis protocols. A stable continuous cell line has been prepared by transforming primary shrimp lymphoid cells with the viral oncogene, SV40-large T-antigen. Although the transformed shrimp lymphoid cells exhibited many of the properties of stable, continuous transformed cell lines, they were found to be non-permissive to some of the shrimp viruses. The transformed cells exhibited antiviral activities.

Detection and diagnosis

At present the detection/diagnosis of shrimp viral diseases is still dependent on the clinical history and light and/or electron microscopical examination of affected tissues showing characteristic cytopathology obtained from infected shrimp. Asymptomatic and latent infections can be detected only through the use of either enhancement or bioassay techniques in sensitive indicator shrimp. However, these traditional methodologies have limited sensitivity, require time (days to weeks), specialized equipment, highly trained personnel and high cost. A number of molecular and immunologically based technologies have been recently developed which have facilitated the rapid, specific, sensitive and cost-effective detection/diagnosis of shrimp viral infections. Various methods, such as the nitrocellulose-enzyme immunoassay (NC-EIA), the Western blot and various modifications of the nucleic acid probe (NAP) and polymerase chain reaction (PCR) procedures have been effectively employed.

Basic Properties of Some Penaeid Shrimp Viruses

In this section, the discussion is limited to those shrimp viruses on which there is adequate information concerning their basic properties.

RNA viruses

Rhabdoviridae   There are two viruses belonging to this family: the rhabdovirus of penaeid shrimp (RPS) and the yellowhead virus (YHV). The YHV is provisionally grouped in this family.

Rhabdovirus of penaeid shrimp   The RPS is the first rhabdovirus to be isolated from penaeid shrimp and also to uniquely infect a continuous fish cell heteroploid line, epithelioma papulosum cyprini (EPS). It was originally isolated from infectious hypodermal and hematopoietic necrosis (IHHN)-diseased and healthy *P. stylirostris* and *P. vannamei* obtained from shrimp farms in Hawaii and Ecuador. However, experimental infections of juvenile penaeids (5–6 g) did not induce histopathological changes characteristically associated with IHHNV infection, nor were clinical or gross manifestations of disease observed. In such animals no mortality occurred and virus replication was demonstrated only in the lymphoid (Oka) organs by plaque assay and immunofluorescence. The affected lymphoid organs, which showed gross cellular changes, were significantly larger in size (6–7 times) than the corresponding organs from uninfected animals and appeared to be the primary target organ of RPS infection. Mortality was observed in younger postlarval (PL) shrimp (0.2 g) experimentally infected by three routes of infection: water-borne (12%), oral feeding (21%) and intramuscular injection (43–50%). The water-borne and oral feeding routes may represent the natural routes of transmission.

Thin-section electron microscopic studies indicated that RPS replicates in the cytoplasm of infected cells and appears to bud from both cytoplasmic vesicles and the plasma membrane. Both thin sections and negative staining studies showed bullet-shaped particles which are enveloped (typical of animal rhabdoviruses). Emanating from the envelope are regularly shaped projections with a knob-like structure at the distal end. Complete virions measured 115–138 × 65–77 nm.

In virus susceptibility studies of several fish cell lines, the heteroploid EPC cell line was determined to be the most susceptible to RPS and had the highest yield of virus. The EPC was found to be especially useful for the primary isolation of RPS. Although several of the other fish cell lines were susceptible, their yields of infectious RPS were much lower (<10%). Single-cycle growth studies of RPS in EPC cells showed an eclipse period of 3 h, followed by a period of exponential growth which was completed by 48 h postinfection (p.i.). Since the virus uniquely replicates in a fish cell line (EPC) causing distinct cytopathic changes, this has enabled the development of a quantitative plaque assay protocol which has greatly facilitated the study of RPS. The efficiency of plating (EOP) of RPS in EPC was determined to be 30 virus particles per infectious unit. The virus was found to be highly fragile, being sensitive to 20% ethyl ether, low pH, repeated freezing and thawing (3 times), to 37°C (12 h), and storage at −10°C (4 weeks) but was stable at −70°C for several weeks. The buoyant density of RPS in sucrose gradients is 1.19 g cm^{-1}.

The molecular weight of the single RNA species of the RPS genome was determined to be 3.6×10^6 Da (∼10.4 kb). The viral RNA has a negative polarity and is sensitive to ribonuclease. Since the replication of RPS in EPC was not inhibited by the DNA antagonist 5-bromo-2′ deoxyuridine (20 µg ml^{-1}), this confirms the RNA genome of the virus.

Analysis by sodium dodecylsulfate–polyacrylamide gel electrophoresis (SDS–PAGE) of RPS proteins revealed the presence of at least four major structural proteins with the following molecular weights (kDa): 165, 65.7, 45.1 and 27.8. The number of structural proteins and the electrophoretic profile of RPS are very similar to those of the prototype rhabdovirus, vesicular stomatitis virus (VSV), and of the fish rhabdovirus carpio (RC) (also named spring viremia of carp virus, SVCV), both of which belong to the genus *Vesiculovirus*. In number of structural proteins and electrophoretic profile, they are different from the lyssatype fish rhabdoviruses, infectious hypodermal necrosis virus (IHNV) and viral hemorrhagic septicemia virus (VHSV). The lyssa variety is easily distinguished from the vesiculo group in that the matrix proteins are composed of two structural polypeptides, M1 and M2, versus a single polypeptide, M, in the vesiculo group. Western blot analysis of the electrophoretically separated RPS structural proteins with anti-RPS polyclonal serum revealed, in addition to the four major proteins, an extra viral protein with a molecular weight of 38 kDa. Based on its molecular weight, this polypeptide was presumed to be nonstructural protein which is present in the vesiculo group of rhabdoviruses. The Western blot technique further revealed that the RPS is partly related to VSV, IHNV and VHSV. The anti-RPS serum identified the G protein of both IHNV and VHSV and the M protein of VSV. Although the anti-RPS serum cross-reacted with the structural proteins of RC, suggesting a close evolutionary relation of these two viruses, the intensity of reaction to RC was much weaker than that observed with RPS. Serologically, RPS is unrelated to IHNV and VHSV and is closely related to but distinguishable from RC when the plaque reduction and neutralization techniques are used.

A solid-phase enzyme-immunoassay protocol, nitrocellulose-enzyme immunoassay/streptavidin–biotin (NC-EIA/SAB), employing a rabbit polyclonal anti-RPS IgG, was developed for the diagnosis and detection of RPS. The NC-EIA/SAB was reported to detect as few as 10 plaque-forming units (PFU) or 300 viral particles (400 pg of viral protein) in experimentally infected shrimp. The protocol has successfully detected natural RPS infections in apparently healthy animals at different stages of development in shrimp farms in Hawaii.

Yellowhead virus The yellowhead virus was named after the disease it caused in the black tiger shrimp, *P. monodon*. Diseased animals showed a characteristic yellow color of the cephalothorax and gills and a pale or bleached appearance. The infection generally resulted in a cumulative mortality of 100% within 3–5 days after the onset of the disease. The etiological agent was initially identified as a baculo-like virus but subsequently was reported to contain RNA and to possess properties not characteristically associated with baculoviruses.

In addition to the original host *P. monodon*, two other penaeid species, *P. stylirostris* and *P. vannamei*, were reported to be highly susceptible to YHV. Intramuscular inoculation of a 10%, w/v, cephalothorax filtrate prepared from naturally infected *P. monodon* Fabricius into subadult (3–10 g) *P. stylirostris* (Stimpson) and *P. vannamei* (Boone) resulted in 100% cumulative mortality within 5–7 days p.i. In such experimentally infected animals, the characteristic light yellowing of the hepatopancreas and gills observed in naturally infected *P. monodon* was not seen. Histopathological examination of naturally and experimentally infected shrimp revealed widespread cellular necrosis in the gills, connective tissues, hemocytes, hematopoietic organs, and lymphoid organ, and strongly indicated a preferential infection of the cells of ectodermal and mesodermal origins.

Primary cultures of shrimp lymphoid cells have been used for the quantitative titration of infectious YHV. This has permitted study of the pathogenesis of YHV in the infected shrimp. The primary targets for infection were the lymphoid organ, gill and head soft tissues, all of which contained 10- to 800-fold higher titers of infectious virus than found in the other tissues and organs tested. Four fish cell lines (fathead minnow or FHM, EPC, chinook salmon embryo or CHSE-214 and brown bullhead or BB) and two insect cell lines (SF9 from *Spodoptera frugiperda* and CRL 1963 from *Drosophila*) were found not susceptible to YHV.

Electron microscopic examination of ultrathin sections of gills and lymphoid tissues from infected animals revealed the presence of numerous enveloped virus particles with bacilliform morphology, measuring $150-200 \times 40-50$ nm in the cytoplasm of infected cells. Virions budding out through the cytoplasmic membrane were frequently observed. Cross-sections of the complete virions showed an electron-dense nuclear core which measured 20–30 nm in diameter, surrounded by a trilaminar envelope.

To prepare purified virus the hemolymph was found to yield the cleanest preparation and the largest number of virus particles. Attempts to purify YHV from the gill and head soft tissue met with difficulty because of contaminating vesicles and other membranous cellular materials which banded nonspecifically with the virus in sucrose gradients. The buoyant density of purified YHV ranged from 1.18 to 1.20 g ml^{-1}. This is comparable to the buoyant densities of known rhabdoviruses.

Electron microscopic examination of uranyl acetate-stained, purified YHV revealed peplomer-containing, enveloped, rod-shaped particles measuring 190–200 × 50–60 nm and resembling the plant rhabdoviruses. As with plant rhabdoviruses, the virus particle is fragile and flexible, often assuming pleomorphic forms. The nucleocapsid is arranged in an orderly helical fashion. The helix consists of a coiled tubular structure layered in a regular fashion at right angles to the long axis of the complete virus particle. YHV does not exhibit the bullet-shaped morphology typical of rhabdoviruses infecting vertebrates. However, it closely resembles the bacilliform (with rounded ends) rhabdo-like viruses infecting the blue crab, *Callinectes sapidus*, and the helical, rod-shaped plant rhabdoviruses. In terms of their dimensions and ultrastructure, these rhabdoviruses are very much alike.

Genome analysis of YHV by agarose gel electrophoresis showed a single band of RNA of mol. wt. 8×10^6 Da (~ 22 kb). The size of the RNA genome is approximately twice that of the rhabdoviruses. The viral RNA is susceptible to ribonuclease (RNase) and is therefore a single-stranded structure. The failure of YHV RNA to be translated in an *in vitro* rabbit reticulocyte translation system strongly indicates that the viral genome possesses a negative polarity.

Structural protein analysis of purified YHV preparations by SDS-PAGE revealed four major bands with the following estimated molecular sizes (kDa): 170, 135, 67 and 22. These bands probably correspond to the large (L), glycoprotein (G), nucleocapsid (N) and matrix (M) proteins of rhabdoviruses. The putative G protein of YHV was determined to be glycosylated.

Western blot analysis of the protein bands using rabbit polyclonal anti-YHV immunoglobulin G (IgG) showed strong reactivity by the antibody with the putative G protein. The proteins of VSV, RPS, and control shrimp tissues did not crossreact with the same antibody preparation. Although the structural protein profile of YHV is similar to that of RPS and other members of the family *Rhabdoviridae*, the molecular sizes of YHV proteins are different. The G protein of YHV is larger (135 kDa versus 90 kDa) and probably accounts for the very prominent peplomers. Furthermore, YHV has a smaller M protein (22 kDa versus 30 kDa), which may account for the high flexibility and fragility of the virus.

In hemagglutination studies, both YHV and VSV were found to agglutinate chicken red blood cells with endpoints of 1:256 and 1:64, respectively. Neither virus was eluted even after 24 h incubation at room temperature, suggesting the formation of a stable complex which lacked receptor-destroying enzymes.

A number of *in vitro* methodologies are available for the detection/diagnosis of YHV infection. An indirect NC-EIA method employing a rabbit polyclonal anti-YHV IgG has been used for the rapid, specific diagnosis and detection of acute and asymptomatic YHV infection of the penaeid shrimp. The solid-phase enzyme immunoassay procedure was capable of detecting as few as 100 TCID$_{50}$ units of virus or an equivalent of 0.4 ng of viral protein. Although gill tissues and lymphoid organs were highly satisfactory sources of YHV antigen for the NC-EIA test, the sampling of the hemolymph which was found to contain a considerable amount of virus, was found to be a more convenient and a less invasive way of monitoring YHV infection in cultured shrimp, particularly invaluable broodstock animals.

Recently a Western blot protocol has been successfully used for the detection of YHV infection in field samples of cultured shrimp from Southeast Asia and the USA. A reverse transcriptase–polymerase chain reaction (RT-PRC) protocol has been used with limited success.

Two of 45 recombinant clones which gave positive hybridization with YHV RNA were negative with the DNA of *P. monodon* and that of the white spot baculovirus. The problem with the probes is that we do not know from which regions of the viral genome they originate. Also, the family of genes making up the YHV genome has not been identified.

Picornaviridae The only member provisionally assigned to this family is the Taura syndrome virus (TSV) which causes a highly infectious disease named Taura syndrome (TS) among the whiteleg shrimp, *P. vannamei*. Epizootics of TS have resulted in extensive economic losses to the shrimp farming industry in the Americas. Several penaeid species have been found to be susceptible to TSV: *P. chinensis, P. aztecus* and *P. duorarum*. In contrast *P. stylirostris* and *P. setiferus* were found to be resistant after experimental challenge with TSV.

Taura syndrome generally occurs in juvenile (0.1–5 g) *P. vannamei*, and its clinical effect is mortality (>90%). As a rule, older animals are more resistant.

There is scant information available concerning the presence or distribution of TSV in feral shrimp populations. Several attempts to demonstrate TSV in captured wild broodstock, spawned eggs or naupli have not been successful.

Little is known concerning the natural transmission routes of TSV. Experimental transmission studies have provided strong evidence that the waterborne-oral feeding route may represent the natural route of transmission. Some evidence has been presented to suggest the role of seagulls as the probable transport vector of TSV among shrimp farms.

The buoyant density of TSV in CsCl gradients is 1.338 g ml^{-1}. The virus is a nonenveloped icosahedron with a diameter of 30–32 nm. It has a single-stranded RNA genome which is polyadenylated at the 3′ end. Viral RNA has a positive sense and is approximately 9 kb in length. The viral capsid is made up of three major (55, 40 and 24 kDa) and one minor (58 kDa) structural proteins.

Shrimp with acute natural and experimentally induced TSV infections show a distinct histopathology that consists of multifocal areas of necrosis in the cuticular epithelium and often in the subcuticular connective tissue. Present in these tissues are numerous variably sized eosinophilic to basophilic cytoplasmic inclusion bodies that give TS lesions a 'buckshot' pattern of necrosis which is typical of the disease. These characteristic changes are used as a means of diagnosis of TS. An *in situ* hybridization method using a complementary DNA (cDNA) probe has been developed as a diagnostic tool for the detection of TSV in fixed tissue preparations.

DNA viruses

Occluded baculoviruses The two occluded baculoviruses that have caused serious disease and economic losses in shrimp farms are: Baculovirus penaei (BP) occluded type A also known as *Penaeus vannamei* single nuclear polyhedrosis virus (PVSNPV) and *Penaeus monodon* baculovirus (MBV) occluded type A also known as *Penaeus monodon* single nuclear polyhedrosis virus (PMSNPV).

Baculovirus penaei BP was first described by light and electron microscopy in naturally infected *P. duorarum* (pink shrimp). Since then the virus has been found in several wild and cultured penaeid species: *P. aztecus*, *P. setiferus*, *P. vannamei*, *P. stylirostris*, *P. penicillatus*, *P. schmitti*, *P. paulensis*, *P. subtilis* and several others. Thus far the virus has been limited in its distribution to the Western hemisphere and Hawaii.

Epizootics of BP can result in high mortality of larval and early postlarval shrimp, particularly in intensive culture systems which facilitate the development and transmission of the disease. However, in larval or late postlarval penaeid shrimp, the effects of BP infection are minimal. Age appears to play a role in susceptibility of the penaeid shrimp to BP.

In the infected animal, BP affects primarily cells of the hepatopancreatic and midgut epithelium. In the hypertrophied nuclei of infected cells in these affected tissues, the newly synthesized progeny may be either free or occluded, with characteristic tetrahedral crystalloid bodies termed occlusion bodies (OBs). The polyhedra are easily seen by light microscopy and may be as large as 17 μm. From one to several polyhedra may occupy a nucleus. The OBs, which are composed primarily of the protein polyhedrin, are used as a diagnostic feature of patent BP infections.

Little is known concerning persistent BP infections in the natural environment. Attempts to demonstrate this phenomenon experimentally in the larvae and postlarvae of *P. vannamei* have not been successful.

A mixed infection involving BP and a reo-like agent has been described. Each shrimp with a reo-like infection also had a BP infection, but the reverse was not always true. Both viruses were observed in the same tissue and occasionally in the same cell.

There is sparse information concerning the biochemical and cellular events involved in the infection cycle of BP. Based on electron microscopical studies the BP virion, presumably after attachment and viropexis or fusion, uncoats or injects its DNA into the host cell nucleus at the nuclear pore. After integration of the virion into the host cell genome, a series of morphologically recognizable sequences of events occur, leading to the eventual production of mature BP and tetrahedral OBs. A distinct intracellular morphological change observed is the appearance of extensive membranous labyrinths (ML) adjacent to the endoplasmic reticulum. The ML appeared to originate from dilated Golgi and endoplasmic reticulum vesicles and from the outer nuclear envelope.

The BP virion is a rod-shaped nucleocapsid surrounded by a trilaminar envelope. Unlike some nuclear polyhedrosis viruses with multiple nucleocapsids per envelope, BP has only one per envelope. The intact, enveloped virions, when banded in CsCl gradient, exhibit a buoyant density of 1.265 g ml^{-1}. On the basis of negative staining, the enveloped virion is $312–320 \times 75–87$ nm and the nucleocapsid is approximately 306–312 × 62–68 nm. The complete enveloped virions appear to possess appendage-like structures at both extremities that are assumed to be loose envelope extensions. Similar structures have also been seen among other shrimp baculoviruses, such as the nonoccluded virions. Thin section measurements of the virion reveal a smaller particle of approximately 270–296 × 54–59 nm with nucleocapsid dimensions of 260 × 44.2 nm.

Sucrose-banded OBs, when analyzed by SDS-PAGE using 12% polyacrylamide gels, revealed one major polypeptide with a molecular weight of 52 kDa. Nothing is known about the structural proteins and glycoproteins that compose the complete enveloped virus.

The BP genome is a double-stranded, circular DNA with a molecular weight of 75×10^6 Da. Analysis by electrophoresis in a 1% agarose gel of extracted BP DNA digested with the restriction endonuclease *Bam*HI revealed seven bands with estimated sizes: ≥ 23, 11.7, 8.2, 4.8, 4.0, 2.9 and 1.1 kb. The largest band probably contained two or more high-molecular-weight bands.

The BP virion is sensitive to a number of physical and chemical conditions. It is completely inactivated under the following conditions: within 30 min at pH 3 but not at pH 11; after 10 min at 60–90°C; after ultraviolet (UV) inactivation for 40 min at a wavelength of 254 nm; and after desiccation for 48 h. On the other hand, it survives 32 parts per thousand sea water at 22°C for 7 days and at 5°C for at least 14 days.

Diagnosis of BP infections has been accomplished in a number of ways: (1) by light microscopic observation of characteristic tetrahedral OBs in wet mount squash preparations of the hepatopancreas, midgut or feces or on histological sections and (2) by the use of the recently developed gene probes that detect BP nucleic acid in infected cells by *in situ* hybridization assay. The latter procedure, which was found to be specific, can also detect BP infections even before the appearance of OBs in wet mount squashes. The probes can detect BP in various species of shrimp from different geographical areas.

More recently, a PCR-based detection procedure was developed for BP. However, this procedure still has, among several caveats, the potential problem of the presence of compounds in shrimp tissues that inhibit the DNA polymerase used in the PCR procedure. It should be added that these recently developed molecular procedures have not been comprehensively evaluated in field studies.

Penaeus monodon baculovirus Since its initial isolation, MBV has been found in a wide variety of both cultured and wild penaeid shrimp species from Asia, Australia, Africa, southern Europe and the Middle East. Reports indicate its presence in shrimp stock in the Americas, but the animals were originally imported from Asia. The virus has been linked to serious diseases and major economic losses in shrimp farms in Southeast Asia and Asia.

A similar agent was found in cultured *P. plebejus* in Australia and was called *Plebejus* baculovirus (PBV). However, on the basis of virus-induced host cell cytopathology and virus morphology, PBV is believed to be a strain of MBV type of viruses rather than a distinct virus type.

MBV is a highly infectious virus that spreads very quickly and causes high larval and juvenile mortality. In adult shrimp the infection is less severe, with the animals showing no significant external signs of disease. In the Indo-Pacific region, MBV has been reported to be a ubiquitous pathogen of cultured *P. monodon*. However, despite its high prevalence and wide distribution, the virion does not appear to be a highly virulent pathogen for *P. monodon*. In disease epizootics, the penaeid shrimp has been frequently found to have mixed infections of MBV and other pathogens. Transmission of MBV is believed to be primarily oral, e.g. from cannibalism. However, other routes of horizontal transmission may occur, such as through contamination of spawned eggs with virus-contaminated feces.

As with all occluded baculoviruses, a principal histopathological and diagnostic feature of MBV infections is the presence of single and multiple, generally spherical OBs, in the hepatopancreas and less often in midgut epithelial cells. The OBs, which have diameters in the range 0.1–20 μm, may be demonstrated in squash preparations of hepatopancreas, midgut, or feces by phase or bright-field microscopy. Different kinds of stains, such as 0.05% aqueous Malachite Green, Acridine Orange, or Phloxine, can be used to enhance visualization of MBV occlusions.

Very little information is available concerning the replication of MBV. A limited ultrastructural study on the morphogenesis of the virions in hepatopancreatic cells revealed certain cytopathic alterations occurring late in the infection, such as nuclear hypertropy, chromatin diminution, loss of nucleolus, formation of virogenic stromata, appearance of many enveloped virions, and appearance and formation of OBs. Another distinct change was the appearance of ML membranes, as was observed in BP infection. Again, the ML was postulated to play two roles in the virion replication cycle: first, as a conduit or transport system for viral structural precursors from the cytoplasm to the nucleoplasm, and second, after this function is completed, as a mechanism for release of virus and OBs.

Primary shrimp lymphoid cell cultures have been used to support MBV replication. As the result of viral replication, cytopathogenic effects occurred as early as 2–3 days p.i. and became more extensive as the infection progressed. The virus was successfully passaged in primary lymphoid cell cultures at least six times. Unfortunately, no further studies were done until the recent report on the use of primary shrimp lymphoid cells for the growth and assay of YHV and the Chinese baculovirus (or white spot baculovirus).

Electron microscopic examination of uranyl acetate-stained MBV revealed enveloped, rod-shaped particles measuring 265–282 × 68–77 nm and nucleocapsids measuring 250–269 × 62–68 nm. The envelope surface appeared to consist of small, uniformly sized granular structures interspersed with small spikes which were more apparent at the vertices. At the extremities of the envelope were appendage-like structures which were believed to be envelope extensions. Each extremity of the nucleocapsid was enclosed with a double-layered structure, or cap, 16–18 nm thick.

When banded in 30–50% CsCl, complete MBV has a buoyant density of 1.28–1.29 g ml^{-1}, and the OBs have a buoyant density of 1.32–1.33 g ml^{-1}.

The polyhedrin subunits of the spherical MBV polydedron were icosahedral-like structures measuring 22–23 nm in diameter. Analysis of purified MBV OBs by SDS-PAGE and Western blot protocols revealed a single protein band of 62 kDa. The molecular size of the MBV polyhedrin appears to be slightly larger than that of BP (53 kDa), the other occluded baculovirus of penaeid shrimp.

Visualization of MBV DNA by electron microscopy revealed large, supercoiled molecules which were not sufficiently relaxed to allow measurement of the total molecular weight of the genome. However, the viral DNA, after digestion with *Bam*HI endonuclease and electrophoresis in 1% agarose gel, yielded five bands with the following estimated sizes: ≥21, 9, 6.5, 3.5 and 2.8 kb. From these studies, the mol. wt. of the MBV DNA was estimated to be 58–110 × 10^6 kDa (80–160 kb), which falls within the DNA size range of insect baculoviruses. In another study, the molecular size of MBV DNA based on *Eco*RI-cleaved fragments was estimated to be 100–200 kb.

Traditional diagnosis/detection of MBV infection is accomplished by histological examination for the presence of characteristic spherical OBs in hypertrophied nuclei of the hepatopancreas and anterior midgut of the infected animal. Still another source of OBs is shrimp feces. However, these methods do not detect MBV infection at early stages, nor are they adequately sensitive.

Molecular-based methods for the early and specific detection and diagnosis of MBV infections have been developed. The PCR procedure and either *in situ* or dot-blot hybridization techniques employing DNA probes can be used for accurate and early diagnosis or detection of MBV infection.

Non-occluded baculoviruses There are several members belonging to this non-occluded baculovirus group; the classification of all of them has not been officially accepted by the International Committee on Taxonomy of Viruses (ICTV). All of these viruses have caused major epizootics and significant economic losses to the shrimp aquaculture industry.

Baculoviral midgut gland necrosis virus (BMNV) nonoccluded type C also named Penaeus japonicus *nonoccluded baculovirus (PJNOB)* The BMNV is a nonoccluded, gut-infecting virus first isolated in *kuruma* shrimp, *P. japonicus*, larvae. It is highly pathogenic in the early life stages of the shrimp, causing heavy mortality in larval production. Although *P. japonicus* is the natural host for BMNV, other penaeid species, such as *P. monodon, P. chinensis,* and *P. semisulcatus*, were found to be experimentally susceptible. Whereas *P. monodon* was found to be highly susceptible, both *P. chinensis* and *P. semisulcatus* showed great resistance to the virus. As with the other shrimp viral pathogens, the waterborne-oral feeding route may represent the natural route of transmission.

Histological examinations of BMNV-infected animals indicate that the midgut and the intestine are the target organs. Infected cells show characteristic nuclear hypertropy and chromatolysis, as well as the absence of OBs which characterize infections by Type A baculoviruses.

Thin-section electron micrographs of the infected nuclei and the midgut lumen reveal numerous rod-shaped, enveloped viral particles, many of which have outer and inner envelopes. The average dimension of the virion was 310 × 72 nm. Purified inner rod-like nucleocapsid structures had capped ends and measured approximately 260 × 50 nm.

No information is available concerning the replication of BMNV at the cellular level.

Viral DNA extracted from purified nucleocapsids was sensitive to digestion with restriction endonucleases *Bam*HI and *Sau*3AI, but not with *Eco*RI, *Pst*I, *Xho*I and *Sal*I. Electrophoretic analysis in agarose gels of the enzyme-digested viral DNA revealed 13 fragments with relative molecular sizes in the range

2.2–27.0 kb. From these results, the mol. wt of viral DNA was estimated to be 85.1×10^6 Da.

Structural protein analysis of nucleocapsid preparation by SDS-PAGE revealed two major proteins with molecular weights of 35 and 14 kDa and three minor bands (mol. wt = 72, 65 and 12 kDa).

Several methods are available for the diagnosis of BMNV infections. Both stained preparations and dark-field microscopic diagnostic methods are used to detect infected, hypertrophied nuclei in squashed preparations of affected tissues such as midgut and intestine. The dark-field microscopic method, because of its simplicity, rapidity, precision and low cost, is the method of choice in shrimp hatcheries in Japan. An immunofluorescent antibody (IFA) procedure has been successfully used to detect BMN-specific virus antigen in smears or sectioned preparations of affected tissues, such as midgut epithelial cells.

White spot baculovirus (WSBV) nonoccluded type C also called systemic ectodermal and mesodermal baculovirus (SEMBV), bacilliform virus (BV), rod-shaped nuclear virus of Penaeus japonicus *(RV-PJ), penaeid rod-shaped DNA virus (PRDV), penaeid hemocytic rod-shaped virus (PHRV) and Chinese baculovirus (CBV)* All these names have been given to the viral isolates obtained from different species of cultured penaeid shrimp from different geographical areas. Until further characterizations of their serological, biochemical and genomic properties are made, the isolates may be considered to be either related strains of the same virus or identical. Although *in situ* hybridization studies have suggested that these nonoccluded baculovirus isolates may be closely related, a recent report has presented evidence to show that they can be distinguished by RFLP (restriction fragment length polymorphism) analyses of the viral genomes. All of these isolates cause epizootics and mass mortality in cultured penaeid shrimp. Diseased shrimp show a characteristically abnormal reddish color together with white spots primarily on the inside surface of the carapace. However, with two experimentally infected penaeid species, *P. stylirostris* and *P. vannamei,* the characteristic white spots were not seen and the reddish color was seen only in the extremities of the appendages. These gross distinctive changes have been used in the diagnosis of WSBV infection. At the cellular level, infected cells showed markedly hypertrophied nuclei. In certain cases, histopathological examination of infected gill tissues may show Cowdry type A nuclear inclusions in hypertrophied nuclei. The natural route of transmission for these virions appears to be the waterborne-oral feeding routes.

Electron microscopical examination of thin sections of affected tissues revealed the presence of large numbers of rod-shaped baculo-like viral particles located primarily in the markedly enlarged nuclei which also showed a loss of integrity of the marginated chromatin material. Viral particles had a multilaminar outer envelope which had a mean size of 265 ± 20 nm in length and 120 ± 10 nm in diameter. The size of the electron-dense nucleocapsid of the virus was 205 ± 12 nm in length and 78 ± 5 nm in diameter. A large number of viruses had double envelopes.

When banded isopycnically in CsCl, the complete virus had a buoyant density of 1.23 g ml^{-1} and the nucleocapsid particle 1.31 g ml^{-1}.

Negatively stained purified CBV particles measured 322–378 nm in length and 130–159 nm in diameter. The inner nucleoprotein core exhibited a unique striated structure and measured 316–350 nm in length and 65–66 nm in diameter. The striations appeared to be the result of the stacking of ring-like structures. These rings consisted of two rows of 12–14 globular units, each measuring 10 nm in diameter.

Genomic analysis of purified CBV revealed a nonsegmented, double-stranded DNA molecule. The reported sizes of the viral DNA genome ranged from 150 kbp to 200 kbp.

Analysis of the structural proteins of purified CBV by SDS-PAGE showed among several, four prominent protein bands with approximate molecular weights of 19, 23.5, 27.5 and 75 kDa. The structural viral proteins were substantiated by Western blot analysis. The 19, 27.5 and 75 kDa structural proteins were found to be nonglycosylated components associated with the viral envelope. The 23.5 kDa protein, also nonglycosylated, was identified with the capsid structure.

For the rapid, sensitive and specific detection/diagnosis of CBV (WSBV) infections both diagnostic probes for *in situ* hybridization and primers for detection by PCR technology have been successfully used. Such studies have also indicated that the gut and the gills of the penaeid shrimp were the primary routes of viral entry and that the lymphoid organ and gills were primary targets for viral replication.

A combined SDS-PAGE/Western blot/EIA protocol has been successfully used for the early detection of CBV in the hemolymph of infected animals. This combination technology has several advantages for the monitoring and surveillance of shrimp populations for virus infections. The sampling of hemolymph is relatively simple and less invasive, particularly for the monitoring of invaluable shrimp broodstocks.

Primary shrimp lymphoid cell cultures have been used in an *in vitro* quantal assay ($TCID_{50}$) for CBV.

Despite limitations associated with primary cell cultures, this assay provides a simple, convenient, reliable and quantitative method for the study of shrimp viruses.

Four fish cell lines (epithelioma papulosum cyprini [EPC]), chinook salmon embryo (CHSE-214), fathead minnow (FHM), and sockeye salmon embryo (SSE-5) and an insect cell line (CRL1963, a *Drosophila* cell line) were resistant to CBV.

A second group of DNA-containing penaeid shrimp viruses causing epizootics are two members of the parvovirus family.

Infectious hypodermal and hematopoietic necrosis virus (IHHNV) The IHHNV is widely distributed, causing severe epizootics and massive mortality in cultured penaeid shrimp, particularly the juveniles of *P. stylirostris*. In other penaeid species, the disease is somewhat less severe. With certain cultured penaeid species, such as *P. vannamei*, a 'runt-deformity syndrome' (RPS) may be the consequence. The affected animals characteristically exhibit greatly reduced growth rates and a variety of cuticular deformities, all of which lessen their market value.

Natural infections by IHHNV have been reported in a number of penaeid species, such as *P. stylirostris, P. semisulcatus* and *P. japonicus*. As with the other shrimp viral pathogens, the waterborne-oral feeding route may represent the natural route of transmission. Survivors of IHHN epizootics apparently harbor the virion for life and transmit it to their progeny by vertical and horizontal routes.

Gross clinical symptoms of acute IHHNV infections are not specific. In the infected animal, certain distinguishable histopathological changes occur. Present in affected cells are intranuclear Cowdry type A inclusion bodies (CAI) contained in hypertrophied nuclei in tissues of ectodermal (epidermis, hypodermal epithelium of foregut and hindgut, nerve cord, and nerve ganglia) and mesodermal (hematopoietic organ, antennal gland, gonads, lymphoid organ, connective tissues, and striated muscle) origin.

Purified IHHNV has been prepared from infected penaeid shrimp and banded in CsCl gradients at a buoyant density of $1.40\,g\,ml^{-1}$. Negatively stained, purified virions are nonenveloped icosahedrons with a diameter of 20–22 nm. The virions possess a linear, single-stranded DNA genome of either negative or positive polarity with an estimated size of 4.1 kb. The purified virion is made up of at least four structural polypeptides, VP1 to VP4, with molecular weights of 74, 47, 39 and 37.5 kDa.

To date no cell lines exist which will support the growth of IHHNV. No information is available regarding viral replication at either the cellular or molecular levels.

Several methods are available for the diagnosis of IHHNV infections. The histopathological examination of affected tissues for the presence or absence of intranuclear CAI has provided a fairly reliable diagnosis. However, the formation of CAI may be induced by rather general types of cell injury not involving viruses. Under certain conditions, both DNA- and RNA-containing viruses have been reported to cause CAI. Another method involves enhancement procedures in which the suspected animals are kept under stressful conditions for 2–3 weeks prior to sampling for histologic examination.

For the detection of asymptomatic IHHNV infections, susceptible small juveniles of *P. stylirostris* have been used as indicator shrimp for the presence or absence of the virus.

Gene probes have been developed for the detection/diagnosis of IHHNV infection. The probes have been used in dot-blot and *in situ* hybridization studies and are currently available commercially as a kit.

Hepatopancreatic parvo-like virus (HPV) The HPV is another parvo-like virus that infects a number of cultured and wild *Penaeus* species (*P. chinensis, P. merguiensis, P. semisulcatus, P. monodon, P. indicus, P. penicillatus, P. esculentus*). It has a wide geographic distribution, including the Indo-Pacific area and the Americas. The relationship between all of these reported HPV-type viruses is not known since identification of these virions was based solely on microscopic or histopathological examinations.

Although HPV has been circumstantially implicated in the cause of major disease epizootics, its role as a serious pathogen remains to be clearly defined. This is because of the relative difficulty of diagnosing HPV infections and also because these infections are often accompanied by other viral pathogens which may obscure its importance. Little is known concerning the natural mode of transmission of HPV, although the waterborne-oral route is the most likely. No cell lines are currently available which support the replication of HPV.

In the infected animal, the principal lesion of the disease is characterized by the necrosis and atrophy of the hepatopancreas, which is common to all the penaeid species. Large, prominent, basophilic, Feulgen-positive intranuclear inclusion bodies were often observed in hypertrophied nuclei of hepatopancreatic tubule epithelial cells. These histological changes were used in the diagnosis of HPV infections.

The HPV and the IHHNV are both parvoviruses, but in the permissive host animal they infect different target tissues: the hepatopancreatic epithelial cells for HPV and all nonenteric tissues for IHHNV.

Electron microscopic analysis of thin sections of HPV-infected cells revealed intranuclear inclusion bodies containing granular virogenic stroma and viral particles 22–24 nm in diameter.

Purified HPV prepared from infected penaeid shrimp and banded in CsCl gradient had a buoyant density of 1.41 g ml^{-1}. Negatively stained, purified virions were nonenveloped, icosahedral particles with a diameter of 22 nm. The virions contained a linear, single-stranded DNA genome of either negative or positive polarity with an estimated molecular size of 5 kb, which, surprisingly, encoded a single protein of 54 kDa.

Gene probes have been used with limited success in *in situ* hybridization assays for the diagnosis of HPV infections. Since the probe did not react positively in the tissues of HPV-infected penaeids from the Indo-Pacific region and the Americas, it is strongly indicated that there are probably several different strains of HPV. The HPV probe did not crossreact with the other shrimp parvovirus, IHHNV. The probe is commercially available as a kit for the diagnosis of HPV.

The following penaeid shrimp viruses have been reported. Most of them remain to be isolated and their relevant properties characterized:

Lymphoidal parvo-like virus (LOV)
Penaeid hemocyte-infecting, nonoccluded baculovirus (PHRV)
Shrimp iridovirus (IRIDO)
Type III reo-like virus (REO-III)
Type-IV reo-like virus (REO-IV)
Lymphoid organ vacuolization virus (LOVV)
Naked star-shaped virus (NSV).

See also: **Baculoviruses (*Baculoviridae*): Granuloviruses, Nucleopolyhedrovirus; Parvoviruses (*Parvoviridae*): Molecular biology, General features; Picornaviruses – insect (*Picornaviridae*); Polioviruses (*Picornaviridae*): General features, Molecular biology.**

Further Reading

Lightner DV (1993) In McVey JP (ed.) *Handbook of Mariculture*, 2nd edn, vol. 1, p. 393. Boca Raton: CRC Press.

Loh PC (1997) Viral pathogens of the penaeid shrimp. *Adv. Virus Res.* 48: 263.

Shope Fibroma Virus   *see* **Poxviruses**

Shope papilloma and bovine viruses   *see* **Papillomaviruses – animal**

SIGMA RHABDOVIRUSES (*RHABDOVIRIDAE*)

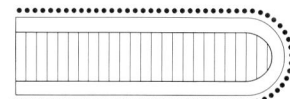

Danielle Teninges, Centre National de la Recherche Scientifique, Institut de Génétique humaine, Montpellier, France

Copyright © 1999 Academic Press

History

The sigma virus of *Drosophila* is a harmless virus of a harmless insect and probably would never have attracted any attention were it not for the fact that geneticists use carbon dioxide (CO_2) as a mild narcotic for the flies they handle. This gas is generally not noxious and flies recover from narcosis within a few minutes after return to a normal atmosphere. Those infected by the sigma virus, in contrast, remain irreversibly paralyzed and die. CO_2 sensitivity in some *Drosophila* strains was first reported in 1937 by L'Heritier and Tessier as a hereditary trait which was not chromosome-linked. The viral etiology was not suspected at first owing to the complete absence of horizontal transmission of CO_2 sensitivity in natural conditions. Later, L'Heritier observed that inoculation of acellular extracts from CO_2-sensitive flies into resistant flies produced the symptom after an incubation period which increased with the dilution of the inoculum. The size of the agent was deduced from the target size to x-ray inactivation. Studies by electron microscopy confirmed this information and identified sigma virus as a member of the rhabdovirus family. It has not been assigned to a genus. With its genetic background, *Drosophila melanogaster* was an ideal host to allow genetic analyses of the host factors involved in a virus–insect association and most efforts have been centered on research of this kind.

Pathology

The CO_2 sensitivity symptom is the only sign of disease observed in infected flies. It affects larvae as well as adults and persists throughout their lives. The range of CO_2 concentrations that are lethal to the flies is not frequently met in nature and this cannot account for any counterselection of infected flies. Among inoculated flies the expression of CO_2 sensitivity is correlated to the appearance of infectious material in the central nervous system. Immunocytochemistry reveals the presence of granular inclusions of viral material in the cortex of the cephalic and thoracic ganglia. In hereditarily infected flies, such inclusion bodies are present in all tissues, except muscle. Wild sigma virus-infected flies have been compared to uninfected flies for egg viability, male and female fertility, female longevity and sexual selection. Sigma virus infection only reduced egg viability; other parameters did not show any systematic or significant variation. Survival of adults under winter conditions in France was also studied and showed that the fitness of infected flies to overwintering was slightly lower. Wild sigma virus clones show a very low multiplication rate, which may account for their relative innocuousness. Laboratory strains selected for high multiplication rates generally affect fertility and egg viability in such proportions that when they appear in natural populations they are probably severely counterselected.

In *Drosophila* cells cultivated *in vitro*, sigma virus multiplies without any evidence of a cytopathic effect and a persistent infection is maintained throughout cell transfers.

Since a number of other rhabdoviruses and a bunyavirus (but no flaviviruses) were shown to induce CO_2 sensitivity after inoculation to *Drosophila* flies or to mosquitoes, exposure to CO_2 was proposed as a fast means of screening infected insects in nature.

Virion and Genome Structure

Sigma virus particles exhibit all the structural details of typical rhabdoviruses: a bullet shape, a coiled nucleocapsid, and an envelope derived from the host cell and covered with surface projections. The diameter is 75 nm and the length 200 nm. The presence of shorter particles has also been recorded. The genome structure of a strain selected for high yields in *Drosophila* cell cultures *in vitro* has been studied. It consists of a single segment of approximately 13 000 nucleotides. It encodes six proteins mapped in the following order on the genome strand: 3′-N-P-X-M-G-L-5′ where N is the nucleoprotein and P a phosphoprotein which is the equivalent of the polymerase-associated protein in vesicular stomatitis virus (VSV); gene 3 (X) encodes a protein of unknown function with many potential phosphorylation sites and showing similarities to some of the retroviral reverse transcriptase motifs; M is the matrix protein, G is the glycoprotein and L is the polymerase. The respective lengths predicted for the polypeptides are 450 amino acids for N, 322 for P, 296 for X, 207 for M, and 499 for G. The exact length of L is still unknown but its electrophoretic mobility corresponds to a protein of 250 kDa. The consensus gene-start and gene-end sequences are respectively, CAACANC and $CAUG(A)_7$ in the mRNA sense and thus conform to the consensus AACA and $AUG(A)_7$ observed in all the rhabdoviruses previously analyzed.

Intergenic sequences are thought to intervene in transcriptional control. Some rhabdoviruses like VSV have constant intergenes, whereas others, such as rabies virus, show variation. Sigma virus belongs to the second category and has 36 untranscribed nucleotides which separate N and P, six which separate P and X and four which separate X and M; then G overlaps M, starting 26 nucleotides upstream of the end of the M gene, so the polymerase has to read through the end sequence of the M gene to transcribe the G gene. In spite of this overlap, the transcription results in the regular synthesis of monocistronic M and G mRNAs. The start signal of the L gene is immediately adjacent to the end signal of the G gene. As deduced from UV target size analyses, the transcription of unsegmented negative-strand viruses proceeds sequentially from the 3′ extracistronic region of the genome to the 5′ end. A gene overlap implies that sites of initiation other than the most 3′ proximal one can be used by newly entered polymerases. Gene overlap could be a means of reducing the expression of the two most distal genes from the 3′ end.

Serology and Taxonomy

Fifty animal rhabdoviruses of diverse origins were screened for antigenic crossreactivity. Most of them could be classified in the two large subgroups – the lyssaviruses and the vesiculoviruses. In this study, sigma virus was shown to crossreact with Tupaia, a vesiculovirus isolated from a shrew, and with

Tibrogargan, Humpty Doo and Parry Creek, three lyssaviruses isolated from mosquitoes; it was thus proposed to bridge the gap between the two subgroups. Considering other criteria, such as the scores of similarity between predicted protein sequences, sigma virus appears almost equally distant from the prototypes of both subgroups. The progress of molecular data on other rhabdoviruses may raise the necessity for the definition of new subgroups more closely related to sigma virus.

Virus–Host Interactions

Hereditary transmission is a very efficient means of propagation but its efficiency varies according to the virus genotype and to the sex and genotype of flies. The so called 'stabilized' females transmit the virus to all their descendants with few exceptions. They issue from oocytes that were infected very early, and in which the virus was able to multiply enough to invade all the germline cells from the outset. Their male progeny may also transmit the virus but with a lower efficiency (infection via a spermatozoid is an efficient means of cloning virus particles). The pattern of virus transmission from flies hatched from spermatozoid-infected eggs is different from that of stabilized females: males do not transmit the virus and females may transmit it but only to a small proportion of their descendants. This is an effect of the low concentration of virus genomes in the spermatozoid-infected eggs: cell differentiation and organogenesis probably result in barriers against the penetration of the virus into some tissues. There could be a race during embryogenesis between the virus invasion and the building up of these barriers. Male germ cells which are not infected at the very early stages of embryogenesis (before segmentation) are not invaded at a later stage of development. Female germ cells may be invaded at any stage, including adults, provided that the virus genotype is g^+ (g^- mutants are normally perpetuated in stabilized maternal lines and virions are infectious to somatic cells but they cannot invade the germinal cysts, once isolated by organogenesis). Some stabilized maternal lines (the ultra-rho lines) perpetuate defective viruses which are not infectious and which do not induce CO_2 sensitivity; the only sign of their presence is an immunity to superinfection by homologous virus – immunity which shows exactly the same inheritance pattern as nondefective viruses.

In other stabilized lines, the rho lines, the same phenotype was observed but a still unexplained genetic instability of the viral genomes infecting these lines resulted in the occasional production of fully infectious virions. Some stabilized maternal lines, infected with temperature-sensitive mutants for maturation functions, express exactly the same phenotype as the ultra-rho lines when bred for several generations at nonpermissive temperature, but the CO_2 sensitivity symptom is restored upon return to the permissive temperature. The persistent infection of germ cells through generations by viruses which are defective (or temperature restricted) proves that only the maturation functions are affected in these mutants, not the genome replication. It also proves that viral information may be transmitted by cellular continuity without a necessity for infectious virus production.

Natural populations of *D. melanogaster* are often polymorphic for alleles of genes that confer resistance to sigma virus infection. These restrictive alleles map to six different loci: *ref(1)H*, *ref(2)M*, *ref(2)P*, *ref(3)O*, *ref(3)V* and *ref(3)D* (the number in parentheses represents the *Drosophila* chromosome carrying the gene, the capital letter is the particular name of the gene, and specific alleles of those genes are indicated by an exponent). The refractory loci (*ref*) do not represent a general antiviral system: not only do they not affect other insect viruses but none of them confers resistance to all strains of sigma virus (with a possible exception for *ref(3)V*; see later).

Restrictive effects have been assessed for several parameters of viral infection, such as the mean incubation time required for the expression of CO_2 sensitivity, the probability of initiating infection, the kinetics of virus production (either in flies or in cells cultivated *in vitro*) and the efficiency of virus transmission either by females or by males. A distinction can be made between restriction during either virus maturation or earlier stages of virus production (i.e. genome replication): since hereditary transmission in stabilized maternal lines does not require the production of infective virus, those alleles restricting this transmission necessarily affect the genome replication steps. The four alleles $ref(1)H^b$, $ref(2)M^m$, $ref(2)P^p$ and $ref(3)D^d$ reduce the probability of initiating infection and increase the incubation time for the manifestation of the CO_2 sensitivity symptom. The transmission through the maternal gametes is also reduced very strongly by $ref(1)H^b$ and $ref(2)P^p$, whereas $ref(2)M^m$ and $ref(3)D^d$ exert a weaker action. This implies that the products of these four genes intervene in the replication of the viral genomes. $Ref(3)O^e$ does not affect the hereditary transmission but increases the incubation time of the viral clones sensitive to its action. The allele $ref(1)H^b$ is the only fully dominant allele; flies heterozygous at all other loci express intermediate phenotypes. The $ref(3)V^p$ restrictive allele does not affect the virus multiplication in somatic cells nor in female germ cells and its unique effect is to prevent transmission by spermatozoa. The specificity of this interaction with sigma virus is still unknown, as to date no viral strains have been found to be resistant. In contrast, the major effects described for the restrictive alleles at other loci apply only to sensitive viral strains.

Flies that are homozygous for either permissive or restrictive alleles are indistinguishable except for the difference in their capacity to permit the multiplication of sigma virus. The most extensively studied refractory gene is *ref(2)P*. Loss of function alleles (*ref(2)P^{null}*) were induced by mutagenesis of a permissive *ref(2)P^o* allele. Homozygous flies for the *ref(2)P^{null}* alleles are all viable and display no phenotype other than male sterility in particular genetic backgrounds. Some alleles of a gene located on the third chromosome suppress the male sterility of *ref(2)P^{null}* homozygotes. Such alleles are present in approximately one-third of the flies in natural populations, which means that *ref(2)P* is essential to male fertility in two-thirds of the flies. The mutation exclusively affects the structure of the spermatozoa in which the organization of the mitochondrion and axonema is perturbed. Nevertheless, *ref(2)P* is expressed in a wide variety of tissues: it is expressed in female germ cells as seen from the strong inhibition of the virus transovarian transmission by restrictive alleles; however females are normally fertile, thus the gene is not essential at the cellular level. It is also expressed in somatic cells, as seen, for instance, from the effects on virus yields and CO_2 sensitivity. This expression is autonomous: in organs transplanted into individuals bearing permissive or restrictive alleles, the action of *ref(2)P* on the virus conforms to the organ genotype.

The effect of restrictive alleles is also observed at the single cell level in permanent *in vitro* cell lines. Homozygotes *ref(2)P^{null}* are permissive to sigma virus infection, thus the *ref(2)P* gene product serves no indispensable function in the virus cycle and hence could be considered as a defense gene. The expression is ubiquitous. All the transcripts found in different tissues result from the same splicing pattern of three exons but different initiation sites are used. As a consequence, the 5′ untranslated region varies in length according to the cell type. The size distribution of the transcripts and their abundance varies according to the tissue, suggesting a tissue-specific regulation of the gene expression at the transcriptional and possibly at the translational level.

The gene encodes a single protein of about 600 amino acids containing a cysteine-rich region resembling a zinc-finger motif. The amino acid sequence is very variable and there is a length polymorphism in the coding region. Restrictive and permissive alleles are codominant, and *ref(2)P* proteins of both types form complexes with the viral P protein. The *ref(2)P* protein crossreacts with antibodies directed against the viral N protein, due to the presence of a common conformation-dependent epitope. The *hap* viral mutants are mutants which escape the restrictive effect of *ref(2)P^p*. In the *hap7* mutant, this epitope is not present and the N protein differs from that of the original virus by a single amino acid substitution.

These data could suggest that the *ref(2)P* protein competes with the N protein by means of this epitope to complex the P protein in a form which is unsuitable for its function in the viral transcriptional complex (which requires the N, P and L proteins). However, the restriction mechanism is certainly more complicated, as a transgene containing only the 91 N-terminal amino acids of a restrictive allele, but not the epitope, is sufficient to confer a restrictive phenotype to transformed *Drosophila* lines in the conditions of artificial inoculation, and not in the hereditary transmission process.

Interestingly, a simultaneous adaptation or disadaptation of a number of *hap* mutants to other *ref* genes, such as *ref(1)H^b*, *ref(3)O^e* or *ref(2)M^m*, was observed. This covariation suggests that the same viral protein interacts with the cellular proteins encoded by these other *ref* genes.

The variability of natural alleles of the *ref(2)P* gene is high and there is a high rate of amino acid replacement to synonymous codon changes. The most recent alleles are the restrictive ones. A possible explanation is that when a restrictive mutant appears and reaches sufficient frequency in a population, the virus evolves rapidly in response to this new allele, which becomes permissive to the adapted virotype; then a new restrictive mutant may arise and be transiently selected.

The time between inoculation and the first detection of virus progeny is about 30 h at 20°C. All the present knowledge about the viral replication process results from the physiological study of temperature-sensitive and host-range mutants. These mutants identify four steps in the growth cycle of the sigma virus. At 20°C, after a rapid phase of adsorption-penetration (1 h), there is a phase lasting about 8 h which corresponds to the temperature-sensitive period of the mutant *hap7*. The next stage, from 4 to 15 h postinfection, is defined by the mutant *ts4*. The mutants *hap7* and *ts4* have been designated early mutants. *Ts4* is defective in hereditary transmission at the restrictive temperature (28°C); *hap7* is not, even at 30°C. The function affected in *hap7* is indispensable before genome replication, and facultative once genome replication has started.

The next stage is defined by mutants such as *ts9*, in which germinal transmission is not temperature sensitive. In such mutants, designated late mutants, the genome replication functions are not affected and their temperature-sensitive period corresponds to a phase of virus assembly and budding. The functions necessary to initiate infection are not affected in *ts*9 (as deduced from analyses of infectious center decay) but the virions are thermolabile. The *ts* mutations have not yet been assigned to any gene. In analogy to the molecular biology of other rhabdoviruses, some predictions can be made. In VSV only the three proteins of the viral nucleocapsid (N, P and L) are required for the synthesis of monocistronic capped and polyadenylated mRNAs and, in the next step, of full genome length RNAs.

The matrix protein M is required for the transport of newly synthesized nucleocapsids toward the membrane patches in which the glycoprotein G is inserted and for the budding of progeny virions. The sigma virus counterparts of these proteins are likely to play the same roles. If so, the proteins modified in early mutants may be N, P or L, while late mutants may bear temperature-sensitive M or G proteins. We have no clues which could permit the prediction of the phenotypes of mutants affected in the additional protein X. Nevertheless, the absence of cytopathogenicity of the virus, even in the most permissive host genotype, and even in the most sensitive stages of host development, strongly suggests that the sigma virus multiplication rate is self-restricted. It is tempting to speculate that the protein of yet unknown function, or the gene overlap, or both, could account for this feature. According to the first hypothesis, mutants with disfunctioning X protein would produce higher virus yields. Paradoxically, clones with temperature-sensitive mutations of X would be more invasive to the host and thus have enhanced temperature resistance. Viral strains with such a phenotype exist. High yield and high-temperature resistance in sigma virus clones are always correlated with a pathogenic effect on the germline and the loss of hereditary transmission. Such characteristics are shared by the vesiculoviruses (which do not have an X gene) when inoculated into *Drosophila*.

Ecology

The specific CO_2 sensitivity symptom makes the identification of infected flies very easy and has allowed significant exploration of *Drosophila* natural populations. CO_2-sensitive flies were found among several *Drosophila* species throughout the world. The viruses carried by the different fruit fly populations share the major characteristics of sigma virus (hereditary transmission, symptom, etc.) but they may be distinct. The data indicate that such viruses are endemic in all the populations of *Drosophila*, the infected flies being the minority (10–20% in French natural populations). The high proportion of uninfected flies does not correspond to a virus-resistant fraction of the populations, as they and their offspring may become infected experimentally in the laboratory.

The genetic approach to the study of an insect–virus relationship performed with sigma virus underlines the complexity of the interactions and the difficulties involved in the control of all the relevant parameters.

See also: **Rabies virus (*Rhabdoviridae*); Rhabdoviruses (*Rhabdoviridae*): Plant rhabdoviruses, Ungrouped mammalian, bird and fish rhabdoviruses; Vesicular stomatitus viruses (*Rhabdoviridae*).**

Further Reading

Dezélée S, Bras F et al (1989) Molecular analysis of ref(2)P, a *Drosophila* gene implicated in sigma rhabdovirus multiplication and necessary for male fertility. *EMBO J.* 8: 3437.

Fleuriet A (1988) Maintenance of a hereditary virus: the sigma virus in populations of its host, *D. melanogaster*. In: Hecht M and Wallace B (eds) *Evolutionary Biology*, p. 2. New York: Plenum Press.

Landes-Devauchelle C, Bras F, Dezélée S et al (1995) Gene 2 of the sigma rhabdovirus encodes the P protein and gene 3 encodes a protein related to the reverse transcriptase of retroelements. *Virology* 213: 300.

Wayne ML, Contamine D and Kreitman M (1996) Molecular population genetics of *ref(2)P*, a locus which confers viral resistance in *Drosophila*. *Mol. Biol. Evol.* 13: 191.

Wyers F, Petitjean AM, Dzu P et al (1995) Localization of domains within the *Drosophila* ref(2)p protein involved in the intracellular control of sigma rhabdovirus multiplication. *J. Virol.* 69: 4463.

Simian Hemorhagic Fever Virus   *see* Encephalitis Viruses and Arteriviruses (*Arteriviridae*)

Simian Herpesvirus   *see* Herpesvirus Saimiri and Ateles

SIMIAN IMMUNODEFICIENCY VIRUSES (*RETROVIRIDAE*)

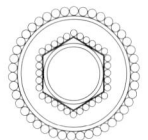

Vito G Sasseville and **Ronald C Desrosiers**, Harvard Medical School, New England Regional Primate Research Center, Southborough, Massachusetts, USA

Hillary G Morrison, Marine Biological Laboratory, Woods Hole, Massachusetts, USA

Copyright © 1999 Academic Press

History

Simian immunodeficiency virus (SIV) was first isolated in 1984 from immunodeficient captive rhesus macaques (*Macaca mulatta*) at the New England Regional Primate Research Center (NERPRC). This virus was originally called STLV-III because of its similar morphology, growth characteristics and antigenic properties to the newly described immunosuppressive virus in humans termed HTLV-III, LAV or ARV. When HTLV-III was renamed human immunodeficiency virus (HIV), STLV-III was appropriately changed to SIV. Retrospective studies show that SIV was introduced to the NERPRC via a group of rhesus monkeys with immunosuppressive disease delivered from another primate center 15 years prior to the initial isolation of SIV in 1985. This original cohort of animals was most likely inadvertently infected with SIV from wild-caught sooty mangabey monkeys housed at the same location. Following this initial isolation of SIV from rhesus macaques, SIV was isolated from other captive macaque species (*M. fascicularis*, *M. nemestrina*, *M. arctoides*) dying of diseases associated with immunosuppression and from feral asymptomatic African nonhuman primates, including African green monkeys (SIVagm), mandrills (SIVmnd), sooty mangabey monkeys (SIVsmm), red-capped mangabeys (SIVrcm), Sykes' monkeys (SIVsyk) and chimpanzees (SIVcpz).

Taxonomy and Classification

SIVs belong to the *Lentivirus* genus of the *Retroviridae* family. This genus includes the classic ungulate lentiviruses (visna virus of sheep, caprine arthritis encephalitis virus and equine infectious anemia virus) and the immunodeficiency viruses of humans (HIV), monkeys (SIV), cats (FIV) and cattle (BIV). The retroviruses can be subclassified by morphologic and morphogenic criteria. Lentivirus particles are approximately 80–110 nm in size and consist of an RNA genome and viral enzymes enclosed in a core of viral proteins that is encased by a cell-derived membrane spiked with viral envelope glycoproteins. Lentiviruses can be distinguished from other subgroups of retroviruses by the presence of a cylindrical or rod-shaped nucleoid in mature particles. In lymphocytes, lentivirus particles bud from the plasmalemma into the extracellular space, but in macrophages particles often bud from the plasma membrane into cytoplasmic vacuoles where they can accumulate. Lentiviruses also share a similarity in certain biological properties and the organization of their genomes. Unlike many of the other retroviruses, they are not oncogenic. Instead, they produce long-term, persistent infections which eventually lead to chronic debilitating disease. All lentiviruses studied to date replicate and persist in cells of the monocyte/macrophage lineage. In addition to the standard *gag*, *pol* and *env* genes that all retroviruses have, lentiviruses possess a number of additional genes not found in other retroviruses.

The SIVs are named according to the primate species of origin, e.g. SIVmac from macaques or SIVsmm from sooty mangabey monkeys. Based on genetic sequence analysis, five discrete groups of primate lentiviruses have been identified (**Fig. 1**, **Table 1** and see later). These are HIV-1/SIVcpz, HIV-2/SIVsmm/SIVmac, SIVagm, SIVmnd and SIVsyk.

Geographic and Seasonal Distribution

African green monkeys (*Cercopithecus aethiops*), Sykes' monkeys (*Cercopithecus mitis*), sooty mangabey monkeys (*Cercocebus torquatus atys*), red-capped mangabey monkeys (*Cercocebus torquatus torquatus*) and mandrills (*Papio sphinx*) have been shown to be infected with SIV in their natural habitats. Serological evidence suggests that SIV infection of African green monkeys is widely distributed in Africa. Between 20 and 50% of African green monkeys in Kenya, Ethiopia, South Africa and Senegal have antibodies to SIV. However, green monkeys which became established in the Caribbean since the seventeenth century are seronegative. Recent data also indicate that sooty mangabey monkeys in their native habitat in the coastal forests of western Africa are infected with their own highly divergent SIVs. These SIVsmm isolates, which differ markedly from

Table 1 Primate lentivirus nonstructural genes

Gene	SIVagm	SIVsmm/SIVmac/HIV-2	SIVmnd	SIVsyk	HIV-1/SIVcpz
vpu	−	−	−	−	+
vpx	+	+	−	−	−
vpr	−	+	+	+	+
tat	+	+	+	+	+
rev	+	+	+	+	+
vif	+	+	+	+	+
nef	+	+	+	+	+

one another, are closely related to HIV-2 subtypes D and E from humans in the same areas. These findings suggest that different HIV-2 subtypes may have originated from multiple cross-species transmissions of divergent SIVsmm strains from sooty mangabeys to humans. Macaque monkeys do not harbor SIV in their native Asian habitat, but became infected presumably via contact with SIV-infected sooty mangabeys while in captivity at Regional Primate Research Centers in the United States. Thus, African nonhuman primates and not Asian macaques are the natural hosts of SIV.

Host Range and Virus Propagation

African green and Sykes' monkeys, sooty and red-capped mangabey monkeys and mandrills appear to be natural hosts for their own discrete SIVs. Other species that are susceptible to infection are restricted to primates including humans (SIVhu) on rare occasions. However, immunosuppressive disease appears to be largely restricted to SIV-infected macaque monkeys. The natural routes of transmission for SIV are in general not known, but most evidence suggests horizontal spread via fighting and biting among group-housed macaques. Experimentally, macaques have been infected via intravenous and intramuscular inoculation and by exposure of the genital mucosa. Some SIVs clearly have the capacity for crossing species barriers. For example, SIVsmm is readily able to infect macaque monkeys. In contrast, numerous attempts to infect macaques and other Old World primates with HIV-1 have met with limited success. Baboons (*Papio cynocephalus*), rhesus and cyno-

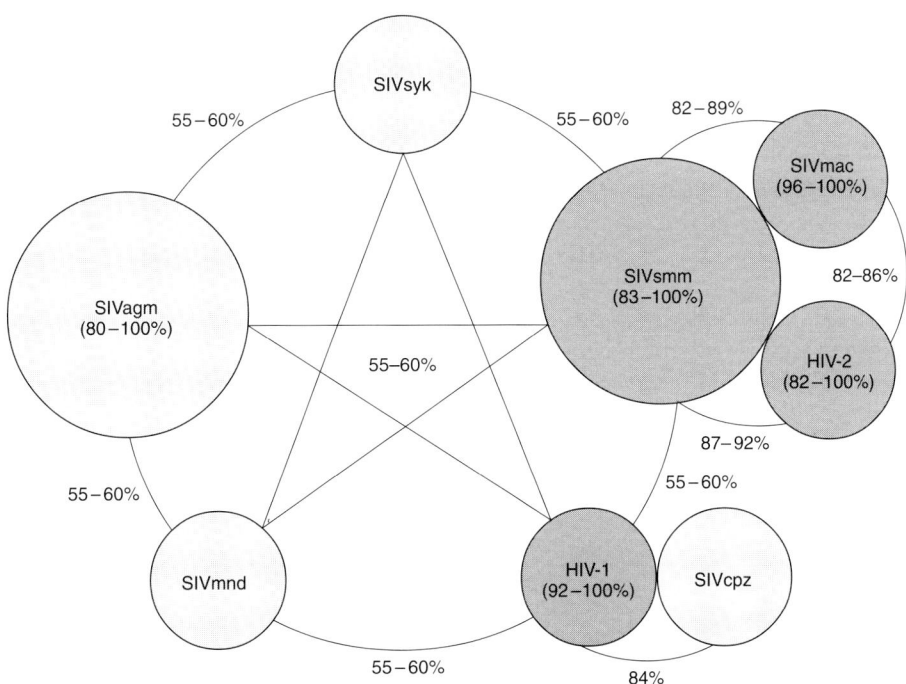

Figure 1 Five groups of primate lentiviruses.

molgus monkeys could not be infected with HIV-1. However, it was discovered that chimpanzees (*Pan troglodytes*) are susceptible to HIV-1 infection, but with the exception of one animal infected for greater than ten years, they have not developed AIDS-like disease. Likewise, pig-tailed macaques (*M. nemestrina*) have been reported to be infected with HIV-1, albeit transiently, but also fail to develop immunosuppression and disease. Although both of these models are important in investigating the interaction of HIV-1 with the host, the lack of clinical disease in most of these animals as well as the expense and endangered species status of chimpanzees limits their usefulness as animal models for AIDS.

SIVs can be propagated in mitogen-stimulated primary peripheral blood mononuclear cells (PBMC), in monocytes/macrophages from primates, and in many cultured cell lines, primarily tumor-derived CD4+ T lymphocytes and monocytes. The acutely pathogenic strains SIVsmmPbj14, SIVmac239YEnef and SIVmac239/R17Y are unusual in their ability to replicate in lymphocytes of resting PBMC cultures without prior lymphocyte activation. In PBMC cultures and many of the cell lines, viral infection results in the fusion of cellular membranes producing large syncytial cells. Syncytium formation, which is mediated by *env*, allows the virus to spread directly from cell to cell. Persistently infected virus-producing cell lines can be established from the cells surviving initial infection. Some isolates also grow well in cultured macrophages derived from lung, blood or bone marrow. As with HIV-1, infection with SIV is predominantly a CD4-mediated event, but CD4 alone is not sufficient to mediate viral entry. Certain chemokine receptors have been shown to be important coreceptors for both SIV and HIV infection. Nonsyncytium-inducing (macrophage tropic) HIV-1 strains predominantly use CCR5, whereas CXCR4 (LESTR/fusin) is utilized primarily by syncytium-inducing (T cell tropic) strains. CCR3, CCR2b, BOB (GPR15) and Bonzo (STRL33) are also utilized by some HIV strains. Similarly, SIV strains have so far been found to utilize CCR5, BOB and Bonzo. As with CD4 interactions with HIV/SIV, coreceptor use is also controlled by *env*. In rare instances, HIV-1 and SIV infection of CD4− cells *in vitro* has been reported. Infection of CD4− cells may be through these or other novel chemokine receptors.

Genetics

Retroviruses contain an RNA genome that replicates via a DNA intermediate. The viral particle contains a diploid genome of single-stranded RNA, linked noncovalently near the 5′ ends of the molecules. The 5′ end of the viral RNA is capped, and the 3′ end is polyadenylated. DNA synthesis by the viral-encoded reverse transcriptase is primed by host tRNA that is base-paired to the viral RNA. The double-stranded (ds) DNA provirus is integrated into the host cell chromosome by a viral-encoded integrase and further events in transcription, translation and assembly are host cell dependent. Particles assemble and bud through the plasma membrane.

All retroviruses possess certain basic features in their genomic organization. Regulatory sequences controlling DNA synthesis, integration, transcription and other functions are located in the long terminal repeat (LTR) at each end of the provirus. LTRs are common to the broader group of eucaryotic transposable elements (retrotransposons) that include the retroviruses. The open reading frames encoding the major structural proteins lie between the LTRs. Genes may be encoded in any of the three possible open reading frames, and overlaps between open reading frames are common. All retroviruses contain genes called *gag* (group-specific antigen) encoding the core proteins, *pol* (polymerase) encoding the viral reverse transcriptase, protease and integrase, and *env* encoding the envelope glycoproteins.

The SIVs similarly contain *gag*, *pol* and *env* genes and use a replication strategy similar to all retroviruses. However, SIVs, HIVs and other lentiviruses contain a number of genes not found in other genera of retroviruses. The SIV genome is approximately 9.6 kb from the 5′ cap to the 3′ polyadenylation site. The sequences of several cloned SIVs have been reported (SIVmac251, SIVmac142, SIVmac239, SIVsmmH4, SIVsmmPBj14, SIVmmGB1, SIVagm-TYO1 and SIVcpz). The envelope gene, encoding gp120 and gp41, often contains a premature translation termination signal, resulting in a truncated transmembrane protein. In addition to the major open reading frames *gag*, *pol* and *env*, the human and simian immunodeficiency viruses contain open reading frames for *tat* (transactivator protein), *rev* (regulator of gene expression), *vif* (viral infectivity protein) and *nef* (originally termed negative factor). The *vpu* open reading frame found in HIV-1 and SIVcpz is not present in HIV-2 nor in any of the SIVs. HIV-1/SIVcpz, SIVsmm/HIV-2/SIVmac and SIVmnd contain an open reading frame called *vpr*, which is not found in SIVagm. SIVagm and SIVsmm/HIV-2/SIVmac contain a gene called *vpx* not found in SIVmnd and HIV-1/SIVcpz. Genes *vpx* and *vpr* share sequence similarity and one probably arose from the other via a gene duplication event. The presence of these additional open reading frames in the five discrete groups of primate lentiviruses is summarized in **Table 1**. Several of these additional genes (specifically *vpx, vpr* and *nef*) can be deleted without abrogating the ability of the virus to replicate in tissue culture cells, but they certainly must contribute to the virus life cycle *in vivo*. Nef has been found to play an important role in maintaining high virus loads *in vivo* and for disease development. These observations have led to the development of molecular clones of SIV with specific deletions in *vpx, vpr* and *nef*, which have been successfully utilized as modified live-virus vaccines in rhesus monkeys.

SIV proteins are translated from a complex population of unspliced, singly spliced and multiply spliced mRNA molecules. The amount of each protein is regulated at least in part by the extent of splicing. The mechanisms that regulate splicing continue to be unraveled, but the interaction of the Rev protein (encoded by fully spliced transcripts) with a region of RNA called the rev-responsive element (RRE) is known to result in the accumulation of full-length transcripts that are translated into the major structural proteins.

SIVs, like other lentiviruses, accumulate genetic changes rapidly *in vivo*, presumably because of errors introduced by the error-prone reverse transcriptase and because of the selective pressures of the host. Lentiviruses may differ from other retroviruses in being able to tolerate greater variation in their envelope glycoproteins and this may contribute to their ability to persist. In one report, the rate of fixation of mutations in the gp120 portion of the envelope gene of SIVmac239 was found to be 8.5×10^{-3} changes per site per year. Mutations in the envelope gene result in antigenic variations that may enable the virus to evade ongoing host immune responses and contribute to its ability to establish persistent infection. Other mutations in the *env* gene appear to affect cell and tissue tropism, for example, by altering the ability of the virus to replicate in macrophages vs lymphocytes. Moreover, recent evidence suggests that env-mediated chemokine receptor usage by HIV changes with time allowing the virus to infect additional populations of leukocytes. Another mechanism that may generate genetic diversity is the production of heterozygous dimer genomes or pseudotype particles in cells that are infected by more than one virus. Endogenous SIV sequences have not been detected in the germ line and gene conversion/recombination events have not been documented.

Evolution

Comparisons of genetic sequences among human and simian immunodeficiency viruses suggest that there are at least five discrete groups of primate lentiviruses in existence (**Figs 1** and **2**): HIV-1 and the closely related SIVcpz; SIVmnd; SIVagm; SIVsmm/SIVmac/HIV-2; and SIVsyk. The evolutionary origin of each of these groups may never be known. It is possible that HIV-1 and HIV-2 evolved from simian viruses and entered the human population by cross-species transmission relatively recently in history. Cross-species transmission between primates in nature or in captivity may have resulted in the generation of new pathogenic variants, with SIVmac infection of macaques possibly being analogous to HIV-2 in humans. However, it is also possible that some of the primate immunodeficiency viruses may have always been present in the corresponding host population but not have been recognized until recently. The SIVs and HIVs are more closely related to one another than to any of the nonprimate lentiviruses. This suggests that the HIVs and SIVs are inherently primate viruses and that they were not derived from rodents, cats, ungulates or other nonprimates via cross-species transmission.

Serologic Relationships and Variability

The *gag* and *pol* genes are the most highly conserved among related primate lentiviruses; sequence comparison of these regions are often used to estimate relatedness rather than serologic tests. Antiserum to the Gag protein is generally crossreactive among different isolates within a group, whereas antiserum to the envelope protein can be used to distinguish between them. Serologic crossreactivity between a member of one group to one in another group is usually weak even to Gag proteins.

Epidemiology

SIV has been found in many species of African nonhuman primates throughout sub-Saharan Africa, but infection does not cause AIDS-like disease. In contrast, SIV infection of Asian macaque monkeys in captivity induces AIDS-like disease similar to that observed in HIV-infected humans. SIV-associated disease has not been seen outside these settings.

Transmission and Tissue Tropism

The routes of transmission of SIV in the wild are not known, but, as with HIV-1, transmission through contact with infected blood seems likely. In nonhuman primates, bite and scratch wounds may be more significant than sexual contact. Macaques can be experimentally infected via intravenous or intramuscular inoculation, or by exposure of the genital mucosa. Like HIV, SIV is tropic for CD4+ cells; both viruses grow preferentially in CD4+ cells, and soluble CD4 or monoclonal antibodies specific to the CD4

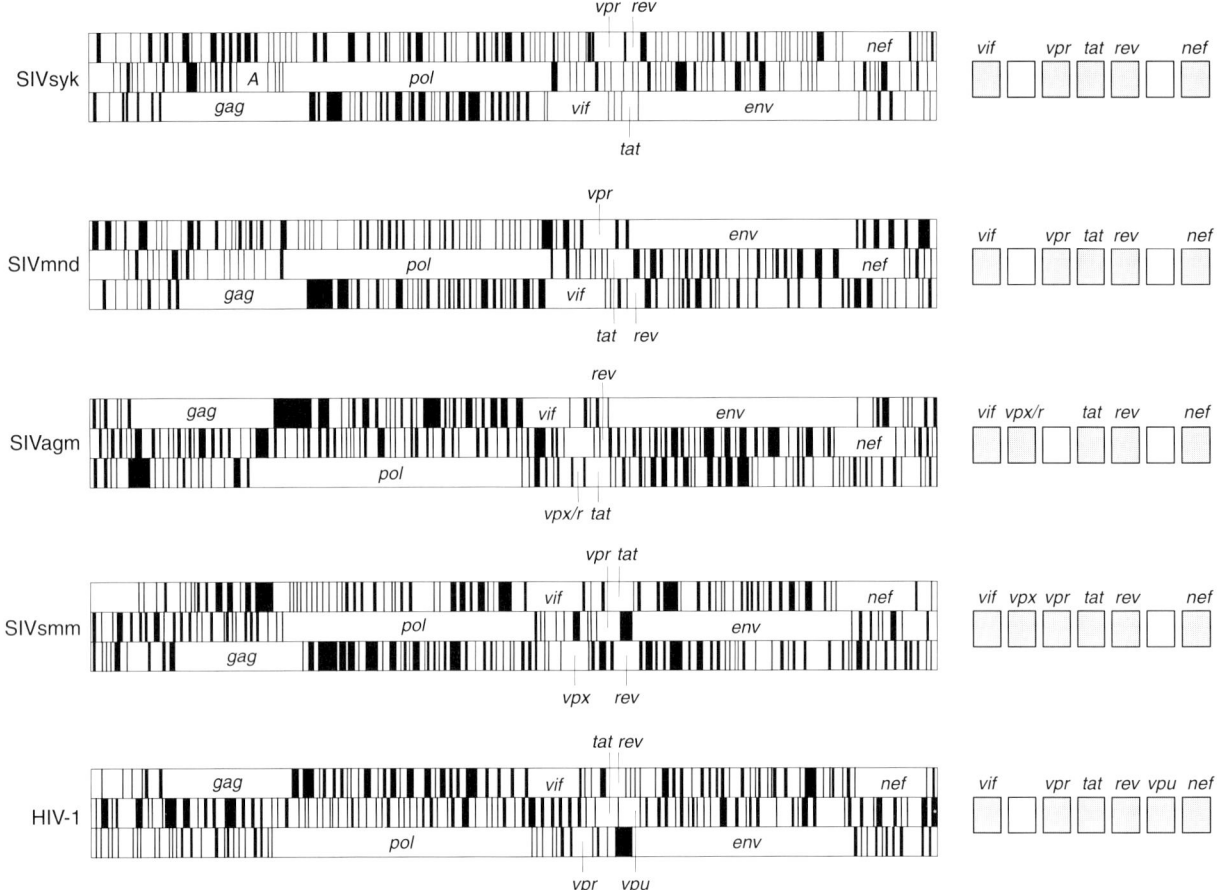

Figure 2 Organization of open reading frames in the five groups of primate lentiviruses. Reproduced from Hirsch VM, Dapolito GA, Goldstein S *et al* (1993) *Journal of Virology*, 67: 1517. Permission granted by American Society for Microbiology.

antigen can block viral infection. Recently, it has been shown that several coreceptors are required for *env*-mediated cell fusion and entry of HIV and SIV into CD4+ cells. These coreceptors are all members of the seven-transmembrane G-protein-coupled receptor family; many serving as chemokine receptors. Of the chemokine receptors used by HIV (CCR5, CCR2b, CCR3, CXCR4, BOB and Bonzo), SIV has so far been found to utilize CCR5, BOB and Bonzo. The primary targets for infection in the macaque are CD4+ helper/inducer T lymphocytes, mononuclear phagocytes, Langerhans cells and dendritic cells of lymphoid organs. Thus, lymphoid tissues (thymus, spleen, lymph nodes, gut-associated lymphoid tissue) are the principal targets of virus infection and replication. Cells of the monocyte/macrophage lineage are also major cell types replicating virus in the infected host. Infection of CD4− cells, such as endothelium, neurons, astrocytes, various epithelial cells and CD34 bone marrow progenitors, has been reported *in vitro*, but infection *in vivo* is controversial.

Pathogenicity

Natural infection of African green and Sykes' monkeys, red-capped and sooty mangabeys and mandrills with their own SIV appears to be nonpathogenic. SIVmac and SIVsmm can be pathogenic in rhesus, cynomolgus, stump-tail (*M. arctoides*) and other macaques. Disease course is dependent on the viral strain used for infection and host immune response to the virus. Acutely pathogenic strains (SIVsmmPBj14, SIVmac239YEnef and SIVmac239/R17Y) can cause death from severe enterocolitis within seven to ten days postinfection. Other strains containing gene deletions (specifically *vpx*, *vpr* and *nef*) are able to replicate *in vitro* and *in vivo*, but are markedly attenuated and rarely cause mortality. However, these clinical outcomes are the exception and most animals infected with a variety of other SIV strains generally succumb within 1–3 years postinfection with immunosuppressive disease. The induction of AIDS-like disease in macaques following infection with SIVmac is currently used as a model for human AIDS to investigate mechanisms of pathogenesis and to evaluate potential vaccines and therapies.

Clinical Features of Infection

Infection of rhesus macaques with SIV induces both acute and chronic disease syndromes similar to that of HIV-infected humans. Within the first few weeks of infecting macaque monkeys with most strains of SIV, animals develop antigenemia and often have lymphadenopathy of the axillary and inguinal lymph nodes and an erythematous maculopapular rash. A CD8+ T cell lymphocytosis and rise in SIV-specific antibodies correlate with decreased antigenemia. Following the onset of an effective immune response (cell-mediated and humoral), animals enter an asymptomatic period of variable duration. During this time, immune abnormalities include gradual declines in the absolute CD4+ lymphocyte count, CD4/CD8 ratio, and responses to mitogens. Animals can also exhibit chronic diarrhea and wasting, with losses of up to 60% of original body weight. Lymphoid changes are profound and include thymic atrophy and hyperplasia or atrophy of lymphoid tissue (lymph nodes, spleen, gut-associated lymphoid tissue) depending on the stage of the disease. End-stage of SIV infection is characterized by a spectrum of diseases that can be divided into four broad categories: SIV-related inflammatory diseases; opportunistic infections associated with immunosuppression; neoplastic diseases; diseases of unknown pathogenesis. Tropism of SIV strains for monocyte/macrophages correlates with pronounced inflammatory and degenerative changes in the central nervous system (CNS), lung, digestive tract, and other organs independent from pathology associated with opportunistic pathogens. The incidence and characteristics of these lentivirus-induced inflammatory lesions in SIV-infected macaque monkeys closely mimics those observed in HIV-infected patients. CNS involvement (SIV encephalitis) is frequent, with the likelihood of brain lesions appearing to depend on the strain of SIV. At necropsy, 30–50% of SIVmac-infected macaques have a characteristic multinucleate giant cell encephalitis similar to that described for HIV encephalitis. Likewise, the opportunistic pathogens observed in SIV-infected macaques are similar to those observed in HIV-infected patients and include *Mycobacterium avium* complex, cytomegalovirus, rhesus Epstein–Barr virus (rhesus lymphocryptovirus), papovavirus (SV40), adenovirus, *Pneumocystis carinii*, *Cryptosporidia* sp. and *Toxoplasma gondii*. Neoplastic diseases in SIV-infected macaques are primarily limited to lymphomas, the occurrence of which varies among the different Primate Research Centers. Epizootics of lymphoma in SIV-infected macaques have been associated with co-infection with rhesus Epstein–Barr virus. Diseases of unknown pathogenesis include a nonneoplastic proliferation of lymphoid tissue (lymphoproliferative syndrome), arteritis and arteriopathy.

The course of disease in pigtailed macaques infected with SIVsmmPBj14 virus and rhesus macaques infected with SIVmac239YEnef and SIVmac239/R17Y is extremely rapid in comparison to most other strains of SIV. Macaques infected with these strains usually develop marked lymphoid proliferation, maculopapular rash and profuse, hemorrhagic diarrhea within one week of infection, and can die from severe fluid and electrolyte loss.

Pathology and Histopathology

Pathologic findings in macaques are varied and depend on the clinical course of disease. Within a few weeks of infecting macaque monkeys with most strains of SIV, an erythematous maculopapular eruption can occur, which is histologically identical to that described in primary HIV-1 infection. Vessels of the superficial dermis are congested and contain perivascular infiltrates of lymphocytes and macrophages. SIV nucleic acid and protein have been observed only in biopsies obtained from rhesus macaques infected with the acutely pathogenic strains SIVmac239YEnef and SIVmac239/R17Y, which induce a rash of greater severity and earlier onset than that observed with other strains of SIV.

Lymphoid tissues are the principal targets for SIV and a range of histologic changes are observed including follicular hyperplasia and dysplasia, follicular involution and hyperplasia of the T cell-dependent areas, and lymphoid depletion. These histologic changes represent successive stages in the reaction of lymphoid tissue to persistent SIV infection. In addition, some animals develop a generalized lymphoproliferative syndrome in which lymphoid tissues throughout the body become enlarged due to a nonneoplastic proliferation of lymphocytes. Multiple nodular aggregates of similar cells frequently are found in other organs and tissues of affected animals, including the salivary gland, kidney, lung, liver, bone marrow, skin and thymus.

Approximately 50% of infected animals develop primary lentiviral-induced meningoencephalitis, which is characterized by perivascular infiltrates of macrophages and multinucleated giant cells localized primarily in the white matter. These perivascular macrophages and multinucleated giant cells contain abundant viral nucleic acid and protein and contain mature lentiviral particles within cytoplasmic vacuoles. These findings are similar to reports on HIV-infected patients with HIV encephalitis. Other SIV-induced lesions in macaques are multinucleate giant cell infiltrates in the lymph nodes, spleen, lung, gastrointestinal tract and other organs.

Other inflammatory lesions, which are histologically distinct from those directly related to SIV, are usually secondary to opportunistic infections. In the CNS, these include SV40-induced progressive multifocal leukoencephalopathy and cytomegalovirus- and *T. gondii*-induced necrosuppurative meningoencephalitis. Rarely, in the absence of a significant inflammatory response to opportunistic infections, the presence of the abnormally large numbers of organisms can cause morbidity and mortality. For instance, *P. carinii* commonly proliferates unabated to the point of filling most alveoli within lung lobes; eventually killing the host.

In SIV-infected macaques, diarrhea can apparently be caused directly by SIV. In these cases, nonspecific enteropathy consisting of blunting of the small intestinal villi, shortening of the crypts of Lieberkuhn, a predominantly mononuclear inflammatory infiltrate within the lamina propria, and attenuation or immaturity of the epithelium is seen. However, diarrhea is most frequently associated with overgrowth of commensal and pathogenic protozoa (i.e. *Cryptosporidia* sp., *Giardia* sp, *Balantidium coli*, *Trichomonas* sp.) and bacteria (*Mycobacterium avium*). *Cryptosporidia* sp. also infects the tracheal, pancreatic and biliary epithelium. Unexplained arterial lesions have been seen in SIV-infected macaques. These most frequently involve medium- to large-sized pulmonary vessels and include a spectrum of histologic patterns from transmural lymphocytic infiltrates to complete occlusion of the lumen secondary to intimal proliferation and thrombosis. Other organs, such as heart and kidney, may also have SIV-induced abnormalities, but these have not been well characterized.

Immune Response

Depending on viral isolate and host immune response, the disease course in SIV-infected macaque monkeys can be quite variable, as in HIV-infected patients. Experimentally infected animals generally fall into two classes: those that develop a high, persistent humoral and cellular immune response, and those with little or no response. Although the early immune response does limit viral replication, it does not control it. In both HIV-infected people and SIV-infected macaque monkeys, viremia is persistent and sustained by continuous rounds of viral replication throughout the course of infection. Animals in the first group remain persistently infected, develop a protracted disease course similar to AIDS in humans, and generally die one year or longer after infection. Viral load in the blood is variable with higher loads being predictive of rapid disease progression. Approximately 25% of animals do not mount a significant immune response to SIV and viral loads in the blood remain high throughout the course of infection. Generally, these animals die within 3–5 months and are termed rapid progressors. In addition to virus factors, unique host factors may also be important for disease susceptibility and progression.

Prevention and Control

Extensive testing programs have essentially eliminated SIV from captive macaque colonies. However, continued vigilance is needed to maintain breeding colonies free from accidental exposure to the virus. Animals can be conveniently tested serologically for evidence of infection. As rare human cases of SIV infection have been documented, SIV is handled with the same precautions as for work with HIV-1. Disposable surgical gloves and gowns are used, all work with live virus is carried out in a biosafety cabinet, procedures creating aerosols are avoided and use of glass and needles is minimized.

Future Perspectives

The most important role of SIV will be its use in basic research relevant to AIDS. The induction of AIDS in macaques by infectious molecular clones of SIV represents the best existing animal model for AIDS in humans. SIVs are the closest known relatives of the HIVs and the disease induced in macaques is remarkably similar to AIDS in humans. Rhesus and other macaque species are not endangered, can be purchased at a reasonable cost and breed well in captivity. This system can be used to dissect the molecular determinants of AIDS pathogenesis; to define the role of the so-called nonessential genes; to map functional regions of the structural genes such as the envelope; and to evaluate the potential of new treatment and vaccine strategies. Finally, the ongoing investigation of 'new' isolates and their genetic relatedness to existing SIV and HIV isolates may shed light on the origins and evolution of the primate immunodeficiency viruses.

See also: **Autoimmunity; Bovine immunodeficiency virus (*Retroviridae*); Feline immunodeficiency virus (*Retroviridae*); Human immunodeficiency viruses (*Retroviridae*): Anti-retroviral agents,**

General features, Molecular biology; Immune response: Cell mediated immune response, General features; Persistent viral infection; Visna-Maedi viruses (*Retroviridae*).

Further Reading

Desrosiers RC (1990) The simian immunodeficiency viruses. *Annu. Rev. Immunol.* 8: 557.

Desrosiers RC and Ringler DJ (1989) The use of simian immunodeficiency viruses for AIDS research. *Intervirology* 30: 301.

Eichberg W (ed.) (1990) Nonhuman primate models for AIDS II. *J. Med. Primatol.* 19: 161.

Gardner MB (1996) The history of simian AIDS. *J. Med. Primatol.* 25: 148.

King NW (1993) Simian immunodeficiency virus infections. In: Jones TC, Mohr U and Hunt RD (eds) *Nonhuman Primates I*, p. 5. Berlin, Heidelberg: Springer.

SIMIAN VIRUS 40 (*PAPOVAVIRIDAE*)

Janet S Butel, Division of Molecular Virology, Baylor College of Medicine, Houston, USA

Copyright © 1999 Academic Press

History

Simian virus 40 (SV40) was discovered in 1960 as a contaminant of poliovaccines. Hundreds of millions of people worldwide were inadvertently exposed to SV40 in the late 1950s and early 1960s when they were administered contaminated virus vaccines prepared in rhesus macaque kidney cells. Infectious SV40 had unknowingly contaminated batches of both the inactivated and live attenuated forms of the poliovaccine, as well as preparations of some other viral vaccines. Although primary cultures of monkey cells were known to be commonly contaminated with indigenous viruses and safety testing was carried out, SV40 had escaped detection because it failed to induce cytopathic effects in rhesus cells. However, when it was inoculated into African green monkey kidney cells, a prominent cytoplasmic vacuolization developed. Originally christened as 'vacuolating virus', the name was later changed to SV40 to conform with a numerical system of designating simian virus isolates.

Concern about the vaccine contaminations heightened considerably when it was found in 1962 that SV40 was tumorigenic in newborn hamsters and could transform many types of cells in culture. Because of the potential risk to public health posed by the previous distribution of contaminated poliovaccines, SV40 became the focus of intensive investigation. Fortunately, the individuals exposed to SV40-contaminated vaccines appear not to be at higher risk of developing cancer than those who received SV40-free vaccines. However, SV40 DNA is sometimes found in tumors arising in persons too young to have been exposed to the contaminated vaccines. For scientists, SV40 has turned out to be an invaluable tool for dissecting molecular details of eukaryotic cell processes. Numerous techniques now commonly used in molecular biology were pioneered in the SV40 system. It continues to serve as a leading model for basic studies of viral carcinogenesis.

Taxonomy and Classification

SV40 is classified as a member of the *Polyomavirus* genus in the *Papovaviridae* family (**Table 1**). The other well-studied member of the genus is polyoma virus of mice. The group also includes the human polyomaviruses, BKV and JCV, as well as isolates from other species, including hamsters, rabbits, cattle, birds and baboons. The papillomaviruses are classified in the other genus, *Papillomavirus*, in the family. The human and animal polyomaviruses are antigenically distinct, and there is only one recognized serotype for each virus.

The polyomaviruses are small and simple and share certain physical and chemical properties. These include an icosahedral capsid about 45 nm in diameter that contains three viral proteins, the lack of an envelope and a double-stranded (ds) circular covalently closed DNA genome about 5 kbp in size. The outstanding biological characteristics of the polyomaviruses are that they establish persistent infections in natural hosts, stimulate cellular DNA synthesis in infected cells, and are tumorigenic in the appropriate hosts.

Properties of the Virion

SV40 particles are small and spherical, with a diameter of approximately 45 nm. Infectious virions

Table 1 Properties of SV40

Classification	Family *Papovaviridae*, genus *Polyomavirus*
Strain variation	Genetically stable; one serotype, multiple strains
Virion	Icosahedral, 45 nm in diameter, no envelope
Genome	Circular covalently closed dsDNA, 5200 bp
Proteins	Three structural proteins, VP1, VP2, VP3; cellular histones condense DNA in virion; nonstructural replication protein, T-antigen, is potent oncoprotein
Replication	In certain primate kidney cells; nucleus; stimulate cell DNA synthesis; long growth cycle
Natural host	Asian macaques, especially the rhesus monkey
Diseases	Asymptomatic persistent infections in natural hosts; neurological disease in immunocompromised hosts; tumors in experimentally infected rodents
Historical note	Contaminant in early poliovaccines administered to millions of people

have a sedimentation coefficient of 240S in sucrose and band at a density of 1.34 g ml^{-1} in CsCl; empty capsids have a density of 1.29 g ml^{-1}. The molecular mass of the SV40 virion has been estimated at 270 kDa. The DNA content is 12.5% (w/w). The major capsid protein (VP1) accounts for 75% of the total virion protein. VP2 and VP3 are minor capsid proteins. Cellular histones (H2A, H2B, H3, H4) are used to condense the viral DNA for packaging and are present in the core of the particle. There is no lipid envelope. SV40 does not agglutinate erythrocytes.

SV40 particles exhibit icosahedral symmetry. The virion is composed of 72 pentameric capsomeres composed of the VP1 protein arranged on a $T = 7d$ icosahedral surface lattice. This puzzling structure (that the hexavalent capsomeres have pentameric substructure) demands nonequivalent contacts between pentamers. This seems to be accomplished by the C-termini of the VP1 polypeptides, which extend as arms from one pentamer and fit into binding sites on adjacent pentamers. The arms can go in different directions, providing the necessary flexibility to build a capsid. The N-terminal arm of VP1 is completely internal in the virus particle. Minor capsid proteins VP2 and VP3 are predominantly internal as well and do not contribute to the basic structure of the virus outer shell.

The virus particles are very resistant to heat inactivation but are relatively labile when heated in the presence of divalent cations. Whereas SV40 is stable at 50°C for hours, incubation in the presence of 1 M $MgCl_2$ at 50°C for 1 h will inactivate the virus. At a higher temperature (60°C), ~99% of infectious virus is inactivated within 30 min in the absence of divalent cations. Purified virions can be disrupted by strong alkaline conditions (pH 10.5), by lower pH (9.2) plus a reducing agent, or by detergent treatment. Intact virus particles are not affected by nucleases, but in the presence of a reducing agent nuclease can enter the virion and cleave the viral DNA. SV40 is efficiently inactivated by UV light irradiation, following single-hit kinetics.

Properties of the Viral Genome

The SV40 genome is a circular covalently closed dsDNA molecule (**Fig. 1**). The native DNA assumes a superhelical configuration (form I) that sediments at 21S in a neutral sucrose gradient. A single-stranded (ss) nick generates relaxed circular dsDNA molecules (form II) that sediment at 16S, whereas a ds break produces linear dsDNA (form III, 14S). Alkaline denaturation of form I DNA produces dense cyclic coils that sediment at 53S. Form II DNA is converted into ss circular (18S) and ss linear (16S) molecules by denaturation. The supercoiled (form I) molecules can be separated from relaxed circular and linear forms by centrifugation of a DNA preparation in CsCl gradients with ethidium bromide. The form I molecules will band in a lower position in the gradient. The DNA forms also separate during electrophoresis in a neutral agarose gel; the supercoiled molecules migrate the fastest, the linear forms move at an intermediate speed, and the relaxed circles migrate the slowest.

The viral DNA both in virions and in infected cells is associated with cellular histones H2A, H2B, H3 and H4. The histones are assembled in 24–26 nucleosomes on the viral DNA. The nucleosome structure and histone composition of the viral minichromosome mimic the chromatin structure of cellular DNA.

SV40 DNA was the first eukaryotic viral genome to be physically mapped by restriction endonuclease analysis (1971) and to be completely sequenced (1978). The DNA of reference strain 776 contains 5243 bp for a calculated molecular weight of 3.5×10^6. The genome is numbered in a clockwise direction from 1 to 5243, the center nucleotide of the unique *BglI* recognition site being assigned as 0/5243. Numbering continues through the late region in the

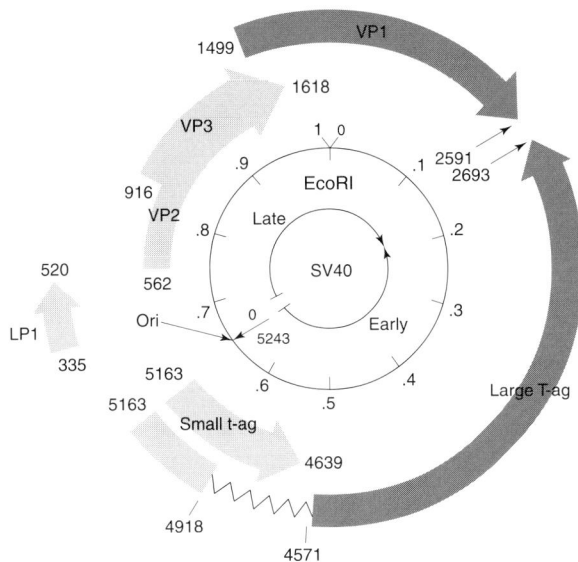

Figure 1 Genetic map of SV40. The thick circle represents the circular SV40 DNA genome. The unique *Eco*RI site is shown at map unit 0/1. Nucleotide numbers begin and end at the origin (*Ori*) of viral DNA replication (0/5243). Boxed arrows indicate the open reading frames that encode the viral proteins. Arrowheads point in the direction of transcription; the beginning and end of each open reading frame is indicated by nucleotide numbers. Various shadings depict different reading frames used for different viral polypeptides. Note that T-ag is coded by two noncontiguous segments on the genome. The genome is divided into 'early' and 'late' regions that are expressed before and after the onset of viral DNA replication, respectively. Only the early region is expressed in transformed cells. (Reproduced with permission from Brooks GF, Butel JS and Ornston LN (1998) *Jawetz, Melnick & Adelberg's Medical Microbiology*, 21st edn. Norwalk, CT: Appleton & Lange.)

sense orientation and the early region in the antisense orientation. The numbering system begins and ends (0/5243) in the middle of the functional origin of DNA replication. The unique *Eco*RI site at nucleotide 1782 was arbitrarily chosen as a point of reference and assigned a value of 0/1.0 on the circular map. Laboratory-adapted strains of SV40 contain a duplication of the 72 bp element in the enhancer region, whereas most natural isolates do not.

SV40 makes maximal use of a limited amount of genetic information, including having compact regulatory sequences and overlapping genes. The genome contains a single origin of replication (core *Ori* = 64 bp in size) embedded within a nontranslated regulatory region. These elements control transcription and replication and span about 400 bp. The SV40 genetic map is divided into two halves, corresponding to regions that are expressed during the early and late stages of infection. These regions represent the 'early' nonstructural genes and the 'late' structural genes, respectively, and are transcribed off opposite strands of the viral DNA.

There is a variable domain at the C terminus of the T-*ag* gene, encompassing about 270 bp. Nucleotide changes within this region can be used to distinguish strains of SV40.

Properties of Viral Proteins

SV40 encodes six gene products: two 'early' nonstructural proteins [large T antigen (T-ag), small t antigen (t-ag)], three 'late' structural proteins (VP1, VP2, VP3) and a maturation protein (LP1 or agnoprotein).

The nonstructural proteins are expressed early in infection, before the onset of viral DNA synthesis. The coding regions of the two T-ags overlap; alternative splicing of viral transcripts determines each protein sequence. Large T-ag of strain 776 (**Table 2**) contains 708 amino acids (~ 90 kDa), and small t-ag contains 174 residues (~ 20 kDa). The large and small T-ags share 82 N-terminal amino acids, whereas the remainder of each protein is unique. The T-ag/t-ag common exon contains a 'J domain,' believed to modulate hsc70 activity in the assembly and disassembly of multiprotein complexes.

Large T-ag is an essential replication protein required for initiation of viral DNA synthesis. It stimulates host cells to enter S phase and undergo DNA synthesis and is the SV40 transforming protein. Large T-ag contains a nuclear transport signal (Pro126-Lys-Lys-Lys-Arg-Lys-Val132) that targets the protein into the nucleus. However, about 10% of the T-ag in the cell is found in the cytoplasm and the plasma membrane. The biology of small t-ag is enigmatic. It is a cytoplasmic protein that is not essential for viral replication in cultured cells. It associates with the regulatory and catalytic subunits (36 kDa and 63 kDa) of protein phosphatase 2A and is believed to cause cellular growth stimulation. Perhaps it is required during natural infections by SV40 in host primates.

Large T-ag is a multifunctional protein that is chemically modified in several ways (**Fig. 2**). Its functions in SV40 DNA replication are regulated by phosphorylation. The sites of phosphorylation are clustered near the ends of the molecule, one region lying between residues 106 and 124 and the other between residues 639 and 701. The majority of the phosphorylated residues are serines, although two threonine residues also become phosphorylated. Unlike many oncoproteins, T-ag is not phosphorylated at tyrosine residues.

T-ag is a DNA-binding protein that recognizes multiple copies of the sequence GAGGC in three T-

Table 2 Properties and functions of SV40 T-ag

Structural properties
1. Size:
   708 amino acids
   82 N-terminal residues shared with t-ag
   81 632 Da
   M_r 90 000–100 000
2. Modifications:
   Phosphorylation
   N-terminal acetylation
   O-glycosylation
   Poly-ADP-ribosylation
   Palmitylation
   Adenylation
3. Supramolecular structure
   Zinc finger
   Nuclear localization signal
   J domain
   Monomers, dimers, higher homooligomers
   Heterooligomers with transcriptional coactivators (CBP, p300, p400)
   Heterooligomers with DNA polymerase α; hsc70; cdc-2, cyclin, and tubulin
   Heterooligomers with tumor suppressor proteins (p53, pRB, p107, p130)

Subcellular distribution
1. Nuclear:
   Nucleoplasmic
   Chromatin bound
   Nuclear matrix associated
2. Plasma membrane:
   Nonidet P-40 soluble
   Nonidet P-40 insoluble (plasma membrane lamina)
   Butanol soluble

Functions
1. Specific DNA binding (viral origin of replication)
2. Initiation of viral DNA replication
3. Autoregulation of viral early transcription
4. Induction of viral late transcription
5. Determination of host range
6. ATPase activity
7. Helicase activity
8. Complex formation with CBP, p300, p400
9. Complex formation with cellular proteins p53, pRB, p107, p130
10. Complex formation with DNA polymerase α
11. Complex formation with heat shock protein hsc70; cdc-2 and cyclin; tubulin
12. Entry of cells into S phase and initiation of cellular DNA replication
13. Induction of cellular gene expression and enzyme synthesis
14. Adenovirus helper function
15. Initiation and maintenance of cellular transformation
16. Induction of immunity to SV40 tumor cells
17. Target for cytotoxic T cells (TSTA)

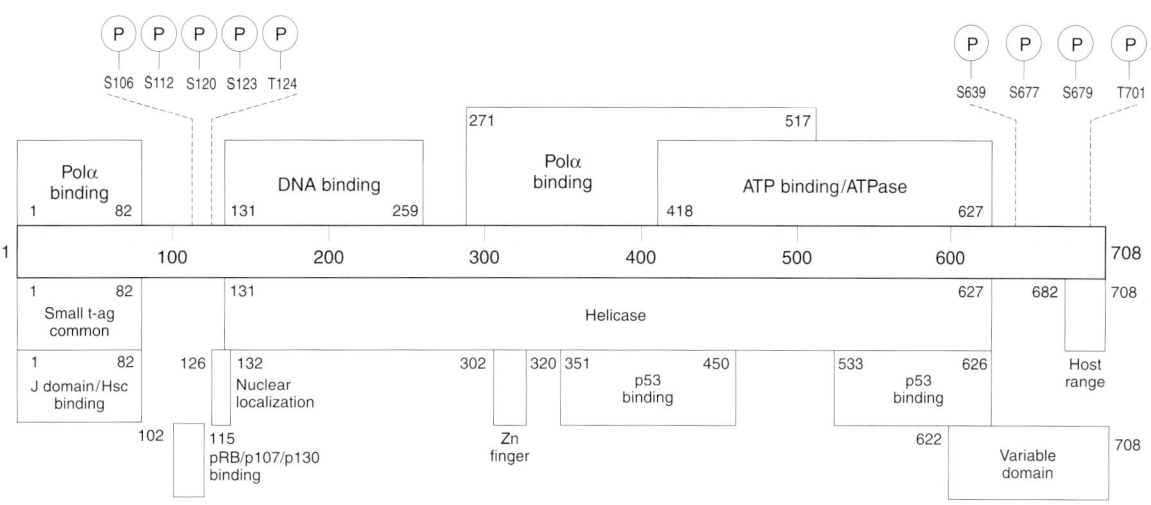

Figure 2 Functional domains of SV40 large T-ag. The numbers given are the amino acid residues using the numbering system for SV40-776. Regions are indicated as follows. Small t-ag common: region of large T-ag encoded in the first exon. The amino acid sequence in this region is common to both large T-ag and small t-ag. Polα binding: regions required for binding to polymerase α-primase. J domain/Hsc binding: region required for binding the heat shock protein hsc70. pRB/p107/p130 binding: region required for binding of the RB tumor suppressor protein, and the RB-related proteins p107 and p130. Nuclear localization: contains the nuclear localization signal. DNA binding: minimal region required for binding to SV40 Ori DNA. Helicase: region required for full helicase activity. Zn finger: region which binds zinc ions. p53 binding: regions required for binding the p53 tumor suppressor protein. ATP binding/ATPase: region containing the ATP binding site and ATPase catalytic activity. Host range: region defined as containing the host range and Ad helper functions. Variable domain: region containing amino acid differences among viral strains. The circles containing a P indicate sites of phosphorylation found on large T-ag expressed in mammalian cells. S indicates a serine and T indicates a threonine residue. (Reproduced with permission from Stewart AR, Lednicky JA, Benzick US, Tevethia MJ and Butal JS (1996) Identification of a variable region at the carboxy terminus of SV40 large T-antigen. Virology 221: 355.)

ag-binding sites in the viral Ori. The phosphorylation of one amino acid, Thr124, is crucial for T-ag to be able to bind to site II and to initiate viral DNA replication. The minimal origin-specific DNA-binding domain of T-ag lies between residues 131 and 259. T-ag is predicted to have a zinc finger motif, typical of DNA-binding proteins, between amino acids 302 and 320. T-ag-specific ATPase and helicase activities are required in addition to DNA-binding activity in order for T-ag to function in initiation of DNA replication. The ATP-binding domain of T-ag is similar in structure to other ATP-binding proteins and is located between residues 418 and 627.

Large T-ag forms complexes with several cellular proteins. Such interactions are involved in T-ag functions in viral DNA replication and induction of cellular DNA synthesis. Target cellular proteins found in heterooligomeric structures with T-ag include transcriptional coactivators (CBP, p300, p400), tumor suppressor proteins (p53, pRB, p107, p130), DNA polymerase α, the molecular chaperone heat-shock protein hsc70, cell-cycle regulatory proteins cdc-2 and cyclin and tubulin. The indicated cellular proteins are not all found in the same T-ag-associated complex; many subpopulations of T-ag exist in a cell.

The variable domain at the C terminus of T-ag encompasses the host range-adenovirus helper function exhibited by SV40 (and mapped to T-ag) in some monkey kidney cell lines. The significance of the variable domain to natural infections by the virus is unknown.

The structural (capsid) proteins are expressed late in infection, after the onset of DNA replication. They are synthesized in much greater abundance than the early proteins. The major capsid protein, VP1, contains 362 amino acids (~ 45 kDa). The minor structural proteins are VP2 (352 residues, ~ 38 kDa) and VP3 (234 residues, ~ 27 kDa). The coding regions for VP2 and VP3 overlap, and they are translated in the same reading frame, so the sequence of VP3 is identical to the C-terminal two-thirds of VP2. VP3 is synthesized by independent initiation of translation via a leaky scanning mechanism. It is not a proteolytic cleavage product of VP2. The N-terminal portion of VP1 is derived from sequences that encode the C-termini of VP2 and VP3. However, VP1 is translated in a different reading frame from a different spliced transcript, so it shares no sequences with VP2 and VP3. VP1 is modified by phosphorylation and acetylation.

The late proteins are required only for the assembly

of progeny virions during lytic infection. They are not involved in the early phases of viral replication. They are synthesized in the cytoplasm and move into the nucleus where particle morphogenesis occurs. The minor capsid proteins contain nuclear transport signals. The VP2/3 signal is Gly-Pro-Asn-Lys-Lys-Lys-Arg-Lys-Leu (VP2, residues 316–324; VP3, residues 198–206). For VP1, two clusters of basic residues within the N-terminal 19 residues are independently important for nuclear targeting. Mutations in VP1 affect capsid assembly and/or virion stability. Mutations in VP2 and VP3 affect the uncoating process, when virions penetrate new host cells.

The agnoprotein LP1 is synthesized late in infection but is not found in virus particles. It is a small (62 residue, ~8 kDa) basic protein involved in particle assembly. It is believed that LP1 interacts with VP1 molecules to inhibit self-polymerization until they interact with viral minichromosomes in the nucleus to form virions.

Replication

Overview of SV40 replication cycle

The SV40 replication cycle is cleanly divided into early and late events, with the onset of viral DNA replication being the dividing landmark. SV40 virions attach to receptors on the cell surface, become internalized, and are transported to the cell nucleus where the viral DNA is uncoated. After uncoating, the half of the genome that contains the early region is transcribed ('early' mRNAs). Viral early proteins (T-ags) are synthesized, cellular genes are expressed, and the cells enter S phase. Viral DNA replication then begins. 'Late' mRNAs are transcribed from the other half of the viral genome (the opposite strand), and viral structural proteins are synthesized. Virus particles are assembled. The majority of progeny virions stay associated with the cell until cell lysis occurs following cell death. The SV40 multiplication cycle is slow, taking 48–72 h. The time course of the virus growth cycle is dependent on the viral multiplicity of infection and the growth state of the host cell at the time of infection.

Strategy of replication of nucleic acid

SV40 DNA is replicated in the cell nucleus as a free unintegrated minichromosome. The only viral components required are the viral origin of replication on the DNA and the T-ag protein; all other factors are provided by the host cell replication machinery. T-ag is required for the initiation of DNA replication. The specific T-ag functions required are its DNA-binding ability and its ATPase/helicase activities. The relative simplicity of the SV40 system has allowed the development of cell-free replication systems and the identification of factors involved in mammalian DNA replication.

T-ag binds to the viral *Ori*, a 64 bp segment that contains binding site II for T-ag. In an ATP-dependent process, T-ag causes localized unwinding of the *Ori* region; cellular single-stranded binding protein is required to stabilize the unwound single strands. The cellular DNA polymerase α–primase complex initiates DNA replication, and replication proceeds bidirectionally, with the two forks advancing at equal rates. The strand growing in the 5′ to 3′ direction is synthesized in a continuous fashion, whereas the strand growing in the 3′ to 5′ direction is synthesized as small pieces (Okazaki fragments). Elongation involves DNA polymerase α, DNA polymerase δ and proliferating cell nuclear antigen. Termination occurs 180° away from the viral *Ori*; topoisomerase II segregates the newly synthesized daughter molecules. Cellular histones are added to the new strands during the process of DNA replication.

Only certain monkey and human cells support SV40 DNA replication. This cell permissiveness seems to depend on the nature of the DNA polymerase α–primase complex.

The onset of viral DNA replication is carefully coordinated with the host cell cycle by the phosphorylation of a specific site on T-ag. The T-ag synthesized soon after viral infection drives the cell to enter S phase. The binding of p53 and pRB cellular proteins is presumably important in this process. A cell cycle-dependent kinase becomes activated and phosphorylates T-ag at Thr124. Only then can T-ag bind to site II in the viral *Ori* and initiate viral DNA replication. This regulation assures that viral DNA does not become unwound for replication until the host cell has entered S phase and the necessary cell replication factors are in place.

Characterization of transcription

Transcription of the viral DNA is carried out by the cellular RNA polymerase II. In the noncoding region of SV40 DNA near the origin of replication are early and late promoter structures and enhancer elements. Early transcription begins at about nucleotide 5237, proceeds in the counterclockwise direction, and ends at the polyadenylation site at nucleotide 2694. The early promoter contains a TATA box about 30 bp upstream of the early RNA initiation site. (This start site is about 70 nucleotides upstream of the initiation codon shared by the early proteins.) There are three G+C-rich regions, the '21 bp repeats,' located 40–103 nucleotides upstream that are binding sites for the Sp1 cellular factor. Even farther upstream are the SV40 enhancer elements, the 72 bp elements, which contain binding sites for other cellular factors that regulate transcription. The primary early transcripts are differentially spliced to generate the mRNAs that code for large T-ag and small t-ag.

There is no requirement for virus-encoded proteins, but early transcription is regulated by T-ag. As the concentration of T-ag increases in the cell, it binds first to site I and then to sites II and III on the viral DNA. Early transcription is repressed when site II is occupied, because the presence of T-ag blocks the binding of RNA polymerase. Therefore, T-ag regulates its own synthesis.

Late transcription begins after viral DNA synthesis is underway. The abundance of late transcripts is much greater than the early transcripts because progeny DNA molecules are utilized as templates. A heterogeneous collection of late mRNAs is made, with late transcription beginning at multiple sites between nucleotides 120 and 482 and proceeding in the clockwise direction, ending at a polyadenylation site at nucleotide 2674. Both the 21 bp repeats and the 72 bp elements have positive effects on late transcription. T-ag *trans*-activates late transcription by an unknown mechanism that does not involve DNA binding. The late transcripts are alternatively spliced into two size classes (19S, 16S). VP1 is synthesized from 16S RNA and both VP2 and VP3 are translated from the 19S species. The agnoprotein is synthesized predominantly from the most abundant species of 16S RNA.

Characterization of translation

Early gene products (T-ag, t-ag) are synthesized from differentially spliced early transcripts. Likewise, the structural proteins (VP1, VP2, VP3) are produced from differentially spliced late transcripts. VP3 is a truncated version of VP2, due to initiation of translation at an internal site on the same species of transcripts. The agnoprotein LP1 is translated from the leader region of late transcripts. The late gene products are produced in much greater abundance than the early proteins, reflecting the relative concentrations of the transcripts.

Post-translational processing

No post-translational cleavages are involved in the production of SV40 proteins. As noted above, T-ag and VP1 are modified in various ways, including phosphorylation.

Uptake and release of virions

SV40 particles attach to receptors on the cell surface. The receptors recognized by virus particles are believed to be the major histocompatibility complex class I molecules.

Attached particles are internalized by endocytosis. Conformational changes are thought to occur that expose the nuclear localization signals on capsid proteins and allow the virions to squeeze through the nuclear pore complex. The capsid disassembles in the nucleus, releasing the viral DNA.

Maturation of progeny virions occurs in the nucleus, where the viral nucleic acid is replicated. Viral proteins are synthesized in the cytoplasm off viral transcripts exported from the nucleus, and the proteins are then transported back into the nucleus. The structural proteins condense around the viral minichromosomes. There is a packaging signal on SV40 DNA that includes the *Ori* and part of the enhancer element. During the maturation process, the agnoprotein is released and is not retained as a component of mature virions. Assembly intermediates that sediment more slowly than extracellular virions have been detected. Certain SV40 T-ag mutants are defective in the assembly of virus particles, but the mechanism is obscure. There are size constraints for packaging DNA; molecules ranging from 3.5 kbp to 5.7 kbp can be encapsidated into SV40 particles.

Some progeny virus is released from the cell by an unknown mechanism, but the majority stays associated with the cell until lysis caused by cell death. Host cells are killed as the result of a variety of effects, including the release of lysosomal enzymes into the cytoplasm and damage to the cell mitochondria. Late in infection, monkey kidney cells develop a characteristic cytopathic effect, cytoplasmic vacuolization. Between 10^4 and 10^5 virus particles are produced by each infected cell.

Geographic and Seasonal Distribution

The geographic distribution of SV40 can only be inferred, as no comprehensive surveys have been conducted. Its distribution in the wild presumably reflects its narrow host range. As far as is known, SV40 is found naturally in wild populations of certain Asian macaque species. Many captive primates can be infected if they have been in contact with an infected macaque. Infections in humans are probably more widespread geographically, as contaminated poliovaccines were broadly distributed. Nothing is known about seasonal effects on natural infections by SV40.

Host Range and Virus Propagation

Papovaviruses, in general, have a narrow host range,

Table 3 Origin of SV40 strains

Virus strain	Year isolated	Source
SV40-776	1960	Adenovirus type 1 seed stock prepared in monkey kidney cells
Baylor	1961	Type 2 Sabin poliovaccine prepared in 1956 in monkey kidney cells
VA45-54	1960	Uninoculated green monkey kidney cells
Rh911	ca. 1960	Uninoculated rhesus monkey kidney cells
A2895	ca. 1961	Tumor from hamster injected with rhesus monkey kidney cells
D-128	1962	Uninoculated rhesus monkey kidney cells (Russia)
SVPML-1	1970	Cultured human brain cells from patient with progressive multifocal leukoencephalopathy
SVMEN*	1984	Human meningioma (cloned directly)
SVCPC*	1995	Human choroid plexus carcinoma
SV40-K661	1997	Brain from rhesus monkey coinfected with simian immunodeficiency virus

Data taken from Stewart AR, Lednicky JA and Butel JS (*J. Neurovirol.* 1998; 4: 182) and from Lednicky JA, Arrington AS, Stewart AR *et al* (*J. Virol.* 1998; 72: 3980).
*SVMEN and SVCPC are identical.

with each virus infecting only one or a few closely related species. Based on antibody surveys of wild populations of primates, the natural hosts for SV40 appear to be a few species of Asian macaque monkeys, especially the rhesus (*Macacca mulatta*). In captivity, several related species are easily infected, including the cynomolgus macaque (*M. fascicularis*) and the African green monkey which belongs to the same family as macaques (Cercopithecidae). The virus grows poorly in more distantly related primates. SV40 can infect humans.

SV40 is propagated in tissue culture in established cell lines derived from kidneys of African green monkeys. Characteristic vacuolated cells appear in response to viral replication. The virus grows in rhesus kidney cell lines in which it establishes a persistent infection but produces no cytopathic effects. The SV40 growth cycle is long, compared with those of other virus families.

SV40 does not cause tumors in its natural hosts. To demonstrate its tumorigenic potential, the virus must be inoculated into experimental animals (newborn hamsters are most susceptible). Many types of cells can be transformed in culture, especially those of rodent origin. Primate cells can be transformed, but only if experimental conditions are manipulated to prevent viral replication.

Genetics

SV40 is genetically stable. Sequence variation exists at the C-terminus of the *T-ag* gene among different isolates. Many point mutations, deletions and substitutions have been introduced into the SV40 genome in the course of experimental studies designed to examine mechanisms of gene regulation, viral replication and cell transformation. Adaptation of natural isolates to tissue culture involves the selection of viruses with duplications or rearrangements in the viral regulatory region. The origins of the most well-characterized SV40 strains are listed in **Table 3**. Serial undiluted passage of virus in cultured cells often results in the accumulation of defective-interfering particles containing DNA with extensive deletions and rearrangements. To produce high-titer stocks of virus, serial passage of undiluted preparations should be avoided.

Evolution

Different strains of SV40 can be distinguished on the basis of nucleotide differences in the regulatory region and in the variable domain of the *T-ag* gene. During natural infections, viruses with heterogeneous regulatory regions but a common *T-ag* gene may be generated. During adaptation to tissue culture, a virus with a duplication in the enhancer will usually be selected. The evolutionary origin of SV40 is obscure. Sequence comparisons have revealed short regions of similarity between portions of SV40-encoded gene products and cellular proteins. It may be that the viral proteins are composites of functional domains pirated from cellular progenitors. Because of size constraints imposed on the SV40 genome by capsid architecture, the bulk of the coding sequence for a cellular protein would have to be jettisoned, making identification of origins difficult. Among the polyomaviruses, SV40 is most closely related to BKV by base sequence homology. When all the polyomaviruses are compared, the lowest homologies are found in the noncoding regulatory sequences.

Serologic Relationships and Variability

Only one serotype of SV40 is known. The virus does not undergo noticeable antigenic variation. Perhaps restrictions imposed by the symmetry of the capsid permit only minimal deviation in amino acid sequence of the structural proteins, making most changes lethal for the virus.

There is a genus-specific antigenic determinant on the major capsid protein, VP1, that is shared by all animal and human polyomaviruses. It is internal in the virion, but antibodies are elicited against it by immunization with disrupted capsids or with purified VP1 protein. The determinant is expressed in infected cells. Antibodies against the shared determinant are not neutralizing, as the site is not exposed on the surface of virus particles. Although the structural proteins of SV40 and the two human polyomaviruses are antigenically distinct (with the exception of the genus-specific determinant on VP1), the T-ags of SV40, BKV and JCV show extensive antigenic cross-reactivity.

Epidemiology

Most adults of the Asian macaque species believed to be natural hosts for SV40 have neutralizing antibodies to the virus. Few of the juvenile animals of those species, in the wild, have antibodies. However, in captivity the young animals are readily infected if they have contact with a virus-positive animal.

Serologic surveys have detected SV40-neutralizing antibodies in humans not exposed to contaminated vaccines, with prevalences of 2–10%. Possible cross-reactivity with BKV and JCV does not explain the presence of such antibodies. This suggests that SV40, or an unknown SV40-like agent, is circulating in the human population.

Transmission and Tissue Tropism

SV40 establishes persistent infections in the kidneys of susceptible hosts. The level of virus present may be very low. Modes of transmission are not known, but transmission probably occurs due to virus shed in the urine. Experiments have established that susceptible animals can be infected by the oral, respiratory or subcutaneous routes. Both viremia and viruria occur in infected animals. SV40 may cause neurologic disease in immunocompromised hosts.

The major known source of human exposure to SV40 was via the administration of contaminated viral vaccines before SV40 was recognized. That risk no longer exists. Human exposure could occur by contact with infected monkeys, a situation limited to small numbers of animal handlers. It is presumed that patterns of tissue tropism and transmission similar to those described in monkeys would be observed in humans infected by SV40.

Pathogenicity and Pathology

SV40 infections in normal monkeys appear to be asymptomatic and harmless. However, SV40 has been associated with a fatal case of pulmonary and renal disease, as well as with cases of progressive multifocal leukoencephalopathy, in unhealthy rhesus monkeys. SV40 can cause widespread infections in monkeys suffering from simian AIDS. No tumors have been found in the natural hosts. Transgenic mice carrying wild-type SV40 DNA develop choroid plexus papillomas and die rapidly because of the physiological importance of the tumor site. When foreign tissue-specific regulatory sequences are substituted for the native promoter-enhancer of the virus, SV40 expression can be directed to other tissues in transgenic animals. Tumors usually appear in the targeted tissue and are lethal. In conventional animals, tumors induced by virus injection tend to stay localized and do not invade or metastasize, but rodents bearing such tumors usually succumb due to the tumor load. SV40-induced tumors are usually classified as undifferentiated carcinomas or sarcomas. Intravenous inoculation of SV40 into weanling hamsters induced leukemia, reticulum cell sarcoma and osteogenic sarcoma. SV40 DNA has been detected in several types of human cancers, including brain tumors (especially those from children in the first decade of life), mesotheliomas, osteosarcomas and kidney tumors. The role SV40 may have played in the induction of those tumors is unknown.

Immune Response

SV40, like other members of the *Polyomavirus* genus, induces an asymptomatic, persistent infection in natural hosts. An antibody response to capsid antigen is elicited that can be detected in neutralization assays. It is well documented with the human viruses BKV and JCV that impaired cell-mediated immunity is associated with virus re-activation, showing that viral replication is under the control of the immune system of the host; the same presumably applies to SV40.

Little is known about the immune response of humans to infection by SV40. Small numbers of individuals exposed to contaminated vaccines were analyzed for neutralizing antibody responses to SV40. Humoral responses were variable and dependent on the size of inoculum and route of inoculation. Recent serological surveys have detected SV40 neutralizing antibody in 2–10% of persons not exposed to SV40-contaminated viral vaccines. Antibodies to SV40 were most often detected in people with some type of immune suppression.

Experimental studies have shown that animals with active infections by SV40 may produce humoral antibodies against the replication oncoprotein, T-ag. The responses were variable and probably reflected the extent of viral replication. It should be noted that a T-ag antibody response could not be used to monitor SV40 infections in humans because of the crossreactivity among the T-ags of SV40 and the human viruses BKV and JCV.

SV40 tumor-bearing animals develop a strong immune response to T-ag. Both humoral and cell-mediated responses occur. No antibodies are produced against capsid antigens, as the structural proteins are not expressed in tumor cells in rodents. Cytotoxic T cells directed against T-ag determinants at the cell membrane help render the animals resistant to the growth of SV40 tumor cells. This system has been an important experimental model for helping to understand the immune response to neoplastic cells in humans.

Interferon is induced only weakly by the polyomaviruses and is not thought to be an important component of the host response to SV40.

Prevention and Control

No control measures are available to prevent SV40 infections.

Future Perspectives

The reports of antibodies to SV40 in humans and the infrequent association of SV40 markers with human tumors suggest that SV40 may be present in the population. If its presence is substantiated, it will be important to determine the natural history of SV40 in humans, including modes of transmission and factors affecting susceptibility to infection. If tumors are produced in humans following exposure to SV40, it will be necessary to develop appropriate control measures to prevent such infections. Because of its small genetic content and dependence on host cell functions, SV40 will continue to be a useful model system for discerning mechanisms of cellular processes, such as mammalian cell DNA replication, cell cycle progression and growth control processes altered in neoplasia.

See also: **Defective interfering viruses; JC and BK viruses (*Papovaviridae*); Persistent viral infection; Polyomaviruses – murine (*Papovaviridae*): General features, Molecular biology; Virus structure: Atomic structure, Principles of virus structure.**

Further Reading

Cole CN (1996) *Polyomavirinae:* the viruses and their replication. In: Fields BN, Knipe DM, Howley PM *et al* (eds) *Fields Virology*, 3rd edn, p. 1997. Philadelphia: Lippincott-Raven.

Liddington RC, Yan Y, Moulai J *et al*. (1991) Structure of simian virus 40 at 3.8-Å resolution. *Nature* 354: 278.

Prives C (1990) The replication functions of SV40 T antigen are regulated by phosphorylation. *Cell* 61: 735.

Shah K and Nathanson N (1976) Human exposure to SV40: review and comment. *Am. J. Epidemiol.* 103: 1.

Stewart AR, Lednicky JA and Butel JS (1998) Sequence analyses of human tumor-associated SV40 DNAs and SV40 viral isolates from monkeys and humans. *J. Neurovirol.* 4: 182.

Tevethia SS (1990) Recognition of simian virus 40 T antigen by cytotoxic T lymphocytes. *Mol. Biol. Med.* 7: 83.

SINDBIS AND SEMLIKI FOREST VIRUSES (*TOGAVIRIDAE*)

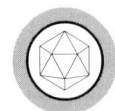

Milton J Schlesinger, Department of Molecular Microbiology, Washington University School of Medicine, St Louis, USA

Copyright © 1999 Academic Press

History

Sindbis (SIN) virus was first isolated in 1952 from a group of *Culex univittatus* mosquitoes captured in a light trap in the Sindbis health district 30 km north of Cairo, Egypt. Isolation was by inoculation of triturated mosquitoes into 3-day-old mice. The diameter of the virus was estimated to be 40–48 nm and, based on its pathogenesis in neonatal but not adult mice, it was initially classified as a coxsackie-type virus. Additional studies showed it to be distinct from these viruses and it was placed into a separate class.

Semliki Forest virus (SFV) was first isolated in Uganda in 1942 from *Aedes (Aedimorphus) abnormalis*. Its diameter was estimated to be 20–67 nm.

Taxonomy and Classification

SIN and SFV are members of the *Alphavirus* genus of the *Togaviridae* family. Based on sequences of the viral genomes, SIN and SFV are grouped separately and both are distinct from another group that includes Eastern equine and Venezualen equine encephalitis viruses. In the SFV group are ten other alphaviruses; in the SIN group are four other alphaviruses plus Western equine encephalitis virus, which is a genetic recombinant with glycoproteins derived from SIN-like sequences and the balance of the genome from Eastern equine encephalitis virus. SIN and SFV are serologically related to Eastern, Western and Venezualan equine encephalitis viruses. They have also been classified as members of the RNA virus superfamily 1.

Geographic and Seasonal Distribution

SIN strains have been isolated worldwide. Two geographical subgroups exist: European–African and Asian–Australian. Sindbis virus has been isolated in the Near East, Africa, Southeast Asia, India, Borneo, Australia, the former USSR and Czechoslovakia. Viruses closely related to SIN have been isolated in Scandinavia, New Zealand, Brazil and Argentina. SFV and closely related viruses have been isolated from Africa, the former USSR, Australia, Japan, Malaysia and South America. As mosquito-borne viruses, they are more prevalent in tropical regions and their presence is amplified during summer months and during periods of precipitation in tropical areas.

Host Range and Propagation

The natural vectors of SIN include *Culex univittatus*, *C. antennatus*, *C. annulirostris*, *C. pseudovishnue*, *C. tritaeniorhynchus*, *C. bitaeniorhynchus* and *Mansonia fuscopennata*. SIN has been isolated also from mites and ticks. Migratory birds are an important host and probably account for the global distribution of these viruses. SIN transmission between birds is from bites of *Ae. albopictus*, *Ae. aegypti* and *C. pipiens*. SFV is propagated by *Ae. abnormalis* and *Aedes* spp. Transovarial transmission occurs in *Aedes* spp. Both viruses exist in an enzootic cycle involving small wild animals, birds, subhuman primates and mosquitoes. They are arthropod-borne viruses.

Virion Structure

SIN and SFV virions are spherical, 70–80 nm in diameter, with icosahedral symmetry and a $T = 4$ lattice. The internal nucleocapsid or core is spherical, 40 nm in diameter, with icosahedral symmetry and a $T = 4$ lattice. The virus particle (molecular mass of 52 MDa) is composed of 30% lipid, 57% protein, 6% carbohydrate and 7% RNA. The sedimentation coefficient is 280 S and the density is 1.22 g ml^{-1} in sucrose-D_2O. The core's sedimentation coefficient is 140 S. Virions of SFV and SIN are stable to storage at 4°C and to repeated freeze–thawing. Infectious particles rapidly lose activity at 56°C ($-1 \log/10$ min, but varies with a particular strain) and are labile to organic solvents, detergents and thiol reducing agents. The RNA in isolated cores is susceptible to RNase.

The external spikes are arranged as 80 trimers, each consisting of stable heterodimers composed of two glycosylated transmembranal proteins. The spikes are embedded in a lipid bilayer which is derived from the plasma membrane of the infected host cell. Curvature of the membrane is such that the outer area is about 40% greater than the inner leaflet. Cryo-electron micrographs of Sindbis virus are presented in **Fig. 1**: a cross-sectional view has been constructed to show the internal core and the lipid bilayer, which appears nonuniform with an average thickness of 4.8 nm. The spike arrangement indicates a cup-like structure for the trimers which form at their base a protein shell around the lipid bilayer with exposed areas of the latter on the virion surface. An atomic structure of the capsid protein has been determined from x-ray diffraction data to a resolution of 0.3 nm and amino acids from 114 to 264 are folded in a manner closely resembling mammalian serine proteases with the catalytic triad of serine, histidine and aspartate surrounding a hydrophobic pocket occupied by tryptophan.

The genome consists of a nonsegmented, single-stranded RNA with a sedimentation coefficient of 49 S. The RNA is capped at its 5' end with m^7G and is polyadenylated at its 3' terminus with average length of 70 A's. Genomic RNA is of the positive orientation and isolated RNA is infectious. The complete sequences of about 12 kb from two strains of SIN and one of the SFV genome have been determined and plasmids containing these sequences in the form of cDNA can be transcribed *in vitro* to yield infectious RNA. The cDNA under control of a eukaryotic promoter is also infectious.

The genome encodes four nonstructural and four

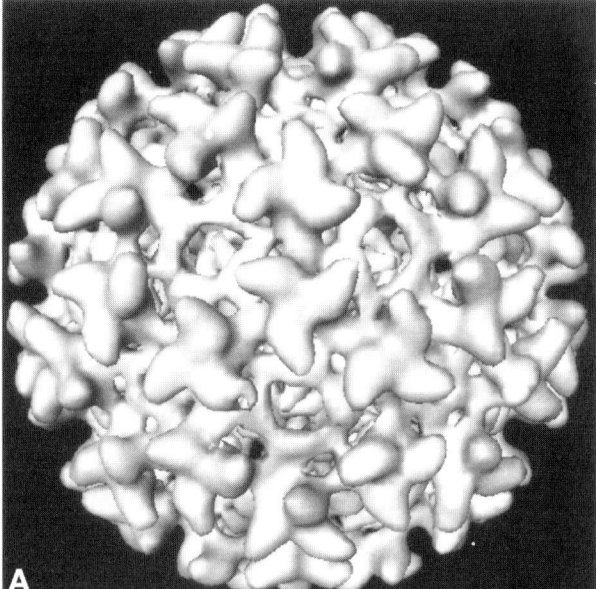
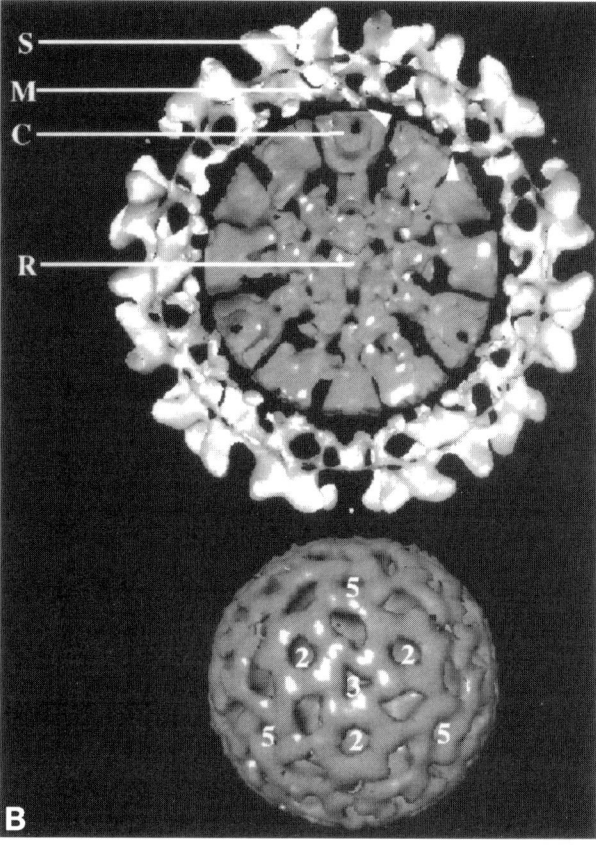

Figure 1 Image reconstruction of Sindbis virus structure based on cryo-electron micrographs. (**A**) Surface view of the virion indicating trimeric spike arrangement. (**B**) Cross-sectional view shows spikes (S), lipid envelope (M), nucleocapsid protein (C) and RNA genome (R). Below, surface of the nucleocapsid with 5, 3 and 2-fold axes of symmetry. (Reproduced with permission from V. Prasad. In: Fields BN et al (eds) (1996).) Fields Virology 3rd edn, p. 76. Philadelphia: Lippincott-Raven.)

structural proteins. Their sizes and functions are listed in **Table 1**. Four regions in the genome contain cis-acting sequences critical to expression and replication of the genome. These include 44 nucleotides at the 5' terminus, 21 nucleotides at the junction between nonstructural and structural genes, 19 nucleotides at the 3' terminus and a sequence of 132 nucleotides near the 5' terminus of the SIN RNA (nt 948) which forms a structure that functions as a packaging signal and selectively binds to the virus capsid. Different sequences in the NSP2 gene appear to serve this function for SFV.

Replication and Molecular Biology

Infection initiates with virus binding to host cell receptors. Attachment is sensitive to ionic conditions and host range mutants can differ in net surface charge of the virion. SIN binds to a highly conserved laminin receptor on mammalian and possibly also on insect cell surfaces. Chicken cells have a high-affinity receptor distinct from laminin and accounting for half of potential receptor sites. Mouse neuronal cells may have two other surface receptors. The virus protein most important for binding to cell receptors is E2, although changes in E1 can affect binding. The E2 sequence between amino acids 170 and 220 is particularly critical. A single amino acid change in SIN at position 55 of E2 from glutamine to histidine confers neurotropism and neurovirulence in rodents. In most cells, the major route for uptake is via clathrin-coated pits and acidified endosomes. Delivery of virus cores into the cell cytoplasm occurs after fusion of the virus membrane with the cell's endosomal membrane, which is mediated by the E1 glycoprotein. At a pH <6, this protein dissociates from the heterodimer to form a homotrimer with a conformation distinct from that on the virion surface. A hydrophobic sequence of amino acids at positions 78–96 has been designated as a fusion domain that is exposed at the lower pH and may initiate formation of a coiled-coiled structure required for fusogenesis. Cholesterol and sphingolipid are essential components in the host cell membrane for virus binding and fusion. Bio-

Table 1 Sizes and functions of SIN and SFV proteins

Protein	SIN	SFV	Properties and function(s)
NSP1	540	537	Methyl and guanyl transferase; 5′ capping activity; specifically required for initiation of (−)RNA transcription; modulation of NSP2 proteinase; membrane associated; palmitylated and mutants lacking fatty acyl groups show different cell membrane distribution
NSP2	807	798	Cysteine protease in the C-terminal half of the protein which functions in *cis* and *trans* cleavages of the NSP polyprotein; nucleoside triphosphatase and RNA helicase motifs in the N-terminal half of the protein; RNA binding activity; specifically required for 26S RNA transcription; accumulates in the nucleolus of infected (or transfected) cells; single site mutations decrease the virus-induced shutoff of host cell protein synthesis
NSP3	556	482	Phosphoprotein (threonine/serine are phosphorylated); variable length in the C-terminus
NSP4	610	614	RNA polymerase; unstable and degraded by the ubiquitin pathway; concentration is tightly regulated
Capsid	264	267	Forms nucleocapsid; folds during synthesis to a serine-like protease that autocatalytically cleaves the capsid from the polyprotein; contains hairpin RNA structure near the N-terminus that enhances translation of virus encoded structural proteins in infected cells; positively-charged N-terminus binds genomic RNA
p62	487	488	Precursor to E2; type 1 transmembrane glycoprotein; palmitylated and glycosylated; cleaved in a *trans*-Golgi vesicle by a furin-type protease; rarely incorporated into virus particles
E3	64	66	N-terminal part of p62 containing the signal sequence; glycosylated; retained on SFV but not on SIN virions
E2	423	422	Component of the heterodimeric virus spike; contains sites for binding to cell receptors and epitopes for neutralizing antibodies; type 1 transmembrane protein with 33 amino acids at its C-terminus in the cytoplasm which forms a motif that binds to the capsid during assembly; glycosylated, palmitylated and, possibly, phosphorylated; amino acid changes in the ecto-domain affect virus assembly, stability, virulence and tropism
6K	55	60	Membrane associated; palmitylated; C-terminus is the signal sequence for E1; small amounts in virions; enhancer for virus assembly and budding
E1	439	438	Component of the heterodimeric virus spike; glycosylated and palmitylated; contains sequences which function in low-pH activated membrane fusion; type 1 transmembrane protein with 2 positively-charged amino acids in the cytoplasm

Values are the number of amino acids in the protein. Note that the p62 protein does not normally appear as a structural protein of the infectious virion.

chemical mechanisms for nucleocapsid uncoating to release RNA are unknown. Within 0.5–1 h postinfection, cells are resistant to superinfection by homologous viruses.

Biosynthetic activities that lead to progeny virions consist of the following steps.

1. Genomic RNA is partially translated to form a polyprotein composed of the four nonstructural proteins, nsP1–4 (**Fig. 2A**). For SIN, most of the polyprotein terminates at the end of the NSP3 gene at an opal stop codon; however, suppression of this codon allows for 20% of the polyprotein to include nsP4. For SFV, the entire nsP1–4 polyprotein is formed. Several stop codons located about two-thirds of the length of the genomic RNA insure that termination of translations stops at the end of the NSP4 gene for both SIN and SFV.
2. A complex consisting of the nsP1–3 polyprotein and nsP4, which has been proteolytically cleaved from nsP1–4 by a *cis*-acting protease encoded in the nsP2 C-terminus, interacts with a 19 nucleotide sequence at the 3′ end of genomic RNA to initiate replication that produces a full length (−)RNA template (**Fig. 2B**). Host cell proteins are also involved in this activity. The replication complex is associated with cellular membranes. Transcription from (−) to (+) RNAs requires modification of the nsP123 complex by the nsP2 protease acting in *trans* to give individual subunits with altered structures (**Fig. 2B**). Proteolytic cleavage of the nsP1–3 complex shuts off (−)RNA synthesis. (−)RNA templates are transcribed into full length (+)RNAs and into a subgenomic species with sequences identical to the 3′ one-third of the virus genomic RNA and a sedimentation coefficient of 26 S (**Fig. 2A**). The minimal promoter for 26S RNA transcription consists of 19 nucleotides upstream and five nucleotides downstream from the transcriptional start site on the (−) RNA. Full-length genome

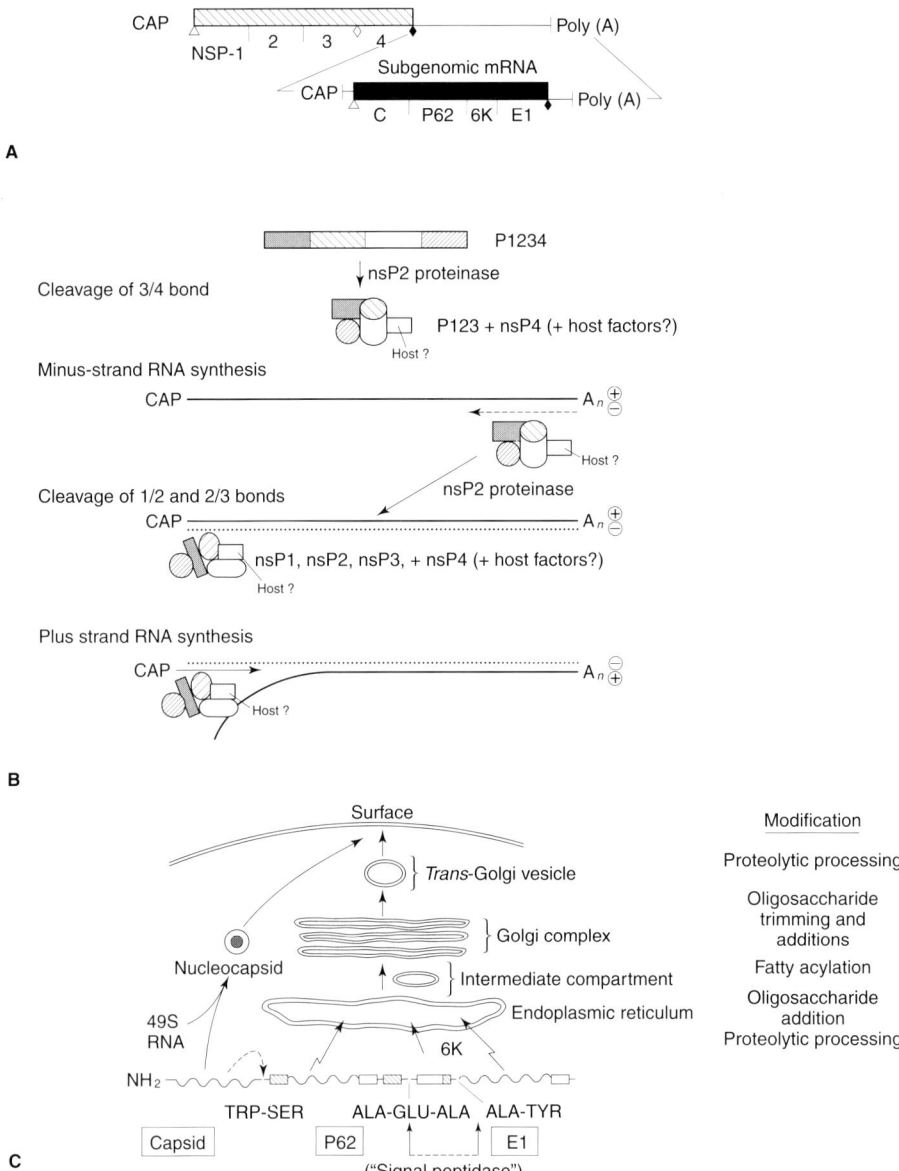

Figure 2 Organization and expression of SIN and SFV genome. (**A**) Order of genes and the sites of initiation (△) and termination (◆) of translation for the genomic and subgenomic mRNAs. In SIN, and opal codon (◇) terminates translation to produce the polyprotein P123. (**B**) Two stages of processing by the nsP2 proteinase of the P1234 polyprotein translated from the genomic mRNA and the function of the different complexes in viral RNA transcription and replication. See text for details. (Reproduced with permission from Strauss and Strauss (1994).) (**C**) Formation, maturation and transport through intracellular membrane vesicles of the viral structural proteins translated from the subgenomic 26S mRNA. Signal sequences for insertion into the membrane are noted by the cross-hatched boxes. (Reproduced with permission from Schlesinger and Schlesinger (1996).)

(+) RNA is packaged with capsid subunits and subgenomic 26S mRNA becomes the predominant RNA translated in the infected cell.

3. 26S RNA encodes the capsid, p62 (E3 + E2), 6K and E1 virus structural proteins and translation initiates at a single site near its 5′ capped end. The first gene translated codes for the capsid protein which folds to form a serine-like protease that autoproteolytically releases capsid protein from the growing nascent polypeptide. A stem–loop structure in the mRNA near the N-terminus of the capsid functions as a translational enhancer in virus-infected cells, yielding very high levels of the virus structural gene products. A transmembranal signal sequence encoded at the N-terminus of the second gene initiates insertion of its protein

product, p62, into the lumen of the endoplasmic reticulum (**Fig. 2C**). Stop-transfer signals followed by additional signal and stop-transfer signals lead to insertion of the C-termini of p62, 6K and E1 and the N-terminus of the 6K into the ER membrane. Host cell signalases cleave at p62–6K and 6K–E1 sites in the ER lumen to give the separate p62, 6K and E1 polypeptides. These three proteins move as a cohort through the intracellular transport vesicles of the host cell where several post-translational modifications occur. The latter include attachment of glycosyl groups to p62 and E1 immediately upon entry into the lumen of the endoplasmic reticulum; a reorientation of the C-terminus of p62 from a transmembranal to a cytoplasmic location, covalent attachment of palmityl groups to cytoplasmically oriented cysteines of p62, 6K and E1 during transport to the Golgi and proteolytic cleavage of the p62 to the E2 glycoprotein in a *trans*-Golgi vesicle by a furin-like protease.

4. Assembly of progeny virus requires two stages: there is the self-association of capsid subunits in the cell cytoplasm to form substructures that bind to specific regions of genomic RNA (nucleotides 945–1076 of SIN and 2737–2993 plus others for SFV) to form nucleocapsids. Capsids can, however, assemble to nucleocapsid-like particles in the absence of RNA. Preformed nucleocapsids bind to arrays of E1–E2 trimers localized to the plasma membrane to initiate the budding process. A motif composed of hydrophobic amino acids in the 33 amino acid cytoplasmic domain of E2 acts as a ligand to bind to a hydrophobic pocket receptor on the surface of capsid subunits. There are 240 such interactions which lead to envelopment of the nucleocapsid by the host cell plasma membrane. Lateral interactions among the glycoproteins are important in the assembly process. The host cell can also influence this assembly; i.e. hyperglycosylated E2 is inhibitory for growth in vertebrate cells but has little effect in assembly in insect cells, and deletion of the 6K protein is relatively nondefective in insect cells but blocks virus assembly in avian cells grown at 40°C. Fusion of the virus lipid bilayer allows for release of progeny virions from the cells. Assembly and budding require cholesterol in the membrane. The process described can occur within 3 h in permissive cells such as chicken embryo fibroblasts and produces thousands of progeny virus which are secreted into the extracellular fluid. Replication is slower in cultured insect cells, with peak production of virus occurring some 15–20 h postinfection.

Pathology and Histopathology

Neither SIN nor SFV are serious pathogens for adult vertebrates unless virus is injected directly into the brain. In rare infections in humans, SIN and SFV produce arthralgia, rash and fever. Human polyarthritis can result from infection by some SIN strains.

SIN is highly pathogenic to embryonated hens' eggs. Within the host organism, the infected cells include neuron and glial cells, striate and smooth muscle cells, cells of lymphoid origin, synovial cells and brown fat cells. Neonatal rodents develop severe neurocytopathology when virus is given intracerebrally or intraperitoneally. In the CNS, focal cystic degeneration, vascular dilatation and neurolysis occur. Strains of SIN that lead to fatal encephalitis after infection of neonatal mice show lesions associated with a severe stress response – including high levels of interferon α/β and toxic cytokines such as tumor necrosis factor α and little evidence of encephalitis. Less virulent strains produce a more classical encephalitis. Adult mice are susceptible to some SIN strains and neuroinvasiveness is attributed to a change in amino acid 55 of the E2 glycoprotein from glutamine to histidine. Other single-site amino acid changes in E2 alter neurovirulence and cytopathology of SIN. Additional changes in the 5′ noncoding region of the genome and at position 190 of the E2 glycoprotein can confer neuroinvasiveness on other isolates. Attenuation of these strains by mutations produces encephalitis but low levels of mortality and low levels of interferon α/β. Comparison of neurological damage in B6 versus SJL mice infected with SFV show more acute encephalomyelitis in the former, which could be correlated with lower levels of several cytokines and higher virus titers early after infection. Cytopathic effects and neurovirulence are dependent also on strains of SFV. Subacute demyelinating disease, chronic benign infection and teratogenesis in pregnant mice have been detected in SFV-infected mice and high mortality for some strains is attributed to replication in the spleen, lymph nodes and liver. Replication in skeletal muscle leads to atrophy, focal necrosis and viremia.

In vertebrate tissue culture, SIN and SFV have a broad host range and are highly cytopathic, inducing apoptosis in many cells. Host cell macromolecular synthesis (protein, DNA and RNA) is shut off early after infection as a result of expression of virus nonstructural genes and high levels of virus RNA. Mutations in the NSP2 gene of SIN can lead to a persistent infection in BHK cells. Blocks in Na^+/K^+-ATPase activity in membranes from SIN-infected cells alters internal ion concentrations and contributes to cell cytolysis. Virus structural protein synthesis and intracellular vesicle transport are associated with cytopathology.

In the mosquito, replication occurs in epithelial cells of the midgut, in the salivary glands, thoracic muscle and respiratory tissue. Persistent infection occurs in the insect hemolymph, hindgut and tracheole-associated cells, as well as in cultured insect cells. An antiviral hydrophobic peptide is induced by virus infection of cultured insect cells and limits infection but leads to persistent virus replication. Infection of the mosquito also leads to persistent infection.

Genetics

The frequency of mutation is about 10^{-4}–10^{-5}, which is similar to other RNA viruses. Specific nucleotide mutations, however, have been noted in which the frequency is much lower, in the range of 10^{-7}–10^{-8}. Low rates of divergence have been found and attributed to the natural infection and growth of the virus in both insects and vertebrate cells with varying temperatures and host cell metabolic activities. Temperature-sensitive and host-range mutants have been isolated and placed into seven complementation groups. A large number of site-directed and deletion mutations in virtually every gene of these viruses have been prepared and analyzed utilizing the infectious cDNA clones of SIN and SFV. Close to 50% of the amino acids in the structural proteins of SFV are identical to SIN, and 64% are identical between the nonstructural proteins of the two viruses. A chimeric virus with SFV capsid gene and SIN glycoprotein genes is infectious but the reciprocal construct is not.

Defective interfering (DI) particles are generated within six to nine passages in tissue culture cells at high multiplicities of infection. Genomes of DI particles are about one-third the size of wild-type genome and contain scrambled and repeated portions of the genome. Three regions of the wild-type virus genome are conserved in the DI particle: the 5′ domain, a packaging site near the 5′ end of the RNA and 19 bases at the 3′ terminus of the genome RNA.

SIN and SFV undergo recombination; homologous, nonhomologous and aberrant homologous crossovers occur.

SIN and SFV vectors have been developed to express a foreign gene inserted in the subgenomic region and expressed from the 26S mRNA. They contain conserved cis-acting sequences and are self-replicating. Helper viruses containing virus structural genes but lacking nonstructural genes and packaging signals are used to package replicon RNA. These virus-like particles can be used to deliver the foreign genes into a susceptible host cell in place of cDNA or RNA.

Evolution

Evolutionary trees have been constructed based on sequences of eight alphaviruses and they show SIN and SFV occupying different subgroupings. SIN-like viruses that were isolated from different geological areas but are related serologically diverge up to 20% in amino acid identity. Western equine encephalitis virus is a recombinant that contains glycoprotein genes derived from a SIN-like virus and the rest of its genome from an Eastern equine encephalitis virus parent. Domains in the SIN nonstructural proteins, nsP1 (methyltransferase), 2 (helicase) and 4 (core RNA polymerase), are homologous to similar domains in tobacco mosaic virus and several other RNA plant viruses in the bromo and tobamo groups. Furthermore, the plant viruses transcribe one or more subgenomic mRNAs, one of which encodes the capsid, in a manner identical to SIN and SFV. There is the suggestion that alphaviruses evolved from recombination with the tobamo group of plant viruses.

Immunological Response

SIN and SFV are highly antigenic and produce high titers of neutralizing antibodies. Humans with antibodies to SIN and SFV have been found worldwide. Cell-mediated immunity and cytokine response also play important roles in clearing virus infections. Benign persistent infections result from infection of *scid* mice, which lack both humoral and cell-mediated immunity.

Two domains of E2 have epitopes to which monoclonal antibodies will bind and block infection (neutralizing). One epitope of E1 generated a monoclonal antibody that is neutralizing and this overlaps with an E2 epitope. Most monoclonal antibodies to E1 are sensitive to the protein's conformation but this is not so with E2, as monoclonal antibodies can react with fragments and denatured protein. Antibodies to some of the latter peptides injected into mice protected them against virus infection.

See also: **Encephalitis viruses (*Flaviviridae*): Encephalitis viruses and related viruses causing hemorrhagic disease; Pathogenesis: Animal viruses; Rubella virus (*Togaviridae*); Viral membranes; Virus structure: Atomic structure, Principles of virus structure.**

Further Reading

Johnston RE and Peters CJ (1995) In: Fields BN, Knipe DM, Howley PM *et al* (eds) *Fields Virology* 3rd edn, p. 843. Philadelphia: Lippincott-Raven.

Schlesinger S and Schlesinger MJ (1995) In: Fields BN, Knipe DM, Howley PM *et al* (eds) *Fields Virology* 3rd edn, p. 825. Philadelphia: Lippincott-Raven.

Strauss JH and Strauss EG (1994) The alphaviruses: gene expression, replication and evolution. *Microbiol. Rev.* 58: 491.

SINGLE-STRANDED RNA PHAGES (*LEVIVIRIDAE*)

J van Duin, Gorlaeus Laboratories, Leiden University, Leiden, The Netherlands

Copyright © 1999 Academic Press

Introduction

Since their discovery in 1961 by Loeb and Zinder, the RNA phages have served as a model system to explore a variety of problems in molecular biology. As a source of homogeneous and readily obtainable messenger RNA, they have been particularly helpful in solving questions on regulation of gene expression at the level of translation. The concepts of translational polarity and translational control by repressor proteins resulted from early studies on bacteriophage RNA.

The RNA phages have also provided us with the best defined RNA replication system, which is currently used to study template recognition, *in vitro* RNA recombination and replication.

Available infectious clones have opened the possibility to explore the compromise between the need to fold in a specific way and the need to encode proteins.

Taxonomy and Classification

The RNA coliphages form the family *Leviviridae*. Within this family two genera can be distinguished, *Levivirus* and *Allolevivirus*. The leviviruses, also known as supergroup A, are subdivided into group I and II, whereas the alloleviviruses (supergroup B) consist of the groups III and IV (**Fig. 1**).

The best characterized phage in group I is MS2. Close relatives are R17, f2, M12 and JP501. Somewhat more distant but still in group I is fr, isolated by Hoffmann-Berling from a dung hill. The genomes of MS2, M12, JP501 and fr are completely sequenced and from the others partial sequences are known. In group II, GA and KU1 have been fully sequenced. Other members of this group are JP34, TH1 and BZ13. The prototype of group III is Qβ which, together with M11 and MX1, has been sequenced. Other members include VK and TW18. In group IV SP and NL95 are sequenced representatives. Other strains belonging to group IV are FI, TW19 and TW28. Most of the phages mentioned here are part of the Watanabe Collection at the Keio University, Japan.

Classification into the four groups (**Fig. 1**) was initially based on serological and physicochemical properties, but is presently being replaced by hybridization with group-specific DNA probes. This test recognizes the nucleic acid sequence as the primary criterion for classification. Serotyping is sometimes ambiguous since a few amino acid substitutions in the major coat protein can change the immunological properties dramatically.

Most research has centered around groups I (MS2) and III (Qβ) but it is assumed that features found for group I also hold for group II. Likewise, properties of group III should also exist in group IV.

Virion Structure

In addition to one molecule of positive-strand RNA, each virion contains 180 copies of the coat protein and one copy of the maturation, or A, protein. The group III phages contain in addition about 12 copies of the read-through protein in their capsid. For this reason, the protein shell of the single-stranded (ss) RNA phages is not isomeric like other icosahedral viruses such as poliovirus or satellite tobacco necrosis virus. The diameter of the phage is 26 nm, and the protein shell is about 2 nm wide (**Fig. 2**). The icosahedral shell has a $T = 3$ surface lattice. Crystals of phage MS2, GA, fr and Qβ have been obtained. The coat protein structure of MS2 has been solved to 2.7 Å resolution by x-ray diffraction. Unfortunately, the RNA and the A protein are not seen in the electron

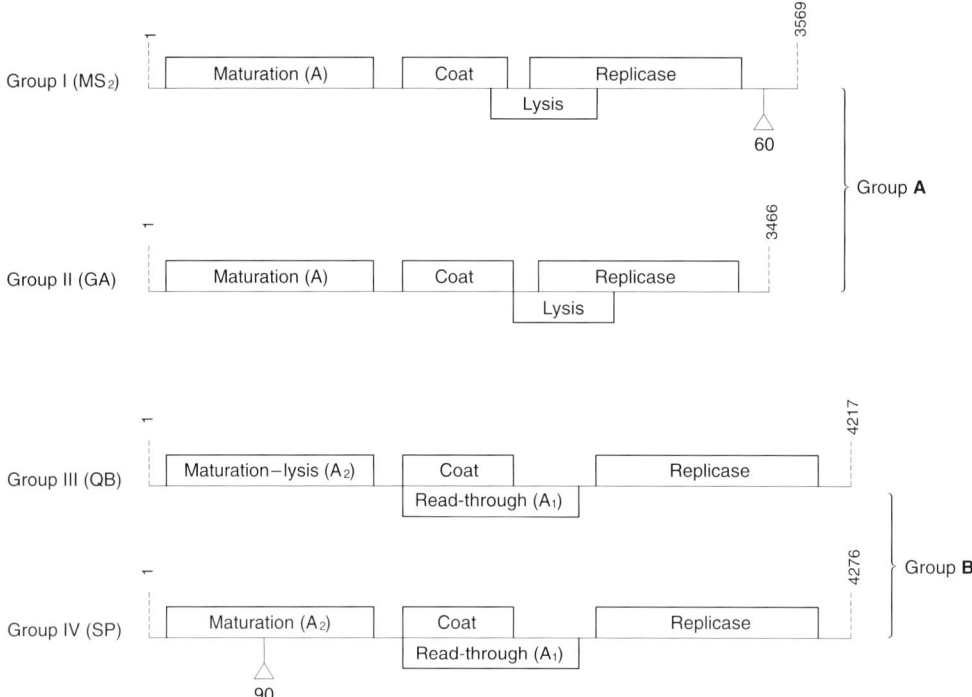

Figure 1 Genetic map of groups I–IV RNA coliphages. Inserts in group I with respect to group II and in group IV with respect to group III are given as triangles.

density map. These molecules are apparently not ordered in the crystal.

The Infection Process

The RNA gains access to the interior of the cell via long, filamentous structures called pili. These can be of various origins and serotypes. In *Escherichia coli*, the sex (or F) pili are employed as vehicle but in *Pseudomonas* and *Caulobacter* polar pili are used for this purpose. Transfer of RNA via pili is not essential for infection, however. Cells that lack pili can be infected if they are converted to spheroplasts.

The attachment of the phage to the sides of the pili proceeds via the maturation (A) protein (**Fig. 3**). The coat protein is dispensable for this process; bacteria can be infected with a binary complex of A protein attached to phage RNA. In group III phages the minimal infection set requires the additional presence of the readthrough (A1) protein.

Contact of the phage with the pilus results in cleavage of the A protein into a 15 kDa and a 24 kDa fragment. This cleavage probably triggers the ordered ejection of the tightly packed RNA from the virus shell. The binding sites of the MS2 A protein on the RNA have been determined at nucleotide regions 400 and 3500, respectively. When cleavage of the A protein occurs between the two RNA binding domains of the protein this would potentially lead to the liberation of the two ends. Conceivably, the 5′ end of the RNA begins to move along the pilus towards the cell. This stage of infection corresponds to the RNase-sensitive step. The two A protein fragments remain associated with the RNA during penetration of the cell envelope. However, it is unlikely that these protein fragments play any further role, since the naked RNA is fully able to generate infectious progeny in spheroplasts. For example, transformation of *E. coli* with phage cDNA containing plasmids leads to productive infection.

Host Range and RNA Phages of Other Genera

RNA phages have also been found in other Gram-negative bacteria. In *Pseudomonas aeruginosa* PP7 and 7S have been characterized and ϕCb5, ϕCb12r, ϕCb8r and ϕCb23r were found in different *Caulobacter* strains. Lately, an *Acinetobacter* RNA phage was identified. As judged by several criteria, these phages must be very similar to the coliphages. They have the same morphology, diameter, and molecular weight range. Sequence comparison shows PP7 to be a member of supergroup A.

Pseudomonas and *Caulobacter* phages enter the cell via polar pili. The dependence of RNA phages on pili

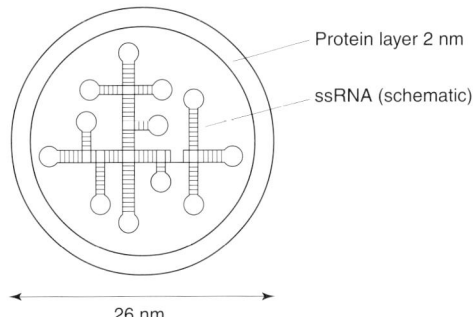

Figure 2 Schematic view of an RNA bacteriophage. The RNA is shown as a highly ordered structure.

as an entry to the bacterial cytoplasm is also reflected in the existence of the ssRNA phage PRR1 that will infect many genera such as *Pseudomonas, E. coli, Salmonella typhimurium*, and *Vibrio cholerae*, provided the host expresses the pili encoded in the drug resistance factor RP (P compatibility group, e.g. RP1, RP4, or R1822). In this connection, it should be mentioned that some members of the *Enterobacteriaceae* have been artificially converted to coliphage sensitivity by introducing the F factor of *E. coli* into *Shigella, Proteus* or *Salmonella*.

Ecology

Furuse has examined and reviewed the geographical distribution of the ssRNA phages as well as their present-day habitat. They are most frequently encountered in sewage and feces of mammals, and their titers in sewage samples may be as high as 10^7 PFU/ml. RNA phages may constitute up to 90% of total coliphages present in these samples, but the number can vary substantially.

The geographical distribution of groups II and III shows a strong bias. In northern Japan, there is a relative abundance of group II over group III (6:1) per sampling site. Moving southward, this ratio drops dramatically until in Southeast Asia group II becomes rare. Furuse has suggested that the north–south gradient is related to differences in climate. Group III (and also groups I and IV) propagates well at 40°C but not at 20°C, whereas for group II the situation is reversed. A problem with this hypothesis is that group II is rare in, for example, The Netherlands where the average temperature is below 20°C.

Although the natural host for ssRNA phages is not known with certainty, it is clear that they survive passing through the gastrointestinal tract of gnotobiotic mice and propagate stably in the intestines if *E. coli* is present as host. Thus *E. coli* can sustain the life cycle of the phage under 'natural' circumstances. In Japan and The Netherlands attempts have been made to determine whether certain phage groups are preferentially associated with certain animal species or with humans. So far, these studies have not been conclusive.

Index Organism

The RNA coliphages and enteroviruses share the same habitat. In addition, because of their structural similarity RNA phages show approximately the same inactivation characteristics as enteroviruses in sewage water treatment processes. For this reason RNA phages can be and are used as index organisms for the possible occurrence of pathogenic enteroviruses.

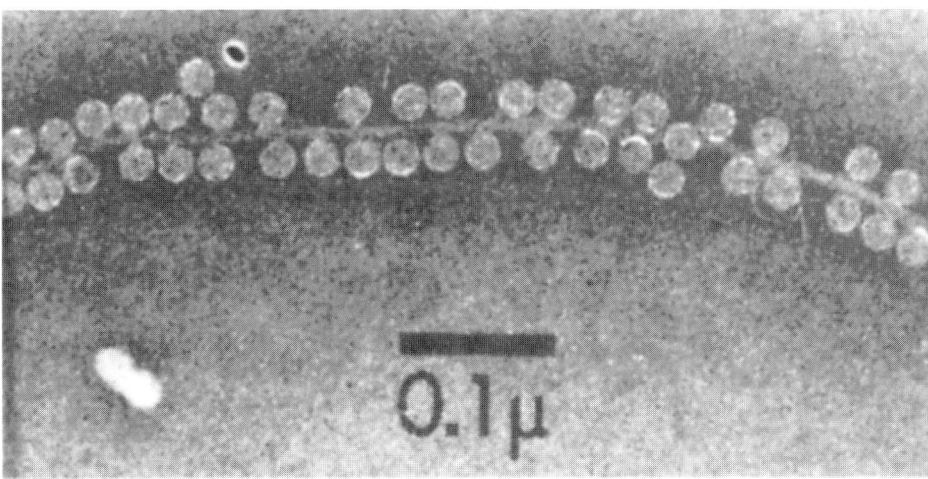

Figure 3 RNA phages attached to the F pilus of *E. coli*. Bar = 0.1 μg. (Reproduced with permission from Zinder ND (1975) Attachment, ejection and penetration stages of the RNA phage infectious process. In: Zinder ND (ed.) *RNA Phages,* p. 89. Cold Spring Harbor: Cold Spring Harbor Laboratory Press.)

RNA phages can be positively identified by specific DNA hybridization probes (see above).

The Genetic Map

A map of the four groups is shown in **Fig. 1**. The conspicuous difference between supergroups A and B is the presence of a readthrough protein in group B. Here, the major coat protein gene ends in a leaky UGA stop codon that is read as tryptophan with a probability of about 5%. This leads to a C-terminally extended coat protein that is incorporated in the capsid and required for infectivity. The other major divergence is the presence of a separate lysis gene in group A. This out-of-frame overlapping gene encodes a hydrophobic peptide about 70 amino acids long, that short-circuits the cytoplasmic membrane of the bacterium. Somehow, loss of membrane potential distorts the balance between components of the bacterial enzyme ensemble that cleaves and extends the peptidoglycan network. This leads to cell lysis.

Genetic differences within the genera are more subtle. In supergroup A the most pronounced one is a 60-nucleotide insertion in the 3' untranslated leader of group I. A 90-nucleotide insertion in the A2 protein gene of group IV represents the major difference with group III in supergroup B.

The Lysing Protein of Group B Phages

The strong similarity in gene arrangement and control of gene expression between the ssRNA phages is fully lost in the way the phages organize their escape from the wasted host. Bacteria that overproduce the Qβ maturation protein lyse. Qβ mutants carrying an amber mutation in the maturation protein gene do not cause bacteriolysis. Thus it is now thought that the maturation protein of supergroup B has a dual function; it is a constituent of the virion and it triggers cell lysis.

Control of Gene Expression

The appearance of the phage-coded proteins in the infected cell is carefully controlled in timing and amount. For instance, replicase is a minor early product, and the amount of coat protein exceeds by far that of the other proteins. Since no DNA intermediates occur in the life cycle of the phage, control is predominantly exerted at the translational level: it is the RNA secondary structure that regulates access of ribosomes to initiation regions.

The maturation protein is needed at only one copy per virion, and its translation is accordingly kept at a low level. In MS2 the maturation gene can only be translated from a growing strand. Its ribosomal binding site is only accessible during a short period when the growing RNA has not yet reached its equilibrium folding. In the equilibrium structure the RNA is inaccessible. For Qβ the mechanism awaits clarification.

In group A, both replicase (R) and lysis (L) gene are under translational control of the coat gene as witnessed by the observation that early nonsense mutations in the coat gene inhibit expression of the R and L genes. For the replicase the underlying mechanism is base-pairing between the start of the R gene and a coding region of the coat gene. Coat protein-synthesizing ribosomes pass through this region, destroy the pairing and temporarily liberate the R start. Coupling of the lysis gene arises by a local hairpin burying the L start. Exposure is brought about by a ribosome that has arrived at the coat gene terminator codon. After releasing the synthesized coat protein this ribosome can, with a low efficiency, reach the L start site by random movements along the RNA.

The real down regulator of replicase is the coat protein. Once present in sufficient concentration, dimers bind to a hairpin structure that contains the R-start, thereby preventing any ribosome binding. The complex between the hairpin and the coat protein dimer has been modeled by x-ray analysis.

Translational coupling of L and R genes, and the temporary expression of the A gene are not only simple ways to cut down on the product levels, but the designs also serve a more sophisticated purpose. On full-sized RNA the only site independently accessible to ribosomes is the start of the coat gene. As discussed below replicase binding also involves this start site. The resulting competition between ribosome and replicase effectuates that the RNA is either used for replication or for translation.

Apart from the occasional competition by the replicase, the coat protein is not negatively regulated.

Replication

Most of our knowledge on replication has been obtained in the Qβ system, but it is assumed that the principles also apply to the other groups. The replicase holoenzyme contains four different proteins called subunits I to IV, or subunits α, β, γ and δ. Subunit I was identified as ribosomal protein S1, and subunits III and IV are the translation elongation factors EF-Tu and EF-Ts. Thus, three proteins that normally function in the synthesis of proteins are recruited by the phage to assist in RNA synthesis. Subunit II is encoded in the viral genome, and these four subunits all occur in the enzyme complex in not more than one copy. Replication proceeds via the synthesis of a free negative strand. Annealed positive and negative strands are not a substrate for the replicase enzyme.

The requirements for copying the positive and the negative strand are different. To copy the negative strand, only subunits II, III and IV are required, whereas positive strand replication also needs subunit I. In addition, copying the positive strand is greatly dependent on the product of the bacterial *hfq* gene, called Host Factor. In the uninfected cell one function of this protein seems to be to promote the accessibility of highly structured messengers. In replication its role may be similar, since replication in the absence of Host Factor proceeds only if the base-pairing occluding the 3′ terminus of Qβ RNA is destabilized by substitutions that introduce mismatches. Supergroup A uses a different host factor for copying the positive strand.

Replicase binds to two internal Qβ RNA sequences, called the S and M site. The interaction with the S site provides for the necessary competition with the ribosome, but it is not required for replication itself. Interaction with the M site is essential. It is supposed that in this binary complex the folding of the RNA places the 3′ terminus in the active site of the enzyme. In this concept then, the specificity of the enzyme is derived from RNA structure and not from sequences. From this point of view it is easy to see that Qβ replicase can multiply group IV RNAs as the RNA foldings in groups III and IV are very similar.

Replication of the negative strand depends on structure elements at both the 5′ and 3′ termini and is thus basically different from positive strand copying.

6S RNA and Qβ RNA Variants

Infection of *E. coli* by Qβ leads, apart from phage multiplication, to the accumulation of what has been termed '6S' RNA. This is a nonhomogeneous collection of RNA molecules that vary in size from about 50 to 200 nucleotides and that together with their negative strands serve as templates for Qβ replicase. They do not code for any protein nor do they contribute to the infection process. These molecules arise either by continuous deletion of Qβ RNA sequences or by RNA recombination events using the plethora of RNA fragments present in each cell. Some show homology with Qβ RNA but others do not. All are characterized by a high degree of secondary structure and like all phage RNA have at least three consecutive Cs at their 3′ ends. 6S RNA is also generated on transformation of *E. coli* with the cDNA for Qβ replicase or by the *in vitro* incubation of Qβ replicase with the four nucleotide triphosphates in the absence of added template. The last experiment showed that Qβ replicase is able to perform uninstructed RNA synthesis.

From an evolutionary point of view, it is interesting that these molecules that are not constrained by a coding sequence quickly respond to selective pressure. It is easy to obtain mutants of 6S RNA that are adapted to *in vitro* replication under adverse conditions, such as the presence of ethidium bromide, T1 ribonuclease or limiting amounts of the building blocks. Abbreviated Qβ RNA variants can be prepared *in vitro* by gradually reducing the time allowed for Qβ replication. After some 70 replication rounds the length of Qβ was reduced to about 12%. There seems no basic difference between such truncated Qβ RNA and the RNA present in the defective interfering (DI) virus particles that accompany, for instance, influenza infection. Also here, the abridged molecules once created by replication errors can survive as long as they are templates for the replicase, and their multiplication does not endanger the survival of the virus population as a whole.

The rapid yield to selective pressure by 6S RNA and the Qβ RNA variants reflects the inaccuracy of the Qβ replicase, which has been estimated at between 10^{-3} and 10^{-4} per nucleotide per replication. The presumed absence of a 3′ → 5′ exonuclease editing activity in Qβ replicase would be consistent with its relatively low copying fidelity. At the same time the frequency with which deletions occur must also be unusually high.

Rigidity and Plasticity of the Genome Structure

Considering the inaccuracy of phage RNA replication one might expect an endless scale of phage sequences, all fit to survive. This turns out not to be true. The sequences of Qβ and MS2 have, despite many years of laboratory cultivation, not or hardly changed. Similarly it has turned out to be quite difficult to find RNA phages in nature whose sequences diverge substantially from the group prototype. For instance, group I representatives like f2, R17, M12, JP501, all isolated independently in different parts of the world, show more than 90% sequence identity. Thus there seem to be very few solutions that are good enough to coexist. It is assumed that the selection pressure, which discards all potential variants (for instance those having synonymous codons), originates from the contribution of the RNA secondary structure (**Fig. 2**) to phage fitness. Such contributions involve regulatory circuits, RNase resistance, delaying the annealing of positive and negative strands and probably many other parameters.

In spite of this apparent rigidity the genome

structure shows a high degree of flexibility under noncompetitive conditions. Laboratory evolution of phages containing a wanton distortion in RNA structure yields many pseudorevertants presenting us with a large spectrum of structural solutions. These solutions all perform well as long as they do not have to compete with their wild-type counterpart. Then they lose and disappear from the population.

Phylogeny of RNA Phages

An interesting but necessarily most difficult question is that of the origin and kinships of the RNA bacteriophages. It is generally assumed that all of them derive from a common ancestor because of the nearly identical genetic organization, the strong resemblance of the replicases, the use of the same host proteins (except Host Factor) as auxiliaries in the copying reaction, and the similarities of several control mechanisms. These properties are more easily explained by divergent than by convergent evolution.

Therapeutic Use of RNA Phages

There is presently renewed interest in DNA phages as combatants of bacterial infections. Early pilot studies showed that *E. coli* adapts to RNA phages by losing its F pili.

Further Reading

Armon, R and Kott Y (1966) Bacteriophages as indicators of pollution. *Crit. Rev. Environ. Sci. Technol.* 26: 299.

Furuse K (1987) Distribution of coliphages in the environment: general considerations. In: Goyal SM (ed.) *Phage Ecology*, p. 87. New York: Wiley.

Havelaar HA (1991) Bacteriophages as model viruses in water quality control. IAWPRC Study Group on Health Related Water Microbiology. *Wat. Res.* 25: 529.

Olsthoorn RCL, Licis N and van Duin J (1994) Leeway and constraints in the forced evolution of a regulatory RNA helix. *EMBO J.* 13: 2660.

Valegård K, Murray JB, Stockley PG, Stonehouse NJ and Liljas L (1994) Crystal structure of an RNA bacteriophage coat protein–operator complex. *Nature* 371: 623.

Van Duin J (1988) In: Fraenkel Conrat H and Wagner RR (eds) *The Bacteriophages*. Series *The Viruses*, p. 117. New York: Plenum Press.

SMALLPOX AND MONKEYPOX VIRUSES (*POXVIRIDAE*)

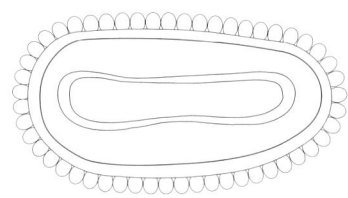

Keith Dumbell, Department of Medical Microbiology, University of Cape Town Medical School, Cape, South Africa

Geoffrey L Smith, Sir William Dunn School of Pathology, University of Oxford, Oxford, UK

Copyright © 1999 Academic Press

Smallpox (Variola) Virus

History

A Chinese account of a disease which was clearly smallpox was written in the 4th century. Over the next two centuries reliable accounts described smallpox in Japan, Korea, India and Egypt. Shortly after this, the Islamic expansion carried smallpox into North Africa and Europe. From the 15th century smallpox was taken to America and southern Africa with the spread of European colonists. According to the Chinese account, smallpox had appeared in China during the first century, but it may have been current in India well before that. A few Egyptian mummies show evidence of a pustular rash which has some resemblance to smallpox, but there are no accounts of such a disease in contemporary Egyptian or Jewish writings.

Taxonomy and classification

Variola (smallpox) viruses belong to the *Orthopoxvirus* genus of the *Chordopoxvirinae* subfamily of DNA viruses in the *Poxviridae* family and have linear, double-stranded DNA genomes of 186 kb. The virions are large (about 250 × 200 nm), brick-shaped particles. Like vaccinia they can be seen as mature, intracellular virions or as enveloped, extracellular virions. When viewed by electron microscopy after dehydration and embedding in Epon, the particles have two lateral bodies and a central core, but the lateral bodies are not evident when orthopoxviruses are observed by cryoelectron microscopy.

Variola virus has a close antigenic relationship to other orthopoxviruses; it is distinguished as a species by its biological characters and by the characterization of its DNA genome.

Virion structure and properties

What is known about the structure, physical properties and replication of variola virus conforms so closely to the much better studied vaccinia that the reader is referred to that entry. One point of difference is that the variola genome has only a short inverted terminal repeat sequence (ITR) of 725 bp, unlike the 10 kb ITR of vaccinia virus.

Geographic and seasonal distribution

The last natural case of smallpox occurred in 1977; and in 1980 the World Health Organization (WHO) declared that the disease had been eradicated. In its heyday smallpox had a worldwide distribution. The development of effective public health services and the routine practice of vaccination gradually eliminated the disease from North America and most of Europe, but outbreaks, apparently endemic in origin, continued in these parts of the world through the first decades of the 20th century. For a variety of reasons, routine vaccination failed to eradicate smallpox from many tropical and subtropical areas. At the start of the global eradication campaign in 1967 there were still 31 countries in which the disease was endemic.

After smallpox eradication was complete, the number of laboratories maintaining stocks of variola virus was rapidly reduced. At present (1998), variola virus is maintained in just two high-containment laboratories situated in Atlanta, USA and in Novosibirsk, Russia. The WHO is coordinating a program to obtain DNA sequences from representative strains of variola. It is intended that these sequence data shall become the permanent record of this virus and all remaining stocks of the virus shall be destroyed before the end of the 20th century.

Smallpox was maintained entirely by transmission from an active case to another human; latency did not occur. Consequently, active search would reveal cases throughout the year in countries where the disease was endemic. Nevertheless, there were low seasons and high seasons. In tropical areas it seems likely that the seasonal changes in incidence were achieved more through the ease or difficulty of traveling about than from direct effects of climate on survival of virus or susceptibility to it.

Host range and virus propagation

Variola virus had a narrow host range and natural infection was confined to humans. The virus was propagated in laboratories on the chick chorioallantois or in cell cultures, usually of human origin. There was no experimental animal model in which inoculation of variola virus produced clinical disease resembling smallpox and in which the pathology could have been studied. The virus produced a mild disease in some species of monkeys and could be propagated, at least for a time, in baby mice and in rabbits.

Genetics

DNA restriction maps of variola from different geographic areas were remarkably uniform and showed little, if any, variation in viruses from different countries. Consistent differences were found between variola major strains and alastrim strains from South America, but this did not apply to strains of variola minor from Africa. The complete DNA sequence of variola virus strains Bangladesh-1975 and India-1967 and the partial sequences of Harvey-1947, Congo-1970, Somalia-1977 and Garcia-1966 have been determined and are deposited in DNA data banks. There are several instances of some of the individuality of variola virus, but there is at present no evidence that variola encodes any gene which has no counterpart in the genome of another poxvirus.

Comparisons of the entire sequence of a variola virus with that of vaccinia virus has revealed that the central two-thirds of the genomes are highly conserved, with >95% nucleotide identity, but towards the termini the sequences diverge and there are sequences unique to either virus. There are several instances of highly related coding sequences being intact in one virus and truncated or fragmented in the other. Surprisingly, in the majority of cases where coding sequences are disrupted, the sequence is intact in vaccinia and broken in variola. Some open reading frames that at first appeared to be unique to variola have been found to be present in other orthopoxviruses. At present it would appear that the virulence of variola virus for humans probably resided in the combination and variation of multiple genes present in several poxviruses, rather then a 'key' unique virulence gene.

Variola viruses readily recombine with other orthopoxviruses: some of the resulting recombinants were characterized biologically, but work with variola virus ceased before these results were correlated with the exchange of particular segments of the parental genomes.

Evolution

The naturally occurring orthopoxviruses: cowpox, monkeypox and camelpox, currently occupy separate geographic and biologic niches in Europe, Africa and the Middle East. The similarities between the genomes of these three viruses, variola and vaccinia are sufficient to imply a common ancestor. Furthermore, there is evidence that several orthopoxvirus genes, for instance those encoding enzymes for virus transcription and DNA replication, have counterparts in other genera of poxviruses, such as leporipox, capripox, avipox and suipox, molluscipox and yatapox. Two orthopoxviruses that have been identified in America, volepox and raccoonpox, are less closely related to other orthopoxviruses.

Camelpox seems to be most closely related to variola, in biological properties, in some features of the genome, and in its natural infection of only a single species. There is, however, no firm evidence that camelpox virus can infect humans, despite much contact between camels and unvaccinated humans. It is possible that both camelpox and variola viruses having found a single species present in numbers adequate to maintain their survival, have lost the presumed primitive ability of orthopoxviruses to utilize a variety of host species – an ability which has been retained for the survival of cowpox and monkeypox.

Serologic relationships and variability

There was never any evidence for antigenic variability in variola viruses. Indeed it was even difficult to separate variola from other orthopoxviruses by serologic tests. Any strain of vaccinia would protect against variola in any part of the world and in different years. In accord with this, the proteins of the envelope of extracellular virions are highly conserved between vaccinia and variola. Several different antigens of variola virus find their way to the surface of the infected cell before virus release. Because of this and also the length of the incubation period, it is unlikely that minor variation in any particular antigen would confer sufficient advantage to be preferentially selected.

Epidemiology and transmission

The vast majority of smallpox was contracted by direct contact with an infected person. There were rare instances of indirect spread via fomites but animals played no part in sustaining or transmitting the variola virus.

Despite occasional startling incidents, smallpox required close contact for effective transmission and spread mainly within households or to other close contacts.

Those infected with smallpox remained well for the 10–12 days of the incubation period and, during this time, were not infectious to others. In natural smallpox (as opposed to variolation) virus was transmitted by droplet infection. The most usual source was the lesions that occurred in the pharynx or mouth (the enanthem). These ulcerated more quickly than the lesions developing in the skin (the exanthem) and were well situated for distribution to close contacts. Primary lesions were presumed to occur in the respiratory tract but were never seen or demonstrated post mortem. Throat swabs from contacts who subsequently developed smallpox were occasionally found to harbor virus during the incubation period, but there was no evidence that transmission occurred before the end of the incubation period. Nor did those who were subclinically infected pass on the disease.

Cases were potentially infectious until all the lesions had completely healed but virus was not so readily dispersed from dried exudate or scabs. There was no evidence of latency and no spontaneous recurrence. Consequently, once an outbreak had run its course or been controlled in a local community, smallpox would not recur unless reintroduced from outside that community.

Outbreaks varied in severity, but even in a severe outbreak there would be some milder cases. At times whole outbreaks of mild smallpox occurred with little or no fatality. This led to the distinction of two varieties of the disease, variola major and variola minor, and to the presumption that the variola minor outbreaks were caused by a distinct strain of variola virus of lower virulence. In some areas the minor form became established as the endemic strain. The variety of variola minor known as alastrim apparently arose towards the end of the 19th century and produced consistently mild disease. This strain was first described in southeast USA and thence spread through North America, to Europe, to South America and to Australasia. Outbreaks of minor smallpox were still occurring in Europe in the 1950s and in Brazil through the 1960s. Isolates from outbreaks of alastrim in Europe and Brazil shared biologic characters and a DNA restriction pattern which distinguished them from variola major viruses. The position in Africa was less well defined. Outbreaks of major and of minor smallpox continued to occur. Although the endemic variola in some African countries was clinically and epidemiologically variola minor in recent years, virus isolates from these cases could not be distinguished from isolates of variola major virus.

Clinical features

The incubation period of 10–12 days was terminated by the abrupt onset of fever and prostration, often with nausea or vomiting. On the 3rd day of illness a macular rash appeared; this became papular and then vesicular and eventually pustular. The rash tended to be more concentrated on the head and limbs than on the trunk. The lesions were firm and raised but also based deeply in the skin. Scabs formed as the ulcerated pustules dried and gradually separated over 2–3 weeks, leaving depigmented areas. Residual facial scarring, due to destruction of sebaceous glands, was a characteristic feature of the survivors of major smallpox. Blindness was another, not uncommon, sequel. The above description applies to classical cases of major smallpox, in which the fatality rate was 16–30%. Prognosis was worse if the rash was slower in development, with the lesions remaining flat and soft or becoming hemorrhagic. Sometimes the initial prostration was severe, generalized hemorrhagic manifestations appeared on the second or third day and no distinctive rash developed. These patients invariably died, usually between the 5th and 7th day of illness. A more favorable prognosis was signified if the rash evolved more quickly and the lesions were more superficial. This was the usual course of events in people who had been vaccinated, but not recently enough to give complete protection.

When the causative virus was variola minor, prostration was notably less than in patients who had a comparable extent of rash following infection with variola major virus.

Pathology and histopathology

The majority of smallpox lesions were in the skin and mucous membranes of the mouth and oropharynx. The small number of postmortem studies that were done showed few specific lesions in internal organs, except in cases of hemorrhagic smallpox. In the absence of obvious damage in the vital organs it was presumed that death had been due to the profound toxemia. Fuller accounts will be found in the texts cited at the end of this entry.

Immune response

Antibody that neutralized intracellular virus and hemagglutination inhibiting (HI) antibody appeared by about the 6th day of the disease, corresponding to the 18th day after infection. This is slower than the antibody response to primary vaccination and may explain partly why vaccination soon after contact with smallpox often ameliorated the outcome. However, experience with the complications of vaccination showed that a failure to develop cell-mediated immunity was more important than failure to develop antibody. It is presumed that cell-mediated immunity also controlled the development and resolution of smallpox lesions, but this was not adequately investigated.

Recovery left a lasting immunity; although second attacks of smallpox were not unknown. Neutralizing antibody persisted for many years; HI antibody was demonstrable for some months to a few years.

Prevention and control

Successful vaccination gave complete protection against smallpox for at least 3 years and probably 5 or more. Immunity waned after longer intervals, but rarely, if ever, did anyone who had been vaccinated contract fatal smallpox. The International Certificate of vaccination against smallpox was given a validity of 3 years, but those at high risk were normally revaccinated at yearly intervals.

Compulsory routine vaccination should, theoretically, have eradicated smallpox in any area where it was practiced. However, in many countries where the disease was endemic, the fraction of the population that escaped the vaccination program sufficed to maintain a chain of active cases and a reservoir of the virus.

The main factors in containing an outbreak of smallpox were the isolation of cases and the tracing of contacts before the end of their incubation period. These measures were supplemented with vaccination or revaccination in the locality of the outbreak, and were effective in the control and elimination of smallpox introduced into a nonendemic area. The eradication of smallpox from endemic areas was achieved by detecting current outbreaks and containing them. This strategy effectively interrupted the local transmission of the virus and progressively reduced the number of chains of transmission which remained.

Future perspectives

In 1980 the World Health Organization certified officially the eradication of smallpox, and no further cases have come to light in the 18 years that have elapsed since then. This major achievement seems to be firmly established. The only remaining viable variola viruses are the two reference collections of variola strains held in high containment laboratories at Atlanta and Novosibirsk and the possibility that virus might have survived in the bodies of any smallpox victims who were mummified or buried in permafrost conditions. Extrapolation from the known rates of decay of variola virus in smallpox scabs indicates that this possibility is unrealistic.

It has been agreed that the two collections of variola virus strains should be destroyed before the end of the twentieth century. The archival record of variola virus will then be the complete DNA sequence of a small number of representative strains and some fragments of variola DNA which have been cloned into recombinant plasmids. Of course much of the gene pool of variola virus will still remain, in the genomes of other, closely related orthopoxviruses. When the genomes of further orthopoxviruses have been sequenced it will be possible to determine what features of the variola genome were unique to that virus. The section on monkeypox includes a discussion of whether variola virus could emerge again from natural sources.

Monkeypox Virus

History

Monkeypox virus was first described as the cause of an apparently spontaneous outbreak of fever and rash in a colony of cynomolgus monkeys held at the State Serum Institute in Copenhagen in 1958. During the next few years similar outbreaks were reported in monkey colonies in the USA. In 1966 monkeypox infection was introduced into the zoo at Rotterdam. Here the first animals affected were giant anteaters from South America, but the disease spread to various species of apes and monkeys. The viruses isolated from these animals were found to be similar and to represent a species of orthopoxvirus that had not been described before 1958. In two separate incidents in 1970 monkeypox virus was found to have caused a smallpox-like illness in humans in the Democratic Republic of the Congo (formerly Zaire) and in Liberia. Sporadic cases have continued to occur in the African rain forest belt, particularly in the Democratic Republic of the Congo. The virology and epidemiology of monkeypox have been intensively investigated because of the possible threat to the success of smallpox eradication.

Taxonomy and classification

Monkeypox virus is a separate species of the *Orthopoxvirus* genus. Biologically it can be differentiated from other species by the morphology and ceiling temperature of its pocks on the chick chorioallantois and by its pathogenicity to rabbits. Antigenically it crossreacts extensively with other orthopoxviruses but produces a few specific antigens which can be detected with suitably absorbed antisera or monoclonal antibodies. The genome, of approximately 190 kb, has a distinctive restriction map, and DNA sequence data are available for parts of the genome.

Virion properties and replication

There is no reason to believe that replication of monkeypox virus differs significantly from the more extensively studied vaccinia virus.

Geographic and seasonal distribution

The reservoir of monkeypox virus is confined to the tropical rain forest belt of Africa. On current information the reservoir hosts are arboreal rodents, from which sporadic transmissions occur to simians and to humans. Human infections are rare events: most of the reported cases have been in the Democratic Republic of the Congo, which harbors more than half of the present African rain forest. There is no marked seasonal incidence, but some correlation with times of maximum agricultural activity (see Epidemiology).

Partial DNA sequence studies of American and European isolates show identity with isolates from West Africa, thus confirming the presumption that the outbreaks in Europe and America were initiated by subclinical infection in monkeys or other animals exported from West Africa. There have been no outbreaks outside Africa since 1968, following a general tightening of regulations concerning exports of animals. DNA sequence data confirm that the outbreaks in Europe and America were caused by a monkeypox virus originating from West Africa rather than Central Africa.

Host range and virus propagation

Under experimental conditions monkeypox virus is capable of infecting most common laboratory animals and many simian species. The resulting disease is usually mild in African monkeys but Asian and South American monkeys suffer moderate to severe disease. Apes, with the exception of chimpanzees, are seriously affected and the wide range of susceptible exotic animals is illustrated by the two South American giant anteaters which became infected while in transit to the Rotterdam Zoo.

In its natural habitat, monkeypox virus has been recovered from many sporadically infected humans and from one sick squirrel (*Funisciurus anerythrus*) and a chimpanzee. Other information comes from serologic surveys; antibody specific to monkeypox has been detected in a significant proportion of squirrels belonging to the genera *Funisciurus* and *Helioscirus*. Specific antibody was also detected in seven species of cercopithecus, and also in cercocebus and colobus monkeys. Monkeypox virus was propagated in laboratories on the chick chorioallantois, where it produced characteristic small pocks with a central hemorrhage. Cell cultures of many different species were susceptible.

Genetics

*Hin*dIII restriction maps of the monkeypox virus genome confirm the conservation of the central part of the orthopoxvirus genome throughout the genus. Although restriction site maps show more variation in the outer quarters of the genome, DNA fragments from these regions crosshybridize strongly with corresponding fragments of other orthopoxviruses and rule out any long region of sequence that could be unique to monkeypox. There must be short unique stretches to account for the monkeypox-specific antigens that have been demonstrated, but few studies of DNA sequence in monkeypox have yet been reported. There is some variation in restriction site maps of monkeypox isolates from different geographical areas but variants with more dramatic changes in genome structure can readily be isolated in the laboratory. These are the 'white pock' mutants, which also have been described among other orthopoxviruses with a hemorrhagic pock phenotype, such as cowpox.

Evolution

Monkeypox virus, like cowpox virus, appears to be sustained by transmission in small rodents. The present distributions of these viruses do not overlap but the antigenic and genetic similarities among all the orthopoxviruses are such that they must share a common ancestor. Each of these two viruses is known to infect a variety of species under natural conditions, including humans. This could have led to the possibility of further speciation. It has been suggested that monkeypox might be the progenitor of variola. This is ruled out because a gene sequence (ORF) which is present in variola (and vaccinia) has been shown to be degenerate and partially deleted in monkeypox DNA. Also it must be remembered that smallpox appeared in East Asia well before it was current in Africa (see the earlier section on variola virus).

Epidemiology and transmission

In the Democratic Republic of the Congo, sporadic cases of monkeypox infection have continued. Most cases occur in small rural villages in the rain forest belt. The age-specific incidence of primary monkeypox (i.e. excluding spread from person to person) is highest in young children between 1 and 8 years, peaking in the 3–4 year age group. Young children have access to the cleared areas between the village and the forest; in this area also are found squirrels of the genera *Funisciurus* and *Heliosciurus* in which monkeypox antibody is prevalent. The age-specific incidence of secondary cases is more evenly distributed. Most outbreaks are believed to be limited to the primary (and sometimes coprimary) cases. Chains of presumed human-to-human transmission have so far been limited but there is concern that the virus may adapt to become more transmissible in humans. Ongoing surveillance is required. Variation in the reported incidence from area to area and from year to year may well depend on natural fluctuations in the wildlife reservoir but will also be affected by the efficiency of surveillance activities. Transmission from person to person is probably from the enanthem via the respiratory route, but the secondary attack rate among unvaccinated household contacts is much lower than that found in smallpox. Based on experience to date, the basic case reproduction rate does not exceed 1.0 and outbreaks would be self-limiting even in an unvaccinated community.

Clinical features

The incubation period of human monkeypox appears to be about 12 days, the same as for smallpox, but there have been only a few instances where it could be accurately determined. The clinical picture of human monkeypox closely follows that of ordinary smallpox. Most cases in unvaccinated children have been severe, but equivalents of the flat or hemorrhagic types of smallpox have not been encountered. The illness begins with fever, followed in 1–3 days by the rash, and an enanthem is usually present on the oral mucosa. Unlike smallpox, most patients develop a generalized lymphadenopathy or, less often, a regional lymphadenopathy. Mortality in the unvaccinated has been about 11%, though somewhat higher than this in children under 2 years of age. Nearly all deaths have been in children under the age of 9 years.

Pathology and histopathology

This has only been studied in experimental infection of monkeys. Histopathology of the lesions resembled that of smallpox. Following intramuscular inoculation, there was an intense local inflammatory response. Virus spread to the regional lymph nodes and thence to spleen, tonsil and bone marrow. Viremia occurred between the 3rd and 14th days and a generalized rash appeared about the 7th or 8th day.

Immune response

The antibody response to infection with monkeypox virus can conveniently be detected by hemagglutination inhibition or by ELISA tests. High titers in straight antibody tests suggest a response to monkeypox rather than to vaccination, but a residual titer after absorption with vaccinia virus is required to demonstrate antibody specific to monkeypox. For this reason radioimmunoassay tests have been most useful because of the high titers obtainable from unabsorbed sera by this technique. More specific tests are in course of development.

Prevention and control

Recent vaccination with vaccinia virus effectively protects against monkeypox, and those who had been vaccinated some years previously were susceptible but were less likely to develop severe illness. Widespread routine vaccination would be necessary to protect all who might come into contact with monkeypox; but the incidence of monkeypox is so low that complications arising from the vaccination program might rival the morbidity to be expected from monkeypox itself.

Future perspectives

The main incidence of monkeypox in humans has been in young children. Although this age group is currently unprotected by vaccination, there has not been any evidence of a rising incidence of monkeypox infections. Until recently monkeypox has not presented a public health problem serious enough to require specific action. Significantly more cases of monkeypox have been reported recently, including longer chains of transmission than had previously been recorded. The situation is being closely monitored and recent isolates of the virus will be rigorously compared to see if significant changes have occurred. At this stage it is hard to forecast future developments.

See also: **Cowpox virus (*Poxviridae*); Immune response: Cell mediated immune response, General features; Vaccines and immune response; Vaccinia virus (*Poxviridae*).**

Further Reading

Fenner F, Henderson DA, Arita I, Jezek Z and Ladnyi ID (1988) *Smallpox and its Eradication*. Geneva: World Health Organization.

Fenner F, Wittek R and Dumbell KR (1989) *The Orthopoxviruses*. New York: Academic Press.

Jezek Z and Fenner F (1988) Human monkeypox. *Monogr. Virol.* 17.

SOBEMOVIRUSES

OP Sehgal, University of Missouri, Columbia, Missouri, USA

Copyright © 1999 Academic Press

History

Southern bean mosaic virus (SBMV) is the archetype of the plant virus genus *Sobemovirus* in the family *Tetraviridae*. SBMV was the subject of intensive biological and physicochemical investigations during the 1940s and was the only virus, other than tobacco mosaic and tomato bushy stunt viruses, that had been well characterized at this early period. In the 1970s through the mid 1980s, SBMV served as a prototype on the applicability of small angle x-ray diffraction and neutron scattering in deciphering virion organization. During the same period, studies with SBMV and turnip rosette virus (TRoSV), yielded vital information on the nature of macromolecular forces that govern virion stability.

Taxonomy and Classification

The International Committee on Taxonomy of Viruses recently established the genus *Sobemovirus* in the family *Tetraviridae* (1995). At present, a number of viruses including SBMV and TRoSV are recognized as members of the sobemovirus genus. These are: blueberry shoe string virus (BSSV), cocksfoot mottle virus (CfMV), lucerne transient streak virus (LTSV), rice yellow mottle virus (RYMV), Rottboellia yellow mottle virus (RoYMV), *Solanum nodiflorum* mottle virus (SNMV), sowbane mosaic virus (SoMV), subterranean clover mottle virus (SCMoV) and velvet tobacco mottle virus (VTMoV). Additionally, seven viruses may be considered as probable members pending availability of additional

Table 1 Geographical distribution, natural hosts and insect vectors of sobemoviruses

Virus	Geographical distribution	Natural hosts	Vectors
SBMV	USA, Central and South America, Africa, Asia	Bean, cowpea	Beetles
BSSV	USA, Canada	*Vaccinium corymbosum, V. angustifolium*	Aphids
CfMV	Europe, New Zealand	Cocksfoot, wheat	Beetles
LTSV	Australia, New Zealand, Canada	*Medicago sativa* (lucerne)	Beetles
RYMV	Tropical Africa	*Oryza sativa* (rice)	Beetles
RoYMV	Nigeria	Itchgrass	Unknown
SNMV	Australia	*Solanum nodiflorum, S. nigrum, S. nitidibaccatum*	Mirid, beetles
SoMV	World-wide	*Chenopodium* spp., apple, grapes, *Atriplex suberecta*	Leafminers, aphids
SCMoV	Australia	Subterranean clover, club clover	Beetles
TRoSV	UK	Turnip, swede	Beetles
VTMoV	Australia	*Nicotiana velutina*	Mirid, beetles
Tentative members			
CYMV	Colombia	*Calopogonium mucunoides* (calopo)	Beetles
CMMV	Europe	Cocksfoot	Aphids
CyMV	Europe, New Zealand	*Cynosurus cristatus*	Aphids
GCFV	Asia, Australia, New Zealand	Ginger	Unknown
PMV	USA, Mexico, Africa	Several grasses	Beetles
RgMV	Japan	*Dactylis glomerata, Lolium multiflorum,*	Unknown
SsbMV	India	*Sesbania grandiflora*	Unknown

information on their properties. These are: calopo yellow mosaic virus (CYMV), cocksfoot mild mosaic virus (CMMV), cynosurus mottle virus (CyMV), ginger fleck virus (GCFV), panicum mosaic virus (PMV), ryegrass mottle virus (RgMV), and sesbania mosaic virus (SsbMV). Olive latent virus 1, a putative sobemovirus, resembles *Necrovirus* species in its genomic organization and expression and should be included in the genus *Necrovirus*. Other tentative virus species are in the genus.

Geographical Distribution, Natural Hosts and Vectors

Most sobemoviruses have somewhat limited distribution, but as a group, they are found throughout the world (**Table 1**). Individual members have few natural hosts but, as a whole, they infect a wide spectrum of plant species. Eight sobemoviruses affect dicotyledonous species, and an equal number affect monocotyledonous species, but none are transmitted to both. Leaf-eating beetles are their most common vectors.

Properties of the Virion

Sobemovirus virions are isometric with a diameter of *ca.* 25–30 nm (**Fig. 1**). Most virions exclude negative stains from penetrating to the core, a reflection of a highly compact capsid organization. SBMV virions exhibit no structural changes even when inactivated (>99%) by exposure to ultraviolet light, heating, freezing and thawing or nitrous acid. However, EDTA treatment, which removes capsid-associated divalent cations, results in virion 'swelling', and such virions are then rendered permeable to negative stains.

Sobemovirions are nonenveloped, and contain *ca.* 21% RNA and 79% protein. SBMV, LTSV and TRoSV virions contain significant amounts of intimately bound divalent cations (calcium, magnesium). The virions sediment sharply as single components in sucrose gradients, with $s_{20,w}$ values ranging from 109S (PMV) to 120S (BSSV). A characteristic feature of most sobemovirions is that they band homogeneously in cesium chloride (densities ranging from 1.34 to 1.39 g ml^{-1}) but heterogeneously in cesium sulfate gradients. The banding heterogeneity in cesium

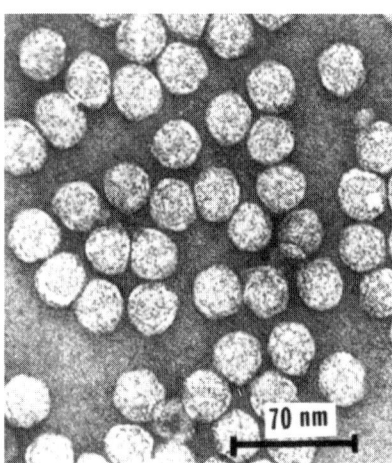

Figure 1 Purified virions of southern bean mosaic virus, bean strain. Uranyl formate was used as the negative stain.

sulfate gradients is a reflection of conformational variations among virions in a population rather than any differences in their chemical composition.

Capsid Organization and Stabilizing Interactions

The sobemovirus capsid is constructed from a protein of about 30 kDa. A proportion of coat protein subunits in SBMV and TRoSV virions exist as stable dimers that are preferentially linked to RNA. The basic SBMV capsid structure is $T = 3$ quasi-symmetry of 180 subunits. High resolution x-ray diffraction has revealed three types of quasi-equivalent subunits, namely A, B and C, which are chemically identical but have different conformations. The A subunits cluster at the fivefold axes, whereas sets of B and C aggregate at the quasi-sixfold vertices. Each subunit consists of a random domain, i.e. the N-terminal 'arm' located towards the virion interior, and the surface domain, which is organized into an eight-stranded antiparallel β barrel and five α helices. Considerable similarity exists between the organization of SBMV capsid with those of tomato bushy stunt, tobacco necrosis, poliovirus type 1 and human rhinoviruses. Sobemovirus virions are extremely stable in vitro in their native state. For SBMV and TRoSV, this stability is derived from strong inter-subunit linkages mediated by hydrophobic interactions, divalent cations and pH-dependent bonds. Additionally, protein–RNA linkages contribute to virion stability. Perturbations in the pH-dependent and divalent cation-mediated bonds cause the capsid to relax, rendering it sensitive to proteases, salt or detergents. Only LTSV and CyMV among the sobemoviruses, are sensitive to detergent in their native states.

Properties of the Genome

Sobemovirus genomes are linear, single-stranded RNAs of positive polarities and range in mol. wt from ca. 1.3×10^6 to 1.5×10^6. The complete sequences of genomic RNAs of SBMV bean strain (4109 nucleotides (nt)), SBMV cowpea strain (4194 nt), RYMV (4450 nt), CfMV (4038 nt) and LTSV (4275 nt) have been determined. A covalently linked protein (VpG) is present at the 5′ terminus in all of these RNAs; VpG is necessary for the infectivity of SBMV, RYMV and LTSV RNAs. The 5′ end sequence motifs for SBMV and LTSV are ACAAA; for RYMV it is ACAA; whereas for CfMV it is AUAAU. Furthermore, SBMV, LTSV and RYMV genomes contain a polypurine sequence, AG(G)AAA, about 8–10 nt downstream from the ACAA(A) element; for CfMV, the comparable sequence is AGAAAGA. The 3′ ends of sobemoviral genomes lack poly(A) tails and, unlike many other plant viral genomes, are not configured into tRNA like structures.

Encapsidated Subgenomic and Satellite RNAs

Virions of SBMV, GCFV, LTSV, SNMV, SCMoV, TRoSV, VTMoV and CMMV encapsidate minor amounts of heterogeneous subgenomic (sg) or putative sgRNAs. VTMoV virions contain two discrete sgRNAs, RNA-1a (0.63×10^6 Da) and RNA-1b (0.25×10^6 Da), besides the genomic RNA (**Fig. 2**). CfMV virions encapsidate a discrete 0.5×10^6 Da RNA and several intermediate-sized putative sgRNAs. Included among the heterogeneous population of SBMV and TRoSV sgRNAs are the autonomized coat protein cistrons. The sgRNAs of SBMV, RYMV and LTSV possess VpG at their 5′ ends followed by the same sequence motifs as their respective genomic RNAs. LTSV, RYMV, SCMoV, SNMV and VTMoV virions encapsidate discrete, viroid-like satellite (sat) RNAs, in addition to the genomic and subgenomic RNAs. These satRNAs exist in linear and circular forms (**Fig. 2**). Complete sequences are known for satRNAs of LTSV (322 nt), RYMV (220 nt), SCMoV (322 nt and 380 nt), SNMV (377 nt) and VTMoV (366 nt). The satRNAs of SNMV and VTMoV exhibit a high degree of sequence homology and are different from those of SCMoV or LTSV. At 220 nt, RYMV satRNA represents the smallest known, naturally occurring viroid-like RNA. A region comprising 19% of the sequence of RYMV satRNA shows about 93% homology to the

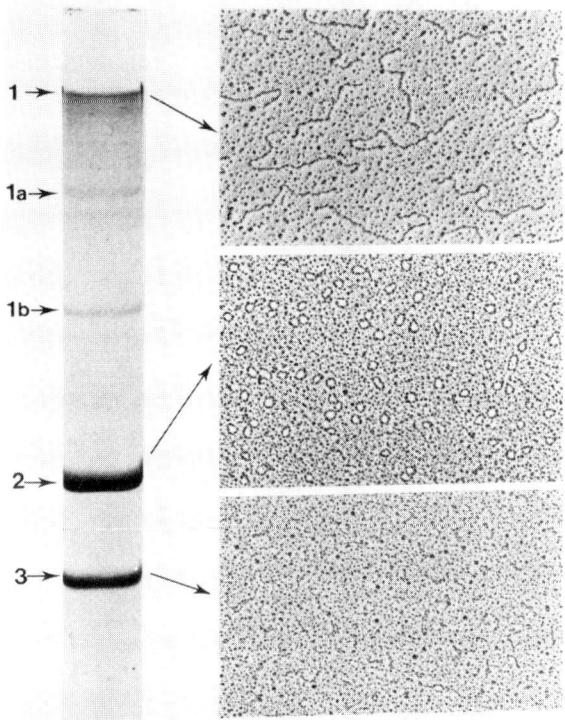

Figure 2 Polyacrylamide gel electrophoresis and electron microscopy of the virion RNAs of velvet tobacco mottle sobemovirus. (Reproduced with permission from Velvet Tobacco Mottle Virus, *AAB Descriptions of Plant Viruses* no. 317, 1986; courtesy of Dr J. W. Randles.)

satRNA of a Canadian LTSV isolate. The sobemoviral satRNAs contain a conserved hammerhead structure which is involved in self-cleavage (ribozyme).

Transmission

Sobemoviruses are transmitted readily with sap inoculation, a reflection of their high endogenous concentration and particle stability. Transmission via contact with leaf abrasion during strong wind is possible, but actual proof is lacking. RYMV exuded with guttation fluid may contaminate irrigation water, which then serves as the inoculum source. Some sobemoviruses, SBMV, SCMoV, SoMV and PMV, are transmitted through the seed.

Insects are the principal vectors of sobemoviruses. SBMV, CfMV, CYMV, PMV, RYMV and TRoSV are transmitted by chrysomelid beetles, whereas SNMV and VToMV are transmitted by coccinellid beetles; SBMV is transmitted also by a coccinellid beetle. The mirid bug, *Cyrtopeltis nicotianae*, is the vector of SNMV and VToMV. Aphids have been implicated in the transmission of BSSV, CMMV and CyMV. SoMV is transmitted by the leafminer fly, *Liriomyza langei*; it is carried mechanically on mouth parts and the ovipositor.

SBMV is acquired by the chrysomelid beetle, *Ceratoma trifurcata*, within a few minutes after feeding and transmitted without a latent period. Virions are present in fairly high concentration in the regurgitant fluid, intestines and hemolymph, but there is no evidence of SBMV multiplication in the vector. The virus persists in beetles for about 5–7 days. It is transmitted through contaminated mouth parts, during regurgitation and with reflexive bleeding. The coccinellid beetle, *Epilachna varivestis*, is an efficient SBMV vector, but the virus is not found in the hemocoel. Obviously, systemic transport within the beetle's body is not a prerequisite for SBMV transmission. CfMV is transmitted by a cereal leaf beetle, *Lema melanopa*. It is excreted in the fecal matter and can cause infection if deposited at freshly damaged feeding sites.

Experimental Host Range and Symptomatology

Most sobemoviruses have restricted host ranges and infect only a few species in one or two plant families. For example, RoYMV infects itchgrass (*Rottboellia cochinchinensis*) and corn (*Zea mays*) in the family Gramineae. The host ranges of SBMV, SCMoV and CYMV are restricted to a few species in the family Leguminosae; CfMV is restricted to the family Gramineae, whereas VToMV is confined to the family Solanaceae. SNMV, LTSV and TRoSV infect a few species in 3–4 different families. Additionally, most sobemoviruses have few hosts in common. For example, of the eight sobemoviruses that affect Gramineae, only PMV and RoYMV are transmitted to corn.

Symptoms induced by sobemoviruses are persistent mosaic, mottle or chlorosis, often accompanied by leaf deformities and stunted plant growth. CYMV produces a striking yellow variegation of leaves. BSSV causes shoestring symptoms in which the leaves are transformed into curled, strap-like structures; additionally, flowers show 'breaking', and immature berries exhibit reddish streaking or vein-banding patterns.

The Infection Process

Sobemoviruses enter through wounds caused by mechanical abrasion or insect feeding and, like other plant viruses, usually establish infection in the directly invaded cells. However, SBMV virions introduced by *E. varivestis* at the feeding site move out rapidly via

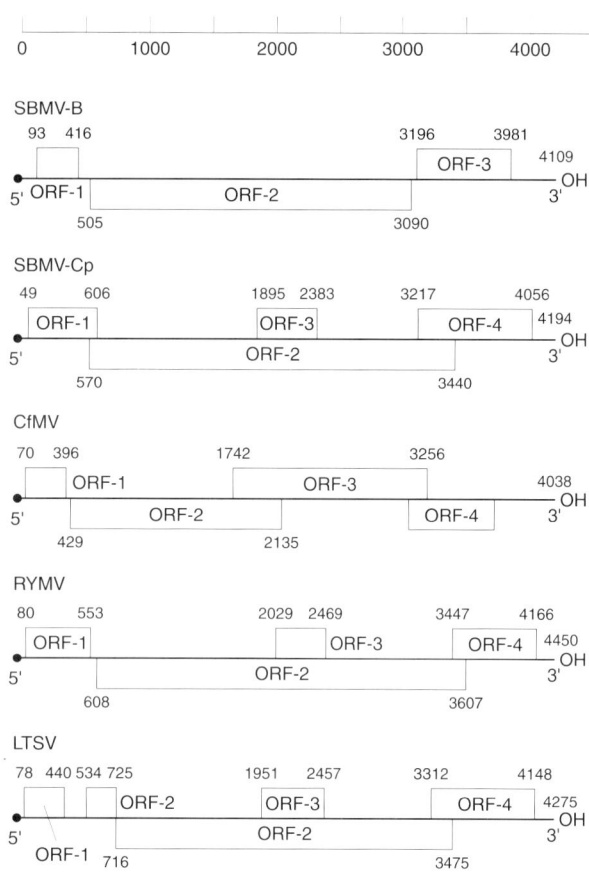

Figure 3 Organization of sobemovirus genomes. The viral RNA is represented by the thick line, and VpG is shown as the solid circle at the 5′ terminus. The open reading frames (ORFs) are shown as boxes.

leaf veins and cause infection in the unwounded cells. Apparently, SBMV virions can enter uninjured cells, although the precise mechanism is unknown. Upon entry into a cell, SBMV virions swell, extruding the 5′ terminus of RNA which is located near the capsid surface. A contact between the exposed RNA region and ribosomes leads to an early translational event, followed by complete capsid disassembly.

Isolated SBMV RNA must exist in a proper configuration to be infective. A marked structural stabilization of SBMV RNA *in situ* occurs when virions are heated, and this altered conformation is retained even when RNA is released from the capsid; this RNA is noninfectious. Upon structural destabilization, however, this RNA regains full infectivity. That SBMV RNA in a conformationally stabilized state is biologically inert, yet is rendered fully competent with denaturation, is a novel and unique phenomenon and underscores the importance of RNA secondary and tertiary structure in the infection process.

Replication and Expression of Virion RNAs

Although details are scanty, the replication mode of sobemoviral genomes appears to be typical of viruses that contain ssRNA of positive polarity, i.e. infection by plus strand RNA leads to the production of an intermediate double-stranded RNA complex from which progeny plus-strand RNAs are transcribed. The presence of genomic RNA replicating structures (approx. mol. wt 2.8×10^6) in SBMV and VTMoV infections have been detected in the cytoplasm where most of the virus-specific RNA polymerase activity is located.

Figure 3 is a schematic representation of the expression strategies of sobemoviral genomes. Each genome has three to four open reading frames (ORFs). The size of ORF 1 differs among these viruses and has a potential to encode a 12 kDa to 18 kDa protein; for LTSV ORF 1, two putative coding regions (ORF 1a and ORF 1b) have been identified. The nature or function of protein encoded by ORF 1 is not known, and little sequence similarity exists in this region among the sobemoviruses. ORF 2 encodes a polyprotein containing VpG, serine protease and polymerase domains. The CfMV polyprotein is encoded by two overlapping frames; ORF 2a codes for VpG and serine protease whereas ORF 2b codes for replicase which is expressed via a ribosomal frameshift event. The ORF 3 product has not been identified, and in SBMV-bean strain a comparable ORF is lacking. The viral coat proteins are encoded in ORF 3 of SBMV bean strain and ORF 4 of the other sobemoviruses; however, these coat proteins are expressed from sgRNAs. The transcription initiation sites for some of these sgRNAs have been tentatively identified and are: nt3241 for SBMV cowpea strain; nt3441 for RYMV and nt3285 for LTSV.

The relationship between sobemoviral coat proteins, based on alignment of their predicted amino acid sequences by clustal algorithm, is shown in **Fig. 4**. Among viruses infecting legumes, the SBMV bean and cowpea strains have coat proteins that are more

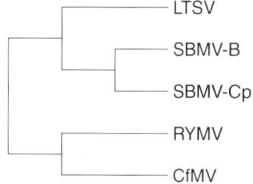

Figure 4 Relationship between coat proteins of sobemoviruses based on alignment by the clustal algorithm of their predicted amino acid sequences.

closely related to each other than to LTSV coat protein. Further, coat proteins of viruses affecting the Gramineae, RYMV and CfMV, appear more closely related between themselves than with the viruses that infect legumes. It will be of interest to ascertain if a similar relationship will hold true when sequence information for coat proteins of other sobemoviruses becomes available.

The replication of sobemoviral satRNAs, which proceeds via the rolling circle model proposed for viroids, is dependent on the presence of a suitable helper sobemovirus. The abilities of sobemoviruses to support satRNA replication, however, differs markedly. LTSV supports replication of satRNAs of SNMV and SCMoV, but SNMV does not support replication of VTMoV satRNA and vice versa. Also, LTSV satRNA replicates in the presence of an appropriate helper sobemovirus in divergent plant species. Thus, it replicates in *Brassica rapa*, *Raphanus raphanistrum* and *Sinapis arvense* (Brassicaceae) and *Chenopodium amaranticolor* (Chenopodiaceae) in the presence of TRoSV, and in *Triticum aestivum* (wheat) and *Dactylis glomerata* (Gramineae) in the presence of CfMV; all of these plants are nonhosts for LTSV. TRoSV fails to support LTSV satRNA replication in *Thlaspi arvense* or *Nicotiana bigelovii* although these plants are susceptible to TRoSV. Apparently, satRNA replication depends not only on the helper virus polymerase but also on some specific host factor(s).

Virion Assembly

The sequence of events leading to sobemoviral assembly *in vivo* is not understood. Under *in vitro* conditions, however, a few SBMV coat protein subunits (dimers?) bind with RNA, generating a complex which then serves to nucleate the capsid assembly. The coat protein amino-terminal arm appears to be the site with which RNA interacts first to generate this complex. Some evidence suggests that a stretch of 25 nucleotides (nt1410 to nt1436 in ORF 2) on the genomic RNA of SBMV cowpea strain is the coat protein recognition site; this region is highly conserved among sobemoviruses and configures into a stable hairpin structure. Since several subgenomic and satRNAs are encapsidated with great efficiency, these also must possess putative coat protein recognition site(s).

In Vivo Distribution and Cytopathology

Sobemoviruses are present in most plant parts including epidermis, mesophyll, meristem, xylem and phloem. Virions occur in cytoplasm and vacuoles,

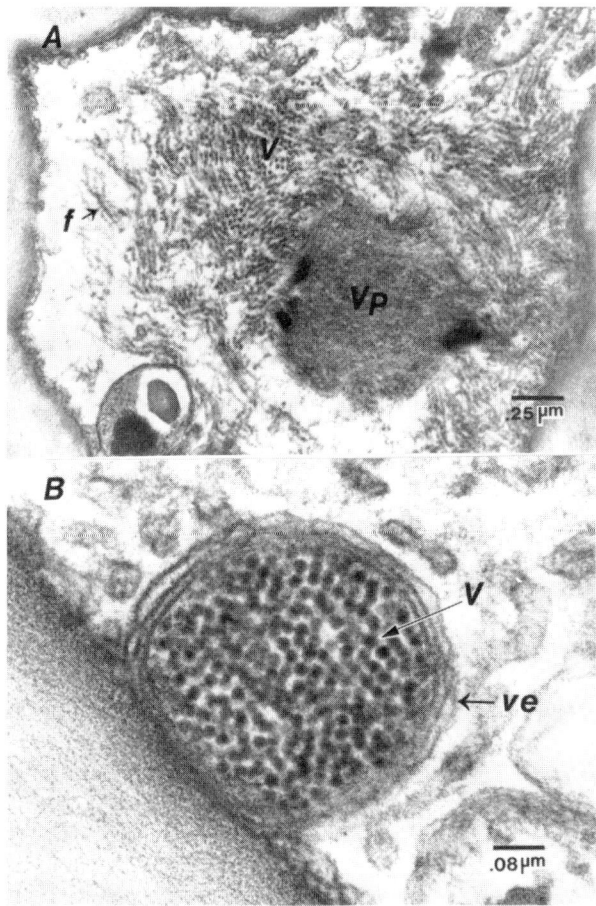

Figure 5 Foliar cells of *Calopogonium muconoides* infected with the calopo sobemovirus. (**A**) Virus-like particles, V, associated with viroplasm, V$_P$, and fibrils, f. (**B**) Virions, V, enclosed in a vesiculated structure, ve. (Reproduced with permission from Morales FJ (1995) A sobemovirus hindering utilization of *Calopogonium muconoides* as a forage legume in the lowland tropics. *Plant Dis.* 79: 1220.

and except for BSSV, RYMV and CyMV infections, also in the nuclei. They are not found, however, in the mitochondria and chloroplasts. The cytoplasm of infected cells may contain fibrillar material resembling double-stranded replicative form of RNA, which is either enclosed in discrete membranous vesicles or distributed in diffused patches. Sometimes, virions are enclosed in discrete vesiculated structures (**Fig. 5**). In other cases they are arranged in a crystalline array in cytoplasm and vacuole. Bundles of microtubules are seen in cells infected with BSSV, RYMV and SNMV, but their nature is not known.

Serology

Sobemoviruses are strongly immunogenic. In general, they are neither serologically crossreactive nor are they related to viruses belonging to other groups.

However, SNMV and VTMoV are serologically related and so are SBMV, SsbMBV and CYMV; SCMoV and LTSV are distantly related.

SBMV bean and cowpea strains are serologically similar but not identical. Likewise, RYMV isolates from Kenya and the Ivory Coast are dissimilar. Isolates of CfMV and CyMV from New Zealand, but not those from Europe, are serologically related. No serological variations have been observed among the naturally occurring isolates of TRoSV, GCFV, SoMV or LTSV.

Epidemiology and Control

SBMV and RYMV often reach epiphytotic proportions under field conditions. For SBMV, seed-borne inocula and weeds serve as the primary sources of infection. RYMV incidence is considerably higher in areas of continuous rice cultivation than those with interrupted plantings. This suggests that locally present RYMV inocula contribute largely to disease initiation. The beetle vectors move rapidly from plant to plant spreading RYMV. During the off-season, RYMV survives in volunteer and wild rice (*Oryza longistaminata*) plants, regrowths of harvested crops and in ratoons. Some sources of germplasm for resistance towards SBMV and RYMV are available. In view of the worldwide importance of rice and bean/cowpeas in the human diet, the applicability of gene engineering techniques for developing virus-resistant cultivars needs to be exploited.

Conclusions

The sobemoviruses constitute a homogeneous group based on their physicochemical parameters, including stability characteristics, and genomic expression strategies. These viruses possess relatively simple organizations, and their genomes are the smallest among the plant viruses. Furthermore, sobemoviruses represent a class of genetically stable viruses because few naturally occurring variants or strains have been identified. Also, the markedly divergent and non-overlapping host ranges underscore a high level of biological specificity and host plant adaptability of sobemoviruses.

Though the primary structures of the coat proteins of SBMV and tobacco necrosis virus are largely similar, there is only a limited resemblance in their polymerase sequences around the GDD motif. However, considerable similarities exist in the amino acid sequence motifs of the putative polymerase and nucleic acid helicase proteins between sobemoviruses and members of luteovirus subgroup II. Moreover, presence of the ACAAAA element at the 5' end of genomic and sgRNAs is a property which sobemoviruses share with members of the dianthovirus group and luteovirus subgroup II. LTSV, RYMV, SCMoV, SNMV and VTMoV can be distinguished from other sobemoviruses because they encapsidate satRNAs. That different sobemoviruses can support replication of a given satRNA is a reflection of the nonspecific nature of such an association. In this regard, LTSV satRNA seems most versatile because it interacts with a suitable helper virus in divergent dicotyledonous and monocotyledonous species. Likewise, LTSV, more than any other sobemovirus, is effective in supporting replication and encapsidation of sobemoviral satRNAs. It is rather interesting that satRNA of RYMV, a virus with host range restricted to the monocotyledons, exhibits structural homology with satRNA of LTSV which affects dicotyledonous species. Finally, RYMV satRNA, the smallest viroid-like RNA associated with a plant virus, possesses retroviroid and viroid-like structures making it a probable candidate as an evolutionary bridge between these classes of subviral plant pathogens. Thus, sobemoviral satRNAs offer attractive possibilities for indepth study of molecular interactions between two distinctive biological entities and on the nature and mode of origin of satRNAs associated with plant viruses.

See also: **Dianthoviruses (*Tombusviridae*); Luteovirus; Necroviruses (*Tombusviridae*); Plant virus disease – economic aspects; Vectors: Plant viruses; Virus structure: Principles of virus structure.**

Further Reading

Brunt A, Crabtree A and Gibbs A (1990) *Viruses of Tropical Plants*. Wallingford: CAB International.

Francki RIB, Milne RG and Hatta T (1985) Sobemovirus group. In: *Atlas of Plant Viruses*, vol 1. Boca Raton: CRC Press.

Hull, R (1988) The Sobemovirus group. In: Koenig R (ed.) *The Plant Viruses*, vol. 3, *Polyhedral virions with monopartite RNA genomes*. New York: Plenum.

Sehgal, OP (1995) Sobemoviruses. In: Singh RP, Singh US and Kohmoto K (eds) Pathogenesis and host specificity in plant diseases; histopathological, biochemical, genetic and molecular bases, vol. 3, *Viruses and Viroids*. Oxford: Pergamon.

SPO1 PHAGE (*MYOVIRIDAE*)

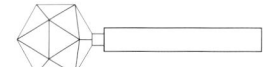

Charles R Stewart, Department of Biochemistry & Cell Biology, Rice University, Houston, Texas, USA

Copyright © 1999 Academic Press

History

SPO1 is a large virulent phage of the Gram-positive bacterium *Bacillus subtilis* and is in the genus 'SPO1-like viruses' of the *Myoviridae* family. Shunzo Okubo isolated it from soil in Osaka, Japan, during the early 1960s, and brought it with him to Chicago, where he collaborated with Bernard Strauss and Marvin Stodolsky on the first published studies of SPO1. Peter Geiduschek, Stodolsky's mentor, saw in SPO1 the opportunity to test the generality of the lessons then being learned about sequential gene action in the *Escherichia coli* phage T4, and began a series of experiments which illuminated the regulation of SPO1 gene action and stimulated the interest of many others.

Taxonomy and Evolution

SPO1 is a member of a family of *B. subtilis* phages, whose distinguishing feature is the presence of the unusual base, hydroxymethyluracil, instead of thymine in the DNA. All members of the family, which also includes SP82, Φe, 2C, SP8, H1 and SP5c, appear to be descended from a common ancestor, since they show many striking similarities in structure, restriction maps, genetic maps, gene products and gene regulation. However, they also show many differences in detail, and thus have had the opportunity for significant divergence. Perhaps the most striking similarity is the presence, in SPO1, SP82, 2C, and Φe, of a group I self-splicing intron, discovered by David Shub and his colleagues by testing RNAs from phage-infected cells for their capacity to incorporate labeled GTP. Each of these introns includes an open reading frame that specifies an endonuclease that catalyzes the substitution of its intron for the homologous intron in a related phage genome. The greater efficiency of the SP82 endonuclease, when acting on the SPO1 genome, permits SP82 DNA to exclude closely linked SPO1 alleles from the progeny of a mixed infection. These are among the very few introns known in procaryotes. The presence of introns both here and in T4 has been cited as an argument for the existence of introns in ancient evolutionary times, before the divergence of Gram-positive from Gram-negative bacteria. SPO1 is similar to T4 in many other ways as well, including size, structure, overall organization of the life cycle, and the presence of an unusual pyrimidine.

Virion Structure and Proteins

An SPO1 particle includes a single linear double-stranded DNA molecule and at least 53 different polypeptides, organized into an icosahedral head about 87 nm in diameter, a short neck, and a contractile tail of 19×140 nm, ending in a complex base plate 60 nm in diameter.

Genome Structure and Gene Function

The single DNA molecule is 145 kb long, with a 12.4 kb terminal redundancy, and with hydroxymethyluracil (hmUra) completely replacing thymine as the base-pairing partner for adenine. The presence of hmUra gives the DNA a CsCl buoyant density substantially higher than that of other DNAs of similar GC content, which has been useful in making experimental distinctions between phage and host DNAs. The two strands of the phage DNA are physically separable on CsCl, a characteristic that has been used extensively to identify the template strand for specific transcripts. Marmur and Greenspan used that property of SP8 to demonstrate for the first time that specific RNAs are complementary to one strand of the DNA from which they were transcribed.

Figure 1 shows a map of the SPO1 genome. Sixty-three genes have been identified by conditional lethal mutations and/or DNA sequencing, and have been mapped into a single linkage group that spans the entire genome. Conditional lethal mutations have permitted analysis of the functions of 40 of the known genes, showing that genes involved in the same function, such as DNA replication, tail formation, head formation, or virion assembly, tend to be clustered together on the map. The 35 genes that have been sequenced, 24 of which, being in the terminal redundancy, are present in two copies, occupy about 31 kb. The genes specifying the 53 known structural proteins are expected to occupy another 61 kb, on the basis of the molecular weight of the proteins, as estimated by gel electrophoresis. The remaining 53 kb may be estimated to include about 56 genes, assuming similar average size and density, for a total of about 144 genes.

Growth Cycle

Under optimal conditions, SPO1 has an eclipse period of 25–30 min, a latent period of 33–40 min, and a

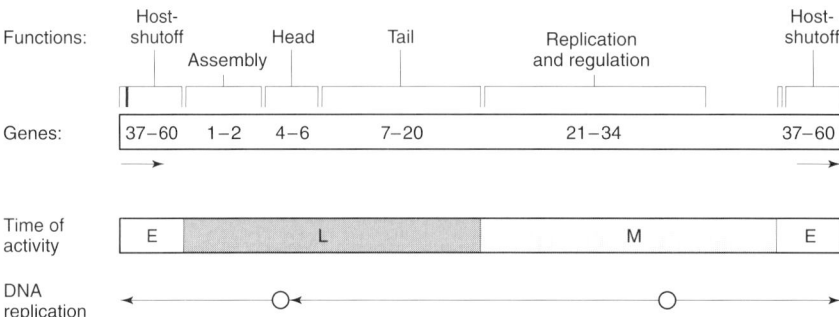

Figure 1 Maps of the SPO1 genome. The 'Genes' box shows the approximate map location of most of the known genes. The position of the terminal redundancy is shown by the arrows under the ends of that box. Genes 37–60, being located in the terminal redundancy, are indicated twice. Genes 35 and 36, located in the small portion of the terminal redundancy to the left of gene 37, are not shown. The clustering of genes according to function is indicated above the 'Genes' box. Most or all of the known genes in each region are believed to specify products involved in the function indicated. Genes for replication and regulation are interspersed among each other, and certain genes are required for both processes. Two genes required for assembly are located in different regions, gene 3 in the head region and gene 35 in the small box to the left of the host-shutoff region. As discussed in the text, the host-shutoff function of genes 37–60 has not been definitively established. Since most of the terminal redundancy has been sequenced, genes 37–60 make up a continuous cluster of known genes. In the rest of the genome, the known genes are interspersed among regions of unknown function, and no genes have been identified between gene 34 and the terminal redundancy. The 'Time of activity' box shows regions predominantly transcribed during early (E), middle (M) or late (L) times, as indicated by the unshaded, lightly shaded and heavily shaded areas, respectively. A minority of each type of transcript is also scattered among the other areas of the genome; for instance, gene 28 is transcribed at early times. The 'DNA replication' line shows the simplest pattern of replication consistent with the data. The two Os represent origins of replication, and the arrows show the directions of replication proceeding from each origin.

burst size of 100–300 phage. Into this brief period is packed a remarkably complex sequence of events. Immediately after infection, some of the SPO1 early genes are turned on, with the others following during the next few minutes. Shortly thereafter occurs the shutoff of host DNA replication and gene expression. By 5 or 6 min after infection, SPO1 middle genes begin turning on and some of the early genes are turned off. The middle genes specify most of the enzymes necessary for SPO1 DNA synthesis, which begins about 10 min after infection. Shortly thereafter, SPO1 late genes begin to function, directing the synthesis of structural proteins, and some of the early and middle genes are turned off. By 25 min after infection, the first infectious phage particles have formed, and lysis begins as early as 33 min, resulting in the destruction of the infected cells. The following sections describe each of these processes in detail.

Regulation of Gene Action

The transitions from early to middle to late gene activity are caused by a cascade of sigma factors. The major host RNA polymerase, with sigma factor A, transcribes from promoters whose -35 and -10 sequences approximate the consensus sequences TTGACA ... TATAAT. The promoters for the SPO1 early genes fit that consensus and thus are transcribed by the host polymerase. One of the early genes, gene 28, specifies another sigma factor, which substitutes for sigma A on the RNA polymerase, changing the specificity of the polymerase so it then recognizes the promoters of the middle genes, whose consensus sequence is AGGAGA ... TTTNTTT. Two of the middle genes, 33 and 34, specify proteins which cause the RNA polymerase to recognize the late gene promoters, with consensus sequence CGTTAGA ... GATATT. The sigma factor specified by gene 34 is essential for all late transcription, whereas the accessory protein specified by gene 33 is required for some, but not all, late transcription.

This sequence of events was put together primarily from a series of elegant experiments done by Jan Pero, Peter Geiduschek and their colleagues. RNA pulse-labeled at early, middle or late times showed completely different patterns of hybridization competition and of hybridization to Southern blots of restriction digests of SPO1 DNA. Mutations in gene 28 prevented the transition from the early to the middle patterns, whereas mutations in genes 33 or 34 prevented the middle to late transition. Three different RNA polymerases, A, B and C, were extracted from SPO1-infected cells and used to transcribe SPO1 DNA *in vitro*, producing RNAs which showed the same hybridization patterns as the pulse-labeled early, middle and late RNAs, respectively. Analysis of the polypeptides associated with the three polymerases showed that A contained sigma

A, B contained (instead) the gene *28* product, and C contained (instead) both the gene *33* and gene *34* products.

Thus, the sequential onset of early, middle and late transcription is explained by the sigma cascade. The mechanisms responsible for other regulatory events in the SPO1 life cycle are not yet understood, although, in some cases, gene products that play essential roles have been identified. One of the most interesting is TF1, a type II DNA-binding protein that is synthesized in large quantities during SPO1 infection, and that binds preferentially to specific sites on DNA containing hmUra, causing bending of the DNA. SPO1 mutants deficient in TF1 fail to shut off transcription of certain middle genes and fail to turn on transcription of certain late genes. The bending caused by TF1 may be, in itself, a cause of these regulatory changes, or may make those genes accessible to other regulatory factors.

Certain mutations in two other genes, *22* and *27*, also prevent activity of certain late genes. The effect of the gene *22* mutation may be an indirect result of its prevention of phage DNA synthesis, suggesting that some change in structure, associated with replication, may be necessary for the activation of certain late promoters. The effect of the gene *27* mutation, however, seems to be independent of its effect on replication.

Other regulatory events whose mechanisms are not yet understood include: the delay in the onset of transcription of some early genes relative to others; the turn-on of translation of certain early mRNAs, requiring the activity of one or more SPO1 gene products; the shutoff of two different groups of early genes at two different times; the shutoff of those middle genes for which TF1 is not required; and probably others that are not yet so well defined.

By hybridization of pulse-labeled RNAs to Southern blots of restriction digests of the SPO1 genome, transcription maps have been prepared showing which regions of the genome are transcribed at which times. A summary of the overall trends revealed by such mapping is included in **Fig. 1**. Detailed analysis of individual transcription units, within certain regions of the genome, has been performed by S1 mapping and by *in vitro* transcription, and the results are summarized in the following paragraphs.

Most early transcription takes place in the terminal redundancy, each copy of which contains at least 13 promoters, most of which are very active and some of which are among the strongest promoters known. This high density of active promoters in a duplicated region may be for the purpose of competing effectively with host promoters for RNA polymerase. All 13 promoters direct transcription toward the middle of the redundant region, where two efficient transcription terminators halt transcription from the left and right sides, respectively. Many of the early transcripts of both SPO1 and SP82 undergo processing, by cleavage with RNase III, and six putative sites for RNase III cleavage have been identified within this region of SPO1. This entire region of early transcription has been sequenced, and the roles of its gene products are discussed below.

Most middle transcription occurs in a 60 kb region that occupies most of the right half of the genome. A 28 kb subset of this region includes all five of the regulatory genes mentioned earlier, as well as all the genes known to be required for SPO1 DNA replication. A total of 13 active middle promoters and three relatively weak early promoters have been identified in this region. Each of the early promoters is in a tandem arrangement with a middle promoter, permitting some sequences to be transcribed by both the early-specific and middle-specific polymerases. Eleven of the genes, including all the regulatory genes, have been sequenced.

Most late transcription occurs in the left half of the unique region of the genome. This region includes nearly all the genes known to be directly involved in head or tail morphogenesis, and it is assumed that most late genes specify structural proteins.

DNA Replication

Conditional lethal mutations have identified 10 SPO1 genes as essential for SPO1 DNA replication. Except for gene *28*, most or all of these are middle genes, whose products begin to appear about 7 min after infection. Thus, the time at which replication is initiated, about 10 min after infection, may be determined simply by the time at which all necessary proteins and precursors have accumulated to a sufficient concentration. Genes *23* and *29* are required for the synthesis of hmUra, *32* and *21a* or *b* for initiation of replication, and *22*, *30* and *31* for elongation. Gene *31* specifies the DNA polymerase and is the site of the intron discussed above. Other SPO1 gene products that play a role in replication, but whose genes have not been identified, include DNA gyrase, dCMP deaminase, dTTPase, dTMPase and an inhibitor of thymidylate synthetase.

There are at least two origins of replication, near the opposite ends of the unique region of the SPO1 genome. One growing point proceeds leftward from the right-hand origin, replicating most of the unique region. Another proceeds leftward from the left-hand origin, replicating from there to the end. There must be at least a third growing point to replicate the right end of the genome, but it is not clear whether that starts above the right-hand origin and replicates rightward or whether there is a third origin, farther to the right, from which replication proceeds bidirectionally. **Figure 1** includes a representation of the simplest interpretation of the data on directions of replication.

As the SPO1 DNA replicates, it forms concatemers of as many as 20 genomes, joined end to end by overlapping terminal redundancies. It has been proposed that concatemer formation is one solution to the inability of DNA polymerase to synthesize the 5' end of a linear DNA molecule. The two daughters of the replication of a linear molecule would each have protruding 3' ends which would be complementary to the opposite terminal redundancy. This complementarity would nucleate annealing of the entire terminal redundancies, to form an end-to-end dimer, a process which would be repeated again and again. When the concatemer was broken back down to unit genomes, cleavage would be staggered so as to produce protruding 5' ends, whose complements could then be synthesized by DNA polymerase. This hypothesis predicts that, after formation of the first dimer, and before the second round of replication has begun, genetic markers in the terminal redundancy should have been replicated only to half the extent of markers in the rest of the genome, a prediction that has been dramatically confirmed, for SPO1, by temperature-shift experiments with temperature-sensitive mutants affected in gene 32.

Morphogenesis

Little is known about SPO1 morphogenesis. Although many of the known genes are required for head or tail formation or for virus assembly, and 53 proteins have been identified as part of the virus particle, only one gene has been identified with a specific viral protein (gene 6 specifies a particular head protein), and only one morphogenetic process has been studied. The proteolytic processing of a precursor polypeptide to produce the mature form of the major head protein requires the activity of both the gene 5 product and TF1. Nothing is known of the biochemical activity of the gene 5 product, and TF1 may have any of several possible roles. Other type II DNA-binding proteins participate in the wrapping of DNA molecules into chromatin-like structures, suggesting that TF1 might play a similar role in folding SPO1 DNA for packaging into the head, and that processing of the head protein might be an integral part of the packaging process. Alternatively, TF1 might be necessary for expression of gene 5, or for some other necessary gene.

Effect on the Host Cell

It is to the selective advantage of a virus to shut off the macromolecular syntheses of the host cells, so they will not compete with the comparable viral syntheses for energy, materials and access to biosynthetic machinery. Most synthesis of host DNA, RNA and proteins is shut off within a few minutes after SPO1 infection. The shutoff mechanisms are highly selective, since not only do they have no effect on the synthesis of the comparable phage macromolecules, they also spare certain host syntheses. Host ribosomal RNA continues to be synthesized at nearly normal rates, which seems sensible since the phage has a use for the host ribosomes. The mechanism by which SPO1 distinguishes between host and phage DNAs is not clear. It must be more subtle than the presence or absence of hmUra, since some host genes are unaffected. Unlike T4, which causes the complete degradation of DNA without hydroxymethylcytosine, SPO1 causes no detectable degradation of *B. subtilis* DNA.

Most or all of the 24 early genes in the terminal redundancy are believed to specify components of the host-shutoff machinery, although this belief still awaits definitive confirmation. About one-third of the 24 genes have been tested individually, by expression in uninfected cells, and nearly all are inhibitory to the bacteria, four or five of them to the point of lethality. They affect different host functions, with the two best-characterized acting specifically on RNA polymerase and cell division, respectively. The nucleotide sequence of this 24 gene cluster shows promoters and ribosome-binding sites that are designed for highly efficient expression, and such efficiency has been shown both *in vivo* and *in vitro*. This duplicated cluster of highly expressed genes seems appropriate for specification of the host-shutoff machinery, which must, within a few minutes, cause the cessation of biosyntheses that are occurring at thousands of sites in each infected cell.

Recombination and Mutagenesis

SPO1 has a very active recombination system, producing frequencies of recombination between nearby genetic markers of about 0.001% per base pair. Nothing is known about the mechanisms of recombination or the gene products involved, but the high frequency facilitates several types of experimentation. Cloned SPO1 restriction fragments, as small as 200 bp, undergo significant recombination with the homologous region of the SPO1 genome, resulting in marker rescue of markers as little as 12 bp from the end of the fragment, permitting efficient fine-structure mapping. Also, new mutations can be constructed *in vitro* and inserted into the SPO1 genome by marker rescue recombination. Mutations of the genes specifying either protein TF1 or F.3 were introduced into *B. subtilis* on cloned fragments less than a kilobase in length, and were allowed to recombine with superinfecting wild-type SPO1. By the criterion of plaque-lift hybridization, the frequencies with which the mutations replaced the wild-type alleles ranged from 5×10^{-4} to 4×10^{-3}.

Recombination is also an integral part of the process of transfection by SPO1 DNA (most studies of the phenomenon have been done with the close relative SP82). When a cell is infected with purified DNA, the DNA is damaged by nuclease activity of the host cell. (This activity is inhibited, and therefore causes no problem, during normal infection.) Production of a single intact genome requires recombination between several of the damaged genomes.

Cloning Vehicle

SPO1 can also serve as a cloning vehicle. Entire plasmids, carrying a short region of homology to the SPO1 genome, can be inserted into the SPO1 genome by Campbell-mode integration. At least 5.6 kb of exogenous DNA can be added to the SPO1 genome in this way without apparent effect on the viability of the phage. Although too cumbersome to be used for routine cloning, this procedure offers a way to test the effect on SPO1 infection of adding specific genes to the genome, and to test the effect of the incorporation of hmUra on the functioning of any DNA of interest.

See also: **Bacillus phage ϕ29 (*Podoviridae*); *Bacillus subtilis* phages; History of virology: Bacteriophages; Phage taxonomy and classification; Phages as cloning vehicles; Phages in soil; Recombination of viruses; T4-like phages (*Myoviridae*).**

Further Reading

Geiduschek EP, Schneider GJ and Sayre MH (1990) TF1, a bacteriophage-specific DNA-binding and DNA-bending protein. *J. Struct. Biol.* 104: 84.

Goodrich-Blair H and Shub DA (1996) Beyond homing: competition between intron endonucleases confers a selective advantage on flanking genetic markers. *Cell* 84: 211.

Losick R and Pero J (1981) Cascades of sigma factors. *Cell* 25: 582.

Stewart CR (1993) SPO1 and related bacteriophages. In: Sonenshein SL, Hoch JA and Losick R (eds) *Bacillus subtilis and Other Gram-positive Bacteria*, p. 813. Washington: American Society for Microbiology.

Spongiform Encephalopathies see **Prions**

SPUMAVIRUSES (*RETROVIRIDAE*)

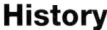

Mel Campbell and **Ayalew Mergia**, Department of Medical Pathology, University of California, Davis, California, USA

Philip C Loh, Department of Microbiology, University of Hawaii at Manos, Honolulu, USA

Paul A Luciw, Department of Medical Pathology, University of California, Davis, California, USA

Copyright © 1999 Academic Press

History

Foamy viruses were first recognized in the 1950s as contaminating viral agents which caused cytopathic effects in cultures of rhesus monkey kidney cells. On the basis of morphological, biochemical and genetic properties, foamy viruses are retroviruses; however, recent studies have demonstrated major differences in the replication strategy employed by these viruses and that of conventional retroviruses. Certain aspects of foamy virus replication are similar to hepadnaviruses. Cytopathology in foamy virus-infected monolayer cell cultures is characterized by extensive formation of intracellular vacuoles in multinucleated syncytial cells. By light microscopy, infected cell cultures have a foamy appearance, and hence the Latin term *spuma* for foamy was coined for this group of retroviruses (i.e. spumaviruses). These viruses, also designated syncytium-forming viruses, have been recovered from various mammals, including cats, cows, hamsters, sea

Table 1 Foamy virus isolates

Species	Viral designation	No. of serotypes
Human	Human foamy virus (HFV)	1
Simian/Great Ape	Simian foamy virus (SFV)	11
Feline	Feline foamy virus (FeFV)	2
Bovine	Bovine syncytium-forming virus (BSFV)	1
Murine	Hamster syncytium-forming virus (HaSFV)	1
Otariidine	Sea lion foamy virus	1

Simian foamy virus (SFV) isolates

Species	Virus serotype
Prosimian	5
Rhesus macaque	1, 2, 3
African green monkey	1, 2, 3
Baboon	1, 2, 3, 10
New World primates	4, 8, 9
Chimpanzee	6, 7
Gorilla	7
Orangutan	11

Adapted from Mergia A and Luciw PA (1991) Replication and regulation of primate foamy viruses. *Virology* 184: 475.

lions, and from various Asian, African and New World primate species (**Table 1**). In some instances, distinct spumavirus serotypes have been obtained from members of a single species (**Table 1**). In 1971, a spumavirus was isolated from a patient with nasopharyngeal carcinoma, and this virus has been designated human foamy virus (HFV), human spumaretrovirus (HSRV) or human spumavirus (HSpV) (**Fig. 1**).

Taxonomy and Classification

Foamy viruses are classified into the genus *Spumavirus* of the *Retroviridae* family. Foamy virus particles are spherical (100–140 nm diameter) and consist of a ring-shaped nucleoprotein core surrounded by a bilayer membrane envelope. The viral genome is dimeric single-stranded RNA that has positive polarity and encodes three genes for virion polyproteins (i.e. *gag*, *pol* and *env*) and additional open reading frames (ORFs). Extra ORFs, or accessory genes, are also a feature of complex retroviruses such as human immunodeficiency virus (HIV) and human T-lymphotropic virus (HTLV). Foamy viruses replicate via reverse transcription and integrate into host cell DNA; long terminal repeats (LTRs) are located at each end of proviral DNA. Viral-coded reverse transcriptase and integrase are packaged into virions. Reverse transcription is largely completed in the virion prior to entry. Although many features are shared with other retroviruses, comparisons of nucleotide sequences and replication strategy indicate that foamy viruses are a unique and distinct group of retroviruses.

Properties of the Virion

Foamy viruses share several morphological features with retroviruses. Extracellular HFV particles are polymorphic. In addition to naked extracellular preassembled cores, two morphologically different types of enveloped particles are observed. The majority of particles are spherical, with a diameter of 100–120 nm, and contain a 40–55 nm pentagon-shaped electron-lucent nucleoprotein core (i.e. nucleoid) with surface spikes, 10–13 nm in length, on the envelope. A second minor population of particles is larger (120–150 nm diameter), with condensed, amorphic cores. It has been suggested that the former type of particle is an immature form, while the second type represents mature virions. While immature in morphology, these particles are highly infectious. Mature virus particles have a bouyant density of 1.16 gm ml^{-1} in sucrose gradients. Immature viral particles in the cell cytoplasm are ring-shaped, measuring 35–45 nm, and consist of an electron-opaque shell and an inner, less dense center. Prominent envelope glycoprotein spikes up to 15 nm long

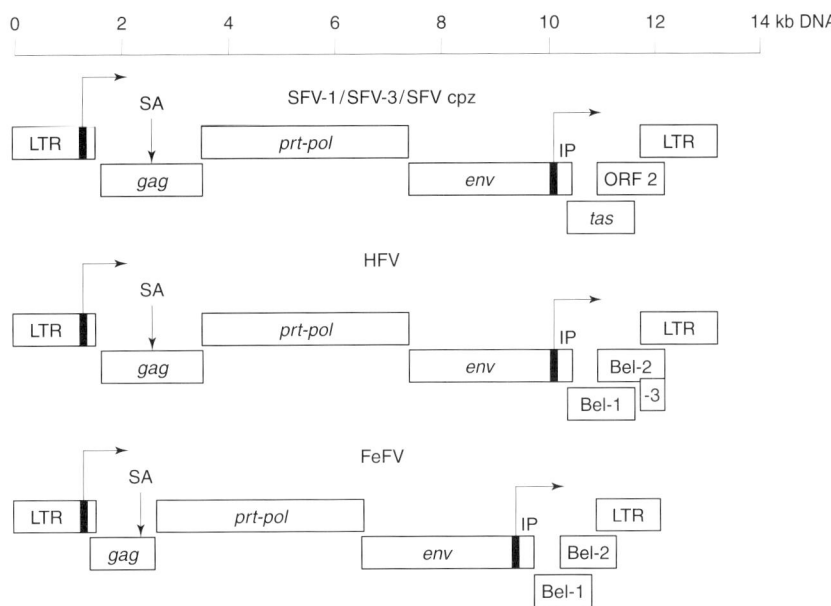

Figure 1 Genetic organization of SFVs, HFV and FeFV. Open reading frames (ORFs) and the long terminal repeats (LTRs) are shown for SFV-1 (rhesus macaque isolate), SFV-3 (African green monkey isolate), SFVcpz (chimpanzee isolate), HFV and FeFV (feline isolate). *tas* and bel-1 are transcriptional transactivators for the respective virus. The genetic organization of SFV-3 and SFVcpz is the same as SFV-1. The horizontal arrows designate viral transcripts that initiate in the 5′ LTR and internal promoter (IP). SA indicates the *prt-pol* splice acceptor.

project out from the virus membrane; the *env* gene encodes the glycoprotein, which has a transmembrane anchor (TM) domain and a surface (SU) domain. The virion core contains two identical copies of single-stranded viral RNA complexed with core proteins derived from the polyprotein precursor encoded by the *gag* gene. Purified extracellular particles contain predominantly unprocessed Gag and Prt-Pol precursor proteins.

Properties of the Genome

Foamy viruses package single-stranded RNA genome in virions. Each virus particle contains two identical copies of genomic RNA; thus, foamy viruses are diploid, as are other retroviruses. Reverse transcription is largely completed in the virion. The retrovirus RNA genome has positive polarity, and the 5′ end contains a cap structure (7-methylguanosine in a 5′–5′ linkage via a triphosphate to a second 2′-O-methylated nucleotide). In addition, a poly(A) tail, from about 100 to 200 nucleotides in length, is found at the 3′ end of retroviral RNA genomes. The 5′ cap structure and the 3′ poly(A) tail are features of virion RNA, subgenomic viral transcripts in infected cells, as well as normal cellular mRNA. Virions also contain small RNA molecules derived from the host cell; a cellular transfer RNA species that charges with lysine is bound to a site near the 5′ end of the viral RNA genome and serves as primer for initiating synthesis of plus-strand viral DNA during reverse transcription. In infected cells, the viral genome consists of both unintegrated linear DNA (double-stranded), covalently closed supercoils, and provirus integrated into the host cell genome. LTRs are located at the ends of linear viral DNA molecules; thus, viral genes lie between the LTRs.

Complete nucleotide sequences have been elucidated for SFV-1, SFV-3, SFVcpz, HFV and FeFV; accordingly, the genetic organizations of these foamy viruses are known (**Fig. 1** and **Table 2**). The proviral lengths in base pairs (bp) of SFV-1 (12 952 bp), SFV-3 (13 111 bp), HFV (12 142 bp), SFVcpz (13 246 bp), and FeFV (11 656 bp) are the largest among retroviruses. Sizes for domains in the LTR (i.e. U3, R and U5) and lengths of ORFs are given in **Table 2**. Foamy viruses encode *gag*, *pol* and *env* genes, each of which specifies a polyprotein precursor for virion proteins. In addition, foamy viruses encode three (SFV-1, SFV-3, FeFV) or two (SFVcpz and HFV) ORFs that extend from the end of the *env* gene into the 3′ LTR (**Fig. 1**). Genomic organizations of SFV-1 and SFV-3 are the same; however, HFV and SFVcpz show an extra ORF (i.e. bel-3; truncated in SFVcpz) (**Fig. 1**). A +1 ribosomal frameshift was presumed to be required for translation through the overlap of the foamy virus *gag* and *prt-pol*

Table 2 Relationships of SFV-1, SFV-3 and HFV[a]

Regions	Length SFV-1/SFV-3/HFV/SFVcpz/FeFV[b]	% amino acid homology[c]		
		SFV-1/HFV	SFV-1/SFV-3	SFV-3/HFV
gag	646/643/648/653/514	48 (66)	67 (78)	46 (65)
prt-pol	1159/1157/1152/1154/1156	76 (85)	84 (91)	73 (83)
env-SU	568/565/567/571/475	64 (80)	66 (80)	62 (78)
env-TM	416/425/415/417/418	73 (88)	84 (92)	73 (85)
bel-1/ORF-1 (tas)	311/301/300/300/209	39 (58)	54 (67)	34 (47)
bel-2/ORF-2	422/395/364/417/357	38 (56)	54 (65)	36 (56)
		% nucleotide homology		
LTR domains	Length SFV-1/SFV-3/HFV/SFVcpz/FeFV[d]	SFV-1/HFV	SFV-1/SFV-3	SFV-3/HFV
U3	1297/1332/777[e]/1423/1070	38	60	34
R	170/217/196/182/134	86	83	81
U5	160/161/150/155/149	84	84	83

[a]Genbank accession numbers for SFV-1 (M33561, M55279, M74039, X58484), SFV-3 (M74895), and HFV (X05591, 05592), SFVcpz (UO4327), FeFV (X98741).
[b]Length in predicted codons.
[c]Comparisons are made on the basis of identical amino acids. The value in parenthesis is the percent homology based on similar amino acids.
[d]Length in nucleotides.
[e]Nonrandom deletions in the HFV LTR U3 region are observed during cell culture; an early passage, nondeleted form of the U3 domain of HFV is the same length as the SFVcpz U3.

translation frames. Translational frameshifting to produce gag-prt-pol polyproteins in other retroviruses is by a −1 ribosomal frameshift event. However, recent studies have demonstrated that foamy virus prt-pol expression is independent of gag synthesis and requires a spliced mRNA which initiates in the 5′ LTR and is subsequently spliced utilizing a splice acceptor in the gag gene; gag determinants are removed from this prt-pol messenger RNA. Predicted protein-coding regions of SFV-1 and SFV-3 show 54–85% homology (**Table 2**). Similar pairwise comparisons of SFV-1 with HFV reveal 38–76% homology, and alignment of SFV-3 and HFV demonstrates 34–78% homology (**Table 2**). In summary, foamy viruses have complex genomes, encoding genes for virion proteins and accessory genes, as do several other retroviruses such as HIV and HTLV. Also, foamy virus prt-pol expression is fundamentally different from that of other retroviruses.

Properties of Viral Proteins

Knowledge of foamy virus proteins is based on direct analysis of virions and infected cells and also on comparisons of predicted protein sequences from other retroviruses. Analysis of HFV cores revealed Gag polypeptides with apparent molecular weight of 78 and 74 kDa and a Prt-Pol precursor protein of 135 kDa. Proteolytic processing of foamy virus Gag precursor proteins is inefficient; only a cleavage event near the C-terminus of Gag, which generates p74 from p78, is observed in infected and in purified virions. Prt-Pol cleavage appears to proceed to a greater extent than Gag processing in infected cells with p80 Pol (reverse transcriptase), p40 (integrase) and p15 (nucleocapsid protein) generated from the p135 Prt-Pol precursor. Domains within the pol gene for reverse transcriptase, RNAse-H, and integrase are identified by alignment with other retroviruses. The matrix (MA) protein derived from the N-terminus of the gag polyprotein precursor has not been identified for foamy viruses. For all other retroviruses, the C-terminus of the gag gene specifies a nucleocapsid (NC) protein which has a conserved motif of several cysteine residues; this motif is a metal-binding finger that mediates the interaction of NC protein to the viral RNA genome. Inspection of the predicted sequences of the foamy virus gag gene does not reveal a domain with a cysteine motif; instead, sequences near the C-terminus of the gag gene encode an NC protein with a high content of glycine and arginine residues (GR boxes). GR boxes are involved in nucleic acid binding and in a transient translocation of the HFV Gag precursor protein to the nucleus of infected cells. This motif is not conserved in FeFV, although there is some conservation of positively charged residues. FeFV Gag protein is considerably smaller than SFV and HFV Gag.

The SFV-1 *env* glycoprotein is a heterodimer composed of a 70 kDa SU domain and a 30 kDa TM domain. In cells infected with HFV, three viral glycoproteins with molecular weights 170 kDa, 130 kDa and 47 kDa have been identified; respectively, these may represent the *env* precursor, SU and TM domains. Comparison of the predicted amino acid sequences of the *env* genes of SFV-1 and HFV reveals that the *env* proteins are very similar in size as well as in structure; all cysteine residues and the majority of potential glycosylation sites are conserved. The external portion of the TM domain of SFV-1 and HFV is almost twice as large as those in other retrovirus subfamilies. Thus, the TM domain of foamy viruses may be folded into a structure which is fundamentally different from the other retroviruses. An endoplasmic reticulum retrieval signal has been identified in the foamy virus envelope and is conserved among all sequenced foamy viruses; however, its significance remains to be determined.

Physical Properties

Spumaviruses possess lipid bilayer membranes; therefore, stability is similar to that of other viruses with membrane envelopes. Heat and extremes of pH inactivate infectivity, and detergents and organic solvents disrupt virion structure. Ionizing radiation and x-rays inactivate the spumavirus RNA genome. Infectivity is lost after repeated cycles of freezing and thawing and after prolonged storage at 4°C, although virus is relatively stable in the frozen state.

In Vitro Cell Cultures

Single cycle growth studies of foamy viruses in cell culture reveal an eclipse period of 24 h and a maximum yield of virus attained by 72 h postinfection. Approximately 10% of the HFV yield in human diploid cells is released into the medium; the remainder is cell associated. The rate of adsorption of HFV to human embryonic fibroblasts (HEFs) at 37°C is maximal at 3 h postinfection. Nothing is known about cellular receptors in this early stage of infection. After attachment, the viral particle enters into the cell by either viropexis or direct entry. Whether a fusion factor is involved in the penetration process, as seen in other enveloped virus families, remains to be determined.

As with other retroviruses, foamy virus replication is related to host cell division. Similar to oncoviruses, such as murine leukemia virus (MLV), but unlike the lentivirus HIV-1, foamy viruses require host cell proliferation for productive infection. Productive infection is observed only if the target cells pass through mitosis. The semipermissiveness of heteroploid epithelial cell lines to infection with HFV or SFV-3 was determined to be the result of the methylated state of viral DNA. Treatment of such cell lines with the inhibitor of DNA methylation, 5-azacytidine, enhances viral production.

Strategy of Replication of Nucleic Acid

The pattern of foamy virus replication in tissue culture generally conforms to that of other retroviruses; however, differences are noted with respect to viral DNA synthesis. In contrast to conventional retroviruses, a high proportion of infectious HFV particles contain double-stranded DNA similar in size to full-length provirus, suggesting that reverse transcription takes place in the virion, before new rounds of infection. Most retroviruses initiate plus-strand DNA at one site, the 5' boundary of the 3' LTR. Foamy viruses utilize this site and may potentially also initiate at an internal site in the *pol* gene; a gap is located in *pol* in the linear duplex viral DNA intermediate. In acutely infected monolayer cells, very large quantities of linear viral DNA molecules are synthesized. These accumulations of viral DNA are presumed to be a consequence of reinfection; permissive cells are presumed to contain numerous cell receptors, and, thus, endogenously synthesized viral *env* glycoprotein may not be present in sufficient amounts to bind to all cell receptors and block superinfection. Several other retroviruses which induce cytopathology in cell culture systems also show large amounts of unintegrated linear viral DNA. Integrated (i.e. proviral) forms of foamy virus DNA have not yet been rigorously identified; however, the fact that these viruses encode an integrase domain in the *pol* gene supports the notion that integration is a critical step in the foamy virus life cycle.

Transcription

The U3 domains of the LTRs of foamy viruses contain *cis*-acting promoter elements (including the TATA box) which are recognized by cellular transcription factors. In addition, a second viral promoter (the internal promoter; IP) is located near the 3' end of the *env* gene (**Fig. 1**). Both promoters are dependent on the viral transactivator for full activity. Simian foamy viruses have U3 domains that are longer than those of all other retroviruses; thus, the potential is high for many *cis*-acting regulatory motifs. In the nuclei of infected cells, viral transcription initiates in the 5′ LTR and in the IP, possibly in a temporally regulated manner. The IP appears to be a stronger promoter in infected cells (basal and trans-activated levels). Transcripts with the potential to code for the ORF region gene products originate predominantly from the IP. Subgenomic transcripts derived from either the 5′ LTR or the IP are subject to complex splicing. All subgenomic viral transcripts which initiate in the 5′ LTR have a short 5′ leader (51 nucleotides) specified by the R region in the LTR. Both foamy virus promoters demonstrate very low basal levels of activity in transient expression assays, involving transfection of plasmids containing either the LTR or IP, into mammalian tissue culture cells. ORF 1 of SFV-1, SFV-3, SFVcpz and FeFV and bel-1 of HFV are transcriptional transactivator (*tas*) genes that act through *cis*-acting targets in the U3 domain of the respective LTR, or through sequences immediately 5′ to the IP TATA box, to augment levels of viral transcripts. Mutational analysis of cloned viral genomes has demonstrated that the *tas* gene is required for viral replication. The target sequences for *tas* for each virus are upstream from the TATA box. SFV-1 Tas and HFV Bel-1 proteins interact directly with DNA target elements in each promoter. Foamy virus LTRs lack any significant homology with the LTRs of lentiviruses and other retroviruses; in addition, the *tas* genes are unrelated to the regulatory genes of other retroviruses. The Tas-responsive elements in the LTR and IP of each individual virus also show little overall homology other than a conserved TATA box. Thus, the mechanism of transactivation in the foamy virus system is fundamentally different from that for other viruses, and may be different for a given transactivator acting at the 5′ LTR versus the IP. Functions for the potential genes encoded by the remaining ORFs (i.e. ORF 2; Bel-2,-3) are not yet known. Foamy viruses do not appear to contain a Rev/Rex axis as in the lentiviruses or oncoviruses. The additional ORFs are dispensable for replication in tissue culture cells; only the viral transactivator is required.

Translation

A subgenomic mRNA encodes the Prt-Pol precursor which lacks Gag determinants. No Gag-Pol precursor can be detected in foamy virus-infected cells or virions. The Env polyprotein precursor is translated from a subgenomic spliced mRNA. The subgenomic mRNA for Env is presumed to be translated on membrane-bound cytoplasmic polysomes, and other viral mRNA species may be translated on free polysomes in the cytoplasm. Proteins encoded by *bel-2* and *bel-3* have been identified in infected cells. An abundant protein containing N-terminal sequences from the *bel-1* gene and C-terminal sequences from the *bel-2* gene has been detected in infected cells; however, the function of this fusion protein, designated Bet, is not known.

Post-translational Processing

In conventional retroviruses, the viral *gag*, *pol*, and *env* genes encode polyprotein precursors that are processed by specific cleavages. Viral protease produces the matrix (MA), capsid (CA) and nucleocapsid (NC) proteins from the *gag* gene precursor. Little processing of the foamy virus Gag precursor is observed in infected cells or in virions. Only a C-terminal cleavage of p78 Gag to generate p74 Gag is readily observed in foamy virus-infected cells or in virions. The putative MA protein of foamy viruses (and several other retroviruses) has a glycine immediately after the initiator methionine; therefore, MA is predicted to be myristoylated at the N-terminus by a host cell enzyme. Reverse transcriptase and integrase are cleaved from the *pol* gene precursor, presumably by the viral protease. The *env* precursor is glycosylated by cellular enzymes and cleaved into the SU and TM domains; this cleavage site at two basic residues is recognized by a host cell endopeptidase.

Assembly Site, Release, Uptake, Cytopathology

Assembly of nucleoprotein cores appears to occur in the cytoplasm. Intracellular viral particles are ring-shaped, 35–50 nm in diameter, and consist of an electron dense shell and an inner electron-lucent center. Particles mature by budding through the cell plasma membrane.

The receptor(s) for these viruses has not been identified, and the entry mechanism (i.e. direct fusion of viral and cell membranes or receptor-mediated endocytosis) has not been studied.

Cytopathology in monolayer tissue culture cells is characterized by extensive formation of intracellular vacuoles in multinucleated syncytial cells. Certain hematopoietic cell lines can produce high levels of virus without obvious cytopathology for an extended period of culture.

Geographic and Seasonal Distribution

Isolates of FeFV, representing two serotypes, have been identified in domestic cats from three continents (**Table 1**), and an isolate has also been obtained from a European wildcat. FeFV has been identified in healthy cats as well as in cats with neoplasms or nonneoplastic diseases. BFV infection in cattle populations also appears to be widespread. Four serotypes of SFV have been isolated from Old World monkeys and three additional serotypes are from New World monkeys (Table 1). Two unique serotypes of SFV were recovered from chimpanzees and one unique serotype from prosimians (Table 1). A recent SFV isolate from orangutan appears to be serologically distinct. In summary, foamy viruses appear to be endemic in some animal species in certain areas. Recent studies have refuted previous seroepidemiological studies which indicated that HFV may infect a small number of individuals in Africa and certain Pacific islands; however, rare zoonotic infection of humans with SFVs has been documented. Nothing is known about the seasonal distribution of foamy viruses in any mammalian species.

Host Range and Virus Propagation

Foamy viruses have a wide host range in cell culture systems. The SFVs replicate and cause cytopathology in epithelial and fibroblastic cells from primates, rodents and chickens. Lymphoid cells can be persistently infected with no visible cytopathic effects on the host cells. Cytopathology in monolayer cells is generally characterized by multinucleated syncytia at early times and extensive vacuolization at later times; inclusion bodies are not observed. HFV replicates in diploid fibroblast-like cell lines but not in heteroploid epithelial-like cell lines. *In vitro*, SFV-1 establishes a carrier state in HEp-2 (human hepatoma) and BHK (baby hamster kidney) cell lines, and a Vero (monkey fibroblast) cell line harboring SFV-3 in a latent state has been described. Manifestation of cytopathology with respect to time after infection *in vitro* depends on the serotype of the virus, titer, passage history and cell type used to propagate virus. Under optimal conditions, SFVs induce cytopathology and reach maximal titers as early as 4–5 days after infection. Virus is spread by the extracellular route and by cell-to-cell transmission.

Genetics

Although the complete sequences of the SFV-1, SFV-3, HFV, SFVcpz and FeFV genomes have been elucidated, the extent of variation within each virus and the potential for recombination between viruses are not known.

Evolution

Foamy viruses are exogenous agents, as uninfected host cells do not contain sequences related to these viruses. Sequence comparisons reveal that SFV-1 (rhesus macaque isolate) and SFV-3 (African green monkey isolate) are more closely related to each other than either is to HFV. HFV and SFVcpz are highly related. A potential progenitor virus(es) for the primate foamy viruses remains to be identified. Evolutionary relationships of the primate foamy viruses with foamy virus isolates from other species are not yet established.

Serologic Relationships and Variability

Serologic relationships have been determined by analyzing properties of virus neutralizing antibodies in sera of naturally infected animals and rabbits immunized with whole virus preparations. Antibodies to foamy virus isolates from primate, feline, bovine or murine (i.e. hamster) species do not crossreact, and these viruses are immunologically unrelated to retroviruses in other genera. At least 11 simian serotypes and two feline serotypes have been identified (Table 1). Serologic patterns of the SFVs are complex, in that a single species may have two or more serotypes, and the same serotype has been isolated from different species (Table 1). Antibodies to HFV apparently crossreact with several SFVs. The genetic and molecular basis for serological crossreactivity (and variability) has yet to be determined; these studies will require sequencing of foamy virus genomes coupled with an analysis of immunologic epitopes on viral proteins.

Epidemiology

SFVs are prevalent in captive and wild-caught primates. Surveys of primates reared in captivity suggest that foamy virus prevalence is extremely high, especially in adults, were rates of infection may approach 100%. Previous seroepidemiological studies revealed that HFV may be present in a small number of humans in parts of Africa and the Pacific islands. Recent re-examination of these populations have been unable to confirm these previous findings, which suggested an association of foamy virus with specific human disease, and also failed to find any evidence of naturally occurring human infection with a foamy virus.

Transmission and Tissue Tropism

Mechanisms which account for spread of foamy viruses are not well defined. Vertical transmission has been described in cats, cows and monkeys. FeFV, BFV and SFV have been isolated from throat washings or nasal swabs from the respective hosts. Thus, it is possible for horizontal transmission to occur by direct contact and, perhaps, by the respiratory route via aerosolization.

SFVs have been isolated from several organs (e.g. brain and lymphoid cells) and fluids of healthy and diseased primates. Analysis of fractionated monkey peripheral blood mononuclear cells indicated foamy virus infection of diverse cell populations, with the highest proviral burden in CD8+ T cells. In their respective hosts, FeFV and BFV are also distributed in many different tissues. A feature of the virus–natural host relationship is that foamy viruses have not been directly observed by electron microscopy or other means in the tissue from which they were isolated. Recovery of virus has always been achieved by culturing cells from the original tissue *in vitro*. The mechanism(s) of virus activation is still unknown.

Pathogenicity

Although several reports provide tentative links between presence of a foamy virus and certain clinical conditions, the vast majority of naturally infected hosts do not display any disease. Epidemiologic studies suggested an association of FeFV with polyarthritis in cats, yet experimentally infected cats remained free of symptoms. HFV has been recovered from several patients with de Quervain subacute thyroiditis, and additional HFVs have been obtained from individuals with other disease conditions; however, none of these viral isolates have been well characterized. The prototype HFV was recovered from an individual in East Africa who had a nasopharyngeal carcinoma. Whether this HFV is a genuine human retrovirus or a simian foamy virus contaminant remains to be resolved by characterization of additional (independent) foamy virus isolates from humans. Sequence analysis of SFVcpz indicated a close relationship between this chimpanzee isolate and HFV, thus HFV may represent a rare zoonotic infection or SFV contaminant. In summary, reports on foamy viruses in humans represent anecdotal observations, and an etiologic role for a putative HFV in human pathology is not yet established.

Seronegative natural hosts experimentally infected with foamy virus develop antibodies to the virus but show no clinical symptoms. Heterologous hosts inoculated with foamy viruses generally do not present with any disease signs. Rabbits experimentally infected with SFV-1 seroconverted and harbored virus in several tissue for 1–3 weeks postinfection. In another study, rabbits infected with SFV-7 by the intravenous route demonstrated transient suppression of cell-mediated immune functions. Progressive encephalopathy and muscular abnormalities were produced in transgenic mice containing a portion of the cloned HFV genome that includes the ORF (or *bel*) region; this region encodes the transcriptional transactivator (*tas*). This observation in the transgenic animal model intimates a pathogenic potential for foamy viruses, perhaps with respect to neurodegenerative diseases. Whether foamy viruses are cofactors for disease for other infectious agents is not known.

Clinical Features of Infection

Naturally and experimentally infected hosts develop antiviral antibodies, and virus is recoverable from a variety of organs by culturing tissue explants *in vitro* to activate viral gene expression. A clear association between foamy avirus infection and disease has not yet been established (see above, Pathogenicity). Extremely rare zoonotic infection of humans, through occupational exposure (animal laboratory workers), has been documented. Infected individuals appear healthy.

Pathology and Histopathology

Currently there is no significant information available on the pathology and histopathology of foamy virus infections in their natural hosts, as clinical disease has not been convincingly associated with these viruses. Histologic analysis of transgenic mice containing portions of the HFV genome reveals patterns of neurological and muscular degeneration (see above, Pathogenicity).

Immune Response

Naturally infected animals have virus-neutralizing antibodies. Accordingly, the presence of these antibodies may account for viral latency or a low-level persistent infection. Other defense mechanisms, such as interferon, may also subdue viral replication in the host. The role of cell-mediated immunity in foamy virus infection remains to be explored.

Prevention and Control of Foamy Viruses

Foamy virus infections of their natural hosts are not known to cause any major clinical disease; consequently, the development of preventive and control measures are not necessary at this time. However, experimental xenotransplants from nonhuman primates to humans raises the possibility of SFV infection in humans.

Future Perspectives

Many fundamental aspects of foamy virus replication

and virus–host interactions remain to be investigated. The emerging picture of foamy virus replication is one with distinct differences from that of conventional retroviruses, with some features reminiscent of hepadnaviruses. The distribution of foamy viruses in a species and the precise modes of transmission are not well established; these studies will be aided by sensitive techniques for detecting viral genomes (e.g. amplification via polymerase chain reaction) and antiviral antibodies (e.g. ELISA systems and immunoblots with genetically engineered viral antigens). The reason(s) for lack of pathology in animals infected with foamy viruses is not known; it is tenable that these viruses may be associated with long-term, chronic degenerative disease(s). In addition, foamy viruses may be cofactors for other infectious agents. In the host, the precise cell types and organs harboring virus and viral genomes are not well defined. Whether infection is 'persistent' or 'latent' remains to be determined. Additional studies are required to elucidate the mechanism of viral transactivation (via tas/bel) and to evaluate the effects of cell-activation signals on viral gene expression. The significance of host immune mechanisms for controlling viral replication and pathogenesis is not determined, and a mechanism(s) which accounts for viral cytopathology has not been elucidated. The extent of strain variation, particularly in the *env* genes of primate foamy viruses, is an area for future study. A cellular receptor for attachment of virus particles has not yet been identified. In addition, the broad host range and apparent lack of pathogenesis are factors which may make foamy viruses useful for the development of retroviral vectors for gene transfer. Transduction of a wide variety of vertebrate cells, including primary hematopoietic progenitor cells, by foamy virus vectors has been reported.

See also: **Human immunodeficiency viruses (*Retroviridae*): Molecular biology, Anti-retroviral agents, General features; Human T-cell leukemia viruses (*Retroviridae*): HTLV-1, HTLV-2; Retroviruses – type D (*Retroviridae*).**

Further Reading

Aguzzi A (1993) The foamy virus family: molecular biology, epidemiology, and neuropathology. *Biochim. Biophys. Acta* 1155: 1.

Aguzzi A, Marino S, Tschopp R and Rethwilm A (1996) Regulation of expression and pathogenic potential of human foamy virus in vitro and in transgenic mice. *Curr. Top. Microbiol. Immunol.* 206: 243.

Hooks JJ and Detrick-Hooks B (1981) *Spumavirinae*: foamy virus group infections. In: Kurstak E and Kurstak C (eds) *Comparative Aspects and Diagnosis of Viral Disease*, p. 599. New York: Academic Press.

Rethwilm A (1995) Regulation of foamy virus gene expression. *Curr. Top. Microbiol. Immunol.* 193: 1.

Rethwilm A (1996) Unexpected replication pathways of foamy viruses. *J. Acquir. Immune Defic. Syndr. Hum. Retrovirol.* 13 (suppl. 1): S248.

Yu S, Baldwin DN, Gwynn SR, Yendapalli S and Linial ML (1996) Human foamy virus replication: A pathway distinct from that of retroviruses and hepadnaviruses. *Science* 271: 1579.

Squirrel Fibroma Virus   *see* **Poxviruses**

St. Louis Encephalitis Virus   *see* **Encephalitis Viruses**

Swine Herpesvirus-1   *see* **Pseudorabies Virus**

Swine Vesicular Exanthema Virus   *see* **Caliciviruses**

Swinepox Virus   *see* **Poxvirus**

SYNERGISM: PLANT VIRUSES

Vicki Bowman Vance, Department of Biological Sciences, University of South Carolina, Columbia, South Carolina, USA

Copyright © 1999 Academic Press

Mixed Virus Infections are Common in Plants

Mixed virus infections occur in both plant and animal systems, and doubly infected organisms commonly display changes in disease symptoms and in the accumulation of one or both of the co-infecting viruses. However, such infections are relatively uncommon in animal hosts where they are generally associated with depression of the immune response. In contrast, higher plants are frequently infected with multiple viruses. In some cases, the virus interaction is antagonistic and infection by one virus interferes with the subsequent replication or spread of the other virus. This type of interaction is the basis for the phenomenon known as 'cross protection', where a plant is protected from a virulent strain of a virus by prior inoculation with a mild or asymptomatic strain of the same virus. Cross protection is limited to closely related viruses.

In other cases of mixed virus infection in plants, the viral interaction is synergistic and co-infection enhances the replication and/or spread of one or both viruses. The co-infection usually results in a much more severe disease than either virus causes in a single infection, and a number of plant disease syndromes are caused by the interaction of two independent viruses in the same host. In contrast to cross protection, synergistic viral interactions almost always occur between unrelated viruses. Such synergistic interactions offer a unique opportunity to investigate the regulation of viral disease because the accumulation and pathogenicity of one virus are altered when it interacts with a relatively simple genetic element, the genome of the co-infecting virus.

Potyvirus-associated Synergisms

Many synergistic diseases involve a member of the potyvirus group of plant viruses. In these *potyvirus-associated* synergisms, the other virus of the pair may be any of a broad range of unrelated viruses, including pararetroviruses, such as cauliflower mosaic virus, and RNA viruses of both the alphavirus supergroup (for example potato virus X [PVX]) and the picornavirus supergroup (for example cowpea mosaic virus). Table 1 lists a number of examples of potyvirus-associated synergisms.

Several such potyvirus-associated synergistic diseases have been examined in some detail, and in each, a dramatic increase in host symptoms has been observed in doubly infected plants compared to singly infected plants. The increase in symptoms in doubly infected plants is correlated with an increase in the accumulation of the nonpotyvirus; however, in general, there is no corresponding increase or decrease in the level of the potyvirus.

The PVX/potyvirus Interaction

A model synergism

The interaction between PVX and potato virus Y (PVY, a potyvirus) in tobacco has been well characterized and serves as a model to understand the underlying molecular basis for potyvirus-associated synergistic disease. Plants mechanically inoculated with both viruses develop synergistic disease, which is characterized initially by severe vein clearing and then necrosis of the first systemically infected leaf tissue. The dramatic increase in symptoms in the first systemically infected tissue is correlated with a large (3–10-fold) increase in the level of PVX compared to

Table 1 Potyvirus-associated synergisms

Potyvirus	Heterologous virus
Potato virus Y	Potato virus X
Tobacco vein mottling virus	
Tobacco etch virus	
Pepper mottle virus	
Blackeye cowpea mosaic virus	Cucumber mosaic virus
Cowpea aphidborne virus	
Bean yellow mosaic virus	
Zucchini yellow mosaic virus	
Soybean mosaic virus	Bean pod mottle virus
	Cowpea mosaic virus
Maize dwarf mosaic virus	Maize chlorotic mottle virus
Wheat streak mosaic virus	
Potato virus Y	Tobacco mosaic virus
Turnip mosaic virus	Cauliflower mosaic virus
Maize dwarf mosaic virus	Barley yellow dwarf virus
Tobacco etch virus	Dodder latent mosaic virus

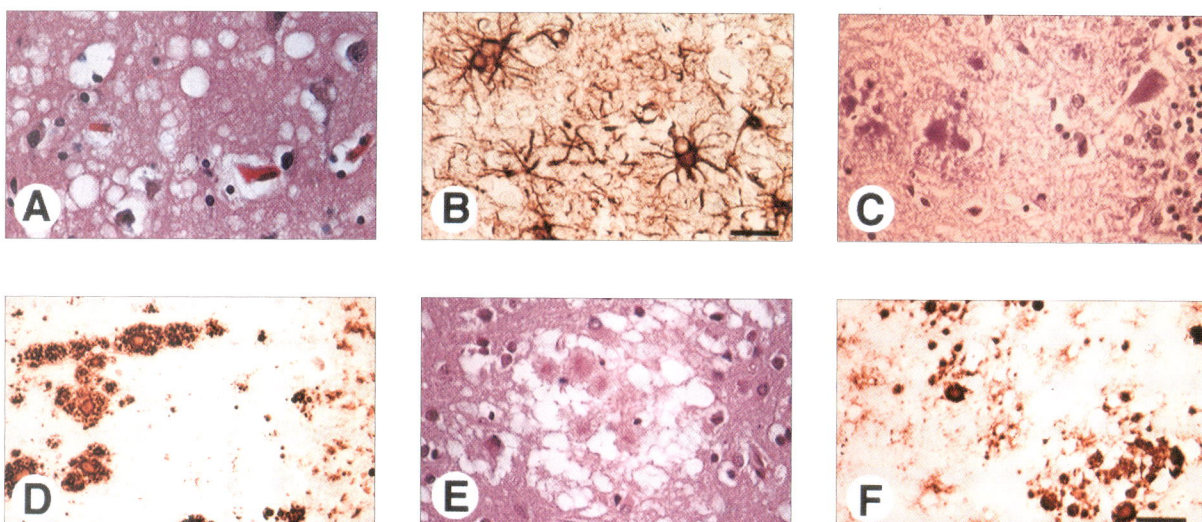

Plate 27 Neuropathology of human prion diseases. Sporadic CJD is characterized by vacuolation of the neuropil of the gray matter, by exuberant reactive astrocytic gliosis, the intensity of which is proprtional to the degree of nerve cell loss, and rarely, by PrP amyloid plaque formation (not shown). The neuropathology of familial CJD is similar. GSS (P102L), as well as other inherited forms of GSS (not shown), is characterized by numerous deposits of PrP amyloid throughout the CNS. New variant CJD (vCJD) has clinical and epidemiological features that suggest it was acquired by infection with prions. The neuropathological features of vCJD are unique among CJD cases because of the abundance of PrP amyloid plaques that are often surrounded by a halo of intense vacuolation. (**A**) Sporadic CJD, cerebral cortex stained with hematoxylin and eosin showing widespread spongiform degeneration. (**B**) Sporadic CJD, cerebral cortex immunostained with anti-GFAP antibodies demonstrating the widespread reactive gliosis. (**C**) GSS, cerebellum with most of the GSS-plaques in the molecular layer (left 80% of micrograph) and many but not all are periodic acid Schiff (PAS) reaction positive. Granule cells and a single Purkinje cells are seen in the right 20% of the panel. (**D**) GSS, cerebellum at the same location as panel C with PrP immunohistochemistry after the hydrolytic autoclaving reveals more PrP plaques than seen with the PAS reaction. (**E**) Variant CJD, cerebral cortex stained the hematoxylin and eosin shows that the plaque deposits are uniquiely located within vacuoles. With this histology, these amyloid deposits have been referred to as 'florid plaques'. (**F**) Variant CJD, cerebral cortex stained with PrP immunohistochemistry after hydrolytic autoclaving reveals numerous PrP plaques often occuring in clusters as well as minute PrP deposits surrounding many cortical nerons and their proximal processes. Bar in B = 50 μm and applies also panels A, C, and D. Bar in F = 100 μm and applies also to panel D. See article **Prions - Human and Animal** for more information.

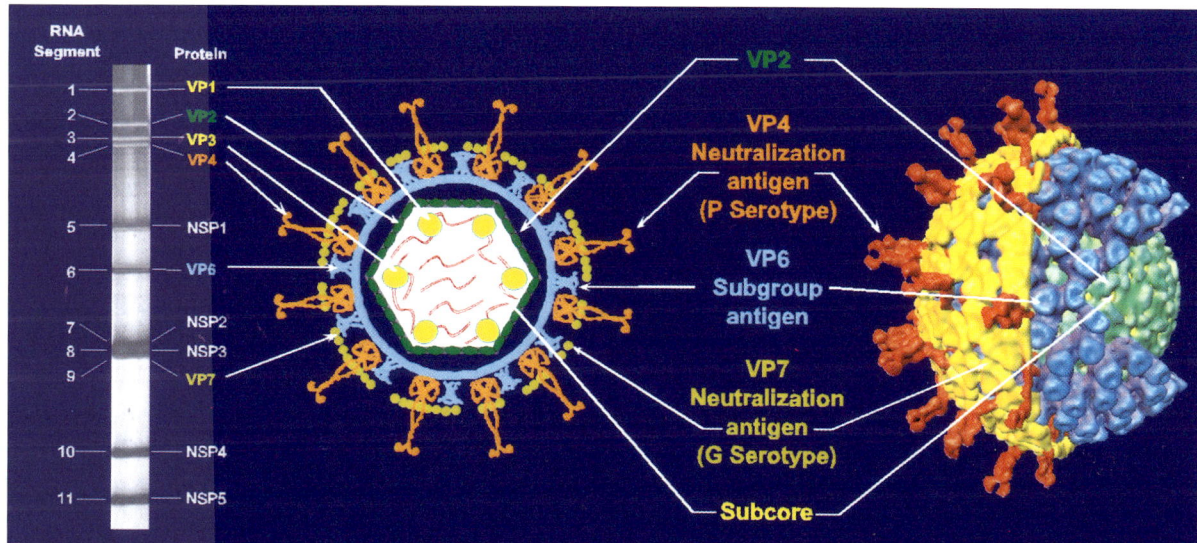

Plate 28 Rotavirus genes, proteins and structure. The left panel shows the RNA segments and the gene coding assignments for the simian rotavirus SA11. See **Table 1** (p. 1586) for details on the genes and proteins. The location of the viral structural proteins in the different shells of the virus particles is shown in the schematic in the center. The major structural proteins that make up the outer shell of particles (VP4 and VP7), the intermediate shell (VP6), the inner shell (VP2) and the subcore region composed of ordered viral RNA are illustrated in the 25 Å three-dimensional structure of particles shown in the right panel. (This reconstruction was kindly provided by B.V.V. Prasad.). See article **Rotaviruses (*Reoviridae*) Molecular Biology** for more information.

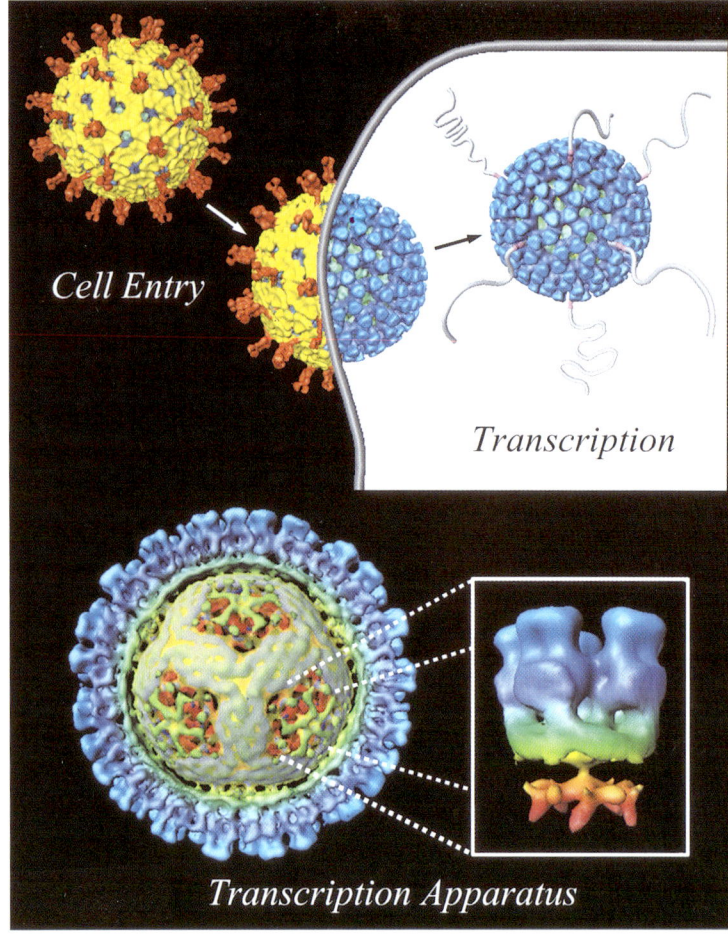

Plate 29 Rotavirus transcription. The top panel illustrates the early changes in rotavirus structure that lead to transcription and release of the mRNA molecules from the double-layered particles. The bottom panel shows the internal structure of rotavirus double-layered particles that are surrounded by trimers of the intermediate shell protein VP6 (blue). The double-stranded RNA genome is organized as a dodecahedral shell inside the particles and the minor internal proteins VP1 and VP3 are organized in a flower-shaped structure at the fivefold axes. The right-hand insert shows a side view of this structure highlighting VP6 (blue), VP2 (green) and the complex of VP1 and VP3 (orange). The newly made transcripts are extruded from these complexes at the fivefold axes (see top panel). (Figure kindly provided by J. Lawton.) See article **Rotaviruses (*Reoviridae*) Molecular Biology** for more information.

Plate 30 An illustration of protein crystallography used to determine protein structure. See article **Virus Structure: Atomic Structure** for more information.

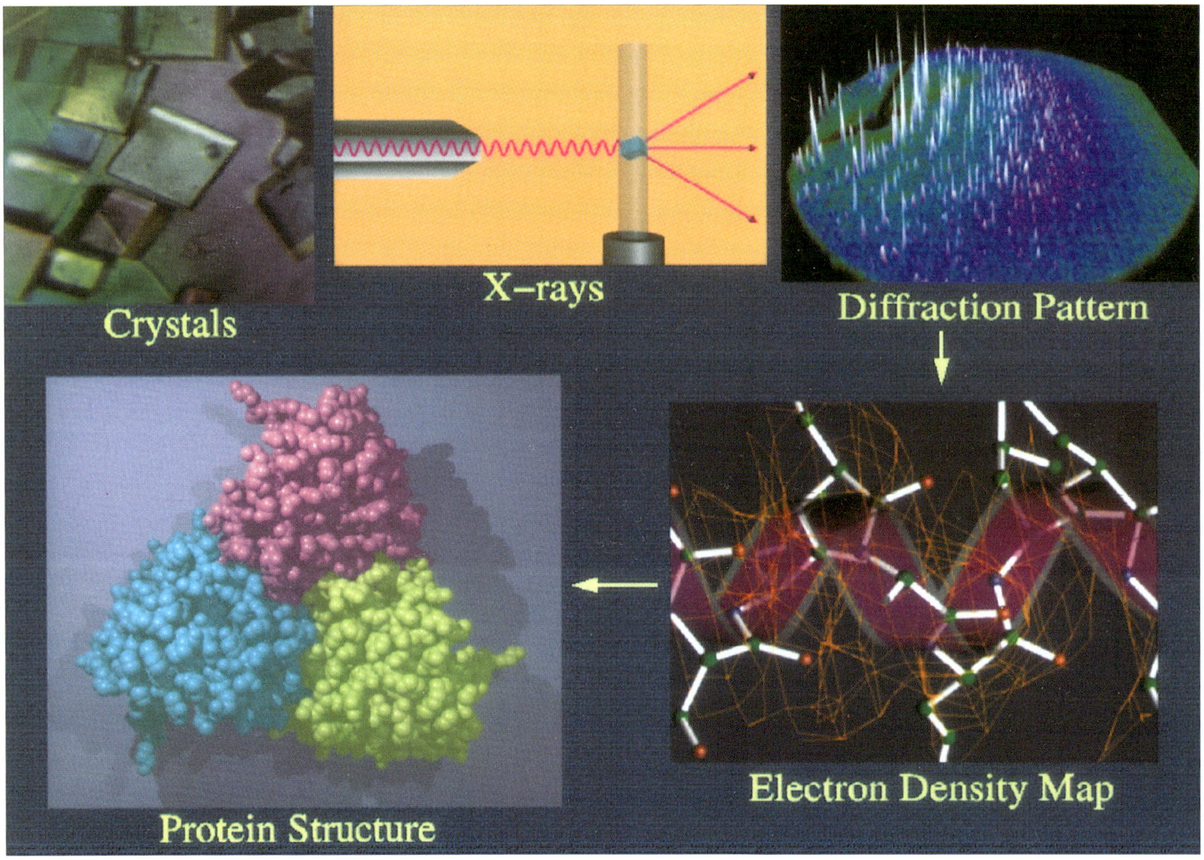

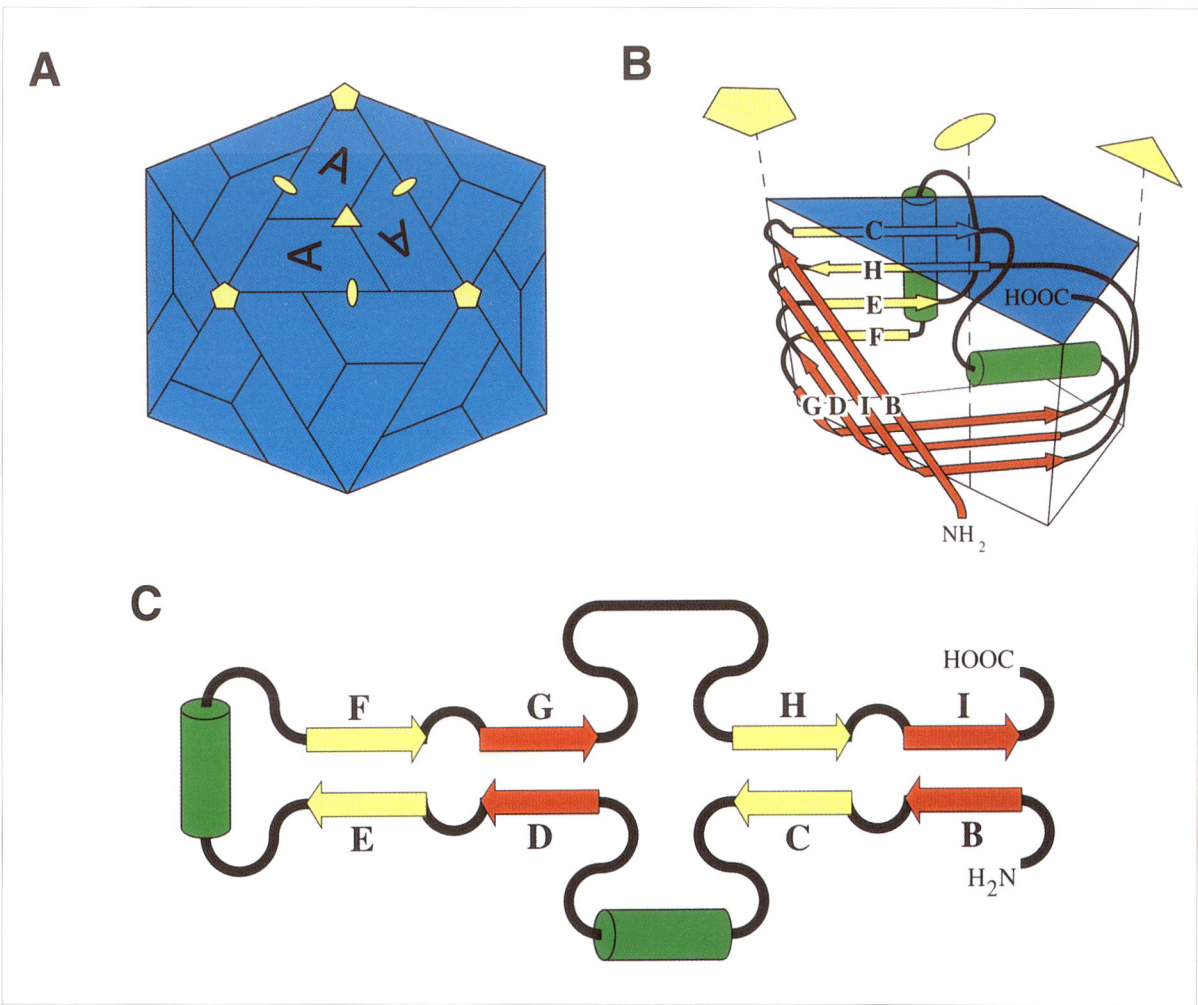

Plate 31 (**A**) The icosahedral capsid contains 60 identical copies of the protein subunit (blue) labeled A. These are related by fivefold (yellow pentagons at vertices), threefold (yellow triangles in faces) and twofold (yellow ellipses at edges) symmetry elements. For a given sized subunit this point group symmetry generates the largest possible assembly (60 subunits) in which every protein lies in an identical environment. (**B**) A schematic representation of the subunit building block found in many RNA and some DNA viral structures. Such subunits have complementary interfacial surfaces which, when they repeatedly interact, lead to the symmetry of the icosahedron. The tertiary structure of the subunit is an eight-stranded β-barrel with the topology of the jellyroll (see (**C**), β-strand and helix coloring is identical to (**B**). Subunit sizes generally range between 20 and 40 kDa with variation among different viruses occurring at the N-and C-termini and in the size of insertions between strands of the β-sheet. These insertions generally do not occur at the narrow end of the wedge (B–C, H–I, D–E and F–G turns). (**C**) The topology of viral β-barrel showing the connections between strands of the sheets (represented by yellow or red arrows) and positions of the insertions between strands. The green cylinders represent helices that are usually conserved. The C–D, E–F and G–H loops often contain large insertions. See article **Virus Structure: Principles of Virus Structure** for more information.

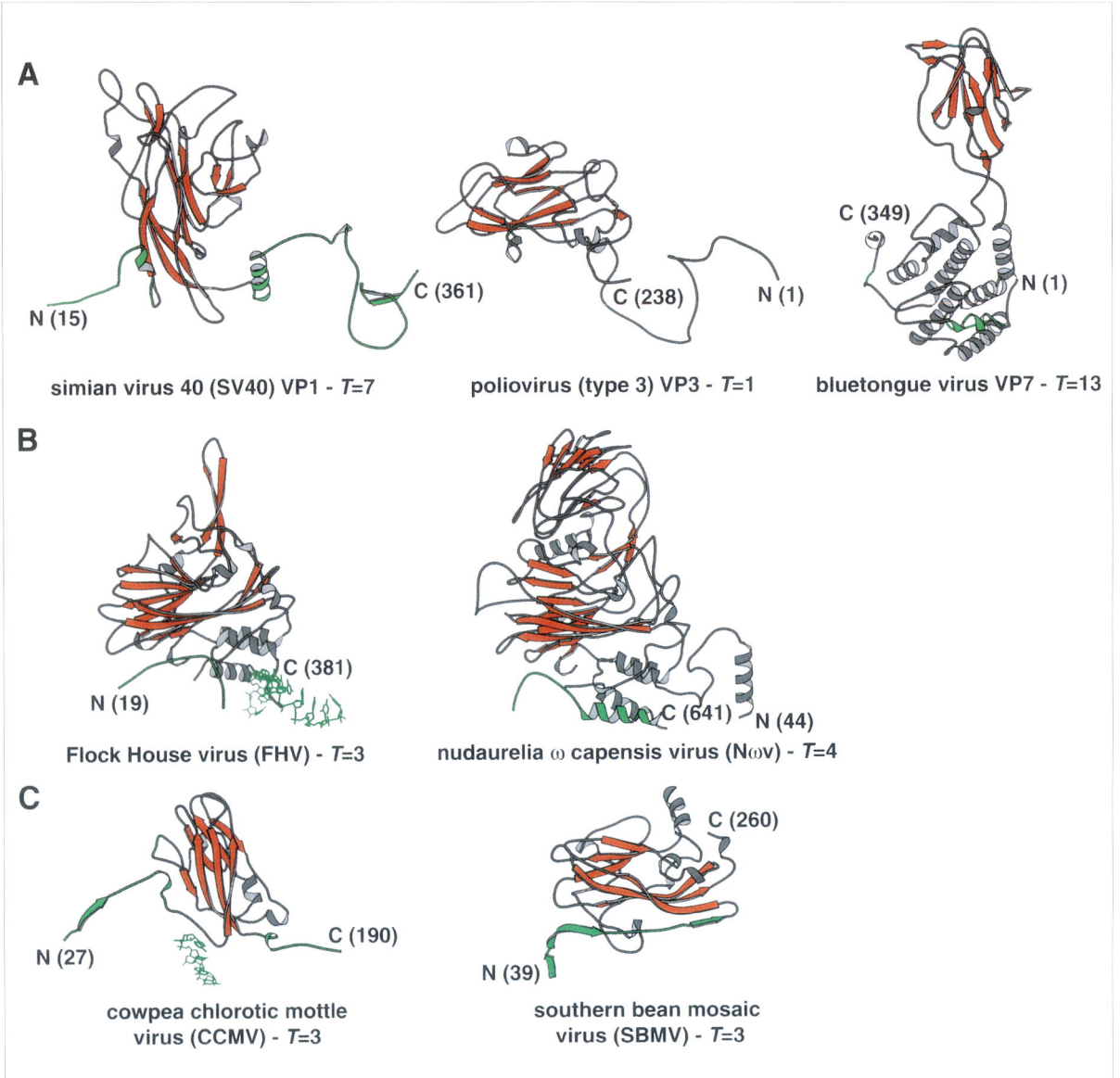

Plate 32 Structure of (**A**) vertebrate, (**B**) insect and (**C**) plant virus protein subunits that assemble into icosahedral shells. The name of the virus appears below the corresponding protein subunit along with the capsid triangulation number T (explained in **Plate 33**). The N- and C-termini are labeled with the residue numbers in brackets. Many virus subunit structures determined to near atomic resolution have the β-barrel fold and/or insertions with nearly all β-secondary structure (colored red, see **Plate 31B, C**). Multiple copies (from 180 to 780) of the single subunit shown for each virus, except for that of poliovirus, form the entire icosahedral protein shell. Assembly of icosahedral virus particles with more than 60 subunits (e.g. see **Plate 31A**) requires quasi-symmetric interactions (nonidentical interactions between neighboring identical subunits, discussed in detail later in this chapter, see **Plates 33** and **34**) often involving subtle to extensive differences in structure at the subunit N- and C-termini. The subunit regions involved in quasi-symmetric interactions critical to virion structure and assembly are colored green (only a single variation is shown for each virus). The 'switch' in structure between identical subunits is a response to differences in the local chemical environment, defined the number of subunits forming the icosahedral shell, in order to maintain similar bonding between neighboring subunits. The structural variations include the presence or absence of highly ordered RNA structure (green stick models) in FHV and CCMV. Poliovirus utilizes multiple copies of two additional subunits highly similar to VP3 to form a complete virion. Thus, there is no quasi-symmetry in poliovirus (note the absence of any green highlights) since neighboring subunits are different proteins. See article **Virus Structure: Principles of Virus Structure** for more information.

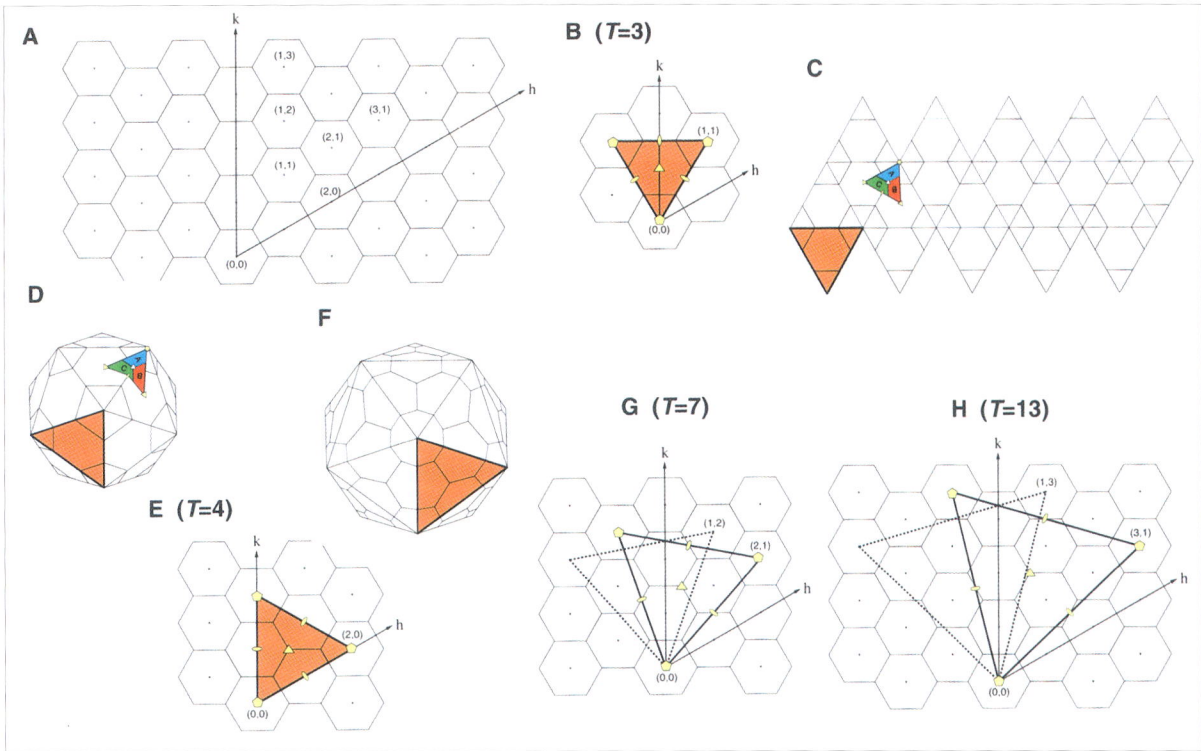

Plate 33 Geometric principles for generating icosahedral quasi-equivalent surface lattices. These four constructions show the relation between icosahedral symmetry axes and quasi-equivalent symmetry axes. The latter are symmetry elements that hold only in a local environment. (**A**) It is assumed in quasi-equivalence theory that hexamers and pentamers can be interchanged at a particular position in the surface lattice. Hexamers are initially considered planar (an array of hexamers forms a flat sheet as shown) and pentamers are considered convex, introducing curvature in the sheet of hexamers when they are inserted. Inserting 12 pentamers at appropriate positions in the hexamer net generates the closed icosahedral shell, composed of hexamers and pentamers. The positions at which hexamers are replaced by pentamers are defined by the indices **h** and **k** measured along the labeled axes. The values of (**h,k**) used in the following examples are labeled. To construct a model of a particular quasi-equivalent lattice, one face of an icosahedron (equilateral triangles colored orange in (**B–F**) is generated in the hexagonal net. The origin (0,0) is replaced with a pentamer, and the (**h,k**) hexamer is replaced by a pentamer. The third replaced hexamer is identified by threefold symmetry (i.e. complete the equilateral triangle). Each quasi-equivalent lattice is identified by a number $T = h^2 + hk + k^2$ where **h** and **k** are the indices used above. T indicates the number of quasi-equivalent units in the icosahedral asymmetric unit (a hexamer contains six units and a pentamer contains five units). For the purpose of these constructions it is convenient to choose the icosahedral asymmetric unit as one-third of an icosahedral face defined by the triangle connecting a threefold axis to two adjacent fivefold axes. Other asymmetric units can be chosen such as the triangle connecting two adjacent threefold axes and an adjacent fivefold axis (see (**C**) and **Plate 35**). The total number of units in the particle is $60T$, given the symmetry of the icosahedron. The number of pentamers must be 12 and the number of hexamers is $(60T - 60)/6 = 10(T - 1)$. (**B**) One face of the icosahedron for a $T = 3$ surface lattice is identified by the orange triangle with the bold outline (this corresponds to a face of the icosahedron in **Plate 31A**). The yellow symmetry labels are the same as those defined in **Plate 31**. The hexamer replaced has coordinates **h** = 1, **k** = 1. The icosahedral asymmetric unit is one-third of this face and it contains three quasi-equivalent units (two units from the hexamer coincident with the threefold axis and one unit from the pentamer). (**C**) Arranging 20 identical faces of the icosahedron as shown can generate the three-dimensional model of the quasi-equivalent lattice. Three quasi-equivalent units labeled A (blue), B (red) and C (green) are shown. These correspond to the three quasi-equivalent units defined in **Plates 34** and **35** rather than the alternative definition used in (**A**) and (**B**). (**D**) The folded icosahedron is shown with hexamers and pentamers outlined. The orange face represents the triangle originally generated from the hexagonal net. The $T = 3$ surface lattice represented in this construction has the appearance of a soccer ball. The trapezoids labeled A, B and C identify quasi-equivalent units in one icosahedral asymmetric unit of the rhombic tri-icontahedron discussed in **Plate 35**. (**E**) An example of a $T = 4$ icosahedral face (**h** = 2, **k** = 0). In this case the hexamers are coincident with icosahedral twofold axes. (**F**) A folded $T = 4$ icosahedron with the orange face corresponding to the face outlined in the hexagonal net. Note that folding the lattice has required that the hexamers have the curvature of the icosahedral edges. (**G**) A single icosahedral face generated from the hexagonal net for a $T = 7$ lattice. Note that there are two different $T = 7$ lattices (**h** = 2, **k** = 1 in bold outline; and **h** = 1, **k** = 2 in dashed outline). These lattices are the mirror images of each other. To fully define such a lattice, the arrangement of hexamers and pentamers must be established as well as the enantiomorph of the lattice. (**H**) A single icosahedral face for a $T = 13$ lattice is shown. The two enantiomorphs of the quasi-equivalent lattice (**h** = 3, **k** = 1 – bold; and **h** = 1, **k** = 3 – dashed) are outlined. The procedure for generating quasi-equivalent models described here does not exactly correspond to the one described by Caspar and Klug (1962). Caspar and Klug distinguish between different icosadeltahedra by a number $P = h^2 + hk + k^2$ where **h** and **k** are integers that contain no common factors but 1. The deltahedra are triangulated to different degrees described by an integer f that can take on any value. In their definition $T = Pf^2$. The description in this figure has no restrictions on common factors between h and k, thus $T = h^2 + hk + k^2$ for all positive integers. The final models are identical to those described by Caspar and Klug. See article **Virus Structure: Principles of Virus Structure** for more information.

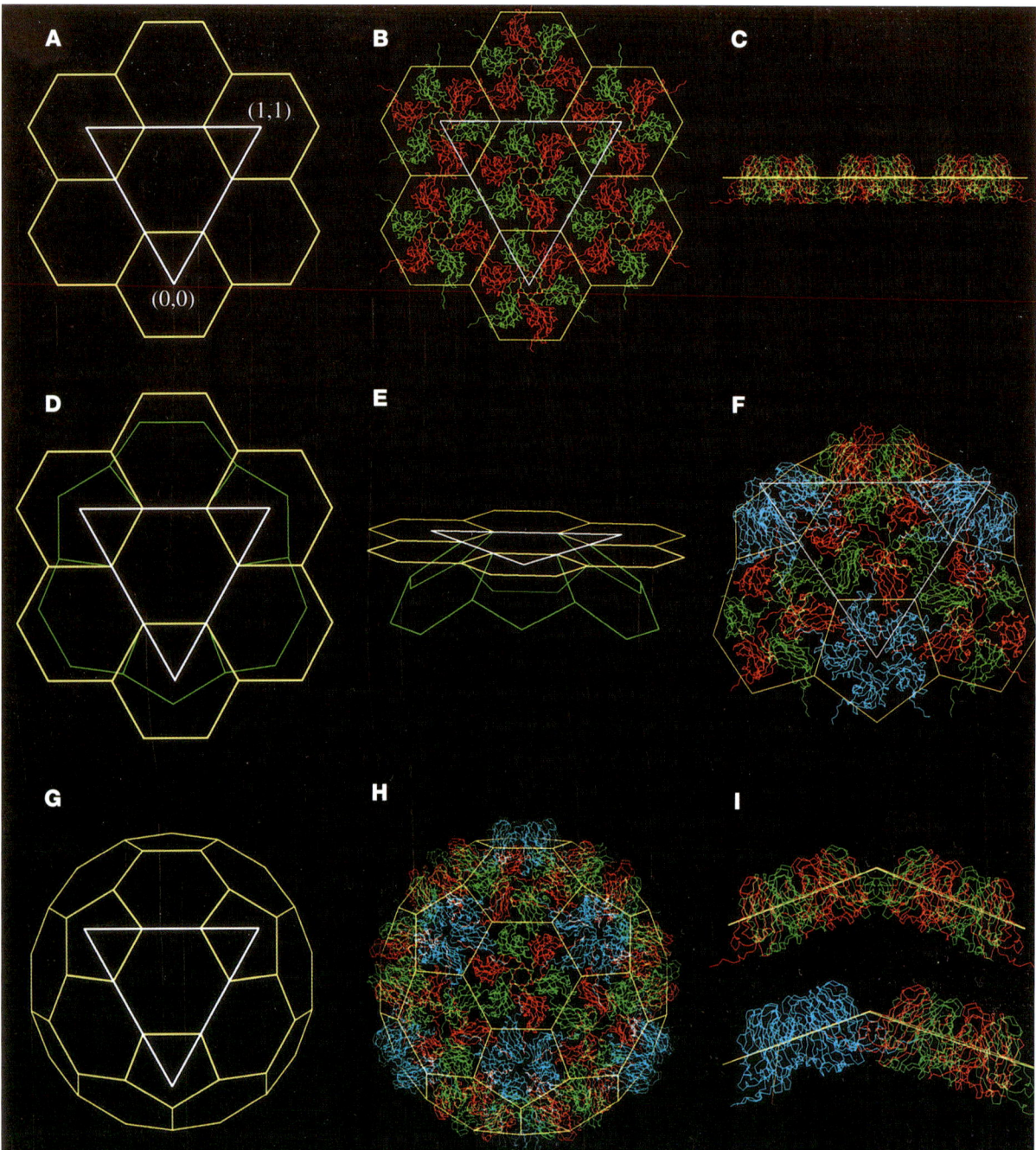

Plate 34 Molecular graphics construction of a $T = 3$ quasi-equivalent icosahedron. (**A**) Hexagonal sheet overlaid with the triangular coordinates (white) for a theoretical $T = 3$ quasi-equivalent icosahedron (**h** = 1, **k** = 1, see **Plate 33B**). The sheet has true sixfold rotational symmetry about axes passing through the hexamer centers, which are normal to the sheet. (**B**) Copies of the hexamer coordinates from the CCMV X-ray structure (colored by asymmetric unit position, see **Plate 35**) can be positioned in the sheet by simple translations. (**C**) A side view of the modeled sheet demonstrates its planarity. (**D**) Hexamers at the corners of the white (**h** = 1, **k** = 1) triangle become pentamers. The planar sheet (yellow model) takes on curvature to maintain contacts between the polygons (green model). (**E**) The magnitude of the pentamer-induced curvature is displayed in the side view of the partial polyhedron. (**F**) Coordinates of the CCMV X-ray structure fit this construction without any manipulation. (**G**) A completed $T = 3$ icosahedral model. The 12 pentamers generate curvature that closes the structure. This cage (a truncated icosahedron) accurately describes the geometric morphology of CCMV (**H**) which is composed of modular, planar pentamers (12) and hexamers (20). Angular pentamer–hexamer and hexamer–hexamer interfaces (**I**) stabilize curvature in the absence of convex pentamers used to construct the soccer ball of **Plate 33D** (see also **Plate 35**). See article **Virus Structure: Principles of Virus Structure** for more information.

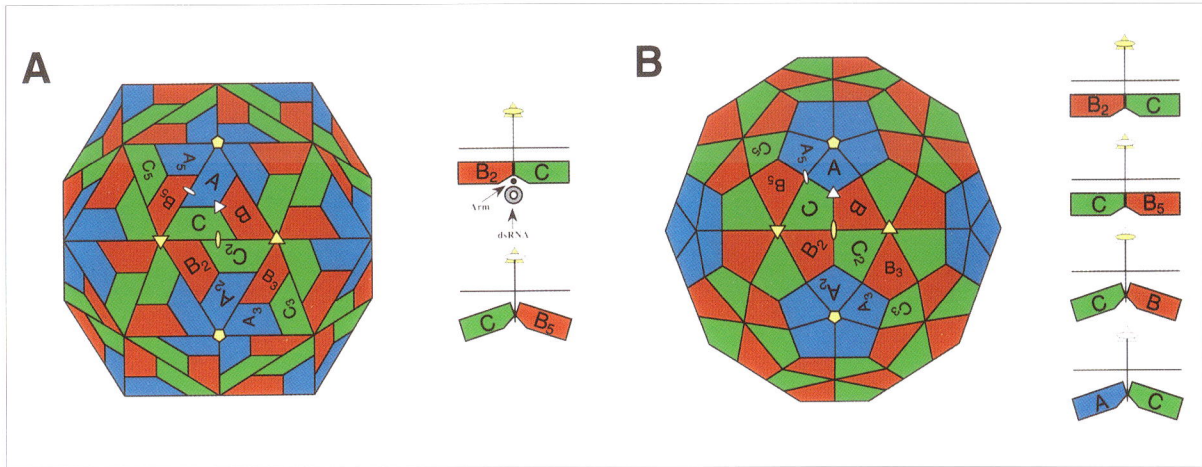

Plate 35 Although quasi-equivalence theory can predict, on geometrical principles, the organization of hexamers and pentamers in a viral capsid, the detailed arrangement of subunits can only be established empirically. High-resolution X-ray structures of $T = 3$ plant and insect viruses show that the particles are organized like the icosahedral rhombic tri-icontahedron or truncated icosahedron (**Plate 34**). A convenient definition of the icosahedral asymmetric unit for both geometrical shapes is the wedge defined by icosahedral threefold axes left and right of the particle center and an icosahedral fivefold axis at the top. The icosahedral asymmetric unit contains three subunits labeled A (blue), B (red) and C (green) (see **Plate 33C, D**). The asymmetric unit polygons represent chemically identical protein subunits that occupy slightly different geometrical (chemical) environments as indicated by differences in their coloring. Polygons with subscripts are related to A, B, and C by icosahedral symmetry (i.e. A to A_5 by fivefold rotation). The shapes of the $T = 3$ soccer ball model in **Plate 33D**, truncated icosahedron in **Plate 34** and rhombic tri-icontahedron are all different; however, the quasi-symmetric axes are in the same positions relative to the icosahedral symmetry axes for all three models. Quasi-threefold and quasi-twofold axes are represented by the white symbols. The quasi-sixfold axes are coincident with the icosahedral threefold axes in $T = 3$ particles as shown in **Plates 33 B–D** and **34**. (**A**) The rhombic tri-icontahedron is constructed by placing rhombic faces perpendicular to icosahedral twofold symmetry axes (yellow ellipse). Thus, the A, B and C polygons are coplanar within each asymmetric unit. The shape of the subunit in $T = 3$ plant and insect viruses is nearly identical to the shape of the subunit in the $T = 1$ virus and they pack in a very similar fashion. The $T = 1$ subunits in one face (**Plate 31A**) are related by an icosahedral threefold axis, while the $T = 3$ subunits in one face are related by a quasi-threefold axis. The dihedral angle between subunits C and B_5 (juxtaposed across quasi-twofold axes) is 144° and is referred to as a bent contact (bottom right image), while the dihedral angle between subunits C and B_2 (juxtaposed across icosahedral twofold axes) is 180° and is referred to as a flat contact (top right image). Two dramatically different contacts between subunits with identical amino acid sequences are generated by the insertion of an extra polypeptide from the N-terminal portion of the C subunit into the groove formed at the flat contact. This polypeptide is called an 'arm'. The flat contact can also be upheld by insertion of nucleic acid structure into the same groove. The N-terminal arms of the A and B subunits are disordered, and nucleic acid structure has not been observed in the groove across the quasi-twofold axis; thus, C and B_5 are in direct contact as in, for example, the X-ray structure of FHV. (**B**) A truncated icosahedron achieves curvature at different interfaces compared to the rhombic tri-icontahedron. Interactions between B_2–C and between C–B_5 polygons are both defined by 180° dihedral angles (side view at top right) whereas bends similar in magnitude occur within the asymmetric unit at the B–C and C–A polygon interfaces (138° and 142°, respectively; side view at bottom right). This creates the planar pentamer and hexamer morphological units characteristic of the truncated icosahedron and the CCMV X-ray structure (**Plate 34H**). See article **Virus Structure: Principles of Virus Structure** for more information.

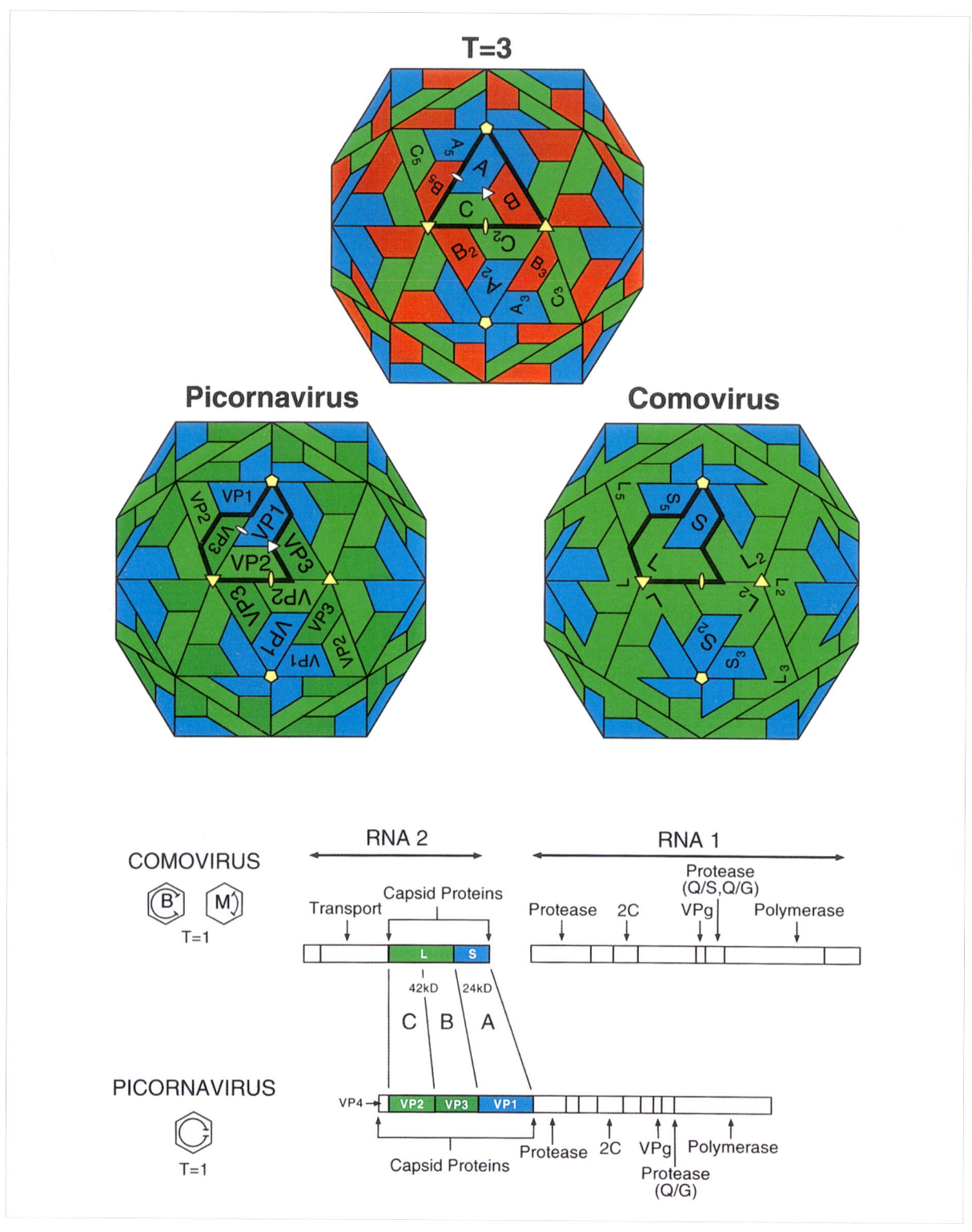

Plate 36 A comparison of $T = 3$, picornavirus and comovirus capsids. In each case, one trapezoid represents a β-barrel and the icosahedral asymmetric units are outlined in bold. The icosahedral asymmetric unit of the $T = 3$ shell contains three identical subunits labeled A, B and C (see **Plate 35**). The asymmetric unit of the picornavirus capsid contains three β-barrels, but each has a characteristic amino acid sequence labeled VP1, VP2 and VP3. The comovirus capsid is similar to the picornavirus capsid except that two of the β-barrels (corresponding to the green VP2 and VP3 units) are covalently linked to form a single polypeptide, the large protein subunit (L), while the small protein subunit (S) corresponds to VP1 (note the similar color shading). The individual subunits of the comovirus and picornavirus capsids are in identical geometrical (chemical) environments (e.g. VP1 and S are always pentamers) making these $T = 1$ capsids. Comoviruses and picornaviruses have a similar gene order, and the nonstructural 2C and polymerase genes display significant sequence homology. The relationship between the capsid subunit positions in these viruses and their location in the genes is indicated by color coding and the labels A, B and C in the gene diagram. See article **Virus Structure: Principles of Virus Structure** for more information.

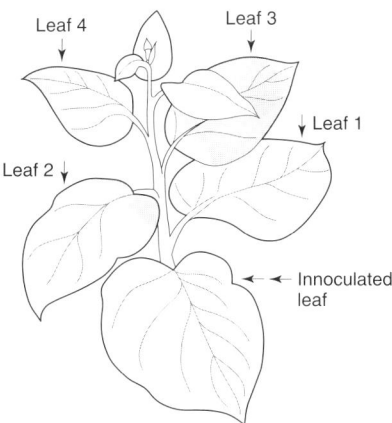

Figure 1 Diagram of a tobacco plant showing the pattern of acute phase synergism symptoms on the bottom of leaf two, all of leaf three and the tip of leaf four above the inoculated leaf. The location of acute phase symptoms is indicated by shading.

the analogous regions of plants singly infected with PVX.

Both the timing of invasion by the two viruses and the developmental state of the host are important for induction of the PVX/PVY synergistic response. PVX must enter the systemically infected cells at a time when PVY is actively replicating and expressing its viral gene products. Outside that window in time, PVX invasion does not lead to the synergistic increase in symptoms or the correlated increase in PVX accumulation. The severe symptoms on first systemically infected leaves are found in a characteristic pattern, confined to the base of the second leaf, over most of the third leaf and at the tip of the fourth leaf above the inoculated leaf (**Fig. 1**). These severely affected tissues are said to be in the acute phase of the synergistic disease. The pattern of acute phase symptoms reflects the developmental state of the plant, since all the affected tissues were at the same level of maturity at the time of viral invasion. The pattern of acute phase disease was one of the first clues that the host may play an important role in the development of synergistic disease. The fact that the timing of PVY invasion was found to be important suggests that an interaction between the potyvirus (or potyvirus gene product) with the host might play a role in mediation of the disease syndrome.

The increase in PVX accumulation in acute phase tissue is due to a change in control of PVX replication. PVX is a (+) strand RNA virus that replicates via production of a complementary RNA, the (−) strand RNA, that is used as a template for production of high levels of the genomic RNA. The genomic RNA encodes five known gene products and serves as mRNA for the 5′-proximal gene product, the 166 kDa putative replicase. The genes that are encoded internally on the genomic RNA are expressed via production of subgenomic mRNAs, each serving as mRNA for the gene encoded at their respective 5′-proximal ends. The virion is rod shaped and consists solely of the genomic RNA encapsidated by the viral coat protein. In the acute phase of PVX/PVY synergism, the levels of infectious PVX particles, PVX genomic RNA, PVX coat protein and PVX coat protein subgenomic mRNA all increase to about the same extent (3–10-fold) over that in the analogous singly infected tissues. In contrast, the level of the PVX complementary RNA, which serves as a template during replication, consistently increases to a level 3-fold above that of the virion and its component parts. Thus, the ratio of (−) strand to (+) strand PVX RNA is increased during synergism and this suggests a change in the regulation of PVX RNA replication. This change in PVX replication does not require replication of the PVY genome, and is mediated by expression of a subset of the PVY genes (see next section).

Although much of the early synergism work centered on the PVX/PVY interaction, a similar synergistic response is induced in co-infections of PVX with several other potyviruses, including the well-studied tobacco vein mottling virus (TVMV) and tobacco etch viruses (TEV). The finding that many different potyviruses could induce the same changes in host response and in PVX replication was important because it was the first hint that the role of the potyvirus in potyvirus-associated synergisms might be the same for all such diseases.

PVX/potyviral synergism is mediated by the potyviral P1/HC-Pro sequence

Two lines of evidence lead to the conclusion that PVX/potyviral synergistic disease does not require replication of the potyviral genomic RNA and that the response is mediated by expression of potyviral sequences in the 5′ proximal one-third of the potyviral genome. The first line of evidence stems from experiments using transgenic plants expressing various subsets of the potyvirus genome. Plants expressing the 5′ proximal region of either the TVMV or the TEV genomic RNA and infected singly with PVX displayed the synergistic increases in symptoms and in PVX RNA replication. These results indicate that the 5′-proximal region of the genomic RNA of either TVMV or TEV is sufficient to mediate synergistic disease.

The second line of evidence stems from experi-

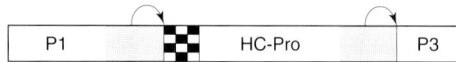

Protein	Domain	Potyvirus function	Synergism △ Replication	Synergism ↑ Symptoms
P1		Replication, polyprotein cleavage	Yes	No
HC-Pro	Zinc finger	Aphid transmission	No	No
	Central	Replication, long distance movement, pathogenicity	Yes	Yes
	Proteinase	Polyprotein cleavage	?	?

Figure 2 Diagram of the potyviral P1/HC-Pro sequence which mediates potyvirus-associated synergisms. Proteinase domains of both P1 and HC-Pro are indicated by shading, whereas the location of the cleavage site for each of these proteinases is indicated by an arrow. The amino terminal zinc finger-like domain of HC-Pro is indicated by a checkerboard pattern. The functions of the P1 and HC-Pro sequences in the potyvirus life cycle, as well as their role in synergism are indicated below the diagram.

ments using PVX as a vector to express this same region of the TEV genome (PVX-5′TEV). An infectious cDNA clone of the PVX genome was engineered to express the TEV sequence under control of a repeated coat protein subgenomic promoter. When inoculated onto tobacco, this engineered PVX induced a characteristic synergistic response with enhancement in both symptoms and in RNA replication. When used to infect tobacco tissue culture cells, expression of the potyviral sequence dramatically prolonged the accumulation of PVX (−) strand RNA over a three-day time-course experiment. This result indicates that the potyviral 5′ proximal sequence induces a synergistic change in PVX RNA replication and confirms that the region is sufficient to mediate synergistic disease.

The region of the potyviral genome that mediates synergism includes the viral genomic 5′ untranslated region (UTR) as well as the coding region for the N-terminal portion of the viral polyprotein, including P1, helper component protease (HC-Pro), and about a quarter of P3 (termed P1/HC-Pro sequence, **Fig. 2**). This region is expressed as polyprotein and subsequently processed by the proteolytic activities of both P1 and HC-Pro.

We can obtain clues for how HC-Pro and P1 might mediate synergism by examining the functions they perform in the TEV infection process (**Fig. 2**). Both HC-Pro and P1 are multifunctional proteins. P1 has proteinase activity that cleaves the potyviral polyprotein, creating the C-terminus of P1 and the N-terminus of HC-Pro. P1 also functions in *trans* as an accessory factor for genome replication and has RNA binding activity. One possibility is that P1 plays a direct role in synergism, perhaps analogous to its role as an accessory factor in TEV replication. Alternatively, it might enhance synergism only indirectly by producing the authentic HC-Pro N-terminus by means of its proteinase activity.

HC-Pro has at least three functional domains: an N-terminal domain required for aphid transmission; a central domain involved in pathogenicity, RNA replication, and leaf-to-leaf movement of the virus through the phloem; and a C-terminal domain required for autoproteolytic processing of the HC-Pro C-terminus. The central domain of HC-Pro is of particular interest because it is involved in the regulation of both pathogenicity and RNA replication of potyviruses, and these are the characteristics that are altered in PVX during synergism.

The potyviral P1/HC-Pro sequence also mediates other potyvirus-associated diseases

The finding that transgenic plants expressing the P1/HC-Pro region of the potyviral genome develop synergistic disease when infected with PVX raised the possibility that many or all potyvirus-associated synergisms might be mediated by this same sequence. To test this hypothesis, two other viruses, tobacco mosaic virus (TMV) and cucumber mosaic virus (CMV), were used to infect transgenic tobacco line U-6B, which expresses the P1/HC-Pro region of the TEV genome. Both viruses can infect tobacco and are known to interact synergistically with a potyvirus. TMV and CMV are both (+) strand RNA viruses in the alphavirus supergroup; however, CMV has a tripartite genome, and many strains also support replication of an associated satellite RNA, whereas the genome of TMV, like that of PVX, is monopartite. The transgenic plants expressing the potyvirus P1/HC-Pro sequence displayed the enhanced symptoms characteristic of synergism when infected singly with either TMV or CMV. **Figure 3** shows enhanced symptoms of PVX, CMV and TMV in the U-6B plants as compared to those in nontransgenic control plants. At the molecular level, infection of the U-6B transgenic resulted in increased accumulation of the genomic RNAs of both of these heterologous viruses. Thus, the response of TMV and CMV to expression of the potyvirus P1/HC-Pro sequence is similar to that previously shown for PVX.

Because both TMV and CMV are capable of

inducing synergistic disease in mixed infections with a member of the potyvirus group, this result supports the hypothesis that all such potyvirus-associated synergistic diseases, which occur in an evolutionarily diverse range of host plants and involve interactions with a large number of viral groups, are mediated by the same potyviral sequence. The fact that expression of this sequence alters disease induction by each of these unrelated heterologous viruses suggests that it affects a step in viral infection that is common to all of these viruses and thus of general significance.

Identification of functional domains within the P1/HC-Pro sequence

The role of P1/HC-Pro in synergism could be mediated by the entire P1/HC-Pro region, either the RNA itself, or the encoded polyprotein. Alternately, the response could be mediated by a part of the RNA sequence or one or a subset of the encoded proteins. Three complementary approaches have been used to delineate the domains of P1/HC-Pro that function in potyviral synergism. The first approach was to use transgenic plants expressing mutant versions of the P1/HC-Pro sequence. Six transgenic lines, three with mutations within the P1 coding region and three with mutations within the HC-Pro coding region, were infected with PVX to assay the ability of the mutant transgene to induce synergism. The three lines with mutations within the P1 coding region all maintained the ability to mediate the synergistic response to PVX. In contrast, two out of three of the mutations within the HC-Pro coding region failed to induce synergistic disease. Both mutations that interfered with the ability to cause synergism were located within the region encoding the central domain of HC-Pro. This result established the importance of the HC-Pro central domain for induction of PVX/potyviral synergistic disease.

A second approach was to use mixed inoculation experiments with a mutant version of TEV. Plants were co-inoculated with PVX and TEV-del-2, a spontaneous deletion mutation of TEV in which the first 65 amino acids of HC-Pro are missing, and assayed for synergistic disease. The mutant TEV interacted with PVX to produce synergistic disease indistinguishable from that produced by mixed infection with wild-type TEV. This result showed that the amino-terminal 65 amino acids of HC-Pro, encoding a zinc-finger-like domain required for aphid transmission of the potyvirus, are dispensable for induction of PVX/TEV synergism.

Although the first two approaches established some sequences required in the induction of synergism, they

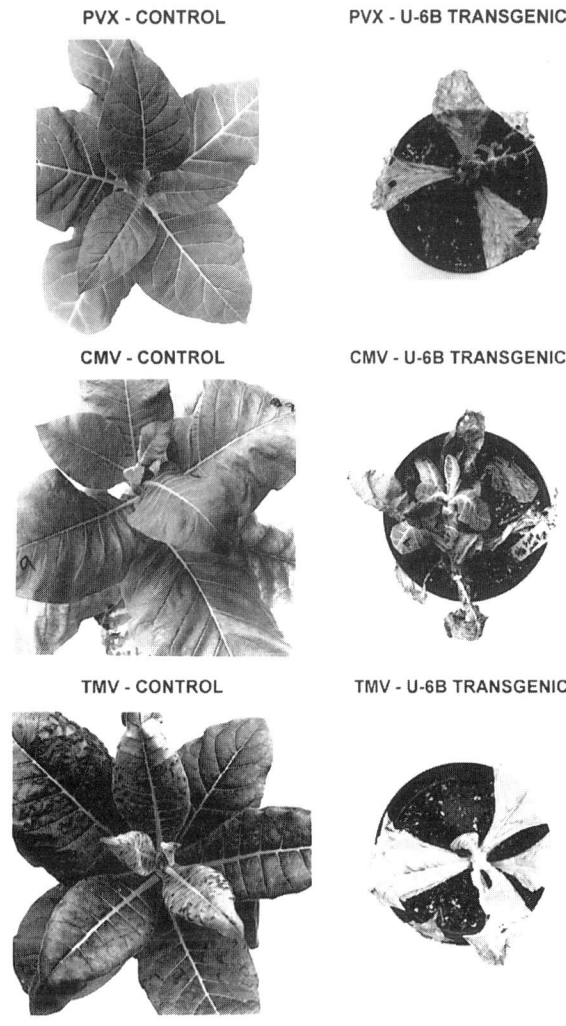

Figure 3 Enhanced pathogenicity of PVX, CMV and TMV in transgenic tobacco expressing high levels of the P1/HC-Pro sequence. The left hand column shows nontransformed tobacco plants infected with PVX (top row), CMV (middle row) or TMV (bottom row). The right hand column shows infection of the P1/HC-Pro expressing transgenic line U-6B infected with the same set of viruses.

did not establish the minimal sequence required for the response. The third approach was to use PVX as a vector to express various parts of the P1/HC-Pro sequence and then assay the engineered viruses for the ability to cause disease symptoms and the change in PVX replication characteristic of synergism. This approach revealed that the HC-Pro protein was both necessary and sufficient to cause the synergistic increase in host symptoms. In contrast the synergistic enhancement of PVX replication required both P1 and HC-Pro. This result suggests that the synergistic increase in symptoms and in PVX replication, although correlated in mixed infections, may be mediated via different pathways.

Possible mechanisms for potyviral-associated synergism

Potyviral-associated synergisms result in increases in both the accumulation of the nonpotyvirus of the synergistic pair of viruses and in the host symptoms. In the case of PVX/potyviral synergism, these two aspects of the synergistic disease are mediated by different functional domains of the P1/HC-Pro sequence, possibly reflecting action via different pathways. The central domain of HC-Pro is required for both enhanced replication and enhanced symptoms. Since this region of HC-Pro has been shown to prolong replication of the potyvirus in plants and because expression of P1/HC-Pro also prolongs PVX (−) strand RNA accumulation in tobacco culture cells, it is possible that the basis of potyvirus-associated synergism is the ability of HC-Pro to prolong replication not only of potyviruses, but also of a broad range of heterologous viruses.

Although it has been shown that P1/HC-Pro acts to alter replication of PVX, the possibility that the potyviral sequence also facilitates viral movement has not been ruled out. In fact, because the central domain of HC-Pro is required for both movement and replication of the potyvirus and the same domain is also required for the synergistic effect on PVX, a role in movement in addition to the role in replication remains quite possible.

The TEV P1/HC-Pro sequence mediates synergistic disease during infection by viruses from three different groups (PVX, potexvirus; TMV, tobamovirus; CMV, cucumovirus). Therefore, it has been proposed that synergism may occur via an indirect mechanism involving an interaction of the TEV-encoded proteins with one or more host factors common to the different viral infections rather than a direct mechanism involving interactions with different RNAs or proteins from three heterologous viruses.

Two different indirect mechanisms could explain transactivation of viral replication by P1/HC-Pro. The TEV sequence might augment viral replication by enhancing the synthesis, activity or availability of a host factor that affects both TEV and the heterologous viruses in a positive way. It has been shown that host factors may be used as part of the virus replication machinery in plant cells. However, there is no evidence for host factors that act as general positive regulators of virus replication.

Alternatively, the potyviral sequence might interfere with the activity or availability of a negative regulator of viral replication, perhaps part of a host defense system that normally limits the viral infection. Post-transcriptional gene silencing has recently been proposed to act as a general defense system against plant viruses and this system is a candidate for a defense system impacted by P1/HC-Pro. In one post-transcriptional gene silencing model, an RNA targeting system is activated by high level expression of a particular RNA sequence, such as an invading virus. Once activated, the system rapidly destroys the RNA target in a sequence specific manner. The same cellular system is also thought to be involved in post-transcriptional gene silencing of nonviral transgenes in plants. In the case of plant viral synergism, the P1/HC-Pro sequence might interfere with the induction or the action of the post-transcriptional silencing pathway and thus allow a broad range of viruses to overstep the normal host imposed limits of RNA accumulation.

Nonpotyviral Synergisms

A number of plant viral synergisms which do not involve a member of the potyvirus group have been reported (Table 2); however, in contrast to the potyvirus-associated synergisms, none of these nonpotyviral synergisms have been well characterized at the molecular level. Probably the best studied of the nonpotyviral synergisms is the interaction of TMV and PVX, which causes the synergistic disease in tomatoes called double streak. This synergistic interaction has been reported to result in an increase in the level of PVX in doubly infected plants. One possibility is that the nonpotyvirus synergisms are mediated by expression of a subset of one viral genome, in a manner similar to that shown for the PVX/potyviral synergism. Interestingly, a high proportion of the nonpotyviral synergisms involve TMV as one member of the pair of interacting viruses, and this raises the possibility that the TMV genome includes a synergism sequence similar in function to the potyviral P1/HC-Pro sequence.

See also: **Vectors: Plant viruses; Potexviruses; Potyviruses (*Potyviridae*).**

Table 2 Nonpotyviral synergisms

Virus pair	
Tobacco mosaic virus	Potato virus X
Tobacco mosaic virus	Cucumber mosaic virus
	Tobacco ringspot virus
Tobacco mosaic virus	Tomato aspermy virus
Cowpea chlorotic mottle virus	Southern bean mosaic virus
Alfalfa mosaic virus	Potato acuba virus

Further Reading

Bennett CW (1953) Interactions between viruses and virus strains. *Adv. Virus Res.* 1: 39.

Dodds JA and Hamilton RI (1976) Structural interactions between viruses as a consequence of mixed infections. *Adv. Virus Res.* 20: 33.

Kassanis B (1963) Interactions of viruses in plants. *Adv. Virus Res.* 10: 219.

Matthews REF (1991) *Plant Virology*, 3rd edn. San Diego, CA: Academic Press.

Rochow WF (1972) The role of mixed infections in the transmission of plant viruses by aphids. *Annu. Rev. Phytopathol.* 10: 101.

Ross AF (1957) Responses of plants to concurrent infection by two or more viruses. *Trans. NY Acad. Sci.* 19: 236.

T1-LIKE PHAGES (*SIPHOVIRIDAE*)

JR Christensen, Rochester, New York, USA

Copyright © 1999 Academic Press

Natural History

T1 is one of the seven phages collected by Delbrück and renamed T1 through T7; they all make clear-centered plaques on *Escherichia coli* B. T1 is unrelated to any of the others. Its latent period at 37°C is 13 minutes, and the burst size is about 100. T1 also infects some other laboratory strains of *E. coli* (e.g. K-12 and C) and *Shigella dysenteriae*. Out of 290 clinical isolates of *E. coli*, T1 could replicate in two and kill a third without producing phage.

T1's best-known relative is the *Shigella* phage, D20, with which it readily hybridizes. T1-like phages can be isolated from sewage, but none has received much study. Among laboratory strains of T1, there are a few minor differences, revealed by restriction analysis.

The virion is highly stable in the dry state, so that careless technique may cause T1 (like other phages with this property) to become airborne in the laboratory, and to unexpectedly lyse cultures contaminated accidentally.

The Virion

In the electron microscope, T1 closely resembles lambda, with a polyhedral head about 55–60 nm across, and a long, flexible tail about 7×150 nm. Fifteen virion proteins have been recognized. One of these, P7, accounts for about 50% of the total protein, and two additional proteins for another 35%.

The genomic molecule is double-stranded DNA with approximately 48 500 bp. Only the four conventional bases are present. About 0.2% of the cytosine residues and 1.7% of the adenine residues are methylated, at the 5 and 6 positions, respectively. The DNA molecule includes a terminal redundancy of about 2800 ± 530 bp (6%), so that the coding capacity is about 46 000 base pairs. Because of the way the genome is packaged during morphogenesis (see below), there is a limited set of cyclic permutations of the nucleotide sequence within a population of virions.

Early Events in Infection

Adsorption of T1 is a two-step process: an initial, reversible interaction with an outer membrane-spanning protein coded by *fhuA (tonA)*, followed by an irreversible interaction involving the *tonB*-coded protein and energy provided by bacterial metabolism.

The exterior loops of FhuA serve as receptor for a variety of ligands, including several iron compounds, phages T1, T5 and ϕ80, and colicin M. Mutation studies indicate that the various ligands bind to non-identical but partially overlapping portions of FhuA.

It has been proposed that TonB serves to transmit inner-membrane energy to FhuA, altering its conformation, and allowing T1 infection (and the transport of certain other ligands, including ϕ80) to proceed. However, a possibly different role for TonB during T1 infection has been proposed (see below). T5 does not require TonB activity, nor indeed does a host-range mutant of T1, T1*hr*.

During the first 1–2 min after infection, there are marked changes in the membrane properties and in the energy state of the bacterium: there is a large efflux of K^+, the proton motive force (PMF) decreases, but does not vanish, and intracellular ATP levels fall, due to the activity of the proton-translocating ATPase. Those transport systems driven by ATP or by the PMF are inhibited, but the activity of the sugar phosphotransferase systems is stimulated. None of these changes requires phage gene activity.

During this same period of time, entry of phage DNA into the cell and shut-off of host protein synthesis occur. A model that puts these observations together has been proposed (though there is some dispute about it): preinfection, at least two cation gradients contribute strongly to the energized state of the membrane – K^+ is higher inside the cell, and H^+ is higher outside. The entry of T1 DNA is effected by a proton symport that involves *tonB*. This process tends to deplete the PMF, but partial activity is maintained by H^+ efflux, driven partially by ATP hydrolysis and partially by K^+ symport. The resulting fall in intracellular ATP leads to a fall in GTP. This, and perhaps other changes in the intracellular ionic environment, produces an inhibition of translation of host proteins at the initiation level. (Presumably the translation of phage proteins is resistant to these changes.)

Within a few minutes, a 'resealing' process occurs, although it is not clear that the membrane is restored exactly to its original condition. Resealing and the continued maintenance of the remaining level of the PMF are necessary for the infectious process to continue.

Another early event is the appearance of a phage-coded DNA methyl transferase. Although the specificity of this enzyme is identical to the host's *dam* enzyme, it is quite distinct in other enzymological properties, and T1 DNA shows no hybridization to that of the cloned host gene. The phage-coded enzyme almost totally methylates the adenines occurring within 5'-GATC sequences, even when the phage is grown in *dam* mutants. The biological role of this methylation is unclear.

Transcription

T1 depends on the host RNA polymerase for transcription throughout its cycle. Both early and late, all or nearly all transcripts are read from the same strand of DNA. All major regions of the genome are transcribed early, but there is a relative shift at later times towards the regions coding for virion proteins. The basis for the shift remains unknown. Considerable transcription (but not translation) of host genes continues after infection.

Protein Synthesis

The synthesis of 31 phage-coded proteins has been documented in infected cells. From their combined molecular weights, these account for about 80% of the coding capacity of the genome. Five temporal patterns of synthesis have been noted: proteins synthesized only early; only late; continuously but at a declining rate; continuously and steadily; continuously and at an increasing rate. As with the synthesis of host proteins, much of this regulation is probably at the transitional level.

DNA Synthesis

Among virulent, double-stranded DNA phages, T1 is unusual in that is depends on the *polC*-coded α subunit of Pol III for DNA synthesis. This is a property typical of temperate phages. It also depends on most of the other host-coded proteins involved in the elongation phase of DNA synthesis, except for *dnaB*, but does not require host proteins involved in the initiation of DNA synthesis.

Host DNA synthesis is stopped very early in infection. This inhibition requires protein synthesis, presumably for the expression of a phage gene, but the gene responsible has not been identified.

Two sets of phage genes are required for DNA synthesis. Mutants in genes 1 and 2 are totally defective in DNA synthesis. Presumably, the products of these genes function in initiation of synthesis on T1 templates. The continuing function of both of these genes is required throughout the growth cycle. Lysis of the host is delayed after infection by these mutants, but most phage-coded proteins are produced normally.

Two other genes, 3.5 and 4, encode a recombination function called Grn (for general *r*ecombi*n*ation – pronounced 'green'). This function is obligatory for phage production (see below) but, once expressed, it becomes progressively dispensable as the infection proceeds. Under some conditions, the host's RecE or lambda's Red recombination system can substitute, at least partially, for Grn. Evidence suggests that gene 4 encodes an exonuclease, but no such enzyme has been isolated.

Early in infection, the products of DNA synthesis are linear, monomeric molecules. Later, under the influence of Grn, linear, concatameric molecules are produced; these have a broad distribution of sizes up to about 8- to 10-mers, presumably produced mainly by 'head-to-tail' recombination between homologous redundant ends on two molecules. In the total absence of Grn function, no concatamers are found, and DNA synthesis ceases prematurely, about 6 min into the infection. Why synthesis stops under these conditions is not clear, particularly since, once Grn has been expressed, synthesis of both monomers and concatamers continues even though further Grn activity is blocked. In the total absence of Grn, the cells lyse at the normal time, but no phage are released.

As with other virulent phages, T1 infection leads to degradation of the host's DNA. The liberated material provided about two-thirds of the precursors for the synthesis of T1 DNA. Mutants in gene 2.5 are deficient in host DNA breakdown, but phage DNA synthesis proceeds normally.

However, while phage DNA synthesis can proceed

in the absence of host breakdown, the converse is not true. In T1 there is an unusual functional dependence of the degradation of host DNA upon ongoing synthesis of phage DNA. If phage DNA synthesis is prevented, whether by use of mutants or of naladixic acid, degradation of host DNA does not occur. If degradation has already begun, and a synthesis block is imposed, degradation stops. Thus, no conditions have been found under which free degradation products can be detected. With T4 and other virulent phages that have been studied, if phage DNA synthesis is blocked, host DNA degradation nevertheless occurs, with released materials leaking into the medium.

Morphogenesis

Relatively little is known about the pathways of T1 capsid assembly. Some virion proteins, including P7, are cleaved from larger precursors, as occurs during capsid assembly with several other phages. Mature, DNA-filled heads can join to tails and form infectious particles *in vitro*.

More is known about the manner in which DNA becomes encapsidated. Linear genomic concatamers are the substrate for packaging. The process is initiated at a site called *pac*, located between gene 1 and gene 2 on the map, and processive head-filling proceeds toward gene 1 (leftward, as the map is conventionally represented). As mentioned above, a 'headful' is about 1.06 genomes worth of DNA. Only two or three particles are produced from a single initiation event, so that a limited set of cyclic permutations is produced. Thus, about 18% of the genome will, in some of the particles, be represented twice, once at each end of the packaged DNA molecule.

A mutation, *pip,* located between markers in genes 2.5 and 3 (and which likely represents a separate gene), has a marked influence on DNA packaging. If the host happens to be a lambda lysogen, T1*pip* has an enhanced frequency of initiating packaging 'mistakenly' at a site, *esp-λ*, located on the lambda prophage (see Transduction, below). The *pip* mutant is also deficient in processive packaging, so that almost all of the packaged molecules are initiated at *pac* even though, judging by the small burst size, the efficiency of initiation at *pac* is probably reduced by the mutation.

Mutants in most of the genes involved in head production are grossly defective in processing concatameric DNA to monomeric DNA, suggesting that nearly-complete head structures are required for the maturing of concatamers into monomeric 'headfuls'. However, mutants in gene 12 process concatamers normally, though they do not produce heads; presumably they fill DNA normally into head precursors that are unstable due to the lack of the gene 12 product. Finally, *am*383, the sole mutant in gene 13.3, which maps in the head region and encodes a virion protein, is only partially defective in processing concatamers. It is not clear whether this mutation is phenotypically 'leaky', or whether this observation points to some special role for this gene in DNA packaging.

Extracts, prepared from cells infected with T1 bearing amber mutations in both gene 1 and gene 2, are capable of packaging either homologous or heterologous DNA added *in vitro*. Two packaging pathways have been identified.

If the extract is given homologous DNA extracted from virions of T1 (or T1-like phages), it produces phage. Presumably, the pathway involves two steps: the production of concatamers, via recombination, followed by packaging, initiated at *pac*.

Given heterologous DNA extracted from T3, T7 or lambda *nin*, all of which are about 80% the length of T1 DNA and lack any known *pac*-like sites (*esp-λ* is in the *nin* region), the extract produces the corresponding phage by a *pac*-independent pathway. DNA from wild-type lambda is packaged less efficiently than that from lambda *nin*, suggesting that the second pathway prefers shorter molecules. (The first pathway does not act on wild-type lambda DNA, despite the presence of *esp-λ*, as there are no redundant ends to facilitate concatamer formation.)

Mutants and Maps

The current genetic map (**Fig. 1**) contains 23 essential genes, identified by complementation tests between conditional-lethal mutants, and the nonessential gene 2.5, identified by *tar* mutants (which enhance transduction frequency). These are in numerical order, with fractional gene numbers for those genes identified since the first 18 genes were mapped.

At the left end are the genes discussed above: 1, 2, 2.5, 3.5 and 4, as well as *pac* and *pip*, all of which have roles in DNA metabolism. Curiously, also within this cluster is gene 3, which has no role in DNA metabolism – rather it is essential for tail formation. Perhaps it has a regulatory role, rather than coding for a virion protein.

Next come eight more genes, 5 through 11.5, that are required for the production of phage tails. The *hr* mutation, which allows T1 to infect *tonB* (but not *fhuA*) mutant bacteria, maps just to the left of the available gene 5 markers, and may be within that gene. Finally come ten genes, 12 through 18, required for the production of phage heads. Probably there are at most a very few undiscovered head or tail genes, judging from the number present in the morphologically similar phage, lambda.

Several tail and head genes, plus the *pac* region, have been cloned in the positive selection vector, pLV59. These clones, which together include about one-third of the total genome, have allowed a comparison of the genetic and physical maps (**Fig. 1**). Genetic markers are relatively far apart at both ends, but especially so at the left end. The occurrence of 'head-to-tail' recombination during concatamer formation would be expected to increase genetic distances between markers at the map ends (this does not mean that the genetic map is 'wrong', merely that it represents a different kind of information). But this effect will not be found to the right of *pac*, and so the wide genetic distances between markers in the region form gene 2 to gene 5 cannot be due to this effect. It is almost certain, however, that more genes remain to be discovered, particularly genes for nonessential functions, as these will not be discovered in collections of conditional lethal mutants. Unless these nonessential genes are scattered among the head and tail genes, which seems highly implausible, their likely location is in the leftward portion of the map.

Restriction and Modification

T1 passes freely among such *E. coli* strains as B, K-12 and C, so it is not subject to either B or K restriction. At one time it was felt that the high level of methylation of T1 DNA might account for this, but as 5'-GATC sequences are the main sequence methylated (at least, the total level of adenine methylation is consistent with the number of such sequences that might be expected on a genome of T1's size), and as this sequence is not part of the recognition sequence for either the B or K restriction enzyme, this seems unlikely.

However, in P1 lysogens, T1 grown in a nonlysogen is subject to restriction and modification; P1-modified T1 plates with full efficiency on both lysogens and nonlysogens. When unmodified T1 infects a lysogen, about 80% of phage DNA is degraded and excreted into the medium within 5 min. After this, degradation stops, and several

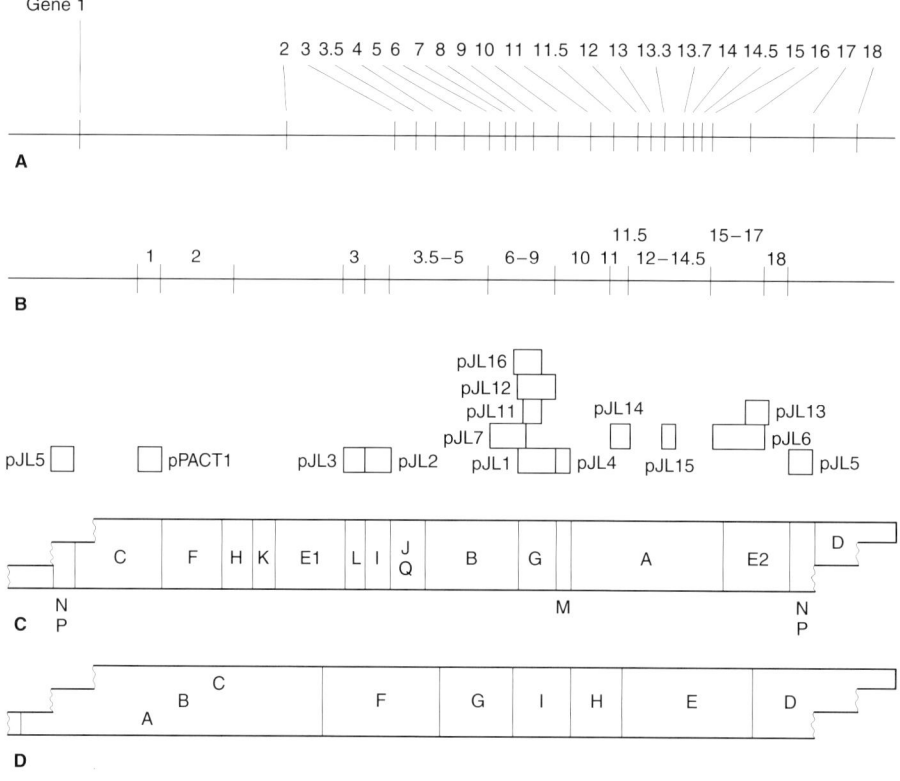

Figure 1 Genetic and physical maps of T1. (**A**) The genetic map, with each gene identified by the *am* or *ts* mutant used to map the gene. (**B**) Positions of the T1 genes on the DNA molecule. Each interval represents the outer limits of the regions occupied by the *am* mutant tested, relative to the physical map below. (**C**) Locations of the T1 cloned fragments relative to the physical map. (**D**) Physical map of T1 DNA with the *Bgl*II (upper) and *Bgl*I (lower) cleavage sites. (Reprinted, with permission, from Liebeschuetz J, Harris RD and Ritchie DA (1987) *J. Gen. Virol.* 68: 2049–2052.)

observations indicate that biologically active fragments of the restricted genome persist in the lysogenic cells for a considerable period of time.

Complementation occurs in 10–25% of the cells when unmodified T1*am* + *hr* and modified T1*amhr* + phage coinfect lysogens. This is true for most of the genes tested but not all. Most of the progeny phage are *amhr* +, so this is not primarily due to marker rescue, though that also occurs (see below). Complementing activity is but little diminished when infection by the modified phage comes 4, or even 9, minutes after infection by the unmodified one.

In co-infection experiments that use plaque-morphology markers to distinguish modified from unmodified phage (no complementation required), recombinational rescue of the alleles of the unmodified parent occurs in a few percent of the cells. Certain markers are rescued more frequently than others are. In three-factor crosses, usually only a single marker is rescued in a given cell. The alleles of the nonmodified phage remain available for rescue for at least 10 min.

In addition, under special conditions, unmodified T1 alone can successfully infect lysogens. The required conditions are high multiplicity of infection (about 10), strong aeration in nutrient medium, and occurrence of protein synthesis during the first few minutes after infection. (These special conditions are not required for the phenomena described above.) Up to 10% of the cells produce phage; this is called cooperative infection. The progeny phage are mostly modified, and they have undergone extensive recombination. Again, dividing the infecting phage into two portions, with up to 6 min intervening, does not interfere with cooperation.

Finally, among the rare (c. 1 in 10^4) lysogens that do yield phage after infection by a single, unmodified T1, individual cells lyse and produce their progeny (most of which are unmodified) over a period of 3–5 h.

Transduction

In common with other phage that package DNA by a headful mechanism, T1 is a generalized transducing phage. To demonstrate this, it is necessary to use T1*am* phage (typically a double *am* stock), permissive donors and nonpermissive recipients; otherwise, potential transductants are killed on the assay plate by the large excess of viable, virulent phage in the transducing lysate. The fact that, for a given marker, transduction frequencies are quite reproducible from experiment to experiment makes T1 a good subject for studying various aspects of the transduction process.

Although all markers tested can be transduced, the frequency of transduction varies widely among different markers. It appears likely that packaging of bacterial DNA can be initiated at many sites in the chromosome that mimic, to varying degrees, T1's *pac* site. This idea is strengthened by the discovery of two specific sites that have a special property: markers to one side of the site, but not the other, are transduced at high frequency; this is what would be expected of transductional 'pick-up' initiated at a *pac*-like site. One of these, *esp*, is located between *att-λ* and *gal* on the bacterial chromosome. From this site, *bio* (but not *gal*) markers in nonlysogens, or lambda plaque-forming units (PFUs) in lysogens, are transduced at relatively high frequency. The second site, *esp-λ*, is within lambda, between genes P and Q, and from this site, PFUs are readily transduced from polylysogens. Experiments with tandem heteroimmune dilysogens show that packaging proceeds leftward from this site. While initiation of packaging at *pac*-like sites probably contributes greatly to T1 transduction, *pac*-independent packaging of heterologous DNA can occur *in vitro* (see above), and a similar process may be involved in the transduction of low-frequency markers.

Small plasmids can also be transduced. The frequency is markedly enhanced by cloning *pac* or *esp-λ* into the plasmid. Transducing particles carry head-to-tail multimers of plasmid DNA; perhaps Grn can stimulate circle-into-circle recombination.

The phage-induced degradation of host DNA would be expected to compete with transduction. It does: most of the transducing particles are formed early in the infectious cycle, and *tar* mutations (gene 2.5), which block degradation, enhance the formation of transducing particles.

See also: **Coliphage lambda (*Siphoviridae*).**

Further Reading

Drexler H (1988) Bacteriophage T1. In: Calendar R (ed.) *The Bacteriophages*, vol. 1, p. 235. New York: Plenum Press.

Figurski DH and Christensen JR (1974) Functional characteristics of the genes of bacteriophage T1. *Virology* 59: 397.

Liebescheutz J, Harris RD and Ritchie DA (1987) Further characterization of phage T1 DNA clones. *J. Gen. Virol.* 68: 2049.

Wagner EF, Auer B and Schweiger M (1983) *Escherichia coli* virus T1: genetic control during viral infection. *Curr. Top. Microbiol. Immunol.* 102: 131.

T4-LIKE PHAGES (*MYOVIRIDAE*)

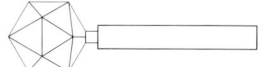

Gisela Mosig, Department of Molecular Biology, Vanderbilt University, Nashville, Tennessee, USA

Copyright © 1999 Academic Press

History and Overview

Bacteriophages T2, T4 and T6 were among the seven *Escherichia coli* phages ('Snow White and the Seven Dwarfs') selected by Max Delbrück to study fundamentals of viral replication. T2, T4 and T6, which are serologically related are called the 'T-even' phages. The genomes of these phages are contained in large (~170 000 bp) linear, double-stranded (ds) DNA molecules, whose termini contain repetitions of 3–5% of the genome, and are randomly permuted over circular maps (**Fig. 1**). The DNA molecules are packaged in elongated 'heads' of quasi-icosahedral symmetry. The heads are connected to tails whose baseplates and attached tail fibers (**Fig. 2**) are instrumental for recognition, adsorption and injection of the DNA into host bacteria. Differences in the tail fiber regions are important for recognition of different receptors in different host strains, which can be used to distinguish different members of the T-even family.

Since the early days of phage research, many phages from different parts of the world have been classified to belong to this family, based on similar genomic organization, regulatory patterns and sequence similarity of their 'essential' genes and on the presence of hydroxymethylcytosine (HMC) instead of cytosine in their DNA. The HMC residues are glycosylated to different extents in different members of the family. The essential roles of these modifications for the developmental strategy of these phages are discussed below (Restriction-Modification and Exclusion).

T-even phages are some of the most successful molecular parasites. Like all viruses, they depend for their propagation on many vital structures and functions of their hosts, e.g. membranes, energy metabolism, transcriptional and translational machines, and they manage to subvert host functions gradually to their own purposes in an exquisite choreography that allows adaptations to different environmental conditions, including different physiological states of the host. In contrast to many other viruses, they encode their own DNA replication, recombination and repair functions, making them particularly suitable for the study of these fundamental biological processes.

The gradual subversion of host functions to phage propagation is achieved at several interconnected levels:

1. A cascade of phage-induced proteins modifies the host RNA polymerase and its accessory proteins (sigma factors) covalently and noncovalently. These modifications together ultimately turn off all host transcription, and allow timed initiation of transcription from different classes of phage promoters and selective processivity of RNA polymerase on HMC-containing DNA.
2. There are no known T4 transcriptional repressors, but RNA processing by phage and host enzymes, translational repressors and still poorly understood modifications of ribosomes modulate T4 gene expression. Translational modulation is thought to be particularly suitable for physiological adjustments during the rapid development of T-even phages: one growth cycle is finished in less than 30 min at 37°C.
3. The host DNA and host mRNA, present at the time of infection, are rapidly degraded, and the breakdown products are efficiently reused to synthesize phage DNA and RNA.
4. The onset of the first phage DNA replication from specific origins requires host RNA polymerase to generate primers and is thereby connected to physiological regulatory processes of the host. Most subsequent initiations of replication forks depend on DNA primers in intermediates of recombination and on phage-encoded recombination proteins, which are entirely phage controlled.
5. During the later stages of development, DNA packaging proteins compete with replication–recombination proteins for the intracellular phage DNA, thereby coordinating replication and packaging.

These processes are interconnected at several levels. For example, late transcription depends on DNA replication, and in turn influences synthesis of and competitions between recombination, replication and packaging proteins. Together with multiple redundant pathways for these processes, the crossconnections allow a flexible development, which is the recipe for the success of the T-even phages.

Most of the recent work with T-even phages has

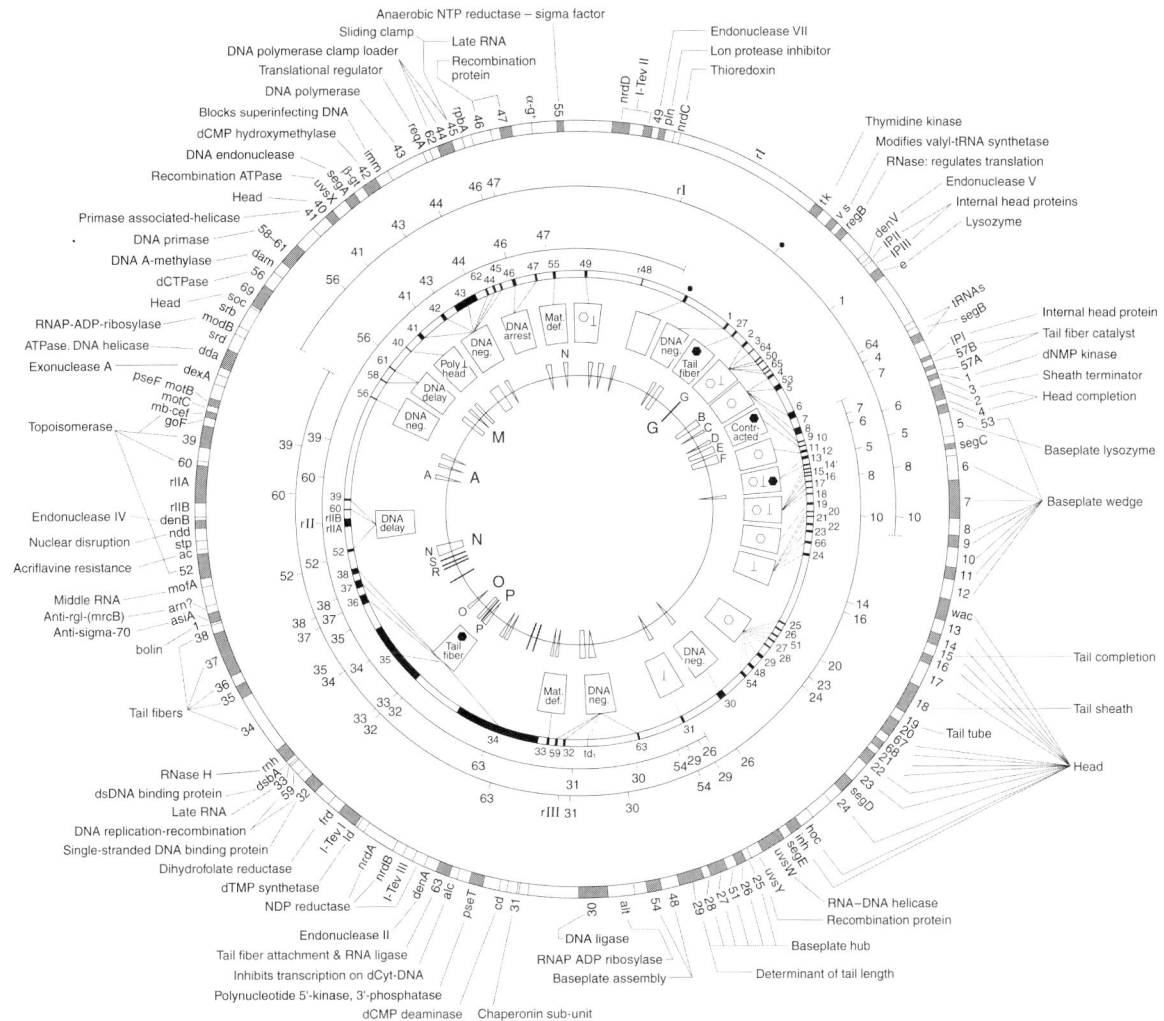

Figure 1 Comparison of several maps of T4 genes. The outermost circle shows the map of known genes and origins of replication, based on the DNA sequence. The next three overlapping circular segments drawn as thin lines show the positions of the indicated genes based on the probability of cutting ends during packaging between these genes and reference markers in rI, rII and rIII. The next circle shows the position of these genes based on recombination frequencies. The rectangles depict mutant phenotypes. The innermost circles represent the heteroduplex loops between T2 and T4 DNA. The substitution loop M is aligned with gene 69 in the outer circle.

been concentrated on T4, mainly because the isolation of a large collection of conditional lethal mutants has provided a powerful impetus for molecular analyses by biochemical and biophysical methods.

Genome Structure and Map

The genome of T4 resides in about 168 000 bp of double-stranded DNA containing glucosylated HMC residues. Using genetic tricks, phage mutants with unmodified cytosine-containing DNA can be isolated. Their DNA has been instrumental in cloning and sequencing the T4 genome.

Mature DNA molecules (chromosomes), packaged into virions, are linear and contain 3–5% of the genome as terminal redundancies at both ends. In contrast, intracellular replicating DNA is highly branched and contains multiple covalently linked (head to tail) copies of the genome. These structures are called 'concatemers'. Mature T4 chromosomes are cut during packaging of intracellular DNA (see below) at nearly random map positions. As a consequence, the ends of different individual chromosomes are almost randomly permuted over the circular genetic map (**Fig. 1**).

Numerous mutations, and their assignments to complementation groups and open reading frames (ORFs) have defined approximately 130 genes with known functions. In contrast to the lambdoid phages, early and late gene clusters and transcription units are

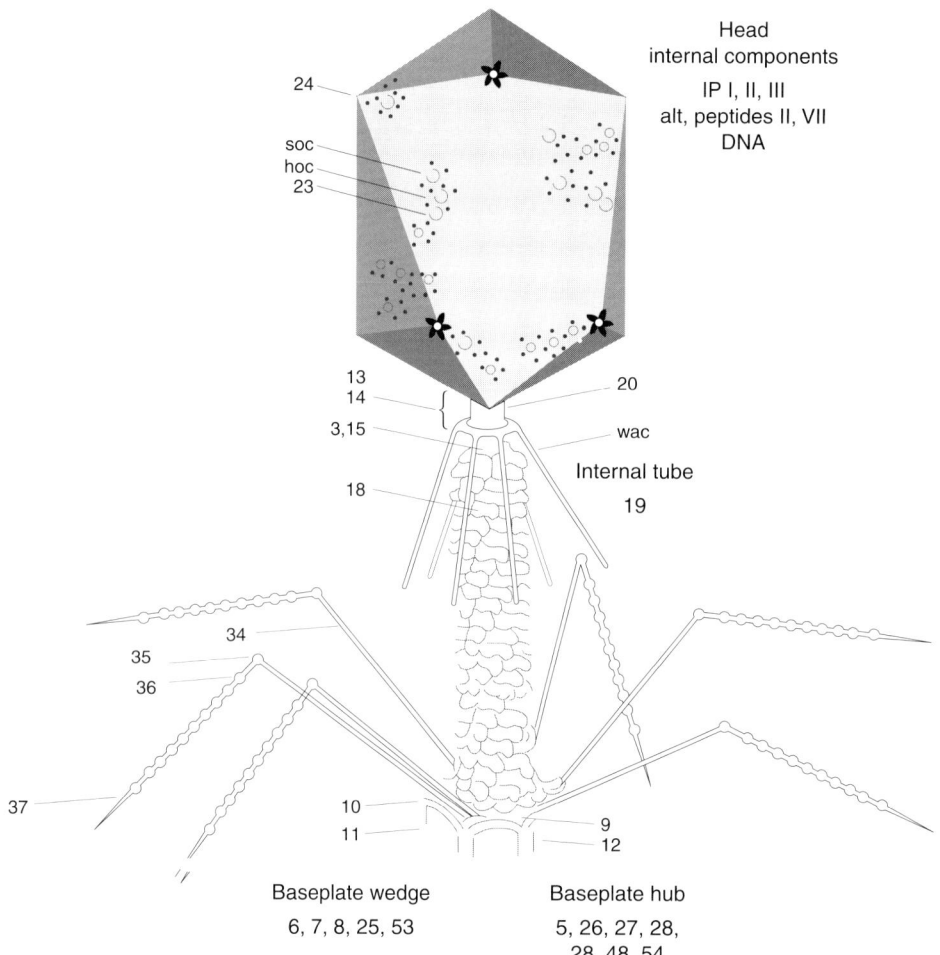

Figure 2 Diagram of the T4 virion, based on electron microscopy at 2–3 nm resolution. Locations of proteins are indicated by the corresponding gene numbers (cf. **Fig. 1**). The portal vertex composed of gp20 is attached to the upper ring of the neck structure inside the head itself. The internal tail tube is inside the sheath and itself contains a structural component in its central channel. The baseplate contains short fibers of gp12; these are shown in stored, folded conformation. (From Karam et al (1994) with permission of ASM Press.)

interdigitated, transcribed from multiple promoters, and genes for related or interacting proteins are not necessarily clustered (**Fig. 1**). In this respect, as well as in sequence similarities of certain proteins with the same functions, the T-even phages resemble more the herpesviruses than other phages.

More than 100 additional ORFs were revealed by DNA sequencing; many of them are still in search of functions. There are many overlapping coding regions, many ORFs are very small, and in some regions the two complementary DNA strands code for different proteins. In spite of the large genome size only a few short regions are devoid of coding capacity. These observations suggest that apparently redundant and 'nonessential' genes confer selective advantage, an inference that is supported by other evidence, discussed below.

Particle Structure and its Relationship to Assembly, Infection and Host Range

T-even phages build some of the most complex virus particles, which resemble lunar landing modules (**Fig. 2**). They devote more than 40% of their genetic information to synthesis and assembly of the protein components of these particles. The importance of host functions during assembly became apparent by 'host defective' (*hd*) mutations and compensating phage mutations and led to the discovery of the first chaperonin, now called GroEL.

The complex assembly pathways, revealed by exquisite mutational and biochemical analyses, accommodate efficient packaging of DNA and efficient genome transmission by allowing two-step adsorption to different receptors in the host's cell wall, and easy release of the DNA during subsequent infection. Complete uptake of phage DNA by a host bacterium is also dependent on membrane potential.

Twenty-four genes are involved in head morphogenesis, more than 25 encode structural components of the tail and tail fibers and five more are needed as morphogenetic catalysts. Heads, tails and tail fibers are assembled in independent pathways and put together after the heads are filled with DNA.

Head shapes and the protein components of heads, tails and baseplates are similar among the T-even phages, except that two nonessential proteins (Hoc and Soc) that decorate and stabilize T4 heads are missing in some members of the family.

Heads

Assembly of heads is complex and has resisted *in vitro* reconstitution. *In vivo* it appears to be initiated on the bacterial membrane. The major head subunits (cleaved gp23) form the bulk of the heads; a related minor cleaved gp24 forms the pentamers at the vertices. Both proteins are converted into an assembly-competent state by a chaperonin composed of a host subunit groEL and a small phage subunit gp31, which takes the place of groES of the bacterial chaperonin. Sequential action of scaffolding proteins and cooperative conformational changes lead to sequential changes in dimensions and shapes of the head precursors while they are being assembled and filled with DNA. Extensive controlled proteolysis by a phage-encoded protease, whose precursor is part of the scaffolding assembly, cleaves head subunits, scaffolding proteins and other packaged proteins, e.g. the ADP-ribosylating Alt protein (see Temporally Controlled Gene Expression During T-even Development, below) and internal proteins bound to the DNA. Together, these processes render head assembly irreversible. Proteolysis *in vivo* is probably triggered by entry of some DNA; *in vitro* it can be achieved by other conditions. In any case, proteolysis is a prelude to rearrangements of the subunits and expansion of the head volume and allows decoration of the heads with Hoc and Soc proteins mentioned above.

Head size is not uniquely determined. The normal T4 head can be described by skewed icosahedral symmetry (T = 13) whose side faces have been elongated (Q = 21). It can accommodate full-length chromosomes with terminal redundancies. Anomalous heads of different sizes and shapes are made in low proportions in wild-type T4 infections, and in higher proportions when infecting phages have mutations in genes for head subunits or scaffolding proteins, or due to incorporation of arginine analogues. Head lengths and shapes are determined at an early assembly stage, prior to formation of the unprocessed proheads.

Small heads ('petites') contain incomplete genomes, which represent nearly random permutations of the genetic map, and recombination between several of them reconstitutes complete genomes with expected frequencies. Most of the larger 'giants' contain oversized chromosomes representing linear concatemers. A small proportion of heads contain more than one DNA molecule; it is not yet known whether these are packaged into the rare anomalous heads containing more than one portal vertex.

The anomalous head sizes and shapes occur because assembly depends on numerous interactions of several proteins, each of which can exist in multiple conformational states and in different concentrations.

Tails

The tails are built like complex cocked mechanical devices with additional catalytic activities. The multifunctional baseplate contains information for building the tail and serves as a perfect valve for DNA entry into bacteria in the next infectious cycle. It consists of a central hub, six outer wedges and six tail spikes, each of these structures being assembled from several different subunits. Baseplate formation combines aspects of catalyzed assembly, self-assembly, concerted conformational changes and proteolysis.

Baseplate components are important for the irreversible second step of phage adsorption. A concerted conformational change of all baseplate components from a hexagon to a star configuration opens a hole in the tail to allow DNA to exit from the particles. It also activates the lysozyme activity of gp5 that actively punctures the host cell wall from the outside.

The tails are of remarkably uniform length, determined by a subunit of the baseplate that acts like a tape measure. Tails have a tubular inner core, through which DNA passes from the head to the baseplate, and an outer sheath that contracts during infection by conformational changes of individual subunits.

Tail fibers

Six bent tail fibers are attached to the tail of each particle. Each fiber consists of two half-fibers whose proteins are joined at an angle. The inner (proximal) half-fibers are attached to the baseplate. The outer (distal) half-fibers contact phage-specific receptors on the surface of the bacterial cell wall during the first, reversible step of adsorption. In many newly formed phage particles this end is transiently attached to the junction of heads and tails, rendering the fibers less fragile.

Tail fibers of different T-even phages appear superficially similar, but the amino acid sequences and genes are different in the different family members, resulting in recognition of different receptors in the host cell wall. These differences are used to distinguish different T-even phages by their host range. Apparently, illegitimate recombination with other DNA sequences, e.g. those of prophages that reside in the host genome, allow rapid evolution and adaptations to different receptors in different hosts' cell walls under selective pressure.

Temporally Controlled Gene Expression During T-even Development

T-even phages inactivate host translation and transcription in many small steps by multiple redundant mechanisms. The temporal regulation of phage gene expression is likewise exerted at many levels: transcript initiation, elongation and termination; stability, conformation and recognition by ribosomes of the transcripts, and combinations thereof.

Different classes of phage genes are distinguished in terms of timing as early (immediate early, IE), middle (delayed early, DE), or late. Operationally, IE genes are distinguished from the other classes in that they can be transcribed by host RNA polymerase without modification by phage proteins. Expression of all other T-even genes requires phage protein synthesis for several reasons. Successive transcription initiations from early, middle and late promoters are accomplished by a cascade of RNA polymerase modifications: the α subunits are covalently ADP-ribosylated and several accessory proteins bind non-covalently. Moreover, RNA polymerase can be attracted to middle promoters by proteins bound to specific DNA sequences, and it can be activated for initiation at late promoters by another protein bound to DNA, and used in both late transcription and DNA replication, the sliding clamp gp45 (see DNA Replication and Recombination In Vivo, below).

Another classification criterion distinguishes all genes that are expressed prior to the onset of DNA replication as 'prereplicative' or 'early' from 'postreplicative' or 'late' genes whose expression depends on DNA replication.

The distinction between different classes is, however, blurred because most T4 genes are under dual or multiple controls and because of overlapping and interdigitated transcriptional, post-transcriptional and translational control signals. Thus, promoters can be classified as early, middle or late, but genes defy this classification. One example (of ten known T4 regions with overlapping early, middle and late transcripts) is shown in **Fig. 4**. The regulation of T4 gene expression is better described by a web of interacting regulatory networks than by simple progression along a linear timed pathway.

Collectively, prereplicative genes encode: (1) nucleases that degrade the host DNA; (2) enzymes of the deoxyribonucleotide biosynthesis complex; (3) proteins of the replication and recombination machines; (4) proteins that modify the T4 DNA to protect it from degradation by its own nucleases and from other restriction enzymes; (5) several tRNAs; (6) proteins that modify structure and function of the host RNA polymerase; (7) at least one RNase (RegB protein) that selectively destroys certain early transcripts; (8) proteins that repress translation (e.g. RegA protein). In addition some prereplicative transcripts serve as primers for leading strand DNA synthesis in origins of replication (see below).

A T4-encoded sigma factor, gp55, associated with host core RNA polymerase, directs transcription from late promoters. Late transcription requires several additional proteins and concomitant DNA replication, further discussed below.

The late genes code for virion components, for some DNA repair and recombination proteins, and proteins that cut and package the complex vegetative DNA into preformed heads. A soluble lysozyme, different from but evolutionarily related to the baseplate lysozyme, lyses the host bacteria to release the progeny phage particles. Late genes that are under multiple controls (e.g. **Fig. 4**) can be expressed early, particularly when the RNA is broken or when infections occur at high temperatures, i.e. conditions that allow access of ribosomes to the translation initiation regions of late genes in the early RNA.

Transcription

The first set of promoters, early promoters, resembles the consensus sequence of *E. coli* promoters with additional information content (**Fig. 3a**). They are recognized by the *E. coli* RNA polymerase containing the major sigma factor σ^{70}, at a time when the host DNA is still largely intact. T4's early promoters are preferred to *E. coli* promoters, apparently not due to gene dosage effects. Several factors are thought to contribute to such preferential transcription of T4 versus *E. coli* genes:

1. Many early T4 promoters contain upstream polyA tracts, functioning as bendable sequences or as 'promoter UP elements'.
2. Arg265 of one α subunit of the host's RNA polymerase is ADP-ribosylated immediately after infection by the T4 Alt protein that is packaged

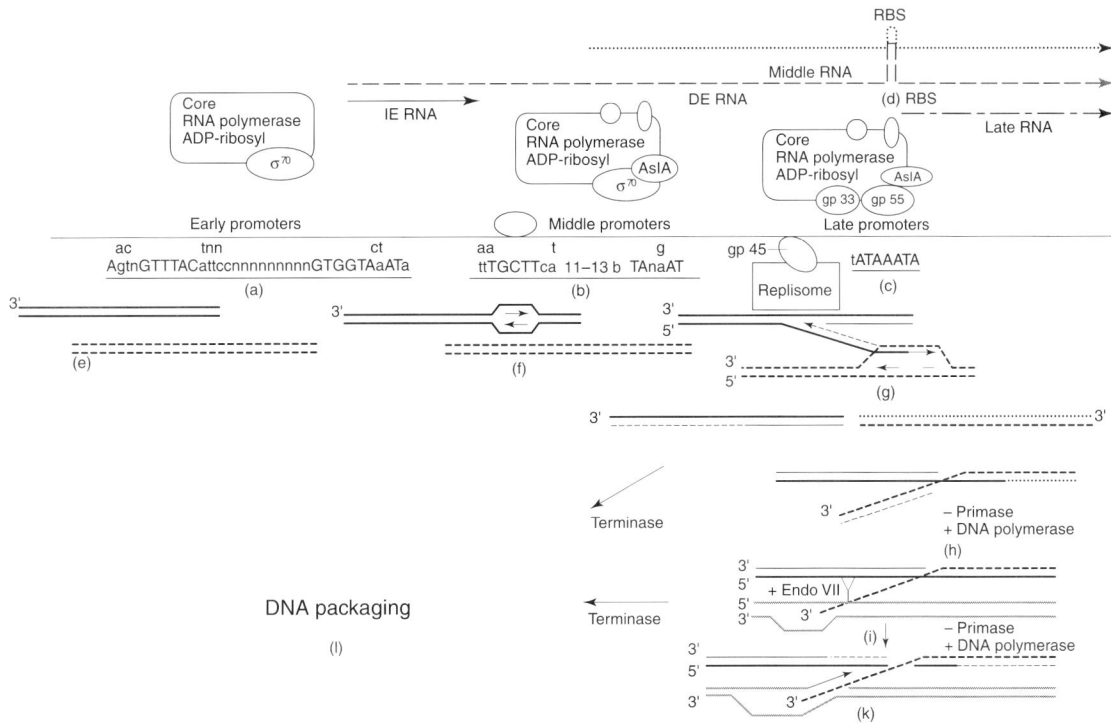

Figure 3 A diagram of transcription, DNA replication, recombination and packaging during T4 development (progressing in time after infection from left to right). The upper panel (a)–(d) shows overlapping early, middle and late transcripts in a 'generic' region, the modifications of host RNA polymerase after infection and the consensus sequences of early, middle and late T4 promoters that are recognized by different forms of the RNA polymerase. Ribosome-binding sites for late proteins in prereplicative transcripts are sequestered in hairpins (d); see also **Fig. 4**. The lower panel shows different stages of DNA replication and recombination. (e) Two infecting permuted T4 chromosomes. (f) Bidirectional origin initiation in one of them. Leading strand synthesis is primed by RNA polymerase-generated transcripts; lagging strand synthesis is primed by short RNAs synthesized by primase. As soon as the first growing point reaches an end (only one is shown), the partially single-stranded 3′ terminus invades the homologous region of another chromosome (g) or the terminal redundancy of the same chromosome (not shown). Join–copy replication is initiated from the invading 3′ DNA end. When an endonuclease cuts at the recombinational junction, join–cut–copy recombination can be initiated from the 3′ ends to allow copying of single-stranded segments of an invading DNA. Together both processes generate branched concatemers, which become increasingly more complex by reiterations. This DNA is processed to mature, unbranched chromosomes during packaging. Parental molecules are drawn as bold lines, filled with different patterns. Newly synthesized DNA is drawn as thin lines. Discontinuous synthesis of Okazaki pieces is indicated by dashed lines, continuous synthesis by solid lines. Arrowheads indicate the directions of RNA or DNA synthesis. (Modified from Mosig et al (1995).)

and injected with the phage DNA. This Arg265 is located at the dimer interface of the two α-subunits and it is important for activation of many strong E. coli promoters including those for ribosomal RNA. Its modification affects transcription in several ways.

3. At the time of infection, the host DNA is associated with nonspecific (e.g. HU, NS) or semi-specific (e.g. IHF, FIS) DNA binding proteins. In contrast, the infecting phage DNA is at first largely free and may be much more readily accessible to the host's RNA polymerase.

Host transcription is further reduced and the transition from host to phage transcription is accelerated by products of several early phage genes. Some of them disrupt the host nucleoid. Alc protein selectively inhibits transcript elongation on the host DNA but allows elongation on phage DNA, whose cytosine residues are hydroxymethylated and glycosylated (see below). The *asiA* product binds to the C-terminal segment of σ^{70}, interfering with transcription from all host promoters with standard −35 regions, as well as from T4 early promoters. However, phage infection can proceed because most prereplicative genes can also be transcribed from middle promoters (**Fig. 3**).

MotA protein bound to mot-boxes in middle promoters (**Fig. 3b**) recognizes Ast-A-modified RNA polymerase and allows initiation from middle promoters and expression of most prereplicative genes after the AsiA protein has inhibited initiation

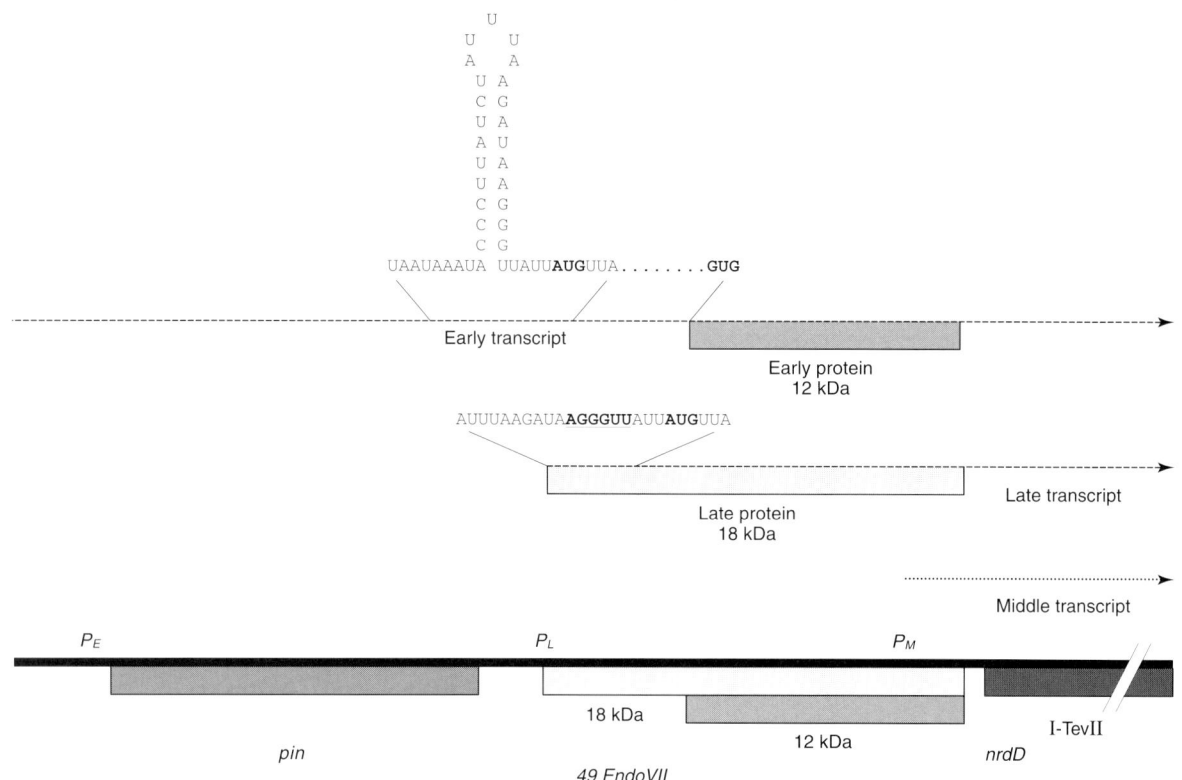

Figure 4 An example of interwoven transcriptional and post-transcriptional controls in the T4 gene *49* region (cf. **Fig. 1**). The locations of early (P_E), middle (P_M), and late (P_L) promoters and the protein-encoding segments of genes *pin*, *49* and *nrdD* are marked. Overlapping transcripts are distinguished by differentially patterned horizontal lined with arrows. The *nrdD* transcripts encode two proteins, one from spliced and the other (a truncated peptide) from unspliced RNA. I-TevII is a self-splicing intron. The late gene *49* transcript is predominantly translated into the 18 kDa EndoVII. In the larger, early transcript the Shine–Dalgarno sequence is sequestered in a hairpin. A shorter 12 kDa protein can be initiated in frame from an internal GUG. (Modified from Karam *et al* (1994).)

from early promoters. Initiation from early and middle promoters can overlap in time, depending on the proportions of RNA polymerase molecules that have been modified. Initiation from late promoters (**Fig. 3c**) requires a phage-encoded sigma factor (gp55), activation by gp45, the sliding clamp of the T4 replisome, and an adapter protein (gp33). In addition it requires concomitant DNA replication, or 'uncoupling' from DNA replication by combinations of certain recombination- and ligase-defective mutations. The critical common aspect of the latter conditions is that single-strand interruptions in the DNA provide entry sites for the sliding clamp, gp45, that is loaded on to the DNA by a complex of gp44 and gp62. The sliding clamp has to track along DNA to activate RNA polymerase bound at late promoters by T4 σ^{gp55}, to form open complexes and initiate transcription.

As indicated in **Figs 3** and **4,** most T4 genes can be transcribed from several promoters belonging to different classes. Genes downstream of any promoter may be poorly expressed because of premature *rho*-dependent transcription termination or because of RNA processing or degradation, or because the ribosome binding sites are sequestered by secondary structures.

Certain *rho* (transcription termination factor) mutations (also called host defective, *hdF* or *nusD*) of *E. coli* prevent growth of wild-type T4 by causing premature termination of many T4 transcripts. Mutations that allow growth in these specific *rho* mutants have been found in three nonessential T4 genes. It was initially thought that the corresponding T4 genes encode transcriptional antiterminators, but current evidence suggests that at least one of them allows T4 growth in the (*nusD*) *rho* mutants, because it stabilizes the few functional transcripts that have not been prematurely terminated.

Several additional phage proteins with unknown functions associate with host RNA polymerase. They are probably important in facilitating transcription initiation and elongation after phage infection under certain stress conditions.

The timing of differential gene expression during

T4 development is modulated by specific nucleases; for example, a T4 *regB*-encoded ribonuclease cleaves early transcripts rather selectively in the ribosome-binding sites of certain early T4 genes, thereby reducing expression of certain early T4 genes, and presumably of some host genes, at the post-transcriptional level. Moreover, several host nucleases and autocatalytic cleavages are important in processing the precursor RNAs for eight T4-encoded tRNAs and two tRNA-like structures of unknown function. The T4 tRNAs supplement host tRNAs during translation and are important for codons that are rare in *E. coli*, but frequent in T4; thereby they help maintain the different codon usages and AT contents of phage and host.

The introns in at least three T4 mRNAs (for thymidilate synthetase, *td*, and aerobic and anaerobic nucleotide reductase genes *nrdB* and *nrdD* respectively, have to be excised by self-splicing. Numerous mutations define the active centers of these ribozymes in exquisite detail.

Translational controls

Due to the interspersion of early and late genes on the T4 map (**Fig. 1**) and the 'sloppiness' of the interdigitated T4 transcription patterns shown in **Figs 3 and 4,** many early and middle transcripts are extended into late genes. Nevertheless, few or no corresponding late proteins are synthesized early at normal growth temperatures of 37°C or below. At higher temperatures there is some early expression of these late genes *in vivo* and early RNA sheared *in vitro* can direct synthesis of these late proteins. It is remarkable that expression of all of ten such late genes investigated so far follows similar patterns: in the long early transcripts a hairpin sequesters the translation initiation region, either the Shine–Dalgarno sequence or the initiation codon, or both. An additional late promoter immediately upstream of the late gene directs synthesis of transcripts that cannot form the hairpin, and these transcripts are efficiently translated (**Figs 3d** and **4**). Remarkably, phage evolution has conserved the early transcription of these late genes, while incorporating other means of preventing their translation. Pausing of RNA polymerase at such hairpins might facilitate access of the T4 σ^{gp55} required for initiation from the late promoters.

Three additional regulatory systems of T4 use translational controls. Expressions of gene *32* for the major single-stranded DNA binding protein (SSB) involved in DNA replication, recombination and repair, and of gene *43* for DNA polymerase, are autogenously regulated by translational repression. A more general, nonessential translational repressor (RegA protein), which binds to several specific transcripts, can reduce translation of several T4 replication proteins and of some host proteins. This repression is most apparent under experimental conditions that prolong early and delay late transcription.

DNA Replication and Recombination *In Vivo*

DNA replication and recombination are tightly interwoven, following several different redundant pathways. The T-even phages provided the first and most compelling evidence for recombination-dependent DNA replication. Redundant alternative modes of replication and recombination ensure that both processes work under many different conditions and during different stages of development. Known interrelationships are shown diagrammatically in **Fig. 3**.

The first round(s) of DNA replication are initiated from one of several potential origins. Because of the circular permutation of chromosomal ends (**Fig. 3e**), in each individual chromosome any origin is located at different distances from the ends. In most chromosomes only one origin is used, perhaps due to limited abundance of replisome components. Different origins share the requirement for transcription from early or middle promoters, generating large transcripts that can serve as primers for leading strand DNA synthesis at one of several sites approximately 1 kb downstream of the promoter. However, each of the four origins that have been closely investigated has a different sequence and overall structure, presumably related to preferred usage under different conditions. Three origins (*A*, *F* and *G*) require transcription from middle promoters, *oriE* depends on an early promoter. **Fig. 3f** depicts initiation from an arbitrary generic origin.

The transition from σ^{70}-dependent prereplicative transcription to T4 σ^{gp55}-dependent late transcription inhibits initiation from these origins, either by default (because the RNA polymerase no longer recognizes origin promoters), or because late protein(s), e.g. UvsW protein, actively prevent transcripts from serving as primers for DNA synthesis, or for both reasons.

Subsequent DNA replication is initiated from intermediates of homologous recombination (**Fig. 3g, i**). The recombinational intermediates are mainly formed by invasion of a single-stranded terminus into the homologous region of another molecule (or at the other end of the same molecule). When T4 chromosomes are broken by radiation damage or by certain nucleases, single-stranded termini of internal breaks can initiate recombination similarly as natural ends of infecting chromosomes. This is a major reason for the recombinogenic effects of radiation damage.

The recombination intermediates can initiate replication from the 3′ ends of the invading single strand (join–copy recombination, **Fig. 3g**), or, after an endonucleolytic cut at the junction from a 3′ end in the invaded strand (join–cut–copy recombination, **Fig. 3i**). The join–copy mode can start as soon as a growing point has reached an end. The join–cut–copy mode requires an additional endonucleolytic cut, which probably depends on one or more late proteins, and therefore occurs later. This mode can bypass the requirement for primase or topoisomerase in T4 DNA replication and can be used when these enzymes are limiting, e.g. late in infection. Ultimately, reiterations of these processes generate a highly branched concatemeric network in which no individual chromosomes can be distinguished.

Of course, not all recombination junctions need to be converted to replication forks. Some T4 recombination can occur, albeit with delay, when DNA replication is inhibited. Electron micrographs of such T4 DNA intermediates provided the first compelling evidence for the importance of branch migration in homologous recombination. Under these conditions, no viable progeny is produced, because no packagable concatemers are formed; there is little, if any, late transcription, and there are no heads to be filled.

DNA Replication *In Vitro*

Virtuoso biochemical and biophysical characterization of replication proteins, in combination with genetic experimentation, has led to an understanding of functions and interactions of the basic replication proteins in the replisome, a biological machine that moves the replication fork, or through which the replicating DNA is passed. Seven proteins, corresponding to genes *43* (DNA polymerase), *44* and *62* (sliding clamp loader), *45* (sliding clamp), *41* (DNA helicase), *61* (primase to synthesize primers for lagging strand synthesis) and *32* (single-stranded DNA-binding protein), form an active complex that replicates model templates with *in vivo*-like speed. Leading and lagging strand synthesis are coupled by interactions of primase-helicase with DNA polymerase. These basic reactions and protein functions are similar in all procaryotic and eucaryotic systems; in fact, some of the T4 proteins can partially substitute in eucaryotic *in vitro* systems.

Recombination-dependent initiation by a join–copy mechanism has also been achieved. Consistent with genetic analyses, these *in vitro* reactions require several recombination proteins in addition to the seven basic replication proteins just mentioned: the T4 RecA analogue gpUvsX, the single-stranded DNA binding proteins gpUvsY and gp59. The latter protein loads the gene *41* helicase, an enzyme that is important for branch migration in addition to its unwinding function at the replication fork. Initiation by the join–cut–copy mechanism and origin initiation have not yet been achieved *in vitro*.

Many of the T4-encoded DNA enzymes, most importantly DNA ligase, kinase and polymerase, are now standard components of cloning procedures and kits.

DNA Packaging

The ends of mature T4 chromosomes are nearly randomly permuted over the map, and 3–5% of the genome is repeated at both ends as so-called terminal redundancies. Mature chromosomes are generated from the branched concatemeric vegetative DNA during packaging by a terminase, a heteromeric protein encoded by genes *16* and *17* that associates with DNA and with gp20 at the portal vertex of the head (**Fig. 1**) and uses ATPase activities for the head-filling process. Gene *17* produces several proteins of different sizes by initiation from in-frame internal initiation codons. Several of these proteins have nuclease activity; the largest one also binds non-specifically to single-stranded DNA segments. There is controversial evidence as to whether T4 has sequence specific *pac* sites or whether it initiates packaging at such random single-stranded DNA segments. Perhaps both processes can initiate packaging. If the first initiation of packaging is a relatively rare event, processive packaging of 103–105% genome lengths to fill the preformed heads can account for the random circular permutation of the ends in mature virion DNA by either mechanism. Endonuclease VII which cuts Holliday and Y junctions and mismatched base pairs *in vitro* is required *in vivo* to trim the branches of vegetative DNA. It can associate with gp20 and retain nuclease DNA ligase, endonuclease V and topoisomerase are also required, presumably to provide uninterrupted double-stranded DNA as packaged chromosomes.

An *in vitro* packaging system has been developed to package large pieces of foreign DNA.

Restriction-Modification and Exclusion

In the following discussion the term 'restriction' is used in its broadest meaning, not limited to type II restriction enzymes. The complex modification and restriction of T4 DNA and of other DNA by T4 can best be rationalized as the result of an ongoing evolutionary process that includes exchanges between the phage, its host and prophages resident in the host.

T-even phages destroy dCTP, synthesize dHMCTP and use the latter for DNA synthesis. This modification protects the T4 DNA against T4-encoded restriction endonucleases II and IV that degrade the host DNA as part of the parasitic strategy to usurp the host. However, HMC residues render DNA susceptible to the Mcr restriction systems of the host. These host functions were the first restriction systems (then called Rgl) discovered. They are now called McrA and McrB, because they restrict DNA containing methylcytosine or hydroxymethylcytosine. These restriction functions are overcome when the HMC residues are glycosylated. In T4 DNA, all HMC residues are modified; 70% with α- and 30% with β-glycosyl linkages. In T2 and T6 DNA, there are no α-glycosyltransferases, and 25% of the HMC residues remain unglycosylated. T6 contains many diglycosylated residues. In addition, a T4-encoded early anti-restriction protein (Arn) protects nonglycosylated T4 DNA against one but not all of these host restriction enzymes.

T2 and T4, but not T6, encode a Dam methylase that methylates 0.5–1.5% of the adenine residues at the N^6 positions, mostly but not exclusively at GATC sequences. These enzymes exhibit patches of similarity at the protein level with the *E. coli* Dam methylase and the *Dpn*II methylase of *Diplococcus pneumoniae*. The only proven physiological role of adenine methylation is protection against the phage P1 restriction system, when there is no HMC glycosylation.

Intriguingly, several other 'host' genes that exclude T4 by various strategies are located in resident prophages or their defective derivatives.

The Mcr A system of K12 mentioned above resides in a cryptic prophage-like element, *e14* that is not present in all *E. coli* strains.

Another protein of *e14*, Lit, in combination with a short internal peptide (*gol*) of the major T4 head protein, gp23, cleaves the host's elongation factor EF Tu, thereby inhibiting translation of all late T4 proteins.

The classical example of phage exclusions by genes of resident prophages is that of T4 *rII* mutants in lambda lysogens by lambda's *rexA* and *rexB* genes. This exclusion was elegantly used in Benzer's classical analyses of structure and function of a gene. It occurs at the time of transition from join–copy to join–cut–copy recombination mentioned in the section on DNA replication and recombination, and it involves several enzymes important in the latter mechanism, as well as a putative ion channel produced by lambda's Rex proteins. Probably the otherwise nonessential RII proteins counteract this restriction, but the molecular mechanism is still unknown.

Another cryptic DNA element of certain *E. coli* strains, *prr*, encodes a PrrC protein that excludes T4 RNA ligase/polynucleotide kinase-deficient mutants. PrrC protein is a cryptic RNA endonuclease that is activated by the small (26 residues) T4 Stp protein to cleave the anticodon loop of an essential host tRNA^{Lys}. T4 RNA ligase/polynucleotide kinase can repair this damage, but in the absence of RNA ligase the cleavage of this tRNA is lethal to T4 protein synthesis. Intriguingly, the *prrC* gene is located between three genes of a type IC restriction cassette. The corresponding proteins are thought to inhibit PrrC RNase activity in uninfected cells.

Phage P2 lysogens exclude T4 by two mechanisms: the Tin protein poisons the single-stranded DNA binding protein gp32 that is essential for all T4 DNA replication and recombination, and the P2 Old protein can degrade DNA from ends, nicks and gaps (although the ends of the infecting T4 chromosomes are probably protected by bound T4 gp2).

Evolution

Sequences and map positions of the 'essential' genes whose products have the same functions of most T-even phages are similar. In contrast, genomes of different members of the family have different 'nonessential' genes interspersed between these essential genes (**Fig. 1**). The heterologies contribute to apparent exclusions of alleles of one phage by another, and to the species barriers between different members of the family. They first became evident as insertion or substitution loops in electron micrographs of heteroduplex DNA prepared *in vitro* by annealing single strands of T2, T4 and T6 DNA, and have been confirmed by sequence comparisons in many cases.

In some cases the sequence divergence reflects gene amplifications and permutations of duplicated sequences. The tail fiber genes of different T-even phages appear to have diverged by illegitimate recombinations with genes of other phages, including prophages residing in the host genome. Substitutions of sequence blocks of individual genes by foreign sequences can account for the variability between different members of the family. In turn, these substitutions allow adsorption to different hosts with different receptors, accounting for the remarkable coevolution of viral and host genomes.

Such illegitimate recombinations are not limited to genes for recognition proteins. Illegitimate pairing of partially homologous sequences and join–copy and join–cut–copy recombination (discussed above) were apparently involved in horizontal gene transfer of nonessential genes adjacent to the essential dCTPase gene, and probably other genes as well. Although inactivating their functions has little or no consequences for phage development in the laboratory, we surmise that these genes are important for viral growth and survival under different physiological conditions, in different hosts with different receptors or containing different prophages, and in the face of various restriction systems imposed by different hosts.

Future Perspectives

The T-even phages have been instrumental in first formulations of several fundamental biological concepts: (1) the unambiguous recognition of nucleic acids as genetic material; (2) the operational distinctions in defining the gene by mutational, recombinational or functional analyses (the concepts of muton, recon and cistron); (3) the demonstration of mRNA; (4) the nature of the triplet code, and the importance of initiation and nonsense codons; (5) homologous recombination as exchange between DNA molecules, and the importance of heterozygotes in this process; (6) the role of homologous recombination in initiating DNA replication; (7) restriction and modification of DNA as important aspects of host–virus interactions; (8) light-dependent and light-independent DNA repair mechanisms; (9) the importance of pathways of macromolecular assemblies (protein machines) in morphogenesis and DNA metabolism; (10) the presence of self-splicing introns and mobile endonucleases in prokaryotes; and (11) the facility of ribosomes to skip unspliced introns in mRNA during translation.

Recent progress towards understanding the importance of redundant pathways and proteins for fundamental processes is bound to lead to better appreciation of the functional significance of web-like interconnections between different processes for development, for virus–virus and virus–host interactions, and for evolution.

See also: **SPO1 phage (*Myoviridae*); History of virology: Bacteriophages; T1-like phages (*Siphoviridae*); Salmonella phage P22 (*Podoviridae*).**

Further Reading

Brody EN, Kassavetis GA, Ouhammouch M *et al* (1995) Old phage, new insights: two recently recognized mechanisms of transcriptional regulation in bacteriophage T4 development. *FEMS Microbiol. Lett.* 128: 1.

Geiduschek, EP (1997) Paths to activation of transcription. *Science* 275: 1614–1616.

Karam JD, Drake JW, Kreuzer KN, *et al* (eds) (1994) *Molecular Biology of Bacteriophage T4*. American Society of Microbiology: ASM Press: Washington, DC.

Kutter E, Gachechiladze K, Poglazov A *et al* (1996) Evolution of T4-related phages. *Virus Genes* 11: 213.

Mosig G (1998) Recombination and recombination-dependent DNA replication in bacteriophage T4. *Annu. Rev. Genet.* 32: 379–413.

Mosig G and Eiserling F (1988) Phage T4: structure and metabolism. In: Calendar R (ed.) *The Bacteriophages*, vol. 2, p. 521. New York: Plenum Press.

Mosig G, Colowick N, Gruidl ME, Chang A and Harvey AJ (1995) Multiple initiation mechanisms adapt phage T4 DNA replication to physiological changes during T4's development. *FEMS Microbiol. Rev.* 17: 83.

T5-LIKE PHAGES (*SIPHOVIRIDAE*)

D. James McCorquodale, Midwestern University, Downers Grove, Illinois, USA

Copyright © 1999 Academic Press

Classification and Morphology

Bacteriophage T5 and its relatives BF23, PB, BG3 and 29-alpha are in the T5-like viruses genus of the *Siphoviridae* family. They have a general morphology that consists of an icosahedral head and a long noncontractile flexible tail. The head of T5 has an average diameter of 90 nm. The tail is attached to one of the head apices via a head–tail linker protein and has three L-shaped tail fibers attached at a site near its distal end. A ring-like structure is formed at this site as a result of the attachment of these tail fibers. The tubular tail undergoes a transition at the tail fiber attachment site to a conical form, which tapers into a single straight tail fiber. The tail has a diameter of 12 nm with a length of 190 nm. The cone (12 nm) plus

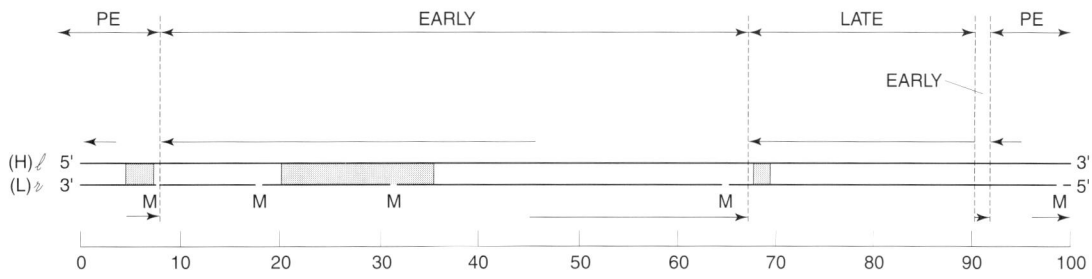

Figure 1 Structure and organization of the genome of T5 and BF23. The heavy double lines represent the two DNA strands of the double-stranded genome. H and L indicate the relative bouyant density of the upper un-nicked strand to that of the lower nicked strand. The script '1' and 'r' indicate leftward transcription from the upper strand and rightward transcription from the lower strand, in agreement with the 3'-5' polarities of the two strands. Major nicks in the lower strand are indicated by gaps in the heavy line and the letter 'M'. Deletable regions are indicated by shaded regions between the two heavy lines. The distribution of pre-early, early and late genes along the genome is indicated by name and by lines with arrowheads at both ends. The direction of transcription for each class of genes is indicated by directional arrows above and below the two heavy lines. The 0–100 scale at the bottom divides the genome into percentages from left to right.

the single straight tail fiber (50 nm) bring the total length of the tail to about 250 nm. The phage protein (Oad) that binds irreversibly to the host receptor (FhuA) is located in the conical region. The tail is hollow from the head to the cone-shaped structure and provides part of the route for transfer of phage DNA from the phage head to the host cell. A total of 15 different polypeptides have been detected in mature T5 phage particles and the number of copies of each polypeptide per particle depends on the part of the phage structure that it forms. For example, the major head polypeptide is present at 730 copies per particle whereas the straight tail fiber polypeptide is present at only five copies per particle.

Structure of the Genome

The DNA within mature T5 or BF23 particles is linear, double-stranded, and about 121 300 bp long (**Fig. 1**). It contains only the four common bases, adenine, guanine, cytosine and thymine, none of which are methylated. Its AT content is 61%. Two features of the DNA stand out. First, it has unusually long direct terminal repetitions of about 10 100 bp and second, it is nicked at precise sites, and all nicks are in one strand only. The nicks consist of a missing phosphoester bond between the 5'-phosphate group of one nucleotide residue and the 3'-OH group of its adjacent nucleotide residue. Thus, these nicks can be ligated with DNA ligase. The nicks are introduced by a site-specific nicking enzyme coded by genes *sciA* and *sciB*, which map at the right end of the 'late' region of the genetic map (see **Fig. 1**). Nicks are classified as 'major' or 'minor', with major nicks occurring in virtually all phage DNA molecules and minor nicks occurring in only a small fraction of these molecules.

The frequency of the major nicks (four per 111 200 bp) predicts a recognition sequence of seven or eight nucleotides. A prominent sequence on the 5' side of nicks in T5 DNA is 5'-GCGCGGTG-3', and the sequence in the unnicked strand around the major nick at 64.8% of the length of DNA from the left end of both T5 and BF23 DNA is 5'-CCCGCGCCC-3'. The left end is defined as the end that always enters the host cell first during normal infections (**Fig. 1**). Thus the sequence most efficiently recognized by the nicking enzyme appears to be

$$\text{intact strand: } 5' \ (C) \ \boxed{CCGCGCC} \ C \ 3'$$
$$\text{nicked strand: } 3' \ G(T) \ \boxed{GGCGCGG} \ G \ 5'$$
$$\uparrow$$
$$\text{nick}$$

The boxed in sequence would generate major nicks whereas minor variations in this sequence would presumably generate minor nicks.

The DNA can be deleted in three regions without affecting viability (**Fig. 1**). The major deletable region is between positions 20.0 and 35.7%. Although this region spans about 19 kb, only about 13.3 kb can be deleted from the DNA and still be packaged. Larger deletions yield DNA too small to be packaged. This deletable region contains genes that code for at least one tRNA for each of the 20 amino acids found in proteins. Another deletable region is between positions 4.1 and 7.1% (about 3.6 kb) and is therefore in the terminal repetition. It follows that most genes in the right half of the terminal repetition are unessential. The third deletable region is between positions 67.8 and 69.5% and is within a nonessential gene that codes for the L-shaped tail fibers of the mature phage. Because regions of the T5 and BF23 genomes can be deleted, these phages could be used as cloning vehicles for inserts up to about 19 kb. However, such use has not been developed. Nevertheless, some T5 promoters, because of their strength (see below), are currently being used in expression vectors.

The nucleotide sequences that have been determined in T5 DNA plus those determined in BF23 DNA (not counting overlapping sequences) come to about 30% of their genomes, or about 36 400 nucleotides. Most of this sequencing has been done in the region from 58.3 to 92.2%, which includes some early but mostly late genes, and includes T5 genes *D7-8-9* (the phage DNA polymerase), *D10* (a putative helicase), *D11*, *D12* and *D13* (nucleoside triphosphate-binding proteins, probably involved with DNA replication, recombination and/or repair), *D14*, *D15* (a 5′-exonuclease), the *dut* gene (dUTPase), the *1tf* gene (L-shaped tail fibers), the *oad* gene, the *11p* gene (lipoprotein), and BF23 genes 25 (equivalent to T5 gene N4) and 24 (tail proteins). Four other interesting regions of T5 or BF23 have been sequenced. About 1000 bp have been sequenced in the region where the first step of DNA transfer stops (see below), which is very close to the right end of the left terminal repetition (positions 7.4–8.3%). Present in this sequence are several direct repeats and palindromes, DnaA-binding sites and simple repeats with a periodicity suggestive of DNA bending. Another sequence of about 1100 bp (positions 2.4–3.3%) defines gene *A2–A3*, an unidentified open reading frame (ORF) on its right, and the beginning of gene *A1* on its left. The third region (positions 22.4–27.8%) that has been sequenced codes for tRNAs, but contains short ORFs interspersed between the tRNA genes. Lastly, a sequence of about 180 bp defining the left end of BF23 DNA (90% homologous to that of T5 DNA) encodes a strong transcriptional stop signal just after the termination codon for the *dmp* gene (5′-deoxyribonucleoside-5′-monophosphatase), which is the leftmost gene in the terminal repetitions.

The genetic maps for both T5 and BF23 have been correlated with their physical genomes such that pre-early genes are located from 0 to 8.3%, and are repeated between 91.7 and 100%, i.e. pre-early genes are in the terminal repetitions. Early genes are located between positions 8.3 and 67.2% as well as in a very short region between 90.5 and 91.5%. Late genes are located between 67.2 and 90.5%.

Restriction maps for T5 DNA have been developed for the restriction endonucleases *Bal*I, *Bam*HI, *Bgl*I, *Bst*EII, *Eco*RI, *Hin*dIII, *Hpa*I, *Kpn*I, *Pst*I, *Sac*I, *Sal*I, *Sma*I, *Sst*I and *Xho*I, and for BF23 DNA for *Bal*I, *Bam*HI, *Eco*RI, *Hpa*I and *Sal*I.

The Infection Process

Attachment of T5 to host cells is facilitated by the L-shaped tail fibers which bind rapidly and reversibly to polymannose O antigens on the outer surface of the outer membrane of the host cell, and move the phage across the outer surface until a receptor is located. The host cell receptor for T5 is *fhuA*, the receptor for ferrichrome, and for BF23 is *btuB*, the receptor for vitamin B_{12}. Irreversible binding occurs between the phage Oad protein and these host receptors, and is accompanied by a covalent cross-linking of three copies of a minor tail protein, pb4. The straight tail fiber, pb2, rearranges to form a channel as does the host cell receptor, thereby providing the route of entry of phage DNA into the host cell. The straight tail fiber is long enough to span the outer membrane, the periplasm, and the inner membrane, but it may also draw the outer membrane to the inner membrane to create contact points where the phage DNA actually enters the host cell through the newly formed channel. Transfer of phage DNA by both T5 and BF23 is unique in that they transfer their DNA in two steps. The left terminal repetition is always transferred first after which DNA transfer stops. DNA transfer resumes only after the pre-early genes in the left terminal repetition have been expressed. The remaining 92% of the phage DNA is then quickly transferred to the host cell such that late genes follow the entry of early genes by only a few seconds.

During transfer of the left terminal repetition (the first step of DNA transfer), the entry channel for DNA is open and low-molecular-weight substances such as K^+ and phosphate leak out of the host cell so that partial depolarization of the periplasmic membrane ensues. After transfer of the left terminal repetition, the channel is closed by Ca^{2+} and the periplasmic membrane repolarizes. When the channel is reopened for transfer of the remaining 92% of the DNA, low molecular weight components of the host cell again leak out and another partial depolarization of the periplasmic membrane occurs. Ca^{2+} again closes the channel, the periplasmic membrane repolarizes, and a successful infection is established. The T5 and BF23 systems therefore both have a Ca^{2+}-requirement, and cannot progress when the concentration of Ca^{2+} is below 0.1 mM.

Pre-early Genes

Since genes in the terminal repetition (**Fig. 1**) are the first phage genes to be expressed in the infected host cell, they have been termed 'pre-early'. Pre-early genes that have been identified include *dmp* (coding for a deoxyribonucleoside-5′-monophosphatase), *A1* (coding for a protein required for completion of DNA transfer, for shutdown of expression of pre-early genes, and for degradation of host DNA), and *A2-A3* (coding for a protein that is also required for completion of DNA transfer and that binds to DNA, lipopolysaccharide, and host RNA polymerase). Other functions induced by genes in the terminal repetition include the inactivation of host restriction endonucleases, of the host cell reactivation system, of host DNA methylases as well as the total inhibition of host DNA, RNA and protein synthesis. The product of gene *A2-A3* (gp*A2-A3*) is also crucially involved in the abortive response that ensues when either T5 or BF23 infects host cells that harbor a ColIb plasmid or, in some cases, a ColIa plasmid.

Effect on Host Cell Metabolism

Infection by T5 or BF23 results in a rapid and complete degradation of host DNA to individual deoxyribonucleotides, and therefore the synthesis of host DNA, RNA and protein ceases soon after infection. Mutations in gene *A1* prevent this degradation and cells infected with *A1* mutants continue synthesis of host proteins for at least 60 min. The deoxyribonucleotides derived from host DNA are partially degraded to ribonucleosides, free bases and deoxyribose-1-phosphate. The free bases and deoxyribonucleosides are secreted by the infected cell so that all deoxyribonucleoside triphosphates used in the synthesis of phage DNA are synthesized via *de novo* pathways of nucleotide anabolism. A possible reason for the clearance of all nucleotides derived from host DNA is that the phage-induced nuclease that degrades host DNA may only attack methylated DNA. Phage DNA is not methylated and so would be protected from attack, but if any methylated bases derived from host DNA were incorporated into phage DNA, it would be attacked. Thus, the elimination of host-derived bases would be a requirement for a successful infection. This suggestion would also require that a phage function inactivate host DNA methylases, which, as stated above, is known to occur after infection by T5.

Another requirement for a successful infection is the inactivation of host cell restriction endonucleases. Neither T5 nor BF23 DNA contain *Eco*R1 or other common restriction sites in their terminal repetitions but do have them in the central nonredundant portion of their genomes. Thus, inactivation of host restriction endonucleases by the product of one or more pre-early genes, and therefore prior to entry of the portion of the genome containing susceptible restriction sites, allows the susceptible portion of the phage genome to escape the action of host restriction endonucleases. If, on the other hand, the terminal repetition contains even a single restriction site that is cleaved by a host restriction endonuclease, the infection is unsuccessful.

Early Genes

After pre-early genes are expressed, phage DNA transfer resumes and early but not late genes begin their expression as soon as the rest of the phage DNA enters the host cell. Early genes code mostly for enzymes and proteins required for biosynthesis of deoxyribonucleotides, replication of phage DNA and regulation of transcription. Early gene expression begins about 5 min after infection at 37°C, and continues in the case of some early genes until about 20 min after infection, but in the case of other early genes until lysis. Thus, early genes can be divided into two subclasses on the basis of their period of expression.

Products of early T5 genes that have been identified include DNA polymerase (*D9*), deoxynucleoside monophosphokinase (*dnk*), dihydrofolate reductase (*B3*), 5′-exonuclease (*D15*), ribonucleotide reductase (possibly *B1* or *B2*), thioredoxin, thymidylate synthase (*thy*), dUTPase (*dut*), tRNAs (genes within the major deletable region), lipoprotein (*11p*), and RNA polymerase modifying proteins (*C2*, *D5* and *14* and *10* in the case of BF23). This array of early gene products enables the infected cell to initiate phage DNA replication, which begins about 8–9 min after infection and continues until lysis.

Late Genes

Expression of late genes begins at 10–12 min after infection and continues until lysis. Most late genes code for structural proteins of the mature phage particle, and when they begin to accumulate, phage morphogenesis begins using the phage DNA that had begun replication earlier. The eclipse period for T5 and BF23 is about 20 min. Thus, there is a well-regulated temporal sequence for the synthesis of phage DNA and of pre-early, early and late proteins which corresponds to the same temporal sequence for the synthesis of mRNAs. Although most late genes code for structural proteins of the mature phage particle, two late genes (*sci*A and *sci*B) code for the protein that introduces nicks into the phage DNA. Lysis of the infected cell presumably depends on a late gene which codes for a lysis protein, but this has yet to be demonstrated for the T5 system. Lysis exposes the progeny phage to phage receptors liberated from the lysed host cells. To counteract the inactivation of progeny phage by these receptors, the product of early gene *11p* (a lipoprotein) combines with liberated host receptors to inactivate them.

Regulation of Transcription

The temporal appearance of phage-specified proteins in T5- or BF23-infected cells is regulated at the level of transcription (**Fig. 1**). However, since all classes of T5 or BF23 genes (pre-early, early and late) are efficiently transcribed *in vitro* by unmodified host RNA polymerase (with sigma-70), and this capacity for transcription is the same whether nicked or ligated phage DNA is used as a template, the temporal expression of phage genes *in vivo* must be regulated by mechanisms that prevent the simultaneous expression of all classes of genes if the phage DNA entered the cell in one step. This regulation appears to be accomplished in part by sequential modifications of the host RNA polymerase. On the other hand, expression of pre-early genes is temporally separated from early and late gene expression because of the two-step mechanism of phage DNA transfer, whereby pre-early genes enter the host cell first and must be expressed before early and late genes are able to enter the cell. Pre-early genes are therefore transcribed *in vivo* by the pre-existing unmodified host RNA polymerase. The first modification to host RNA polymerase is the binding of the pre-early proteins coded by gene *A2-A3* (gpA2-A3) and gene *A1* (gpA1). The modification by gpA1 causes shutdown of pre-early gene transcription, whereas the modification by gpA2-A3 prevents the premature transcription of late genes when the phage DNA carrying early and late genes enters the host cell after pre-early genes are expressed. It follows that early genes, but not late genes, can be transcribed by host RNA polymerase modified by gpA2-A3 and gpA1. Transcription of late genes would then require a further modification of RNA polymerase by early gene products, and for T5 they are gpC2 and a 15 kDa protein, whereas for BF23 they are gp10 and gp14. GpA2-A3 is then displaced from the RNA polymerase and late transcription proceeds with the resulting gpC2-15 kDa (for T5) or gp10-gp14 (for BF23) modified RNA polymerase.

DNA Replication

T5 DNA contains multiple origins of replication, which suggests that its DNA is replicated linearly. However, T5 DNA is found in a circular form in infected cells, and the length of such circles is equal to a genome length minus one terminal repetition. Formation of these circles could therefore arise from a recombinational event between the terminal repetitions of a single incoming parental DNA. The occurrence of circles suggests a rolling circle model of DNA replication. Sedimentation studies of replicating T5 DNA from infected cells shows a fast-sedimenting fraction, which could be linear concatemers or the rolling circle intermediate, and a slow-sedimenting fraction that corresponds to genome-length T5 DNA. These findings suggest that excision of genome-length DNA from larger precursors and packaging of phage DNA into immature heads proceed independently of one another.

Morphogenesis

Morphogenesis follows two separate pathways, head formation and tail formation. The immature head is filled with a genome length of phage DNA that is cut from a linear concatemer consisting of phage genomes minus the length of one terminal repetition. The most likely mechanism for excising exactly one genome from such a linear concatemer is by means of two staggered single-strand cuts at each internal terminal repetition in order to generate genome-length DNA with each terminal repetition having a 3'-recess. Filling of each 3'-recess would then generate full, completely double-stranded phage DNA.

Both head and tail morphogenesis involve cleavage of polypeptides that contribute to the formation of these structures. Tails can be connected to heads *in vitro*, but packaging of T5 or BF23 DNA *in vitro* has not yet been accomplished.

Abortive infection in ColIb Hosts

If T5 or BF23 infects a host cell harboring the colicinogenic plasmid, ColIb (or some ColIa plasmids), the infection is abortive. In such infections, the phage adsorbs to the host cell normally, and the phage DNA is transferred into the host cell in the usual two-step manner without being degraded. Pre-early genes are expressed and shutdown normally, but early genes barely begin expression before the host cell prematurely lyses, resulting in death of both the host cell and the infecting phage. Gene products from the phage, the host cell and the plasmid are necessary for this abortive response. The phage gene is pre-early gene *A2-A3*, which binds to both DNA and host RNA polymerase. The host cell genes involved are *cmrA* and *cmrB*, which map suspiciously close to *trkA* and *trkB*, respectively, which code for potassium transport proteins located in the cell membrane. The plasmid gene is *abi* (*ab*ortive *i*nfection), which could code for a polypeptide of 114 amino acids that is strongly hydrophobic and may therefore interact with cell membranes. The putative Abi protein, however, has not yet been detected and is presumably synthesized in very small amounts. How the gene products from three sources interact to cause the abortive response has yet to be elucidated.

Transfection

Transfection of spheroplasts by naked T5 or BF23 DNA provides a means to assess the functional importance, other than that of phage DNA transfer, of the two pre-early proteins, gpA1 and gpA2-A3, which are normally required for transfer of phage DNA into the host cell. Transfection bypasses the normal mechanism, and by so doing, phage DNA with an amber mutation in either gene A1 or A2-A3 can produce intact phage (still with the original amber mutation) when transfected into su^- spheroplasts. The efficiency of such phage production is considerably lower than that produced from wild-type phage DNA, but still much higher than that produced from phage DNA with an amber mutation in an essential gene such as T5 DNA polymerase. For a DNA with an amber mutation in gene A2-A3, the efficiency was 16%, for one in gene A1 it was 1.4%, and for one in the essential gene D9 it was 0%. It thus appears that the role of gpA2-A3 in preventing premature transcription of late genes is important, but not as important as the role of gpA1 in shutting down host macromolecular synthesis by degrading host DNA plus shutting off pre-early transcription.

Interestingly, transfection by T5 or BF23 DNA is a two-hit process in wild-type spheroplasts. Since in transfection, the entire DNA molecule enters the spheroplast in one step, the first DNA molecule to enter inactivates hostile host functions but its nonredundant region is largely degraded. However, such a spheroplast should now be able to accept a second DNA molecule without degradation and a successful infection would follow. One hostile host function appears to be the RecB nuclease since transfection is a one-hit process in $recB^-$ hosts.

Cloning Genes from T5 or BF23

Many restriction fragments from T5 or BF23 DNA are not directly clonable because they either code for lethal products or contain such strong promoters that the cells harboring them cannot survive. The strength of some T5 promoters has prompted their use in expression vectors, some of which are commercially available. Fragments that have been cloned are largely from the region from 58 to 92%, which includes mostly late structural genes with some early genes, and from 21 to 36%, which includes all the tRNA genes that are expressed during the early period. A small fragment from 2.1 to 3.4% in the pre-early region has also been cloned.

T5 genes that have been overproduced from an expression vector include gene D7-8-9 (coding for T5 DNA polymerase), gene D15 (coding for T5 5'-exonuclease), and 11p (coding for a lipoprotein that inactivates host cell receptors). BF23 genes 24 and 25 (coding for a minor and major tail protein, respectively) have also been cloned, sequenced, and expressed.

Future Perspectives

Contributions from the T5 and BF23 systems include the identification and use of some of their gene products. Pre-early gene products that inactivate specific host functions, including restriction endonucleases and DNA methylating enzymes, should show interesting mechanisms of action and prove experimentally useful. Similarly, the availability of the 'nicking' enzyme would add to our battery of enzymes for manipulation of DNA. The nucleotide sequence of all T5 and BF23 promoters and their strength of binding to unmodified and modified forms of host RNA polymerase should sharpen our understanding of promoter function. The elucidation of the mechanims by which the two-step transfer of phage DNA to host cells and the ColIb-directed abortive response is accomplished will probably reveal some unique cellular interactions. Finally, the complete nucleotide sequence of T5 and BF23 genomes would greatly help our understanding of this system.

See also: **Host-controlled modification and restriction; Phage taxonomy and classification; Phages as cloning vehicles; Replication of viruses.**

Further Reading

Bonhivers M and Letellier L (1995) Calcium controls phage T5 infection at the level of the *Escherichia coli* cytoplasmic membrane. *FEBS Lett.* 374: 169.

Bujard H, Niemann A, Brevnig K *et al* (1982) The interaction of *E. coli* RNA polymerase with promoters of high signal strength. In: Rodriguez RL and Chamberlin MJ (eds) *Promoters Structure and Function*, p. 121. New York: Praeger.

Decker K, Krauel V, Meesmann A and Heller KJ (1994) Lytic conversion of *Escherichia coli* by bacteriophage T5: blocking of the FhuA receptor protein by a lipoprotein expressed early during infection. *Mol. Microbiol.* 12: 321.

Duckworth DH, Glenn J and McCorquodale DJ (1981) Inhibition of bacteriophage replication by extrachromosomal genetic elements. *Microbiol. Rev.* 45: 52.

McCorquodale DJ and Warner HR (1988) Bacteriophage

T5 and related phages. In: Calendar R (ed.) *The Bacteriophages*, p. 439. New York: Plenum.

Nakayama S-I, Kaneko T, Ishimaru H, Moriwaki H and Mizobuchi K (1994) Cloning, sequencing, and expression of bacteriophage BF23 late genes 24 and 25 encoding tail proteins. *J. Bacteriol*. 176: 7280.

T7-LIKE PHAGES (*PODOVIRIDAE*)

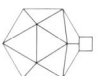

Ian J Molineux, Department of Microbiology, University of Texas, Austin, Texas, USA

Copyright © 1999 Academic Press

General Properties, Ecology and Evolution

Bacteriophage T7 is the prototype of a group of virulent phages having a $T=7$ icosahedral head approximately 60 nm in diameter, a stubby, noncontractile tail (about 20 nm in length and 10 nm wide) plus six thin tail fibers. It is the type species of the genus 'T7-like phages' in the *Podoviridae* family. The distinguishing characteristic of the group is the synthesis of an RNA polymerase that is both resistant to the antibiotic rifampin and highly specific for phage promoters. T7-like phages that infect one of a variety of Gram-negative bacteria have been described, but none are yet known that infect Gram-positive hosts. Most studies have been performed on the coliphage T7 and properties of other phages are usually described relative to those of T7.

T7 does not form plaques on most *Escherichia coli* strains newly isolated from nature because it does not adsorb to smooth or capsulated bacteria. In *E. coli* B the primary receptor for T7 is the R-core portion of the lipopolysaccharide (LPS) of the outer membrane; in smooth strains the R-core is inaccessible to the phage gp17 tail fibers, which specify the adsorption host-range. The precise adsorption component may be different on *E. coli* K-12 or C strains, on which T7 grows equally well. T7-like phages are known that grow on smooth bacteria; virion-associated hydrolases may degrade cell surface polysaccharides to allow a gp17 homologue to access the primary receptor.

T7 and T3 were isolated in 1945 as phages that grew on *E. coli* B. Similar coliphages have been isolated from different parts of the world and about 60 representatives are known that can be subdivided by the promoter specificity of the phage-coded RNA polymerase. Recombination between phages in a subdivision is very efficient, recombination between those in different subdivisions is extremely rare but undoubtedly highly significant in the evolution of specific phages. Electron microscopic analyses of heteroduplexed DNA of T7-like phages showed varying degrees of homology, some regions exhibiting >90% sequence identity and others with no apparent similarity. These observations suggest that a given phage is the result of multiple recombination events between many T7-like phages.

Genetic Structure

The genetic map of T7 is based on the nucleotide sequence of 39 937 bp. Numbers define genes, ordered sequentially from the genetic left end of the DNA (**Fig. 1**). Three classes of genes have been identified: class I, or early, genes are expressed until about 8 min after infection at 30°C; class II genes are expressed from about 6 to 15 min after infection; and class III genes are expressed from about 8 min until lysis (about 25 min at 30°C). Fifty-six known or potential T7 genes have been described – less than half are essential for phage growth on usual laboratory strains but mutant hosts have allowed the functions of several other genes to be elucidated. There are indications that a few genes may be remnants of homing endonucleases or other mobile elements. More than 90% of the genome is coding and most of the remainder contains recognizable genetic signals. Little overlapping of genes occurs; by means of an internal in-frame initiation gene *4* specifies two distinct polypeptides and programmed ribosomal frameshifting yields two products from gene *0.6*, gene *5.5* (yielding a 5.5–5.7 fusion), and gene *10*. Only the gene *10* frameshift has been well characterized; both gp10A and the longer, −1 frameshifted, gp10B are assembled into wild-type particles but either alone suffices for viability. The frameshifted protein may be biologically significant since a comparable T3 gp10B exists even though the frameshifting sequences have diverged from T7. Other T7-like phages are also thought to contain two forms of their major capsid protein.

Genetic signals include promoters and terminators

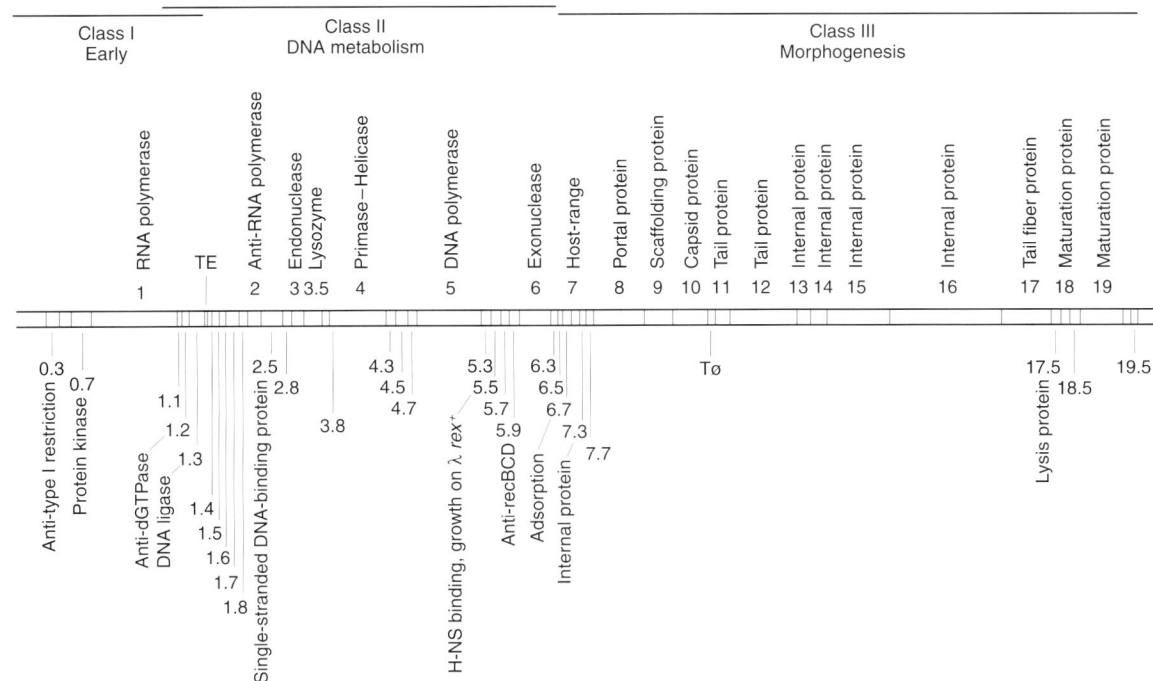

Figure 1 Genetic map of bacteriophage T7.

for the host and phage RNA polymerases, RNase III recognition sequences, the primary origin of DNA replication, and a terminal repetition of 160 bp used in forming concatemers during replication. The terminal repeat of different T7-like genomes is different in both length and sequence. The sequence GATC (a major regulatory sequence in *E. coli*) is distinctly underrepresented; this sequence, statistically expected 156 times in a 40 kb genome, occurs only six times in T7, 10 times in T3, and not at all in BA14. T7 and T3 inactivate type I restriction enzymes but remain susceptible to cells harboring type II and III enzymes. However, susceptibility to the latter enzymes may not be universal among the T7 group: some members contain restriction sites in their genomes but grow despite the presence of the cognate enzymes. The phage gene(s) responsible for type II and III enzyme inactivation are unknown.

Class I genes

Class I genes are those transcribed by *E. coli* RNA polymerase immediately after infection; the biochemical functions of five gene products are known. Type I restriction enzymes are inactivated by gp0.3 (which, for some T7-like phages, also harbors *S*-adenosyl methionine hydrolase activity). gp0.7 is a serine–threonine protein kinase that phosphorylates many host proteins, including RNA polymerase, RNase III, some ribosomal proteins and several translation factors. gp0.7 is also responsible for shut-off of host-catalyzed transcription, although this function is separable from kinase activity. Since host-catalyzed transcription is inactivated and the upstream T7 promoter ϕOL is poorly utilized during infection, early phage genes are also shutoff. Although class I mRNAs are stable, their translation (and those of residual host mRNAs) abruptly ceases about 8 min after infection; how inhibition is achieved is unknown.

gp1 is the T7 RNA polymerase, gp1.2 inhibits *E. coli* dGTPase, and gp1.3 is DNA ligase. Of class I genes, only gene *1* is essential, the remainder are required only in certain hosts or under adverse conditions. In the first few minutes of infection, T7 gene products thus inactivate some potentially deleterious host enzymes and, via inhibition of *E. coli*, and synthesis of T7, RNA polymerase, subsume all intracellular nucleotides and the translation machinery for the exclusive benefit of phage development.

Class II and class III genes

Class II and III genes are transcribed by T7 RNA polymerase; they are distinguished by a selective shut-off of class II transcription and translation about 15 min after infection. Class II genes function primarily in T7 DNA metabolism; they comprise the last three class I genes, *1.1–1.3*, plus genes *1.4–6.3*. In addition to their role in concatemer formation and resolution, the gp3 endonuclease and the gp6 exonuclease also degrade host DNA to mononucleotides; these are subsequently utilized for T7 DNA synthesis. More than 80% of the nucleotides in progeny phage originated from the host chromosome. *In vitro*, gp3 and gp6 degrade T7 DNA and their activities must be regulated *in vivo*; regulation may involve gp2 but the mechanism is not well understood. The gene 3.5 lysozyme is also multifunctional: its location among the class II genes reflects its role in replication and transcriptional regulation rather than in cell lysis.

Expression of the late class III genes is independent of DNA replication; times of appearance, rates of synthesis and final accumulation of class III proteins are unaffected by preventing phage replication. Essentially all class III genes are involved in phage morphogenesis and maturation or in cell lysis.

Phage Particle

The phage capsid is composed of 415 copies of gp10A or gp10B. At one vertex of the icosahedron, 12 molecules of gp8 form a portal through which the phage genome can pass. The portal also serves as the connector for the phage tail, consisting of six copies of gp12 and 12 or 18 copies of gp11. Six tail fibers, each comprised of gp17 trimers, are attached to the tail just below its junction with the capsid. The particle also contains several internal proteins – three forming a hollow cylindrical core structure, coaxial with the tail, that is attached to the inner surface of the capsid and the portal. This internal core is important during both DNA packaging and ejection. Functions of other particle proteins are incompletely understood, although gp6.7 is essential for adsorption and gp13 for an early stage of infection. Cryoelectron microscopy shows the 40 kb T7 genome spooled around the tail-specified axis in a close-packed, quasi-crystalline array.

T7 Infection Cycle

Aside from lysis, the T7 infection cycle has been modeled as a linked set of differential equations, directly derived from experimental data. The computer simulation accurately displays genome translocation into the cell, gene expression and its regulation, DNA replication and morphogenesis.

DNA Ejection

Following adsorption to *E. coli* K-12 the infection is initiated by degradation of the internal head proteins gp7.3 and gp13. The stubby T7 tail cannot directly penetrate the cell cytoplasm and a channel across the outer envelope must form to allow DNA translocation. The internal core of the head dissociates and its constituent proteins enter the cell (**Fig. 2**). gp14 localizes to the outer membrane; the N-terminal region of gp16 shares homology with a bacterial lytic transglycosylase and may enlarge a hole through the peptidoglycan. This presumed activity of gp16 is important only when cells are at high density or low temperature, conditions likely favoring increased crosslinking of the peptidoglycan. Much of the 143 kDa gp16 presumably spans the periplasm but the protein also penetrates the cytoplasmic membrane to complete the DNA translocation channel. gp15 appears to be cytoplasmic at this stage of infection but its function is unknown.

Only when channel assembly is complete does the phage genome exit the capsid. gp16 appears to be one component of an enzymatic motor, fueled by the proton motive force, that ratchets T7 DNA at a constant rate from the capsid into the cell. About 850 bp enters the cytoplasm by this mechanism; in the absence of transcription DNA translocation normally aborts at this stage. Therefore, neither the classic syringe model for phage DNA ejection nor the concept of packaged DNA resembling a compressed coiled spring apply to T7. It should be noted that these two widely held ideas have no direct experimental support in any phage–host system.

Within the 850 bp that enter the cell lie three *E. coli* RNA polymerase promoters. Transcription from these promoters causes 19% of the genome to be pulled into the cell, simultaneously causing expression of the nine early genes. One of these codes for T7 RNA polymerase, responsible not only for translocating the remaining 81% of the genome but also for all class II and class III gene expression. Complete internalization of the T7 genome occupies one-third of the latent period; the slow transcriptional mode of entry both ensures gp0.3 synthesis with consequent inactivation of type I restriction enzymes before cognate sites enter the cell, and may also help regulate temporal gene expression.

Transcription

All transcription of T7 DNA *in vivo* goes from left to right on the genetic map (**Fig. 3**). The three *E. coli* RNA polymerase promoters are all active, the A1 promoter being among the strongest known. Additional minor promoters identified by *in vitro* transcription studies or predicted from the nucleotide sequence are not known to be biologically significant except for mutant phages. Transcription from the major promoters usually terminates at the early terminator TE to produce three RNAs differing at

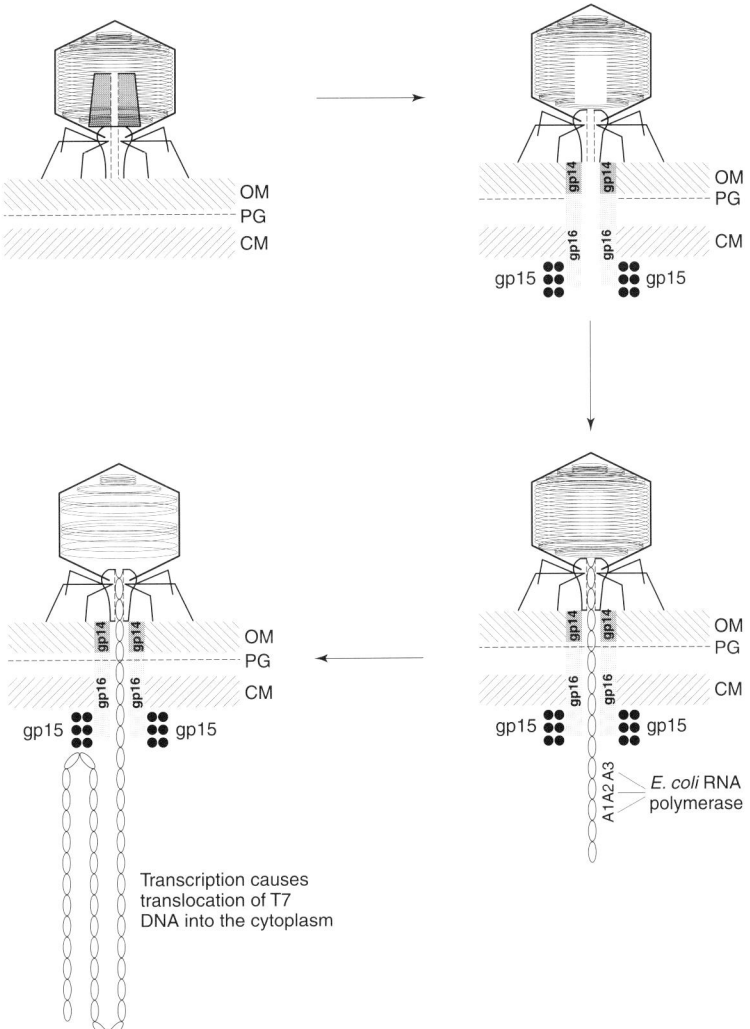

Figure 2 T7 DNA translocation into the bacterial cytoplasm. OM, outer membrane; PG, peptidoglycan; CM, cytoplasmic membrane.

their 5' ends but containing identical coding information. Transcription that reads through TE terminates inefficiently near the 3' end of gene *3.5*, distal to gene *10* at the T7 RNA polymerase terminator, or at the genome end.

Processing of primary transcripts by the host enzyme RNase III is a major feature of T7-infected cells, although nonessential for phage development. Early RNAs are processed into a noncoding initiator RNA and five mRNAs, only one of which is monocistronic. Processing of late transcripts also occurs but all RNase III-generated RNAs remain polycistronic. The stability of T7 RNAs during infection is likely due, in part, to the formation of base-paired structures at their 3' ends by RNase III processing.

T7 RNA polymerase promoters consist of a highly conserved 23 bp segment that runs from −17 to +6, relative to the transcription start. Seventeen promoters exist in the T7 genome, ten expressing class II and class III genes and five expressing only class III genes. The ϕOL and ϕOR promoters may function more in replication or maturation than in mRNA synthesis but neither are essential for phage viability. T3 contains a similar, though not identical, set of promoters.

Transcription from class II promoters and the first three class III promoters terminates distal to gene *10* at Tϕ and results in a nested set of polycistronic RNAs that differ at their 5' ends. Termination at Tϕ is about 80% efficient – in T7 the essential genes *11* and *12* are expressed only from readthrough RNAs; these, together with transcripts from $\phi 13$ and $\phi 17$, terminate near the genome end.

The significance of synthesizing such a complex array of transcripts, in particular over the class II

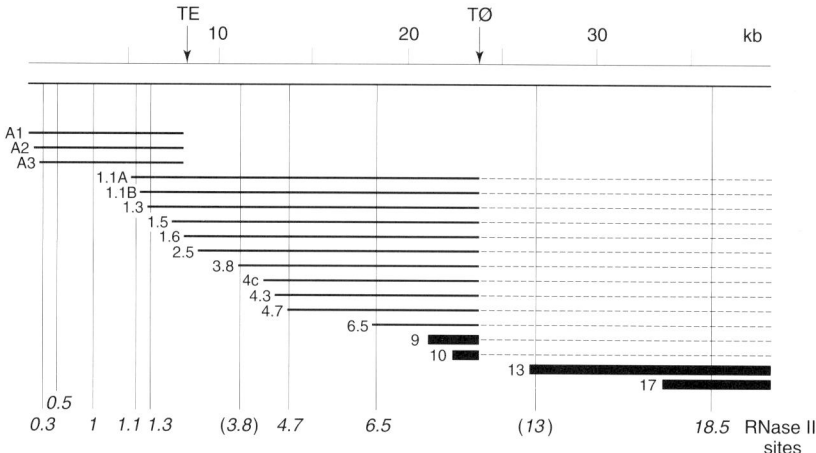

Figure 3 T7 RNAs. Promoters are indicated at the 5' ends of transcripts. Horizontal dashed lines represent the major readthrough RNAs. Vertical lines indicate the positions of cleavage by RNase III; sites are named by the gene following the site. Sites where cleavage is inefficient are in parentheses.

region, is unclear; however, it does provide a means of selectively producing large quantities of gene 9 and especially gene *10* RNAs. These are partly responsible for the high levels of gp9 and especially gp10 in the infected cell. A leader sequence on gene *10* mRNA and the initial gene *10* codons both also appear designed to maximize gp10 synthesis: during infection perhaps 100 000 gp10 molecules can be made from a single T7 genome in about 20 min.

The sequences of the five class III promoters are identical; these promoters are stronger than class II promoters, whose sequences differ from consensus at 2–7 positions. Promoter strength differences are manifest by the frequency of abortive initiation, which is higher at class II than at class III promoters. gp3.5 lysozyme also complexes with T7 RNA polymerase to inhibit the conformational change necessary for polymerase to switch from the initiation to the processive elongation mode of synthesis. One consequence of gp3.5–gp1 complex formation is then to effect the selective shut-off of class II transcription. Since gp3.5 is itself a class II product, its synthesis is autoregulating and high-level expression of gene *3.5* inhibits phage growth. gp3.5–gp1 complex formation also stimulates DNA replication, perhaps by providing primers via abortive transcription initiation over an origin sequence or by facilitating replication complex assembly on the separated strands of the transcription bubble. Transcripts originating from ϕOR encounter a strong transcriptional pause site that is prolonged by gp3.5 on concatemeric DNA immediately 3' of the terminal repeat. Enhanced pausing at this site may aid assembly of the machinery for DNA packaging. Gene *3.5* is thus central to several aspects of T7 development.

Promoter specificities

The RNA polymerases coded by other T7-like phages are similar to that of T7. A single amino acid change allows T7 RNA polymerase to specifically recognize T3 promoters, and *vice versa*. RNA polymerases coded by *Salmonella* phage SP6 and *Klebsiella* phage K11 have diverged more extensively from the T7 enzyme, although their respective promoters retain substantial homology to T7. However, there is little recognition of these enzymes for noncognate promoters. Of likely evolutionary significance is the homology between these phage-coded enzymes and the *Saccharomyces cerevisiae* mitochondrial RNA polymerase.

DNA Replication

Replication *in vivo* requires T7 RNA polymerase, DNA polymerase, primase/helicase, single-stranded DNA binding protein (gp2.5), endonuclease and exonuclease. There is no requirement for topoisomerase activity as no closed circular species of the T7 genome form. Even though *E. coli* RNA polymerase is transcriptionally inactive when replication begins, it can interfere with DNA maturation and packaging and gp2 is required to alleviate inhibition. Other than thioredoxin, which forms a 1:1 complex with gp5 in T7 DNA polymerase, no host proteins are known to be required for phage replication. A crystallographic structure of T7 DNA polymerase, bound to a primer-template and nucleoside triphosphate, has been reported.

Replication *in vivo* is normally initiated at an A+T-rich region located 15% from the left end,

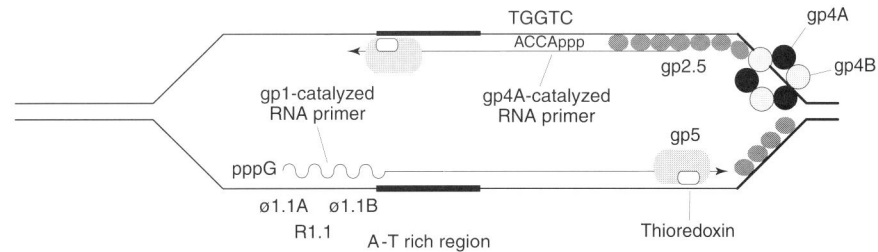

Figure 4 Initial events at the primary origin of DNA replication. Not all protein:proteins are indicated.

although deletion mutants lacking this origin grow well in most laboratory hosts. Replication is bidirectional on the linear genome, the replication 'bubble' enlarges, providing a Y-shaped molecule, before further elongation yields two linear molecules (**Fig. 4**). Replicated linear molecules necessarily contain unreplicated 3′ ends; T7 circumvents replicated genome erosion by forming linear concatemers via its terminal 160 bp repeats. As replication proceeds, fast-sedimenting DNA molecules appear that consist mainly of linear concatemers and branched, recombining molecules. The fast-sedimenting DNA complex, containing >100 genome equivalents, is ultimately converted by the gp3 resolvase into concatemeric molecules that are substrates for the packaging machinery. Although incorporation of thymidine into T7 DNA can be detected for about 20 min, the >200-fold increase in T7 DNA mass resulting from replication is achieved much more rapidly, fluctuations in nucleotide pool sizes as bacterial DNA is degraded and reutilized confound analyses of precursor incorporation data. The rate of T7 DNA mass increase is suggestive of numerous replication forks, consistent with the idea that recombination intermediates may be converted into replication forks, as is the case with T4. Recombination rates in T7-infected cells are very high; wild-type recombinants have been detected between mutants altered in adjacent nucleotides. Recombination is independent of the host RecA but requires most T7 replication proteins. Single strands may be formed by gp6 exonuclease or during replication; strand exchange is catalyzed by gp2.5 and the gp4 helicase, and gp3 resolves Holliday junctions.

Plasmid-based assays *in vivo* have revealed secondary replication origins that may function in later stages of phage replication. Plasmids containing the promoters $\phi6.5$ and $\phi13$ are replicated following T7 infection as efficiently as plasmids containing $\phi1.1A$ or $\phi1.1B$ and the primary origin; those containing ϕOR are replicated even more. Furthermore, plasmids containing both ϕOR and a packaging signal are packaged after replication, yielding particles that transduce the plasmid DNA. Plasmids containing other promoters are, at best, poorly replicated after infection, but what makes a promoter functional in DNA replication is not understood.

In vitro, bidirectional replication from the primary origin has been achieved using purified T7 RNA and DNA polymerases, gp2.5, and the heterohexameric primase–helicase complex of gp4A and gp4B. RNA polymerase synthesizes primers of 10–60 nucleotides from both promoters immediately upstream of the origin. The gp4 hexamer forms a sliding clamp that translocates 5′ to 3′ to unwind unreplicated DNA using ribo- or deoxy-NTP (preferring dTTP *in vitro*) hydrolysis for energy. The clamp also interacts with both gp2.5 and DNA polymerase, making DNA synthesis more processive. Whereas gp4B has only helicase activity, gp4A also serves as a primase; the N-terminal 63 residues not present in gp4B contain a zinc-finger motif that interacts with the sequences 3′-CTGG(G/T)-5′ or 3′-CTGTG-5′ in single-stranded DNA. Primers, 5′-ACC(A/C) or 5′-ACAC are synthesized that initiate lagging strand DNA synthesis. gp2.5 interacts with both DNA polymerase and primase–helicase to stimulate lagging strand synthesis and to promote bidirectional replication from the primary origin. Although *E. coli* SSB stimulates T7 DNA polymerase activity *in vitro*, it cannot substitute for gp2.5 for bidirectional replication from the primary origin and T7 SSB is an essential protein.

Capsid Assembly and DNA Packaging

Detailed information on morphogenesis has been obtained with both T7 and T3. It is assumed that the mechanism of particle assembly is common to both phages.

Packaging of T7 DNA starts with the assembly of a DNA-free procapsid. The major capsid protein gp10 assembles around a gp9 scaffold in a reaction that has been accomplished *in vitro* using purified proteins. One vertex of the icosahedral procapsid is modified by the addition of gp8 to form the portal. In addition, the procapsid contains the internal protein core, and also the maturation protein gp19. The latter is likely outside the procapsid, as it recognizes the gp8 portal

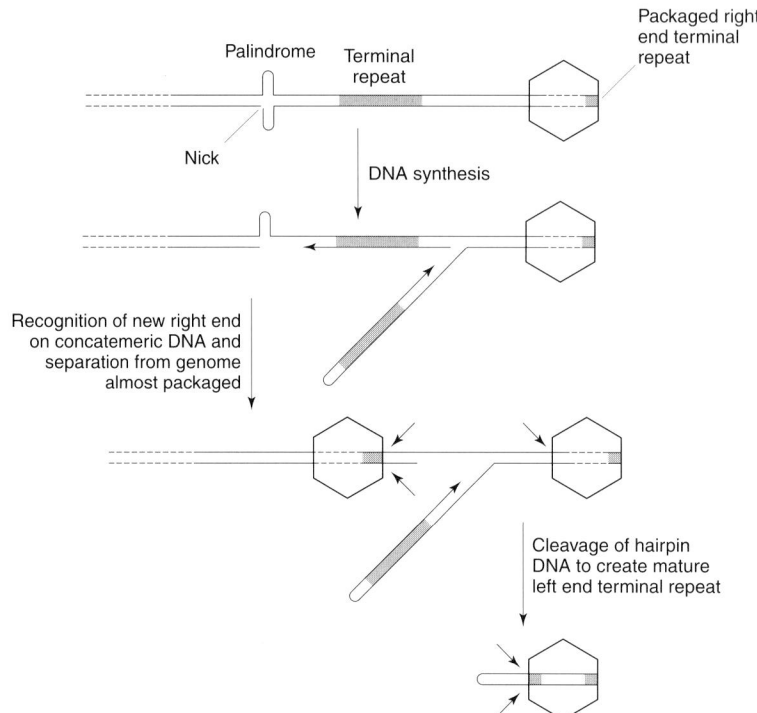

Figure 5 Pathway for duplication of the terminal repeat during packaging from concatemeric DNA.

protein and, perhaps in conjunction with gp18, interacts with concatemeric DNA before packaging. Both gp18 and gp19 are required for packaging, though neither are found in the mature phage particle. Packaging of a single genome from concatemeric DNA is estimated to take about 90 s, a rate that has been achieved *in vitro*.

During packaging of DNA, the procapsid undergoes a conformational change characterized by an increase in size and a conversion from rounded to icosahedral morphology. The gp9 scaffolding protein likely exits the procapsid as these changes occur. After association of the procapsid with concatemeric DNA, packaging proceeds from a genomic right end leftwards in an incompletely understood process. A series of reactions is necessary for duplication of the 160 bp terminal repeat that in concatemers is present in only one copy between genomes. The DNA is nicked by an unknown nuclease at a palindromic sequence located to the left of the right terminal repeat, creating a hairpin primer for DNA polymerase (**Fig. 5**). Extending the hairpin through the terminal repeat and into the genome being packaged provides duplex DNA that could be converted into a mature left end. On the remaining concatemeric DNA, primase-initiated synthesis on the displaced strand proceeds through the terminal repeat, providing sequences that could be converted into the mature right end of the next genome to be packaged. However, the nicking site and palindromic sequences are nonessential, although the obligatory alterations in the packaging mechanism are unknown.

The nuclease recognizing the termini of mature T7 DNA is unknown, although gp19 possesses a nonspecific endonucleolytic activity that is suppressed by gp18, and both proteins are required to create the mature termini. T7 RNA polymerase is also required for DNA packaging; it seems likely that gp3.5-enhanced pausing of transcription near the concatemer junction may recruit gp19 for initiation of packaging.

The final stage of phage development is lysis of the host cell, a process poorly understood. Genes 3.5 and 17.5 are required, perhaps together with another component (gp18.5 and/or nucleic acid?). gp17.5 may be a holin that disrupts the cell membrane, allowing gp3.5 lysozyme to lyse the cell or to release phage from cell debris. The potential role of DNA in lysis is unclear, but replication-defective mutants are as lysis defective as gene 3.5 amber mutants, even though replication does not affect gene expression.

Host Functions in T7 Development

A number of natural *E. coli* or other enterobacterial hosts are nonpermissive for many members of the T7 group of phages. In most cases the host genes involved are unknown. Several prophages or resident plasmids are known to have the potential to inhibit growth of T7 by a process(es) distinct from adsorption or DNA restriction; however, the incoming phage often contains a gene that prevents inhibition. The λ *rex* genes exclude certain missense mutants of T7, perhaps by a comparable (but unknown) mechanism to that of exclusion of T4 *r* II mutants. The Col Ib plasmid inhibits growth of *0.7* mutants; the basis of exclusion is not understood but may involve the failure to inactivate *E. coli* RNA polymerase. Most T7-like phages are also excluded from growth in F plasmid-containing cells, although T3 is an exception. The *pifA* gene of F interferes with the normal functions of T7 genes *1.2* and *10*; interaction of either gene with *pifA* causes inhibition of all macromolecular synthesis and membrane functions. The rapid loss of metabolic potential of the abortively infected, F-containing *E. coli* suggests that some key cellular component(s) is inactivated by the interaction of T7 and *pif* genes. This component is unidentified but can be protected from PifA and gp10 (or gp1.2) by increased synthesis of the *E. coli* membrane protein FxsA, a protein with no known independent function.

Expression Systems Based on T7 RNA Polymerase

The specificity of T7 RNA polymerase for its promoter has allowed the development of high-level, regulated expression systems for cloned DNA in both procaryotes and eucaryotes. Typically, the gene *10* promoter is employed, with or without gene *10* translational start sequences; T7 RNA polymerase is supplied from the cloned gene or by phage infection. Epitope-tagged expression vectors to aid in product purification are available. A phage display system based on the capsid protein accommodating both high and low levels of display has also been developed.

Future Perspectives

The utility of the expression and display systems alone will ensure continued research on bacteriophage T7. Our understanding of, in particular, mechanisms of DNA replication and transcription will continue to be furthered using T7 as a model. The mechanisms of DNA translocation across membranes and the morphogenesis and structure of complex nucleoprotein assemblages are two additional fields of research where the T7 model can be expected to make significant contributions.

Further Reading

Cerritelli ME, Cheng B, Rosenberg AH *et al* (1997) Encapsidated conformation of bacteriophage T7 DNA. *Cell* 91: 271.

Chung Y-B, Nardone C and Hinkle DC (1990) Bacteriophage T7 DNA packaging. *J. Mol. Biol.* 216: 939.

Dunn JJ and Studier FW (1983) Complete nucleotide sequence of bacteriophage T7 DNA and the locations of T7 genetic elements. *J. Mol. Biol.* 166: 477.

García LR and Molineux IJ (1996) Transcription-independent DNA translocation of bacteriophage T7 DNA into *Escherichia coli*. *J. Bacteriol.* 178: 6921.

Kong D and Richardson CC (1996) Single-stranded DNA binding protein and DNA helicase of bacteriophage T7 mediate homologous DNA strand exchange. *EMBO J.* 15: 2010.

Molineux IJ (1991) Host–interactions: recent developments in the genetics of abortive phage infections. *New Biol.* 1991 3: 230.

Tanapox Virus   *see* **Yabapox Viruses**

TAXONOMY, CLASSIFICATION AND NOMENCLATURE OF VIRUSES

Claude M. Fauquet, The Scripps Research Institute, Division of Plant Biology, La Jolla, California, USA

Copyright © 1999 Academic Press

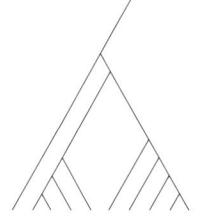

History of Virus Classification and Virus Nomenclature

Humans feel the need to classify natural entities and the viruses are no exception. As in other biological systems, virus classification is an approximate and imperfect exercise. Like any other type of classification, it is a totally artificial and human-driven activity without any natural base. However, science requires workable descriptions of living systems and their constituent parts, and, when achieved properly, classifications are extremely useful for showing similar characteristics and properties across populations. Unfortunately for virus taxonomy no fossil record exists and so evolutionary relationships are very speculative, meaning that only a logical and precise virus classification can provide indications of the evolution of viruses. Appropriately chosen classification criteria are also informative in the case of newly discovered viruses. In theory, nomenclature and classification are totally independent, but for viruses both issues are often considered at the same time. As a result, taxonomic names for the viruses have always been the subject of passionate discussions and the taxonomic status of viruses is a sensitive and critical issue.

Virus classification is a relatively new exercise, as the first evidence for existence of a virus was only presented at the end of the nineteenth century by Beijerinck in 1898. It was not until 1927 that Johnson, a plant virologist, drew attention to the need for a system of virus nomenclature and classification. First efforts to classify viruses utilized a range of ecological and biological criteria, including pathogenic properties in the case of human and animal viruses, and symptoms for plant viruses. For example, viruses sharing the pathogenic properties causing hepatitis (e.g. hepatitis A virus, hepatitis B virus, yellow fever virus, and Rift Valley fever virus) were grouped together as 'the hepatitis viruses'. Virology developed substantially in the 1930s and early classifications for the viruses reflected these advances. In 1939, Holmes published a classification of plant viruses dependent on host reactions and differential host species, using a binomial-trinomial nomenclature based on the name of the infected plant; however, only 89 viruses were described and classified in this way. With the development of electron microscopy and biochemical studies in the 1950s, the first virus groupings based on common virion properties emerged: like the Herpesvirus group described by Andrewes in 1954, the Myxovirus group by Andrewes *et al*, in 1955, and the Poxvirus group by Fenner and Burnet in 1957. During this period there was also an explosion of newly discovered viruses; in response, several individuals and committees independently proposed virus classification systems but none was widely adopted by the scientific community. It became obvious that only an international association of virologists could propose a comprehensive and universally acceptable system of virus classification.

At the 1966 International Congress for Microbiology held in Moscow, the International Committee on Nomenclature of Viruses (ICNV) was established by an international group of 43 virologists. An international organization was set up with the aim of developing a taxonomy and nomenclature system for all viruses that would be recognized worldwide. The name of the ICNV was changed in 1974 to the more appropriate International Committee on Taxonomy of Viruses (ICTV), which remains active today. ICTV, the unique official committee of the Virology Division, is now considered the international official body for all matters related to taxonomy and nomenclature of viruses.

Since the founding of the ICTV, all virologists have agreed that the hundreds of viruses isolated from different organisms should be classified together in a unique system, but separate from other microorganisms such as fungi, bacteria and mycoplasma. However, there was much controversy on the way to do it. Lwoff, Horne and Tournier argued for the adoption of a system classifying viruses into subphyla, classes, orders, suborders and families. Descending hierarchical divisions would have been based on nucleic acid type (DNA or RNA), strandedness (single or double), presence or absence of an envelope, capsid symmetry, and so on. The hierarchy of this system has never been recognized by the ICTV; nevertheless, the types of criteria used became the basis of the universal taxonomy system now in place, and all ICTV reports have used this scheme. Until 1990, no hierarchical classification level higher than the family was used, however, the system has recently begun to move in this direction. A first order, *Mononegavirales*, was accepted in 1990, and another two, *Caudovirales* and *Nidovirales*, were adopted in 1996. In its nonlinnean structure, the scheme is quite different from that used in the taxonomy of bacteria and other organisms. Nevertheless, the usefulness of the scheme is being demonstrated by its wide application. It has replaced all competing classification schemes for all viruses and no one would now dispute with the ICTV the international mandate to name and classify viruses.

Since its establishment, a total of seven virus taxonomic reports (also known by the names of the ICTV Presidents acting as Editors in Chief of the reports) have been published by the ICTV: Wildy in 1971; Fenner in 1976; Matthews in 1979; Matthews in 1982; Francki *et al* in 1991; Murphy *et al* in 1995; and van Regenmortel *et al* in 1999. At the first meeting in Mexico City in 1970, two families with a corresponding two genera and 24 floating genera were adopted to begin the grouping of the vertebrate, invertebrate and bacterial viruses. In addition, 16 plant virus groups were designated, as reported by Matthews in 1983. The fifth ICTV report, edited by Francki *et al* in 1991, described one order, 40 families, nine subfamilies, 102 genera, two floating genera and two subgenera for vertebrate, invertebrate, bacterial and fungal viruses, and 32 groups and seven subgroups for plant viruses. While most virologists shifted to placing viruses in families and genera, plant virologists retained the term 'groups' until 1993. It was only in 1995, as described in the sixth ICTV report, that the ICTV proposed a uniform system for all viruses, with two orders, 50 families, nine subfamilies, 126 genera, 23 floating genera and four subgenera encompassing 2644 assigned viruses. Most recently, at the 28th meeting of the ICTV in March 1998 in San Diego, California, the Universal Virus Classification was adopted; this comprises three orders, 56 families, nine subfamilies, 203 genera, 30 floating genera and a total of 3954 species, strains and/or serotypes of species and tentative species. It is a general trend that the number of described taxa and the number of species of viruses is increasing steadily, easily explained by the increasing complexity of the virus classification and by the amount of data available to demarcate viruses.

With precise and complete descriptions available for a large number of virus families, this classification now constitutes a valuable source of information for new 'unknown' viruses. Therefore, the ICTV classification is not only a taxonomic exercise for virus evolutionists but also a valuable diagnostic tool and educational system for virologists, teachers, medical doctors and epidemiologists.

How does the ICTV operate?

The ICTV is a committee of the Virology Division, which is in turn part of the International Union of Microbiological Societies. The ICTV is a nonprofit-making organization composed of prominent virologists representing countries from throughout the world who work to designate virus names and taxa through a democratic process. The ICTV operates through a number of committees, subcommittees and study groups consisting of more than 492 eminent virologists with expertise in viruses infecting humans, animals, insects, protozoa, archaea, bacteria, mycoplasma, fungi, algae, yeasts and plants. Taxonomic proposals are initiated and formulated by individuals or by the study groups. These proposals are revised and accepted by the corresponding subcommittees and presented for executive committee approval. All decisions are then ratified at a plenary session (or also now by postal vote) held at each Virology Congress where all members of ICTV and more than 50 representatives of national microbiological societies are represented. At present, there are 47 study groups working in concert with six subcommittees – namely, the vertebrate, invertebrate, plant, bacteria, fungus and virus data subcommittees. The ICTV does not impose any taxonomic terms or taxa but ensures that all propositions are compatible with ICTV rules for homogeneity and consistency. The ICTV regularly publishes reports describing all existing virus taxa with a list of classified viruses as well as descriptions of virus families and genera. An Internet web site, where the most important information relative to virus taxonomy is made available, is updated regularly. The sixth report was published by Murphy *et al* (1995) and the seventh by van Regenmortel *et al* (1999).

The increasing number of virus species and virus strains being identified, together with the explosion of data on many descriptive aspects of viruses and viral diseases, and particularly sequence data, has led the ICTV to launch an international virus database project. This project, termed ICTVdB, is scheduled to be fully operational and accessible to the scientific community around the year 2000. The ICTVdB, in addition to the taxonomic descriptions of all the taxa, will comprise all the information available about each virus species, and later each virus strain, for all the descriptors necessary to identify and recognize all viruses.

A Universal System for Virus Classification

There are currently two systems in use for classifying organisms: the linnean and the adansonian systems.

The former is the monothetic hierarchical classification applied by Linnaeus to plants and animals, while the adansonian is a polythetic hierarchical system initially proposed by Adanson in 1763. In 1984 Maurin and collaborators suggested applying the linnean classification system to the viruses. Although convenient to use, this system has shortcomings when applied to the classification of viruses. Firstly, it is difficult to appreciate the validity of a particular criteria. For example, it may not be appropriate to use the number of genomic components as a hierarchical criteria. Secondly, there are no obvious reasons for prioritizing criteria, and in consequence it is difficult to rank all the available criteria. For instance, is the nature of the genome (DNA/RNA) more important than the sense of the coding sequence of the genome or the shape of the virus particles?

The adansonian system considers all available criteria at once and makes several classifications, taking the criteria into consideration successively. The criteria leading to the same classifications are considered as correlated and are therefore not discriminatory. Subsequently, a subset of criteria are considered, and the process is repeated until all criteria can be ranked to provide the best discrimination of the species. This system has not been used frequently in the past owing to its labor-intensive nature, but this situation has changed as a result of the power and availability of today's computer technology. Furthermore, qualitative and quantitative data can be simultaneously considered when generating such a classification. In the case of viruses, it was determined by Harrison and collaborators in 1971 that at least 60 characters could be used for a complete virus description (**Table 1**). Thus, the limiting factor for applying the adansonian system is now not its labor-intensive nature but the lack of data for many of the viruses.

In addition, the increasing number of viral nucleic acid sequences being reported, in combination with the appropriate computer software, allows the comparison of viruses to generate different phylogenetic trees, according to the gene or set of genes used, as for example proposed by Koonin in 1991, Dolja and Koonin in 1991 and Dolja et al in 1991. However, to date, none of them has satisfactorily provided a clear classification of all viruses. A multidimensional classification, taking into account all the criteria necessary to describe viruses, would probably be the most appropriate way of representing a virus classification, but again the shortcomings of data for some viruses would prevent the use of this system in the foreseeable future.

For almost 25 years, the ICTV has been classifying viruses essentially at the family and genus levels using a nonsystematic polythetic approach. Viruses were clustered first in genera and then in families. A subset of characters, including physicochemical, structural, genomic and biological criteria, is then used to compare and group viruses. This subset of characters may change from one family to another, according to the availability of the data and the importance of a particular character for a particular family. It is obvious that there is no homogeneity in this respect throughout the virus classification and that virologists weigh the criteria differently in this subjective process, leading to the generation of a nonhomogeneous classification. Nevertheless, over time we can see stability of the current ICTV classification at the genus and family level. When sequence, genomic organization and replicative cycle data are subsequently used for taxonomic purposes, they usually confirm the actual classification. It is also obvious that hierarchical classifications above the family level will encounter conflicts between phenotypic and genotypic criteria and that virologists will have to consider the entire classification process in order to progress in this direction.

Currently, and for practical reasons only, virus classification is structured according to the presentation indicated in **Tables 2** and **3**. This 'Order of Presentation of the Viruses' does not reflect any hierarchical or phylogenetic classification but only a convenient order of presentation of the virus taxa. Since a taxonomic structure above the level of family (with the exception of the orders *Mononegavirales*, *Caudovirales* and *Nidovirales*) has not been developed extensively, any listing must be arbitrary. The order of presentation of virus families and genera follows four criteria: (1) the nature of the viral nucleic acid; (2) the strandedness of the nucleic acid; (3) the use of a reverse transcription process (DNA or RNA); and (4) the positive or negative sense of gene coding on the encapsidated genome. These four criteria give rise to six clusters comprising the 86 families and floating genera of viruses. In the past, two other criteria were also taken in account: the presence or absence of a lipid envelope and the segmentation of the genome as mono-, bi-, tri-, tetra- or multipartite. However, it has become clear that the presence of an envelope was entirely related to the nature of the host and that families could comprise genera having viruses with segmented or nonsegmented genomes, but sharing all other properties, including genome organization and sequence homology. These criteria have been therefore abandoned.

The Virus Species Concept and its Application

In 1991 the ICTV accepted the concept that viruses

Table 1 Virus family descriptors used in virus taxonomy

I Virion properties
A Morphology properties of virions
    1 Size
    2 Shape
    3 Presence or absence of an envelope and peplomers
    4 Capsomeric symmetry and structure

B Physical properties of virions
    1 Molecular mass
    2 Buoyant density
    3 Sedimentation coefficient
    4 pH stability
    5 Thermal stability
    6 Cation (Mg^{2+}, Mn^{2+}) stability
    7 Solvent stability
    8 Detergent stability
    9 Radiation stability

C Properties of genome
    1 Type of nucleic acid DNA or RNA
    2 Strandedness: single-stranded or double-stranded
    3 Linear or circular
    4 Sense: positive, negative or ambisense
    5 Number of segments
    6 Size of genome or genome segments
    7 Presence or absence and type of 5′ terminal cap
    8 Presence or absence of 5′ terminal covalently linked polypeptide
    9 Presence or absence of 3′ terminal poly(A) tract (or other specific tract)
    10 Nucleotide sequence comparisons

D Properties of proteins
    1 Number
    2 Size
    3 Functional activities (especially virion transcriptase, virion reverse transcriptase, virion hemagglutinin, virion neuraminidase, virion fusion protein)
    4 Amino acid sequence comparisons

E Lipids
    1 Presence or absence
    2 Nature

F Carbohydrates
    1 Presence or absence
    2 Nature

II Genome organization and replication
    1 Genome organization
    2 Strategy of replication of nucleic acid
    3 Characteristics of transcription
    4 Characteristics of translation and post-translational processing
    5 Site of accumulation of virion proteins, site of assembly, site of maturation and release
    6 Cytopathology, inclusion body formation

III Antigenic properties
    1 Serological relationships
    2 Mapping epitopes

IV Biological properties
    1 Host range, natural and experimental
    2 Pathogenicity, association with disease
    3 Tissue tropisms, pathology, histopathology

Table 1 Continued

4 Mode of transmission in nature
5 Vector relationships
6 Geographic distribution

Adapted from ICTV guidelines for family descriptions.

exist as species, in a similar manner to other organisms, and adopted a definition for a virus species proposed by van Regenmortel in 1990: 'A virus species is a polythetic class of viruses that constitutes a replicating lineage and occupies a particular ecological niche.' This simple definition and the position taken by the ICTV has already had, and will continue to have, a profound effect on virus classification. Effectively, in the sixth ICTV report virus names were indicated in 'List of species' but they were in fact a 'List of virus names' with undefined taxonomic status. In the seventh ICTV report, according to the polythetic nature of the species definition, a 'List of species-demarcating criteria' is provided for each genus, indicating how virus species can be identified in this particular genus. Viruses are then differentiated in species and tentative species according to this list of criteria and the availability of information to demarcate the species.

First, it is intended to define for each genus the criteria demarcating a virus species, and, second, to compare these criteria from one genus to the next, searching for homogeneity throughout the virus classification. Naturally this list of criteria should follow the polythetic nature of the species definition and more than one criteria should be used to determine a new species. It is obvious that most of the criteria in the list of demarcating criteria are shared amongst the different genera, within and across families; namely, host range, serological relationships, vector transmission type, tissue tropism, genome rearrangement and sequence homology (**Table 4**). However, if the types of criteria are similar, the levels of demarcation clearly differ from one family to another. This may reflect differences in appreciation from one family to another but also the differential ranking of a particular criterion in different families. The huge differences (up to 30%) in sequences among nucleoproteins of species of lentiviruses does not have the same biological significance as small differences in capsid protein sequences (1–10%) of species of potyviruses, and therefore universal levels of sequence identity for similar genes may not exist for viruses! The levels of demarcation may even change from one gene to another within the same family. Homogenization of the application of the species definition concept throughout the virus definition will be the next challenge of ICTV for the eighth report to be published by 2002. This, in turn, will contribute to homogeneity of the genus and family demarcation criteria (**Table 4**) and will permit creation of new families or merging of existing families. However, it is important to note that the nature of the demarcating criteria at the genus level will probably not change as these have passed the test of time. Despite the fact that they were mostly established using biochemical and structural criteria, they remained valid when correlated with genome organization and sequence data.

The Universal Virus Classification

The present universal system of virus taxonomy is set arbitrarily at hierarchical levels of order, family (in some cases subfamily), genus and species. Lower hierarchical levels, such as subspecies, strain, serotype, variant, pathotype and isolate are established by international specialty groups and/or by culture collections, but not by the ICTV. However some of them may be indicated in the ICTV report for information or because in the past these names were listed as 'viruses' in previous reports.

Virus species

The species taxon is always regarded as the most important taxonomic level in classification but it has proved to be the most difficult to apply to the viruses. ICTV definition of a virus species was long considered to be 'a concept that will normally be represented by a cluster of strains from a variety of sources, or a population of strains from a particular source, which have in common a set or pattern of correlating stable properties that separates the cluster from other clusters of strains' as stated by Matthews in 1982 and by Francki et al in 1991. This was a general definition, which was in fact not very useful for practically delineating species in a particular family. Furthermore, this definition directly addressed the definition of a virus strain, which had never been attempted in the history of virus taxonomy. In 1991, the ICTV Executive Committee accepted a definition proposed by van Regenmortel in 1990 (see above). This definition states: 'A virus species is a polythetic class of viruses that constitutes a replicating lineage

Table 2 Continued

Order	Family	Subfamily	Genus	Type species	Host
	Parvoviridae	Parvovirinae	Parvovirus	Mice minute virus	Vertebrates
			Erythrovirus	B19 virus	Vertebrates
			Dependovirus	Adeno-associated virus 2	Vertebrates
		Densovirinae	Densovirus	Junonia coenia densovirus	Invertebrates
			Iteravirus	Bombyx mori densovirus	Invertebrates
			Brevidensovirus	Aedes aegypti densovirus	Invertebrates

The DNA and RNA reverse transcribing viruses

Order	Family	Subfamily	Genus	Type species	Host
	Hepadnaviridae		Orthohepadnavirus	Hepatitis B virus	Vertebrates
			Avihepadnavirus	Duck hepatitis B virus	Vertebrates
	Caulimoviridae		Caulimovirus	Cauliflower mosaic virus	Plants
			"PVCV-like viruses"	Petunia vein-clearing virus	Plants
			"SbCMV-like viruses"	Soybean chlorotic mottle virus	Plants
			"CsVMV-like viruses"	Cassava vein mosaic virus	Plants
			Badnavirus	Commelina yellow mottle virus	Plants
			"RTBV-like viruses"	Rice tungro bacilliform virus	Plants
	Pseudoviridae		Pseudovirus	Saccharomyces cerevisiae Ty1 virus	Yeast, Plants
			Hemivirus	Drosophila melanogaster copia virus	Yeast, Invertebrates
	Metaviridae		Metavirus	Saccharomyces cerevisiae Ty3 virus	Yeast, Plants, Invertebrates
			Errantivirus	Drosophila melanogaster gypsy virus	Invertebrates
	Retroviridae		Alpharetrovirus	Avian leukosis virus	Vertebrates
			Betaretrovirus	Mason-Pfizer monkey virus	Vertebrates
			Gammaretrovirus	Mouse mammary tumor virus	Vertebrates
			Deltaretrovirus	Bovine leukemia virus	Vertebrates
			Epsilonretrovirus	Walleye dermal sarcoma virus	Vertebrates
			Lentivirus	Human immunodeficiency virus 1	Vertebrates
			Spumavirus	Human spumavirus	Vertebrates

Table 2 Continued

Order	Family	Subfamily	Genus	Type species	Host
		Gammaherpesvirinae	Lymphocryptovirus	Human herpesvirus 4	Vertebrates
			Rhadinovirus	Ateline herpesvirus 2	Vertebrates
			"Ictalurid herpes-like viruses"	Ictalurid herpesvirus 1	Vertebrates
	Adenoviridae		Mastadenovirus	Human adenovirus 2	Vertebrates
			Aviadenovirus	Fowl adenovirus 1	Vertebrates
			Rhizidiovirus	Rhizidiomyces virus	Fungi
	Polyomaviridae		Polyomavirus	Murine polyomavirus	Vertebrates
	Papillomaviridae		Papillomavirus	Cottontail rabbit papillomavirus	Vertebrates
	Polydnaviridae		Ichnovirus	Campoletis sonorensis virus	Invertebrates
			Bracovirus	Cotesia melanoscela virus	Invertebrates
	Ascoviridae		Ascovirus	Spodoptera frugiperda ascovirus	Invertebrates

The ssDNA viruses

Order	Family	Subfamily	Genus	Type species	Host
	Inoviridae		Inovirus	Coliphage fd	Bacteria
			Plectrovirus	Acholeplasma phage L51	Mycoplasma
	Microviridae		Microvirus	Coliphage φX174	Bacteria
			Spiromicrovirus	Spiroplasma phage 4	Spiroplasma
			Bdellomicrovirus	Bdellovibrio phage MAC1	Bacteria
			Chlamydiamicrovirus	Chlamydia phage 1	Bacteria
	Geminiviridae		Mastrevirus	Maize streak virus	Plants
			Curtovirus	Beet curly top virus	Plants
			Begomovirus	Bean golden mosaic virus	Plants
	Circoviridae		Circovirus	Chicken anemia virus	Vertebrates
			Nanovirus	Subterranean clover stunt virus	Plants

Table 2 Continued

Order	Family	Subfamily	Genus	Type species	Host
			Leporipoxvirus	Myxoma virus	Vertebrates
			Suipoxvirus	Swinepox virus	Vertebrates
			Molluscipoxvirus	Molluscum contagiosum virus	Vertebrates
			Yatapoxvirus	Yaba monkey tumor virus	Vertebrates
		Entomopoxvirinae			
			Entomopoxvirus A	Melolontha melolontha entomopoxvirus	Invertebrates
			Entomopoxvirus B	Amsacta moorei entomopoxvirus	Invertebrates
			Entomopoxvirus C	Chironomus luridus entomopoxvirus	Invertebrates
	Asfarviridae		Asfivirus	African swine fever virus	Vertebrates[b]
	Iridoviridae				
			Iridovirus	Chilo iridescent virus	Invertebrates
			Chloriridovirus	Mosquito iridescent virus	Invertebrates
			Ranavirus	Frog virus 3	Vertebrates
			Lymphocystivirus	Flounder virus	Vertebrates
	Phycodnaviridae				
			Chlorovirus	Paramecium bursaria Chlorella virus 1	Algae
			Prasinovirus	Micromonas pusilla virus SP1	Algae
			Prymnesiovirus	Chrysochromulina brevifilum virus	Algae
			Phaeovirus	Ectocarpus siliculosus virus 1	Algae
	Baculoviridae				
			Nucleopolyhedrovirus	Autographa californica nucleopolyhedrovirus	Invertebrates
			Granulovirus	Cydia pomonella granulovirus	Invertebrates
	Herpesviridae				
		Alphaherpesvirinae			
			Simplexvirus	Human herpesvirus 1	Vertebrates
			Varicellovirus	Human herpesvirus 3	Vertebrates
			"Marek's disease-like viruses"	Marek's disease virus	Vertebrates
			"ILTV-like viruses"	Infectious laryngotracheitis virus	Vertebrates
		Betaherpesvirinae			
			Cytomegalovirus	Human herpesvirus 5	Vertebrates
			Muromegalovirus	Mouse cytomegalovirus 1	Vertebrates
			Roseolovirus	Human herpesvirus 6	Vertebrates

Table 2 Order of presentation of the viruses

Order	Family	Subfamily	Genus	Type species	Host
The DNA viruses					
The dsDNA viruses					
Caudovirales	Myoviridae		"T4-like viruses"[a]	Enterobacteria phage T4	Bacteria
			"P1-like viruses"	Enterobacteria phage P1	Bacteria
			"P2-like viruses"	Enterobacteria phage P2	Bacteria
			"Mu-like viruses"	Enterobacteria phage Mu	Bacteria
			"SP01-like viruses"	Bacillus phage SP01	Bacteria
			"φH-like viruses"	Halobacterium virus φH	Archaea
	Siphoviridae		"λ-like viruses"	Enterobacteria phage λ	Bacteria
			"T1-like viruses"	Enterobacteria phage T1	Bacteria
			"T5-like viruses"	Enterobacteria phage T5	Bacteria
			"L5-like viruses"	Mycobacterium phage L5	Bacteria
			"c2-like viruses"	Lactococcus phage c2	Bacteria
			"ψM1-like viruses"	Methanobacterium virus ψM1	Archaea
	Podoviridae		"T7-like viruses"	Enterobacteria phage T7	Bacteria
			"P22-like viruses"	Enterobacteria phage P22	Bacteria
			"φ29-like viruses"	Bacillus phage φ29	Bacteria
	Tectiviridae		Tectivirus	Enterobacteria phage PRD1	Bacteria
	Corticoviridae		Corticovirus	Alteromonas phage PM2	Bacteria
	Plasmaviridae		Plasmavirus	Acholeplasma phage L2	Mycoplasma
	Lipothrixviridae		Lipothrixvirus	Thermoproteus virus 1	Archaea
	Rudiviridae		Rudivirus	Sulfolobus virus SIRV1	Archaea
	Fuselloviridae		Fusellovirus	Sulfolobus virus SSV1	Archaea
			"SNDV-like viruses"	Sulfolobus virus SNDV	Archaea
	Poxviridae	Chordopoxvirinae	Orthopoxvirus	Vaccinia virus	Vertebrates
			Parapoxvirus	Orf virus	Vertebrates
			Avipoxvirus	Fowlpox virus	Vertebrates
			Capripoxvirus	Sheeppox virus	Vertebrates

Table 2 Continued

Order	Family	Subfamily	Genus	Type species	Host
The RNA viruses					
The dsRNA viruses					
	Cystoviridae		Cystovirus	Pseudomonas phage φ6	Bacteria
	Reoviridae		Orthoreovirus	Reovirus 3	Vertebrates
			Orbivirus	Bluetongue virus 1	Vertebrates
			Rotavirus	Simian rotavirus SA11	Vertebrates
			Coltivirus	Colorado tick fever virus	Vertebrates
			Aquareovirus	Golden shiner virus	Vertebrates
			Cypovirus	Bombyx mori cypovirus 1	Invertebrates
			Fijivirus	Fiji disease virus	Plants
			Phytoreovirus	Wound tumor virus	Plants
			Oryzavirus	Rice ragged stunt virus	Plants
	Birnaviridae		Aquabirnavirus	Infectious pancreatic necrosis virus	Vertebrates
			Avibirnavirus	Infectious bursal disease virus	Vertebrates
			Entomobirnavirus	Drosophila X virus	Invertebrates
	Totiviridae		Totivirus	Saccharomyces cerevisiae virus L-A	Fungi
			Giardiavirus	Giardia lamblia virus	Protozoa
			Leishmaniavirus	Leishmania RNA virus 1-1	Protozoa
	Partitiviridae		Partitivirus	Gaeumannomyces graminis virus 019/6-A	Fungi
			Chrysovirus	Penicillium chrysogenum virus	Fungi
			Alphacryptovirus	White clover cryptic virus 1	Plants
			Betacryptovirus	White clover cryptic virus 2	Plants
	Hypoviridae		Hypovirus	Cryphonectria hypovirus 1-EP713	Fungi
			Varicosavirus	Lettuce big-vein virus	Plants
The negative-stranded ssRNA viruses					
Mononegavirales					
	Bornaviridae		Bornavirus	Borna disease virus	Vertebrates

Table 2 Continued

Order	Family	Subfamily	Genus	Type species	Host
	Filoviridae		"Ebola-like viruses" Zaire	Ebola virus	Vertebrates
			"Marburg-like viruses"	Marburg virus	Vertebrates
	Paramyxoviridae	Paramyxovirinae			
			Respirovirus	Human parainfluenza virus 1	Vertebrates
			Morbillivirus	Measles virus	Vertebrates
			Rubulavirus	Mumps virus	Vertebrates
		Pneumovirinae			
			Pneumovirus	Human respiratory syncytial virus	Vertebrates
			Metapneumovirus	Turkey rhinotracheitis virus	Vertebrates
	Rhabdoviridae				
			Vesiculovirus	Vesicular stomatitis Indiana virus	Vertebrates
			Lyssavirus	Rabies virus	Vertebrates
			Ephemerovirus	Bovine ephemeral fever virus	Vertebrates
			Novirhabdovirus	Infectious hematopoietic necrosis virus	Vertebrates
			Cytorhabdovirus	Lettuce necrotic yellows virus	Plants
			Nucleorhabdovirus	Potato yellow dwarf virus	Plants
	Orthomyxoviridae				
			Influenzavirus A	Influenza A virus	Vertebrates
			Influenzavirus B	Influenza B virus	Vertebrates
			Influenzavirus C	Influenza C virus	Vertebrates
			Thogotovirus	Thogoto virus	Vertebrates
	Bunyaviridae				
			Bunyavirus	Bunyamwera virus	Vertebrates
			Hantavirus	Hantaan virus	Vertebrates
			Nairovirus	Nairobi sheep disease virus	Vertebrates
			Phlebovirus	Sandfly fever Sicilian virus	Vertebrates
			Tospovirus	Tomato spotted wilt virus	Plants
			Tenuivirus	Rice stripe virus	Plants
			Ophiovirus	Citrus psorosis virus	Plants
	Arenaviridae		Arenavirus	Lymphocytic choriomeningitis virus	Vertebrates
			Deltavirus	Hepatitis delta virus	Vertebrates

Table 2 Continued

Order	Family	Subfamily	Genus	Type species	Host
The positive-stranded ssRNA viruses					
	Leviviridae		Levivirus	Enterobacteria phage MS2	Bacteria
			Allolevivirus	Enterobacteria phage Qβ	Bacteria
	Narnaviridae		Narnavirus	Saccharomyces cerevisiae 20S narnavirus	Yeast
			Mitovirus	Cryphonectria parasitica NB631 virus	Yeast
	Picornaviridae		Enterovirus	Poliovirus 1	Vertebrates
			Rhinovirus	Human rhinovirus 1A	Vertebrates
			Hepatovirus	Hepatitis A virus	Vertebrates
			Cardiovirus	Encephalomyocarditis virus	Vertebrates
			Aphthovirus	Foot-and-mouth disease virus O	Vertebrates
			Parechovirus	Human echovirus 22	Vertebrates
			"Cricket paralysis-like viruses"	Cricket paralysis virus	Invertebrates
	Sequiviridae		Sequivirus	Parsnip yellow fleck virus	Plants
			Waikavirus	Rice tungro spherical virus	Plants
	Comoviridae		Comovirus	Cowpea mosaic virus	Plants
			Fabavirus	Broad bean wilt virus 1	Plants
			Nepovirus	Tobacco ringspot virus	Plants
	Potyviridae		Potyvirus	Potato virus Y	Plants
			Rymovirus	Ryegrass mosaic virus	Plants
			Macluravirus	Maclura mosaic virus	Plants
			Ipomovirus	Sweet potato mild mottle virus	Plants
			Bymovirus	Barley yellow mosaic virus	Plants
			Tritimovirus	Wheat streak mosaic virus	Plants
	Caliciviridae		Vesivirus	Swine vesicular exanthema virus	Vertebrates
			Lagovirus	Rabbit hemorrhagic disease virus	Vertebrates

Table 2 Continued

Order	Family	Subfamily	Genus	Type species	Host
			"Norwalk-like viruses"	Norwalk virus	Vertebrates
			"Sapporo-like viruses"	Sapporo virus	Vertebrates
			"Hepatitis E-like viruses"	Hepatitis E virus	Vertebrates
	Astroviridae		Astrovirus	Human astrovirus 1	Vertebrates
	Nodaviridae		Alphanodavirus	Nodamura virus	Invertebrates
			Betanodavirus	Striped jack nervous necrosis virus	Vertebrates
	Tetraviridae		Betatetravirus	Nudaurelia capensis β virus	Invertebrates
			Omegatetravirus	Nudaurelia capensis ω virus	Invertebrates
			Sobemovirus	Southern bean mosaic virus	Plants
			Marafivirus	Maize rayado fino virus	Plants
	Luteoviridae		Luteovirus	Barley yellow dwarf virus – MAV	Plants
			Polerovirus	Potato leafroll virus	Plants
			Enamovirus	Pea enation mosaic virus 1	Plants
			Umbravirus	Carrot mottle virus	Plants
	Tombusviridae		Avenavirus	Oat chlorotic stunt virus	Plants
			Aureusvirus	Pothos latent virus	Plants
			Carmovirus	Carnation mottle virus	Plants
			Dianthovirus	Carnation ringspot virus	Plants
			Machlomovirus	Maize chlorotic mottle virus	Plants
			Necrovirus	Tobacco necrosis virus	Plants
			Panicovirus	Panicum mosaic virus	Plants
			Tombusvirus	Tomato bushy stunt virus	Plants
Nidovirales	Coronaviridae		Coronavirus	Avian infectious bronchitis virus	Vertebrates
			Torovirus	Berne virus	Vertebrates
	Arteriviridae		Arterivirus	Equine arteritis virus	Vertebrates

Table 2 Continued

Order	Family	Subfamily	Genus	Type species	Host
	Flaviviridae		Flavivirus	Yellow fever virus	Vertebrates
			Pestivirus	Bovine diarrhea virus	Vertebrates
			Hepacivirus	Hepatitis C virus	Vertebrates
	Togaviridae		Alphavirus	Sindbis virus	Vertebrates
			Rubivirus	Rubella virus	Vertebrates
			Tobamovirus	Tobacco mosaic virus	Plants
			Tobravirus	Tobacco rattle virus	Plants
			Hordeivirus	Barley stripe mosaic virus	Plants
			Furovirus	Soil-borne wheat mosaic virus	Plants
			Pomovirus	Potato mop-top virus	Plants
			Pecluvirus	Peanut clump virus	Plants
			Benyvirus	Beet necrotic yellow vein virus	Plants
	Bromoviridae		Alfamovirus	Alfalfa mosaic virus	Plants
			Bromovirus	Brome mosaic virus	Plants
			Cucumovirus	Cucumber mosaic virus	Plants
			Ilarvirus	Tobacco streak virus	Plants
			Oleavirus	Olive latent virus 2	Plants
			Ourmiavirus	Ourmia melon virus	Plants
			Idaeovirus	Rasberry bushy dwarf virus	Plants
	Closteroviridae		Closterovirus	Beet yellows virus	Plants
			Crinivirus	Lettuce infectious yellows virus	Plants
			Capillovirus	Apple stem grooving virus	Plants
			Trichovirus	Apple chlorotic leaf spot virus	Plants
			Vitivirus	Grapevine virus A	Plants
			Tymovirus	Turnip yellow mosaic virus	Plants
			Carlavirus	Carnation latent virus	Plants

Table 2 Continued

Order	Family	Subfamily	Genus	Type species	Host
			Potexvirus	Potato virus X	Plants
			Allexivirus	Shallot virus X	Plants
			Foveavirus	Apple stem pitting virus	Plants
	Barnaviridae		Barnavirus	Mushroom bacilliform virus	Fungi

Unassigned viruses
The subviral agents: viroids, satellites and agents of spongiform encephalopathies (prions)

Subviral agent	Family	Genus	Type species	Host
Viroids	Pospiviroidae	Pospiviroid	Potato spindle tuber viroid	Plants
		Hostuviroid	Hop stunt viroid	Plants
		Cocadviroid	Coconut cadang-cadang viroid	Plants
		Apscaviroid	Apple scar skin viroid	Plants
		Coleviroid	Coleus blumei viroid 1	Plants
	Avsunviroidae	Avsunviroid	Avocado sunblotch viroid	Plants
		Pelamoviroid	Peach latent mosaic virus	Plants
Satellites				Plants
				Invertebrates
				Fungi
Prions				Vertebrates
				Fungi

[a] Quotes are used to denote taxon names that are not approved ICTV international names, and are thus temporary until formal names are approved.
[b] Vertebrate arthropod-borne viruses are listed according to their vertebrate hosts.

Table 3 Orders, families and floating genera of viruses according to the seventh ICTV report (1999)

Criteria	Order	Family	Floating genus	Morphology	Genome configuration	Genome size (kb)	Virus host	Number of species			
								Species	Strains/ serotypes	Tentative	Total
dsDNA	Caudovirales	Myoviridae		Tailed phage	1 linear	336	Bacteria, archaea	15	23	117	155
		Siphoviridae		Tailed phage	1 linear	53	Bacteria, archaea	7	0	137	144
		Podoviridae		Tailed phage	1 linear	40	Bacteria, archaea	8	12	66	86
		Tectiviridae		Isometric	1 linear	16	Bacteria	4	0	38	42
		Corticoviridae		Isometric	1 circular supercoiled	10	Bacteria	1	0	2	3
		Plasmaviridae		Pleomorphic	1 circular	12	Mycoplasma	1	0	7	8
		Lipothrixviridae		Rod	1 linear	16	Archaea	2	0	0	2
		Rudiviridae		Rod	1 linear	33–36	Archaea	2	0	1	3
		Fuselloviridae		Lemon-shape	1 circular supercoiled	15	Archaea	1	0	0	1
			"SNDV-like viruses"	Droplet-shape	1 circular	20	Archaea	1	0	0	1
		Poxviridae		Ovioid	1 linear	130–375	Vertebrate, invertebrate	62	8	23	93
		Asfarviridae		Isometric	1 circular	170–190	Vertebrate	1	0	0	1
		Iridoviridae		Isometric	1 linear	160–400	Vertebrate, invertebrate	17	4	3	24
		Phycodnaviridae		Isometric	1 linear	250–350	Algae	27	0	38	65
		Baculoviridae		Bacilliform	1 circular supercoiled	90–230	Invertebrate	17	6	7	30
		Herpesviridae		Isometric	1 linear	120–220	Vertebrate	56	0	65	121
		Adenoviridae		Isometric	1 linear	32–48	Vertebrate	26	102	35	163
			Rhizidiovirus	Isometric	1 linear	27	Fungus	1	0	0	1
		Polyomaviridae		Isometric	1 circular	5	Vertebrate	12	4	0	16
		Papillomaviridae		Isometric	1 circular	6.8–8.4	Vertebrate	7	0	88	95
		Polydnaviridae		Rod, fusiform	1 circular supercoiled	2–28	Invertebrate	59	0	0	59
		Ascoviridae		Ovoid and bacilliform	1 circular	100–180	Invertebrate	3	0	1	4
								330	159	628	117

Table 3 Continued

Criteria	Order	Family	Floating genus	Morphology	Genome configuration	Genome size (kb)	Virus host	Number of species - Species	Strains/serotypes	Tentative	Total
ssDNA		Inoviridae		Rod	1 circular	7–20	Bacteria, mycoplasma	36	7	5	48
		Microviridae		Isometric	1 circular	6	Bacteria, spiroplasma	7	0	33	40
		Geminivirus		Isometric	1 or 2 circular	3–6	Plant	94	2	10	106
		Circoviridae		Isometric	1 circular	1.7–2.3	Vertebrate	3	0	1	4
			Nanovirus	Isometric	6–9 circular	6–9	Plant	4	0	1	5
		Parvoviridae		Isometric	1 – strand	6–8	Vertebrate, invertebrate	38	0	16	54
								182	**9**	**66**	**257**
ssDNA RT		Hepadnaviridae		Isometric	1 circular – strand	3	Vertebrate	5	0	2	7
dsDNA RT		Caulimoviridae		Isometric, bacilliform	1 circular	8	Plant	26	0	8	34
ssRNA RT		Pseudoviridae		Ovoid	1 linear	5–8	Yeast, plant	15	0	0	15
ssRNA RT		Metaviridae		Isometric	1 linear	4–10	Yeast, fungus, Invertebrate	18	0	1	19
ssRNA RT		Retroviridae		Spherical	dimer 1 + segment	7–10	Vertebrate	59	44	2	105
dsRNA		Cystoviridae		Isometric	3 segments	17	Bacteria	1	0	0	1
		Reoviridae		Isometric	10–12 segments	19–62	Vertebrate, invertebrate, plant	62	256	39	357
		Birnaviridae		Isometric	2 segments	6	Vertebrate, invertebrate	4	21	1	26
		Totiviridae		Isometric	1 segment	5–7	Fungus, protozoa	18	0	5	23
		Partitiviridae		Isometric	2 segments	3–10	Fungus, plant	30	0	15	45
		Hypoviridae		Pleomorphic	1 segment	9–13	Fungus	3	0	2	5
			Varicosavirus	Rod	2 segments	14	Plant	1	0	3	4
								119	**277**	**65**	**461**
Negative ssRNA	Mononegavirales	Bornaviridae		Spherical	1 – segment	9	Vertebrate	1	0	1	2
		Filoviridae		Bacilliform	1 – segment	13	Vertebrate	5	19	0	24

Table 3 Continued

Criteria	Order	Family	Floating genus	Morphology	Genome configuration	Genome size (kb)	Virus host	Number of species			
								Species	Strains/ serotypes	Tentative	Total
		Paramyxoviridae		Helical	1 − segment	15–16	Vertebrate	31	5	2	38
		Rhabdoviridae		Bacilliform	1 − segment	10–13	Vertebrate, plant	37	0	142	179
		Orthomyxoviridae		Helical	8 − segments	13–14	Vertebrate	5	1	0	6
		Bunyaviridae		Spherical	3 − segments	12–23	Vertebrate, plant	93	236	66	395
			Tenuivirus	Filaments	4 −?segments	15–19	Plant	6	0	5	11
			Ophiovirus	Filaments	3 − segments	12	Plant	3	0	0	3
		Arenaviridae		Spherical	2 − segments	11	Vertebrate	19	27	2	48
			Deltavirus	Spherical	1 circular − strand	1.7	Vertebrate	1	0	0	1
								201	**288**	**218**	**707**
Positive ssRNA		Leviviridae		Isometric	1 + segment	3–4	Bacteria	4	18	35	57
		Narnaviridae		Ribonucleic complex	1 + segment	2.5	Yeast	3	0	0	3
		Picornaviridae		Isometric	1 + segment	7–8.5	Vertebrate	16	105	137	258
			"CrPV-like viruses"	Isometric	1 + segment	9–10	Invertebrate	5	0	0	5
		Sequiviridae		Isometric	1 + segment	9–12	Plant	5	0	0	5
		Comoviridae		Isometric	2 + segments	9–16	Plant	50	0	9	59
		Potyviridae		Rod	1 or 2 + segments	8–12	Plant	106	0	92	198
		Caliciviridae		Isometric	1 + segment	8	Vertebrate	6	40	8	54
			"HEV-like viruses"	Isometric	1 + segment	7	Vertebrate	1	0	0	1
		Astroviridae		Isometric	1 + segment	7–8	Vertebrate	6	13	0	19
		Nodaviridae		Isometric	2 + segments	5	Vertebrate, invertebrate	14	0	0	14
		Tetraviridae		Isometric	1 + segment	5	Invertebrate	9	0	0	9
			Sobemovirus	Isometric	1 + segment	4	Plant	11	0	3	14
			Marafivirus	Isometric	1 + segment	6–7	Plant	3	0	0	3
		Luteoviridae		Isometric	1 or 2 + segment	6–9	Plant	8	0	11	19
			Umbravirus	No particles	1 + segment	4	Plant	7	0	15	22
		Tombusviridae		Isometric	1 or 2 + segment	4–5.5	Plant	38	0	11	49

Table 3 Continued

Criteria	Order	Family	Floating genus	Morphology	Genome configuration	Genome size (kb)	Virus host	Number of species Species	Strains/ serotypes	Tentative	Total
	Nidovirales	Coronaviridae		Pleomorphic	1 + segment	28–33	Vertebrate	16	5	1	22
		Arteriviridae		Spherical	1 + segment	13–16	Vertebrate	4	0	0	4
		Flaviviridae		Isometric	1 + segment	10–12	Vertebrate	57	47	6	110
		Togaviridae		Isometric	1 + segment	10–13	Vertebrate	23	6	0	29
ssRNA Positive sense			Tobamovirus	Rod	1 + segment	6	Plant	16	0	3	19
			Tobravirus	Rod	2 + segments	9–11	Plant	3	0	0	3
			Hordeivirus	Rod	3 + segments	10	Plant	4	0	0	4
			Furovirus	Rod	2 + segments	9–11	Plant	1	0	4	5
			Pomovirus	Rod	3 + segments	12	Plant	4	0	0	4
			Pecluvirus	Rod	2 + segments	10	Plant	2	0	0	2
			Benyvirus	Rod	4 (or 5) + segments	14–16	Plant	2	0	0	2
		Bromoviridae		Isometric, bacilliform	3 + segments	8–9	Plant	28	0	0	28
			Ourmiavirus	Bacilliform	3 + segments	4–5	Plant	3	0	0	3
			Idaeovirus			8	Plant	1	0	0	1
		Closteroviridae		Rod	1 or 2 + segments	15–19	Plant	18	0	16	34
			Capillovirus	Rod	1 + segment	7	Plant	3	0	1	4
			Trichovirus	Rod	1 + segment	7.5	Plant	3	0	1	4
			Vitivirus	Rod	1 + segment	7.5	Plant	4	0	1	5
			Tymovirus	Isometric	1 + segment	6	Plant	20	0	1	21
			Carlavirus	Rod	1 + segment	7–8	Plant	31	0	29	60
			Potexvirus	Rod	1 + segment	6	Plant	26	0	18	44
			Allexivirus	Rod	1 + segment	9	Plant	6	0	3	9
			Foveavirus	Rod	1 + segment	8–9	Plant	2	0	1	3
		Barnaviridae		Bacilliform	1 + segment	4	Fungus	1	0	1	2
								565	**234**	**403**	**1202**
	Unassigned viruses				—	—	All	30	0	0	30
								1550	**1011**	**1393**	**3954**
	Viroids				—	—	Plant	27	0	8	35
	Satellites				—	—	Plant	33	0	6	39

Table 4 List of criteria demarcating different virus taxa

I Order
- Common properties between several families including:
  - Biochemical composition
  - Virus replication strategy
  - Particle structure (to some extent)
  - General genome organization

II Family
- Common properties between several genera including:
  - Biochemical composition
  - Virus replication strategy
  - Nature of the particle structure
  - Genome organization

III Genus
- Common properties within a genus including:
  - Virus replication strategy
  - Genome size, organization and/or number of segments
  - Sequence homologies (hybridization properties)
  - Vector transmission

IV Species
- Common properties within a species including:
  - Genome rearrangement
  - Sequence homologies (hybridization properties)
  - Serological relationships
  - Vector transmission
  - Host range
  - Pathogenicity
  - Tissue tropism
  - Geographical distribution

and occupies a particular ecological niche.' The major advantage in this definition is that it can accommodate the inherent variability of viruses and is not dependent on the existence of a unique characteristic. Members of a polythetic class are defined by more than one property and no single property is absolutely essential and necessary. Thus in each family it might be possible to determine the set of properties of the class 'species' and to check if the family members are species of this family or if they belong to a lower taxonomic level. The ICTV is currently conducting this exercise throughout all virus families. This exercise should ultimately result in an excellent evaluation of a precise definition of each virus species in the entire classification.

Several practical matters are related to the definition of a virus species with the goal of improving the usefulness of virus classification. These include: (1) homogeneity of the different taxa; (2) diagnosis-related matters; (3) virus collections; (4) evolution studies; (5) biotechnology; (6) sequence database projects; (7) virus database projects; and now (8) intellectual property rights.

Virus families and genera

There is no formal definition for a genus, but it is commonly considered as: 'a population of virus species that share common characteristics and are different from other populations of species'. Although this definition is somewhat elusive, this level of classification seems enduring and useful; some genera have been moved from one family to another over the years, but the composition and description of the genera has remained stable. The characters defining a genus differ from one family to another and there is a tendency to create genera with fewer differences between them. Upon examination, there is more and more evidence that the members of a genus have a common evolutionary origin. The use of subgenera has been abandoned in current virus classification.

Notwithstanding the creation of the ICTV, plant

virologists continued to classify plant viruses in 'groups', refusing to place them in genera and families. However, owing to obvious similarities, plant reoviruses and rhabdoviruses had been integrated into the families *Reoviridae* and *Rhabdoviridae* (**Table 2**). This position was mostly due to plant virologists' refusal to accept binomial nomenclature. Since this form of nomenclature was withdrawn from the ICTV classification rules in 1995, they subsequently accepted the placing of plant viruses into species, genera and families as shown in the sixth ICTV report. However, there are still 30 of so-called 'floating genera' that do not pertain to any family. This is mostly due to the fact that plant virologists prefer to accumulate data on virus species and genera before clustering appropriate genera in families. It is remarkable that this attitude has also been adopted by other virologists as a convenient way of classifying viruses, without having to move genera out of families when it becomes apparent that they are part of a distinct family. For example, the members of the floating genus 'cricket paralysis-like viruses' share enough properties with picornaviruses to be included in the family *Picornaviridae*; however, they also possess properties that would justify their classification in a separate family. Only new data or new viruses will permit a definitive position, therefore for the time being it remains a floating genus. Similarly the same strategy is used to create a floating genus 'ictalurid herpes-like viruses', within the family *Herpesviridae*, although in this case it is a floating genus within the family because of uncertainty as to whether the members of this genus should be classified in one of the existing subfamilies or to a new subfamily.

Virus orders

As mentioned above, the higher hierarchy levels for virus classification are extremely difficult to establish. Despite several propositions in the past, only three have been accepted: *Caudovirales*, *Mononegavirales* and *Nidovirales*. The first virus order, *Mononegavirales*, was established in 1990 and comprises the nonsegmented single-stranded RNA negative-sense viruses, namely the families *Bornaviridae*, *Filoviridae*, *Paramyxoviridae* and *Rhabdoviridae*. This decision was taken because of the great similarity of many criteria between these families, including their replication strategy. A second order, *Caudovirales*, contains all the families of double-stranded DNA phages possessing a tail, including the families *Myoviridae*, *Podoviridae* and *Siphoviridae*. A third order, *Nidovirales*, comprising the families *Coronaviridae* and *Arteriviridae*, was accepted in 1996 because of the impossibility of grouping together these two taxonomic entities, which share many properties and yet are so different, as a single family. Many members of the ICTV advocate the creation of many more orders, but it has been decided to proceed cautiously to avoid creation of short-lived orders. The creation of formal taxa higher than the orders, for example, kingdoms, classes and subclasses, has not been considered by the ICTV.

Virus Taxa Descriptions

Virus classification continues to evolve with the technologies available for describing viruses. The first wave of descriptions, those before 1940, mostly took into account the visual symptoms of the diseases caused by viruses, along with their modes of transmission. A second wave, between 1940 and 1970, brought together an enormous amount of information from studies of virion morphology (electron microscopy, structural data), biology (serology and virus properties) and physicochemical properties of viruses (nature and size of genome, number and size of viral proteins). Since 1970, the third wave of virus descriptions has included genome and replicative information as well as molecular relationships with virus hosts. There is a correlative modification of the list of virus descriptors and **Table 1** lists the family and genera descriptors which are used in the current ICTV report. **Figures 1–5** are diagrammatic representations of families and genera of viruses infecting vertebrates, invertebrates, plants, fungi, yeasts, protozoa and bacteria. The most recent wave of information used to classify viruses is naturally nucleotide and amino acid sequences. It is becoming more and more prevalent in virus taxonomy, as exemplified by the presence of a significant number of 'phylogenetic trees' in the seventh ICTV report, and by the huge number of scientific publications on this topic. Some scientists promote the concept of 'quantitative taxonomy' aimed at demonstrating that virus sequences contain all the coding information required for all the biological properties of the viruses. This is in complete agreement with the polythetic concept of the virus species definition, as demonstrated for example by Padidam *et al* in 1995, van Regenmortel *et al* in 1997, Hyppia *et al* in 1998, and Aleman *et al* in 1999.

The impact of descriptions on virus classification has been particularly influenced by electron microscopy and of the negative staining technique for virions. This technique had an immediate influence on diagnostics and classification of viruses. With negative staining, viruses could be identified from poorly purified preparations of all tissue types, and informa-

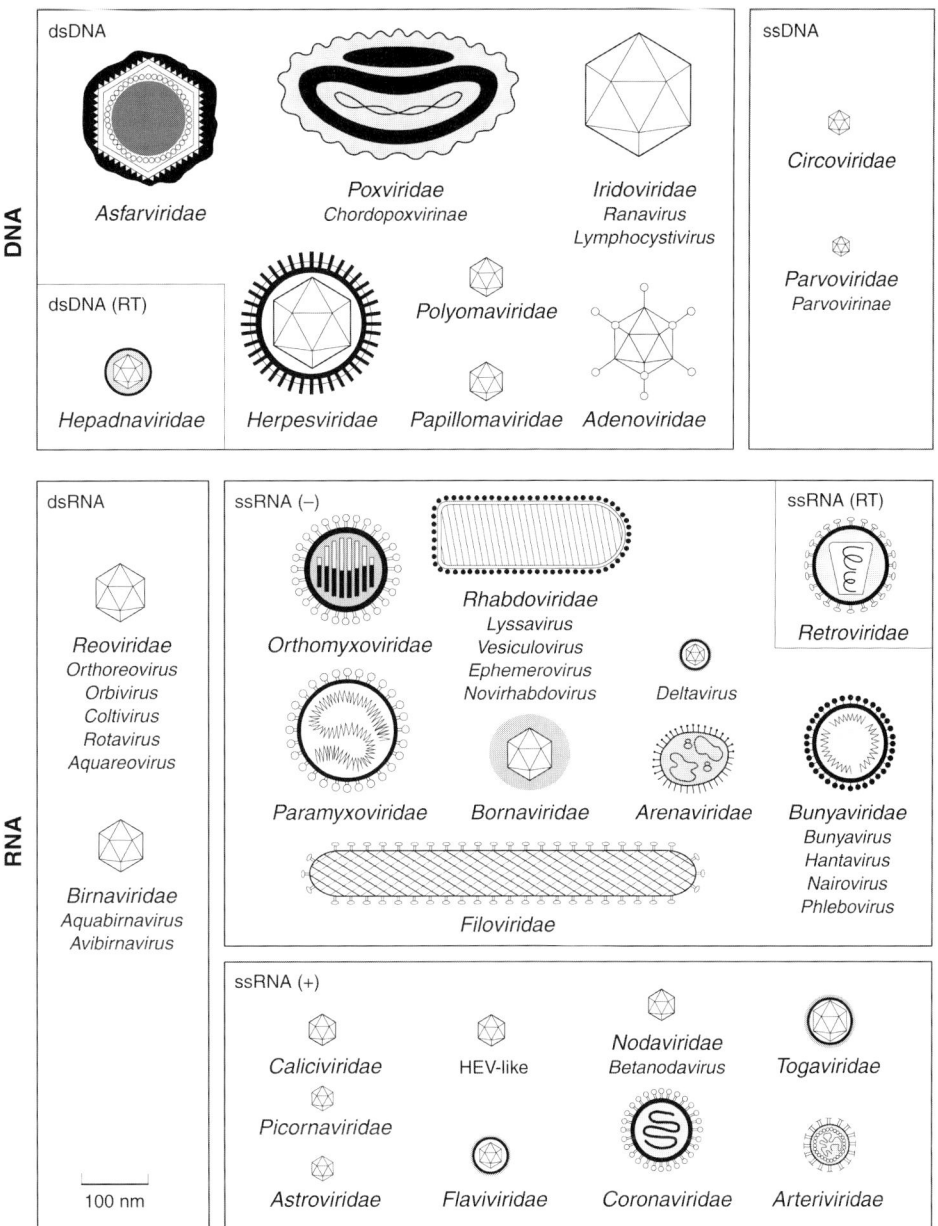

Figure 1 Families and genera of viruses infecting vertebrates.

tion about size, shape, structure and symmetry could be quickly provided. As a result, virology progressed simultaneously for all viruses infecting animals, insects, plants and bacteria. Thin sections of infected tissues brought a new dimension to virus classification by providing information about virion morphogenesis and cytopathogenic effects. These techniques, in conjunction with the determination of the nature of the genome, provided a major source of information for the system of virus classification established in the 1980s, as shown by the large number of viruses listed in the fifth ICTV report in 1989.

In many instances the properties of viruses belonging to the same genus are correlated. Thus, the classification of a few of them will likely be sufficient to allow the classification of a new virus into an established genus. For example, a plant virus with filamentous particles of 700–850 nm and transmitted by aphids is likely to be a member of the genus *Potyvirus*. Establishment of new genera in the future will require more information. Most of the properties listed in **Table 3** will have to be precisely analyzed to warrant the formation of a new genus.

Table 3 lists 45 different categories of properties but each category includes many items. Lists of virus descriptors usually comprise 1000–2000 descriptors.

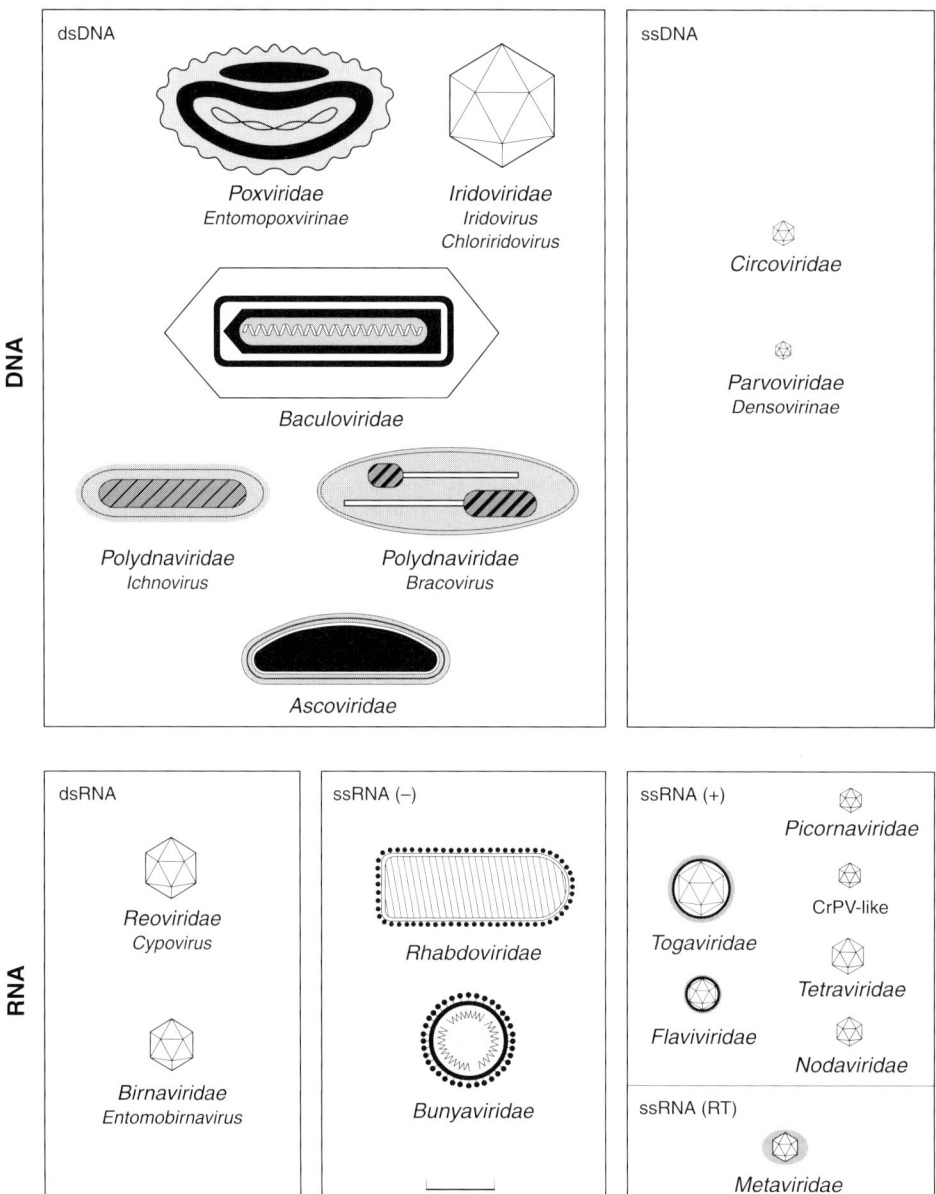

Figure 2 Families and genera of viruses infecting invertebrates.

The establishment of a universal list of virus descriptors is under way and should be adopted by ICTV around 2000 with the establishment of the ICTVdB. It will contain a common set of descriptors for *all* viruses and subsets for specific viruses in relation to their specific hosts (human, animal, insect, plant and bacterial).

A Uniform Nomenclature of Viral Taxa

When a genus is approved by ICTV, a type species is designated. However, none of these type species have received a new international name and only English names are used. Latinized binomial names for virus names have been supported by animal and human virologists of ICTV for many years, but have never been implemented. This suggestion was in fact withdrawn from ICTV nomenclature rules in 1990 and consequently such names as *Herpesvirus varicella* or *Polyomavirus hominis* should not be used. For several years, plant virologists have adopted a different nomenclature, using the vernacular name of a virus but replacing the word 'virus' by the genus name; for example, *Cucumber mosaic cucumovirus* and *Tobacco mosaic tobamovirus*. Though this usage is favored by many scientists, and examples of such practice can

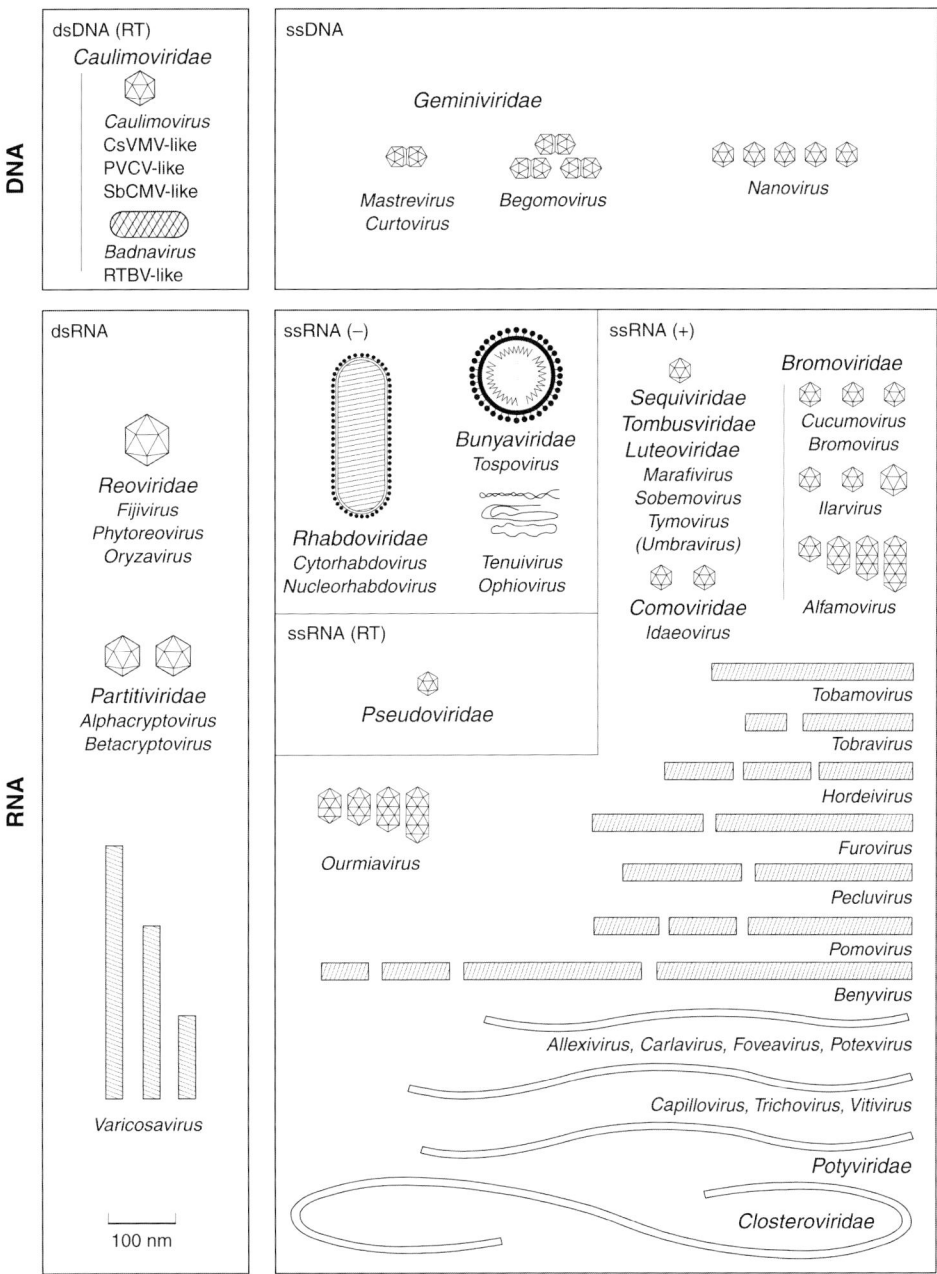

Figure 3 Families and genera of viruses infecting plants.

be found for human, animal and insect viruses (e.g. *Human rhinovirus*, *Canine calicivirus*, *Acheta densovirus*...), it has not been universally adopted by the ICTV.

The ICTV has set rules for virus nomenclature and orthography of taxonomic names that are regularly revisited and improved. The last word of international virus species names is 'virus', the international genus names universally end in '...virus', the international subfamily names end in '...virinae', the international family names end with '...viridae', and the international order names are ending in '...virales'. In formal taxonomic usage, the virus order, family, subfamily, genus and species names are all printed in italics (or underlined) and the first letter is capitalized. For all taxa except the species names, new names are created *de novo* following ICTV guidelines, but in the case of virus names English vernacular form is used. In formal usage, the name of the taxon precedes the name of the taxonomic unit; for example, 'the family *Picornaviridae*' or 'the genus *Rhinovirus*'. In informal vernacular usage, order,

1754 TAXONOMY, CLASSIFICATION AND NOMENCLATURE OF VIRUSES

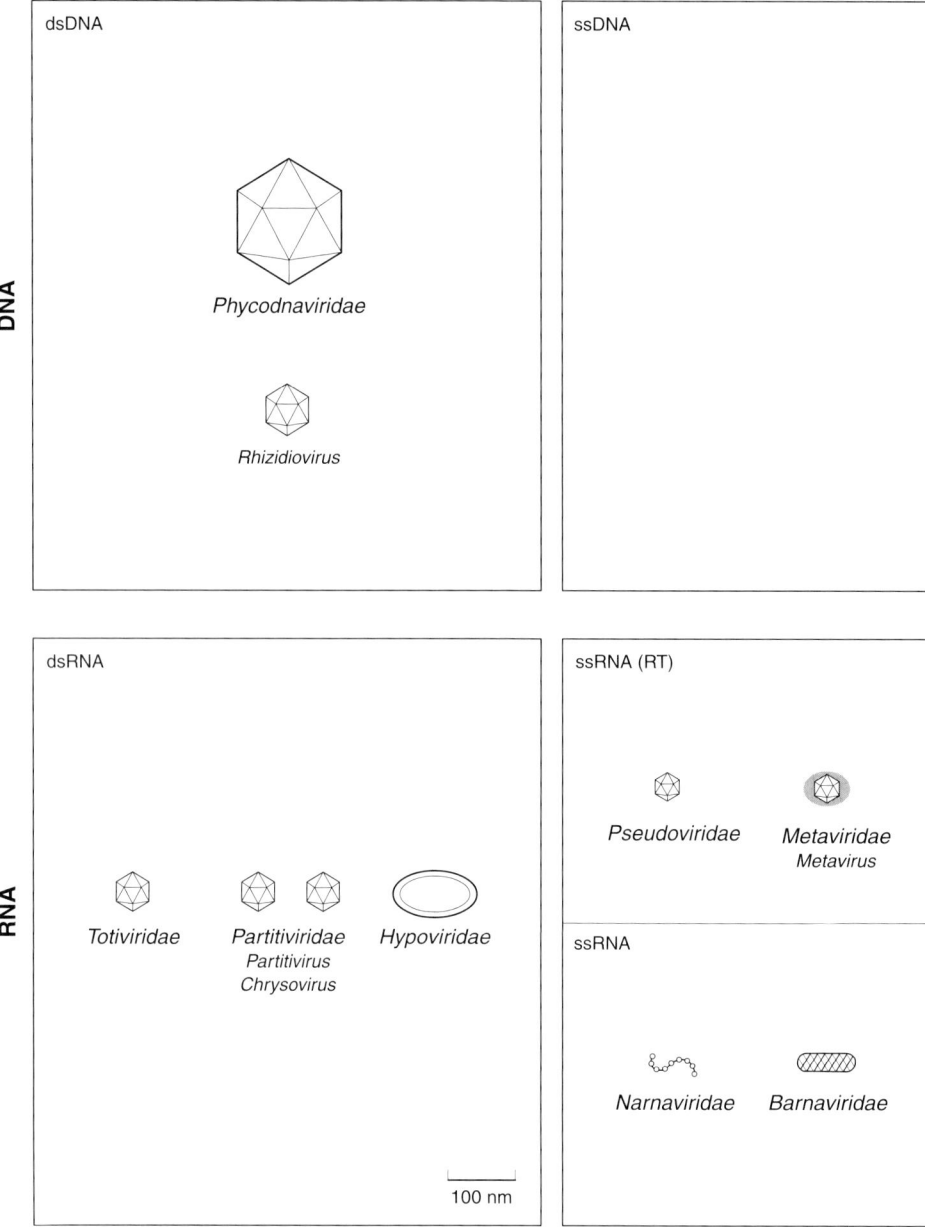

Figure 4 Families of viruses infecting algae, fungi, yeasts and protozoa.

family, subfamily, genus and species names are written in lower case Roman script; they are not capitalized nor italicized (or underlined). Additionally, in informal usage, the name of the taxon should not include the formal suffix, and it should follow the term for the taxonomic unit; for example, 'the mononegavirales order', 'the adenovirus family', 'the avihepadnavirus genus' or 'the tobacco mosaic virus' species. Virus names are often abbreviated for convenient reasons, but ICTV has not set up guidelines to generate such abbreviations. The ICTV reports list abbreviations most commonly used by specialists and the ICTV reports help virologists to identify duplicates of abbreviations in order to decrease the number of such duplicates. In 1988 plant virologists initiated the publication of such lists and have indicated guidelines for the creation of new virus names and new abbreviations. These guidelines were last published in 1991 by Fauquet and Martelli and will be updated again in 1999.

To avoid ambiguous virus identifications, it has been recommended to journal editors that published papers follow ICTV guidelines for proper virus identification and nomenclature, and that viruses should be cited

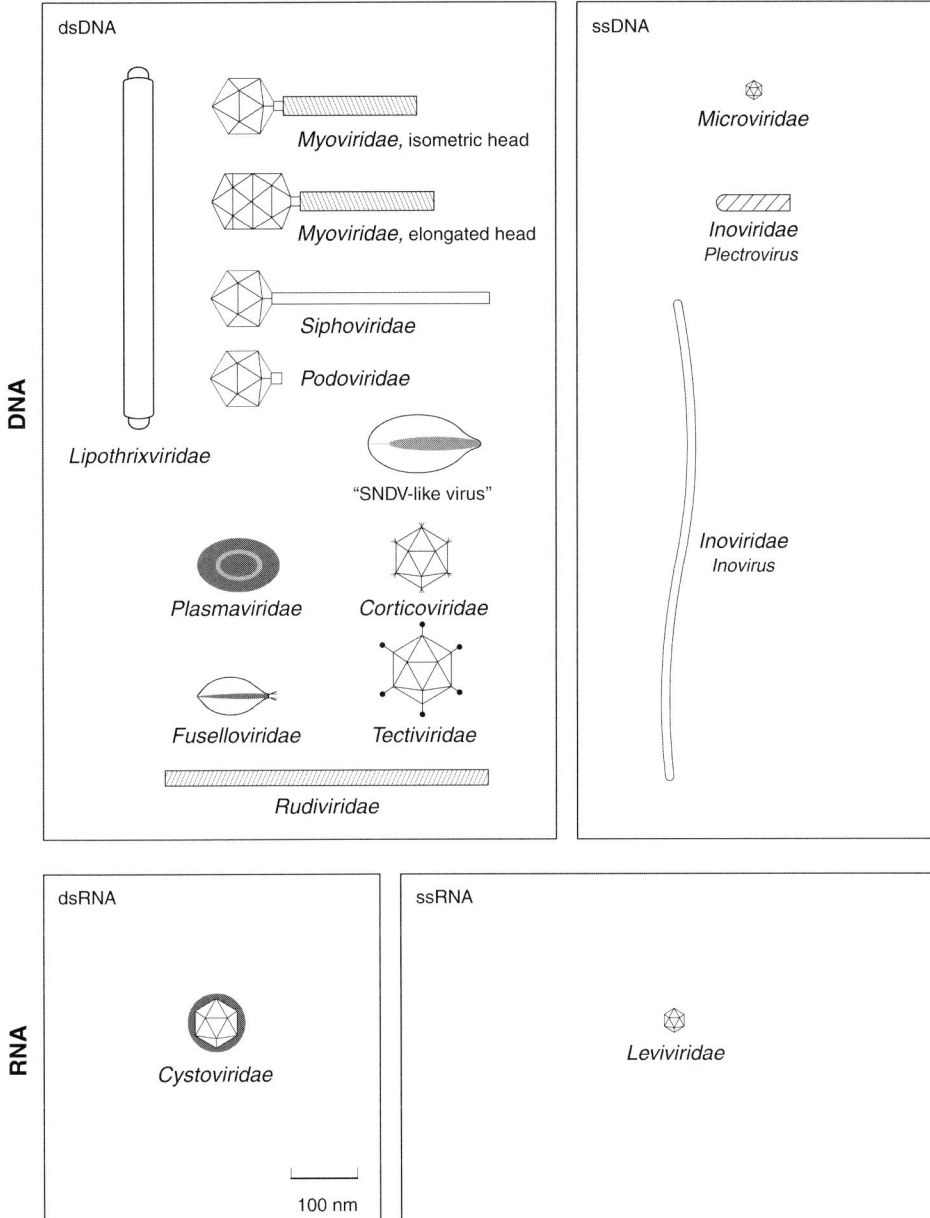

Figure 5 Families and genera of viruses infecting bacteria.

with their full taxonomic terminology when they are first mentioned in an article. For example:

- Order *Caudovirales*, family *Podoviridae*, genus 'T7-like viruses', species *Enterobacteria phage T7*.
- Order *Mononegavirales*, family *Paramyxoviridae*, subfamily *Paramyxovirinae*, genus *Rubulavirus*, species *Mumps virus*.
- Order *Nidovirales*, family *Coronaviridae*, genus *Coronavirus*, species *Avian infectious bronchitis virus*.
- Family *Iridoviridae*, genus *Iridovirus*, species *Chilo iridescent virus*.
- Family *Picornaviridae*, genus *Enterovirus*, species *Poliovirus*, serotype Human poliovirus 1.
- Genus *Tobamovirus*, species *Tobacco mosaic virus*.

See also: **Phage taxonomy and classification; Virus structure: Atomic structure, Principles of virus structure.**

Further Reading

Fauquet CM and Martelli GP (1995) Up-dated ICTV list of names and abbreviations of viruses, viroids and satellites infecting plants. *Arch. Virol.* 140: 393.

Francki RIB, Milne RG and Hatta T (1985) *Atlas of Plant Viruses*. Boca Raton, CRC Press.

Francki RIB, Fauquet CM, Knudson DL and Brown F (1991) *Classification and Nomenclature of Viruses*. Fifth Report of the International Committee on Taxonomy of Viruses. Vienna: Springer.

Lwoff A, Horne R and Tournier P (1962) A system of viruses. Cold Spring Harb. Symp. Quant. Biol.

Matthews REF (1983) *The History of Viral Taxonomy. A Critical Appraisal of Viral Taxonomy*, pp 1–35. Boca Raton: CRC Press.

Murphy FA, Fauquet CM, Bishop DHL *et al* (eds) (1995) *Virus Taxonomy*. Sixth Report of the International Committee on Taxonomy of Viruses. Vienna: Springer.

van Regenmortel MHV, Bishop DHL, Fauquet CM *et al* (1997) Guidelines to the demarcation of virus species. *Arch. Virol.* 142: 1505.

van Regenmortel MHV, Fauquet CM, Bishop DHL *et al* (eds) (1999) *Virus Taxonomy*. Seventh Report of the International Committee on Taxonomy of Viruses. New York: Academic Press.

TENUIVIRUSES

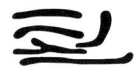

Bryce W. Falk, Department of Plant Pathology, University of California, Davis, California, USA

Copyright © 1999 Academic Press

History

The viruses in the genus *Tenuivirus* (tenuiviruses) have been recognized as important plant pathogens since the early 1900s. However, in 1977 it was first recognized that rice stripe virus (RSV)-infected rice (*Oryza sativa* L.) plants contained unusual fine-stranded particles. These appeared as circular or branched filaments and were distinctly different from particles associated with other plant viruses. Subsequent work showed that plants infected by several other viruses contained similar particles. This and the somewhat unique biological properties shared by these viruses led to the early grouping together of RSV and other plant viruses, including maize stripe virus (MSpV) and rice hoja blanca virus (RHBV). Since 1995, RSV and related viruses have been grouped together by the International Committee on Taxonomy of Viruses (ICTV) as members of the genus *Tenuivirus* (tenuiviruses).

Taxonomy and Classification

There are currently six species within the genus *Tenuivirus*, and at least five tentative species (**Table 1**). The definitive tenuiviruses are: rice stripe virus (RSV; the type species of the genus); MSpV; RHBV; rice grassy stunt virus (RGSV); *Echinochloa* hoja blanca virus (EHBV) and *Urochloa* hoja blanca virus (UHBV). All tenuiviruses exhibit similar properties, and in recent years molecular biological analyses have shown that they are quite distinct from other currently recognized plant viruses. The genus *Tenuivirus* is not placed within a formally recognized virus family; however, tenuiviruses appear in some ways to be more closely related to viruses in the genus *Phlebovirus* of the family *Bunyaviridae*, than they are to other plant viruses.

Biology, Host Range and Vector Transmission

The plant host ranges of all tenuiviruses are limited to monocotyledenous plant species within the family Poaceae, including many plants which are important food crops (i.e. rice (*Oryza sativa* L.) and maize (*Zea mays* L.)). The symptoms induced in infected plants are generally similar for the different tenuiviruses and includes general leaf striping, a distinct white coloring of the leaf stripes and stunting (**Fig. 1**).

Tenuiviruses generally are not mechanically transmissible to their plant hosts; however, mechanical transmission has been reported in limited instances but only under specific conditions. All tenuiviruses are transmitted to plants by specific planthoppers (Homoptera: Delphacidae, see **Table 1** and **Fig. 2**). Transmission of a given tenuivirus is specific and may be limited to planthoppers of a single species. Compared to other vectors of plant viruses (i.e. aphids or whiteflies), delphacid planthoppers are not generally thought of as common vectors; however, they are perfectly adapted to be vectors of tenuiviruses. Delphacid planthoppers which vector tenuiviruses

Table 1 Tenuiviruses, their planthopper vectors and plant hosts, and geographic range

Virus	Vector[a]	Plant hosts[b]	Range[c]
Rice stripe virus (RSV)	*Laodelphax striatellus*	Rice (*Oryza sativa*)	Asia, Far East
Maize stripe virus (MSpV)	*Peregrinus maidis*	Maize (*Zea mays*)	Worldwide tropics and subtropics
Rice grassy stunt virus (RGSV)	*Nilaparvata lugens*	Rice	Asia, Far East
Rice hoja blanca virus (RHBV)	*Tagosodes oryzicola*	Rice	American tropics and subtropics
Echinochloa hoja blanca virus (EHBV)	*Tagosodes cubanus*	Rice, *Echinochloa colona*	American tropics and subtropics
Urochloa hoja blanca virus (UHBV)	*Caenodelphax teapae*	*Urochloa* spp.	—

[a] All Tenuivirus insect vectors are planthoppers in the Delphacidae. The name indicates the main vector.
[b] Indicates the primary economically important host. All tenuiviruses have more extensive experimental host ranges (Falk and Tsai, 1998).
[c] Indicates the main natural geographic distribution.

are phloem feeders, and colonize plants within the family Poaceae. The planthopper vector can acquire the corresponding tenuivirus by feeding from a virus-infected plant and, once acquired, the planthopper generally retains the ability to transmit the corresponding tenuivirus for the remainder of its life. Immediately after acquisition there is a defined incubation period before subsequent transmission to new host plants is possible. This incubation period is fairly long, measured in days, and is suggestive that viral multiplication in the planthopper is a prerequisite before the tenuivirus can subsequently be transmitted to new plant hosts. Further evidence supporting the replication of tenuiviruses in their planthopper vectors is that RHBV, RSV and MSpV can be transovarially transmitted from viruliferous female planthoppers to their progeny, and RHBV can be paternally transmitted to offspring.

Proof for multiplication of tenuiviruses in their planthopper vectors has been demonstrated by using different approaches. For example, RHBV has been maintained in *Tagosodes orizicola* planthoppers for up to ten generations, and RSV has been maintained in *Laodelphax striatellus* planthoppers for 40 generations. Serological analyses have been used to show definitively that MSpV antigens increase over time in *Peregrinus maidis* planthoppers after MSpV acquisition (either by plant feeding or intrathoracic injec-

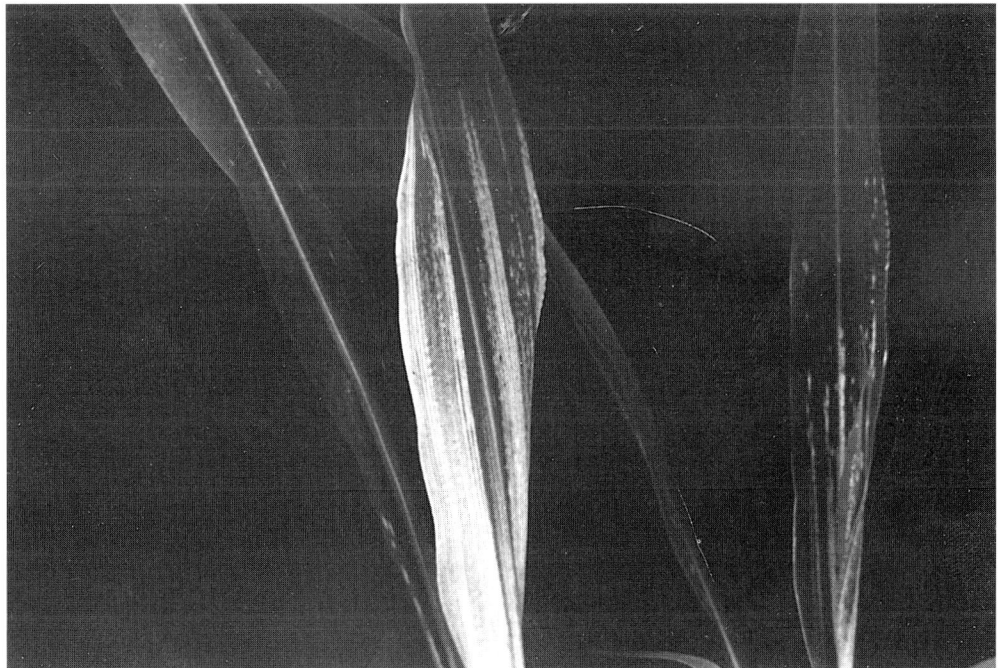

Figure 1 Two *Zea mays* plants showing late and early symptoms, respectively, of infection by the tenuivirus maize stripe virus (MSpV). Leaves in late infections can turn completely white, while in early infections white stripes begin to appear along veins. (With permission, from the *Annual Review of Phytopathology*, Volume 36, copyright 1998, by Annual Reviews.)

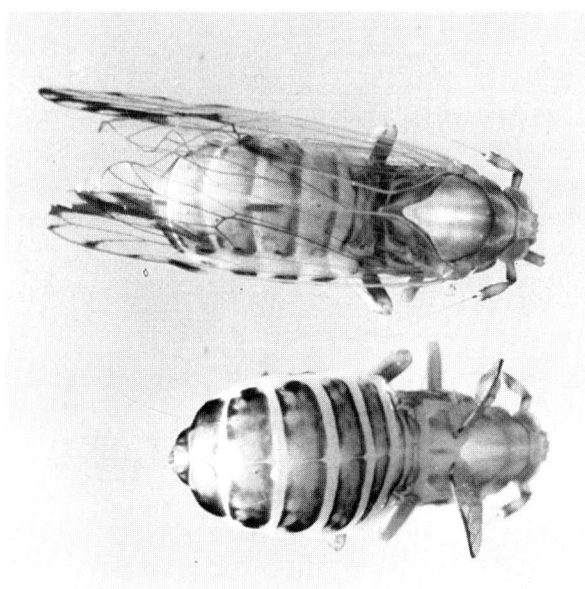

Figure 2 *Peregrinus maidis*, the delphacid planthopper vector of MSpV. The upper planthopper is the long-wing adult form; the lower insect is the short-wing adult. (With permission, from the *Annual Review of Phytopathology*, Volume 36, copyright 1998, by Annual Reviews.)

tion), providing conclusive evidence that MSpV replicates in *P. maidis*.

Even though transmission of a given tenuivirus is specific, it appears that vector specificity may be even further affected by the genetic composition within the vector species population. There are 'transmitters' and 'nontransmitters' for RHBV within *T. oryzicola* populations. The transmitters are competent RHBV vectors, while the nontransmitters are not, and transmitters are capable of supporting RHBV replication, whereas nontransmitters are not. By making crosses between individuals of these two types, the ability to support RHBV replication, and thus transmit RHBV to plants, was shown to be due to a single recessive gene. The above characteristics show that Tenuivirus transmission by planthopper vectors can be classified as circulative-propagative, and is highly specific. Furthermore, the host ranges of tenuiviruses include plants and animals, the latter being their planthopper vectors.

Geographic and Seasonal Distribution

Tenuiviruses are not universally common plant viruses, but they are generally somewhat limited in their geographical distribution, probably due in part to limits for the natural geographical ranges of their planthopper vectors. RSV and RGSV appear to be limited to rice growing areas of Asia, and RHBV and EHBV are limited to tropical and subtropical rice growing regions of the Americas. Only MSpV is found in both the New and Old Worlds. MSpV has been reported from North, Central and South America, Australia and parts of Africa. However, MSpV and its planthopper vector, *Peregrinus maidis*, are limited to subtropical and tropical maize-producing regions in these areas.

Even though they are somewhat limited in their natural incidence, the tenuiviruses are still of considerable economic importance. Their primary host plants are important food crops including rice (*Oryza sativa*) and maize (*Zea mays*), and disease incidence can be severe. For example, RHBV, which causes the only virus disease of rice in the western hemisphere, has sporadically affected rice production in many tropical and subtropical rice production areas of the Americas, and yield losses of 25–50% have been reported. When RHBV was identified in Florida, USA, in the 1950s, a quarantine on Florida rice production was implemented in hopes of preventing RHBV spread into rice producing areas of nearby states. Rice production in southern Florida did not resume until the late 1970s, and now it is a minor crop. RHBV is still of considerable importance in the rice growing regions of Latin America. In their respective geographic regions, RSV and RGSV cause similarly important diseases in rice. RSV has been reported to affect as much as 19% of the total rice acreage in Japan. MSpV causes annual losses in maize in various regions, and losses of 80% have been reported in specific maize growing regions.

Virus Structure and Composition

The name tenuivirus is derived from the nature of the slender (tenuous), filamentous ribonucleoprotein particles (RNPs) associated with the tenuiviruses. RNPs have been identified by electron microscopy in cells of tenuivirus-infected plant and insect hosts. The RNPs also have been purified from plants infected by several different tenuiviruses, including MSpV, RSV, RGSV, EHBV and RHBV. Electron microscopic analysis has shown the RNPs to be threadlike, very thin in diameter (8–10 nm; **Fig. 3**) and often without defined lengths. Frequently the RNPs appear circular, but under various conditions they can exhibit varying degrees of supercoiling.

Rate-zonal sucrose density gradient centrifugation analysis has shown that RNP preparations for specific tenuiviruses can be resolved into four or five distinct RNPs. The sedimentation coefficients of the five MSpV RNPs range from about 70 to 190 S for the slowest to fastest sedimenting RNPs, respectively. Biochemical analyses have shown that RNPs are composed of single-stranded RNA encapsidated

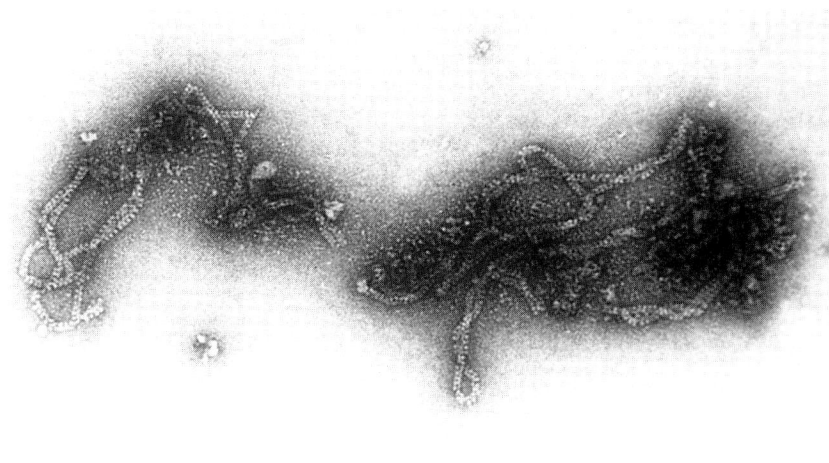

Figure 3 Transmission electron micrograph showing purified rice hoja blanca virus (RHBV) RNPs. Note circular filamentous nature of the particles. Bar = 50 nm. (Courtesy of Dra. A. M. Espinoza Esquivel, University of Costa Rica.)

essentially by a single protein species, the nucleocapsid (N) protein. The N proteins for all tenuiviruses are similar in size, about 32 000–35 000 mol.wt. In addition to the N protein, purified RNP preparations often contain small amounts of a large protein of greater than 200 000 mol.wt which is believed to be the tenuivirus RNA-dependent RNA polymerase.

Four or five distinct genomic RNAs have been isolated from purified RNPs of different tenuiviruses. The overall pattern and sizes of the RNP RNAs for different tenuiviruses, as determined by denaturing agarose gel electrophoresis, are very similar. For MSpV, sizes are estimated to be about 8.3, 3.3, 2.4, 2.2 and 1.3 kb for RNAs 1–5, respectively. Northern hybridization and nucleotide sequence analyses have shown that each of these RNAs is largely distinct, and representative of a single genome segment. Thus the multipartite genomes of tenuiviruses like MSpV are among the largest ($c.$ 18 kb) genomes for the plant viruses.

Analysis of individually purified MSpV and RSV RNPs has shown that the different sized genomic RNAs are separately encapsidated in different RNPs. The smallest RNA (RNA 5) can be isolated from the slowest sedimenting RNP, with larger RNAs being found in faster sedimenting RNPs, respectively. Furthermore, careful studies with RSV have shown that the circumference of the filamentous, circular RNPs is proportional to the size of the encapsidated RNA. The five RSV RNPs are estimated to be $c.$ 290 nm, 510 nm, 610 nm, 840 nm and 2110 nm in circumference for RNPs 1–5, respectively.

The RNP RNAs are believed to be single-stranded. However, under appropriate conditions, both single- and double-stranded RNAs have been detected in RNAs extracted from purified RNPs of MSpV, RGSV, EHBV and RSV. This was somewhat surprising when originally discovered, as it seemed unlikely that both single- and double-stranded RNAs would be contained within the RNPs. It is now believed that only single-stranded RNAs are encapsidated, but that for each size RNA (e.g. RNA 1), complementary molecules are separately encapsidated in different RNPs. This is supported by data which show that mostly single-stranded RNAs are detected when MSpV RNPs are disrupted with detergent and the RNAs immediately analyzed by gel electrophoresis. However, when RNP RNAs for MSpV and RSV are isolated using SDS and phenol, concentrated by ethanol precipitation, and subsequently analyzed by nondenaturing gel electrophoresis, both single- and double-stranded RNAs are detected. The double-stranded RNAs presumably arise *in vitro* by hybridization of complementary strands for each RNA.

Nucleic acid hybridization data support the above observations. Opposite polarity, complementary molecules for each of the five MSpV RNAs have been identified from purified RNPs. However, unequal amounts of the complementary molecules for all five MSpV RNAs are present. Northern hybridization studies of denatured and nondenatured MSpV RNP RNAs suggested that each of the five RNP RNAs is represented primarily as one polarity; however, smaller amounts of the complementary polarity molecules for each RNA are also present. Thus, upon annealing *in vitro*, some double-stranded RNA is formed while the RNA in excess then remains as single-stranded RNA. For a given genomic segment, that polarity which is most abundant is referred to as vRNA, while that which is less abundant is referred to as vcRNA (viral complementary RNA).

The above characteristics are consistent and characteristic features of the tenuiviruses; however, the properties of the RNPs and the molecular biology of tenuiviruses (see below) suggest that the circular RNPs may not be true virions, but possibly they are components of a more complex virion. At this time the exact nature of tenuivirus virions remains in question.

Genome Composition and Structure

The different sized Tenuivirus RNAs are distinct genome components. Infectivity experiments demonstrating whether or not all five of the tenuivirus RNAs are necessary for competent infections have not been done. However, nucleic acid hybridization analyses have shown that for a given tenuivirus the genomic RNAs do not have a high degree of nucleotide sequence homology with each other, and nucleotide sequence analyses show that the individual genomic RNA segments have distinct organizations encoding different proteins.

The genomic RNAs of several tenuiviruses have been sequenced and characterized. While the terminal structures on the Tenuivirus genomic RNAs have not been definitively identified, the 5′ termini do not contain a VPg, nor are they capped. Genomic RNAs of both RSV and MSpV can be readily radiolabeled *in vitro* by using polynucleotide kinase. Similarly, the 3′ ends of the RSV genomic RNAs have been labeled using T4 RNA ligase, suggesting that the 3′ terminus is an OH group. Nucleotide sequence analyses also have shown that the tenuivirus genomic RNAs have conserved and complementary 5′ and 3′ termini. There are 11 nucleotides at the 5′ termini and ten nucleotides at the 3′ termini, which are largely conserved not only among the five genomic RNAs of a given tenuivirus, but also between different tenuiviruses (**Fig. 4**). The minor exceptions are that RSV RNA 1 and MSpV RNA 5 have only 9 of the 10 conserved nucleotides at their 3′ termini. It is also of interest that the terminal eight nucleotides at both the 5′ and 3′ termini are identical to those found in the vertebrate-infecting viruses of the genus *Phlebovirus* (family *Bunyaviridae*). The genomic RNA 5′ and 3′ terminal nucleotide sequences also are complementary (**Fig. 4**). The 3′ 17 terminal nucleotides are complementary to 17 of the 18 5′ terminal nucleotides. A model has been proposed for RSV which allows the 11th nucleotide from the 5′ end to bulge out so that the 17 complementary nucleotides at each terminus could base pair and form a hairpin structure.

RNA 1

5′-**ACACAAAGUCC**
3′-**UGUGUAUCAG***

RNA 2

5′-**ACACAAAGUCC**
3′-**UGUGUUUCAG***

RNA 3

5′-**ACACAAAGUCC**UGGGUAA
3′-**UGUGUUUCAG***ACCCAUU

RNA 4

5′-**ACACAAAGUCC**AGGGCAU
3′-**UGUGUUUCAG***UCCCGUA

RNA 5

5′-**ACACAAAGUCC**UGGCAC
3′-**UGUGUAUCAG*** AACCGUG

Phlebovirus

5′-**ACACAAAG**ACC
3′-**UGUGUUUC**UG

Figure 4 Terminal nucleotide sequences of *Tenuivirus* and *Phlebovirus* RNAs. For the conserved and complementary 5′ and 3′ nucleotide sequences for tenuivirus genomic RNAs, the nucleotides shown in bold are conserved among the RNA sequences determined so far. For the *Phlebovirus* sequence, the nucleotides shown in bold are those which are identical to those found for tenuiviruses. The asterisk (*) in the 3′ terminal sequences represents a space inserted so as to align 5′ and 3′ nucleotides for complementary base pairing.

Such complementarity of RNA terminal nucleotide sequences is largely unique among the plant viruses, with the exception that the genomic RNAs of tomato spotted wilt virus (genus *Tospovirus*, family *Bunyaviridae*) also exhibit this feature. The feature is common among vertebrate-infecting viruses with segmented, negative-sense RNA genomes in the families *Bunyaviridae*, *Arenaviridae* and *Orthomyxoviridae*.

It is of interest to note that for La Crosse virus (genus *Bunyavirus*, family *Bunyaviridae*) the complementary genomic RNA termini exist in infected cells and in RNPs as base paired, stable panhandle structures. It is believed that because the La Crosse virus RNA termini are base paired within the RNPs, this could play a role in determining the circularity of the RNPs. Interestingly, the tenuivirus circular filamentous RNPs are morphologically very similar to those of La Crosse virus, and it is tempting to speculate that the tenuivirus RNA 5′ and 3′ termini are also base paired, and that this feature, at least in part, contributes to the circular nature of the characteristic tenuivirus RNPs.

Nucleotide sequence analyses have shown that the different tenuivirus genomic RNAs exhibit different genetic organizations and encode different proteins. RSV vRNA 1 is 8970 nt and of negative polarity. The vcRNA1 potentially encodes for a protein of 336 860. The smallest tenuivirus genomic RNA, RNA 5

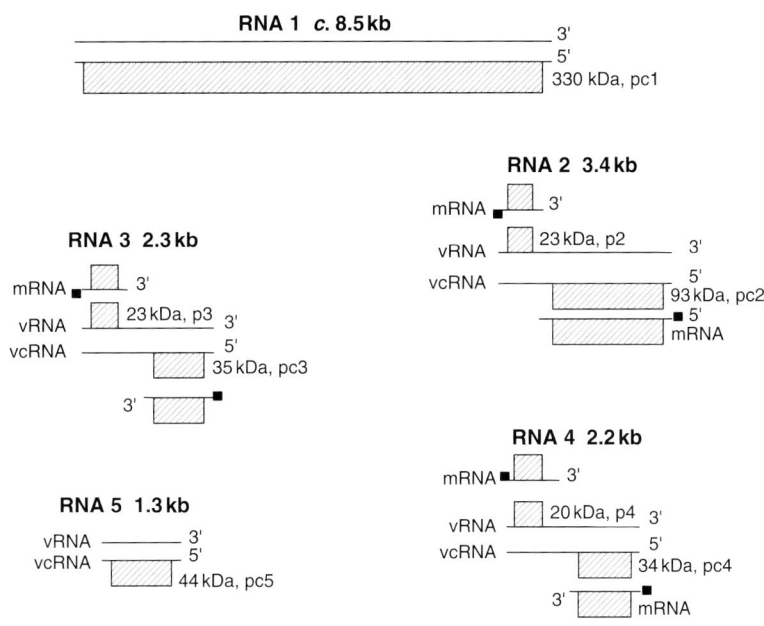

Figure 5 Generic genome map and expression strategy for viruses in the genus *Tenuivirus*. Five tenuivirus genomic RNAs and their approximate sizes (kb) are indicated. vRNA and vcRNA indicate the viral and viral complementary RNAs, respectively. Hatched boxes indicate ORFs. For the ambisense RNAs (RNAs 2, 3 and 4), mRNAs are indicated below or above the vRNA or vcRNA. Black boxes indicate capped 5′ termini on these mRNAs. No caps are shown on the monocistronic RNAs, but it is likely these mRNAs are also capped. Names and sizes of proteins (kDa) are shown.

(1317 nt) is also of negative polarity. MSpV vcRNA 5 encodes a protein, pc5, of 44 000 mol.wt. Analyses of pc5 show it to be highly basic in nature, containing 21% arginine and lysine, but as yet its function is unknown.

The organizations of tenuivirus genomic RNAs 2, 3 and 4 is more complex. Both the vRNA and vcRNAs for each genomic segment encode proteins, thus the coding strategy is ambisense (**Fig. 5**). MSpV vRNA 2 encodes a small hydrophobic protein (23 500 mol.wt) while vcRNA 2 encodes a 93 900 mol.wt protein. Because the vRNA and vcRNA each encode proteins, the terminology used to refer to the respective proteins is determined by whether they are encoded by vRNA or vcRNA. The vRNA 2-encoded protein is designated p2, while the vcRNA 2-encoded protein is pc2 (the c for a protein encoded by the vcRNA). Thus, for the remaining ambisense MSpV genomic RNAs, RNAs 3 and 4, p3 is 22 700 mol.wt, pc3 is 35 000 mol.wt, p4 is 19 800 mol.wt and pc4 is 31 900 mol.wt.

The functions of all of the tenuivirus-encoded proteins are not known. The pc1 is believed to be the RNA-dependent RNA polymerase (RDRP). Amino acid sequence analyses have shown that pc1 contains features characteristic of RDRPs, and it exhibits significant similarity to the RDRPs (L proteins) found for viruses in the genus *Phleobvirus*. The function of p2 is unknown, but computer predictions suggest it to be membrane-associated within infected host cells. The second RNA 2-encoded protein, pc2, exhibits significant similarity to the virion membrane glycoproteins found for viruses in the genus *Phlebovirus*. Interestingly, so far no membrane-bound virions have yet been identified for tenuiviruses. The pc2 is c. 94 000 mol.wt and for MSpV contains the proteolytic cleavage sequence conserved among the glycoproteins for Phleboviruses. VcRNA 3 encodes the c. 35 000 mol.wt nucleocapsid (N) protein. The vRNA 3 encodes p3, a protein of c. 23 000 mol.wt and for which no function is yet identified. The vRNA 4 encodes p4, a protein of c. 20 000 mol.wt. P4 is the most abundant protein found in tenuivirus-infected plants (see below). The vcRNA 4 encodes pc4, a protein of c. 32 000 mol.wt and of unknown function. Some of these proteins are discussed in more detail below, under Virus–Host Relationships or Serological and Nucleic Acid-Based Relationships.

Gene Expression Strategies

The tenuivirus full-length genomic RNAs are not mRNAs. During tenuivirus infection and replication, specific subgenomic mRNAs are generated for the ambisense genomic RNAs (RNAs 2, 3 and 4; see **Fig. 5**), and for MSpV, with the exception of that for p4, subgenomic mRNAs have been identified both in MSpV-infected plants and planthoppers. As tenuivirus genomic RNAs 1 and 5 are monocistronic, it is likely that mRNAs for pc1 and pc5 are essentially full-length, but probably are modified from those found in RNPs.

The subgenomic mRNAs representing the RNA 2, RNA 3 and RNA 4 open reading frames (ORFs) have been detected in MSpV-infected tissues, but not in purified RNPs. The sizes of the RNA 2, RNA 3 and RNA 4 subgenomic mRNAs are c. 700 and 2600 nt for p2 and pc2; 650 and 1350 nt for p3 and pc3; and c. 950 and 1000 nt for p4 and pc4, respectively. In agreement with the polarities of the ORFs contained in each of the ambisense genomic RNAs, the subgenomic mRNAs for a given RNA segment are of opposite polarity to each other, and it is likely that subgenomic mRNAs for a given genomic RNA are not overlapping. The opposing ORFs on a specific genomic RNA are separated by relatively large A-U rich intergenic regions (>350 nt). Whether or not these intergenic regions play a role in mRNA transcription termination is not yet known.

The subgenomic mRNAs correspond in nucleotide sequence with the 5′ regions of the genomic RNA segments; however, the 5′ terminal nucleotide sequences for a given genomic RNA (i.e. vRNA 4) and the corresponding mRNA (i.e. that for the p4 ORF) are not identical. The 5′ termini for several tenuivirus mRNAs have been shown to contain short leader sequences of heterogeneous nucleotide composition, and these are immediately 5′ of the viral RNA sequence. Furthermore, and in contrast to the tenuivirus genomic RNAs, the mRNAs have a 5′ cap. It is believed that these capped leader sequences are generally of host mRNA origin and originate by 'cap snatching'.

Cap snatching is a feature which was first described for influenza virus, and which was subsequently shown to occur for other vertebrate-infecting viruses such as those in the families *Orthomyxoviridae*, *Arenaviridae* and *Bunyaviridae*. During mRNA transcription, host mRNAs are recruited and a virus-encoded cap-specific endonuclease cleaves the host mRNA several nucleotides downstream of the 5′ cap. The resulting 5′-capped sequence is then used as a primer for mRNA synthesis. A few of the 3′ nucleotides base pair with the mRNA template (the 3′ end of the full-length RNAs) and the short, capped ribonucleotide serves as a primer for transcription. Thus, the mRNA gains the 5′ cap and short leader sequence of the donor mRNA. The specificity of donor RNAs that can serve as mRNA primers is not yet known, but generally the capped leader sequences are short, only 10–16 nt.

Virus–Host Relationships

One of the most diagnostic features of tenuivirus infections of plants is the presence of large amounts of the tenuivirus-encoded p4 protein in plant tissues. P4 is the most abundant protein in MSpV-infected plant tissues and can be found at levels exceeding 10 mg g^{-1}. P4 can easily be detected from tenuivirus-infected plants by using serological methods, or directly by light and/or electron microscopy. Within infected plant cells, p4 aggregates into large crystalline structures or inclusion bodies which can occupy significant portions of the plant cell (**Fig. 6**). Similar p4 aggregates can be formed *in vitro*. The inclusion bodies found in the cell cytoplasm are not viroplasms or sites of tenuivirus replication, and p4 is not associated with Tenuivirus RNAs or the RNPs. As such, p4 has been referred to as the major noncapsid protein (NCP). The p4-containing inclusion bodies are detectable by light and/or electron microscopy and are of various morphological types. Light microscopic analysis has shown inclusion bodies to be needle-shaped, ring-like and even in figure-of-eight amorphous structures. Transmission electron microscopy has revealed that these structures can have two types of substructure. The amorphous, semielectron opaque inclusion bodies are the most abundant, sometimes appearing to fill almost the entire cytoplasm. Filamentous, electron-opaque bodies also can be seen but are generally less abundant. All of the above seem to be composed only of p4, and thus the various types may represent different developmental stages. Despite its abundance in tenuivirus-infected plants, p4 has not been detected in MSpV-infected *P. maidis*, the MSpV planthopper vector. The reason for the differential abundance of p4 in plant as opposed to insect hosts is not known; however, RNA hybridization analyses have shown that the p4 ORF subgenomic RNA is highly abundant in MSpV-infected plants, but has not been found in MSpV-infected *P. maidis*. In contrast, other tenuivirus-coded proteins, such as the nucleocapsid protein (N protein; pc3), and their respective subgenomic RNAs can be detected both in MSpV-infected plant and insect hosts.

Serological and Nucleic Acid-Based Relationships

Antibodies to two tenuivirus proteins, p4 (the NCP) and pc3 (N protein), have been generated for most tenuiviruses, and some serological comparisons have been done. Using stringent serological tests, antibodies to each of these proteins have generally shown positive reactions only with corresponding proteins of

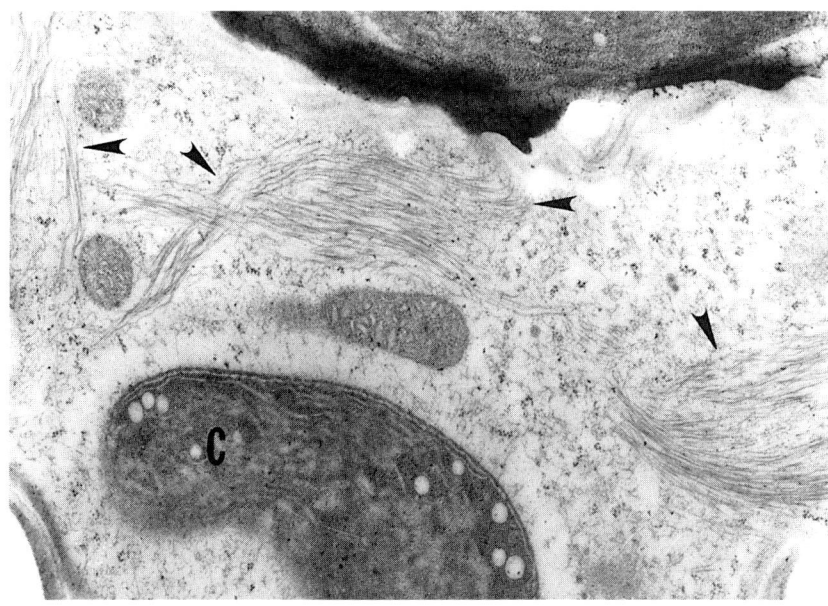

Figure 6 Transmission electron micrograph of a cell of a MSpV-infected *Zea mays* plant. C indicates a chloroplast. Arrows indicate the MSpV typical p4 (NCP) needle-shaped inclusions.

their respective tenuivirus. However, by using less stringent serological tests, slight serological cross-reactions have been obtained between similar proteins encoded by different tenuiviruses. The N proteins of RSV and MSpV are distantly serologically related, as are those of RSV and RGSV. However, the MSpV N protein does not show a serological relationship to those of RGSV or RHBV. Only slight serological crossreactions were detected when the MSpV and RHBV NCPs were compared. Thus, current data suggest that these respective Tenuivirus-encoded proteins are generally serologically distinct from each other.

More recently, computer-based comparisons of tenuivirus genomic RNA nucleotide sequences, and comparisons of deduced amino acid sequences for tenuivirus-encoded proteins have shown that the tenuiviruses are closely related, and they have some specific similarities with some vertebrate-infecting viruses. The genome organizations are similar for all tenuiviruses, and the respective encoded proteins exhibit detectable degrees of similarity. However, some of the tenuivirus-encoded proteins exhibit similarity to related proteins of other viruses. Tenuivirus pc1, pc2 and pc3 all show similarities with proteins encoded by the genomes of viruses within the genus *Phlebovirus*. The RSV pc1, the putative RDRP, shows c. 30% identity, between residues 493–2026, with the L protein of viruses in the genus *Phlebovirus*. RSV pc1 also contains other features found in phlebovirus L proteins, including the four conserved polymerase motifs. The MSpV pc2 shares features found for the phlebovirus glycoproteins, including a putative conserved cleavage site, and pc3 (the N protein) showed significant similarity to the N proteins for two viruses in the genus *Phlebovirus*.

Biologically the viruses in the genera *Phlebovirus* and *Tenuivirus* are distinct, but still have some general similarities. Phleboviruses infect their invertebrate vectors as well as their vertebrate hosts, while tenuiviruses infect their invertebrate vectors (planthoppers) and plants. Distinct membrane-bound spherical virions are typical for phleboviruses. Within these are three RNPs containing the three genomic RNAs. No similar virions are yet found for tenuiviruses, but RNPs similar to those of the phleboviruses are common, and these separately contain the five tenuivirus genomic RNAs. The genomic RNAs of tenuiviruses and phleboviruses have eight identical nucleotides at their 5' and 3' termini. Finally, viruses in these two genera exhibit somewhat similar genome organizations, coding arrangements and expression strategies, and some of their gene products show significant similarity. Thus, tenuiviruses and phleboviruses appear to have a common evolutionary lineage.

Epidemiology and Control

Tenuivirus epidemiology is determined in part by the biology and behavior of their planthopper vectors. Delphacid planthoppers are wing dimorphic, having both short- and long-winged adult forms (**Fig. 2**). Short-wing forms are capable of spreading tenuiviruses over short distances by walking from plant to plant. Long-winged forms can disperse by active flight and as such can spread tenuiviruses over long distances (several kilometers). Planthopper vector populations fluctuate seasonally, and corresponding tenuivirus-induced diseases also fluctuate seasonally and from year to year. However, when crop incidence corresponds with high planthopper populations or activity, diseases caused by tenuiviruses often result. For example, in Florida MSpV disease in *Z. mays* occurs in fall-planted maize crops. *P. maidis* populations build up on alternate grasses during the summer months. As the fall-planted maize plants emerge, planthoppers move into the young succulent plants and severe disease can result. Later fall, or winter or spring plantings are not as severely affected. A similar situation has been reported from Japan for RSV, and when high planthopper populations coincide with young plants, resulting disease can be severe.

Tenuivirus disease control strategies based upon epidemiological data (i.e. late planting to avoid planthopper activity) may offer some help in controlling diseases caused by tenuiviruses; however at present, forecasting tenuivirus epidemics has not proven to be reliable, and thus this has hampered using tactics such as delayed planting. Both plant-derived and genetically engineered forms of resistance to tenuiviruses in plants have been described. Genetic resistance seems to be the most useful and effective strategy for attempting to control RHBV, RGSV and RSV in rice. Continued plant breeding efforts will probably be necessary to provide long-term tenuivirus disease control.>

See also: **Bunyaviridae**: General features; Influenza viruses (*Orthomyxoviridae*): Molecular biology; Tospoviruses (*Bunyaviridae*).

Further Reading

Falk BW and Tsai JH (1998) Biology and molecular biology of viruses in the genus *Tenuivirus*. *Annu. Rev. Phytopathol.* 36: 139–163.

Ramirez B-C and Haenni A-L (1994) Molecular biology of tenuiviruses, a remarkable group of plant viruses. *J. Gen. Virol.* 75: 467.

Toriyama S (1995) In: Singh RP, Singh US and Kohomoto K (eds) *Pathogenesis and Host Specificity in Plant Diseases*. Vol. 3: *Viruses and Viroids*. Oxford: Pergamon Press.

TETRAVIRUSES (*TETRAVIRIDAE*)

Terry N Hanzlik and **Karl HJ Gordon**, CSIRO Entomology, Canberra, Australia

Copyright © 1999 Academic Press

Introduction and History

The *Tetraviridae* are a family of viruses isolated exclusively from lepidopteran insects (moths, butterflies) that have a positive-sense, single-stranded (ss) RNA genome encased in an icosahedral capsid. They were initially isolated and characterized in Australia and South Africa in the 1960s from cadavers of emperor moths. The extensive work on the viruses isolated from the South African *Nudaurelia capensis cynterea* (pine emperor moth) led them to being known for a while as the *Nudaurelia β*-like group. The distinctive T = 4 quasi-symmetry of the capsid's icosahedral structure focused initial attention on the group and engendered the family's present name (from the Greek *tettares*, four). Tetraviruses have been difficult to study because of their limited availability, which was restricted to field-collected insect cadavers, and because of the inability to culture them in cell lines. These difficulties, combined with a perceived lack of economic importance, served to hinder work on the group until new strategies allowed new ways of looking at, and working with, tetraviruses. These studies indicate that the virology of tetraviruses has general implications and that it can be exploited in exciting new ways for agriculture and medicine.

Taxonomy and Serology

Earlier, viruses were classified as members of the family on the basis of a positive serological reaction to sera raised against a few well-characterized tetraviruses. Most of the members noted in **Table 1** have been classified on this basis. Now, however, analysis of physical characteristics is the favored approach, with serology usually used at a later stage. Once an icosahedral capsid containing an ssRNA genome has been ascertained, two strong indicators of tetraviruses

Table 1 Members of the *Tetraviridae*

Virus	Acronym	Family of host	Geographic location
Genus: Betatetravirus			
Nudaurelia capensis β virus[a]	NβV	Saturniidae	South Africa
Antheraea eucalypti virus[b]	AeV	Saturniidae	Australia
Darna trima virus	DtV	Limacodidae	Malaysia
Dasychira pudibunda virus[c]	DpV	Lymantriidae	UK
Philosamia cynthia × ricini virus	PxV	Saturniidae	UK
Pseudoplusia includens virus	PiV	Noctuidae	USA
Thosea asigna virus[d]	TaV	Limacodidae	Malaysia
Trichoplusia ni virus	TnV	Noctuidae	USA
Genus: Omegatetravirus			
Nudaurelia capensis ω virus[a]	NωV	Saturniidae	South Africa
Helicoverpa armigera stunt virus	HaSV	Noctuidae	Australia
Unassigned possible members[e]			
Acherontia atropas virus	AaV	Sphingidae	Canary Islands
Agraulis vanillae virus	AvV	Nymphalidae	Argentina
Callimorpha quadripuntata virus	CqV	Arctiidae	UK
Eucocytis meeki virus	EmV	Cocytiidae	Papua New Guinea
Euploea corea virus	EcV	Danadidae	Australia/Germany
Hypocritae jacobeae virus	HjV	Arctiidae	UK
Lymantria ninayi virus	LnV	Lymantriidae	Papua New Guinea
Nudaurelia ε virus[f]	NεV	Saturniidae	South Africa

[a]Type virus for genus.
[b]Serological evidence shows identity to NβV.
[c]Host renamed *Calliteara pudibunda*.
[d]Host renamed *Setothosea asigna*.
[e]Viruses showing serological relationship to a known β-like tetravirus (excluding NεV), but otherwise uncharacterized.
[f]NεV resembles the tetraviruses but is serologically unrelated to any known member.

are a particle diameter of 35–41 nm and a density in CsCl of <1.30 g mL^{-1}. These characteristics are not definitive, however, and so the International Committee on the Taxonomy of Viruses distinguishes them in its key from similar RNA viruses, such as caliciviruses, on the basis of their being an insect virus, having a major coat protein component of M_r >60 000, and the production of a coat protein from a separate RNA.

The family is unique for positive-strand icosahedral viruses in having two genera, *Betatetravirus* (β-type viruses) and *Omegatetravirus* (ω-type viruses), distinguished by the number of ssRNAs comprising their genomes. The ω-type genus has a bipartite genome and has the Nudaurelia ω-virus (NωV) as the type virus; the β-type genus has its complete genome on a single RNA strand and has the Nudaurelia β-type (NβV) virus as its type virus. Some confusion about classifying β-type viruses can result when a second RNA is extracted from their purified virions; this proves to be a coencapsidated subgenomic RNA, corresponding to the 3′ region of the genomic RNA. Particle morphology viewed from high-resolution electron micrographs may also be used to distinguish virus particles from the two genera on a tentative basis. Reconstructed images at 32 Å resolution may show three distinct pits in planar faces of β-like particles, which are not visible in the ω-like particles (**Fig. 1**).

Serological relationships among the viruses belonging to the two groups show a contrasting pattern. The β-type viruses show a wide relationship, with each member having a positive serological reaction to at least one other member of the genus. This is despite low sequence similarity, as viewed by hybridization at low stringency. However, the two known ω-type viruses do not show a serological relationship, even though they are highly similar at the sequence level.

Physical Properties

Properties of the structural proteins

As is apparent in **Table 2**, data obtained for many tetraviruses show only one major protein, usually with an M_r of >60 000. However, these data were

TETRAVIRUSES (TETRAVIRIDAE)

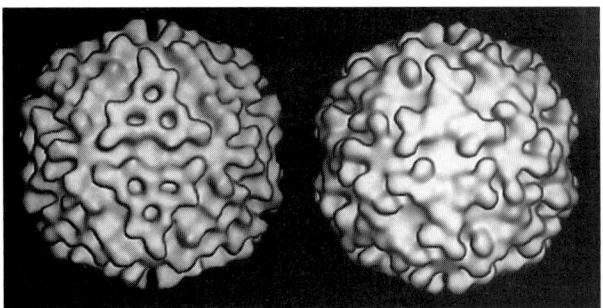

Figure 1 Image reconstructions of frozen hydrated particles of NβV (left) and NωV (right) analyzed by electron microscopy. (Courtesy of Norman Olson and Tim Baker).

obtained before more precise measurements on some tetraviruses showed the equimolar presence of a minor protein with an M_r of 7000–8000. Virions of all tetraviruses are now believed to have this protein constituent. While the minor protein is unmodified, the major protein has an N-terminal block of unknown structure. Also seen in SDS-PAGE profiles of tetravirus proteins extracted from purified virions are small amounts of a protein slightly larger than the major protein. This is a residual amount of an uncleaved protein that is the precursor to both the major and minor proteins. The cleavage takes place upon assembly of the capsid by a mechanism believed to be similar to that detailed for nodavirus capsids. The cleavage occurs towards the C-termini of the precursor proteins between Asn and Phe residues in ω-type tetraviruses and between Asn and Gly residues in β-type tetraviruses.

Properties of the genome

RNAs found encapsidated in tetravirus particles have the lengths shown in **Table 2**. As noted previously, a second species of subgenomic RNA of 2–3 kb in length may be found in minor amounts in β-type RNA, even though this group has a monopartite genome. The genomic RNA strands are capped on their 5′ ends, similarly to most mRNAs, but are not polyadenylated at the 3′ end. However, strong evidence indicates an intriguing tRNA-like secondary structure with a valine anticodon located at the 3′ terminus. The tetraviral tRNA-like structures are the only ones known for an animal virus and are distinct from the plant virus tRNA-like structures by not having a pseudoknot in the aminoacyl stem. Extensive secondary structure elsewhere on the tetraviral genomic RNAs is also likely.

Properties of the virion

Biophysical characteristics of tetravirus particles are listed in **Table 2**. The most precisely measured particle diameters are those of the type viruses, 39.7 nm for NβV and 41.0 nm for NωV. Measurements for other tetraviruses vary slightly below these values, which may be due to less precise measurements in photomicrographs. The equilibrium densities are generally at the low end of the range of densities (<1.30 g ml^{-1}) displayed by unenveloped icosahedral viruses with ssRNA genomes. Tetraviral particles appear to be robust. They are resistant to chloroform extraction and retain stability upon exposure to a wide range of pH (3–11).

The distinctive structure of the tetraviral capsid has drawn much attention to the family, for it is the only capsid solely organized with $T = 4$ quasi-symmetry which allows 240 protein subunits to comprise the capsid. Other, more complex viruses have only substructures organized with this motif, while most other viruses with unenveloped icosahedral capsids have $T = 3$ quasi-symmetries that allow only a 180 subunit composition. Low-resolution studies from image reconstructions of electron micrographs show the 240 protein subunits are arranged in Y-shaped trimers on the surface of the particle (**Fig. 1**). Four each of the trimers compose the irregular triangles seen in **Fig. 1**, which have planar faces separated by deep grooves. The planar faces of the two β types studied in this manner (NβV and TeV) show the three distinct pits apparent in **Fig. 1**.

Further details of the unique character of the tetravirus capsid emerge from the high resolution (2.8 Å) structure of the NωV capsid determined by x-ray diffraction methods (**Fig. 2**). The protein subunit has three distinct domains located on the interior, middle and exterior of the capsid. The conformation of exterior domain is that of a c-type immunoglobulin-like (Ig-like) domain, making the tetravirus capsid the only known example of this structure found in an unenveloped icosahedral virus (one other Ig-like structure has been found on the more complex, enveloped dengue fever virus). The Ig-like structure and its association with binding, as well as its prominent location on the capsid's exterior, suggest that this domain is as least partly responsible for the tropism of NωV. The middle region of the NωV capsid protein is the canonical 'jelly-roll' possessed by all proteins forming icosahedral capsids and forms the contiguous shell of the capsid. The interior domain consists of the cleaved minor protein and the termini of the major protein. The minor protein is mostly helical in structure and appears to interact with the genomic RNAs, as does the N-terminus of the major protein. A hypothesis has been formed in which the helix of the minor protein forms a conduit at the fivefold axis for RNA to exit the capsid through a membrane during the uncoating process.

Table 2 Biophysical properties of tetraviruses

Virus	Diameter (nm)	Density (g/ml⁻¹)	Sedimentation coefficient (S)	$e_{260/280}$	Capsid protein (M_r)	RNA ($M_r \times 10^3$)
Genus: Betatetraviruses						
NβV	39.7	1.295	210	1.45	60 572; 7975[a]	1800 (6.5 kb)[a]
AeV	32	ND	215	ND	ND	ND
TnV	35–38	1.3	200	ND	67 000–68 000	1900
DtV	35–38	1.289	199	1.44	62 000–66 000	ND
TaV	35	1.275	194	1.32	60 800	ND
PxV	35	1.275	206	1.36	62 400	ND
DpV	38	1.31	ND	1.43	66 000	1800
PiV	40	1.33	190	1.42	55 000	1900
Genus: Omegatetraviruses						
NωV	41.0	1.285	ND	ND	62 019; 7817[a]	RNA1=5300 bp RNA2=2448 bp[a]
HaSV	38	1.296	ND	1.22	63 378; 7309[a]	RNA1=5312 bp RNA2=2478 bp[a]
Unassigned possible members						
NεV	40.1	1.285	217	ND	ND	ND

ND, not determined.
[a]Data derived from sequence analysis.

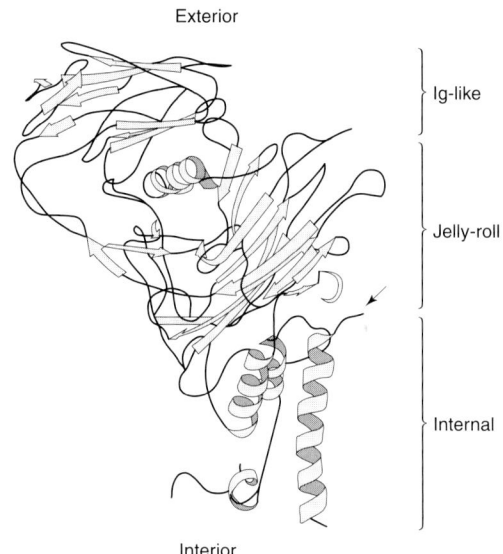

Figure 2 Schematic of the NωV coat proteins resolved to 2.8 Å. (Courtesy of Jack Johnson.) The three domains discussed in the text are noted on the right. The arrow points to the site of the assembly-dependent cleavage that produces the two coat proteins.

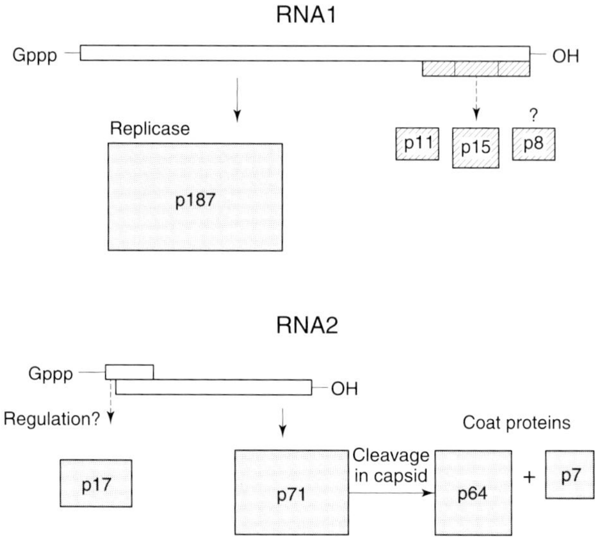

Figure 3 Genome organization and replication strategy of the ω-like tetravirus, HaSV. The genomic RNA1 and RNA2 with their ORFs are represented as open boxes above arrows leading to their functional protein products, represented as shaded rectangles enclosing their molecular weights. Dotted arrow indicates little, if any, production; question mark indicates incomplete understanding, while crosshatched rectangles indicate no evidence for expression.

Molecular Biology

Complete sequences are available for both β-type (NβV) and ω-type (HaSV) viruses. Comparison between the two sequences indicate a clear but distant relationship between the two genera. Detailed analysis of certain domains within the tetraviral sequences indicate the *Tetraviridae* belong to the α-like superfamily of RNA viruses. Analysis of the sequences give the major insights into how tetraviruses replicate, as experimental work is made difficult due to the lack of a cell culture system. However, new strategies for producing viral mutants and studying replication and coat protein assembly have given some insights into tetravirus virology.

ω-like genome organization

The complete sequence of the two RNA strands (RNA1 and RNA2) of the ω-like virus, HaSV, is available, while only RNA2 and a partial sequence of RNA1 exist for the only other known member of this genus, NωV. This information shows the gene products of the two viruses to be highly similar, except at certain key areas of the primary sequences of the coat proteins, as discussed below. Nearly the full length of HaSV RNA1 is accounted for by a single open reading frame (ORF) of 1704 codons encoding the 187 kDa replicase (**Fig. 3**). Experimental evidence exists for the function of this protein through its expression with recombinant baculoviruses (described below). It is not known whether the protein is processed into smaller fragments. Three smaller ORFs exist at the 3' end of RNA1 out of frame with the replicase ORF which could encode proteins of 99, 140 and 73 amino acids. However, there is no evidence for a subgenomic RNA which could express them, nor is there a discernible relationship to other proteins to indicate their function, if any.

RNA2 of HaSV has two out-of-frame ORFs that overlap each other, with a 'leaky scanning' mechanism for ribosomal translation as the likely means of expressing both genes from the same RNA. The first gene has its initiating AUG at base 283 in poor context for translation initiation, which would allow most ribosomes to scan through to the second AUG in good context at base 366, which initiates the second gene. The function of the 16 522 Da product of the first gene remains unclear, although there is experimental evidence to suggest it is involved in the regulation of strand synthesis. The second gene encodes the 647 residue, 70 670 Da precursor protein for the major and minor coat proteins of HaSV. The coat protein gene for NωV encodes a slightly smaller protein than that of HaSV (644 residue) but the two are highly homologous (>67% overall identity) except for three regions of the primary sequence. The

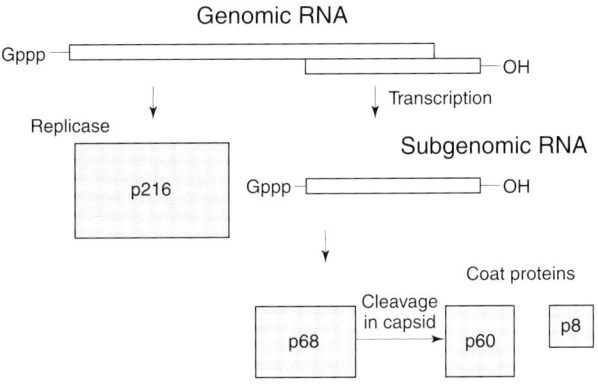

Figure 4 Genome organization of the β-like tetravirus, NβV. The NβV genomic RNA and its subgenomic RNA with their ORFs are represented as open boxes above arrows leading to their functional protein products, represented as shaded rectangles enclosing their molecular weights.

two terminal regions (amino acids 1–48 and 601–647) have 40% and 53% identity and correspond to the interior domain, while the 145 amino acid region in the middle of the primary sequence (amino acids 274–419) has only 33% identity and corresponds to the exterior Ig-like region. These dissimilar sequences in otherwise highly similar coat proteins are consistent with the putative functions of their corresponding structural domains, i.e. binding a different host cell for the exterior domain and interacting with a different RNA sequence for the interior domain.

β-like genome organization

The sequence of the NβV genomic RNA shows it to have only two genes which overlap each other (**Fig. 4**). The larger gene located at the 5′ end produces a 1925 amino acid protein with a calculated molecular weight of 216 kDa and is the RNA-dependent RNA polymerase (replicase), as determined by homologies to those of other viruses. It is not known at present whether further processing of the product of the replicase gene into smaller proteins occurs. The smaller gene located towards the 3′ end of the NβV genome encodes the 68 549 Da coat protein precursor which is cleaved upon capsid assembly to the major and minor coat proteins. This gene is able to be translated by scanning ribosomes through the production of a subgenomic RNA encoding 2.5 kb of the 3′ end of the genomic strand. This subgenomic strand is not capable of being replicated as only one species of double-stranded RNA with the length of the genomic strand is extracted from NβV infected larvae.

Genetic manipulation of tetraviruses

The lack of a cell culture system necessitated the development of a novel means of producing and examining effects of specific mutations in the genomes of tetraviruses. The strategy for producing HaSV mutants exploits its inactivity outside a host gut cell and the ability of the components of many simple icosahedral viruses like HaSV to assemble into virions in a wide variety of environments. Thus, by arranging the presence of the three main component types of HaSV (RNA1, RNA2 and coat protein) inside a plant cell where the virus is inactive, the two RNAs are able to assemble with coat protein to form a virion capable of infecting larvae. This is accomplished in a transient plant protoplast expression system (*Nicotiana plumbiganofolia*) by transfecting three plasmids, two producing the RNA strands by *in vivo* transcription off a modified plant promoter and the other expressing the coat protein precursor. The RNA-producing plasmids are constructed with cDNA copies of the viral RNAs behind a modified cauliflower mosaic virus 35S promoter designed to produce capped transcripts starting at the first viral base. An intact 3′ terminus for the RNA strand is achieved with a *cis*-acting ribozyme engineered to cleave the transcribed RNA after the last 3′ viral base. The third plasmid is engineered to express the coat protein precursor ORF behind an unmodified 35S promoter and without a ribozyme. Upon transfection of the three plasmids, the protoplasts are incubated for 3 days to allow assembly of the components and then fed to insect larvae to replicate and amplify the virus. Virus mutants are produced by site-directed mutagenesis upon the RNA-producing plasmids.

Replication

To counter the difficulty of the lack of a cell culture system to study the replication of HaSV, a system dependent on expressing tetraviral components with two different recombinant baculoviruses was developed. The first baculovirus expressed the HaSV replicase in Sf9 cells behind the polyhedrin promoter to the degree it was readily detected on an immunoblot of Sf9 cells. The high quantity of enzyme apparently compensated for a low level of activity, as replication of RNA2 templates presented to it by a second co-infected baculovirus was detected. The second baculovirus was engineered to produce precise transcripts of RNA2 using a similar strategy to the protoplast expression of tetraviral RNAs with the use of the same ribozyme and a modified *Drosophila* hsp70 promoter. Indicating replication was occurring with this system was the observation that no RNA2 transcript occurred on Northern blots unless the

RNA1 virus was present. By examining the effect of specific deletions of RNA2, this system is being used to examine which elements on RNA2 are important for its replication.

Studies of coat protein assembly

Similar to the coat proteins of many other small icosahedral viruses, assembly of virus-like particles (VLPs) occurs upon expression of only the tetraviral coat protein ORF in nonhomologous expression systems (yeast and baculoviruses). Of particular interest, however, are the observations indicating that the tetravirus coat proteins, without any other viral proteins, are able to perform all four generic functions of viral coat proteins: (1) binding each other to form a stable particle; (2) binding and incorporation of specific RNAs; (3) binding of host cells with subsequent entry; and (4) uncoating of RNA for translation. Experimentation has shown that VLPs display the assembly-dependent cleavage of the precursor, they are able to incorporate RNAs with viral sequences, and they bind specifically to a larval midgut receptor similar to native virions. Furthermore, purified VLPs can carry mRNAs of the reporter genes into gut cells of larvae where the reporter gene shows activity. VLPs carrying reporter gene mRNAs can be produced from Sf9 cells co-infected with two baculoviruses, one expressing the coat protein ORF and the other expressing a transcript having the reporter gene ORF in front of RNA2 sequences which allowed the transcript's encapsidation into the VLPs.

Pathobiology

Host range

Lepidopteran insects are the only known hosts for tetraviruses. A systematic survey of approximately a thousand diseased insects from different orders showed tetravirus hosts were confined largely to noctuid, saturniid and lymacodid moths of the Heterocera suborder of the Lepidoptera. Tetraviruses appear to differ in the breadth of the range of species they are able to infect. HaSV appears unable to infect species outside the subfamily Heliothinae, while *Tricoplusia ni* virus (TnV) and *Dasychira pudibunda* virus (DpV) are able to infect insects outside the family of their nominal host. Closely related viruses may have very distinct host ranges, as exemplified by NωV and HaSV. The former is able to infect a saturniid host, yet is unable to infect the noctuid heliothine host of the latter, despite having a high degree of relationship (>90% for the replicase).

No replication in other animals has been detected. Numerous animals injected with high titres of tetraviruses for antibody production have failed to show any abnormal response or disease symptoms. A detailed pathological study of mice injected with TaV showed no evidence that the virus was in any observable way harmful to them. Transfection of vertebrate cell lines with HaSV genomic RNA also showed no activity. However, studies on serological reactions by vertebrates (including humans) towards particles of tetraviruses, done in the 1970s, suggested that tetravirus specificity was more broad as positive reactions were noted. However, these reactions are believed to be nonspecific, owing to the type of serological test involved and indications that the reaction is not due to replication. Further work is required to consolidate these findings, especially in view of the large body of evidence showing the specificity of tetraviruses for insects and their potential widespread use in agriculture (see below).

Transmission and symptoms

Horizontal transmission via ingestion by larvae has been demonstrated for several tetraviruses. Interestingly, the range of symptoms from this means of transmission varies greatly. Few or no symptoms (only slight growth retardation at high doses) can be seen upon infection of several hosts by TnV. On the other hand, NβV displays a marked pathological effect upon larvae 7–9 days postinfection, with infected larvae in all stages ceasing to feed, becoming moribund, discolored and flaccid, and, upon death, remaining hanging by their prolegs. The cadavers are distinct from those infected with baculoviruses because an internal liquefaction occurs which leaves the integument intact. A dependence upon the larval life-stage can also be seen. HaSV is highly active against neonate larvae, with as little as 5000 particles causing them to cease feeding within a day and to die within 4 days. Surprisingly, HaSV infection of later instar larvae shows little effect. It has not been clearly demonstrated whether adults or pupae are capable of being infected by tetraviruses, although NβV was reported to be isolated from these stages.

Vertical transmission of tetraviruses is also believed to occur. It has been impossible to remove HaSV from a laboratory-bred colony of its host despite stringent sanitation procedures. Evidence from studies of HaSV pathology in early instar larvae show subpathogenic, low-level infections exist for this virus, which is highly virulent at higher doses. TnV appears to be vertically transmitted under artificial conditions and there is evidence for vertical transmission of the more virulent DpV. Symptoms of infection from this route are difficult to detect, with the most obvious being slow-growing larvae. The evidence for vertical transmission, however, remains undefinitive and further work needs to be done to establish it. The most likely mechanism for vertical transmission, should it occur, is transovum, as tetraviruses appear to infect only midgut cells (see below).

Histopathology and tropism

All the available evidence points to the larval midgut as the exclusive site of infection of tetraviruses. Examinations by light and electron microscopy for several viruses have shown their particles only in midgut tissues. In a definitive experiment showing this phenomenon, Northern blots of RNA extracted from infected larvae showed the presence of HaSV RNA only in midgut tissue, even after infection by injection into the hemocele. This experiment also shows that the tissue tropism of HaSV is not due to the lack of exposure to the virus by other host tissues. The marked tropism of HaSV which prevents its culture in continuous cell lines appears to be a function of both the abilities of the particles to bind and enter cells and a restriction on the activity of the replicase in cells other than those of the midgut. Binding studies using the histochemical detection of HaSV particles on cross-sections of larval midguts show exclusive binding to outer cell membranes, particularly the goblet cell apical membrane. However, even when cellular uptake mechanisms for particle entry are bypassed in cultured cells (including those of the cotton bollworm host, *Helicoverpa armigera*) by transfection of HaSV genomic RNA, no replication activity is seen.

In the most detailed pathology study for a tetravirus, HaSV was seen to infect all three major cell types of the lepidopteran midgut: goblet, columnar and regenerative stem cells. Infected cells showed crystalline arrays of particles, which were associated with a massive increase in the rate of cells detaching from the basal membrane and shedding into the lumen. Cells were shed to the extent that few, if any, remained in midguts of insects with advanced infections; this phenomenon was correlated to an increased rate of apoptosis. Hence the rapid loss of infected gut cells may be a cellularly mediated defense that protects the insect against more extensive viral infection.

Ecology

Only informal reports are available to describe the broader interactions between tetraviruses and their hosts in the wild. Hence much must be surmised and inferred from laboratory studies and the limited reports of agricultural use. The broad range of disease symptoms and possible dual means of transmission suggest a complicated picture.

Tetraviruses are readily found in insect hosts with other tetraviruses and other virus types, including cytoplasmic polyhedrosis viruses, baculoviruses and other small RNA viruses. Persistence in wild populations of *Nudaurelia* for decades in South Africa has been described for NβV and NωV, with the latter succeeding the former in prevalence in recent times. This succession may have contributed to the recent decline of the host population to the point where few moths have been observed in areas formerly inundated. The persistence of tetraviruses is probably due to their ability to initiate sublethal infections and to be transmitted vertically, as well as the apparent robust nature of the particle, which would favor its vertical transmission.

At high densities of host populations, horizontal transmission is the main mode of viral spread through dispersed cadavers and frass in which tetraviruses have been shown be present. The *Nudaurelia* populations recorded large-scale epizootics at high densities, at times displaying up to 90% mortality nearly every year for at least four decades. In contrast, no HaSV epizootics have been observed in the low density *H. armigera* populations in closely scrutinized Australian cotton fields, and yet the virus clearly has the capacity for virulence. The few infected *H. armigera* larvae found in the wild are likely to be the result of vertical transmission.

Economic Use and Future Perspectives

Tetraviruses, as well other small RNA viruses of insects, have been little used in Western agriculture as biological control agents for pests. However, SaV and DtV have been used to great effect in Malaysian oil palm plantations to control limacodid caterpillar pests, which can reach very high densities. Production and dispersal of these viruses was accomplished by suspension of naturally infected cadavers in water and spraying. Laboratory tests with purified HaSV on larvae of *H. armigera* strongly indicate their potential for the control of this major pest. Furthermore, the association of NωV with the decline of *Nudaurelia* populations indicates that long-term effects on pest populations with the use of tetraviruses are possible.

There is more interest in the economic use of tetraviruses, however, when the group is looked at through the lens of biotechnology. One major obstacle to their use for insect control has been the difficulty of producing them. However, the simplicity of the tetraviral genome makes production of viral particles in nonhost cells feasible (see above, Molecular Biology). The assembly of HaSV in plant

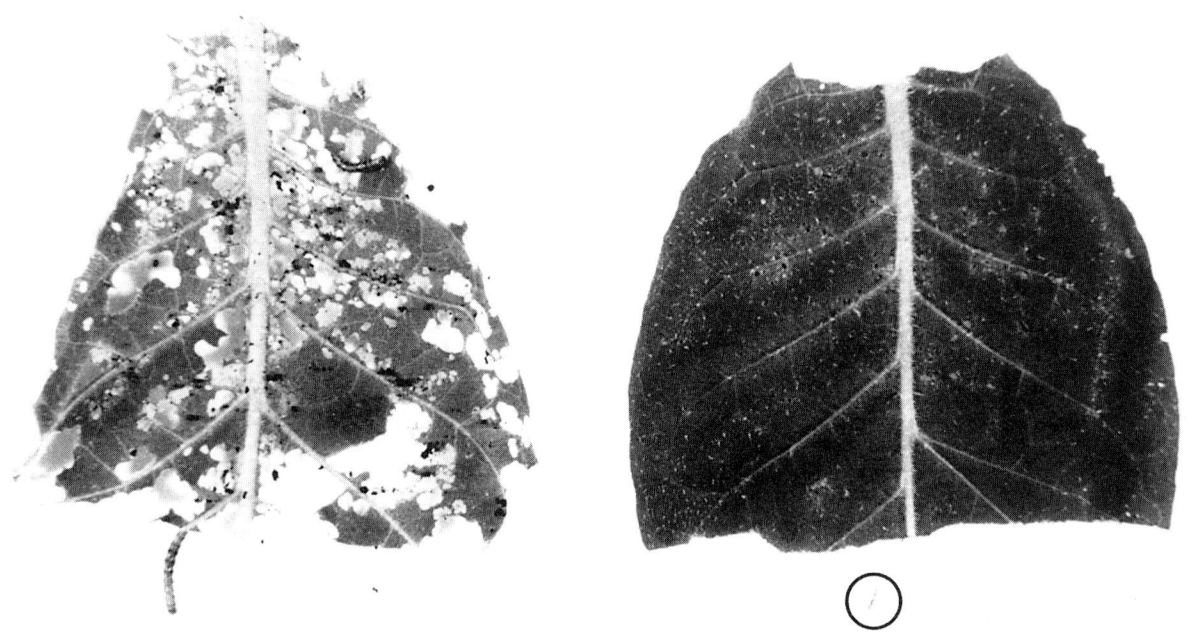

Figure 5 Tobacco made transgenic with genes that produce a tetravirus. The genes introduced into the transgenic tobacco plant on the right were designed to produce the protein and RNA components of the tetravirus, HaSV. These components were able to assemble into infectious virions, as indicated by the stunted, HaSV infected larva encircled below the leaf on the right. The larger larvae feeding on the control leaf on the left were not infected.

protoplasts described above suggested that transgenic crop plants could also accomplish the same feat. To test this hypothesis, the three genes required for HaSV assembly were placed into the genomes of tobacco plants by *Agrobacterium*-mediated transgenesis. The plants were screened for antifeeding activity and several showed they could induce stunted larvae, which subsequently were shown to be infected with HaSV (**Fig. 5**). This experiment indicates a new approach to the control of the world's most economically important group of insect pests, the heliothine caterpillars. Assembly of HaSV is also being tested in yeast with the same three gene strategy. Production of tetraviruses by yeast fermentation would make the virus available cheaply for spraying purposes.

Biotechnology may have another use for tetraviruses that may impact on medicine as well as agriculture. Their particles have the potential to be used as versatile vehicles for the targeted delivery of nonviral RNAs to new cell types. The tetravirus virion can be viewed as a delivery vehicle for viral genes that employs an Ig-like domain to bind specifically to a particular cell surface epitope, allowing its entry into midgut cells. This suggests that its exchange for another Ig-like domain having affinity towards another surface epitope of another cell type would change the destination of the particle's RNA contents to the other cell type. This potential targeting ability, combined with the already demonstrated ability to produce functional VLPs with nonviral mRNAs (described above), makes for a potentially versatile system for delivering transient gene activities to specific cells. Possible medical uses include a novel form of gene therapy or immunotoxins where toxin mRNAs are delivered to cancer cells, allowing more specific expression of toxicity than the present forms. In agriculture, mRNAs for insect-specific toxins could be targeted more quickly to a particular insect. This approach would preclude the use of a virus for every pest insect, and such a system could be made more acceptable to consumers and regulatory authorities.

See also: **Vectors: Plant viruses; Nodaviruses (*Nodaviridae*).**

Further Reading

Gordon KHJ, Johnson KN and Hanzlik TN (1995) The larger genomic RNA of *Helicoverpa armigera* stunt tetravirus encodes the viral RNA polymerase and has a novel 3'-terminal tRNA-like structure. *Virology* 208: 84.

Hanzlik TN and Gordon KHJ (1997) The *Tetraviridae*. *Adv. Virus Res.* 48: 101.

Hendry DA, Hodgson V, Clark R and Newman J (1985)

Small RNA viruses coinfecting the pine emperor moth *Nudaurelia cytherea capensis*. *J. Gen. Virol.* 66: 627.

Moore NF (1991) The Nudaurelia β family of insect viruses. In: Kurstak E (ed.) *Viruses of Invertebrates*, p. 277. New York: Marcel Dekker.

Munshi S, Liljas L, Cavarelli J et al (1996) The 2.8 Å structure of a T = 4 animal virus and its implications for membrane translocation of RNA. *J. Mol. Biol.* 261: 1.

Service R (1996) Arming plants with a virus. *Science* 271: 145.

THEILER'S VIRUSES (*PICORNAVIRIDAE*)

Howard L Lipton, Division of Neurology, Evanston Hospital, Evanston, Illinois, USA

Copyright © 1999 Academic Press

History, Geographic Distribution and Host Range

The mouse encephalomyelitis viruses are enteric pathogens of mice. Discovered by Max Theiler in the early 1930s and originally called murine polioviruses, these agents are frequently referred to as Theiler's murine encephalomyelitis viruses (TMEV). Theiler initially recovered isolates from mice with spontaneous paralysis housed in a research colony; subsequently the TMEV have been found in virtually all nonbarrier mouse colonies, where they cause asymptomatic intestinal infections. While the TMEV are widely distributed throughout the world in mouse colonies, their host range is quite narrow, and includes only mice and rats. Serological evidence indicates that *Mus musculus*, the feral house mouse, is the natural host, but several other species of voles and possibly rats may also serve as hosts. As is the case for other picornaviruses, following peripheral routes of infection, TMEV spreads to the central nervous system (CNS) producing encephalitis, or more commonly, spontaneous paralysis, i.e. poliomyelitis. The incidence of spontaneous paralysis is low, around one paralyzed animal per 1000–5000 mice in a colony reported in the older literature. Since the TMEV may go undetected unless appropriate serological tests for the virus are performed, these agents are a potential hazard for investigators using mice in biomedical research.

In recent years, this group of viruses has assumed additional importance because TMEV infection in mice provides one of the few available experimental animal models for multiple sclerosis. TMEV-induced demyelinating disease is a relevant animal model for multiple sclerosis because: (1) chronic pathological involvement is virtually limited to the CNS white matter; (2) myelin breakdown is accompanied by mononuclear cell inflammation; (3) demyelination results in clinical disease, e.g. spasticity, from involvement of upper motor neuron pathways; (4) myelin breakdown is in part immune-mediated; and (5) the disease is under multigenic control with a strong linkage to certain major histocompatibility complex (MHC) genes.

Classification and Serologic Relationships

Based on the complete nucleotide sequence and genome organization, TMEV have been classified in the genus *Cardiovirus* of the family *Picornaviridae* along with encephalomyocarditis virus (EMCV) and Mengo virus (**Table 1**). TMEV are a separate serological group of cardioviruses, as polyclonal antisera show no crossneutralization between TMEV and EMCV or Mengo virus. Because the coat proteins share a high level of amino acid sequence identity with the other cardioviruses, crossreactions are seen on ELISA when disrupted virions are used as antigens and on complement fixation tests.

Table 1 Classification of TMEV in the family *Picornaviridae*

Human enteroviruses: polioviruses, coxsackieviruses, echoviruses
Human rhinoviruses
Hepatitis A viruses
Aphthoviruses: foot-and-mouth disease viruses
Cardioviruses
    Group A: EMCV, Mengo, MM, Columbia-SK, Maus–Elberfeld
    Group B: TMEV – GDVII, FA, BeAn8386, DA, WW, TO4, TO(B15)
    Group C: Viliuisk virus[a]

[a] Viliuisk virus is either a divergent TMEV or it belongs in a separate group as shown here.

Three-dimensional Virion Structure

Picornavirions have a relative molecular mass of $\sim 8.5 \times 10^6$ Da, of which $\sim 30\%$ is RNA. The spherical virus particles have an external diameter of about 30 nm. The capsid proteins are arranged in icosahedral symmetry with 60 protomers, each composed of a single copy of VP1, VP2, VP3 and VP4.

The three-dimensional structures of the GDVII, BeAn and DA strains have been determined at ~ 0.3 Å resolution by x-ray crystallography. The overall architecture is quite similar to that of other picornaviruses whose structures have been determined, and closely resembles that of Mengo virus. Each of the three major capsid proteins VP1, VP2 and VP3 consist of a wedge-shaped eight-stranded antiparallel β barrel, as demonstrated for other picornaviruses. The N-termini of the capsid proteins form an extensive, intertwined network on the inner surface of the protein shell. The loops connecting the β strands form the outer surface features of the protein shell and provide the surface differences with Mengo virus. The pit which has been proposed as the viral receptor is a broad depression on the virion surface at the junction between VP1 and VP2 along the twofold axis. The TMEV surface structures can be differentiated from that of Mengo virus in having: (1) a larger VP1 CD double loop, with loop I containing an extra five residues and shifted more toward the VP2 EF puff at the twofold axis, while loop II points more toward the fivefold axis; (2) an 11 residue insertion in the VP2 EF puff forming a double loop in which the inserted loop interacts with the VP1 FMDV GH loop; and (3) the tip of the VP3 knob (a loop inserted in βE) points straight outward on the rim of the pit.

Properties of the Genome

The genetic component of the virion is a positive-sense, single-strand RNA molecule that has a sedimentation coefficient of 35 S and is 8100 nucleotides long. Virion RNA has a poly(A) tract on the 3′ end and a small basic protein, VPg, covalently linked to the 5′ end. The complete genomes of the GDVII, DA and BeAn strains have been cloned and sequenced. With the notable absence of a poly(C) tract in the 5′ noncoding region, the organization and sequence of the TMEV genome is remarkably similar to that of EMCV. The polyprotein of the BeAn strain, a typical TMEV, initiates at the AUG codon at nucleotide 1065 and extends for 6909 nucleotides (or 2303 codons), ending at the single UGA termination triplet at base 7972. The polyprotein-coding region is flanked by 5′ and 3′ noncoding sequences of 1064 and 125 nucleotides, respectively. In BeAn the 5′ noncoding region contains a stretch of 11 pyrimidines interrupted by a single purine before the AUG at nucleotide 1065. In picornaviruses, the 5′ noncoding region mediates cap-independent translation and also serves as an internal ribosome entry site (IRES), e.g. when experimentally present in the intercistronic region in a bicistronic mRNA. The TMEV 5′ noncoding sequences have been predicted to form stable secondary structures, which in the 500 nucleotides upstream of the authentic AUG (at 1065) are nearly identical to those predicted for EMCV and foot-and-mouth disease virus. In BeAn, eight AUGs precede the initiator AUG, but none of them has an optimum Kozak context sequence. Hence, it could be argued that selection of the authentic initiator AUG after binding of ribosomes to TMEV RNA does not involve internal ribosome binding. However, BeAn nucleotides $\sim 500–1065$ determine a structure that serves as an IRES in bicistronic mRNAs both *in vitro* (rabbit reticulocyte lysate) and *in vivo* (BHK-21 cells). A poly(A) tail of indeterminate length is present on the 3′ end of the viral genome.

Polyprotein and Post-translational Processing

As is the case for other picornaviruses, the final TMEV gene products are the result of post-translational cleavages of the polyprotein. The 2303 amino acid polyprotein has a calculated molecular weight of 255 990. (This applies to BeAn virus; the polyprotein of GDVII virus contains no insertions or deletions; however, two VP1 amino acids are deleted in that of DA virus.) The processing scheme follows the standard L–4–3–4 picornavirus polypeptide arrangement, i.e. the leader peptide (L), four capsid polypeptides in part one (P1) of the genome, three polypeptides in P2 and four polypeptides in P3 (**Fig. 1** and see below). The coding limits of individual polypeptides have been predicted by analogy with those of EMCV, as the only confirmation to date of the deduced sequence is that of the N terminus of 1D. The eight amino acids flanking the putative cleavage sites are highly conserved for the two viruses. All of the cleavage sites in the polyprotein except for two, 1A/1B and 2A/2B, are processed by the viral protease 3C. The TMEV 3C protease therefore processes Q–C, as well as Q–S and Q–A, dipeptides and, in addition, the E–N dipeptide at the 1D/2A cleavage. However, only 6 of 8 Q–G, 2 of 13 Q–S and 1 of 7 Q–A dipeptides in the polyprotein are cleaved by 3C, indicating that involvement of secondary, tertiary, or both types of structure is also important for recognition of these particular dipeptides. The 2A/2B site is probably autocatalytically cleaved, as in EMCV.

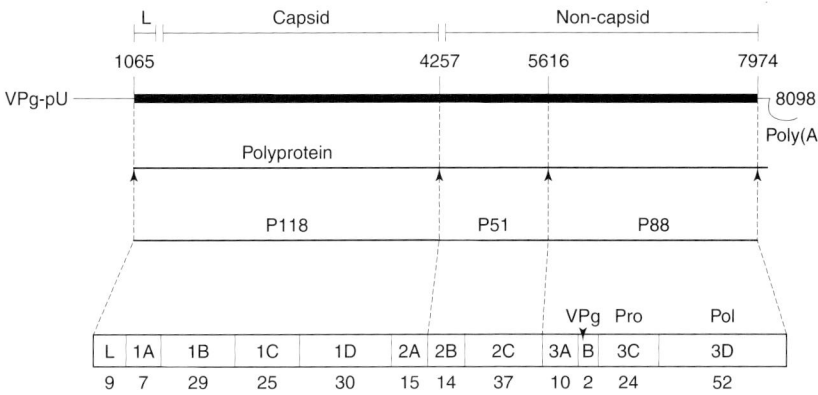

Figure 1 TMEV-specific protein cleavage scheme. The intermediate cleavage products are not shown. The numbers below the 11 final gene products are the molecular weights (in thousands) of each of the proteins as calculated from their predicted amino acid sequences.

Cleavage of the polyprotein gives rise to three primary products, the first of which (116 530 mol. wt) contains the leader protein (8593 mol. wt), the P1 capsid proteins, and the first P2 polypeptide 2A (15 353 mol. wt). Thus, the initial precursor released from the polyprotein is like that of the other cardioviruses and differs from that of other groups of picornaviruses. The capsid proteins are arranged in the following order: 1A (VP4; 7102 mol. wt), 1B (VP2; 29 433 mol. wt), 1C (VP3; 25 463 mol. wt), and 1D (VP1; 30 457 mol. wt). The second processing precursor (2BC) is 51 708 mol. wt and gives rise to 2B (14 863 mol. wt) and 2C (36 845 mol. wt). The P2 proteins 2A, 2B and 2C have not been assigned functions as yet for the cardioviruses. The third or C-terminal precursor protein is 87 950 mol. wt and is processed into the four mature proteins 3A (9934 mol. wt), 3B (2169 mol. wt), 3C (23 612 mol. wt) and 3D (52 235 mol. wt). Protein 3B, also designated VPg, is a small basic protein which is 20 amino acids in size and is found covalently linked to the 5' end of viral RNAs. This peptide may be important in viral replication. By analogy with other picornaviruses, the 3C polypeptide is a viral protease and 3D is the viral polymerase.

Physical Properties

Since the TMEV do not have an envelope they are more resistant than lipid-containing viruses to chemicals and physical agents. They are insensitive to chloroform, ether, nonionic detergents (such as deoxycholate, NP40 and Tween-80) and the ionic detergent sodium dodecyl sulfate, but are inactivated by 0.3% formaldehyde and HCl 0.1 mol l^{-1}. TMEV are rapidly destroyed at temperatures over 50°C and lose some infectivity upon lyophilization. Purified virions can be stored for long periods of time at $-70°C$ without loss of infectivity, but slowly lose infectivity on storage at $-20°C$.

As enteroviruses the TMEV require stability at low pH to pass through the acidic conditions of the stomach. The TMEV are stable over the entire pH range from 3 to 9.5. However, in contrast to the other cardioviruses, such as Mengo virus and EMCV, they are not highly thermolabile in the presence of 0.1 mol l^{-1} chloride or bromide in the pH range 5 to 7.

Theiler's virions have a sedimentation coefficient of 150 S by velocity centrifugation in sucrose and a buoyant density of 1.34 g ml^{-1} by isopycnic centrifugation in cesium salts.

Replication

The reader is referred to entries on human poliovirus and cardioviruses for the strategy of picornavirus RNA replication as no information is available on this topic for the TMEV.

Mapping Genomic Determinants Important in Pathogenesis

The existence of two distinct TMEV neurovirulence groups makes the TMEV particularly useful for molecular pathogenesis studies. The difference in virulence (LD_{50}) between the highly virulent and less virulent TMEV groups is of the order of 10^5 plaque-forming units. Further, full-length cDNA clones of the highly virulent GDVII and the less virulent DA and BeAn viruses have been assembled in different laboratories, and viral RNA transcribed from these cDNAs has been demonstrated to be infectious upon transfection of mammalian cells. To identify the

Table 2 Two TMEV neurovirulence groups

	Highly virulent	Less virulent
TMEV isolated	GDVII, FA, ASK1 VIE 415$_{HTR}$	DA, BeAn 8386, Yale, WW TO(B15), VL, TO4
Disease	Encephalitis	Polio/demyelination
Incubation period[a]	1–10 days	7–20 days/>30 days
CNS target cell[b]	Neurons	Motor neurons/macrophages and oligodendrocytes
Mean LD$_{50}$	10 PFU	10^6 PFU
Persistent infection	No	Yes
Temperature sensitive[c]	No	Yes

[a]Incubation period following experimental infection by the intracerebral route of inoculation.
[b]Preferential site of virus replication in the central nervous system (CNS).
[c]Inability to replicate at 39.8°C compared to 33 or 37°C.
PFU, plaque-forming units.

determinants important in pathogenesis, e.g. virulence and persistence, recombinant viruses between parental cDNAs have been assembled and analyzed *in vitro* and after inoculation of mice.

Neurovirulence and persistence have been mapped primarily to the P1 region encoding the leader and the coat proteins. These results suggest that the mechanism for the pathogenetic properties of virulence and persistence are likely to involve the exterior surface of the virus, and immunological or receptor-mediated events may be involved. Chimeric virus constructs in the coat protein region, resulting in the interaction of potentially disparate protomeric subunits of two parental viruses, have been found to be prone to assembly defects. Such chimeric viruses may exhibit compromised growth *in vitro*. Thus, the pathogenetic phenotypes of chimeric viruses need to be interpreted with caution and require analysis of their growth properties *in vitro*.

Transmission and Tissue Tropism

TMEV are transmitted by the fecal–oral route but can be separated into two biological groups based on neurovirulence (**Table 2**). The first group, consisting of three isolates, GDVII, FA and Ask-1, is highly virulent and causes a rapidly fatal encephalitis in mice. The other TMEV, some 10–20 isolates, that include viruses recovered from the CNS of spontaneously paralyzed mice and from the feces of asymptomatic mice, form a second, less virulent group. Experimentally, the less virulent viruses produce poliomyelitis (early disease) followed by demyelinating disease (late disease). When cell culture-adapted less virulent TMEV are used to inoculate mice, the poliomyelitis phase is subclinical; brain-derived stocks produce both of the less virulent disease phases.

Pathogenesis

Little information is available about the pathogenesis of TMEV infection following peripheral routes of infection, including feeding of virus. In general, isolates from either of the TMEV neurovirulence groups do not readily produce CNS disease following peripheral routes of inoculation, with the exception of one strain, TO(B15). TO(B15) is a mutant selected for its invasiveness from the intestinal tract. When mice are inoculated intracerebrally with the highly virulent strains, the virus replicates throughout the brain and spinal cord, causing encephalitis or encephalomyelitis. Thus, neurons as well as glial cells (astrocytes and probably oligodendrocytes) are infected in the cerebral cortex, hippocampus, basal ganglia, thalamus, brainstem and spinal cord. Affected mice develop a hunched posture and hind limb paralysis. The rapid demise of these animals is the result of widespread lytic infection. The following sections focus on the pathogenesis of the biphasic disease produced by the less virulent TMEV, which provides a model system for multiple sclerosis.

Clinical Features of Infection

Although TMEV are enterically transmitted, the pathogenesis of the infection has been primarily studied using the intracerebral route of inoculation which maximizes the incidence of neurological disease. Following intracerebral inoculation, the less virulent strains produce a distinct biphasic CNS disease in susceptible strains of mice, characterized by poliomyelitis during the first few weeks postinfection, followed by chronic, inflammatory demyelination that begins during the second or third week postinfection and becomes manifest clinically between 1 and 3 months postinfection. Mice with poliomyelitis develop flaccid paralysis, usually of the hind limbs; only one limb may be affected, or paralysis may spread to involve all limbs and lead to death. In contrast to the fatal outcome of paralysis produced by the Lansing strain of human poliovirus type 2, complete recovery from TMEV-induced poliomyelitis is usual. Occasionally, residual limb deformities are seen as the result of extensive anterior horn cell infection and severe paralysis (early disease).

Gait spasticity is the clinical hallmark of the demyelinating or late disease. Late disease is first manifest by slightly unkempt fur and decreased activity, followed by an unstable, waddling gait. Subsequently, generalized tremulousness and ataxia develop, and the waddling gait evolves into overt paralysis. Incontinence of urine and priapism are commonly seen. As the disease advances, prolonged extensor spasms of the limbs can be induced followed by difficulty in righting. Weight loss is not seen until mice are severely paralyzed. The clinical manifestations of late disease are progressive and lead to an animal's demise in several to 14 months.

Pathogenesis and Histopathology

Motor neurons in the brainstem and spinal cord are the main targets of infection during poliomyelitis (early disease), but sensory neurons and astrocytes are also infected. TMEV do not replicate in endothelial and ependymal cells. A brisk microglial reaction is elicited, with the appearance of numerous microglial nodules, particularly in the anterior gray matter of the spinal cord. Examples of neuronophagia are quite frequent at this time, but very little lymphocytic response is seen. The poliomyelitis phase lasts 1–4 weeks, after which time little residual gray matter involvement is apparent other than resolving astrocytosis.

As early as 2 weeks postinfection, inflammation of the spinal leptomeninges begins to appear, followed by involvement of the white matter. Initially, the inflammatory infiltrates are almost exclusively composed of lymphocytes, but at later times plasma cells and macrophages are numerous. The influx of macrophages is in close temporal and anatomic relationship with myelin breakdown. Both light microscope and ultrastructural studies show that myelin breakdown is related to the presence of mononuclear cells, which either actively strip myelin lamellae from otherwise normal-appearing axons or are found in contact with myelin sheaths undergoing vesicular disruption. Foci of inflammation and myelin destruction extend from the perivascular spaces into the surrounding white matter, leading to sharply demarcated plaques of demyelination. The ultrastructure of oligodendrocytes during the initial phase of myelin breakdown has not shown alterations in oligodendroglial loops, which are in close apposition with naked but otherwise normal axons, suggesting that myelin injury may not be directly related to oligodendrocytopathology.

Sites of TMEV persistence

The sites of TMEV persistence are still disputed; however, TMEV persistence clearly involves active virus replication, as infectious virus can be readily isolated from the CNS of infected mice. *In situ* hybridization has revealed two populations of CNS cells positive for viral genomes. Virus replication in the majority of these cells (>90%) appears to be highly restricted, as they contain <500 viral genomes. A small percentage of CNS cells contain >1500 genomes, possibly as many as 10^4–10^5, and are probably productively infected. Highly restricted virus production has been demonstrated in macrophages isolated from the CNS of diseased mice; therefore, macrophages appear to be the primary target for persisting virus. It is also possible that some of the cells with restricted infection are astrocytes. The kinetics of virus replication in the CNS cells with restricted infection remains to be elucidated, such as the length of the replicative cycle and whether the cells are lysed or continue to produce infectious virus for longer times. *In vitro*, TMEV infection only occurs in monocytes once they have differentiated into macrophages. The infection of macrophage cell lines is highly restricted but with normal levels of viral translation, as substantial amounts of viral antigen are produced; ultimately infected macrophages undergo apoptosis. In contrast, oligodendrocytes appear to be productively infected, as an ultrastructural study has shown crystalline arrays of virions in oligodendrocytes in demyelinating lesions. Oligodendrocytes may correspond to the CNS cells containing large numbers of viral genomes by *in situ* hybridization. These data suggest that a lytic infection of oligodendrocytes contributes to demyelination along with immune-mediated mechanisms of damage.

Immune Response

During the first week, TMEV-infected mice mount a virus-specific humoral immune response that reaches a peak by 1 to 2 months postinfection and is sustained for the life of the host. Neutralizing and other virus-specific antibodies have been measured. The majority of the antiviral IgG response in persistently infected, susceptible mice is of the IgG2a subclass, with little antiviral IgM detected by day 14 postinfection, whereas IgG1 antiviral antibodies appear to predominate in resistant and immunized mice. Murine CD4+ T cells of the Th1 subset mediate delayed-type hypersensitivity (DTH) and regulate IgG2a production via interferon γ production, whereas CD4+ Th2 cells regulate IgG1 and IgE production via interleukin 4. Thus, the predominant IgG2a antiviral response in susceptible mice may be an *in vivo* measure of preferential stimulation of a Th1-like pattern of cytokine synthesis. Recently, virus-specific CD8+ cytolytic T cell responses have also been shown help in virus clearance during the acute phase of the infection, and may be responsible for the resistance of certain strains of mice to the demyelinating disease.

When infected, susceptible mice also produce substantial levels of virus-specific CD4+ T cell responses. T cell proliferation and DTH appear by 2 weeks postinfection and remain elevated for at least 6 months. Both DTH and T cell proliferation have been shown to be specific for TMEV and mediated by CD4+ class II restricted T cells. A temporal correlation has also been found between the onset of demyelination and the appearance of these virus-specific T cell responses, as well as for high levels of virus-specific DTH and the susceptibility of mice of different genetic backgrounds and mixes. DTH and T cell proliferative responses in infected and immunized SJL mice (a susceptible strain) are directed toward immunodominant regions (peptides) in each of the three major coat proteins. T cell responses to these epitopes in VP1 and VP2 are believed to participate in the immunopathology (see below).

Although mice mount virus-specific humoral and cellular immune responses early in the infection and peak virus titers fall by 100–1000-fold, TMEV somehow evade immune clearance to persist at low levels indefinitely in the CNS of the host, as described above. Extraneural persistence has not been observed. Current dogma holds that humoral immunity is more important than cellular immunity in clearing infections by nonenveloped viruses, such as picornaviruses, but this has not been established for TMEV; evidence has been presented for a role for both neutralizing antibodies and cytolytic T cells in TMEV clearance. The precise mechanism by which TMEV evade immune surveillance is not known but does not appear to involve antigenic variation. Although complement and virus-antibody deposition in the CNS parenchyma have not been detected, extracellular transport of virus as infectious virus-antibody complexes, in aggregates, or contained or enveloped within cell membranes are means whereby virus could be protected from TMEV-specific immune responses and continue to replicate. This is an area for further study to enable a better understanding of how TMEV evade immune surveillance.

Immune-mediated Mechanism of Demyelination

Appropriately timed immunosuppression can prevent the clinical signs and pathological changes of TMEV-induced demyelinating disease, indicating that the immune response participates in myelin breakdown. A number of different immunosuppressive modalities have proven to be effective, including cyclophosphamide, antilymphocyte serum, antitumor necrosis factor antibodies, and monoclonal anti-IA, CD4+ and CD8+ antibodies. If given too early in the course of early disease, the infection in neurons is potentiated and results in encephalitis and a high mortality rate. Thus, immunosuppression may be most effective when administered after the first week of infection. The incidence of demyelinating disease is increased in SJL mice infected with a dose of virus that normally produces a low incidence of disease and adoptively

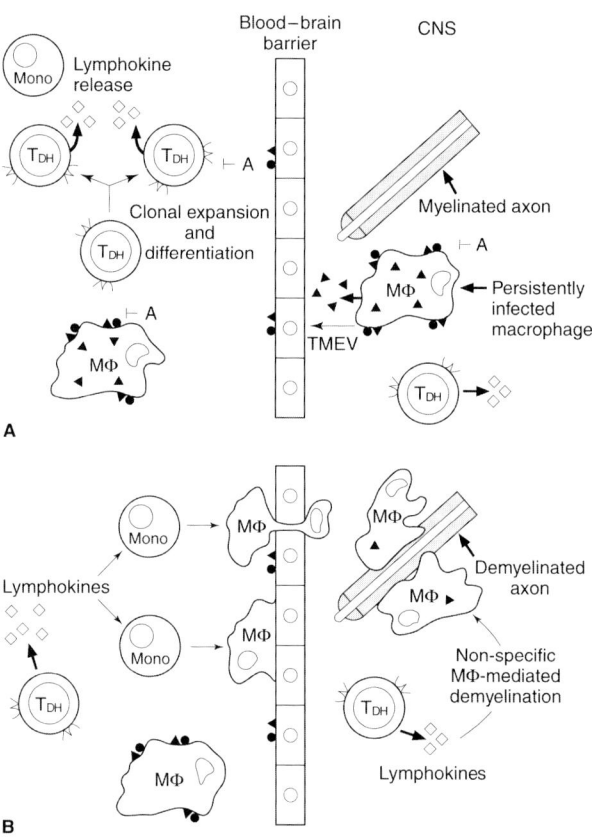

Figure 2 Proposed DTH-mediated mechanism of TMEV-induced demyelination. (**A**) Virus antigen presentation to Th1 lymphocytes, here designated T_{DH} cells, by antigen-presenting cells in either systemic lymphoid organs (left) or inside the blood–brain barrier (right). (**B**) Th1 lymphocyte response resulting in the recruitment of monocytes into the CNS and their differentiation into macrophages (MΦ) which then mediate demyelination.

immunized with TMEV VP2-specific T cell line. This observation supports a role for CD4+ T cells in mediating TMEV-induced demyelinating disease.

The effector mechanism by which a nonbudding virus, such as TMEV, might lead to immune-mediated tissue injury is unknown. Because TMEV antigens have been primarily found in macrophages, it has been proposed that myelin breakdown results from an interaction between virus-specific T cells trafficking into infected areas of the CNS and the virus. Thus, myelinated axons may be nonspecifically damaged as a consequence of a virus-specific immune response, i.e. an 'innocent bystander' response. In this circumstance, cytokines produced by MHC class II-restricted, TMEV-specific T_{DTH} cells primed by interaction with infected macrophages lead to the recruitment and activation of additional macrophages in the CNS, resulting in nonspecific macrophage-mediated demyelination (**Fig. 2**). This hypothesis is consistent with the CNS pathology observed in mice exhibiting TMEV-induced demyelinating disease and the fact that antigen-specific T cells and T cell lines have been shown to cause bystander CNS damage via macrophage activation in other model systems. Alternatively, in the case of extensive infection of oligodendrocytes, demyelination might result from immune injury to these myelin-maintaining cells expressing TMEV antigens in conjunction with H-2 class I determinants. CD8+ T cells would then be the likely T cell to kill infected oligodendrocytes; however, widespread degeneration of oligodendrocytes has not been observed.

See also: **Cardioviruses (*Picornaviridae*)**; **Immune response: Cell mediated immune response, General features**; **Persistent viral infection**; **Polioviruses (*Picornaviridae*): General features, Molecular biology**; **Virus structure: Atomic structure, Principles of virus structure**.

Further Reading

Adami C, Pritchard AE, Knauf T, Luo M and Lipton HL (1998) Mapping a determinant for central nervous system persistence in the capsid of Theiler's murine encephalomyelitis virus (TMEV) with recombinant viruses. *J. Virol.* 71: 1662.

Borson ND, Paul C, Lin X *et al* (1997) Brain-infiltrating cytolytic T lymphocytes specific for Theiler's virus recognize H2D^b molecules complexed with a viral VP2 peptide lacking a consensus anchor residue. *J. Virol.* 71: 5244.

Dethlefs S, Brahic M and Larsson-Sciard EL (1997) An early, abundant cytotoxic T-lymphocyte response against Theiler's virus is critical for preventing viral persistence. *J. Virol.* 71: 8875.

Grant RA, Filman DJ, Fujinami RS, Icenogle JP and Hogle JM (1992) Three-dimensional structure of Theiler virus. *Proc. Natl Acad. Sci. USA* 89: 2061.

Luo M, He C, Toth KS, Zhang CX and Lipton HL (1992) Three-dimensional structure of Theiler's murine encephalomyelitis virus (BeAn strain). *Proc. Natl Acad. Sci. USA* 89: 2409.

Monteyne P, Bureau JF and Brahic M (1997) The infection of mouse by Theiler's virus: from genetics to immunology (review). *Immunol. Rev.* 159: 163.

Penna-Rossi C, Delcroix M, Huitinga I *et al.* (1997) Role of macrophages during Theiler's virus infection. *J. Virol.* 71: 3336.

Peterson JD, Waltenbaugh C and Miller SD (1992) IgG subclass responses to Theiler's murine encephalomyelitis virus infection and immunization suggest a dominant role for Th1 cells in susceptible mouse strains. *Immunology* 75: 652.

Simas JP and Fazakerley JK (1996) The course of disease and persistence of virus in the central nervous system varies between individual CBA mice infected with the BeAn strain of Theiler's murine encephalomyelitis virus. *J. Gen. Virol.* 77: 2701.

Yauch RL, Palma JP, Yahikozawa H, Chang-Sung K and Kim BS (1998) Role of individual T-cell epitopes of Theiler's virus in the pathogenesis of demyelination correlates with the ability to induce a Th1 response. *J. Virol.* 72: 6169.

Tick-Borne Encephalitis see Encephalitis Viruses

TOBAMOVIRUSES

Dennis J. Lewandowski and **William O. Dawson**, Department of Plant Pathology, Citrus Research and Education Center, University of Florida, Lake Alfred, Florida, USA

Copyright © 1999 Academic Press

Introduction

Early research in the late 1800s on the causal agent of the mosaic disease of tobacco led to the discovery of the phenomenon of viruses. Thus tobacco mosaic virus (TMV), the type member of the tobamovirus group, became the first virus to be discovered, and since then has had a central role in many fundamental discoveries in virology. The first quantitative biological assay for plant viruses was the use of *Nicotiana glutinosa*, which produces necrotic local lesions when inoculated with TMV. TMV was the first virus to be purified and crystallized, which led to the discovery of the nucleoprotein nature of viruses and determination of the atomic structure of the coat protein and the virion. TMV was the first virus to be visualized in the electron microscope, confirming the predicted rigid rod shape. The genetic material of TMV was shown to be RNA, a property previously thought to be restricted to DNA. TMV was the first virus to be mutagenized. The first viral protein for which an amino acid sequence was determined was the coat protein of TMV. Subsequent determination of coat protein sequences from a number of strains and mutants helped to establish the universality of the genetic code. Methods of infecting plant protoplasts with viruses were developed with the tobacco–TMV combination, creating a synchronous system to study events in the infection cycle.

Taxonomy and Classification

Tobamoviruses are in the genus *Tobamovirus*; they have not been assigned to a family. There are 15 members within the *Tobamovirus* genus (**Table 1**). Although tobamoviruses are one of the most intensively studied groups of viruses, the taxonomy is often confused. Historically, plant viruses with rigid virions of approximately 18 × 300 nm were classified as a strain of TMV. Many viruses originally referred to as strains of TMV are now recognized as distinct tobamoviruses. For example, the tobamovirus that has been referred to as the tomato strain of TMV, and which is approximately 80% similar to TMV at the nucleotide sequence level, is actually tomato mosaic tobamovirus. Different tobamoviruses for which the entire nucleotide sequence is known are less than 90% identical similar to TMV at the nucleotide level.

Virus Structure and Composition

Tobamovirus virions are straight tubes of approximately 18 × 300 nm with a central hollow core 4 nm in diameter. Virion composition is approximately 95% protein and 5% RNA. Approximately 2100 individual subunits of a single coat protein are arranged in a right-handed helix around a single RNA molecule, with each subunit associated with three nucleotides.

Purified coat protein and viral RNA assemble into infectious particles *in vitro*. Protein–protein associations are the essential first event of virion assembly. Coat protein subunits assemble into several types of aggregates. Coat protein monomers and small heterogeneous aggregates of a few subunits are collectively referred to as 'A-protein'. The equilibrium between A-protein and larger aggregates is primarily dependent upon pH and ionic strength. The larger aggregates that have been characterized are disks, which are composed of two individual stacked rings of coat protein subunits, and protohelices. Protohelices contain approximately 40 coat protein subunits arranged in a spiral around a central hollow core, similar to the arrangement within the virion.

A sequence-specific stem-loop structure in the RNA, the 'origin of assembly', initiates encapsidation and prevents defective packaging which could result from multiple initiation events on a single RNA

Table 1 Definitive tobamoviruses

TMV	Tobacco mosaic virus
ToMV	Tomato mosaic tobamovirus
TMGMV	Tobacco mild green mosaic virus
ORSV	Odontoglossum ringspot virus
PMMV	Pepper mild mottle virus
CGMMV	Cucumber green mottle mosaic virus
SHMV	Sunn-hemp mosaic virus
RMV	Ribgrass mosaic virus
Ob	Tobamovirus Ob
TVCV	Turnip vein clearing virus
YMV	Youcai mosaic virus
FrMV	Frangipani mosaic virus
MaMV	Maracuja mosaic virus
SOV	Sammon's Opuntia virus
UMMV	Ullucus mild mosaic virus

molecule. The origin of assembly is located within the open reading frame (ORF) for the movement protein of most tobamoviruses and within the coat protein ORF of sunn-hemp mosaic (SHMV) and cucumber green mottle mosaic (CGMMV) tobamoviruses. Subgenomic mRNAs containing the origin of assembly are encapsidated into shorter virions that are not required for infectivity. The level of expression of a particular subgenomic mRNA containing the origin of assembly determines the relative proportion of that particular virion species. Consequently, in most tobamoviruses, in which the origin of assembly is located within the movement protein ORF, subgenomic mRNAs account for only a minor fraction of the total virion population. In contrast, where the origin of assembly is located within the highly expressed coat protein subgenomic mRNA, as in SHMV and CGMMV, a significant proportion of smaller virions are produced. Hybrid nonviral RNAs containing an origin of assembly will also assemble with coat protein into virus-like particles of length proportional to that of the RNA.

Virion assembly initiates as the primary loop of the origin of assembly is threaded through a coat protein disk or protohelix with both ends of the RNA trailing from one side. The conformation of the coat protein protohelix changes as the RNA becomes embedded within the groove between the two layers of subunits. Elongation is bidirectional, proceeding rapidly towards the 5' end of the RNA as the RNA loop is extruded through the elongating virion and additional coat protein disks are added. There is disagreement about the mechanism of elongation towards the 3' end of the RNA, but it appears that this slower process involves the addition of smaller protein aggregates.

Genome Organization

The tobamovirus genome consists of one single-stranded (ss) positive-strand RNA of approximately 6400–6600 nucleotides (**Fig. 1A**). There is a methylguanosine cap at the 5' terminus, followed by an AU-rich leader approximately 70 nt in length. The 3' nontranslated end of the RNA consists of sequences that can be folded into a series of pseudoknot structures, followed by a tRNA-like terminus. The tRNA-like terminus can be aminoacylated *in vitro*, and in most cases specifically accepts histidine. The exception is SHMV, which accepts valine and appears to have arisen by a recombination event between a tobamovirus and a tymovirus.

Four ORFs that are contained within the tobamovirus genome (**Fig. 1A**) correspond to the proteins found in infected tissue. Two overlapping ORFs begin

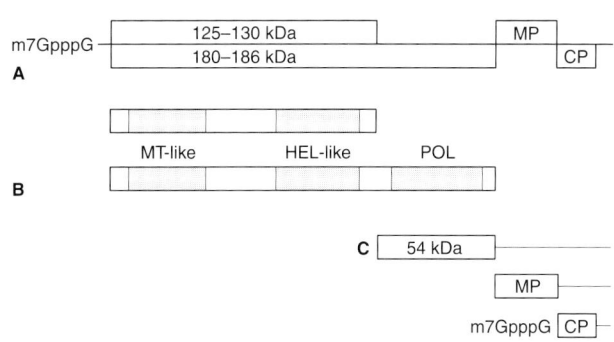

Figure 1 Tobamovirus genome organization and gene expression strategy. (**A**) Tobamovirus genome organization. ORFs designated as open boxes. Untranslated regions designated as solid lines. (**B**) Nonstructural proteins involved in tobamovirus replication. Domains of amino acid sequence similarity to viruses within 'alphavirus supergroup' are designated as hatched boxes. (**C**) Subgenomic mRNAs with 5' proximal ORF labelled. MP, movement protein; CP, coat protein; MT, methyltransferase; HEL, helicase; POL, polymerase.

at the 5' proximal start codon. Termination at the first inframe stop codon produces a 125–130 kDa protein. A 180–190 kDa protein is produced by readthrough of this termination codon approximately 5–10% of the time. Both proteins are necessary for efficient replication.

The remaining proteins are expressed from individual 3' coterminal subgenomic mRNAs, from which only the 5' proximal ORF is expressed (**Fig. 1C**; **Fig. 2**). The next ORF encodes the movement protein, which has RNA binding activity and is required for cell-to-cell movement of the virus. The 3' most ORF encodes the coat protein (17–18 kDa). A subgenomic mRNA containing an ORF for a 54 kDa protein that encompasses the readthrough domain of the 180–190 kDa ORF has been isolated from infected tissue, although no protein has been detected.

Within the protein-coding regions of the genome, there are nucleotide sequences that have additional functions as *cis*-acting elements, such as subgenomic mRNA promoters and the origin of assembly. The promoter elements for subgenomic mRNA synthesis are located on the genomic length complementary RNA, presumably upstream from the respective initiation sites. Gene expression from subgenomic mRNAs is regulated both temporally and quantitatively. The movement protein is produced early and accumulates to low levels, whereas the coat protein is produced late and in massive quantities. Several factors are probably involved in regulation of gene expression from the various subgenomic mRNAs. The subgenomic mRNA for the movement protein is not capped and has a long 5' leader, whereas the coat protein

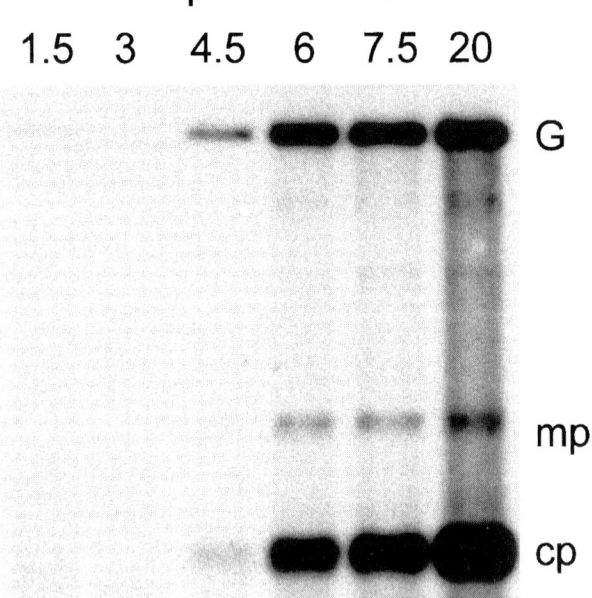

Figure 2 Northern blot of accumulation of TMV positive-stranded RNAs in tobacco protoplasts. Total RNA was extracted from tobacco protoplasts transfected with in vitro RNA transcripts of an infectious TMV cDNA clone at the times indicated. G, genomic RNA; mp, subgenomic mRNA for movement protein; cp, subgenomic mRNA for coat protein.

subgenomic mRNA is capped, has a short AU-rich leader, and is an efficient mRNA. Also, the levels of movement protein and coat protein production in TMV mutants are directly related to distance from the 3' terminus. There are no obvious sequence similarities between the promoters for the movement and coat protein subgenomic mRNAs, suggesting that secondary structure may be important for recognition.

Viral Proteins

The TMV 126/183 kDa proteins are involved in efficient viral replication. Both are contained in crude replicase preparations, and temperature-sensitive replication-deficient mutants map to these ORFs. There are three domains of amino acid sequence similarity shared with replicase proteins from other ssRNA plant and animal viruses (**Fig. 1B**). The N-terminal domain of the 126/183 kDa proteins has sequence similarity with a domain having methyltransferase activity associated with viral RNA capping. The C-terminal domain of the 126 kDa protein (also shared with the 183 kDa protein), is proposed to have helicase activity, based upon conserved sequence motifs. The third domain, which has a signature sequence for RNA polymerase function, is located within the readthrough region of the 183 kDa protein. Additionally, the 126/183 kDa proteins are symptom determinants, as mutations in mild strains map to these ORFs.

The movement protein has a plasmodesmatal binding function associated with its C-terminus and a single-stranded nucleic acid-binding domain associated with the N-terminus. The movement protein–host interaction determines whether the virus can systemically infect some plant species.

Although principally a structural protein, the coat protein is also involved in other host interactions. Coat protein is required for efficient long-distance movement of the virus. Coat protein is also a symptom determinant in some susceptible plant species and an elicitor of plant defense mechanisms in other plant species.

Interactions between Viral and Host Proteins

Available evidence suggests that the interactions of viral proteins with host factors are important determinants of viral movement and host ranges. Amino acid substitutions in the movement protein can alter the movement function in different hosts. Some viruses, including tobamoviruses, can assist movement of other viruses that are incapable of movement in a particular plant species. These interactions suggest that there are more precise associations of viral proteins with host factor(s) than with viral RNA. Additionally, precise coat protein–plant interactions are required for movement to distal positions within the plant.

Virus Replication

Virions or free viral RNA will infect plants or protoplasts. Since tobamoviruses have a genome consisting of messenger-sense RNA that is infectious, one of the first events is translation of the 5' proximal ORFs to produce the proteins required for replication of the genomic RNA and transcription of subgenomic mRNAs. When virions are the infecting agent, the first event is thought to be cotranslational disassembly, in which the coat protein subunits at the end of the virion surrounding the 5' end of the RNA loosen, making the RNA available for translation. Ribosomes then associate with the RNA, and translation of the 126/183 kDa ORFs is thought to displace coat protein subunits from the viral RNA.

After the formation of an active replicase complex, a complementary minus-strand RNA is synthesized from the genomic positive-stranded RNA template. Minus-strand RNA serves as template for both genomic and subgenomic mRNAs. Negative-stranded RNA synthesis ceases early in infection, while positive-stranded RNA synthesis continues. This results in an asymmetric positive- to negative-stranded RNA ratio. Early in infection, genomic RNA functions as template for minus-strand RNA synthesis and as mRNA for production of the 126/183 kDa proteins. Later in the infection cycle, most of the newly synthesized genomic RNA is encapsidated into virions. Subgenomic mRNAs transcribed during infection function as mRNA for the 3' ORFs that are not translated directly from the genomic RNA.

Within an infected leaf, replication proceeds rapidly between approximately 16 and 96 h postinfection within a cell, after which replication ceases. Even though the infected cells become packed with virions, these cells remain metabolically active for long periods of time. During the early stages of infection of an individual cell, the infection spreads through plasmodesmatal connections to adjacent cells. This event requires the viral movement protein that modifies plasmodesmata to accommodate larger molecules. Movement through plasmodesmata does not require the coat protein. A second function of the movement protein appears to be binding to the viral RNA to assist its movement through the small plasmodesmatal openings. The movement protein also appears to associate with the cytoskeleton. As the virus spreads from cell to cell throughout a leaf, it enters the phloem for rapid long-distance movement to other leaves and organs of the plant. This process requires the coat protein.

Cis-acting Sequences

The 5' nontranslated region contains sequences that are required for replication. This region has also been shown to be an efficient translational leader. The 3' nontranslated region contains *cis*-acting sequences that are involved in replication. Certain deletions within the pseudoknots are not lethal, but result in reduced levels of replication. Exchanges of 3' nontranslated regions between heterologous tobamoviruses result in viable viruses, suggesting that these are structural elements. The 3' nontranslated region appears to be a translational enhancer, both in the viral genome and when fused to heterologous reporter mRNAs. Sequences encoding the internal ORFs for the movement and coat proteins are dispensable for replication.

The coat protein subgenomic mRNA promoter is better defined than the movement protein subgenomic promoter. Duplication of the coat protein subgenomic promoter results in transcription of an additional new subgenomic mRNA. Subgenomic promoters from heterologous tobamoviruses are recognized and are active. Foreign sequences inserted behind tobamovirus subgenomic mRNA promoters can be expressed in plants and protoplasts.

Satellite Tobacco Mosaic Virus

Satellite tobacco mosaic virus (STMV), a tobamovirus-dependent satellite virus, has been isolated from *Nicotiana glauca* infected with the tobacco mild green mosaic tobamovirus (TMGMV). The genome consists of one plus-sense ssRNA of 1059 nucleotides. The 240 3' nucleotides share approximately 65% sequence similarity with TMGMV and TMV, contain two pseudoknot structures and have a tRNA-like terminus. No sequence similarity to tobamoviruses exists over the remainder of the genome. Two overlapping ORFs that are expressed in *in vitro* translation reactions are present in the genomic RNA of most STMV isolates. The 5' proximal ORF encodes a 6.8 kDa protein that has not been detected *in vivo*. The second ORF encodes the 17.5 kDa coat protein, which is not serologically related to any tobamovirus coat protein. The 17 nm icosahedral virions are composed of a single STMV genomic RNA encapsidated within 60 STMV coat protein subunits. Replication of natural populations of STMV is supported by other tobamoviruses, but at lower levels than with the natural helper virus, TMGMV. The host range of STMV parallels that of the helper virus. No effects on symptom expression by any of the helper tobamoviruses have been observed.

See also: **Plant virus disease – economic aspects; Satellite RNAs and Satellite viruses.**

Further Reading

Buck KW (1996) Comparison of the replication of positive-stranded RNA viruses of plants and animals. *Adv. Virus Res.* 47: 159.

Dawson WO (1992) Tobamovirus–plant interactions. *Virology* 186: 359.

Dawson WO and Lehto KM (1990) Regulation of tobamovirus gene expression. *Adv. Virus Res.* 38: 307.

Gibbs AJ (1977) Tobamovirus group. *CMI/AAB Descriptions of Plant Viruses*, No. 184.

Matthews REF (1991) *Plant Virology*, 3rd edn. New York: Academic Press.

Turpen TH and Dawson WO (1992) Amplification, movement and expression of genes in plants by viral-based vectors. In: Hiatt A (ed.) *Transgenic Plants: Fundamentals and Applications*. New York: Marcel Dekker.

van Regenmortal MHV and Fraenkel-Conrat H (eds) (1986) *The Plant Viruses*. Vol. 2: *The Rod-Shaped Plant Viruses*. New York: Plenum Press.

TOBRAVIRUSES

Peter B Visser, **Alexander Mathis** and **Huub JM Linthorst**, Institute of Molecular Plant Sciences, Gorlaeus Laboratories, Leiden, The Netherlands

Copyright © 1999 Academic Press

Taxonomy and Classification

The tobraviruses (type virus: tobacco rattle virus) are bipartite plant viruses which are members of the genus *Tobravirus* (a family has not been assigned). These are (1) tobacco rattle viruses (TRV), (2) pea early browning viruses (PEBV) and (3) pepper ringspot virus (PRV), which was formerly known as the CAM strain of TRV. The first two viruses contain several to numerous distinguishable strains or isolates, whereas only one PRV has yet been identified. Their classification into one genus of tobraviruses was originally based on common properties such as particle morphology, transmission vector and the unusual ability to cause a systemic infection in plants with only part of the genome. Recently this grouping has been supported by molecular studies. Comparisons based on molecular characteristics have also indicated that the tobraviruses are members of the supercluster of Sindbis-like viruses. Another plant virus member of this superfamily is the tobamovirus tobacco mosaic virus (TMV), which, both in morphology and genome organization, closely resembles the tobraviruses.

Virus Structure

The tobravirus genome is composed of two single-stranded RNA molecules of positive polarity, which are capped at the 5′ termini and which fold into a tRNA-like tertiary structure at the 3′ termini. However, this tRNA-like structure cannot be aminoacylated, as is the case in other viruses showing such a structure at the 3′ terminus.

The RNAs, designated RNA1 and RNA2, are separately encapsidated by coat protein subunits. The structure of the virions is determined by a helical array of coat protein molecules surrounding the RNA helix, which is very similar to that of tobacco mosaic virus. The virions are rigid rod-shaped particles with similar diameter (20–23 nm) but with a different length. The L (large) particles of TRV, PEBV and PRV have a similar size (180–210 nm); they encapsidate RNA1. The length of the S (small) particles varies considerably (50–110 nm), even between different strains in one subgroup. This difference in size of the S particles reflects the difference in length of the encapsidated RNA2.

During a normal infection cycle, both L particles and S particles are generated, and homogenates of infected plants are highly infectious (M-type infections, where 'M' stands for 'multiplying'). However, sometimes a second type of natural infection is apparent in which no particles are formed (NM-type infections, 'non-multiplying'). While homogenates of plants with NM-type infections are not or hardly infectious, infectious RNA is produced, as is evident after phenol extraction. The recent advancement of our knowledge of plant viruses has made it possible to explain this unique property of the tobraviruses in molecular genetic terms and to relate it to the specific way in which the genes are separated over the two genome segments.

Genome Organization and Molecular Biology

RNA1 molecules are highly homologous between isolates within the same subgroup, but little homology was identified between TRV, PEBV and PRV. RNA2 molecules are very variable in size. Generally, RNA2 of different isolates shows little sequence homology, except for the 3′-terminal region, which is also homologous to the 3′ terminus of RNA1 (**Fig. 1**).

For each of the three tobraviral subgroups, cDNA clones corresponding to the two genomic segments have been characterized. Both RNA1 of TRV strain SYM and RNA1 of PEBV strain SP5 were completely sequenced and shown to encode four open reading frames (ORFs). The first ORF of TRV strain SYM terminates at a UGA stop codon and encodes a protein of 134 kDa. Suppression of this UGA termination codon results in a readthrough protein of 194 kDa. Also, the first two ORFs of PEBV strain SP5 are fused by a UGA termination codon, which, upon suppression, allows the translation of two partially overlapping polypeptides. *In vitro* translation studies have indeed shown that both TRV RNA1 and PEBV RNA1 code for two polypeptides with sizes corresponding to the ones deduced from the nucleotide sequences. Similar mechanisms of genome expression via readthrough translation have been found with viruses belonging to several groups, among which are plant viruses from the tobamo-, luteo-, tymo- and carmovirus groups. The 3′-terminal one-third of tobraviral RNA1 contains two ORFs encoding smaller proteins (29 kDa and 16 kDa for TRV, and 30 kDa and 12 kDa for PEBV), which are probably expressed via subgenomic mRNAs.

These data, supplemented with partial sequence data from other tobraviruses, have indicated that extended similarities exist between the various proteins encoded by the different members of the tobravirus group and even with viruses from other plant virus groups. For instance, the 134 and 194 kDa TRV-SYM proteins contain regions with high homology with similar regions in the TMV 126 and 183 kDa proteins and in the proteins encoded by RNA1 and RNA2 of the tricornaviruses. Based on these similarities, functions have been inferred for the different encoded proteins. The second half of the 134 kDa TRV RNA1-encoded peptide contains a nucleotide-binding motif present in helicases, whereas the readthrough portion of the 194 kDa protein accommodates a so-called 'GDD box', which is present in the catalytic subunit of RNA-dependent RNA polymerases. The presence of these motifs is a strong argument in favor of the involvement in genome replication of the large tobravirus RNA1-encoded proteins.

The 29 kDa protein encoded by TRV RNA1 has homology with the TMV 30 kDa movement protein. The functional homology of these two proteins was proven by mutation analysis. A TRV mutant with a defect in the gene for the 29 kDa protein could not infect whole tobacco plants completely. This defectiveness can be complemented by transgenic expression of the TMV 30 kDa protein. The TRV 29 kDa protein may also play a role in symptom induction as this same mutant, complemented with TMV 30 kDa protein, did not produce necrotic spots on test plants, as does the wild-type TRV.

The small proteins encoded by the 3'-terminal ORF in RNA1 of PEBV (12 kDa) and TRV (16 kDa) are homologous. Both polypeptides contain a cysteine-rich putative zinc-finger structure but lack homology with proteins encoded by other plant viruses. TRV infected protoplasts accumulate large amounts of the 16 kDa protein. Infectious transcripts of TRV RNA1 containing mutated 16 kDa ORFs indicated that this protein is not required for replication. While combinations of infectious transcripts of PEBV RNA1 and RNA2, lacking an intact 12 kDa ORF, were highly infectious and the resulting virus accumulated to high levels in leaves and pods, virus could not be detected in pollen grains and ovules, and seed transmission of the mutant was less than 1% of that of the wild-type virus.

Thus, the combination of replication and movement functions allows RNA1 to replicate and spread on its own to give rise to the NM-type infections.

In contrast to similarity in size of RNA1, RNA2 is more variable in both size and nucleotide sequence. However, in all instances the 5'-proximal gene encodes the coat protein. The coat protein of TRV strain TCM is over 90% similar to the coat protein of known isolates of PEBV at the amino acid sequence level. Likewise, coat protein genes of TRV strains PLB, PSG and PpK20 share over 90% homology, whereas the similarity between coat proteins of TCM and PLB is about 40%. The PRV coat protein cistron has only 40% homology with coat proteins of both TCM and PLB.

The variability in length of RNA2 is due both to the presence of additional genes on the larger molecules and to a variable sized 3'-terminal region homologous with that of the corresponding RNA1 (**Fig. 1**). Northern blot hybridization using probes complementary to different regions in RNA2 of TRV strain PpK20 showed that various subgenomic RNAs are produced which enable separate translation of the three RNA2-derived proteins, including the 5'-proximal coat protein. Similarly, ORFs of PEBV strain SP5 also appear to be produced from subgenomic RNAs.

Computer database analysis revealed that the 29.6 kDa product of PEBV RNA2 has 35% overall

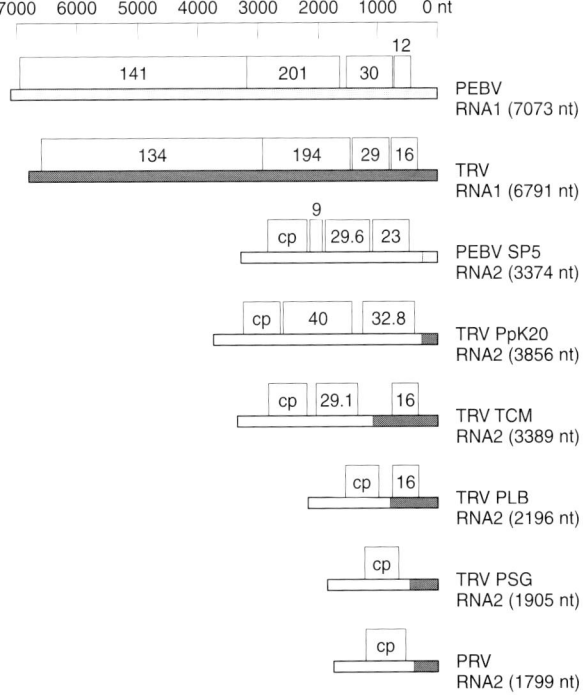

Figure 1 Genomic organization of TRV and PEBV RNA 1 and six tobraviral RNA2 molecules. Relative positions are given of the coat protein and other ORFs (with numbers indicating the molecular weight of their potential products). Shaded bars at the 5' termini of RNA2 correspond with nucleotide sequences homologous with RNA1.

amino acid sequence homology with the 29.1 kDa putative protein of TRV strain TCM. Apart from that, no other homologies with previously described proteins were found for the other putative proteins encoded by RNA2.

Since TRV strain PSG is infectious by mechanical inoculation and its RNA2 does not contain any ORF in addition to that of the coat protein, the extra genes present on RNA2 of other strains probably have no function in replication. However, strain PSG (but also PLB and TCM which do contain extra ORFs in RNA2) lack the ability to be transmitted by any known nematode vector. Recently, infectious cDNA clones of nematode transmissible isolates became available: PEBV TPA56 and TRV PpK20. Sequencing PEBV TPA56 revealed that this isolate is nearly homologous with the nontransmissible PEBV SP5 strain, with only 11 differences out of 3374 nucleotides. Deletions or frameshifts in the nonstructural genes of PEBV TPA56 RNA2 abolished the transmission of this virus by its associated vector nematode *Trichodorus primitivus*. Also, mutations that affected the 40K gene of TRV strain PpK20 abolished nematode transmission by *Paratrichodorus pachydermus*, whereas a large deletion in the 32.8K gene had no effect on transmission. None of the mutations in the nonstructural genes interfered with encapsidation or replication of the virus. From these experiments it could be concluded that at least some of the RNA2 encoded nonstructural proteins of the tobraviruses are involved in transmission by their vector nematodes. Functions of the other nonstructural proteins encoded by RNA2 remain unknown, but it was suggested that they might play a role in the transmission of tobraviral strains by as yet unidentified species of nematode vectors.

Virus Genetics

In all tobraviruses sequenced up till now, very high homology at the 3′ terminus between both genomic RNAs of each isolate was found. The homologous sequence varies between about 500 and 1100 nucleotides (TRV isolates) and was found to be 266 nucleotides in PEBV-SP5 and 459 in PRV. Whereas these sequences are identical in the RNAs of the TRV strains and in PRV, there are nine differences in the PEBV-SP5 homologous stretch. In tobraviruses, the acquisition of the 3′ terminus of RNA1 by RNA2 is thought to have occurred by recombination based on a copy-choice mechanism of the viral replicase. The junction between RNA2- and RNA1-specific sequences shows a sequence that closely resembles the one that occurs at 5′ termini of subgenomic TRV RNAs.

The nature of the selection pressure that leads to perfect or almost perfect homologous 3′-terminal sequences between RNA1 and RNA2 is not known. Earlier work with pseudorecombinants, which are the experimental combination of RNA1 (or RNA1-containing L particles) from one strain with RNA2 (or S particles) from another, suggested that identical 3′-terminal sequences of the two genomic RNAs are essential for virus stability, maybe by playing a role in template recognition of the viral replicase. It was found that the ability to form pseudorecombinants is independent of serological relationship between the strains used, but is only possible within one subgroup, e.g. between different TRV strains but not between a TRV strain and a PEBV strain. However, replication studies on recombinant tobraviruses showed that only the 5′-noncoding region of TRV RNA2 or PEBV RNA2 is sufficient in hybrid RNAs to permit their replication by, respectively, TRV RNA1 or PEBV RNA1, regardless of the origin of the 3′-terminal region. Thus, the specificity of template recognition is determined by the 5′-noncoding, but not by the 3′-noncoding region and, at least under laboratory conditions, nonhomologous 3′ termini between RNA1 and RNA2 do not affect virus stability.

The susceptibility of TRV RNA2 for recombination was demonstrated by analyzing the so-called 'anomalous' isolates. These isolates combine properties of TRV (symptom expression, ability to create pseudorecombinants with other TRV isolates) and PEBV (serological relationship). The genome of the 'anomalous' isolates was shown to consist of an RNA1 molecule with extensive similarity to that of other TRV isolates, whereas RNA2 appeared to contain PEBV-like coding regions with 3′- and/or 5′-terminal sequences homologous with TRV RNAs.

Thus, by maintaining the terminal homology with TRV RNA1 and capturing internal (coding) sequences of PEBV RNA2 by recombination, it seems that TRV has evolved a flexible mechanism to adapt itself to environmental changes. Laboratory experiments confirm TRV RNA2's proneness to recombination. When the RNA of strain PpK20 was serially passed in tobacco plants by using phenol-extracted RNA as the inoculum in each transfer, several defective interfering (DI) RNAs rapidly accumulated. All DI RNAs were found to have deletions in the coding sequences of the RNA2. In most cases the coat protein gene and the 40K gene was lost completely, whereas part of the 32.8K gene remained translatable, sometimes as a fusion protein with coat protein sequences (**Fig. 2**). Two DI RNAs were found to be recombinants containing a 5′ sequence derived from RNA2 and a 3′ sequence derived from RNA1, which emphasizes the importance of the noncoding terminal

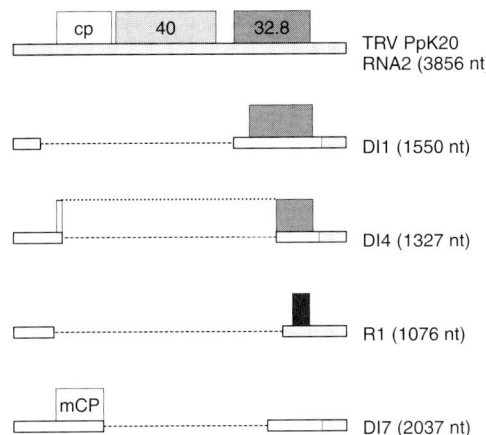

Figure 2 PpK20 defective interfering RNAs and wild-type PpK20 genomic RNA2. The relative positions of the ORFs are shown. Shaded bars at the 5' termini of the RNAs correspond with nucleotide sequences homologous with RNA1. The dashed lines represent the deleted sequences. The dotted line in DI4 joins the N-terminal and C-terminal regions of a potentially encoded fusion protein. The mutated coat protein encoded by DI7 has been designated mCP (Hernández *et al*, 1996).

sequences for virus stability. When serial passage of TRV strain PpK20 was carried out using leaf homogenates as inocula in each transfer, accumulation of a single DI RNA with a truncated but functional coat protein gene was observed (DI 7). This DI RNA rapidly outcompeted the full-length RNA2, resulting in loss of nematode transmissibility. RNA recombination may explain why most laboratory strains, which have been maintained through the years by mechanical passages, have lost their nematode transmissibility and contain RNA2 molecules of widely varying lengths.

Diseases Caused

Tobraviruses have wide host ranges, infecting herbaceous and a few woody plant species. They cause several types of disease. One of the diseases led to the name of this virus group: when the wind blows through a heavily infected tobacco field a rattle-like sound is produced by the TRV-infected dried-out leaves.

Among tobraviruses, TRV has by far the widest host range, probably the widest of any plant virus. TRV infects more than 100 species in nature, including several common weed species (e.g. *Stellaria media*, *Capsella bursa-pastoris*, *Senecio vulgaris*). Experimentally, it was shown that more than 400 plant species in over 50 families can be infected with TRV by inoculation with sap. In about half of these infected plant species, the virus can spread systemically.

In many naturally infected species the virus remains localized at the initial site of infection. Other species are invaded systemically but remain symptomless (as *Stellaria media*) or may develop a wide variety of symptoms. On leaves, symptoms range from necrosis to all kinds of yellow markings (blotching, mottling, mosaic, ringspot), often accompanied by a variable degree of distortion. Of economic importance is the damage caused in bulbous ornamental crops such as tulip, narcissus, lily and crocus, in which leaves become mottled, and gladiolus, which develops notched leaves. Symptoms on underground plant parts include corky arcs in potato tubers (spraing), which lowers the value of the crops, and necrotic spots (malaria) in hyacinth bulbs. Furthermore, vigor and yield are decreased in tomato, sugarbeet, spinach, tobacco, artichoke, celery, pepper and lettuce.

The PEBV subgroup includes the tobravirus isolates that systemically infect leguminous plants. Only four crop species (pea, bean, broad bean and lucerne) are reported to become naturally infected. Symptoms caused by PEBV include large necrotic spots on pea leaflets, leaf distortion with chlorotic V-shaped markings in lucerne and mosaic in bean leaves. Only early browning of pea is known to be a widespread disease. PEBV probably also has hosts among weed species, but these have not been well studied.

No extensive data are available for PRV. This virus is of local concern in Brazil and was reported to cause leaf markings in artichoke and tomato. In addition, wild plants are known to be hosts.

Tobraviruses, especially TRV and PEBV, exist as many serological variants and are known to be very variable in type and severity of symptoms produced. This variability in symptoms may be the result of the specific transmission of tobraviruses by trichodorid nematodes (see below), with different viral strains being transmitted by different nematode species. Furthermore, variation in symptom expression on one host species is well known to occur independently of antigenic variation of the viruses. Experimentally, it was shown that 14 TRV isolates of the same serotype which are naturally transmitted by the same nematode species produced symptoms ranging from severe systemic malformation to mild chlorotic spots on the mechanically inoculated leaves only.

Detection and identification of tobraviruses is further complicated by the existence of NM-type isolates (in which only RNA1 replicates without RNA2). Such infections rapidly spread from cell to cell but only slowly systemically; the symptoms caused are usually more severe than those induced by M-type isolates (in which both RNA1 and RNA2 are present).

Geographic Distribution

TRV is the most widespread of the tobraviruses and has been recorded throughout Europe, in North America, New Zealand and in Japan. PEBV is known to occur in Europe and North Africa, whereas PRV has only been described in South America (Brazil).

Virus Transmission

Nematode transmission

Tobraviruses are naturally transmitted by root-feeding nematodes of the genera *Trichodorus* and *Paratrichodorus*. At present, seven species within the genus *Paratrichodorus* and four within *Trichodorus* are known to be vectors of tobraviruses.

Acquisition of virus particles takes place together with ingestion of the cytoplasm when the vector nematode is feeding on root cells of infected plants. Nematodes remain viruliferous for long periods of time, for example, more than 1 year in *Trichodorus* spp., but not after molting. There is no evidence for multiplication of tobraviruses in the nematodes, nor for passage to progeny nematodes.

Release of the virus particles from the nematode feeding apparatus is thought to occur by a change in pH caused by saliva flow produced when the nematode starts feeding on a new plant.

In nematodes, TRV particles have been observed throughout the length of the esophageal lumen adsorbed to the cuticular lining of the lumen. This particular region has been shown to stain for carbohydrate, suggesting that lectin-like structures are involved in binding the virus particles to the nematode pharynx. Nuclear magnetic resonance studies on tobraviral particles revealed that protruding, flexible elements are present at the particle surface. Further studies indicated that these flexible elements are formed by a number of amino acid residues at the extreme C-terminus of each coat protein subunit, and that the length and amino acid composition of these flexible ends is strain-specific. Therefore, it is assumed that differences between the C-terminal sequences may reflect differences in transmissibility between virus strains. However, there is genetic evidence that, in addition to the coat protein, other viral proteins are involved in the transmission process. Deletions and frameshifts in the reading frames of RNA2 coding for the nonstructural proteins of the transmissible isolate PEBV TPA56 showed that the 29 kDa and 23 kDa proteins, and possibly the 9 kDa protein, are necessary for virus transmission by *Trichodorus primitivus*. Similar experiments with TRV isolate PpK 20 showed that the 40 kDa non-structural protein, but not the 32.8 kDa protein plays a role in the transmission of this virus by *Paratrichodorus pachydermus*. It is suggested that these nonstructural proteins might link the nematode surface to virus particles, perhaps by bridging between the carbohydrate-containing material and the protruding C-terminal part of the virus coat protein. These nonstructural proteins could then be considered as helper components, functionally similar to the helper component of potyviruses or the aphid transmission factor of caulimoviruses.

The factors that determine the specificity of viral transmission have hardly been elucidated. A highly specific relationship has been found between TRV strains and the nematode species involved in their transmission: individual species of *(Para)Trichodorus* transmit serologically distinct isolates of tobraviruses. In addition, certain species are able to transmit more than one virus within the tobravirus group.

Seed transmission

Seed transmission of TRV is not known to occur in crop plants but is possible in several weed species. PEBV and PRV are reported to be seed-borne in pea and tomato, respectively. As described above, there is evidence that the RNA1 encoded 3′-terminal ORF of PEBV is involved in seed transmission, perhaps by allowing passage of the virus over the border between nongenerative and generative tissue.

Virus Epidemiology and Control

The occurrence of tobraviruses depends on the distribution of their nematode vectors, which tend to be prevalent on lighter, sandy or loamy soils. Tobraviruses can survive at sites in three main ways: they can persist in the nematode vector, in perennial plants and in infected seeds.

Viral spread at a site depends on the number, activity and transmitting efficiency of vector nematodes. The number of trichodorids depends mainly on the type of previous crops and on the degree and type of weed infestation (as nematodes multiply differently on different host plants). Weed infestation is also of importance in determining the proportion of nematodes that carry viral particles. A wide range of weed species (e.g. *Stellaria media*) can harbor TRV, with a high incidence of systemic infection. Such plants are a constant source of viral particles to transmitting nematodes. Tests on naturally occurring *Stellaria media* plants are a reliable indication of whether or not TRV occurs at a site.

The activity of nematodes is mainly determined by

soil water content as nematodes need a water film on soil particles to be able to move through the soil. Therefore, incidence of tobravirus-caused diseases is increased after wet periods or in irrigated crops. Optimum temperature for transmission was found to be 15–20°C with little transmission occurring at 4°C.

In Scotland it was shown that 80% of the trichodorid populations in arable land were carrying TRV. The rate of viral transmission by populations of viruliferous nematodes was found to be rather low. This probably reflects the small proportion of virus-carrying individuals. Experiments with single nematodes, however, revealed that, once a nematode has acquired viruses, subsequent transmission to healthy plants can be very efficient.

Another factor affecting the spread of tobraviruses is the vertical and horizontal distribution of vector nematodes. Infected plants typically are patchily distributed in crops. These patches do not necessarily represent the horizontal distribution: as trichodorid nematodes seem to occur in considerable numbers in somewhat deeper soil layers (below the depth of cultivation) but above hard layers, such patches may occur where the topsoil is shallow.

As nematodes move only small distances laterally (probably less than 50 cm per year), spread of virus-carrying nematodes to new sites occurs by agricultural activities. Transport of vector nematodes in wind-blown soil is probably inefficient, as the nematodes are very susceptible to desiccation. Virus-infected seed and vegetative plant material can also be carried for long distances to sites with previously virus-free populations of vector nematodes. Thus it could be observed that trichodorids appeared soon after colonization of a sand dune by grasses but TRV was not recorded until the flora included *Viola tricolor*, in which the virus is seed-borne.

The control of tobraviruses depends largely on the use of tolerant or resistant cultivars (potato, pea) and on the application of expensive nematode-controlling chemicals to vector-infested land. Weeds are both a virus source and a vehicle for virus spread (via seeds). Rigorous control of weeds in order to eliminate virus sources, however, can actually increase TRV infections because virus-carrying trichodorids that may prefer to feed on weed roots are then obliged to feed on crop plants.

Virus dissemination can be minimized by using virus-free planting material (pea, flower bulbs).

See also: **Sindbis and Semliki Forest viruses (*Togaviridae*); Potyviruses (*Potyviridae*); Plant pararetroviruses (*Caulimoviridae*): Caulimoviruses: general features, Caulimoviruses: molecular biology, Legume caulimoviruses; Tobamoviruses.**

Further Reading

Brown DJF, Robertson WM and Trudgill DL (1995) Transmission of viruses by plant nematodes. *Annu. Rev. Phytopathol.* 33: 223.

Harrison BD and Robinson DJ (1986) Tobraviruses. In: Van Regenmortel MHV and Fraenkel-Conrat H (eds) *The Plant Viruses*. Vol. 2: *The Rod-Shaped Plant Viruses*, p. 339. London: Plenum Press.

Hernández C, Carette JE, Brown DJF and Bol JF (1996) Serial passage of tobacco rattle virus under different selection conditions results in deletion of structural and nonstructural genes in RNA 2. *J. Virol.* 70: 4933.

MacFarlane SA (1997) Natural recombination among plant virus genomes: evidence from tobraviruses. *Semin. Virol.* 8: 25.

Wang D, MacFarlane SA and Maule AJ (1997) Viral determinants of pea early browning virus seed transmission in pea. *Virology* 234: 112.

TOMBUSVIRUSES

DM Rochon, Agriculture and Agri-Food Canada, Pacific Agri-Food Research Centre, Summerland, British Columbia, Canada

Copyright © 1999 Academic Press

Taxonomy and Classification

Tombusviruses are 30 nm nonenveloped isometric plant viruses which consist of a monopartite positive-sense RNA genome of about 4.7 kb and 180 copies of an approximate 41 kDa coat protein. The *Tombusvirus* genus presently consists of 13 type species. These are listed in **Table 1** along with a brief description of the geographic distribution and transmission of each member.

Table 1 Natural hosts and geographic distribution of definitive and tentative tombusvirus species[a]

Virus	Acronym	Natural host(s)	Geographical distribution	Transmission[b]
Definitive species				
Artichoke mottled crinkle virus	AMCV	Artichoke	Mediterranean	+M
Carnation Italian ringspot virus	CIRV	Carnation, sweet cherry	UK, Italy, USA, Germany	+G, +M
Cucumber necrosis virus	CNV	Cucumber	Canada	+C, +F (*Olpidium bornovanus*), +M, +So
Cymbidium ringspot virus	CyRSV	Cymbidium, white clover	UK	+C, +M, −Se
Eggplant mottled crinkle virus	EMCV	Eggplant, *Solanum capsicastrum*	Lebanon, India	+G, +M
Grapevine Algerian latent virus	GALV	Grapevine, pear, plum	Algeria, Italy, Germany	+M, found in river water in Germany and Sicily
Lato river virus	LRV	Unknown	Unknown	+M, found in water in Lato River, Italy
Moroccan pepper virus	MPV	Pepper, tomato, eggplant, pelargonium	Morocco, Germany	+G, +M,
Neckar river virus	NRV	Unknown	Unknown	+M, found in water in River Neckar, Germany
Pelargonium leaf curl virus	PLCV	Pelargonium	Eurasia, Mediterranean, N. America	+G, +M, −S
Petunia asteroid mosaic virus (=TBSV-Ch)	PAMV	Petunia, cherry, spinach, grapevine, hop, pepper, plum, privet, tomato	Eurasia, Czechoslovakia, Germany, Spain, Switzerland, UK, former Yugoslavia, Korea	+M, +P, +Se (some hosts)
Sikte waterborne virus	SWBV	Unknown	Unknown	From water from River Sitke, Germany
Tomato bushy stunt virus	TBSV	Tomato, pepper, eggplant, lettuce, spinach, tulip, apple, pear, fringe tree	Europe, Mediterranean, N. and S. America	+M, +G, +Se (some hosts)
Tentative species				
Cucumber leaf spot virus	CLSV	Cucumber	Germany, Greece, Jordan, UK	−C, +F (*O. bornovanus*), +M, +Se
Pothos latent virus	PoLV	Pothos(?)	Southern Italy	+M, found in hydroponic solution

[a]Represents a summary of information from original papers, Martelli *et al* (1988) and the VIDE database on plant viruses (*http://biology.anu.edu.au/research-groups/MES/VIDE/refs.htm*)
[b]Abbreviations for modes of transmission: C, contact between plants; F, fungus transmitted; G, graph transmission; M, mechanical transmission; P, pollen transmitted; Se, seed transmission; (+) indicates known means of transmission; (−) indicates that this means of transmission has been ruled out. Note that most tombusviruses are assumed to be soil-transmitted (see text).

Complete nucleotide sequences have been obtained for the genomic RNAs of artichoke mottled crinkle virus (AMCV), carnation Italian ringspot virus (CIRV), cucumber necrosis virus (CNV), Cymbidium ringspot virus (CyRSV) and the cherry strain of tomato bushy stunt virus (TBSV-Ch). The genomes of these viruses have highly similar structures (see **Fig. 1**) and considerable sequence identity exists between comparable regions at both the nucleic acid and protein level (see **Table 2**). The high level of similarity has prompted the suggestion that some of the tombusviruses currently classified as separate species should instead be classified as strains.

Recently, genome sequences of two other potential tombusviruses, cucumber leaf spot (CLSV) and pothos latent virus (PoLV), have been determined. The predicted genome structures are similar to the genome structures of the definitive species (**Fig. 1**). A high level of sequence identity exists between the protein products of these two viruses, however, three of the five viral encoded proteins share only limited similarity with the corresponding proteins of definitive tombusviruses (**Table 2**).

The family *Tombusviridae* encompasses the genus *Tombusvirus* and seven other distinct genera including *Carmovirus*, *Dianthovirus*, the monotypic *Machlomovirus* and *Necrovirus*. The oat chlorotic stunt virus is in the genus *Avenavirus* and panicum mosaic

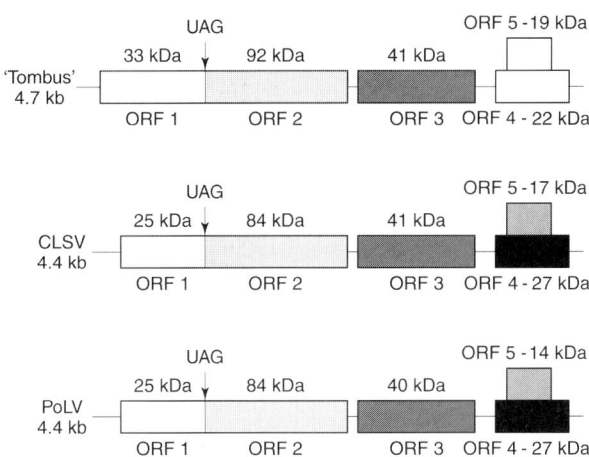

Figure 1 Comparison of the genomic structures of tombusviruses, CLSV and PoLV. The typified 'tombusvirus' genome structure is described in **Fig. 5** legend. The CLSV and PoLV genomic structures are shown individually. Similarly shaded ORFs indicate that the encoded proteins have greater than 30% amino acid sequence identity.

virus in the genus *Panicovirus*. Shared features of the *Tombusviridae* include similar particle morphology, similar genome organizations and expression strategies and also a significant level of amino acid sequence identity in the RNA-dependent RNA polymerase (RdRp) and coat proteins. **Figure 2** shows a dendogram depicting relationships among the RdRps of several members of the *Tombusviridae*. Phylogenetic trees derived from RdRp sequence alignments of *Tombusviridae* are generally reliable indicators of the taxonomic positions of individual members as defined by other criteria. This is in contrast to phylogenetic trees obtained using aligned coat protein

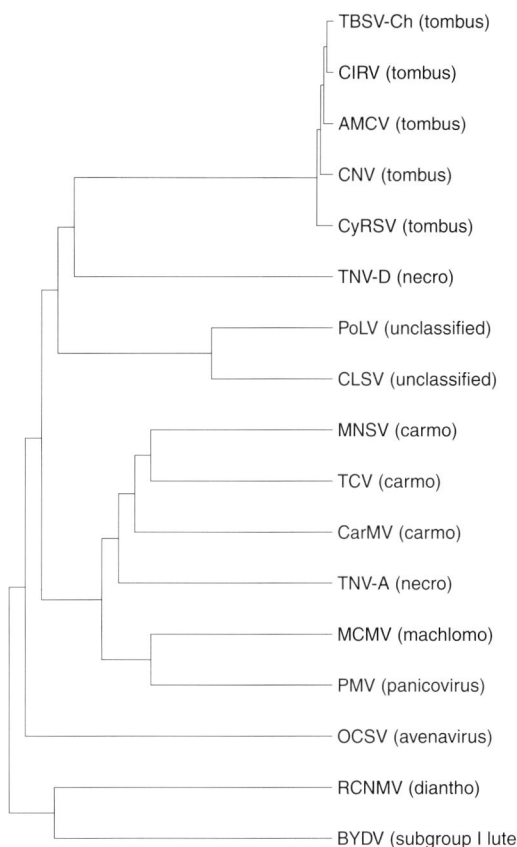

Figure 2 Dendrogram depicting relationships among the RdRps of several definitive and tentative *Tombusviridae* members. Only the readthrough or frameshifted region is aligned. The genus to which the virus belongs is indicated in parentheses. PoLV and CLSV are unclassified. Abbreviations: TBSV-Ch, tomato bushy stunt virus; CIRV, carnation Italian ringspot virus; AMCV, artichoke mottled crinkle virus; CNV, cucumber necrosis virus; CyRSV, Cymbidium ringspot virus; TNV-D, tobacco necrosis virus strain D; PoLV, pothos latent virus; CLSV, cucumber leaf spot virus; MNSV, melon necrotic spot virus; TCV, turnip crinkle virus; CarMV, carnation mottle virus; TNV-A, tobacco necrosis virus strain A; MCMV, maize chlorotic mottle virus; PMV, panicum mosaic virus; OCSV, oat chlorotic stunt virus; RCNMV, red clover necrotic mosaic virus; BYDV, barley yellow dwarf virus.

(CP) sequences (**Fig. 3**). *Tombusvirus* CP sequences (and notably the P domains, *see also* **Virus Structure**) are the most variable in the genome. This hypervariability likely accounts for antigenic distinctions observed between otherwise very closely related viruses.

A phylogenetic study of the RdRp sequences encoded by several positive-strand RNA viruses has shown that tombusviruses (and other *Tombusviridae* genera) group together with members of the animal pesti- and flaviviruses and the bacterial leviviruses forming one of three major supergroups of RNA viruses.

Table 2 Percentage of identical amino acid residues in pairwise comparisons of proteins encoded by ORFs 1–5 of several tombusviruses, CLSV and PoLV

	ORF 1[a]	ORF 2	ORF 3[b]	ORF 4	ORF 5
Tombus/Tombus[c]	53–94	93–97	34–87	84–98	72–92
Tombus/CLSV or PoLV[d]	21–25	43–45	30–53	19–20	12–20
CLSV/PoLV[e]	60	80	33	71	61

[a]The CIRV alignments gave unusually low identity scores. All other alignments gave values between 80 and 94%.
[b]The PLCV CP sequence is included in pairwise alignments.
[c]Shows the range of values obtained in all pairwise comparisons of AMCV, CIRV, CNV, CyRSV, and TBSV-Ch.
[d]Shows the range of values obtained in all pairwise comparisons of AMCV, CIRV, CNV, CyRSV, TBSV-Ch and either CLSV or PoLV.
[e]Shows the values obtained in pairwise comparisons of CLSV and PoLV.

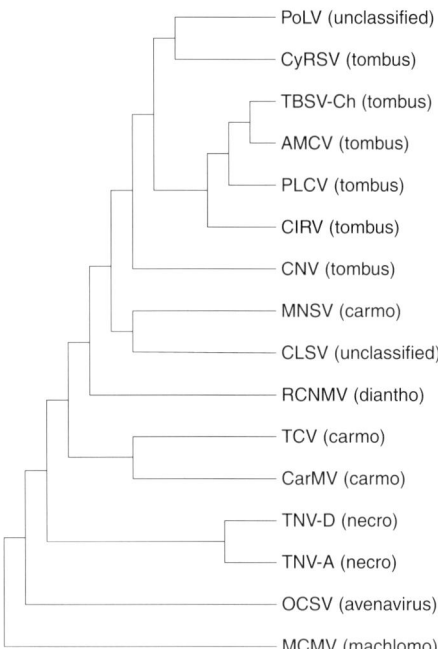

Figure 3 Dendrogram depicting relationships among the coat proteins of several definitive and tentative *Tombusviridae* members. See **Fig. 2** legend for details and abbreviations.

Symptomatology, Host Range and Geographic Distribution

Table 1 summarizes the natural host range, geographic distribution and modes of transmission of the definitive tombusviruses and also PoLV, CLSV and Sikte waterborne virus (SWBV). Tombusviruses as a whole share a wide geographic distribution having been reported in North and South America, several locations in Europe and the Mediterranean and also in Algeria. Individual members of the tombusvirus group, however, generally have a restricted geographic distribution with the exception of TBSV and pelargonium leaf curl (PLCV) which was likely spread internationally through infected pelargoniums. Most tombusviruses naturally infect only a single or a few hosts. This is in contrast to their experimental host range which is wide and diversified. Tombusviruses systemically invade naturally infected plants but remain localized in the majority of experimentally infected plants; common exceptions to this rule are the experimental hosts *Nicotiana clevelandii* and *N. benthamiana*. Tombusvirus-infected crops generally show stunting and diffuse mottling and malformation of leaves. Characteristic lesions associated with the indicator plants basil, globe amaranth and *Chenopodium quinoa* can be used to identify tombusviruses. Further verification can be obtained using antisera or cloned cDNA probes which are widely available. Several tombusviruses have been found associated with defective interfering (DI) RNAs in laboratory infections raising the possibility that DI RNAs can modulate symptoms in natural infections. Finally, many tombusviruses can be inactivated *in vivo* by growing plants at elevated temperatures (ca. 36 °C).

Recent studies have shown that the protein products of open reading frames (ORFs) 4 and 5 are important symptom determinants (see below, Molecular Biology).

Serologic Relationships

Most tombusvirus members are serologically interrelated with cross reactivities ranging from strong to nearly undetectable. CNV and SWBV are the only members which show no detectable serological reaction with other tombusviruses. The tentative species, CLSV, is also serologically unrelated to all tested tombusviruses.

Transmission

Tombusvirus particles are very stable and reach high concentrations in infected tissues. In addition, tombusviruses are efficiently spread and can become established in diverse environments. Different tombusviruses have been shown to be spread in nature by a number of means (see **Table 2**) including seed and pollen transmission, transmission through propagation material and possibly mechanical transmission. Experimentally, tombusviruses are readily sap transmissible and infected leaf extracts retain infectivity after freezing for several years. It is very likely that several tombusviruses are spread through the soil and probably also through irrigation water but attempts to transmit them (except CNV, see below) by soil-borne vectors have not been successful. In addition, attempts to transmit different tombusviruses using aphids, whiteflies or mites have also been unsuccessful.

Several reports have identified tombusviruses in association with rivers and lakes throughout the world and there is evidence suggesting that tombusviruses can enter a field through irrigation water. TBSV is infectious after passage through the human alimentary tract suggesting that tombusviruses may possibly enter rivers through sewage treatment of infective feces.

CNV is the only definitive member of the *Tombusvirus* genus which has been demonstrated to have a specific soil-borne vector. The tentative member, CLSV, is similarly transmitted. Transmission of these viruses is facilitated by zoospores of the Chytrid fungus, *Olpidium bornovanus* (formerly *Olpidium radicale*). Transmission is mechanistically similar to that demonstrated for the transmission of tobacco necrosis necrovirus by *Olpidium brassicae*. Virus particles and *Olpidium* zoospores are released independently into the soil from roots of infected plants and virus particles adsorb to the axonemal sheath of the zoospore flagellum. Virus gains entry into plants following zoospore infection of plant roots. Different *O. bornovanus* isolates transmit CNV and other viruses in a highly specific manner suggesting that a specific recognition mechanism exists between particles and zoospores. It is possible that this high specificity has precluded the identification of fungal vectors for other tombusviruses.

Molecular studies of CNV transmission by *O. bornovanus* have shown that the CNV coat protein contains determinants which specify transmission. Further studies have shown that a single amino acid change in the coat protein shell domain significantly reduces transmission without altering infectivity, particle stability or viral RNA accumulation. This mutation also affects the level of binding of virus particles to zoospores *in vitro* suggesting that the reduction in transmissibility is at least partly due to less efficient recognition between virus particles and a putative zoospore receptor.

Cytopathology

Cytopathic inclusions known as multivesicular bodies (MVB) and virus-containing bleb-like evaginations of the tonoplast are associated with infection by tombusviruses (**Fig. 4**). MVB are composed of vesicles intermingled with or surrounding granular electron-dense material and are believed to originate from either mitochondria, peroxisomes and/or chloroplasts depending on the virus/host combination examined. Clumps of densely staining amorphous material found scattered or loosely aggregated in the cytoplasm of systemically infected cells (dense granules) are also found in tombusvirus-infected cells but not in all virus–host combinations tested. MVB are believed to be sites of RNA replication and dense granules to be accumulations of excess CP subunit.

Experiments using hybrid genomes created between CyRSV and CIRV, which induce MVB from peroxisomes and mitochondria, respectively, have delineated the MVB-inducing region to a portion of the protein encoded by ORF 1.

Particle Structure

The structure of TBSV has been determined by x-ray crystallography and is diagrammatically represented in **Fig. 5**. The particle is a $T = 3$ icosahedron

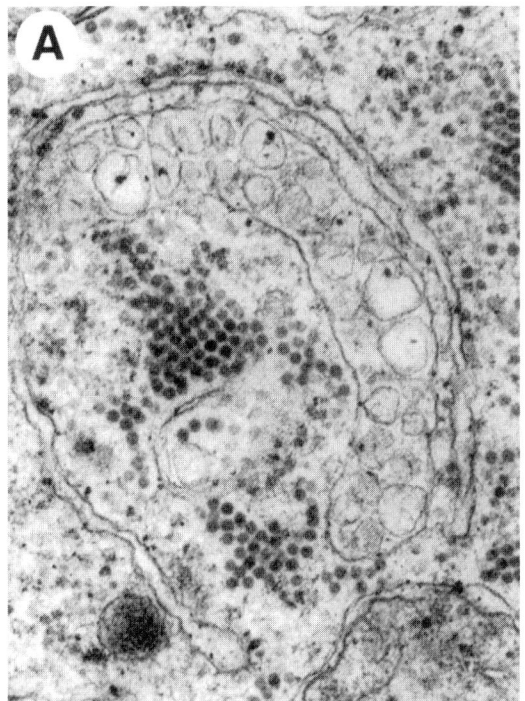

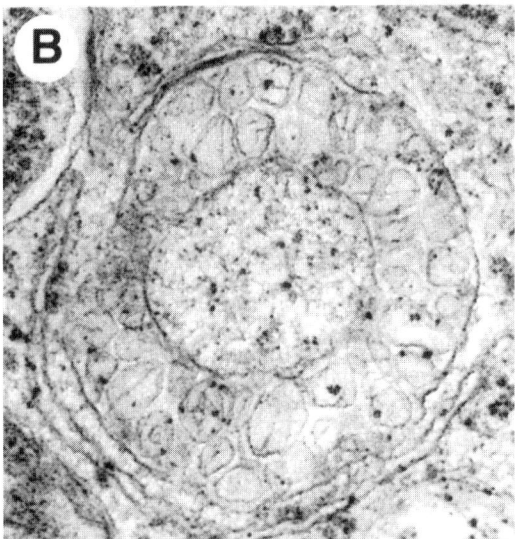

Figure 4 Electron micrographs showing multivesicular bodies formed in CNV-infected *N. clevelandii*. Magnification (**A**) 65 000×; (**B**) 75 000×.

approximately 30 nm in diameter which consists of 180 identical CP subunits. Each of the subunits folds into three major domains: an N-terminal highly basic inward-facing RNA binding domain (R); a tightly bonded globular shell domain (S) and a C-terminal outward facing protruding domain (P). The R domain is connected to the S domain by the arm (a) and a five amino acid hinge connects the S and P domains. The P domain projects from the surface of the particle in 90

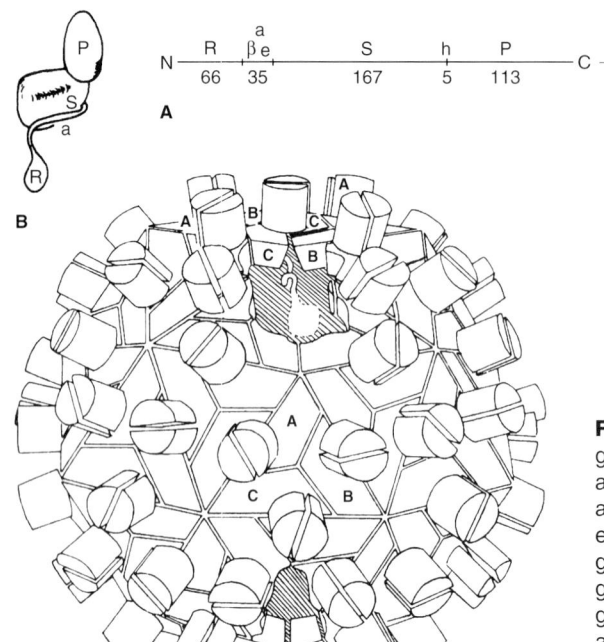
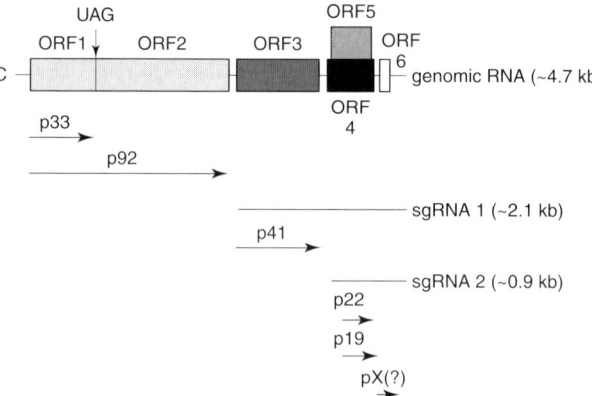

Figure 5 Architecture of the TBSV particle. (**A**) linear arrangement of domains (designated R, a, S, h and P) in the subunit polypeptide. The number of amino acid residues comprising each domain is indicated. (**B**) Schematic diagram of the folding of the polypeptide chain. (**C**) Arrangement of subunits in the virus particle. A, B and C denote the three packing environments of the subunit. (Reprinted with permission from Olson AJ, Bricogne C and Harrison SC (1983) Structure of tomato bushy stunt virus IV. *J. Mol. Biol* 171: 61–93.).

Figure 6 Structure and expression of the tombusvirus genome. The similar structure and expression strategies adopted by tombusviruses is shown. The five major ORFs are indicated by open boxes and the proteins encoded by each ORF by horizontal arrows beneath the ORF. Subgenomic RNA is indicated by a bar beneath the portion of the genome it is derived from. The approximate sizes, in kb, for genomic and sgRNA is indicated. Sizes of proteins may be approximate since they vary slightly from tombusvirus to tombusvirus (i.e. the CIRV 'p33' is actually p36, the CIRV 'p92' is p95, the CNV 'p22' is p21 and the CNV 'p19' is p20).

pairwise clusters. The subunit adopts three conformational states (A, B, C) in the particle due to flexion of the hinge and either an ordered or disordered arm.

TBSV swells at alkaline pH in the absence of calcium ions due to repulsive forces of adjacent negatively charged carboxylate groups. Calcium ions may be important in the release of virion nucleic acid in an infected cell. P domain dimer contacts may also contribute to tombusvirus particle stability. *In vitro* mutagenesis studies show that viral particles do not accumulate when the CNV P domain is deleted. These observations are consistent with a role for the tombusvirus P domain in particle stability. The P domain may also be involved in aggregate formation during particle assembly.

The tombusvirus CP subunit and particle structure shares features in common with several small spherical plant and animal virus particles including those of picornaviruses, black beetle virus, southern bean sobemovirus, turnip crinkle carmovirus and cowpea mosaic and bean-pod mottle comoviruses. Similarities include overall subunit architecture (jelly-roll topology), subunit packing, role of arm domain in coordinating assembly and transition to an expanded virion. The P domain, however, is a feature unique to tombusviruses, carmoviruses and dianthoviruses.

Tombusvirus Molecular Biology

Genome structure

The *Tombusvirus* genus represents one of the most extensively characterized plant virus genera. The genome is a monopartite, plus sense, single-stranded RNA of ~4.7 kb. The genomic sequences of five tombusviruses (AMCV, CIRV, CNV, CyRSV, TBSV-Ch) have been completed and highly infectious transcripts are available for AMCV, CNV, CyRSV and TBSV-Ch. The genomic structure and expression strategy utilized by tombusviruses is highly similar and is summarized in **Fig. 6**. The genome contains five long ORFs (ORFs 1–5) and encodes proteins with approximate molecular weights of 33, 92, 41, 22 and 19 kDa (designated p33, p92, etc.). The sizes of these proteins vary slightly from tombusvirus to tombusvirus (see **Fig. 6** legend) but these designations will apply hereafter. An additional small ORF (ORF 6) located at the 3′ terminus of the genome has been suggested as a possible protein-encoding region. Short

```
                         ****** *******
CNV      ggugcagguuGUGUAAAUUAGGGGCUUCUUGAAUCUaac
AMCV     UAAUUUAGUGAGUCCUGUGAGGGGCCUCUUGAACUAGAC
CIRV     ACAUGAUAUAGUACCAUUGAGGGGCCUCUUGAACAAGAC
CyRSV    GUAGUUGCAUUGCACAGGAAGGGGCUUCUUGAACCUAAC
TBSV-Ch  UAAUUUAGUGUGUCCUGCGAGGGGCCUCUUGAACAAGAC
                                              ^
```

Figure 7 Sequences surrounding the CNV sgRNA2 promoter and comparison to the putative promoters of other tombusviruses. Sequences comprising the core CNV sgRNA promoter are shown in capital letters. Asterisks indicate identity in all five tombusviruses. The sgRNA start site is indicated with a caret and the underlined sequences correspond to the upstream coat protein terminator codon.

intercistronic regions separate ORFs 2 and 3 and ORFs 3 and 4. The 5′ noncoding region ranges in size from 77 to 180 nucleotides (nt) and the 3′ noncoding region (which includes ORF 6) from 338 to 351 nt. The 3′ terminus of the tombusvirus genome does not contain a poly(A) tail and it is presently uncertain as to whether the 5′ end contains a cap structure or some other modification. It is noted that highly infectious transcripts of the tombusvirus genome can be obtained *in vitro* without capping.

Genome expression

ORF 1 initiates with the first AUG codon at the 5′ terminus and terminates with an amber codon to produce p33. The amber codon can be readthrough to produce p92. ORF 2 encodes the CP (p41) and is expressed from the first AUG codon at the 5′ terminus of a ~2.1 kb subgenomic mRNA (sgRNA 1). ORF 5 is nested within ORF 4 in a different reading frame. The respective p19 and p22 translation products are both produced from a single bifunctional ~0.9 kb sgRNA (sgRNA 2; see below).

Genomic plus and minus strand synthesis Most of the data on *cis*-acting sequences required for genomic RNA synthesis rely on studies using defective interfering RNAs (see below, Defective Interfering RNAs).

sgRNA synthesis Subgenomic RNAs accumulate to high levels during tombusvirus infection and are assumed to arise through internal initiation on (−) sense genomic RNA. In CNV and AMCV, synthesis of sgRNA 2 occurs before that of sgRNA 1. A sgRNA which could encode pX is easily detected in CNV-infected plants and protoplasts. Sequences comprising the core promoter for CNV sgRNA 2 have been determined. The promoter lies within a region located 20 nucleotides upstream and six nucleotides downstream of the sgRNA start site. Comparison of sequences within the CNV promoter with the analogous region of other tombusviruses shows strict conservation of 13 of 26 nucleotides (**Fig. 7**). There is little similarity between the sgRNA 2 promoter and the 5′ terminus of the genome or the region surrounding the sgRNA 1 start site. In addition, sequences similar to the ICR2-like motifs found in the promoters of several alphavirus-like (supergroup III) plant and animal viruses are not apparent.

Leaky scanning sgRNA 2 is a bifunctional mRNA capable of encoding distinct proteins *in vitro* and *in vivo* from nested ORFs (ORFs 4 and 5). In CNV, ORF 4 initiates with the first AUG codon on sgRNA 2 16 nt from the 5′ end. ORF 5 initiates at the second AUG codon 29 nt downstream of the ORF 4 AUG. Mutations which increase or decrease the ability of ribosomes to recognize the ORF 4 AUG codon have an inverse effect on ORF 4 expression suggesting that its AUG codon is accessed by leaky ribosomal scanning. Further studies showed that longer sgRNA 2 leader lengths increased expression of ORF 4 relative to ORF 5.

Protein function

p33 and p92 The readthrough portion of p92 contains the canonical 'GDD' motif and surrounding amino acids present in the polymerase domains of positive-strand RNA viruses. Although direct biochemical evidence that these proteins form part of the replicase is absent, genetic evidence is convincing. Methyltransferase, nucleotide binding or helicase motifs have not been identified in either of these two proteins or in any other tombusvirus-encoded protein. The absence of a helicase motif in tombusviruses suggests that a host component may fulfill this function during viral RNA replication.

Immunological analyses of CyRSV- and TBSV-Ch-infected cells have shown that both p33 and p92 accumulate during infection with p33 being approximately 20-fold more abundant than p92. Both proteins are associated with the membrane fraction consistent with a proposed role in viral RNA replication. Mutational analyses of p33 and p92 suggest that both proteins are required for RNA replication but strict evidence for the involvement of p33 is still lacking. Protoplasts from transgenic plants expressing CyRSV p33 and p92 support replication of CyRSV-defective interfering RNAs. In addition, CyRSV deletion mutants lacking ORFs 3, 4 and 5 can replicate in protoplasts. These results provide evidence that ORFs 1 and 2 are the only virus-encoded proteins necessary for viral RNA replication. Tombusviruses are believed to replicate in the membranous structures of MVBs formed during virus infection. Evidence exists that p33 is involved in determining the origin of MVB (see Cytopathology).

CP Mutational analyses of the CNV, CyRSV and TBSV-Ch *CP* genes indicate that the *CP* gene is dispensable for viral cell-to-cell and systemic movement. However, systemic spread of coat-protein mutants is not as efficient as wild-type virus as exhibited by delays in the onset of systemic symptoms, a lower percentage of systemically infected plants, or a reduction in the severity of systemic invasion. It is possible that virion formation is required for efficient entry into the vascular system.

The CP P domain (see Virus Structure) is a feature unique to tombusviruses, carmoviruses and dianthoviruses. Deletion of all or part of the P domain coding sequence in CNV (see Particle Structure) results in the absence of particle formation suggesting a role for the P domain in virus particle stability and/or in the formation of particle assembly intermediates. Interestingly, CNV P domain deletion mutants (but not shell domain mutants) rapidly further delete most of the remaining viral CP sequences during infection. The deletion derivatives likely arise through RNA recombination. It is possible that the deletion derivatives have a higher capacity for cell-to-cell movement due to increased production of the cell-to-cell movement protein.

The CNV CP has been found to contain elements involved in the specificity of fungus transmission (see Transmission for additional details).

p22 Several lines of evidence show that the tombusvirus ORF 4 product (p22) encodes the cell-to-cell movement protein. p22 is not required for RNA replication but is required for accumulation of viral RNA in inoculated plants. In addition, histochemical assays of plants inoculated with TBSV-Ch p22 mutants which contain the GUS gene in place of the CP gene show that infection is limited to single cells. Amino acid sequence comparisons of tombusvirus p22 proteins with known and putative viral movement proteins has shown limited but significant similarity. Finally, TBSV-Ch p22 has been found associated with the membrane fraction of plant cells, consistent with its role in viral cell-to-cell movement.

Potato virus X (PVX) derivatives which express the TBSV-Ch p22 gene produce local lesions in *Nicotiana glutinosa* and *N. edwardsonii* rather than the mild mosaic symptoms typical of PVX. These results indicate that p22 is the primary determinant responsible for local lesion formation in these two host plants. As described below, TBSV-Ch p19 and its analogue in other tombusviruses is the primary symptom determinant in other hosts.

p19 Mutations which affect ORF 5 expression in CNV, CyRSV and TBSV-Ch cDNA result in an attenuated phenotype without affecting viral accumulation in plants. In addition, expression of p19 using a heterologous viral vector, PVX, showed that p19 induced a generalized necrosis on infection of *N. benthamiana* and *N. clevelandii* and local necrotic lesions in *N. tabacum*. These symptoms occurred in place of the mild mosaic associated with PVX infection. These results provide evidence that p19 is a major symptom determinant in tombusviruses and further suggest that p19 may interact with host-specific resistance genes present in related *Nicotiana* species.

Start and stop codon mutations which abolish production of the p19 analogue in CNV (p20) lead to loss of necrotic symptoms on inoculated leaves as well as a highly accelerated rate of defective interfering RNA production in plants. The basis for the enhanced rate of *de novo* DI RNA production requires further investigation.

pX Computer assisted analyses of the 3′ terminal regions of several tombusviruses has suggested the existence of a possible sixth small ORF (ORF 6) in tombusviruses leading to production of a small protein (pX) which is between 3.5 and 7.6 kDa. Mutational analyses of the CyRSV ORF 6 have shown that if pX is produced during infection it is not essential for viral infectivity. However, certain mutations in ORF 6 result in nonviable mutants, suggesting that the pX ORF may harbor important *cis*-acting replication signals. A role for pX in viral infection remains to be established.

Defective Interfering (DI) RNAs

DI RNAs

DI RNAs have been found in association with CIRV, CNV, CyRSV and TBSV-Ch and have been extensively characterized in terms of structure, mechanism of formation and mode of interference. DI RNAs occur naturally in plants infected under laboratory conditions and are also generated *de novo* from genomic RNA. DI RNAs are associated with a marked attenuation of the severe symptoms typical of tombusvirus infections.

DI RNA structure DI RNAs correspond to conserved, noncontiguous portions of the tombusvirus genome and range in size from approximately 400 to

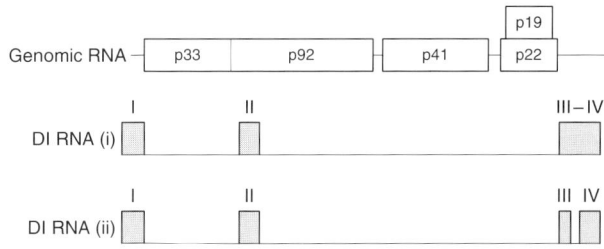

Figure 8 Structure of a prototypical tombusvirus DI RNA. The tombusvirus genome structure is at the top and the two major types of DI RNAs are shown below. Genomic RNA sequences retained in the DIs are indicated by boxes in the DIs whereas horizontal lines correspond to deleted sequences. The four major regions (I–IV) found in DI RNAs are indicated. (Adapted from White (1996).)

800 nt. A prototypical tombusvirus DI RNA consists of four segments of the viral genome designated regions I through IV (**Fig. 8**). Region I corresponds to the 5′ terminal noncoding region and regions III and IV correspond to contiguous or noncontiguous segments at the 3′ terminus of the genome. Region II corresponds to an internal portion of the genome. DI RNAs differ from each other in the amount of sequence deleted between different regions, in the extent of internal deletions within regions, or through duplications of regions or portions of regions. In CNV and CyRSV, head-to-tail dimers of complete monomeric DI RNA units have been observed in plants. The significance of the dimers is not known but dimers can be formed from monomers and it is possible that dimers are templates for the formation of monomers during DI RNA replication.

DI RNA formation A stepwise deletion model for the formation of DI RNAs from genomic RNA has been proposed. In this model, DI RNAs are formed following a series of deletion events as a result of a copy choice mechanism of RNA recombination. Both primary and secondary sequence elements as well as selection for replication competence contribute to the final structure.

Sequences/structures involved in DI replication The smallest DI RNA molecules (∼400 nt) tolerate little sequence or structural change suggesting that the retained sequences contain the minimal essential elements for replication/accumulation. A putative stem–loop structure contained within the 3′ terminal 77 nucleotides of CyRSV RNA has been suggested to be important in negative strand synthesis of DI RNA as well as genomic RNA.

Interference DI RNAs are associated with reductions in virus-induced symptoms and virus accumulation. At least two mechanisms account for the observed symptom attenuation. One is that DI RNAs compete with genomic RNA for the viral replicase resulting in reduced viral RNA synthesis. The other is that the presence of DI RNA results in preferential suppression of sgRNA 2 levels relative to genomic RNA. This suppression leads to lower levels of p22 and p19 and consequently reduces symptoms.

Satellite RNAs

A satellite RNA associated with CyRSV has been characterized and found to be composed of 621 nucleotides. Two regions of the satellite RNA show homology to genomic RNA: 9 of the first 14 nt are shared and 49 of 53 nt of the satellite RNA are similar to a segment in the 5′ noncoding region of genomic RNA. These conserved regions are also present in tombusvirus DI RNAs suggesting an important role of these particular sequences in the replication process.

Virus-Resistant Transgenic Plants

Plants transformed with portions of viral genomes often show resistance to viral infection in a specific manner. Transgenic *N. benthamiana* plants expressing the CyRSV CP are resistant to infection but only at very low virus inoculum concentrations. No resistance occurs at higher inoculum concentrations or when plants are inoculated with RNA. Selected transgenic plant lines expressing CyRSV p92 show resistance when inoculated with RNA or virus. Resistance is specific and inversely correlated with the level of expression of transgene mRNA suggesting resistance is RNA-mediated. Transgenic plants expressing CyRSV DI RNAs were found to be protected from the apical necrosis and subsequent plant death normally associated with infection by this virus. Interestingly, transgenic plants expressing CyRSV satellite RNAs actually increased symptom severity. It was suggested that the expressed satellite RNA sequences may interfere with the ameliorating effects of naturally occurring DI RNAs.

See also: **Carmoviruses (*Tombusviridae*); Defective interfering viruses; Plant virus disease – economic aspects; Satellite RNAs and Satellite viruses; Virus structure: Atomic structure, Principles of virus structure.**

Further Reading

Harrison SC (1983) Virus structure: high resolution perspectives. *Adv. Virus Res.* 28: 175.
Martelli GP, Gallitelli D and Russo M (1988) Tombus-

viruses. In: Koenig R (ed.) *The Plant Viruses*, vol. 3, p. 13. New York: Plenum.

Russo M, Burgyan J and Martelli GP (1994) Molecular biology of Tombusviridae. *Adv. Virus Res.* 44: 381.

Scholthof HB, Scholthof K-BG and Jackson AO (1995) Identification of tomato bushy stunt virus host-specific determinants by expression of individual genes from a potato virus X vector. *Plant Cell* 7: 1157.

White KA (1996) Formation and evolution of tombusvirus defective interfering RNAs. *Semin. Virol.* 7: 409.

TOROVIRUSES *(CORONAVIRIDAE)*

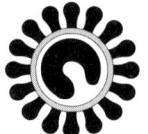

Marian C Horzinek, Virology Unit, Veterinary Faculty, Utrecht, The Netherlands

Copyright © 1999 Academic Press

History

Toroviruses were defined in the early 1980s as a result of a trilateral, partly collaborative study between groups in Berne, Switzerland (isolation in cell culture), Ames/Iowa, USA (discovery of Breda virus and propagation in calves) and Utrecht, The Netherlands (biologic and molecular characterization).

An equine torovirus (ETV), originally referred to as Berne virus, was accidentally isolated in equine kidney cells in 1972 from a rectal swab taken from a horse with diarrhea. Upon post-mortem examination pseudomembranous enteritis and miliary granulomas and necrosis in the liver were diagnosed; Salmonella Lille (O, 6, 7, Z_{38}) was considered to be the causative agent. ETV can be propagated in lines of equine dermis or embryonic mule skin cells, where it causes a cytopathic effect that results in cell lysis. The virus was not neutralized by antisera against known equine viruses. Serologic crossreactions were observed in neutralization and ELISA with sera from calves that had been experimentally infected with morphologically similar particles, the Breda viruses.

A bovine torovirus (BTV), first described as Breda virus was discovered in 1979 during investigations in a dairy herd in Breda (Iowa), in which severe neonatal calf diarrhea had been a problem for three consecutive years. Despite repeated attempts, BTV has not been adapted to growth in cell or tissue culture, which has hampered its biochemical, biophysical and molecular characterization. The pathogenesis and pathology of BTV infections have been studied in gnotobiotic calves.

Torovirus-like particles have been seen in EM preparations from fecal samples of pigs and humans (children and adults); proof that the observed structures are not artefacts was obtained when toroviral RNA sequences were found in the feces of piglets and in stools from humans with diarrhea.

Taxonomy and Classification

The name of the viruses assembled in this genus is derived from the term *torus* (Latin) which designates the lowest convex molding in the base of a column or pilaster. It refers to the biconcave disk or doughnut shape of the virion that is determined by a tubular capsid of helicoidal symmetry, which is surrounded by a peplomer-bearing envelope. In addition to the unique toroid form, virions may also appear as straight or bent rod-shaped particles.

Analysis of the genetic information and replication mode of the prototype ETV showed that toroviruses are evolutionarily related to the *Coronaviridae* and, to a lesser extent, to the *Arteriviridae*. However, the lack of sequence homology in the structural genes and the absence of antigenic relatedness with coronaviruses justify their separate taxonomic position as a genus, *Torovirus*, in the *Coronaviridae* family.

The families *Coronaviridae* and *Arteriviridae* form the Order *Nidovirales* (from *nidus*, Latin for 'the nest' – alluding to the nested set of subgenomic RNAs transcribed during replication), the second order recognized in animal virus taxonomy so far.

Virion Properties

Extracellular ETV particles possess a helical nucleocapsid coiled into a hollow tube (diameter 23 nm, average length 104 nm, periodicity 4.5 nm) which is either straight or bent into an open torus. A tightly fitting envelope, 11 nm thick, surrounds this structure. Consequently, the virion may assume an erythrocyte-like or a kidney shape, depending on whether the envelope follows the small curvature of the nucleocapsid or not. The largest diameter of ETV is estimated at 120–140 nm. Club-shaped projections (average length 20 nm) are present on the particle surface.

In the cell, predominantly rod-shaped particles are encountered. Cross-sections through tubular virions appear as three concentric circles of high electron density with an electron-lucent center.

Negatively stained BTV virions appear to be either kidney- or C-shaped, measuring 30–120 nm, or approximately circular, measuring 75–90 nm in diameter. Their envelope bears prominent drumstick-shaped peplomers (17–24 nm), and a fringe of shorter spikes 8–10 nm in length. The short projections represent the hemagglutinin esterase protein, which is present on the surface of bovine torovirions. In intestinal cells of calves killed 48–96 h after infection, tubules of 21 nm diameter and indeterminate length were found both in the cytoplasm and in nuclei.

In thin-sectioned preparations, intracellular torovirions show a bacilliform morphology (rods with both ends rounded – in contrast to the circular outline of coronavirions); extracellular particles may reveal twin circular structures resulting from cross-sections through both limbs of the C-shaped tubular nucleocapsid.

A model of a torovirion is given in **Fig. 1**.

Genome

ETV virions (sedimentation coefficient 380S) contain one species of polyadenylated RNA of positive polarity; in agarose gel electrophoresis its length appears as ≥20 kb. When assayed under hypertonic transfection conditions genomic RNA is found infectious and RNase-sensitive.

Proteins

Proteins with molecular weights of 20 kDa, 22 kDa, 37 kDa, and 80–100 kDa are identified in labeled ETV virions. Detergent treatment releases the 22, 37 and 80–100 kDa species from the virion, which indicates their association with the envelope. Only the 20 kDa protein is present in purified ETV nucleocapsids and was accordingly named nucleocapsid (N) protein. The heterogeneous, N-glycosylated 80–100 kDa protein is recognized by both neutralizing and hemagglutination-inhibiting monoclonal antibodies and is therefore identified as the peplomer (P) protein. Another membrane-associated polypeptide is the non-glycosylated envelope protein (E; 22 kDa); the 37 kDa molecule also occurs in close association with the viral membrane, but its virus specificity could not be established.

From the deduced amino acid sequence of the nucleocapsid (N) protein gene a basic protein of 18.3 kDa is predicted. *In vitro* transcription and translation, followed by immunoprecipitation, were

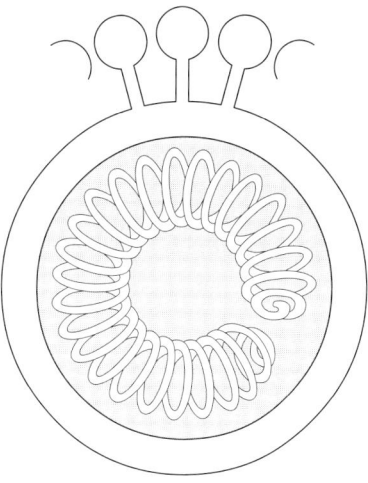

Figure 1 A schematic model of a torovirion. Illustration by Ank Klein-Willink.

used to identify the gene. Identification was confirmed by metabolic labeling, using the knowledge that cysteine residues are absent from the amino acid sequence of the N protein. Smaller N-related polypeptides encountered in ETV-infected cell lysates are products of aberrant translation, due to initiation on AUG codons further downstream in the N protein gene.

The 26.5 kDa product of the ETV membrane (M) protein gene was identified by *in vitro* transcription and translation. Computer analysis revealed the characteristics of a class III membrane protein lacking a cleaved signal sequence but containing three successive transmembrane α-helices in the N-terminal half. Only small portions of either end of the polypeptide are exposed on opposite sides of the vesicle membranes; the C-terminus protrudes at the cytoplasmic side of the membrane. The M protein accumulates in intracellular membranes, predominantly those of the endoplasmic reticulum.

The nucleotide sequence of the peplomer or spike (S) protein gene encodes an apoprotein of 1581 amino acids with an M_r of about 178 kDa. The deduced amino acid sequence contains domains typical for type I membrane glycoproteins: an N-terminal signal sequence, a putative C-terminal transmembrane anchor, and a cytoplasmic tail.

Since BTV has not been labeled in cultured cells, its protein composition was studied by means of surface radioiodination of purified virus. Polypeptide species of 105, 85, 37, and 20 kDa were identified, of which the former two probably represent the BTV peplomeric surface structures. Rabbit antisera raised against purified BTV recognize the ETV S protein in immunoprecipitation experiments.

Physical Properties

Buoyant densities of 1.16, 1.18 and 1.14 g ml^{-1} are reported for ETV, BTV serotype 2 and human toroviruses, respectively.

Under experimental conditions ETV is remarkably stable, even to the action of phospholipase C or deoxycholate; Triton X-100 and organic solvents destroy its infectivity. BTV1 appears to be less stable than ETV, as changes in its sedimentation behavior and density have been observed after prolonged storage at $-70°$C. The infectivity of a fecal preparation containing BTV1 was lost completely after 3 weeks at 4°C whereas ETV in cell-free supernatant remained stable for 92 days. Two cycles of freeze–thawing of purified BTV2 resulted in loss of peplomers.

Replication

Equine torovirus (strain Berne) replication occurs in the cytoplasm via a 3′-coterminal nested set of five subgenomic mRNAs. Preformed tubular capsids bud through membranes of the Golgi stack and of the endoplasmic reticulum. A host cell nuclear function seems to be required since UV preirradiation of cells, actinomycin D and α-amanitin reduce virus yields.

Transcription

In ETV-infected cells five virus-specific polyadenylated RNA species are found with >20.0, 7.5, 2.1, 1.4, 0.8 kb.

Northern (RNA) blot hybridizations with restriction fragments from cDNA clones showed that the five ETV mRNAs form a 3′-coterminal nested set. Sequence analysis revealed the presence of four complete open reading frames of 4743, 699, 426 and 480 nucleotides, with initiation codons coinciding with the 5′ ends of ETV RNAs 2 through 5, respectively; RNA 5 is contiguous on the consensus sequence. ETV RNAs 1, 2 and 3 are transcribed independently, as shown by UV transcription mapping. Upstream of the AUG codon of each open reading frame a conserved sequence pattern is encountered, probably a core promoter sequence in subgenomic RNA transcription. In the area surrounding the core promoter region of the two most abundant subgenomic ETV RNAs, a number of homologous sequence motifs occur.

Translation

The 7.5, 2.1 and 0.8 kb RNAs encode a 151 kDa product (possibly the precursor to the S protein), the M protein, and the N protein, respectively, as shown by *in vitro* translation.

The 3′ part (8 kb) of the polymerase gene of ETV contains at least two open reading frames (designated ORF 1a and ORF 1b) which overlap by 12 nucleotides. The complete sequence of ORF 1b (6873 nucleotides) is known. Like corona- and arteriviruses, ETV expresses its ORF 1b by ribosomal frameshifting during translation of the genomic RNA; also the predicted tertiary RNA structure (a pseudoknot) in the frameshift-directing region is similar. The amino acid sequence of the predicted ETV ORF 1b translation product contains homologies with the ORF 1b product of coronaviruses. Four conserved domains are present: the putative polymerase domain, an area containing conserved cystein and histidine residues, a putative helicase motif, and a domain apparently unique for toro- and coronaviruses.

Post-translational Processing

The N-glycosylated peplomer protein is derived from processing of a 200 kDa precursor present in infected cells but not in virions. Eighteen potential N-glycosylation sites, two heptad repeat domains, and a possible 'trypsin-like' cleavage site exist in the peplomer gene. The mature S protein consists of two subunits and their electrophoretic mobility on endoglycosidase F treatment suggests that the predicted cleavage site is functional *in vivo*. The heptad repeat domains are probably involved in the generation of an intra-chain coiled-coil secondary structure; similar interchain interactions can play a role in the formation of the observed S protein dimers. The intra- and interchain coiled-coil interactions may stabilize the elongated ETV peplomers.

Assembly

About 10 h after infection ETV particles are seen within parts of the unaltered Golgi apparatus and extracellularly. At that time, tubular structures of variable length, diameter and electron-density appear in the cytoplasm and in the nucleus of infected cells, probably representing preformed nucleocapsids. It is unknown whether the accumulation of nucleocapsids in the nucleus reflects a nuclear phase in the replication of ETV or some sort of defective assembly.

Viruses predominantly bud into the lumen of Golgi cisternae. The preformed nucleocapsid tubules approach the Golgi membrane with one of both rounded ends and attach to it along one side. During budding the nucleocapsid is apparently stabilized, leading to a higher electron density and a constant diameter (23 nm).

Intracellular BTV virions are rod-shaped with rounded ends; they measure 35–40 nm in diameter and are 80–100 nm long.

Defective Interfering Virus

Defective interfering (DI) genomes of ETV can be generated by serial undiluted passages. Isokinetic sucrose gradient analysis showed that they are packaged into virus-like particles with lower S values than standard virions. DI RNAs contain sequences from the presumed 5' end and the proven 3' end of the ETV genome. Using probes from the 5' end, a consensus nucleotide sequence of about 800 nt and the 5' end of the putative ETV polymerase gene were identified. A conserved sequence motif, probably involved in subgenomic RNA transcription, is situated immediately downstream of the 5' end of the DI RNAs. There is no evidence for the presence of a common leader sequence in ETV RNAs.

In the gut of a BTV-infected calf, a wave of simultaneous infections progresses through a population of susceptible cells. In view of the immense particle numbers encountered in the feces, enteroabsorptive epithelial cells are probably infected at high multiplicities; DI particles may also be generated *in vivo* and may play a role in modulating the pathogenesis of torovirus infections.

Geographic and Seasonal Distribution

Toroviruses in cattle have been evidenced by ELISA serology in Europe, North America and Asia. Seasonal patterns of infection have been described in calves in relation to herd management (pasture/stable). Most adult horses in Switzerland possess neutralizing antibodies to ETV. Possible human toroviruses have been found in France, Great Britain, The Netherlands and the USA.

Host Range and Virus Propagation

By using the neutralization assay, antibodies to ETV were found in sera from horses, cattle, goats, sheep, pigs, rabbits and feral mice, but not in humans or in carnivores. Torovirus-like particles have been seen in fecal samples of cats with a transmissible diarrhea, but neither serologic nor molecular identification was obtained.

By electron microscopy, pleomorphic virions have been observed in the feces of children and adults with diarrhea; the particles were coated and aggregated after the addition of anti-BTV calf sera. The stool specimen reacted in an ELISA for the detection of BTV antigen in calves, and possessed a low titer of hemagglutinin for rat erythrocytes, which was blocked by antisera to BTV.

Toroviral RNA sequences have been evidenced in the stools from humans with diarrhea. The use of fresh material (avoiding freeze/thawing) is essential for obtaining unequivocal results. Sequence analysis of RNA extracted from specimens of pediatric patients and amplified by reverse transcriptase–polymerase chain reaction (RT-PCR) showed a high degree of identity with the corresponding ETV sequence. This is surprising in view of the observation that the divergence between porcine and bovine/equine torovirus sequences is greater than between human and bovine/equine torovirus sequences. If confirmed, this would indicate occasional spillover of the infection from ungulates to humans, rather than human-to-human transmission.

Cultured cells of equid origin (horse, mule) can be infected with ETV; no other cell species tested supports viral growth. Bovine toroviruses could not be propagated in any culture of primary cells or permanent lines and had to be passaged in gnotobiotic calves. Putative torovirus isolations from young calves with respiratory symptoms (pneumonia) in MDBK cells have been challenged, and a bovine coronavirus was identified in the culture.

Genetics

No information is available.

Evolution

Toroviruses and coronaviruses are ancestrally related by divergence of their polymerase and envelope proteins from common ancestors. In addition, their genome organization and expression strategy, which involves the synthesis of a 3'-coterminal nested set of mRNAs, are comparable. Four domains of amino acid sequence homology exist in the product of ORF 1b of the *POL* gene, which underlines the existence of an evolutionary relationship. In view of these findings, toro- and coronaviruses have been classified as separate genera in the family *Coronaviridae*, which, together with the *Arteriviridae* forms the order *Nidovirales*.

Nucleotide sequence analysis of the ETV genome has revealed the results of two independent nonhomologous RNA recombinations: ORF 4 encodes a protein with significant sequence similarity (30–35% identical residues) to a part of the hemagglutinin esterase proteins of coronaviruses and of influenza virus C. Although this gene is truncated in ETV, it is intact and translated into a functional, enzymatically active protein in BTV; this product is visible as a second fringe of (short) projections on the viral envelope.

The sequence of the C-terminal part of the predicted ETV polymerase ORF 1a product contains 31–36% identical amino acids when compared with the sequence of a nonstructural 30/32 kDa coronavirus protein. The cluster of coronaviruses which contains this nonstructural gene does not express it as a part of their polymerase, but by synthesizing an additional subgenomic mRNA.

Serologic Relationships and Variability

One strain of ETV has been isolated (and re-isolated from the same material), but all attempts to obtain a second equine isolate were fruitless.

Two strains of BTV have been reported in addition to the original isolate by Woode and colleagues: one had been detected in feces from a 5-month-old diarrheal calf in Ohio, and a second Iowa strain was recovered from a 2-day-old experimental animal. On the basis of their reactivity in ELISA, immune electron microscopy and hemagglutination/hemagglutination inhibition assays using rat erythrocytes the three isolates were assigned to two serotypes: BTV1, represented by the Iowa 1 isolate, and BTV2 comprising the Ohio and the second Iowa isolate.

The occurrence of antigenically different toroviruses is not unlikely. Two serotypes of BTV have been described and more probably exist. It is anticipated that serologically unrelated toroviruses will be identified with the aid of nucleic acid probes.

Epidemiology

The high prevalence of BTV antibodies in cows cannot be explained by the few infections found in calves and cows with diarrhea. The viruses may circulate in herds through inapparently or chronically infected animals, as described for rota- and coronaviruses. The level of maternal BTV-specific antibodies influences the clinical outcome of the infection, as differences in the severity of diarrhea were observed between colostrum-fed and colostrum-deprived animals.

With the aid of solid-phase immune-electron microscopy, torovirions can be identified in fecal material; without this selection, virion pleomorphism makes diagnosis by electron microscopy ambiguous.

Transmission and Tissue Tropism

Toroviruses probably spread through feco-oral contact. In feces samples from experimentally BTV-infected calves HA titers in excess of 10^7 units ml^{-1} are measured which would correspond to particle concentrations of $>10^{11}$. Therefore, once an outbreak is under way the infection spreads rapidly, especially when highly susceptible animals are on the premises (e.g. in the calving season).

Using RT-PCR, torovirus sequences were obtained from fecal samples of weaning piglets; an association with weaning diarrhea has not been established.

Pathogenicity

Torovirus infections play a role in diarrhea of breeding calves up to two months of age, and in winter dysentery of adult cattle. Torovirus was detected four times more often in diarrheal calves than in healthy animals. Torovirus-associated diarrhea of calves started later (average 12.7 days of age) than enteritis due to rota- or coronaviruses (average 7.7 and 8.3 days, respectively). Seroconversion was found significantly more often after winter dysentery outbreaks than on farms without a disease history; coronavirus seroconversion was less common.

Clinical Features of Infection

Seroconversions to ETV occurred in all horses between 10 and 12 months of age, but without symptoms. Experimentally infected animals (intravenous route) seroconverted without clinical signs. To the author's knowledge oral infection experiments in horses have not been reported so far.

All BTV strains are pathogenic – although with varying virulence – for newborn gnotobiotic and nonimmune conventional calves after oral infection. Most calves develop anorexia, a watery, yellow–green diarrhea that lasts 4–6 days, and shed virus for 3–4 days. In some calves the diarrhea is preceded by a mild temperature reaction (40°C). In the calves with a normal intestinal flora the diarrhea is generally more severe than in gnotobiotic calves. Reduction of D-xylose resorption may reach 65% in severely affected calves. In some animals depression and dehydration is observed, occasionally with shivering, hyperpnea and watery eye discharge. Mortality in experimental infections approaches 25%.

Pathology and Histopathology

Target organs of BTV in calves are the lower half or two-thirds of the small intestine and the entire large intestine, particularly the spiral colon. There is little macroscopic evidence of the infection. Histological examination shows villous atrophy and epithelial desquamation from the mid-jejunum to the lower small intestine, and areas of necrosis in the large intestine. Both crypt and villus epithelial cells contain antigen as shown by immunofluorescence. The watery diarrhea is probably a result of loss of resorptive capacity of the colonic mucosa, combined with malabsorption in the small intestine. Infection of crypt epithelium may affect the duration of diarrhea, as regeneration of villus epithelium starts in the crypts. The germinal centers of the Peyer's patches are depleted of lymphocytes and may occasionally show fresh hemorrhage. The dome epithelial cells, including the M cells, display the same cytopathic changes as seen in the absorptive cells of villi. Virions are found in cells of both the small and large intestine. Extracellular virus is closely associated with microvilli of absorptive cells and in the coated pits between microvilli, indicating receptor-mediated endocytosis. In addition, virions are found between enterocytes at the basal and lateral plasma membranes. Virions in various stages of degradation are found within macrophages in the lamina propria.

Antigen is detected as early as 48 h after infection in epithelial cells of the lower half of the villus and of the crypts of the affected areas, as well as in dome epithelium. Fluorescence is cytoplasmic (although a few nuclei may be faintly stained) and generally most pronounced in the intestines with the least tissue damage. The mid-jejunum is infected first, the infection eventually reaching the large intestine. Diagnosis by immunofluorescence test (IFT) should be performed preferentially on sections of the large intestine from calves killed after the onset of diarrhea (i.e. several days after the infection of epithelium).

Immune Response

Up to the age of 4 months, all calves in a sentinel experiment regularly excreted BTV in the feces. They showed early serum IgM responses despite the presence of IgG1 isotype maternal antibodies, but no IgA seroconversion. Antibody titers then decreased below detection, persistent IgG1 titers developed in only a few animals. After introduction into the dairy herd at 10 months of age, all calves developed diarrhea and shed virus. Seroconversion for all antibody isotypes was observed at this stage, indicating lack of mucosal memory. In contrast, coronavirus infection in the presence of maternal antibodies leads to isotype switch and a memory response.

Prevention and Control

No control strategies have been implemented.

Future

The pathogenic significance of toroviruses for animals and humans, also as agents of nonenteric infections needs to be established. Diagnostic procedures for the discovery of more distantly related viruses of this cluster will have to include procedures for the recognition of nucleotide sequence motives.

See also: **Arteriviruses (*Arteriviridae*); Defective interfering viruses.**

Further Reading

Cavanagh D and Horzinek MC (1993) Genus Torovirus assigned to the *Coronaviridae. Arch. Virol.* 128: 395.

Cornelissen LA, Wierda CM, van der Meer FJ *et al* (1997) Hemagglutinin-esterase, a novel structural protein of torovirus. *J. Virol.* 71: 5277.

Koopmans M and Horzinek MC (1994) Toroviruses of animals and humans: a review. *Adv. Virus Res.* 43: 233.

Snijder E and Horzinek MC (1993) Toroviruses: replication, evolution and comparison with other members of the coronavirus-like superfamily. *J. Gen. Virol.* 74: 2305.

Snijder E and Horzinek MC (1995) The molecular biology of toroviruses. In: Siddell S and ter Meulen V (eds) *Coronaviruses.* New York: Plenum Press.

Vries AAF de, Horzinek MC, Rottier PJM *et al* (1997) The genome organization of the Nidovirales: similarities and differences between arteri-, toro-, and coronaviruses. *Semin Virol.* 8: 33.

TOSPOVIRUSES (*BUNYAVIRIDAE*)

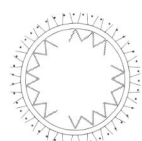

James W. Moyer, Department of Plant Pathology, North Carolina State University, Raleigh, North Carolina, USA

Copyright © 1999 Academic Press

History

Diseases incited by tomato spotted wilt virus (TSWV) were first reported in 1915 and were considered to be of viral etiology by 1930. This taxon of plant viruses was categorized as a monotypic virus group consisting of a single virus (tomato spotted wilt virus; TSWV) until the report of Impatiens necrotic spot virus (INSV) in 1990. Thus, most of the characteristics on which the *Tospovirus* genus is defined were obtained through investigations of TSWV. Although TSWV was originally associated with tomato (*Lycopersicon esculentum*), by the 1950s it had one of the largest known host ranges of any plant virus. By 1998 the known natural and experimental host range exceeded 900 plant species and spanned both monocotyledonous and dicotyledonous plant species. TSWV was known by 1930 to be insect vectored by thrips. It was not until the mid 1960s that the enveloped virion morphology was revealed and the molecular characterization and genome organization did not occur until after 1990. In addition, understanding of the virus–vector biology, cytopathology of both the plant and insect hosts and virus genetics have developed rapidly since 1990. However, efficient *in vitro* cell culture systems for either plant or thrips systems are not available nor is there a system for reverse genetics.

Taxonomy, Classification and Serological Relationships

Tospovirus constitutes the only plant-infecting genus in the *Bunyaviridae*. Tospoviruses are characterized by a quasi-spherical, enveloped virion containing a tripartite RNA genome typical of the family. A single open reading frame (ORF) in the viral complementary-sense (negative) is located on the large RNA (L) and two ORFs in an ambisense (see Molecular Biology) orientation are on both the middle (M) and small (S) segments. The presence of two ambisense RNAs is the defining molecular characteristic that distinguishes this genus from the other genera in the *Bunyaviridae*. Biologically, the tospoviruses multiply in plants and in their insect (thrips) vectors. However, their individual host ranges are highly variable. Some tospoviruses have an extremely large host range (e.g. TSWV) whereas others such as iris yellow spot virus (IYSV) are known to infect only a small number of plant species.

The discovery of INSV led to the current scheme for classifying viruses within the *Tospovirus* genus that is based on nucleic acid sequence homology between nucleocapsid genes. New viruses are named consistent with rules of the International Committee on Taxonomy of Viruses with each virus equivalent to a species. Newly discovered tospoviruses were classified in serogroups, e.g. serogroup I, II etc., and this system was used in the literature. However, the proliferation of viruses and number of monotypic serogroups prompted the abandonment of the numerical system. Distinct viruses are not classified as a group until more than one virus is identified in that group. The serogroup is then identified by the type virus, e.g. tomato spotted wilt virus serogroup (**Table 1**). This system currently distinguishes at least 12 different viruses (**Table 1**). Although the sequence homology between tospoviruses varies with the gene, sequence differences between the nucleocapsid genes are accepted as a measure of overall relatedness. The nucleocapsid protein was chosen not only because it is abundant, but also because of its putative role in regulating the switch from transcription to replication, function in the replication complex and encapsidation of the genome based on viruses with negative strand genome organization. Serological relatedness based on ELISA or Western blot analysis of the nucleocapsid protein is used to classify viruses within serogroups and, as expected, is generally consistent with homology of the nucleocapsid genes. This is distinct from the serological relatedness in other genera of the *Bunyaviridae* that have been measured by neutralization or hemagglutination assays that are indicative of functions mediated by viral glycoproteins which reside in the envelope.

Isolates in the *Tospovirus* genus with greater than 90% nucleocapsid sequence homology are classified as strains of the same virus. Serologically related isolates with 80–90% sequence homology are subjectively classified as strains or as distinct viruses depending on additional criteria. Isolates with less than 80% homology to all of the other known viruses are classified as distinct viruses or species. Those viruses exhibiting serological relatedness are classified in the same serogroup. For example, groundnut chlorotic spot virus is a distinct virus with 78%

Table 1 List of tospoviruses and serogroups

Tospovirus species	Abbreviation
TSWV serogroup:	
Tomato spotted wilt virus	TSWV
Groundnut ringspot virus	GRSV
Tomato chlorotic spot virus	TCSV
WMSV serogroup:	
Watermelon silver mottle virus	WSMV
Watermelon bud necrosis virus	WBNV
Groundnut bud necrosis virus	GBNV
Serologically unrelated	
Chrysanthemum stem necrosis virus	CNSV
Impatiens necrotic spot virus	INSV
Iris yellow spot virus	IYSV
Peanut yellow spot virus	PYSV
Peanut chlorotic fan-spot virus	FCFV
Physalis severe mottle virus	
PSMV Zucchini lethal chlorosis virus	ZLCV

homology to TSWV and a distant serological relationship, was formerly classified in serogroup II, but is now classified as a member of the TSWV serogroup. Homology with TSWV for distinct viruses range from about 60% for INSV to less than 40% for watermelon silver mottle virus (WSMV).

Properties of Virion

Tospovirus virions are quasi-spherical, enveloped particles 80–120 nm in diameter. Two viral-coded glycoproteins, G1 and G2, are embedded in the viral envelope. Ribonucleoprotein (RNP) particles consisting of the viral RNA encapsidated in the nucleoprotein and a small number of polymerase molecules are contained within the envelope. Intact virions as well as carefully prepared RNPs retrieved from sucrose or $CsSO_4$ gradients are infectious. There are several reports of TSWV and INSV isolates that are defective for virion formation, but remain infectious.

Properties of Genome

Tospoviruses have a single-stranded, tripartite RNA genome with segments designated as L, M and S in order of decreasing length. The termini of each of the RNA segments consist of an eight nucleotide sequence (5′ AGAGCAAU 3′) that is conserved throughout the genus on each segment of the viral genome. The first 12 to 15 nucleotides at the termini of each segment are complementary with a high degree of complementarity extending throughout the terminal untranslated regions. The base pairing at the termini results in a panhandle structure that may initiate encapsidation and regulation of transcription. The L RNA is approximately 8.9 kb and codes for the RNA-dependent RNA-polymerase (RdRp) that is translated from the viral complementary sense RNA. The M RNA is approximately 4.8 kb with two ORFs in an ambisense arrangement. The ORF nearer the 5′ terminus codes for the 33.6 kDa nonstructural protein (NSm) in the viral sense and is followed by an A-U rich, 200–250 nucleotide intergenic region. The second ORF codes for the G1/G2 precursor protein in the viral complementary sense. The S RNA is 2.9–3.0 kb with two ORFs in a similar ambisense arrangement. A nonstructural protein (NSs) is coded from the ORF nearer the 5′ terminus in the viral sense and the nucleocapsid gene from the ORF in the viral complementary sense located near the 3′ terminus. The two ORFs are separated by an A-U rich intergenic region of variable length. The S segment from isolates of TSWV may vary in length by as much as 100 nucleotides and is due entirely to insertions and deletions in the intergenic region. In addition, highly conserved sequences are embedded within the intergenic region. In one group of isolates, a 33 nucleotide duplicate sequence was associated with reduced competitiveness of the S RNA from those isolates.

Full-length molecules of the M and S ambisense RNA segments are found in infected tissue and purified virions in both the viral and viral complementary sense (approximate ratio of 10:1) which is consistent with ambisense segments from other viruses. Defective interfering RNAs (DIs) associated with attenuated symptoms are also frequently observed. DIs in TSWV infected tissue are the result of a single deletion event in the L RNA. The formation of DIs is favored by repeated passage in certain hosts, high inoculum concentration and low temperatures. Available evidence supports the hypothesis that secondary structure rather than sequence is the primary determinant of the site of deletion as is viral RNA recombination. There is also a high frequency of DIs that maintain the original reading frame resulting in translation of truncated proteins whose existence was confirmed in nucleocapsid preparations.

Properties of Proteins

A 330 kDa protein encoded by the L RNA has been identified as the putative RdRp through sequence homology. RdRp activity has been associated with TSWV virions. Full length and truncated RdRp molecules have been associated with virions containing DIs. The 33.6 kDa NSm protein encoded by the M RNA has been shown to induce tubule structures from protoplasts and cell surfaces from plants and insects, respectively. Induction of tubules and association with the plasmodesmata in plant cells is evidence that this protein is involved in cell-to-cell movement. The G1/G2 precursor protein is also coded for by the M RNA. These proteins occur in the viral envelope and have been associated with recognition by the thrips. The NSs protein (54 kDa) encoded on the S RNA accumulates to high levels as loose aggregates or paracrystalline arrays of filaments, but has not been linked with any function. The nucleocapsid (N) protein, also encoded by the S RNA, ranges in size from 29 to 31 kDa depending on the virus. This protein encapsidates the viral RNA segments and has been demonstrated to have RNA binding properties. It is highly abundant and is the predominant protein detected in serological assays.

Replication

The RNA of this virus, similar to other negative strand viruses is not infectious and recombinant DNA techniques have not been applied to elucidate genome function. As yet there are no efficient systems for detailed molecular investigations of tospoviruses, although there are reports of infection of plant protoplasts and insect cells. It is known that replication of viral RNA and assembly of virions occurs in the cytoplasm. The RNP containing the L RNA is hypothesized to replicate similar to other negative-strand viruses. The viral RNA is the template for replication and the viral complementary strand serves as the template for translation of the RdRp protein. The S and M ambisense RNAs also replicate similar to negative-strand RNAs. However, translation of these proteins probably occurs from subgenomic mRNAs. Subgenomic mRNAs of appropriate size for each of the ORFs on these two RNAs, have been detected in infected plants. The subgenomic RNAs are capped at the 5′ terminus with 12–20 nucleotides of nonviral origin indicating that tospoviruses utilize a cap-snatching mechanism to regulate transcription. Virions are assembled in the cisternae of the endoplasmic reticulum. Initially they are double-membraned particles that soon coalesce to become groups of virions with a single membrane surrounded by another membrane.

Geographic Distribution

Tospoviruses are found worldwide. However, individual viruses may have limited distribution. In general, they are found in temperate regions colonized by their thrips vector. Exceptions are the viruses (e.g. watermelon silver mottle group) transmitted by *Thrips palmi*, that is found in subtropical regions. TSWV has the most extensive host range and is found worldwide. Conversely, INSV has been of greatest concern in greenhouse-grown floral crops in North America, Central America and Europe. Viruses in the watermelon silver mottle serogroup have been identified in India, Japan and Taiwan, although their vector is found in other parts of the world. IYSV has been reported in Israel, Brazil and western North America. Collectively, tospoviruses have been included among the 'emerging viruses' due to their wide and rapid distribution and the severity of the diseases they incite.

Host Range and Virus Propagation

TSWV has one of the most diverse host ranges of any plant-infecting virus. The virus infects over 900 plant species which include both monocotyledonous and dicotyledonous plants. Other tospoviruses have much narrower host ranges and thus the broad host range of TSWV is not characteristic of the genus. Tospoviruses also replicate in their thrips vectors but distinct from viruses in other genera of this family, are not transmitted transovarially or by plant seeds. These viruses can be transmitted mechanically for experimentation or by their thrips vector. There are no robust plant or insect culture systems for these viruses. However, plant protoplasts have been successfully inoculated.

Genetics and Evolution

The knowledge base for genetics and evolution of tospoviruses has been derived almost exclusively from TSWV. TSWV is unusually adept at adapting to new hosts as well as losing phenotypic characters following repeated passage in experimental hosts, especially *Nicotiana benthamiana*. The virus occurs in plants as a heterogeneous mixture of isolates that have been distinguished by symptom phenotype and more recently with molecular markers. As many as five stable variants have been isolated from a single thrips inoculation site. TSWV has also been shown to form new phenotypes from the mixture. These complex populations provide a reservoir of genetic information that could account for the rapid adaptation. Recombination (sensu reassortment) was shown via classical genetics to be a possible mechanism for reassembling the genetic information among isolates in 1961. TSWV has now been shown to use reassortment of genome segments as a mechanism for adaptation to resistant hosts. The determinants of adaptation to resistance in tomato and pepper have been mapped to the M and S segments, respectively.

Transmission and Epidemiology

Tospoviruses are transmitted from plant to plant by a small number of thrips species. Among the more common vectors are *Frankliniella occidentalis*, *F. fusca*, *F. schultzei*, *Scirtothrips dorsalis*, *Thrips palmi*, *T. setosus* and *T. tabaci*. Thrips feed on the cytoplasm of plant cells. The contents of infected cells are ingested and the virus is transported along the lumen of the digestive tract to the midgut. The virus is then transported by endocytosis across the membrane of endothelial cells which line the midgut of the thrips. This process of acquisition only occurs in thrips in the larval stage of development. Evidence for replication of the virus in the insect vector is based on the accumulation of nonstructural protein (NSs) and the visualization of other inclusions in endothelial cells, muscle cells and the salivary glands. Viral inoculum is introduced into plants in the insect saliva coincident with feeding on the plant. Although the virus is maintained trans-stagially throughout the life of the insect, there is no evidence for transovarial transmission. Thus, each generation of thrips must acquire the virus during the larval stage of development.

The primary mechanisms for virus increase in plant populations is by the thrips vector and dissemination of infected somatic tissue in vegetatively propagated crops. Transmission of the virus through plant seed is not recognized as a significant factor in the epidemiology of tospoviruses. These viruses are thought to move long distances in thrips carried by wind currents. They may also survive in commercial agricultural systems in weeds that serve as a bridge between crops. Secondary spread within a crop can only occur in crops that support virus infection and reproduction of the vector as only the larval stage can acquire the virus for transmission. The recent emergence of these viruses as serious pathogens in crops has been attributed to the increased prevalence of thrips as agricultural pests on a worldwide basis. For example, *F. occidentalis*, the western flower thrips, is a highly efficient vector of several tospoviruses. Its emergence in the floral crop industry was closely followed by the emergence of INSV in the late 1980s.

Pathogenicity and Histopathology

Tospoviruses are noted for the severity of the diseases they cause in plants. Symptoms include chlorotic or necrotic lesions or line patterns on inoculated and systemically infected leaves. Systemic invasion of plants is frequently nonuniform. Many plants exhibit chlorotic, concentric rings as a characteristic symptom. Stems and petioles may exhibit necrotic lesions. Symptoms are sufficiently severe and atypical that many syndromes observed on many plants mimic disease and injury caused by other stresses such as bacterial or fungal pathogens or chemical injury. Infection of younger plants result in severely stunted plants and are frequently lethal. The pathology of infected thrips has not been thoroughly examined, however, preliminary studies indicate that infected thrips have reduced reproductive rates and longevity.

Although tospoviruses also induce characteristic cytopathic structures, it should be noted that the occurrence of these structures, even virions, vary from plant to plant and virus to virus. In addition to virions, inclusions or viroplasms consisting of the nonstructural protein (NSs) and nucleocapsid proteins may be abundant in the cytoplasm. NSs accumulates as a filamentous structure that may aggregate in loose bundles (e.g. TSWV) or in highly ordered paracrystalline arrays (e.g. INSV). Excess nucleocapsid protein occurs in granular electron-dense masses. NSs and nucleocapsid protein inclusions have been observed in infected plant and insect cells.

Prevention and Control

Tospoviruses can be effectively managed in well-defined cropping systems such as glasshouses by obtaining plant propagules known to be free of the virus, implementing a preventative thrips control program in high risk areas together with constant monitoring of production areas for infected plants and the vector. However, these strategies are costly and require intensive management. Control of the viruses in field crops is problematic due to the array of external sources of inoculum. Vector control is generally ineffective against the introduction of virus from external sources, however, it may be more effective against secondary spread within the field. Deployment of resistant cultivars has provided temporary benefits. Although little is known about the benefits of host resistance against most of the tospoviruses, TSWV defeated nearly every resistance gene deployed against it in many crops. Pathogen-derived resistance utilizing the nucleocapsid and NSm genes has been effective in some greenhouse and field tests. However, isolates have recently been obtained that overcome nucleocapsid-mediated resistance. The impact of these viruses on agricultural production is in large part due to the absence of highly effective control measures.

See also: **Bunyaviridae: General features; Replication; Plant virus disease – economic aspects.**

Further Reading

Best RJ (1968) Tomato spotted wilt virus. *Adv. Virus Res.* 13: 65.

De Avila AC, de Haan P, Kormelink R *et al* (1993) Classification of tospoviruses based on phylogeny of nucleoprotein gene sequences. *J. Gen. Virol.* 74: 153.

German TL, Ullman DE and Moyer JW (1992) Tospoviruses: diagnosis, molecular biology, phylogeny, and vector relationships. *Annu. Rev. Phytopathol.* 30: 315.

Prins M and Goldbach R (1998) The emerging problem of tospovirus infection and nonconventional methods of control. *Trends Microbiol.* 6: 31.

Ullman DE, Sherwood JL and German TG (1997) Thrips as vectors of plant pathogens. Lewis TL (ed.) *Thrips As Crop Pests*, p. 539. Wallingford: CAB International.

TOTIVIRUSES (*TOTIVIRIDAE*)

Contents
General Features
Ustilago Maydis Viruses

General Features

Said A Ghabrial, Department of Plant Pathology, University of Kentucky College of Agriculture, Lexington, Kentucky, USA

Jean L Patterson, Department of Virology and Immunology, Southwest Foundation for Biomedical Research, San Antonio, Texas, USA

Copyright © 1999 Academic Press

Introduction

The discovery of the killer phenomenon in the 1960s in the yeast (*Saccharomyces cerevisiae*) and in the smut fungus (*Ustilago maydis*) eventually led to the discovery of the isometric double-stranded (ds) RNA mycoviruses with undivided genomes, presently classified in the family *Totiviridae*. Yeast or smut killer strains secrete a protein toxin to which they are immune, but which is lethal to sensitive cells. The killer toxin is encoded by a satellite dsRNA which is dependent on a helper virus with undivided dsRNA genome (totivirus) for encapsidation and replication. Unlike the helper totiviruses associated with the yeast and smut killer systems, the member viruses in the family *Totiviridae* that infect filamentous fungi and parasitic protozoa are not known to be associated with killer phenotypes. However, purified preparations of some of these viruses are often associated with dsRNA species suspected of being satellite or defective dsRNAs. Viruses with nonsegmented dsRNA genomes of approximately 5200 bp in length have been identified in over 13 strains of the new world parasitic protozoa, *Leishmania braziliensis* and in one strain of the old world parasite, *L. major*. These viruses have recently been placed in the genus *Leishmaniavirus* in the family *Totiviridae*.

The yeast and smut totiviruses and associated killer systems, as well as the totiviruses infecting the parasitic protozoa *Giardia lamblia*, are considered in separate entries in this text. This entry will focus on the totiviruses infecting filamentous fungi and parasitic protozoa, with special emphasis on *Helminthosporium victoriae* 190S virus (Hv190SV) and the totiviruses infecting the protozoa *Leishmania* spp.

Taxonomy and Classification

The family *Totiviridae* comprises three genera, *Totivirus*, *Giardiavirus* and *Leishmaniavirus* (**Table 1**). Viruses in the genus *Totivirus* infect fungi, whereas those belonging to the genera *Giardiavirus* and *Leishmaniavirus* infect parasitic protozoa. The isometric dsRNA totiviruses are unique among dsRNA viruses in that their genomes are undivided, whereas the genomes of all other dsRNA viruses are segmented.

Virion Properties

The sedimentation coefficients $s_{20,w}$ (in Svedberg units) for members of the totivirus genus are in the range of 160–190 S. Particles lacking nucleic acid sediment at the rate of $s_{20,w} = 98–113$ S. Buoyant density in CsCl = 1.40–1.43 g ml^{-1}. Isolates of ScV-L-A and UmV-H1 may have additional components, containing satellite or defective dsRNAs, with different sedimentation coefficients and buoyant densities.

Virion Structure and Composition

The totiviruses have isometric particles, approximately 40 nm in diameter, with icosahedral symmetry. The capsids are single-shelled and comprised of a single major polypeptide. The capsids consists of 120 capsid protein (CP) subunits of molecular mass in the range of 69–88 kDa, arranged in $T = 1$ lattices.

Although the capsid of Hv190SV, like other totiviruses, is encoded by a single gene, it is comprised of two closely related major CPs, either p88 and p83 or p88 and p78. The capsids of all other totiviruses so far characterized appear to contain only a single major CP. Purified Hv190S virion preparations contain two types of particles, 190S-1 and 190S-2, that differ in sedimentation rates and capsid composition. The 190S-1 and 190S-2 virions are believed to represent different stages in the virus life cycle. The 190S-1 capsids contain p88 and p83, occurring in approximately equimolar amounts, and the 190S-2 capsids are comprised of similar amounts of p88 and p78. p88 and p83 are phosphoproteins, whereas p78 is nonphosphorylated.

The virions of totiviruses encapsidate a single mol-

Table 1 Virus members in the family Totiviridae

Genus	Virus (Alternative name)	Abbreviation	Accession number
Totivirus	Saccharomyces cerevisiae virus L-A	ScV-L-A	J04692
	(Saccharomyces cerevisiae virus L1)	ScVL1	X13426
	Saccharomyces cerevisiae virus La	ScV-La	U01060
	(Saccharomyces cerevisiae virus L-BC)	ScV-L-BC	
	Ustilago maydis virus H1	UmV-H1	V01059
	Helminthosporium victoriae 190S virus	Hv190SV	U41345
	Aspergillus foetidus virus S[a]	AfV-S	
	Aspergillus niger virus S[a]	AnV-S	
	Gaeumannomyces graminis virus 87-1-H[a]	GgV-87-1-H	
	Mycogone perniciosa virus[a]	MpV	
Giardiavirus	Giardia lamblia virus	GLV	L13218
	Trichomonas vaginalis virus[a]	TVV	U08999
Leishmaniavirus	Leishmania RNA virus 1-1	LRV1-1	M92355
	Leishmania RNA virus 1-4	LRV1-4	U01899
	Leishmania RNA virus 2-1	LRV2-1	U32108

[a]Tentative member.

ecule of dsRNA 4.7–6.7 kbp in size. Some totiviruses may additionally contain satellite dsRNAs or defective dsRNAs, which are encapsidated separately in capsids encoded by the totivirus genome. The complete nucleotide sequences of eight totiviruses belonging to three genera have been published and the GenBank accession numbers are listed in **Table 1**.

Genome Organization and Expression

The genome organization and expression strategy of the totiviruses infecting fungi and protozoa are similar: each virus genome contains two large open reading frames (ORFs); the 5′ proximal ORF encodes a CP and the 3′ ORF encodes an RNA-dependent RNA polymerase (RDRP). Except for LRV2-1, the RDRP ORF overlaps the CP ORF and is in the −1 frame (ScV-L-A, ScV-La, Hv190SV and GLV) or in the +1 frame (LRV1-1, LRV1-4 and TVV) with respect to the CP ORF. The RDRP ORF of LRV2-1 does not overlap the CP ORF, and is separated from it by a stop codon.

Expression of RDRP as CP-RDRP (*gag-pol*-like) fusion protein via −1 ribosomal frameshifting has been well documented only for ScV-L-A. Virion-associated CP-RDRP has been detected as a minor protein in the case of ScV-L-A, ScV-La (L-BC) and GLV. The RDRP of Hv190SV (and possibly that of LRV1-4) is present as a nonfused separate virion-associated minor protein. Although CP-RDRP fusion proteins were not detected *in vivo*, nor associated with virions of TVV, LRV1-1, LRV1-4 or LRV2-1, expression of RDRP as a fusion protein by +1 ribosomal frameshifting (TVV, LRV1-1 and LRV1-4) or ribosomal hopping (LRV2-1) has been proposed.

The overlap region (16 nt) between the two ORFs of Hv190SV dsRNA (**Fig. 1**) is considerably smaller than that in ScV-L-A (130 nt), LRV1-1 and LRV1-4 (71 nt), and GLV (122 nt). The overlap region of these totiviruses contain sufficient information (structures necessary for ribosomal frameshifting, including a slippery site and a pseudoknot structure involving a predicted stem–loop structure) to promote fusion of ORF1 and ORF2 *in vivo*. The overlap region in the Hv190SV dsRNA genome, on the other hand, lacks a heptamer slippery site and a potential pseudoknot structure cannot be predicted from the secondary structure of the sequences flanking the 3′-terminal region of the CP gene. These observations suggest that expression of RDRP occurs by a mechanism different from translational frameshifting. The finding that the termination codon of the CP ORF (nucleotide position 2605-AUG-2607) overlaps with the predicted

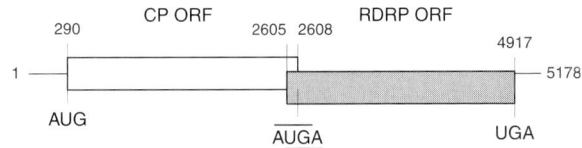

Figure 1 Genome organization of Helminthosporium victoriae 190S virus (Hv190SV) dsRNA. Two large overlapping open reading frames (ORFs) with the 5′ ORF encoding a capsid protein (CP) and the 3′ ORF encoding an RNA-dependent RNA polymerase (RDRP). Note that the termination codon of the CP ORF overlaps the initiation codon of the RDRP ORF in the tetranucleotide sequence AUGA.

TOTIVIRUSES (TOTIVIRIDAE): GENERAL FEATURES

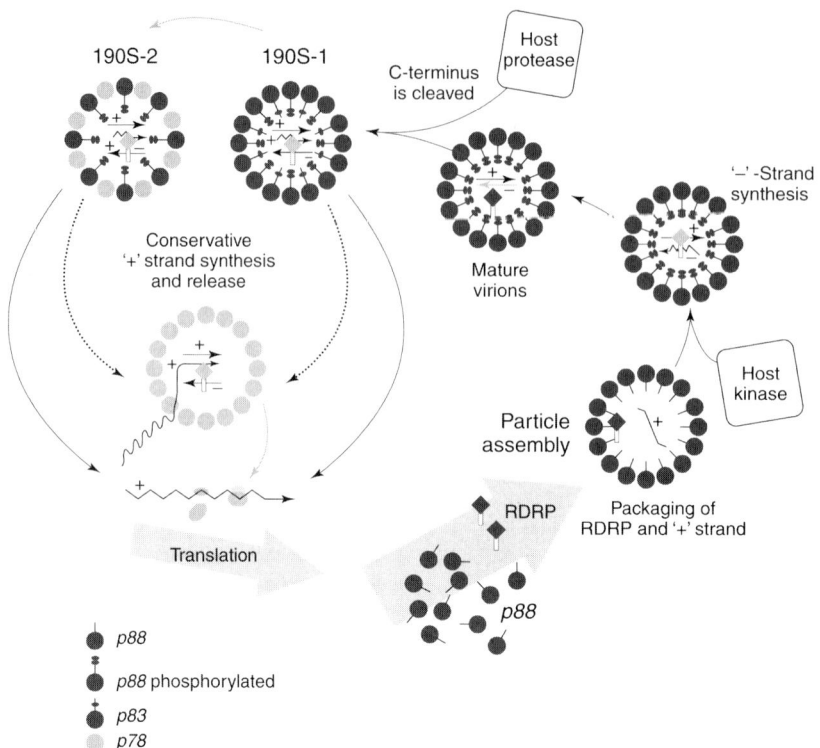

Figure 2 Life cycle of Hv190SV. Mature virions contain a single dsRNA molecule and their capsids are composed entirely or primarily of the capsid protein (CP) p88. Virions representing different stages of the virus life cycle can be purified from the infected fungal host *Helminthosporium victoriae* including the well-characterized 190S-1 and 190S-2 virions. These two types of virions differ in sedimentation coefficient, phosphorylation state and CP composition; 190S-1 capsids contain p88 and p83, whereas the 190S-2 capsids contain p88 and p78 (p88 is the primary translation product of the *CP* gene; p83 and p78 represent post-translational proteolytic processing products of p88 at the C-terminus). p88 and p83 are phosphorylated, whereas p78 is nonphosphorylated. The virions with phosphorylated CPs (p88 + p83) have significantly higher transcriptase activity *in vitro* than those containing the nonphosphorylated p78. Transcription occurs conservatively and the newly synthesized (+)-strand RNA is released from the virions. Phosphorylation of CP is catalyzed by a host kinase, and is proposed to play a regulatory role in transcription/replication. A host-encoded protease catalyzes the proteolytic processing of phosphorylated p88; this occurs in two steps, leading first to p83 (the generation of the 190S-1 virions) and then to p78 (190S-2 virions). The conversion of p88 → p83 → p78 is proposed to play a role in the release of the (+)-strand RNA transcripts from virions. The released (+)-strand RNA is the RNA that is translated into CP and RNA-dependent RNA polymerase (RDRP) and packaged in capsids assembled from the primary translation product p88. It is not known whether p88 is phosphorylated before or after assembly. Synthesis of (−)-strand RNA occurs on the (+)-strand RNA template inside the virion; phosphorylation may be involved in turning on the replicase activity.

start codon for the RDRP ORF (2606-UGA-2608) in the sequence AUGA (**Fig. 1**) suggests that RDRP is translated by an internal initiation mechanism.

Double-stranded RNA Replication

Information on the replication cycle of totivirus dsRNA has mainly been derived from *in vitro* studies of virion-associated RNA polymerase activity and the isolation of particles representing various stages in the replication cycle. In *in vitro* reactions, the RNA polymerase activity associated with virions of the fungal totiviruses ScV-L-A, UmV-H1 and HvV-190S, isolated from lag phase cultures, catalyzes end-to-end transcription of dsRNA, by a conservative mechanism, to produce mRNA for capsid polypeptide, which is released from the particles. Purified ScV-L-A virions, isolated from log phase cells, contain a less dense class of particles which package only (+)-strand RNA. In *in vitro* reactions, these particles exhibit a replicase activity that catalyzes the synthesis of (−)-strand RNA to form dsRNA. The resultant mature particles, which attain the same density as that of the dsRNA-containing virions isolated from the cells, are capable of synthesizing and releasing (+)-strand RNA.

A proposed life cycle of Hv190SV is depicted in **Fig. 2**. Host-encoded protein kinase and protease have been shown to be involved in post-translational modification of CP. Phosphorylation and proteolytic

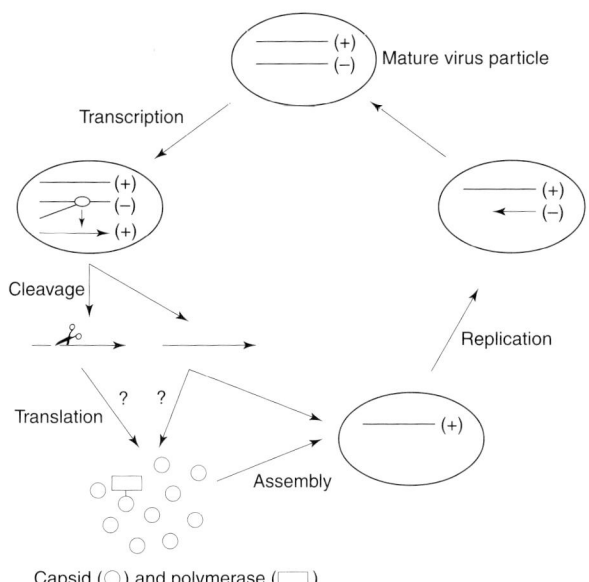

Figure 3 Replication cycle of leishmaniaviruses.

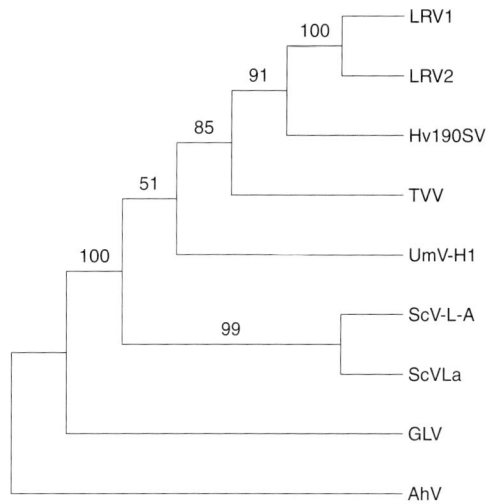

Figure 4 Phylogeny estimates of totiviruses derived from aligned deduced amino acid sequences of RDRP. The resulting consensus tree of 100 bootstrap replicates is shown; the number above each node indicates the percent of bootstrap replicates in which that node was recovered. Tree was outgroup-rooted to the partitivirus Atkinsonella hypoxylon virus (AhV). See **Table 1** for abbreviations of totivirus names.

processing are proposed to play a role in the virus life cycle; phosphorylation of CP may be necessary for its interaction with viral nucleic acid and for subsequent assembly into virions, and/or phosphorylation may regulate dsRNA transcription/replication. Proteolytic processing and cleavage of a C-terminal peptide, which leads to dephosphorylation and the conversion of p88 to p78, may play a role in the release of the (+)-strand RNA transcripts from virions (**Fig. 2**).

Leishmaniaviruses have a slight variation in their life cycle from the other totiviruses. The CP has endoribonuclease activity which is responsible for cleaving 320 nt from the 5' end of the full-length single-stranded (+)-sense RNA. It has been hypothesized that the cleavage activity generates the functional message by removing translation inhibitory sequences. The proposed life cycle is depicted in **Fig. 3**.

Evolutionary Relationships among Totiviruses

Sequence comparison analysis of the predicted amino acid sequences of totivirus RDRPs indicated that they share significant sequence similarity and characteristically contain eight conserved motifs. This sequence similarity was common to the totiviruses that infect the yeast and smut fungi as well as those infecting parasitic protozoa. The RDRP of Hv190SV, a recently characterized totivirus that infects a filamentous ascomycetous fungus, was also found to contain the same eight conserved motifs. The sequence similarity among the RDRPs of these viruses infecting simple eucaryotes extends beyond the highly conserved eight motifs. Of the 70 amino acid positions contained in these conserved motifs, the Hv190SV RDRP is identical in 48, 47, 46, 40, 38 and 21 positions, respectively, to the RDRPs of LRV1, TVV, ScV-L-A, UmVH1, ScV-La and GLV.

Phylogeny estimates derived from multiple alignments of totivirus RDRP ORFs (**Fig. 4**) indicated that the two leishmaniaviruses LRV1 and LRV2 (percent sequence identities of 46%) are most closely related to each other. This is also true for the two yeast viruses ScV-L-A and ScV-La (identity of 32%). It is of considerable interest that Hv190SV, a mycovirus infecting a filamentous fungus, was found to be a sister clade to the leishmaniaviruses and not to the yeast viruses (**Fig. 4**).

Transmission and Host Range

There are no known natural vectors for the transmission of the fungal totiviruses. They are transmitted intracellularly during cell division, sporogenesis and cell fusion. Although the yeast viruses are effectively transmitted via ascospores, the totiviruses infecting the ascomycetous filamentous fungi, e.g. GgV-87-1-H, are essentially eliminated during ascospore formation. The leishmaniaviruses are not infectious and are propagated during cell division. Like other totiviruses, the leishmaniaviruses have no extracellular phase to their life cycles. Successful transfection of the protozoa *Giardia lamblia*, however, has been accomplished via electroporation with (+)-strand RNA transcribed *in vitro* from GLV dsRNA.

There are no known experimental host ranges for the fungal totiviruses because of the lack of suitable infectivity assays. As a consequence of their intracellular modes of transmission, the natural host ranges of totiviruses are limited to individuals within the same or closely related vegetative compatibility groups. Furthermore, mixed infections with two or more unrelated viruses are common, probably as a consequence of the ways by which fungal viruses are transmitted in nature. Dual infection of yeast with ScV-L-A and ScV-L-BC is an example of mixed infection involving totiviruses. Leishmaniaviruses have been found in *L. braziliensis*, *L. guyanensis* and *L. major*.

Virus–Host Relationships

The yeast killer system, comprised of a helper totivirus (ScV-L-A) and associated satellite dsRNA (M-dsRNA), is one of a very few known examples where virus infection is beneficial to the host. The ability to produce killer toxins by immune yeast strains confers an ecological advantage over sensitive strains. The use of killer strains in the brewing industry provides protection against contamination with adventitious sensitive strains.

Totiviruses maintain only the genes that are essential for their survival (*RDRP* and *CP*), but make efficient use of host proteins. The host cells have evolved to support only a defined level of virus replication, beyond which virus infection may become pathogenic. Because of amenability to genetic studies, the yeast–virus system has provided significant information on the host genes required to prevent viral cytopathology. A system of six chromosomal genes, designated superkiller (or *SKI*) *SKI2*, *SKI3*, *SKI4*, *SKI6*, *SKI7* and *SKI8*, negatively control the copy number of the ScV-L-A totivirus and its satellite M-dsRNAs. The only essential function of these genes is to block virus multiplication. Mutations in any of these *SKI* genes lead to the development of the superkiller phenotype as a result of the increased copy number of M-dsRNA. The *SKI* genes affect primarily the initiation of translation rather than the stability of mRNA, and are thus part of a cellular system that specifically blocks translation of nonpolyadenylated mRNAs (like the (+)-strand transcripts of totiviruses). About 30 chromosomal genes, termed *MAK* genes (for maintenance of killer), are required for stable replication of the satellite M-dsRNA. Only three of these *MAK* genes are necessary for the helper virus (ScV-L-A) multiplication. Mutants defective in any of 20 *MAK* genes show a decreased level of free 60S ribosomal subunits. Since the *mak* mutations affecting 60S subunit levels are known to be suppressed by *ski* mutations, and since the latter are now known to act by blocking translation of nonpolyadenylated mRNAs, the level of 60S ribosomal subunits is believed to be also critical for translation of nonpolyadenylated mRNAs.

The Hv190S totivirus that infects the plant pathogenic fungus *Helminthosporium victoriae* utilizes host-encoded proteins (a protein kinase and a protease) for post-translational modification of its CP. Phosphorylation and proteolytic processing of CP may play a role in regulating transcription and the release of (+)-strand transcripts from virions (**Fig. 2**).

See also: Cryptoviruses (*Cryptoviridae*); Hypoviruses (*Hypoviridae*); Partitiviruses – fungal (*Partitiviridae*); Giardiaviruses (*Totiviridae*); *Ustilago maydis* viruses; Yeast RNA viruses (*Totiviridae*).

Further Reading

Ghabrial SA (1994) New developments in fungal virology. *Adv. Virus Res.* 43: 303.

Ghabrial SA (1998) Origin, adaptation and evolutionary pathways of fungal viruses. *Virus Genes* 16: 119.

Ghabrial SA, Bruenn JA, Buck KW et al (1995) Totiviridae. In: Murphy F et al (eds) *Virus Taxonomy: Sixth Report of the International Committee on Taxonomy of Viruses*. p. 245. New York: Springer.

Patterson JL (1990) Viruses of protozoan parasites. *Exp. Parasitol.* 70: 111.

Patterson JL (1993) The current status of leishmania RNA virus 1. *Parasitol. Today* 9: 135.

Ustilago Maydis Viruses

Jeremy Bruenn, Department of Biological Sciences, SUNY/Buffalo, Buffalo, USA

Copyright © 1999 Academic Press

Taxonomy

The *Totiviridae* is a remarkable family of fungal and protozoan viruses. These viruses have a single essential double-stranded RNA (dsRNA) and are recognizably related to each other as viewed by comparison of their RNA-dependent RNA polymerases (RDRPs). They have been discovered in at least four genera of protozoans (*Leishmania*, *Eimeria*, *Giardiavirus* and *Trichomonas*) and nine genera of fungi (*Saccharomyces*, *Ustilago*, *Helminthosporium*, *Gaeumannomyces*, *Mycogone*, *Yarrowia*, *Aspergil-*

lus, Thielaviopsis, and probably *Agaricus*). *Ustilago maydis* viruses are in the *Totivirus* genus of the *Totiviridae* family.

Characteristics of the Host Fungus

The fungus *Ustilago maydis* belongs to the class Basidiomycetes and the family Ustilaginaceae. Its life cycle has three phases: diploid, haploid and dikaryon. While dikaryon formation and development is restricted to host tissue, the diploid and haploid mycelia may grow rapidly in a yeast-like manner in laboratory media. A transient dikaryon (or heterokaryon) may be formed between compatible strains on laboratory medium. *U. maydis* is heterothallic. Sexual reproduction between two haploid strains depends on two unlinked genes. The *a* gene has two alleles and the *b* gene has multiple alleles. Cells with opposite *a* alleles will fuse under appropriate conditions to form a heterokaryon which will infect the host and allow the completion of the life cycle only if the *b* alleles are also different. The *a* gene can, therefore, be regarded as the mating type locus homologous to the simple two-allele mating systems of most yeasts, whereas the *b* gene controls the development of the dikaryon in infected host cells, which is the only place that sexual development can proceed.

Virion Structure and Composition

All the dsRNA viruses are now known to have at least one capsid polypeptide present in 120 copies per virion. This is unique among icosohedral viruses and superficially appears to violate the Caspar and Klug rules for assembly of isometric virus particles. However, in the one case where the x-ray crystal structure of the virion has been determined (Bluetongue virus, or BTV), this apparent $T = 2$ symmetry is really a twofold $T = 1$ symmetry, in which 60 of the subunits adopt one configuration and 60 another. Hence, even though there are 120 copies of the virion protein, half of them are in one conformation and half in the other.

The totiviruses are small icosohedral viruses. *Ustilago maydis* virus (UmV) is about 41 nM in diameter, sedimenting at 172 S and with a buoyant density in CsCl of 1.42 g ml^{-1}. In UmV the capsid polypeptide is about 75 kDa, but no accurate estimate of its size is available. In the one case where the sequence of its coding RNA is known (P1H1), the C-terminus of the protein appears to be generated by cleavage, and the cleavage site has not been determined. Electron microscopy, in the case of UmV and *Saccharomyces cerevisiae* virus (ScV), has demonstrated that there are 120 copies of a single polypeptide in their capsids, arranged as 12 pentamers of dimers of the capsid polypeptide. Presumably, as in BTV, these adopt two configurations in equal numbers in the capsid. In ScV, two of the capsid monomers are thought to be the N-terminal portions of a capsid polypeptide–RDRP fusion protein. Since the P1H1 capsid polypeptide is initially synthesized as such a fusion prior to (presumed) cleavage, this is likely for UmV as well.

Ustilago Maydis Viruses

Most fungal dsRNA viruses do not confer on their host cells any characteristic phenotype. They are persistent, segmented dsRNA viruses whose segments are separately encapsidated and whose only means of transmission is mitosis or meiosis. However, ScV and UmV are known to encode killer toxins, which are thought to provide a selective advantage to cells harboring the responsible viruses.

Interstrain inhibition (the killing phenomenon) in *U. maydis* was discovered by Puhalla during heterokaryon experiments. The inhibitory factor (killer toxin) was shown to be a secreted protein or proteins. Crosses and heterokaryon transfer experiments showed that the inhibitory effect is caused by cytoplasmically inherited factors, which are now known to be single dsRNA segments present in some multisegmented dsRNA viral genomes (see below). A small proportion of *U. maydis* cells (about 1%) can produce killer toxins, to which they are resistant; sensitive cells are the majority in wild populations. There are also some cells that do not have killing ability but are resistant to one toxin. Killer toxins are known in eight genera of yeasts, but the killer toxins of *Ustilago* are the only ones known in a filamentous fungus. The *U. maydis* killer toxins are effective against species in the family Ustilaginaceae, including those that are known as pathogens to wheat, oats and barley.

There are three killer types: KP1, KP4 and KP6, which secrete KP1, KP4 and KP6 toxins, respectively. Correspondingly, there are three groups of resistant cells, in which the resistance is determined by three independent recessive nuclear genes: *p1r*, *p4r* and *p6r*. In KP1, cytoplasmically inherited factors also confer immunity to the KP1 killer toxin. KP4 probably has no cytoplasmically determined immunity, and recent experiments show that KP6 has no cytoplasmically determined immunity. Cells cannot produce the KP6 toxin unless they have the *p6r* gene, and the same is probably true of KP4. The *p1r*, *p4r* and *p6r* genes are thought to encode cellular (membrane, or membrane–cell wall) receptors for the toxin. Since these putative receptors are different in each case, there is no crossresistance to the toxins. The KP6 receptor is apparently recognized by cytoplasmic toxin polypeptides as well as by toxin in the medium. There are no single resistance alleles that confer simultaneous resistance to all three toxins.

Structure and Function of the Killer Toxins

KP6

The three-dimensional structures of two of the *Ustilago* toxin polypeptides have been determined. The crystal structure of KP6α (space group $P6_322$, a = 48.3 Å, c = 124.8 Å) was determined by use of heavy atom isomorphous techniques and by selenomethionine substitution (R-factor = 0.169, resolution 1.8 Å). The monomer has a three finger structure similar to neurotoxins and cardiotoxins and is composed of a four stranded antiparallel β sheet with two α helices on one side, an additional β strand, and a small α-helix segment at the N-terminus. Three intermolecular salt bridges link monomers of KP6α into trimers organized around a threefold segment axis. The trimer has a funnel shape that is wide across the mouth and narrows to a 3.2 Å opening just large enough to permit an ion to pass.

The trimer has many structural features that have been postulated to be critical elements in pore domains of mammalian ion channels, including a solvent-filled funnel lined with charged amino acid residues that could be a selectivity screen for specific ions and a network of salt bridges that stabilize the timer. The 3.2 Å funnel bore is lined by six phenyl rings. These phenyl rings arise in part from a GFG sequence in KP6α that may correspond to a G(Y/F)G sequence that is conserved in K^+ channels. These phenyl groups in KP6α form a cage similar to one postulated to be responsible for K^+ selectivity relative to Na^+ on the basis of *ab initio* calculations. In crystals two trimers are related by a twofold axis perpendicular to the funnel axis, generating a symmetric pair of funnels. The hexamer has dimensions and characteristics that suggest it is a self-assembling ion pore closely resembling the pore (H5) commonly found in voltage-gated and inwardly-rectifying ion channels. The open ends of the two funnels would lie on the bilayer surface and the narrow bore would be at the center of the bilayer. The salt bridges that hold the trimers together are separated by 30 Å and portions of the funnel would extend well out of the membrane.

KP6β may be a functional analogue of the transmembrane strands that are thought to flank the pore in mammalian ion channels and facilitate entry of the pore into the membrane. The structure of KP6β has been modeled upon that of KP6α by examining sequence similarities. Examination of the stereochemical topology of the KP6α hexamer and the KP6β monomer and the charge distribution on their surfaces suggested a model for a dodecamer composed of six molecules of KP6α (as observed in the crystal structure) surrounded by six molecules of KP6β. The resultant $KP6\alpha_6\beta_6$ dodecamer has an outer surface that is essentially neutral and compatible with membrane insertion. The interface between the observed hexamer of KP6α and the modeled hexamer of KP6β exhibits excellent complementarity in surface charge and stereochemistry. Preliminary experiments with planar lipid bilayers are consistent with the KP6 toxin functioning as a channel-former.

KP4

The structure of KP4 was determined to 1.9 Å resolution and is now refined to 1.4 Å using a single isomorphous derivative, with phases improved using real space averaging. KP4 belongs to the α/β sandwich family of proteins and has a double split β-α-β motif. The toxin has a total of seven β strands and three α helices, with the major secondary structure elements consisting of five antiparallel stranded β sheets ($\beta1$, $\beta3$, $\beta4$, $\beta6$, $\beta7$) with two antiparallel α helices ($\alpha2$, $\alpha3$) lying at approximately 45° to the strands in the β sheet. The *U. maydis* KP4 killer toxin and the *Pichia farinosa* KK1 toxin have no evident primary sequence similarity, but their tertiary structures are essentially identical even though KP4 is a single polypeptide and KK1 is two polypeptides. Thus KP4 appears from its structure to be a tandem duplication of one sequence which has subsequently diverged, and it could easily have arisen from two polypeptides processed by Kex2p by a single deletion of the genomic sequence encoding the intervening sequence and the cleavage sites in the prepropolypeptide. This would conveniently explain the absence of Kex2p processing of KP4.

The scorpion toxins are a family of neurotoxins with some interesting similarities to KP4. Albeit about half the size of KP4, the long toxins are similar to KP4 in that they are all highly basic proteins that are stabilized by an extensive network of disulfide bonds. The core motif of the α and β neurotoxins are quite similar and the functional differences between them may lie in the length and orientation of protruding loops extending from this core region. In light of this tenuous similarity to the scorpion toxins, KP4 killing efficacy was tested on sensitive *Ustilago* cells. Cells were rescued by very small concentrations of Ca^{2+} but not with similar concentrations of monovalent cations.

These rescue experiment results strongly suggested

that KP4 affects Ca^{2+} channels. Therefore, the effect of KP4 was tested on mammalian cells lines where more is known about the types and kinetics of cationic channels. Standard whole-cell patch clamp techniques were used to examine the effects of KP4 on voltage-activated Na^+, K^+, Ca^{2+} currents in PC12, GH_3 and adrenal chromaffin cells, and the prevalent action of KP4 was inhibition of voltage-activated Ca^{2+}-channel currents.

Genome Structure and Translation

The UmV viral genomes consist of three distinct size groups of dsRNAs. They are heavy (H), medium (M) and light (L). Three original isolates (named after the killer toxins they encoded) were named P1, P4 and P6. Cells may have as few as three viral dsRNAs (some isolates of P6 strains) or as many as seven viral dsRNAs (some isolates of P4 strains). The H segments appear to encode the essential viral polypeptides: a capsid polypeptide and an RDRP. One of the H1 segments has been sequenced: P1H1 is 6099 bp, and encodes on one open reading frame (540–5999) a polypeptide of 1820 amino acids with a putative capsid polypeptide in the N-terminal region and a typical RDRP sequence in the C-terminal thousand amino acids. P1H1 and P6H1 are nearly identical in sequence, while P1H1 and P1H2 share about 31% amino acid sequence identity in the RDRP region. This is consistent with there being at least two totiviruses in *Ustilago* (H1 and H2), which is similar to the ScVL1 (ScVL-A) and ScVLa (ScVL-BC) viruses in *S. cerevisiae*. Processing of the P1H1 polypeptide is proposed to occur by self-cleavage.

One or more of the M segments in each subtype encode the toxin. By sequence analysis of both the toxin polypeptides and P6M2 and synthesis of toxin in heterologous (yeast and tobacco) and homologous cDNA expression vectors, as well as immunological evidence, the KP6 coding region in P6M2 has been completely defined. P6M2 is 1234 bp, encoding a preprotoxin of 219 amino acids, which is subsequently processed by signal peptide cleavage after residue 19, Kex2p cleavage after residues 27, 108 and 138, and Kex1p cleavage after residue 137 to yield two polypeptides, α of 79 amino acids (8.6 kDa), and β of 81 amino acids (9.1 kDa).

Similarly, P4M2, of 1006 bp, encodes the KP4 preprotoxin of 127 amino acids, which is processed solely by signal peptidase cleavage after residue 22, yielding a toxin of 105 amino acids (11.1 kDa). The KP4 toxin has been expressed from cDNA clones in yeast, tobacco and *Pichia pastoris*.

P1M2, of 1034 bp, encodes the KP1 toxin, which is synthesized as a preprotoxin of 291 amino acids. The KP1 preprotoxin is processed by signal peptidase (24), Kex2p (142 and 173), and Kex1p (141), resulting in an α peptide of 117 amino acids and a β peptide of 118 amino acids (13.4 kDa). Only β is necessary for activity.

All the *Ustilago* toxin peptides are small, highly stable proteins in which all the cysteines appear to be in disulfides. KP6α has four disulfides, KP6β three, KP4 five, and KP1β three. None of the *Ustilago* toxin polypeptides is glycosylated, although KP6α and KP1β have possible N-linked glycosylation sites, and the KP6α site is utilized in *S. cerevisiae*. None of the M segments (including P1M1) have detectable sequence similarities at either the nucleotide level or the protein level, except in the 3′ region of the plus strand, from which the L segments are derived.

The L segments (355 bp) are derived from the 3′ ends of the plus strands of M segments: P6L from P6M2, P1L from P1M1, and P4L from P4M2. Neither the mode of synthesis of these segments nor their function is understood. All the L segments share a great deal of sequence identity (50–95% at the nucleotide level). In general, homologous P1 and P4 segments are very close in sequence (the L segments are 95% identical), while the homologous P6 segments are more divergent. The highest conservation of sequence among P6M2, P1M1 and P4M2 is within 20 bases on either side of the region of M encoding the 5′ end of the L plus strand. This suggests that the L segments are derived by replication of cleavage products of M plus strands (see below).

Complete sequences are known for the following *Ustilago* dsRNAs: P1H1 (6099 bp), P6M2 (1234 bp), P6L (355 bp), P4M2 (1006 bp), P4L (354 bp), P1M1 (1504 bp), P1M2 (1034 bp) and P1L (354 bp). Partial sequences are available for P6H1 and P4H1. P1M1 could encode two secreted polypeptides of 81 amino acids and 143 amino acids after signal peptidase and Kex2 cleavage, but neither peptide has been detected as a component of the P1 toxin (**Fig. 1**).

Replication and Transcription

All dsRNA viruses separate transcription from replication by packaging. Viral plus strands are synthesized in viral particles and extruded into the cell cytoplasm. These have two fates: translation and packaging. Viral plus strands that are packaged into nascent particles are subsequently replicated (by synthesis of the minus strand) after packaging is complete. In ScV, the packaging signal is a small (20 base) sequence. The identity of the packaging signal in UmV is unknown. However, all sequenced UmV

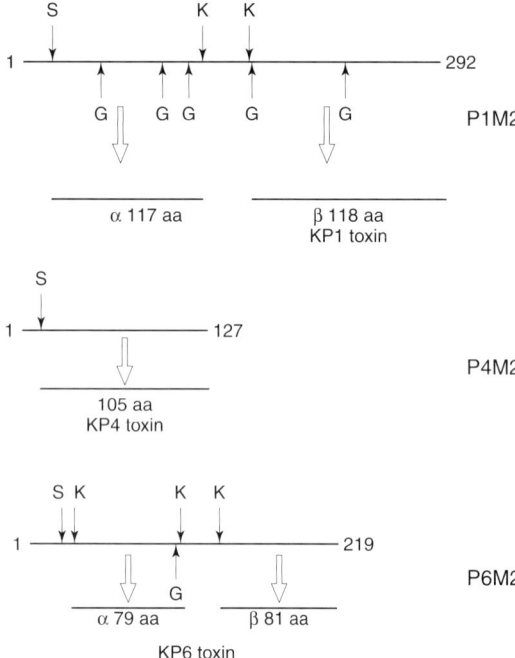

Figure 1 Processing of the KP1, KP4 and KP6 killer toxins, encoded by P1M2, P4M2 and P6M2 respectively. Processing by signal peptidase is indicated by S and processing by Kex2 by K. Possible sites of N-linked glycosylation are shown by G, but none of these sites is glycosylated in the mature peptides.

RNAs have the sequence GAAAAA at the 5' end and AUGCA$_{OH}$ at the 3' end of the plus strand, except for the L segments. These have the sequence UCCG at the 5' end of the plus strand. Since the 5' sequence GAAAAA is common among the fungal dsRNA viruses, and since the complementary region of the minus strand is required for transcriptase activity at least in ScV, this has been taken to be the required start for transcription.

The absence of this sequence in the L segments and their highly conserved sequences around the position of the 5' end of the L plus strand within M probably indicate that the L segments are generated by cleavage of the M plus strand followed by replication. This hypothesis is further supported by the presence of a long putative double-stranded region (a stem) immediately adjacent to the putative site of cleavage. In P4M2, this stem is a remarkable 23 uninterrupted base pairs in length.

Replication and transcription in dsRNA viruses may be either conservative or semiconservative. That is, the plus strand extruded during transcription may be either the parental strand (semiconservative) or the newly synthesized strand (conservative). Replication is conservative in ScV, but for at least one UmV segment, the M2 dsRNA, replication is semiconservative.

Evolution

Due to the extant similarities among totiviruses present in divergent phyla, ranging from protozoans parasitic to animals (*Leishmania*) to fungi parasitic to plants (*Ustilago*), and the fact that these viruses are not infectious but have only vertical transmission, they are thought to have originated very early in evolution, prior to the differentiation of multicellular from single-celled eucaryotes. Sequence relationships among the totivirus RDRPs support this model. For instance, the closest relative of UmVP1H2 is ScVLa, even though UmVP1H1 and UmVP1H2 are present in the same *Ustilago* cells while ScVLa and ScVL1 are present in the same *S. cerevisiae* cells. Similarly, another fungal totivirus (from *Helminthosporium*) is more closely related to the protozoan totiviruses than to the other fungal totiviruses. Although the totiviruses are noninfectious, the closely related *Giardiavirus* is infectious, and both ScV and UmV have been shown to be infectious, albeit very inefficiently, to spheroplasts. These experiments have selected for transformation by *S. cerevisiae* or *U. maydis* DNA plasmids in the presence of purified virus, using recipient cells lacking the viruses. A small percentage of the selected transformants carry the virus. Hence the cell wall (in fungi) or the cell membrane (in protozoans) seems to limit infection.

Geographic Distribution

The same UmV isolates are present in *Ustilago* from Mexico, the USA, the UK, Poland and China. So far only three toxin specificities have been found. Protein purification and sequencing has demonstrated a toxin with the same N-terminus as KP4 in Korea.

Economic Significance

Ustilago is a pathogen on a number of grain crops, the most important of which is maize. It does cause major crop losses of sweet corn. Although UmV has no apparent effect on the virulence of its host, it may be possible to introduce the viral killer toxin genes into the plants, making them resistant to the fungus. The UmV toxins of *U. maydis* are particularly attractive as biological control agents because they have no known effects when ingested. The UmV toxins can be effective against a wide range of *Ustilago* species known to be crop pathogens, including pathogens of maize, wheat, oats and barley. The UmV toxins should therefore be very useful as a means of introducing novel resistance to the ustilaginales into plants, provided the toxins can be expressed at high levels, are correctly processed, and end up in cellular or extracellular compartments where they can inhibit growth of the fungus.

The KP6 and KP4 toxins have been successfully expressed in transgenic tobacco plants, so this may be a possible strategy. Tobacco plants are capable of correctly synthesizing, processing and secreting KP6 toxin polypeptides with the same activity and specificity as the authentic KP6 toxin produced by *U. maydis*. The activity of toxin produced is rather low (about 200-fold lower than in *Ustilago*), possibly due to incorrect processing of the C-terminus of α. Tobacco plants produce about 500 times as much KP4 activity from the same expression vector as that used for KP6. Toxin activity is easily detected at the surface of leaves of transgenic KP4 tobacco plants. Transgenic maize plants expressing genes for both KP4 and KP6 toxins could be resistant to all but a fraction of a percent of the natural *U. maydis* population. Since ingested UmV toxins have no toxic effects on human cells, they would be safe for consumption and have less environmental impact than the fungicides currently used to deter fungal pathogens.

See also: **Cypoviruses (*Reoviridae*); Giardiaviruses (*Totiviridae*); Totiviruses (*Totiviridae*): General features; Partitiviruses – fungal (*Partitiviridae*); Phage ϕ6 (*Cystoviridae*); Reoviruses (*Reoviridae*): General features, Molecular biology, Plant reoviruses; Virus structure: Atomic structure; Yeast RNA viruses (*Totiviridae*).**

Further Reading

Bruenn JA (1993) A closely related group of RNA-dependent RNA polymerases from double-stranded RNA viruses. *Nucleic Acids Res.* 21: 5667.

Gu F, Khimani A, Rane S *et al* (1995) Structure and function of a virally encoded fungal toxin from *Ustilago maydis*: a fungal and mammalian Ca^{2+} channel inhibitor. *Structure* 3: 805.

Kinal H, Park C-M, Berry JO, Koltin Y and Bruenn JA (1995) Processing and secretion of a virally encoded antifungal toxin in transgenic plants: evidence for a Kex2p pathway in plants. *Plant Cell* 7: 677.

Park C-M, Bruenn JA, Ganesa C *et al* (1994) Structure and heterologous expression of the *Ustilago maydis* viral toxin KP4. *Mol. Microbiol.* 11: 155.

Park C-M, Banerjee N, Koltin Y and Bruenn JA (1996) The *Ustilago maydis* virally encoded KP1 killer toxin. *Mol. Microbiol.* 20: 957.

Tao J, Ginsberg I, Banerjee N *et al* (1990) The *Ustilago maydis* KP6 killer toxin: structure, expression in *Saccharomyces cerevisiae* and relationship to other cellular toxins. *Mol. Cell. Biol.* 10: 1373.

TRANSFORMATION – ANIMAL VIRUSES

Ron Wisdom, Department of Biochemistry, Vanderbilt University School of Medicine, Nashville, Tennessee, USA

Inder M Verma, The Salk Institute, San Diego, California, USA

Copyright © 1999 Academic Press

Introduction

The observation that certain viruses rapidly and reproducibly induce tumors in the host was first made nearly a century ago. The ability to accurately duplicate this process in tissue culture has made possible the investigation of neoplastic transformation *in vitro*. This, in turn, has allowed the techniques of molecular biology and genetics to be applied to the problem of cancer, especially cancer induced by viruses. Much of our current knowledge of the molecular mechanisms of cancer today is derived from the study of virally induced tumors. Virus-induced tumors are not only important as laboratory tools for investigation of the fundamental mechanisms of tumor formation; some human cancers, including hepatocellular carcinoma, cervical carcinoma, Burkitt's lymphoma and acute T-cell leukemia, appear to have a viral etiology.

The types of viruses that are capable of inducing tumors are remarkably diverse, and include viruses with RNA and DNA genomes. Nonetheless, certain common features have emerged from the study of neoplastic transformation by different viruses. The first is that tumor formation induced by viruses is the result of the acquisition by the host cell of the viral genome. In all cases of virally induced tumors so far described, at least a part of the viral genome is present. Furthermore, the continued expression of at least a part of the viral genome is required for the transformed phenotype to be present. In the case of the transforming RNA viruses, the viral genome is present in the form of a DNA provirus integrated into the host genetic material. An important consequence of the presence of the viral genetic material is the fact that the transformed phenotype induced by the virus is heritable.

Cancer cells show many properties that distinguish them from normal cells. The hallmark of malignant cells is their ability to grow in the absence of appropriate signals from the extracellular environment. While the extracellular signals that are either not sensed or not required may vary from tumor to tumor, the property of malignancy is cell autonomous, that is, it is a property of the transformed cell and not the surrounding normal tissue. Genetic events that give rise to cancer, then, alter the cellular response to external stimuli. The investigation of cancer over the last decade has served to outline a cell signaling pathway that allows cells to respond to changes in the external environment. Support for the idea that this signaling pathway is the direct target for cancer-inducing mutations has been found in a wide range of both viral and nonviral tumors.

Retroviruses

The study of retroviruses has contributed more to our understanding of cancer than the study of any other group of viruses. The relevant features of the retroviral life cycle involve reverse transcription of the RNA genome into double-stranded proviral DNA, integration of the proviral DNA in the host genome, and expression of the viral genome from the chromosomal site of integration. The retroviruses have been of particular importance for several reasons. First, the small size of the retroviral genome and the small number of proteins expressed from the retroviral genome (a transforming retrovirus frequently encodes only one protein) has made them experimentally favorable for molecular analysis. Second, the proteins that produce neoplastic transformation are not required for the virus to complete its life cycle. Third, the retroviral transforming genes are mutated forms of normal cellular genes, giving their study direct relevance to nonviral forms of tumor formation.

Retroviruses can be divided into those that induce transformation acutely (in days to weeks) and form polyclonal tumors, and those that induce transformation over long periods of time (months) and form monoclonal or oligoclonal tumors. The distinction is important because the mechanism of tumorigenesis is fundamentally different in the two cases. Acutely transforming retroviruses consist of a mixture of replication-defective viruses that contain the transforming activity, and replication-competent non-transforming (helper) viruses that serve to propagate the transforming virus. The transforming virus in these cases often encodes only a single protein, and it is this protein that has the oncogenic activity. These transforming viruses are potent carcinogens, in the sense that the infection of a cell is sufficient to induce transformation with a very short latency. The transforming viral genes are transduced mutated copies of cellular genes, and the transforming proteins correspond to mutant versions of the corresponding cellular proteins. Structural and functional analyses of the viral and cellular forms of transforming proteins allow elucidation of the features that convert a normal cellular protein into an oncogenic one.

In contrast to the acutely transforming retroviruses, the retroviruses that induce tumors only after long latency have several important distinctions. They are replication-competent viruses that have not transduced cellular genes and so do not contain a transforming gene. Tumor formation by these viruses is often the result of the mutation of cellular genes during the integration process. Expression of cellular proto-oncogenes may be transcriptionally activated by the occasional nearby integration of retroviral promoter and enhancer elements, as in the case with c-*myc* activation by avian leukosis virus (ALV) and murine leukemia virus (MLV). As retroviruses integrate into a wide range of sites in the host DNA, only rare integration events will give rise to the activation of a protooncogene, explaining the long latency and the monoclonal nature of the tumors. In addition to being potentially tumorigenic, the juxtaposition of the retroviral transcriptional control signals with cellular protooncogenes may be of importance for a second reason. It is likely that production of a fusion virus–oncogene mRNA is the first step in the viral transduction event that results in the generation of an acutely transforming retrovirus through an aberrant viral recombination event.

Cell signaling

The ability of cells to respond to their external environment is mediated by the interaction of factors outside the cell (peptide and nonpeptide hormones and growth factors, cell matrix and other cells) with specific receptors located on the cell surface. These cell surface receptors contain at least two distinct functions. First, they contain a ligand-binding function which allows sensing of the presence or absence of the appropriate factor in the external environment, and second, they contain or control some type of enzymatic activity that generates an intracellular change in response to the presence of the ligand. Often, this signal is in the form of reversible phosphorylation in response to ligand. The initial signal frequently generates a cascade of intracellular events, which include the generation of small molecule second messengers, such as cyclic nucleotides, calcium ions, and phospholipids, the activation of signals generated by the small GTP-binding proteins, and the activation of other protein kinases. Any long-lasting change in cell behavior, such as growth, requires new gene expression, and an important consequence of the signaling cascade is the activation of a set of transcription factors that directly influence the expression of genes required to alter cell behavior. Theoretically, it should be possible to generate mutant cells defective in the response to extracellular changes by alteration or mutation in any part of the signaling pathway, and the last ten years has witnessed the experimental confirmation of this idea. Thus, neoplastic transformation can be due to mutations in proteins that function as autocrine growth factors, growth factor receptors, membrane-bound and cytoplasmic components of the cell signaling apparatus, and transcription factors, all the normal activities of which are subject to control by changes in the external environment.

Growth factors and receptors

The simian sarcoma virus (SSV) contains a single open reading frame and encodes a single protein (v-Sis). This protein is a fusion protein between the retroviral *env* gene product and the product of a gene derived from the c-*sis* gene of the SSV host, the woolly monkey. The *env* sequences comprise little besides the signal sequence of the Env protein, and the remainder of the protein is the product of the transduced c-*sis* gene. Nucleotide sequence analysis has shown that c-*sis* is the platelet-derived growth factor (PDGF) B chain gene. The v-Sis protein is therefore a form of PDGF, a peptide mitogen for a number of cell types. That the v-*sis* gene product functions as an autocrine growth factor to induce transformation is supported by several lines of evidence. Transformation by v-Sis is limited to cells that express the PDGF receptor. The PDGF receptor is a protein tyrosine kinase the activity of which is dependent on the presence of ligand. In v-Sis-transformed cells, there is increased activity of the PDGF receptor and an increase in total cellular phosphotyrosine-containing proteins when compared to nontransformed cells. As both the v-Sis protein and the PDGF receptor are present in the endoplasmic reticulum, binding and activation of the receptor may occur at sites other than the cell surface. That this is the case is suggested by the observation that activated intracellular forms of the receptor can be found in v-Sis-transformed cells, but not in cells exposed to PDGF. Therefore, the v-*sis* gene product functions as an autocrine growth factor in susceptible cells.

A second class of oncogenic mutations predicted from the cell signaling model outlined above are mutations that separate activation of growth factor receptors from the binding of ligand. The first described example of such a mutation was the v-*erbB* gene of avian erythroblastosis virus (AEV). The v-*erbB* gene is a virally transduced mutant form of the cellular epidermal growth factor (EGF) receptor. AEV infection of chickens results in the rapid induction of erythroblastosis, and although AEV carries a second gene (v-*erbA*), expression of v-*erbB* is necessary and sufficient for the induction of erythroblastosis. The EGF receptor is typical of many growth factor receptors in its molecular architecture. It contains an extracellular domain involved in ligand (EGF) binding, a hydrophobic membrane-spanning domain, a cytoplasmic domain that contains protein tyrosine kinase activity and a C-terminal region involved in regulation of the kinase activity. Several observations suggest that the v-ErbB protein is a constitutively active form of the EGF receptor. In comparison to the EGF receptor, v-ErbB has suffered several structural changes. These include deletion of the extracellular ligand-binding domain and alterations of the C-terminal regulatory region. Molecular analysis has shown that both of these alterations are important for the transforming activity of the protein. Consistent with its proposed function, v-ErbB shows protein tyrosine kinase activity in the absence of EGF, and AEV-transformed cells show increased phospho-tyrosine-containing proteins when compared to non-transformed cells. All mutations that impair the kinase activity of v-ErbB impair the transforming activity of the virus in a coordinate manner. Thus, the v-*erbB* oncogene product is a ligand-independent form of the EGF receptor.

Intracellular signal transduction molecules

A number of retroviral oncogenes have been identified that function as intracellular effectors of changes in the external environment. The v-Src protein of Rous sarcoma virus (RSV) is a cytoplasmic tyrosine kinase anchored to the inner surface of the plasma membrane by an N-terminal modification by myristic acid addition. The v-Src protein contains several mutations when compared to c-Src. Important among these is mutation of a C-terminal tyrosine in c-Src that serves as a negative regulator of the c-Src tyrosine kinase activity. Although it is not known what the physiologic mechanisms are for activating c-Src tyrosine kinase activity, v-Src functions as a constitutively activated enzyme, and RSV-transformed cells contain increased amounts of phosphotyrosine-containing proteins. An additional important feature in the Src protein is the presence of regulatory sequences known as SH2 and SH3 domains. These domains were initially recognized as conserved motifs in other proteins, first in tyrosine kinases and then in other molecules, including the v-crk oncogene and a number of substrates for tyrosine kinase enzymes, such as phospholipase C, phosphatidylinositol 3'-kinase (PI3 kinase), and the ras GTPase-activating protein (GAP). The investigation of the v-crk oncogene has been particularly instructive. The transforming protein, v-Crk, is composed only of SH2 and SH3 sequences, without any tyrosine kinase catalytic domain. However, v-Crk-transformed cells contain elevated levels of phosphotyrosine-containing proteins. Investigation of this phenomenon has led to the realization that SH2 domains function as ligands for proteins containing phosphotyrosine. As all active tyrosine kinase enzymes are themselves phosphorylated on tyrosine, potential substrates may bind through their SH2 domains to the active phosphotyrosine-containing forms of the enzymes. This may be a way of controlling availability of substrates for these enzymes, and the presence of SH2 domains on the substrates of tyrosine kinases is likely to accelerate the identification of substrates, a process that until now has been frustratingly slow.

A second class of cytoplasmic signaling molecule that can be rendered oncogenic by mutation is the Ras family of proteins. Initially identified as v-Ras, the transforming proteins of Harvey murine sarcoma virus (Ha MuSV), the Ras proteins have been conserved as essential functions from yeast to man, with very little sequence variation. The Ras proteins are small GTP-binding proteins with GTP-hydrolyzing activity. The GTPase activity is essentially a way to control the signaling activity, as only the GTP-bound form is active. Recent genetic and biochemical evidence suggests that at least one function of Ras proteins is to mediate the signals generated by protein tyrosine kinases. In contrast to the normal cellular form of Ras, the oncogenic v-Ras contains two point mutations that impair the GTPase activity and so trap the molecule in an 'on' or signal-generating state. Unfortunately, the nature of the signals generated by active Ras remains elusive.

Studies of the regulation of Ras GTPase activity have revealed a second mechanism of oncogenic activation through the Ras signaling pathway. The intrinsic GTPase activity of Ras proteins is augmented by GTPase-activating proteins, or GAPs. The GAP molecules increase the hydrolysis of GTP, and so convert active Ras to inactive Ras. An important observation has been the realization that the gene that confers predisposition to neurofibromatosis (NF1), an inherited form of cancer, encodes a GAP. Inactivating mutations in NF1 GAP are associated with a decrease in GAP activity, a consequent increase in the amount of Ras protein in the active (GTP-bound) state and the formation of tumors.

Cell signaling through transcription factors

The generation of second messengers and cytoplasmic signals by external factors eventually results in changes in gene expression. Several retroviral oncogenes are transduced forms of cellular transcription factors involved in regulating the response to external factors. The transcription factor AP1 is a heterodimeric transcription factor with sequence-specific DNA-binding activity composed of peptides derived from the Fos and Jun families of proteins. The fos family of genes was identified as the cellular homologues of v-fos, the transforming gene of FBJ MuSV, while the jun family was identified by homology to v-jun, the transforming gene of avian sarcoma virus (ASV) 17. AP1 activity is tightly regulated, and is rapidly and transiently induced by a wide variety of mitogens, including the peptide mitogens PDGF and EGF. The induction of AP1 activity requires de novo protein synthesis, and is a consequence of the early induction of the fos and jun genes in response to mitogens. Several lines of evidence suggest that transformation by v-Fos is due to overexpression of AP1 activity. Overexpression of either c-Fos or v-Fos protein is sufficient to result in neoplastic transformation, and mutant proteins that are unable to bind AP1 target DNA sequences are nontransforming. Cells transformed by Fos protein show increased levels of AP1 activity compared to nontransformed cells, consistent with the idea that transformation is the result of activation of a specific set of genes that contain AP1 regulatory sequences in their upstream regions. The identification of the relevant genes the activation of which is important for transformation has proven to be difficult.

A somewhat different situation is represented by the transforming gene, v-rel, of the reticuloendotheliosis virus (REV-T). The Rel family of proteins constitute a large family of proteins with NF-KB activity. NF-KB is a transcription factor that is involved in the response of lymphoid cells to a variety of external stimuli. NF-KB activity is regulated by a number of complex mechanisms, but an important form of regulation appears to be retention in the cytoplasm through its interaction with specific inhibitor proteins. External stimuli then result in the dissociation of the inhibitor and allows translocation of NF-KB to the cytoplasm. An usual feature of transformation by v-Rel is that mutant v-Rel proteins that are localized in the cytoplasm can induce transformation. This suggests that direct transcriptional activation by v-Rel is not the mechanism of neoplastic transformation, and suggests that v-*rel* may function as a dominant negative allele of c-*rel*, and this idea has received some experimental support. According to this model, NF-KB activity would function to promote cellular differentiation and inhibit cell growth, and oncogenesis would be the consequence of decreasing NF-KB activity.

Oncogene cooperation

Spontaneously occurring tumors are recognized to be the result of a multistage process in which multiple mutations arising at different times conspire to produce a tumor. On the other hand, neoplastic transformation due to infection with the acutely transforming retroviruses usually occurs as the result of the introduction of a single gene. Yet even the acutely transforming retroviruses contain examples of cooperativity among oncogenes. AEV contains two genes, v-*erbA*, a transduced mutant form of the thyroid hormone receptor gene, and v-*erbB*, a constitutively active form of the EGF receptor gene. Although v-*erbB* is sufficient to direct neoplastic growth of infected erythroid cells, the expression of v-*erbA* is required for growth of the erythroid cells under some culture conditions. Thus, the fully transformed phenotype is the product of a cooperative interaction between the two genes. This theme of cooperation between various oncogenic proteins has been extensively documented in the process of neoplastic transformation of primary cells.

Transformation by human retroviruses

Retroviruses may acquire transforming activity by transduction of cellular proto-oncogenes, they may activate cellular proto-oncogenes by insertional mutagenesis, or they may transform through the action of regulatory genes required for the viral life cycle to proceed. The causative agent of acute T-cell leukemia, human T-cell leukemia virus (HTLV-1), appears to operate through the last type of mechanism. The viral gene *tax* is a regulator of transcription from the viral long terminal repeat, as well as from certain cellular promoters. Interestingly, Tax activates both the interleukin 2 (IL-2) promoter and the IL-2 receptor promoter, generating a loop with potential autocrine activity in T cells. The mechanism of Tax activation of transcription remains unclear. It is able to activate transcription directed by NF-KB and cyclic AMP-responsive sites, although there is no evidence that Tax itself binds DNA. The mechanism of transformation induced by HTLV-1 is likewise unclear; the tumors arise only after a long latency, sometimes 20 years, and are monoclonal.

DNA Tumor Viruses

Several classes of DNA viruses are able to induce neoplastic transformation in culture. In contrast to the situation with transforming retroviruses, in which transformation is the result of the activation of a gene that is not required for the completion of the viral life cycle, transformation by DNA viruses is the result of expression of proteins intimately involved in the replication of the viral genome.

Simian virus 40 (SV40)

Transformation by SV40 is associated with nonproductive infection and is the result of the expression of a single viral protein, the SV40 large T antigen (T Ag). In contrast to productively infected cells in which the SV40 genome is episomal, in transformed cells the viral genome is integrated into the host DNA in a manner which allows for expression of T Ag. T Ag is a multifunctional protein that forms noncovalent interactions with a number of cellular proteins. Key among these are the products of the cellular tumor suppressor genes p53 and Rb. Oncogenic activation of the p53 and Rb genes is associated with loss, rather than gain of function. p53 was initially identified as a protein stably associated with T Ag in transformed cells. The normally rapid turnover of p53 in uninfected cells is greatly reduced by virtue of complex-formation with T Ag, giving rise to increased levels of the protein in transformed cells. The net result of this interaction is not to increase p53 function, however, but rather to sequester it in an inactive complex. The protein product of the retinoblastoma susceptibility gene, pRb, is also noncovalently associated with T Ag, and this complex results in loss of pRb function. Transformation by T Ag has therefore served as the mechanism of identification of one tumor suppressor gene (p53), and has been the entry point for biochemical investigation of another (pRb).

Adenovirus

Transformation by the human adenoviruses has been observed only *in vitro*. As is the case with transformation by SV40, transformation by adenovirus is the result of a nonproductive infection. DNA transfection experiments reveal that the expression of two different viral genes, E1a and E1b, is required for full transformation. E1a is a multifunctional protein with a bewildering array of activities. The important feature for transformation appears to be the ability to interact with pRB. Expression of the E1a gene alone is sufficient for immortalization of primary cells, but not for full transformation, which requires expression of the E1b gene. The product of the E1b gene is complexed physically with p53. Thus, the combined activities of E1a and E1b are reminiscent of the activities of SV40 T Ag.

Human papilloma virus

Investigation of the transforming activities of the human papillomaviruses (HPV) is of interest for reasons of medical importance as well as scientific interest. Nearly all human cervical carcinomas are associated with the presence of DNA from either HPV 16 or HPV 18. Completion of the life cycle of the HPVs is unusual in that the early and late stages of the life cycle appear to take place in different stages of epithelial cell differentiation, and complete viral replication takes place only in benign papillomas, or warts. This feature has so far made it impossible to grow the HPVs in culture, a problem that has slowed analysis. However, molecular analysis has been informative. Cervical carcinomas are associated with the presence of the viral genome integrated into the host DNA in a manner that allows for expression of the early region of the viral genome. This region is quite complex, with at least eight open reading frames; there is evidence that at least five are involved in generating the transformed phenotype. In a scenario reminiscent of adenovirus, the products of the E6 and E7 open reading frames are physically associated with p53 and pRB respectively. These interactions result in the functional inactivation of p53 by accelerated proteolysis, and pRb by sequestration.

Hepatitis B virus

The hepadnaviruses should be mentioned because of their potential role in human cancers. The hepatitis B virus, especially when acquired by vertical transmission, is associated with the development of hepatocellular carcinoma. At this point, there is no decisive evidence that this association is causal, but strong circumstantial data are present. Experimental evidence suggests two potential mechanisms: activation of cellular oncogenes by integration in a manner similar to insertional mutagenesis by retroviruses, and repetititive mitogenic stimulation due to the toxic effects of chronic exposure to the surface antigen proteins.

Epstein–Barr virus

Nonproductive infection with Epstein–Barr virus (EBV) is associated with Burkitt's lymphoma, a malignancy of B lymphocytes. Once again, there is no decisive evidence for a causal role, but the ability of the virus to immortalize human B lymphocytes suggests a potential mechanism. Infection with EBV may result in the generation of a large pool of preneoplastic cells that are predisposed to further oncogenic mutations.

Future Perspectives

Much of what we understand about the molecular mechanisms of cancer is the result of investigation of virus-induced tumors. This area of investigation has demonstrated, clearly and convincingly, that cancer is a disease caused by mutations in specific genes. We have learned the identity of many of these genes, whether they are carried by the virus, activated by viral insertion, or inactivated by the physical association of their products with viral proteins. The products of these genes form a network of signaling elements that allows cells to respond to the external environment. Where understood, oncogenic mutations result in the production of proteins that propagate mitogenic signals in the absence of appropriate monitoring of the extracellular environment, a result consistent with the proposed normal functions of these proteins. Although many oncogenes were initially identified by virtue of their presence in viral genomes, it is now clear that these genes are also the targets of oncogenic mutations in tumors of nonviral origin. It seems certain that future investigations of virus-induced transformation will further contribute to our understanding of cancer, an understanding that does not appear to be as elusive as a decade ago.

See also: **Adenoviruses (*Adenoviridae*): General features; Avian type C retroviruses (*Retroviridae*); Epstein-Barr virus (*Herpesviridae*): General features; Hepatitis E virus; Human T-cell leukemia viruses (*Retroviridae*): HTLV-1; Murine leukemia viruses (*Retroviridae*); Retroviral Oncogenes; Papillomaviruses – human (*Papovaviridae*): General features; Reticuloendotheliosis viruses (*Retroviridae*); Simian virus 40 (*Papovaviridae*); Tumor viruses – human.**

Further Reading

Hoppe-Seyler F and Butz K (1995) Molecular mechanisms of virus-induced carcinogenesis: the interaction of viral factors with cellular tumor suppressor proteins. *J. Mol. Med.* 73(11): 529.

[This article is reproduced from the 1st edn (1994).]

TRANSPLANTATION AND VIRUS INFECTIONS

Robert A Krance, **Helen E Heslop** and **Malcolm K Brenner**, Stem Cell Transplantation Program, Shell Center for Cell and Gene Therapy, Baylor College of Medicine, Houston, Texas, USA

Copyright © 1999 Academic Press

Introduction

Organ transplantation is being used to correct an ever broader range of medical abnormalities. In large part the expanding application and success of transplantation has been based on improved methods of producing immunosuppression in the recipient, which allow acceptance of a genetically disparate graft. This is particularly true following bone marrow transplantation (BMT), where immunosuppression must be especially profound, since the aim is not only to prevent rejection of the graft by the host but to prevent the incoming immune system from 'rejecting' the recipient to produce graft-versus-host disease (GVHD).

Unfortunately, the immunosuppression required by transplant recipients has a number of adverse consequences. Among the most important of these is the suppression of host immune responses directed against endogenous and exogenous microorganisms. Suppression of immune surveillance allows invasion by opportunist fungi and by protozoa and permits recrudescence of those endogenous viruses which are usually maintained in the latent state. Immunosuppression may also increase the severity of infection after exposure to exogenous viruses. All transplant recipients are vulnerable to virus infections, but bone marrow transplant recipients who are the most intensely immunosuppressed, are the most vulnerable of all. Notwithstanding, the introduction of a number of different therapeutic agents, viral disease remains one of the leading causes of morbidity and mortality after transplantation.

Herpesviruses

The herpes viruses, *Cytomegalovirus*, Epstein–Barr virus, herpes simplex and varicella/zoster represent the greatest potential threat to transplant recipients. All four are present in the latent state in a high proportion of individuals, and all four can cause serious or fatal disease in the immunocompromised host.

Cytomegalovirus (CMV)

Background In a normal individual, defense against CMV is mediated by specific cytotoxic T lymphocytes, by production of specific antibody and perhaps also by MHC unrestricted cellular effector mechanisms. In the transplant recipient, immunosuppression-mediated impairment of these defense mechanisms places the recipient at risk of CMV disease. Depending on location and socioeconomic status, 40–90% of transplant recipients have a past history of primary CMV infection and are at risk of viral reactivation. The remaining seronegative recipients are at risk of acquiring primary infection, either from the donor tissue or from blood products required during the post-transplant period. CMV reactivation or infection does not always lead to CMV disease in the transplant recipient and it is important to distinguish between these phenomena.

Although detection of CMV is not always predictive of disease, there may be a high probability that disease will subsequently occur in patients receiving intensive immunosuppression. Following solid organ grafts, the risk of CMV disease rises with the intensity of the immunosuppression administered and is especially increased by the use of monoclonal anti-T cell antibodies, such as OKT3. Bone marrow recipients who have had their own immune system ablated as part of the conditioning regimen and who have not yet regenerated a donor-derived system are particularly likely to develop CMV disease.

Incidence of CMV infection/reactivation and CMV disease *From blood product support* The risk of a seronegative recipient of seronegative donor tissue acquiring CMV infection from blood product support was previously significant, but the incidence of this mode of transmission has been substantially reduced by the use of CMV seronegative or, more commonly, leukocyte poor blood products and is now less than 5%.

From solid organ grafts Seropositive recipients have a 50–80% chance of developing evidence of viral reactivation, and 10–25% of these individuals will develop evidence of CMV disease. The donor organ is also a source of infection and 50–100% of seronegative recipients will develop infection if they receive a transplant from a seropositive donor. Disease occurs in up to one-half of such patients.

From BMT About 50–60% of both allograft and autograft recipients who are seropositive or have a seropositive donor will have evidence of either primary infection or reactivation, with a peak incidence in the first three months post-transplant. Patients receiving autologous marrow have a low incidence of disease with less than 5% of seropositive recipients developing pneumonitis. By contrast, half of the allograft recipients who develop a primary infection or reactivation will, in the absence of treatment, develop pneumonitis which is fatal in 80–90%. The presence of moderate to severe graft-versus-host disease markedly increases the risk of CMV disease, especially pneumonitis and some studies have shown a reduced incidence of CMV in allograft recipients who receive more effective graft-versus-host disease prophylaxis.

Pathogenesis CMV initially infects a variety of cells including fibroblasts, marrow stromal cells and hemopoietic progenitors. The mechanism of latency is not well understood, but reactivation results in viral shedding. In some situations, such as in AIDS patients, viral replication alone results in disease, but in the transplant patient an immunopathological component is implicated, and both host-versus-graft and graft-versus-host reactions correlate with CMV disease. For example, a host-versus-graft relationship is seen in recipients of liver transplants, who are particularly likely to develop CMV hepatitis. In allogeneic bone marrow transplant recipients, there is evidence that damage to the lungs in CMV pneumonitis results from an abnormal response to antigen, and that this is exacerbated by graft-versus-host disease. The activated immune system may also damage or destroy uninfected 'bystander cells', since antiviral agents which eliminate viral shedding and prevent antigen expression have limited effect on disease progression (see below under Treatment).

Diagnosis CMV infection may be diagnosed either by serological means or by direct isolation of the virus or its DNA. The virus is generally cultured from blood, throat, urine or tissues. CMV is cultured on human fibroblasts and it usually takes 1–4 weeks for the characteristic cytopathic effect to become evident. The use of monoclonal antibodies directed at early or intermediate antigens in conjunction with centrifugation of the specimen on to monolayers of fibroblasts – the shell vial technique – allows diagnosis within 24–48 h. The presence of the virus can be diagnosed even more rapidly by the use of the polymerase chain reaction (PCR) to amplify CMV DNA and RNA, but how accurately detection of viral infection/reaction by such sensitive methodology predicts subsequent CMV disease remains in dispute.

Serological evidence of infection is usually obtained using ELISAs or indirect fluorescence. Diagnosis requires a fourfold rise in titer and may be problematic after BMT when patients are so severely immunocompromised that antibody production is impaired.

Clinical aspects CMV infection in the immunosuppressed host ranges from an asymptomatic illness similar to that in normal individuals to disseminated disease. However, there is a higher incidence of diffuse organ involvement which may present with a variety of clinical manifestations including hepatitis, enteritis, pneumonitis, fever and bone marrow suppression. Disease presentation may also vary according to the organ transplanted. In recipients of renal transplants, pneumonitis is rare and patients are more likely to present with mononucleosis-like symptoms or hepatitis. Recipients of lung, heart or liver transplant have a higher risk of more severe CMV infections such as pneumonitis. Liver transplant recipients are particularly at risk of CMV hepatitis which is more common after primary infection and may be difficult to distinguish from rejection. Finally, following allogeneic bone marrow transplantation, pneumonitis is the most common presentation of CMV disease and will occur in 40–50% of recipients with evidence of infection on blood culture. Pneumonitis presents with fever, cough dyspnea and chest radiograph shows an interstitial pattern. About 80–90% of BMT recipients who develop CMV pneumonitis will die of this complication.

Treatment A number of measures have been used to treat established CMV disease. All are of most benefit after solid organ grafting, and of least value after BMT. Interferon has antiviral activity and may reduce morbidity in renal transplant recipients, but has little effect in BMT patients. Similarly, acyclovir and gancyclovir may reduce viral shedding and may be effective in CMV disease in solid organ recipients, but given alone they do not significantly modify morbidity and mortality from CMV disease in allogeneic BMT recipients.

Intravenous immunoglobulin (IVIg) as a single agent is also ineffective in most studies. However, the combined use of gancyclovir and IVIg in allogeneic BMT recipients with CMV pneumonitis results in disease resolution in around 50–70%. This response rate appears significantly better than the 10% response rate of historical controls, though no

Table 1 Effect of prophylaxis in preventing CMV reactivation/disease

Prophylactic regimen	Effect on Reactivation/Infection	Disease	Mortality
CMV-negative blood products	+	+	+
Acyclovir (low dose)	+/−	+/−	−
Acyclovir (high dose)	+	+	+/−
Gancyclovir	− (see text)	+	+
Intravenous immunoglobulin	−	+	+/−

randomized trials have been performed and the improved survival may in part reflect changes in diagnostic criteria and techniques. Indeed, subsequent studies where the drug combination was administered to patients who were ventilated yielded lower response rates.

Prophylaxis (Table 1) The most effective preventative measure is to use CMV-negative blood products for seronegative recipients who receive seronegative organ grafts. Several studies have convincingly shown that this policy can almost completely eliminate CMV disease. Seronegative recipients of seropositive allogeneic marrow also benefit from seronegative blood products. It has been suggested that seropositive recipients should also receive CMV-negative products to reduce exposure to new strains. In practice most blood banks do not have enough CMV-negative products to supply all these populations and leukocyte-poor products – prepared by filtration of blood – are used instead. It appears that leukocyte-poor products are just as effective – at least in low risk patients.

Antiviral agents have also been explored as prophylactic agents. Acyclovir in renal transplant recipients reduces the rate of CMV infection and disease but did not improve survival. Neither α-interferon nor low-does acyclovir have any convincing effect in BMT recipients. Some studies suggest that acyclovir may reduce the incidence of both CMV infection and invasive disease, but these results are not confirmed in other studies. Gancyclovir effectively reduces the incidence of CMV disease in allograft recipients with CMV infection detected by shell viral technique or by PCR, and more recent studies using prophylactic or pre-emptive gancyclovir have shown that the drug may be used to prevent viral reactivation. Unfortunately, resistant strains of CMV are now beginning to be detected, and CMV disease may also occur once gancyclovir prophylaxis has been stopped. Foscarnet may be an acceptable, non-cross-resistant, substitute for gancyclovir, although the relative efficacy of this drug in BMT patients remains uncertain.

IVIg administered after BMT, resulting in passive transfer of specific antibody, does not reduce the rate of viral reactivation or infection but does decrease the incidence of pneumonia and death. Such treatment may therefore be justified in seropositive recipients. The expense of IVIg does not appear to be justified in seronegative recipients receiving seronegative blood products, in whom risk of CMV infection and disease is negligible. Similarly, in seronegative renal recipients receiving a seropositive graft, IVIg reduces the incidence of CMV disease though not the rate of viral isolation or seroconversion. Neutralizing human monoclonal antibodies are currently being evaluated in phase III trials.

Immunomodulation Several studies have correlated the pattern of CMV infection in allogeneic BMT recipients with the ability to generate CMV specific $CD8^+$ cytotoxic T lymphocytes, which may allow the host to control CMV infection. These observations suggested that adoptive transfer of specific cytotoxic T lymphocytes (CTLs) (expanded *in vitro*) to high risk patients may allow long term protection from overt disease, without the risk of developing chemoresistant strains of virus. Initial studies of this approach have produced promising results.

Epstein–Barr virus (EBV)

Background Even though more than 90% of adults have serological evidence of EBV infection, disease produced by reactivation of this herpesvirus has, until recently, been less prevalent in transplant recipients than disease produced by CMV. However, the development of more aggressive and effective techniques for immunosuppression has not only increased the success of tissue transplantation, but has also substantially increased the incidence of the lymphoproliferative syndrome associated with uncontrolled EBV reactivation in the immunocompromised host.

This complication is particularly common in patients receiving mismatched or unrelated donor BMT, in seronegative neonatal recipients of seropositive liver and in patients receiving small bowel transplants.

Incidence Following solid organ grafting, up to 60% of patients may show evidence of EBV reactivation or infection, assessed on the basis of rising antibody titers to viral proteins. Less than one-third of these patients will develop the clinical features of a viral illness. The incidence of lymphoproliferative syndrome is between 1 and 13%, and is lowest in patients receiving renal allografts and highest in those receiving heart–lung double transplants. Within each group, patients receiving the most intensive immunosuppression, with CSA, antilymphocyte globulin or anti-T cell monoclonal antibody (e.g. OKT3), have the highest incidence.

After BMT the incidence is even more variable. At one extreme, adult patients receiving major histocompatibility complex (MHC) identical sibling allografts as treatment for leukemia have an incidence of 0.25%. At the other extreme, children transplanted for congenital immunodeficiency syndromes who receive marrow from an MHC nonidentical or unrelated donor have a 100-fold greater incidence of lymphoproliferative disease, which occurs in up to 25% of such recipients. This wide variation is in part attributable to the increased immunosuppression required by recipients of mismatched/unrelated marrow, but probably also reflects the long delay in immune reconstitution exhibited by patients receiving a genetically disparate immune system. Because the numbers of mismatched/unrelated donor BMT are steadily rising, some recent BMT series show that death from EBV-induced lymphoproliferation now exceeds that from CMV disease.

Pathogenesis and diagnosis The primary pathologic process is uncontrolled proliferation of mature B lymphocytes. Analysis of proliferating lymphoblasts following solid organ transplant using restriction fragment length polymorphisms (RFLPs) or minisatellite probes, has shown that EBV lymphoproliferation in these patients almost always arises from recipient B cells. In contrast, lymphoproliferation after BMT commonly arises from cells of donor origin. In all cases, the transformed B cells closely resemble morphologically and phenotypically, the lymphoblastoid cell lines generated *in vitro* when human B cells are exposed to EBV in the absence of T cells. The infected lymphocytes may have an immunoblastic or plasmacytoid appearance and are usually CD19, CD20, CD21 and CD24 positive (see below under Treatment). Like Burkitt lymphoma cells, the lymphoblasts are positive for EBV nuclear antigens 1 (EBNA1) but unlike Burkitt lymphoma cells they usually express all of the five other virus-encoded latent cycle nuclear antigens and are positive for most latent membrane proteins. Again in contrast to Burkitt lymphoma cells, lymphoblasts in transplant patients express a number of cell adhesion molecules and ligands. All these phenotypic features would make them intensely vulnerable to cytotoxic T cell killing in a normal individual, and it is only the profound suppression of the immune system after transplantation which permits their outgrowth.

The B cell proliferation may be oligoclonal or monoclonal, and may be associated with production of oligoclonal or monoclonal peaks of immunoglobulin which can be detected by serum electrophoresis. Within the B cells, the virus may be present in linear (replicative) or circular (latent) form. Analysis of these attributes may predict the response to therapy.

Clinical manifestations Early in the illness, fever, malaise and circulating atypical lymphocytes are usually seen. The proliferating lymphoblasts may then produce a number of disease patterns. They may diffusely infiltrate a number of different organ systems, including lungs, liver, kidney, gut, bone marrow and central nervous system. Infiltration may be so extensive that organ failure results. Alternatively, a classical 'lymphoma' pattern is observed, with lymphadenopathy, hepatosplenomegaly, and a biopsy appearance of a diffuse immunoblastic lymphoma. Rarely, a predominantly leukemic picture occurs. Although these distinctive clinical patterns may be seen in isolation, a combination of features often evolves (**Fig. 1**).

Clinical course Initial reactivation of EBV, associated with an 'infectious mononucleosis'-like illness, may resolve spontaneously. But once viral induced-lymphoproliperative syndrome (LPS) has occurred, the course is generally rapidly progressive. Death may result from renal, hepatic or pulmonary failure, from hemorrhage due to ulceration of bowel tumor, or from central nervous system (CNS) involvement.

Treatment Withdrawal of immunosuppression is associated with spontaneous remission of the tumors in up to 50% of recipients of solid organ grafts; regression is more likely to occur in oligoclonal then in monoclonal tumors. Withdrawal of immunosuppression alone is rarely effective when the LPS has occurred after BMT.

Acyclovir may disrupt the replicative lytic cycle of the (linear) virus and interferon may prevent infection of fresh lymphocytes, but neither approach can signi-

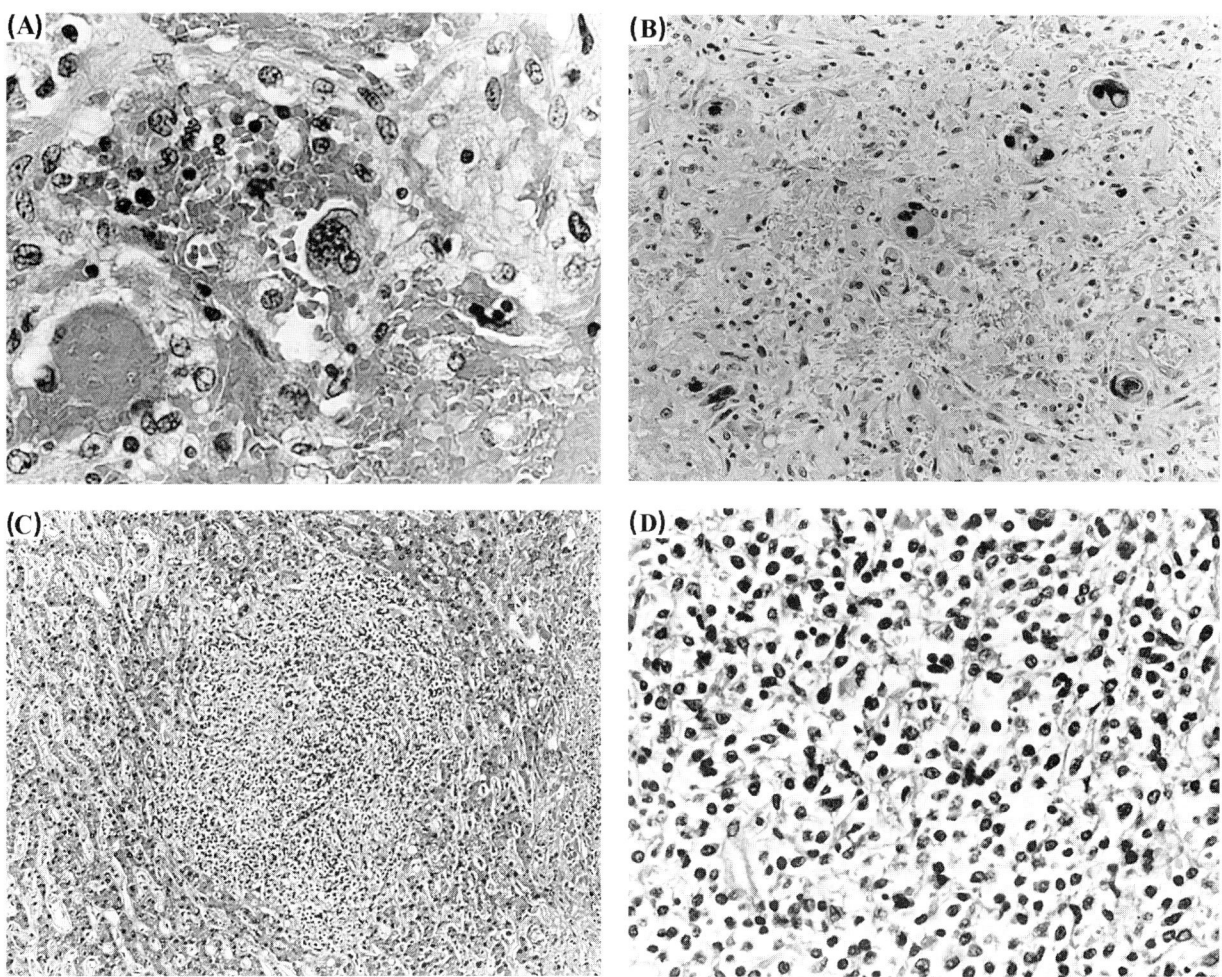

Figure 1 (**A**) Section of lung, infected with CMV, containing intraalveolar hemorrhage and multinucleated giant cell. This is a histologically atypical infection producing only scattered cells with relatively small intranuclear and intracytoplasmic inclusions and no large cells with 'owls-eye' nuclei (hematoxylin and eosin stain; ×315). (**B**) Same infection as in (A) demonstrating numerous cells positive for CMV antigen using monoclonal antibody and immunoperoxidase technique (avidin–biotin complex technique; ×315). (**C**) (EBV low power) Section of liver with lymphoid infiltrate (EBV infection) causing portal expansion (hematoxylin and eosin stain; ×80). (**D**) Same infection as in (C). The portal infiltrate is polymorphous and contains cells ranging from small mature lymphocytes to larger immunoblasts (hematoxylin and eosin stain; ×315).

ficantly modify the growth of already transformed B cells which contain nonreplicating (circular) virus. Nonetheless, remissions have been reported in response to both drugs, although these are more likely in recipients of solid organ grafts and if the tumor is oligoclonal. More recent reports suggest that infusion of monoclonal antibodies to CD21 and CD24 – molecules present on lymphoblasts – may rid the patient of infected B lymphocytes. As with other treatments, this approach seems most effective in solid organ recipients with oligoclonal LPS.

At present the most satisfactory approach to prophylaxis and treatment in BMT recipients is to attempt to restore immunocompetence to EBV by the adoptive transfer of immune T cells. The majority of individuals are EBV seropositive, and between 1 in 1000 and 1 in 10 000 of their circulating CTLS are EBV specific. Transfer of marrow donor T cells therefore regularly produces disease response in patients with uncontrolled lymphoproliferation. Unfortunately, because donor T cells also contain significant numbers of alloreactive CTLs, response may be associated with the development of severe graft-versus-host disease. More recently, it has proved possible successfully to prevent and treat EBV disease by transferring virus-specific CTLs, without the development of graft-versus-host-disease. Alternative approaches have used bulk T cell populations genetically modified to include a thymidine kinase suicide gene. Should graft-versus-host disease develop, these modified cells may be destroyed by administration of gancyclovir.

Finally, the development of mouse models in which proliferating human lymphoblasts can be studied may help in the development and assessment of novel therapeutic strategies.

Varicella Zoster virus

Incidence Reactivation of herpes zoster virus (VZV) infection occurs in 5–25% of solid organ transplant recipients and in as many as 50% of bone marrow transplant patients. Primary infection develops only rarely, and usually in children.

Epidemiology and pathogenesis Like other herpesviruses, the probability of VZV reactivation is increased when cell-mediated immunity is compromised. In solid organ transplant recipients, the eruption of clinical shingles often follows the initiation or increase of medications to prevent graft rejection. The risk of VZV reaction in bone marrow transplant patients is even greater because the attendant immune deficiency is more severe and prolonged than that of solid organ transplant patients. Unlike herpes simplex virus (HSV) reactivation where patients with high HSV antibody titer are more likely to develop reactivation, pretransplant VZV antibody titer does not predict post-transplant infection.

Although VZV infection may develop in the first weeks after transplantation, the median time to reactivation is four to five months for patients not receiving prophylactic acyclovir. Late graft rejection requiring aggressive immunosuppressive measures is frequently accompanied by VZV reactivation in solid organ transplant patients. In allogenic bone marrow transplantation, VZV infection may be more common in patients with graft-versus-host disease, whereas for autologous transplantation VZV infection is more common in patients with Hodgkin's disease or non-Hodgkin's lymphoma.

Manifestations and treatment Classical cutaneous herpes zoster (shingles) is the most common manifestation of VZV infection among transplant patients. Depending on the dermatome affected, VZV reactivation may cause post-herpetic neuralgia, cutaneous scarring or corneal opacification. Solid organ transplant recipients rarely develop disseminated or invasive VZV infection.

In bone marrow transplant patients, VZV infection may present as typical dermatomal herpes zoster, as herpes zoster with cutaneous dissemination, or even as varicella. Serology in these patients indicates past VZV infection. Prior to the availability of acyclovir, cutaneous zoster infection progressed to invasive disease in up 50% of patients, and 10% died. The consequences of visceral dissemination included hepatitis, pancreatitis, and encephalitis; however, VZV pneumonia was the usual cause of death.

Intravenous acyclovir is the most effective and least toxic therapy for VZV infection in transplant patients. In bone marrow transplant patients, prophylactic administration of acyclovir can prevent VZV reactivation, but reactivation is common upon discontinuing the drug. Consequently, prophylactic administration of acyclovir to prevent VZV infection is not recommended. Vidarabine and α-interferon are effective against VZV infections but they are secondary treatments since they are more toxic and less efficacious. Their use is limited to situations when VZV resistance to acyclovir is suspected.

In those patients without prior VZV infection, varicella zoster immune globulin administered within 72 h of VZV exposure may prevent or modify illness. Varicella vaccine is a promising therapy for children who may require transplantation but have not yet acquired their primary immunity.

Herpes Simplex virus

Incidence Reactivation of latent herpes simplex virus (HSV) infection has occurred in 30–90% of seropositive transplant patients. The majority have suffered a mild, usually self-limited illness, with fever accompanied by lesions of the oral or genital mucosa. However, in patients undergoing bone marrow transplant HSV disease has been more severe.

Epidemiology and pathogenesis Less than 5% of HSV illness following transplantation has been due to primary HSV infection. There are two possible sources of primary HSV exposure: intimate contact with an individual shedding HSV or transfer of HSV through the transplanted organ. Transfer of HSV by liver, pancreas, heart and kidney transplantation has been documented. Presumably, the virus, latent in neural tissue within the organ, became reactivated and initiated primary HSV illness in the host.

Between 30% and 100% of adults are HSV seropositive, and 15–30% of these experience recurrent vesicular eruptions. Although the events leading to HSV reactivation are incompletely understood, the combination of high prevalence of HSV seropositivity and iatrogenic immunosuppression have undoubtedly promoted HSV illness among transplant patients. Interestingly, a high antibody titer to HSV pretransplant has been linked to a high risk of viral reactivation.

Clinical manifestations and treatment The incidence of HSV infection peaks during the first weeks after transplantation when cell-mediated immunity is most suppressed. The classic perioral vesicular eruption is the typical manifestation of HSV infection in solid organ transplant recipients. Genital HSV infection is also common. In bone marrow transplant patients, the diagnosis of HSV infection may be problematic because the classic lesions are often superimposed on mucositis caused by the pretransplant chemotherapy and/or radiotherapy.

Visceral dissemination of HSV has been rare following kidney and liver transplantation, more frequent following heart, lung and heart–lung transplantation, and most common following bone marrow transplantation. Manifestations of visceral dissemination include esophagitis, pneumonia, hepatitis and encephalitis; HSV esophagitis and pneumonia are thought to develop from contiguous spread of oral/perioral disease. HSV has been isolated from 5% of bone marrow transplant patients with pneumonia. Often a co-isolate with cytomegalovirus (CMV), the role of HSV in the pathogenesis of pneumonia is unclear.

The incidence of hepatitis or encephalitis due to HSV has been less than 0.5%. Unlike HSV pneumonia or esophagitis, the onset of hepatitis has not always followed oral/perioral lesions. In the first weeks after liver transplantation, immediate liver biopsy is recommended for patients who develop hepatic dysfunction, since prompt initiation of acyclovir has arrested the progression of HSV hepatitis to fulminant and usually fatal liver failure.

Treatment Acyclovir is the principal treatment for HSV infection. It is effective for prophylaxis as well as treatment of established infection. Because the likelihood of disseminated HSV disease is enhanced by immunosuppression, acyclovir prophylaxis may be used routinely in seropositive recipients of bone marrow transplantation, although gancyclovir (given primarily for prophylaxis of CMV as described above) may be substituted. In solid organ transplantation, where immunosuppression is neither as intense nor as prolonged, opinion is divided on the necessity for prophylaxis. If prophylaxis is used, HSV reactivation often occurs once acyclovir is discontinued. In addition, approximately 10% of patients develop HSV reactivation even while receiving prophylaxis.

Disconcerting reports of acyclovir-resistant HSV, particularly among human immunodeficiency virus (HIV)-infected patients, have been confirmed. Vidarabine and foscarnet, an investigational agent, may be effective alternatives.

Other Herpesviruses

In the last few years several new herpesviruses, HHV-6, HHV-7 and HHV-8, have been identified. Only HHV-6 has so far been recognized as a pathogen in transplant patients. HHV-6 is an endemic virus with over 90% of healthy adults seropositive. It infects CD4 cells and therefore also predisposes to the reactivation of other viruses. Infection occurs in 30–60% of transplant recipients usually in the early post-transplant period. Many patients are asymptomatic and marrow suppression, pneumonitis and encephalitis are the most common disease manifestations. The antiviral susceptibility of HHV-6 is similar to CMV and the organism is sensitive to foscarnet and gancyclovir.

Hepatitis Viruses

Hepatitis A virus or hepatitis delta and epsilon viruses have been uncommon sources of hepatitis in transplant patients. In contrast, infections with hepatitis B virus (HBV) or hepatitis C virus (HCV) have been frequent. Transplant patients may be more susceptible to the complications of HBV and HCV infection, but the uncertainty regarding epidemiology and pathogenesis of these infections complicates decisions regarding the suitability of patients with hepatitis for transplant.

There have been many impediments to an understanding of the consequence of hepatitis. Until the recent development of the anti-HCV assay, the course of patients with HCV infection could not be distinguished from the course of patients with other hepatic abnormalities. Even though patients with HCV can now be identified, the current assay is insensitive. Meanwhile, assays for HBV infection, long considered sensitive and specific, do not adequately detail the potential for HBV reactivation and infectivity. Thus, the outcome of patients previously infected with HBV or HCV and reexposed to one or both of these viruses during transplantation is presently hard to predict on an individual basis, although it is evident that their overall risk of continued and progressive liver dysfunction is increased fourfold or more over uninfected patients. Transplant patients may also have serologic evidence of infection by both viruses and distinguishing the active agent by serologic assays is difficult. Finally, liver dysfunction in the post-transplant patient is a common event and other sources of hepatic injury are often present concurrently.

Incidence

The incidence of hepatitis B surface antigen (HBsAg) positivity varies widely. In Taiwan where 15–20% of the population are HBsAg positive, 93% of bone marrow recipients were positive prior to transplant. In the USA and Italy, 0.1% and 6% of bone marrow transplant patients, respectively, were antigen positive. Among renal dialysis patients, 3% in the USA and 46% in France were chronically infected. The prevalence of HBsAg seropositivity among liver transplant recipients is skewed by the particular admission requirements to transplant centers. Because of the high rate of HBV reactivation and subsequent hepatic failure, HBsAg-positive patients are not accepted for liver transplantation in some programs. Nonetheless, HBV chronic active hepatitis with hepatic failure is among the most common indications for liver transplantation.

Non-A, non-B chronic active hepatitis with cirrhosis is the most commonly diagnosed condition in patients undergoing liver transplantation. Anti-HCV has been identified in half of these patients. In addition, 37% and 27% of patients undergoing transplant for Laennec's cirrhosis and chronic HBV infection, respectively, were seropositive for HCV. Among kidney transplant patients, up to 26% tested positive for anti-HCV before transplantation. The incidence of HCV infection in bone marrow recipients is uncertain. The widespread use of intravenous immunoglobulin preparations has been blamed for the prevalence (up to 100% of bone marrow transplant patients) of anti-HCV seropositivity; however, immunoglobulin concentrates have not been implicated as a source of HCV transmission.

Epidemiology and pathogenesis

HBV or HCV infection during transplantation is either due to transmission through infected blood or transplanted organ in a previously uninfected patient or more commonly to reactivation or progression of illness in a previously infected patient. There is little evidence that prognosis differs following either primary or secondary infection. Virus reactivation is fomented by the immunosuppression required to establish the allograft. Reactivation does not immediately lead to changes in liver function, and indeed laboratory evidence of hepatocellular injury may not emerge until withdrawal or reduction of immunosuppression.

Within the HBV-infected group, patients at greatest risk for reactivation are asymptomatic HBsAg-positive carriers. Anti-HBs-positive but HBsAg-negative patients are considered immune. However, the intensive immunosuppression administered for bone marrow transplantation, has promoted HBV reactivation in 'immune' patients.

Transmission of HCV by allograft has also been documented, but the frequency of this event has not yet been established. Transfusion of contaminated blood has been assumed to be a major source of HCV infection in transplant patients. Infection by other routes is possible.

Details of HCV pathogenesis are largely unknown. The assay for anti-HCV antibody has not proved enlightening in that regard, since anti-HCV does not appear for weeks to months after infection, and seropositivity may persist for years without evidence of clinical disease. Alternative assays may provide the missing details. For example, serum HCV RNA can now be measured and its presence correlates with infectivity. Although prolonged viremia is common in patients with chronic hepatitis, it remains to be determined whether clearance of HCV viremia indicates permanent immunity or merely a subclinical state capable of reactivation.

Clinical manifestations and treatment

Hepatitis B virus The reported incidence of HBV reactivation following bone marrow transplantation has been 5–12%. However, these figures undoubtedly underestimate the true incidence of reactivation.

Most HBsAg-positive bone marrow transplant recipients develop transient abnormalities in liver function tests, but clinically significant hepatic dysfunction is uncommon. Patients who were HBsAg positive pretransplant rarely cleared antigenemia post-transplant, whereas antigenemia appearing post-transplant persisted for months but almost always resolved. Regardless of whether HBsAg was cleared, intermittent elevation of liver enzymes persisted in over half these patients. The long-term prognosis for these patients is presently unknown. Currently, HBsAg seropositivity is not an absolute contraindication to bone marrow transplantation.

By eight years after kidney transplant, 25–40% of HBsAg-positive patients have developed chronic active hepatitis, cirrhosis, or hepatocellular carcinoma. Data from one study in which HBV reactivation was documented by PCR showed that HBV DNA was detected post-transplant in the 20% of HBV immune patients. Although these patients remained HBsAg negative, their incidence of chronic hepatitis was equivalent to HBsAg-seropositive patients.

Following orthotopic liver transplantation, more than 80% of HBsAg-positive patients will develop reinfection. Overall survival in these patients was significantly reduced compared to other liver transplant patients. HBV-immune patients have not developed reinfection, and this has led to therapies designed to eradicate HBsAg antigenemia: passive immunization with anti-HBs immunoglobulin, active immunization with HBV vaccine, combined active and passive immunization, and α interferon. It appears that HBV reinfection can be delayed by passive and combined immunization, but late reinfection has occurred. Non-hepatic reservoirs of HBV have been implicated as the cause of reinfection.

Hepatitis C virus There are few reports that document the course of HCV infection in transplant patients. In one, 22% of renal transplant recipients tested repeatedly positive for anti-HCV; 50% of these developed chronic hepatitis. Cirrhosis would be the expected outcome in half of the patients developing chronic hepatitis. Transplantation of solid organs from HCV-seropositive donors has infected over half the recipients. Typically, liver disease progressed to subfulminant hepatic failure or became chronic. At present, transplantation of organs from anti-HCV-positive donors is contraindicated.

Therapy

Some patients with chronic hepatitis secondary to HBV or HCV infection have responded to α-interferon therapy, and this response was occasionally sustained once therapy was completed. Whether α-interferon will improve survival is unknown. Vidarabine and acyclovir have also been effective in a proportion of patients with chronic HBV although their activity was less predictable and vidarabine was more toxic than α-interferon. α-Interferon may enhance graft-versus-host mechanisms in bone marrow transplant recipients. Limited use of α-interferon in patients undergoing orthotopic liver transplantation has failed to prevent HBV reinfection. More recently, the antiretroviral agent lamivudine has been used successfully in small series of transplant patients, where it reduced antigen load and appeared to prevent progression of liver disease due to HBV.

Prevention

Prevention of HBV and HCV infections is the single most effective means of controlling post-transplant hepatitis. In France, immunization against HBV infection has not been the common practice; 46% of chronic dialysis patients are HBsAg positive and 71% of the HBsAg-negative patients are anti-HBs positive. In the USA, measures to prevent HBV infection including isolation of infected patients and HBV immunization have reduced the prevalence to 2.7% and 12% for HBsAg and anti-HBs, respectively. The ability to test blood for anti-HCV will further reduce the incidence of transmitted hepatitis.

Polyomavirus

Primary and usually clinically undetected infections with BK virus (BKV) and JC virus (JCV) occur during childhood, since measurable antibodies to JCV and BKV are present in 70% and 90% of adults, respectively. Such persistence of seropositivity suggests equal persistence of infection, and autopsy studies have identified the viral genome – presumably in a latent state – in various tissues including the kidney. Thus most infections with JCV or BKV in transplant patients are attributed to viral reactivation. However, seronegative renal transplant recipients have acquired primary infection from the transplanted kidney.

Situations in which host immunity, especially cell-mediated immunity, are compromised favor the reactivation of BKV and JCV. Four to eight weeks following kidney transplantation, 26–44% of patients develop viruria. The incidence is higher in patients treated with antilymphocyte serum to prevent graft rejection. Up to half of bone marrow transplant patients also develop viruria with BKV or JCV. Viruria onset has been noted between weeks 2 and 8 and typically persisted for 3–4 weeks. JCV was isolated from 6.7% of seropositive patients, and 55% of BKV seropositive patients excreted the virus. This disparity between the frequency of JCV viruria and BKV viruria is unexplained and contrasts with the experience in renal transplant patients where the incidence of viruria is similar.

BKV or JCV reactivation has been associated with stenosis of the ureteral anastomosis in kidney transplant patients, since virus has been identified in the tissue at the stenosis site. In bone marrow transplant patients, BKV has been linked to hemorrhagic cystitis, with more than 80% of viruric patients developing this complication, an incidence four times that of patients who were not viruric. Compared to autologous or syngeneic transplants, the likelihood of hemorrhagic cystitis was markedly increased among viruric patients undergoing allogeneic bone marrow transplantation. The explanation for this is not apparent. Presumably the more profound immunosuppression that occurs with allogeneic transplantation contributes to the virulence of BKV reactivation.

BKV/JCV have also been identified in the lesions of multifocal leukoencephalopathy, a progressive encephalitis which occurs in a minority of patients on long-term immunosuppression. The contribution of these viruses to the disease state is unclear, but responses to intrathecal cytosine arabinoside have been reported. In general, however, there is no effective therapy identified for BKV or JCV.

Respiratory Viruses

Respiratory syncytial viruses

Infection with parainfluenza and respiratory syncytial virus (RSV) can lead to severe, even fatal, pulmonary disease in transplant patients. Although RSV is a common pathogen among children, infection confers only transient resistance; most adults will be susceptible at the time of transplant. About 20–50% of patients exposed to RSV in the hospital will be nosocomially infected and RSV infection in transplant patients has coincided with community outbreaks of RSV disease. The communicability of RSV emphasizes the need for stringent isolation measures.

Pneumonia is the most serious consequence of RSV infection. RSV pneumonia has seldom been fatal in solid organ transplant recipients, but the mortality rate among bone marrow transplant patients has been 50%. The importance of RSV as a pathogen appears to be increasing. In one transplant center, RSV was identified in 27% of patients with pulmonary disease.

After BMT, the onset of pneumonia is early in the post-transplant course, usually before bone marrow engraftment. Sinusitis and otitis media often precede the pulmonary symptoms, an important diagnostic clue, since other viral pneumonias are not accompanied by these upper respiratory tract findings. Diagnosis of infection before the onset of pneumonia has been made by finding RSV antigen in upper airway secretions. RSV infections that occur after 100 days post-transplant have not been fatal.

Identification of RSV prior to the onset of pulmonary symptoms and treatment with nebulized ribavirin has arrested disease progression. Once the lower respiratory tract is clinically involved, ribavirin treatment has been less effective. Improved methods of drug delivery, including intravenous ribavirin, may improve the outcome in this latter group.

Adenovirus

Incidence

Adenovirus has been isolated in 5–10% of patients after solid organ transplantation and in 5–25% of patients undergoing allogeneic bone marrow transplantation. Less than half the patients in whom adenovirus was isolated had symptoms of viral infection and in some that were ill, cytomegalovirus or herpes simplex virus was isolated concurrently, confusing the assignment of cause. Nonetheless there is undeniable evidence that adenovirus has caused invasive and fatal disease in transplant recipients.

Pathogenesis and epidemiology

Most patients are seropositive for adenovirus prior to transplant. Tonsils, adenoids, other lymphoid tissue and kidneys are recognized as latent virus reservoirs. This plus the absence of a contagious source suggest that reactivation of latent virus may often be the cause of adenovirus infection following transplantation. Rarely latent virus residing in the transplanted tissue has been implicated as an infectious source.

Although many adenovirus serotypes have been isolated post-transplant, not all isolates have been associated with invasive disease. Several serotypes, notably types 11, 12, 34 and 35, which rarely cause community outbreaks, have been isolated in immunosuppressed patients with pneumonia. Adenovirus type 5, implicated as a cause of intussusception and sporadic cases of hepatitis, has commonly been recovered from liver transplant recipients with adenovirus-associated hepatitis. The disproportionate representation of certain serotypes in transplant patients with invasive disease is unexplained.

Immunosuppression promotes adenovirus infection. In liver transplant patients, invasive disease has been most common when additional therapy was needed to prevent graft rejection. Severe graft-versus-host disease, which is immunosuppressive in itself and is managed by immunosuppressive agents, has been noted to promote adenovirus infection in bone marrow transplant patients. The frequency of adenovirus infection has also increased with increasing numbers of alternative donor stem cell transplants.

Clinical manifestations and treatment

Adenovirus infections have occurred as early as the second week or as late as several months after transplantation. The virus has been isolated from the throat, stool, urine, blood and from tissue parenchyma. Manifestations include gastroenteritis, hemorrhagic cystitis, hepatitis, pneumonia, meningoencephalitis and hemophagocytic syndrome. In some circumstances, infections have been mild and recovery complete. Renal dysfunction suggestive of kidney allograft rejection has followed adenovirus viruria and hemorrhagic cystitis. Renal failure requiring dialysis has complicated the course of bone marrow transplant patients, and in these patients adenovirus was isolated from the renal parenchyma. Adenovirus hepatitis following liver transplantation and pneumonia following bone marrow transplantation have been almost uniformly fatal.

At present there is no specific therapy for adenovirus infection. Treatment consists in aggressive support. There are anecdotal reports of successful management of disseminated adenovirus infection with immunoglobulin, ribavirin, gancyclovir or with adoptive transfer of immune lymphocytes (see EBV disease above). One patient, after undergoing liver transplant, developed adenovirus hepatitis and liver failure and was successfully retransplanted. Undoubtedly measures such as these will prevail until adenovirus specific treatment is available.

Immunization
Vaccination

Although viral illnesses occur with high frequency and often devastating effect in transplant recipients, vaccination presently has only a limited role in disease prevention. There are a number of reasons why this should be so. Transplant patients are heavily immunosuppressed, and make poor antibody or T cell responses to killed/subunit vaccines. Administration of live attenuated vaccines, which are potentially more immunogenic, is fraught with peril, since the immune response may be so feeble that even attenuated viruses may produce fatal disease. Finally, effective vaccines to herpes viruses in humans are simply not available. Since it is precisely that virus group which is responsible for most viral-related morbidity and mortality after transplantation, vaccination can at best have a limited impact on outcome. For example, several studies have examined the effect of attenuated Towne strain in renal transplant recipients. Unfortunately, the vaccine induces minimal specific cytotoxic T lymphocytes in seronegative renal transplant recipients, many of whom also fail to make antibody. In clinical trials there was no benefit to seropositive recipients, and no change in the incidence of infection in seronegative recipients. Morbidity was, however, decreased in seronegative recipients.

Despite these limitations, vaccination should still be considered for all transplant patients. In particular, killed or subunit vaccines to poliomyelitis and hepatitis B are readily justified and often produce protective levels of antibody. After BMT, antibody responses to vaccines may be greatly enhanced by immunizing both donor and recipient pre-BMT to allow adoptive transfer of high titer responses. In contrast, live vaccines should be withheld while patients are receiving immunosuppression. After BMT especially, such vaccines should not be given for at least two years; in the presence of chronic graft-versus-host disease this time period may need to be extended indefinitely.

Passive immunization

Although vaccination has a limited role after transplantation, it has been repeatedly suggested that passive immunization with pooled immunoglobulins reduces the incidence or severity of disease associated with viral infection or reactivation after transplantation in general and after BMT in particular (see section on CMV above). These claims have yet to be fully substantiated.

See also: **Adenoviruses (*Adenoviridae*): Animal viruses, General features, Malignant transformation and oncology, Molecular biology; Antivirals; Cytomegaloviruses (*Herpesviridae*): Animal cytomegaloviruses, General features (human), Molecular biology (human), Murine cytomegaloviruses; Epstein-Barr virus (*Herpesviridae*): General features, Molecular biology; Hepadnaviruses (*Hepadnaviridae*): Hepatitis B Virus: General features, Molecular biology; Hepatitis C virus (*Flaviviridae*); Herpes simplex viruses (*Herpesviridae*): General features, Molecular biology; Immune response: Cell mediated immune response, General features; Polyomaviruses – murine (*Papovaviridae*): General features, Molecular biology; Respiratory viruses; Varicella-Zoster virus (*Herpesviridae*): General features, Molecular biology.**

Further Reading

Heslop HE, Rooney CM (1997) Adoptive cellular immunotherapy for EBV lymphoproliferative disease. *Immunol. Rev.* 157: 217.

Hibberd PL, Snyder DR (1995) Cytomegalovirus infection in organ transplant recipients. *Infect. Dis. Clin. North Am.* 9: 863.

Hierholzer JL (1992) Adenovirus infection in the immunocompromised host. *Clin. Microbiol. Rev.* 5: 262.

Riddell SR (1995) Pathogenesis of cytomegalovirus pneumonia in immunocompromised hosts. *Semin. Respir. Infect.* 10: 199.

Shelhamer JH, Gill VJ, Quinn TC et al (1996) The laboratory evaluation of opportunistic pulmonary infections. *Ann. Intern. Med.* 124: 585.

Singh N, Carrigan DR (1996) Human herpesvirus-6 in transplantation – an emerging pathogen. *Ann. Intern. Med.* 124: 1065.

Terrault NA, Wright TL, Pereira BJ (1995) Hepatitic C infection in the transplant recipient. *Infect. Dis. Clin. North Am.* 9: 943.

Walter EA, Bowden RA (1995) Infection in the bone marrow transplant recipient. *Infect. Dis. Clin. North Am.* 9: 823–847

Transportable Bacteriophages   see Mu-like Phages (Myoviridae)

TREE SHREW HERPESVIRUSES (*HERPESVIRIDAE*)

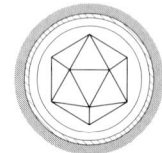

Christian A Tidona and **Gholamreza Darai**, Institute for Medical Virology, University of Heidelberg, Heidelberg, Germany

Copyright © 1999 Academic Press

History

The tree shrews (*Tupaia* sp., family Tupaiidae) belong to a group of primitive higher mammals (*Proteutheria*) and are classified as a separate order (*Scandentia*). The first discovery of herpesvirus-like particles in the tree shrew was reported by Mirkovic in 1970. This *Tupaia* herpesvirus (THV-1), which was isolated from a spontaneously degenerating lung tissue culture from an apparently healthy animal, was characterized by McCombs in 1971 by electron microscopy. Subsequently six additional THV isolates (THV-2 to -7) were obtained and characterized. THV-2 was isolated in 1979 from a degenerating lymphoma cell culture which had been established from a moribund 8-year-old tree shrew. Similarly, THV-3 was isolated from a degenerating cell culture of a Hodgkin's sarcoma (Hodgkin's disease, lymphocytic depletion type) from a moribund 9-year-old tree shrew. The other four THVs (THV-4 to -7) were isolated from spleen tissues of moribund animals aged 4–11 years.

Taxonomy and Classification

THVs are still-unclassified members of the family *Herpesviridae*; however, the recent analysis of the primary structure of the THV-2 genome clearly indicates that these viruses belong to the beta-subfamily of herpesviruses.

Properties of the Virion

Naked viral capsids have a diameter of about 100 nm. Extracellular herpesvirus particles comprise an envelope studded with small surface projections (**Fig. 1A**). Beneath this envelope, an electron dense area is detectable. Some of the enveloped particles contain several viral capsids. The diameter of the envelope usually ranges from 200 to 350 nm (**Fig. 1B**).

Properties of the Genome

THV genomes have attracted attention because they consist of a unique linear double-stranded DNA molecule without any detectable long inverted repeat sequences greater than 40 bp within or at either end of the viral genome. The DNAs of the THV isolates 1–4 were subjected to analytical ultracentrifugation and a specific buoyant density of 1.724 g ml^{-1} was determined. From the UV-absorbance/temperature profile of the viral DNA in 15 mmol l^{-1} NaCl, 1.5 mmol L^{-1} sodium citrate a melting temperature (T_m) of $81.2 \pm 0.8°C$ was calculated. This corresponds to an overall G+C content of $64.5 \pm 1.9\%$, which is in agreement with results obtained from DNA nucleotide sequence analysis.

Measurement of the contour length of viral DNA molecules by electron microscopy revealed molecular sizes of about 194.8 ± 5, 200.8 ± 3, 196.3 ± 3 and 196.3 ± 5 kbp for THV isolates 1, 2, 3 and 4, respec-

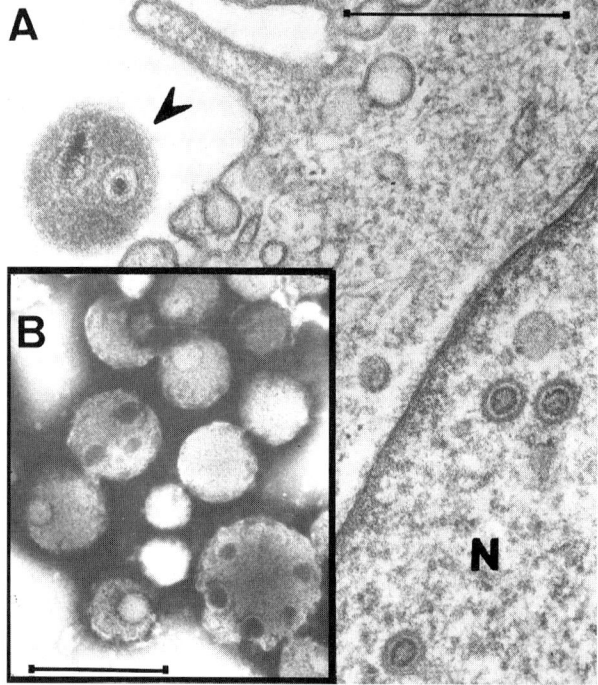

Figure 1 Electron micrographs of *Tupaia* herpesvirus 2 particles. Bars = 500 nm. (**A**) Ultrathin section of a *Tupaia* embryonic fibroblast cell 5 days after infection with THV-2. In the nucleus (N) three virus capsids are present and the mature extracellular virion (arrow) contains two capsids. (**B**) Negative staining of pellets of THV-2 infected tissue culture supernatants using 2% phosphotungstic acid at pH 7.2 reveals the relatively high purity of such materials. Envelope structures are remarkably stable and contain different numbers of capsids.

tively. Physical maps of the THV-2 genome have been constructed.

THV-2 DNA synthesis reaches a maximum between 24 and 36 h post infection, preceded by a transient stimulation of host cell DNA synthesis. Linear concatemeric and circular viral DNA molecules are found during DNA synthesis. The nucleotide sequence of terminal DNA regions of the molecularly cloned THV-2 genome is characterized by a relatively high G+C content of about 75%. Furthermore, the termini contain numerous short repeat elements. A sequence ($A_3C_8AAAGGCAC_6G_5$), postulated to be a consensus signal for site-specific endonucleolytic cleavage in terminal regions of the genomes of herpes simplex virus 1 and 2 (HSV-1, HSV-2), Epstein–Barr virus (EBV) and varicella-zoster virus (VZV), is present at the terminal region of the THV-2 genome. It was found that the signal sequences of HSV and THV-2 are located at similar distances from the genomic termini (at nucleotide positions 432 and 470 bp). This consensus sequence, in combination with several short repeats, which are asymmetrically bracketed by GC-rich arrays, may play a role in forming the mature ends of the THV DNA. Alternatively, this consensus sequence could be the target site for the processing of concatemeric viral DNA molecules into unit-length segments and for the packaging of the processed unit-length molecules into viral capsids.

It was found that THV-1 to -4 genomic DNAs cause infections in tree shrew embryonic fibroblasts.

Viral Proteins

The polypeptide patterns of THV-1 to -3 are remarkably similar, each consisting of at least 35 polypeptides with similar apparent molecular masses ranging from 120 to 230 kDa. While the majority of analogous polypeptides of the three viruses are of indistinguishable electrophoretic mobility, some (e.g. 82–86 kDa polypeptides) showed small differences in apparent molecular mass which were characteristic of the viral strain. By comparative sodium dodecyl sulfate polyacrylamide gel electrophoresis (SDS-PAGE) it is possible to distinguish the THV isolates from each other. At least five glycoproteins are found in purified THV virions. Two-dimensional electropherograms reveal at least 47 discernible protein spots, some of which are specific for a given THV isolate and which are detectable in lysates of THV-infected cells.

Viral Enzymes

A protein kinase activity is associated with THV. Divalent cations such as Mg^{2+} or Mn^{2+} are necessary as well as ATP. The predominant sites of phosphorylation are the free hydroxyl groups of serine and threonine residues. Distinct THV polypeptides (molecular masses of 100, 82, and 53 kDa) were found to be targets of phosphorylation in the presence of 5 mmol l^{-1} Mg^{2+}. At a higher Mg^{2+} concentration (20 mmol l^{-1}), additional viral proteins (220, 71, 31 and 20 kDa) were phosphorylated. The gene encoding the viral DNA polymerase was identified by nucleotide sequence analysis.

Geographic and Seasonal Distribution

THV infection of tree shrews is endemic only to south and southeast Asia, corresponding to the geographic distribution of the animal. Seasonal dependence for viral isolation has not been documented.

Host Range and Virus Propagation

The host range of the different THV strains *in vitro* clearly shows that tree shrew embryonic fibroblasts are the most susceptible cells for viral replication. Primary rabbit kidney cells, human foreskin fibroblasts and marmoset skin fibroblasts are less susceptible than tree shrew cells, whereas THVs do not replicate in rodent cell lines. Tree shrew embryonic fibroblasts are the cells of choice for propagation of THVs.

Genetics

A high degree of DNA sequence homology between the different THV isolates has been detected using DNA/DNA hybridization, heteroduplex mapping of the viral DNA molecules, and generation of intratypic recombinant viruses. This indicates the close genetic relationship between the individual THV strains. The seven isolates of THV are genetically grouped into five strains according to DNA fragmentation patterns. THV strains 1, 2, 3 and 5 comprise isolates 1, 2, 3 and 7 respectively, whereas isolates 4, 5 and 6 together represent THV strain 4. However, minor differences between the individual members of THV strain 4 are detectable in respect of slight size variations of specific restriction fragments.

Evolution

The tree shrew, which is the original host of THVs, is thought to have diverged at the basis of the evolutionary tree of mammals. THVs may therefore be fundamental representatives of mammalian herpesviruses. This is supported by the fact that the THV genome does not contain complex terminal repeat elements and does not occur in different isomeric forms such as modern herpesviruses (e.g. herpes simplex virus).

Serologic Relations and Variability

Serological crossreaction between different THV strains can usually be demonstrated. Crossreaction is sufficiently strong and can be detected with antisera against individual viral strains; however, it is possible to distinguish THV strains from each other in neutralization tests by significant differences in the resulting titers.

Epidemiology

THV epidemiology has not been the subject of intensive studies but analysis of the sera of a limited number of apparently healthy animals in captivity reveals that less than 1% of tree shrews have neutralizing antibodies against THVs.

Transmission and Tissue Tropism

The natural route of transmission of THVs is probably the same as for other herpesviruses. Most infections occur as a result of contact between open lesions and/or moist surfaces; however, spontaneous reactivation of latent virus should also be considered. The target organ for latent THVs is the spleen, as this is the only organ from which infectious viruses can be recovered even after a long period of chronic infection of tree shrews (24 months) and rabbits (14 months). Analysis of the genomes of recovered viruses by different restriction enzymes shows the same DNA fragment patterns when compared to the DNA of the originally inoculated viruses.

Pathogenicity

The pathogenicity of THV-1 to -4 for tree shrews as their indigenous host was studied using juvenile, young adult and adult animals inoculated intravenously or intraperitoneally. *In vivo* pathogenicity studies show that the tree shrew is highly susceptible to these viruses. Intravenous inoculation is always lethal (lethality 100%). In contrast, the majority of intraperitoneally inoculated animals survive the infection (lethality 25%). The major pathology is inflammatory hemorrhagic necrosis of the lungs. High virus titers are detectable in the tissues and whole blood of the infected animals.

It is remarkable that two of the five known THV strains were directly isolated from metastasizing tumors, in one case from a malignant lymphoma and in the other case from a Hodgkin's-like disease. However, only one malignant lymphoma has been induced experimentally in a tree shrew using THV-2. The tumor developed 3.5 years after intraperitoneal administration of the virus. Infectious virus that was genetically identical to the original inoculum was recovered from cultured tumor cells. The failure to routinely induce malignant lymphomas in the tree shrew after experimental inoculation with THV-2 and -3 is probably due to the short period of observation, as tree shrews can reach an age of 14 years.

The response of rabbits to THV-1, -2, -3 and -4 infections is well documented. THV-2 and -3 induce hyperplasia of the thymus in newborn New Zealand rabbits (80%), which in 8% of all cases develop malignant thymomas. Infectious virus can be recovered only from established spleen cultures of the infected rabbits. The spontaneous degeneration of the rabbit splenocyte cultures always develops by the first or second tissue culture passage. The genomes of the recovered viruses are identical when compared with the genome of the originally inoculated viruses.

Clinical Features of Infection

Clinical illness usually appears in juvenile animals infected with THV-1 to -4 on the second day after inoculation. The general symptoms worsen. Intravenous inoculation of these viruses leads to death of the infected animals. Death occurs from day 5 to day 18 post infection as a result of inflammatory hemorrhagic necrosis of the lungs. High virus titers are detectable in the tissues and whole blood of infected animals.

Pathology and Histopathology

It is of particular interest that THV-2 and -3 were isolated from degenerating cultured tumor cells from a high-grade malignant lymphoma and a Hodgkin's-like sarcoma, respectively. The lymphoma was detected in an adult (8-year-old) female tree shrew. Histopathological investigations revealed a discordant hyperplasia of lymphoreticular tissues with formation of nodal follicle-like proliferates. Two types of cells were observed. The first was small with polymorphic nuclei of clear appearance and small nucleoli; the second was of medium to large size with large rounded nuclei. The chromatin showed marginal aggregations with marginal nucleoli. Mitosis was relatively frequent. Several thick reticulin fibers were sparsely distributed after silver staining. Tumor cell infiltration was observed in the parenchyma of the pancreas, the peribronchial lymph follicles, the connective tissue of the pelvis of the kidney, the subserous membrane of the duodenum, and the cerebral meninges.

A generalized lymphoproliferative disorder resembling human Hodgkin's disease was observed in a female tree shrew of 9 years of age. Histological examination revealed hyperplasia of the lymphoreticular tissue with a polymorphic cellular population consisting of immunoblasts, numerous Hodgkin-like cells and Reed–Sternberg-like cells, eosinophilic granulocytes, and a marked lymphocytic depletion. The spleen showed a diffuse infiltration pattern; liver and peripelvic tissue of kidneys were likewise infiltrated.

Future Perspectives

Many interesting aspects of THV replication, such as transcription, post-transcriptional and post-translational processing, viral enzyme activity, etc., are still not understood and deserve intensive study in the future. Furthermore, genetic analysis of other tree shrew viruses, such as tree shrew retro-, rhabdo-, paramyxo- and adenovirus, is necessary for the final determination of their evolutionary roles.

See also: **Cytomegaloviruses (*Herpesviridae*): Animal cytomegaloviruses, General features (human), Molecular biology (human), Murine cytomegaloviruses; Epstein-Barr virus (*Herpesviridae*): General features, Molecular biology; Herpes simplex viruses (*Herpesviridae*): General features, Molecular biology.**

Further Reading

Darai G, Flügel RM, Matz B and Delius H (1981) DNA of *Tupaia* herpesviruses. In: Becker Y (ed.) *Herpesvirus DNA*, p. 345. The Hague: Nijhoff.

Darai G, Zöller L, Matz B *et al* (1982) Tupaia herpesviruses: characterization and biological properties. *Microbiologica* 5: 185.

Koch H-G, Delius H, Matz B (1985) Molecular cloning and physical mapping of the *Tupaia* herpesvirus genome. *J. Virol.* 55: 86.

TRICHOVIRUSES

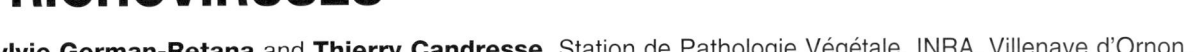

Sylvie German-Retana and **Thierry Candresse**, Station de Pathologie Végétale, INRA, Villenave d'Ornon, France

Copyright © 1999 Academic Press

History

The genus *Trichovirus* was established for plant viruses characterized by an elongated very flexuous and open particle morphology and a small genome size (<8.5 kb) as compared to other members of the *Closteroviridae* family which share an essentially similar particle morphology but have much larger genomes, in general in excess of 15 kb. The name 'tricho' is derived from the Greek 'thrix' meaning hair. The genus was approved by the International Committee of Taxonomy of Viruses in 1993, at the 9th International Congress of Virology, in Glasgow and has recently been placed in the family *Closteroviridae*.

Apple chlorotic leaf spot virus (ACLSV), the type member of the *Trichovirus* genus, had been previously classified in the subgroup A of closteroviruses, according to the morphology of its flexuous and filamentous viral particle. ACLSV was the first clostero-like virus whose genome was completely sequenced and genomic organization determined.

When molecular information became available on other closteroviruses, it became evident that there were very significant differences in genome properties and structure between ACLSV and beet yellows virus (BYV) the type member of the *Closterovirus* genus. These molecular differences, when added to the differences in particle and genome length, vector transmission, tissue tropism and cytopathic effects, led to the splitting of the *Closterovirus* genus and to the establishment of a new viral genus typified by ACLSV and for which the name *Trichovirus* was coined.

Taxonomy and Classification

The genus *Trichovirus* contains nine viral species (including seven tentative members) with similar biological, morphological, and ultrastructural properties. ACLSV and potato virus T (PVT) are definitive members of the genus, whereas grapevine virus A (GVA), grapevine virus B (GVB), grapevine virus C

Table 1 Properties of definitive and tentative trichoviruses

Virus	Particle length (nm)	Coat protein (kDa)	Genome (nt)	Mechanical transmissibility from natural host	Tissue localization in natural host	Vector
Definitive species						
ACLSV	720	22	7555	Easy	Parenchyma	Unknown
PVT	640	27	c. 7600	Easy	Parenchyma	Unknown
Tentative species						
GVA	800	22.5	7349	Difficult	Phloem	Mealybugs
GVB	800	23	7599	Difficult	Phloem	Mealybugs
GVC	725	25.7	nd	Difficult	Phloem	Mealybugs
GVD	825	20.5	c. 7600	Difficult	Phloem	Mealybugs
GBINV	740	22	c. 7600	Easy	Parenchyma	Unknown
HLV	730	22	nd	Easy	nd	Aphids
CMLV	760	20.5	c. 8200	Easy	nd	Mites

nd = not determined.

(GVC), grapevine virus D (GVD), grapevine berry inner necrosis virus (GBINV), cherry mottle leaf virus (CMLV) and heracleum latent virus (HLV) have properties that qualify them as tentative members of the genus (Table 1 and see below).

Note added in proof: GVA, GVB, GVC, GVD, CMLV and HLV have recently been split from trichoviruses to create a new genus, Vitivirus. ACLSV, PVT and GBINV thus remain as the only members of the trichovirus genus (see below).

Geographic Distribution and Host Range

Trichoviruses differ in the extent of their geographical distribution. ACLSV, GVA and GVB are found worldwide, whereas PVT has been reported only in the Andean region of South America, GBINV in Japan and HLV in Scotland. CMLV appears to be distributed over North America, but the precise identity of European isolates of CMLV remains to be evaluated. Information is still lacking on the extent of the geographical distribution of GVC and GVD. The natural host range of trichoviruses is restricted to either a single host (PVT, HLV, GVA, GVB, GVC, GVD, GBINV), or to a somewhat wider host range in the case of ACLSV which naturally infects most temperate rosaceous fruit crops.

The experimental host range for ACLSV includes dicotyledonous hosts from a few families and includes 'general purpose' hosts such as *Chenopodium quinoa*, *C. amaranticolor*, *Phaseolus vulgaris* and *Nicotiana occidentalis*. Experimental host reactions to GBINV inoculation are quite similar to those of ACLSV except that *C. amaranticolor* is not infected by GBINV. PVT shows a similarly rather restricted experimental host range. The experimental host range for HLV contains hosts corresponding to over nine families and includes also one monocotyledonous host, *Zea mays*. GVA, GVB and GVD and CMLV have a very narrow experimental host range including only *Vitis* and a few *Nicotiana* in the case of the grapevine viruses and *Prunus* and *Chenopodium* for CMLV.

Particle Structure and Composition

Although resembling that of some other flexuous elongated plant viruses such as potex- and carlaviruses, the very flexuous and open particle structure is the most conspicuous characteristic of trichoviruses. This unusual morphology is, however, shared with members of the *Closterovirus* and *Capillovirus* genera. Particles have, in general, a diameter of about 12 nm, with a length of 640–825 nm, depending on the virus considered. The RNA content is usually 5–6% and a single type of coat protein subunit is observed with a molecular weight of 20.5 kDa (CMLV)–27 kDa (PVT), although the calculated weight has been found to be as low as 17.6 kDa in the case of GVD.

The pitch of the primary helix, which can usually be measured from the obvious crossbanding of the particle, has been found to be in the range 3.4–3.8 nm, giving estimated ratios of four nucleotides per protein subunit and of about 10 protein monomers per turn of the helix. However, PVT particles differ slightly from those of ACLSV in having a slightly larger diameter (13–14 nm) with a pitch of the helix (3.4 nm) at the lower end of the range for trichoviruses. Correlated with the very open structure of the particle, the genomic RNA of several of these viruses, such as ACLSV and HLV, has been found to be sensitive to RNases in their encapsidated forms. Genome size has been found to be directly correlated with particle length and is reported to vary from 7.3 kb to about 8.2 kb.

An unusual property of the coat proteins of ACLSV, HLV, GBINV, GVA, GVB and GVD, is that they are devoid of tryptophan. This probably explains the high (1.4–1.8) A_{260}/A_{280} absorbance ratios of the corresponding viruses.

Genome Structure

In all cases examined, the genome of trichoviruses has been found to consist of a single molecule of single-stranded (ss) RNA. The genomic RNA of ACLSV is infectious and those of ACLSV, GVA and GVB have messenger activity *in vitro*. Thus, trichoviruses should be regarded as having monopartite ssRNA genomes of positive polarity. The genomic RNAs of the type member ACLSV (in fact, four strains of ACLSV differing in their original host and geographical origin), and two tentative members, GVA and GVB, have been totally sequenced, and the sequences of the 3′ terminal regions of PVT, GVD and GBINV genomes have been determined. Relevant sequence database accession numbers are: ACLSV-P863 (M31714), ACLSV-Ba11 (X99752), ACLSV-P205 (D14996), GVA (X75433), GVB (X75448), PVT (D10172), GVD (Y07764) and GBINV (D88448). The genomic RNAs have a polyadenylated 3′ terminus and are capped at their 5′ end.

Genome Organization and Expression: Affinities with other Virus Groups

Genomic organization of the trichoviruses for which sequence information is available is shown in **Fig. 1**. The ACLSV RNA (7.5 kb) contains three open reading frames (ORFs) encoding proteins with approximate molecular weights of 216 kDa, 50 kDa and 22–28 kDa. The partial sequences available for PVT and GBINV fit the same pattern: the extremity of the large replication-associated protein is followed by two smaller ORFs of 39 kDa (GBINV) or 40 kDa (PVT), and 22 kDa (GBINV) or 27 kDa (PVT).

The large, 5′-located ORF 1 codes for a protein that contains three signature sequences, typical of replicase-associated proteins of the 'Alpha-like' super group of plant viruses: the methyl transferase (MT), the nucleotide binding site of the helicase (HEL) and the RNA-dependent RNA polymerase (RdPd) signatures. Homologies with putative papain-related proteinases of positive-strand RNA viruses such as tymo- and furoviruses, are also found in a block of amino acids preceding the HEL domain (**Fig. 1**).

The ORF 2 of ACLSV shares distant similarities with the cauliflower mosaic virus gene I and TMV 30K movement proteins. The ORF 2-encoded protein has been included in the proposed family I of movement proteins (MP), which also includes the MPs of tobamoviruses, tobraviruses, comoviruses, caulimoviruses and geminiviruses. Furthermore, it has been shown that the ORF 2 protein of ACLSV can be detected in both cell wall and cell membrane fractions prepared from infected *Chenopodium quinoa* tissues, and is phosphorylated *in vivo*. All these properties fit with the assignment of this protein as the movement protein of the virus.

The capsid protein (CP) ORF is located at the 3′ terminus of the genomic RNA. The CP contains amino acids that are highly conserved in the CP of filamentous virus, and hypothesized to be involved in the formation of a salt bridge, assumed to play a key role in structure formation.

As shown in **Fig. 1**, the complete sequences of GVA and GVB contain five ORFs, including two that are absent from ACLSV, PVT and GBINV. ORF 1 which is the large replication-associated protein shows clear homologies and a similar arrangement of the conserved signature sequences with the ORF 1 of ACLSV. ORF 2 codes for a 20 kDa polypeptide with unknown function and for which no significant homology has been found in protein databases. ORF 3 encodes a 36.5 kDa (GVB) or 31 kDa (GVA) protein possessing the conserved motifs of the family I of movement proteins, and recent results show that

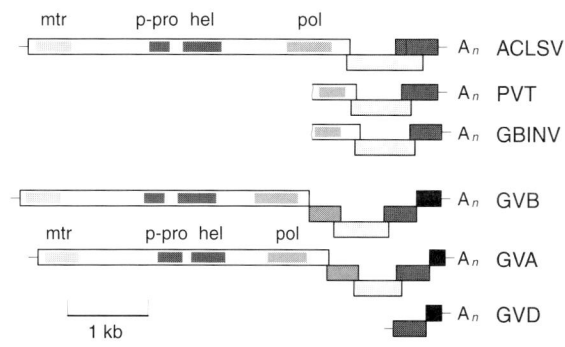

Figure 1 Genomic organization of trichoviruses. ACLSV, apple chlorotic leaf spot virus; PVT, potato virus T; GBINV, grapevine berry inner necrosis virus; GVA, grapevine virus A; GVB, grapevine virus B; GVD, grapevine virus D. mtr, methyl transferase domain; p-pro, papain-like proteinase domain; hel, helicase domain; pol, RNA-dependent RNA polymerase domain.

these proteins are associated with the cell wall, sometimes at the level of plasmodesmata, supporting the hypothesis of their role in the cell to cell movement of the virus. ORF 4 (21.5–21.6 kDa) is the CP cistron showing again low but clear homologies with the CPs of ACLSV, PVT and GBINV. ORF 5 codes for a small (10–14 kDa) protein homologous to the small cystein-rich nucleic acid binding-proteins found in the genome of other plant viruses, such as hordeiviruses and carlaviruses. In the 3′ end of the GVD genome, two ORFs were identified, encoding a cystein-rich 10 kDa protein and the 17.6 kDa CP, respectively; the genome of GVD is thus assumed to follow the same organization as that of GVA and GVB.

Subgenomic messenger RNAs (sgRNAs) have been observed for ACLSV and allow the expression of the ORFs located downstream of the 5′-most ORF. Although there is conflicting evidence for proteolytic processing of the 216 kDa protein of ACLSV, a possible proteolytic maturation of the 216 kDa protein is hypothesized, from the presence of the conserved papain-like protease signature sequence. In vitro translation experiments using the genomic GVB RNA as a template have tentatively shown that the 195 kDa viral replicase could undergo proteolytic cleavage.

Comparative analysis of proteins of definitive and tentative trichoviruses showed that they are all phylogenetically related. However, distinct clusters can be observed, in particular, when analyzing the movement and capsid proteins. In particular, GVA, GVB and GVD are much closer to each other than to ACLSV, PVT and GBINV.

Virus Host Relations: Cytopathic Effects

All trichoviruses can be experimentally transmitted by sap inoculation and by grafting. Mechanical transmission from natural host is easy for ACLSV, PVT, HLV, GBINV and CMLV, whereas sap inoculation is difficult for GVA, GVB, GVC and GVD. It is not surprising that the viruses that are easiest to transmit mechanically are also those that do not appear to be phloem-restricted. GVA, GVB, GVC and GVD are phloem-restricted in their natural host, grapevine, whereas ACLSV, PVT and GBINV seem to multiply primarily in parenchyma cells. However, GVA and GVB can invade the parenchyma of artificially infected herbaceous hosts and become mechanically transmissible under these circumstances. Most trichoviruses are not seed-borne, but PVT has been reported to be transmitted rather efficiently in this manner from a number of hosts and ACLSV may be seed-transmitted at a low frequency in apricot.

The cells of plants infected by GVA, GVB and GVD show conspicuous alterations. Virions accumulate in large bundles or paracrystalline aggregates in infected cells. The vascular bundles of systemically infected leaves of N. occidentalis have a strongly affected cytology with some cells in stage of necrosis. The cytoplasm shows membrane proliferation, vesiculation, and secondary vacuolation. Vesicular evaginations of the tonoplast contain finely fibrillar material. Mitochondria are damaged and chloroplasts are rounded and swollen, with a disrupted lamellar system and enlarged starch grains.

GBINV particles are found in vascular parenchyma and mesophyll cells. Particles exist as aggregated masses in the cytoplasm, but not in the nucleus or vacuole. No virus-specific inclusion bodies are observed. These modifications are comparable to those observed with ACLSV, except that ACLSV particles are sometimes found in the nucleus.

Viral Transmission

The mode of natural transmission differs substantially between the species of Trichovirus. No natural vectors are known for ACLSV, PVT and GBINV, natural dissemination probably being mediated by vegetative multiplication of propagation material.

In the case of HLV, aphid-transmission in a semipersistent manner is assisted by a helper closterovirus [Heracleum virus 6 (HV6)]. Cherry mottle leaf virus (CMLV) is transmitted by the scale mite Eriophyes inaequalis. Grapevine trichoviruses appear to be transmitted by several species of mealybugs in a nonspecies-specific manner. Both GVA, GVB and GVD are transmitted in nature by several species of the pseudococcid mealybug genera Pseudococcus and Planococcus (Planococcus ficus, Pseudococcus longispinus, Pseudococcus citri and Pseudococcus affinis). Studies of the acquisition and transmission of GVA by Ps. longispinus, showed that Ps. longispinus can acquire GVA in a short time (15 min) when feeding on N. clevelandii. The virus can be retained for up to 48 h when the insect is fasting. There is no latent period for the inoculation of GVA to N. clevelandii after a 30 min feeding. Such properties are consistent with a semipersistent mode of transmission.

Diseases and their Economic Significance

The economic importance of ACLSV is largely due to its worldwide distribution. Although it is more or less symptomless in pome fruits, it is responsible for serious diseases in stone fruit trees such as pseudopox (false plum pox) and bark split of plum, butteratura and viruella of apricot. In addition ACLSV includes incompatibility problems and bud failure following grafting of infected material, which can result in important losses in nurseries.

Infection by PVT or HLV induces little or no symptoms. The main disease for PVT has been reported only for potato (*Solanum tuberosum*) in which it is usually latent, but can produce a mild leaf mottle. HLV occurs commonly in Scotland in wild *Heracleum sphondylium* (hogweed) plants, without causing any symptoms.

Cherry mottle leaf virus (CMLV) is associated with a disease of both economic and quarantine importance in sweet cherry. The symptoms are irregular chlorotic mottling and distortion of the terminal leaves. In some cultivars, both the quality and the quantity of fruits are affected, the fruits being tasteless, and showing delayed ripening.

GVA, GVB, GVC and GVD are currently thought to be involved in the etiology of the rugose wood complex of diseases, an economically important problem in grapevine. At least four different disorders participate (corky bark, Rupestris stem pitting, Kober stem grooving and LN33 stem grooving). Individual disorders can be distinguished by indexing on specific *Vitis* indicators, but not in the field, due to the absence of specific symptoms. Rugose wood-affected vines are less vigorous, show a more or less pronounced swelling at the bud union and a marked difference between the diameter of scion and rootstock. The affected vines may decline and die within a few years. The major characteristic features of the disease are symptoms of pitting and grooving in the woody cylinders of the scion, rootstock, or both. There are cases in which the scion also shows an atypical production of corky tissues, just above the graft union, called 'corky rugose wood'. Unraveling the etiology of rugose wood appears to be a very complex problem that has not yet been solved. Circumstantial evidence points to GVA and GVB being the probable agents of, respectively, Kober stem grooving and corky bark diseases.

Grapevine berry inner necrosis, reported in Japan, and originally called mosaic disease, is one the most economically important virus diseases of grapevines in Japan. The diseased grapevines grow less vigorously, sprout late in spring, and show inner necrosis in shoots, shortened internodes and various mosaic patterns on leaves. Berries are small, show external discoloration and interior necrosis.

Serological Relationships and Molecular Variability

Very limited serological relationships have been detected between the trichoviruses. It has been recently reported that GVA, GVB and GVD are distantly serologically related, the shared antigenic determinant between GVA and GVD corresponding probably to a cryptotope. GVA and HLV have also a distant serological relationship. No other serological relationship has been reported between other members of the genus.

The type member of the genus, ACLSV, is characterized by a large biological diversity. Polymerase chain reaction (PCR) has been used to study the variability of ACLSV in the region of overlap between the 50 kDa movement protein and the coat protein genes. Extensive variability is observed between isolates at the nucleotide sequence level, most isolates evaluated showing divergence rates in the 10–20% range from each other. However, at the protein level, the CP is highly conserved between the isolates and variations in the 50 kDa movement protein explain most of the variations in the nucleotide sequence. These results are in keeping with the large biological diversity and the low serological diversity observed between ACLSV isolates. No information on the molecular variability of other trichoviruses has been reported so far.

Virus Epidemiology and Control

In most cases, natural transmission by vectors is not the main cause of long-distance dispersion of the viruses, which is mostly due to human distribution of contaminated material. In regions from which a given virus is absent, quarantine measures are the best protective measure. In affected regions, viral infection is usually controlled through the production and use of virus-free propagation material, along with control of insect vector populations and destruction of virus reservoirs. The most frequently used detection techniques for certification of propagation and planting material include bioassays on susceptible hosts and enzyme-linked immunosorbent assays (ELISA). In addition, detection of dsRNAs associated with viral infection (ACLSV, GVA, GVB, GVD), immunoelectron microscopy (IEM), molecular hybridization and PCR detection methods have been reported for several of these viruses. In the case of ACLSV, it has been possible to obtain virus-free plants through the use of meristem tip culture, thermotherapy or a combination of both, eventually coupled with chemotherapy using agents such as virazole (ribavirin, a cap structure analogue). For GVA and GVB, it is possible to eliminate the viruses from grapevine with the use of meristem tip culture, although with great difficulty, as these viruses are among the hardest to eliminate from the grapevine.

Future Perspectives

Differences in molecular organization, biological and epidemiologic behavior, between definitive (ACLSV, PVT) and tentative (GVA, GVB, GVC, GVD) trichoviruses, seem to be wide enough to warrant the splitting of the *Trichovirus* genus. The creation of a new genus named *Vitivirus*, which would contain GVA, GVB, GVC, GVD, HLV and CMLV, has recently been approved by the Executive Committee of the ICTV.

See also: **Capilloviruses; Closteroviruses (*Closteroviridae*); Plant virus disease – economic aspects.**

Further Reading

Bar-Joseph M and Murant AF (1982) Closterovirus group. *CMI/AAB Description of Plant Viruses*, no. 260.

Brunt A, Crabtree K, Dallwitz M, Gibbs A and Watson L (eds) (1996) *Viruses of plants, Descriptions and Lists from the VIDE Database*. Wallingford: CAB International.

Martelli GP, Candresse T and Namba S (1994) *Trichovirus*, a new genus of plant viruses. *Arch. Virol.* 134: 451.

TUMOR VIRUSES – HUMAN

Herbert Pfister, Institute for Virology, University of Koln, Koln, Germany

Bernhard Fleckenstein, Institute for Clinical and Molecular Virology, Friedrich-Alexander University, Erlangen, Germany

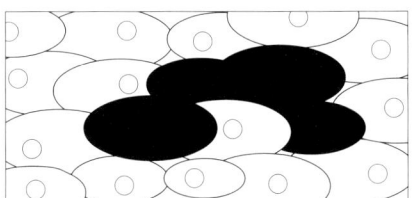

Copyright © 1999 Academic Press

Criteria for Causal Relationship between Virus and Cancer

Although there are numerous animal models for viral oncogenesis, only in rare cases is the virus sufficient by itself for tumor induction. In those systems, experimental infection may lead to sizeable tumors within a few weeks, thus leaving no doubt about the etiologic role of the particular pathogen. In humans, none of the viruses incriminated as being oncogenic appear to be independent of other factors. Many years, and often several decades, pass by before tumors develop from primary infection in a small number of infected individuals. Monoclonal tumors arise from the pool of virus-infected cells. This suggests that the virus is, at best, one of several factors that together increase the probability of a cell undergoing malignant transformation. Possible cofactors are chemical or physical carcinogens. Furthermore, the oncogenic activity of the virus may be restricted to a specific genetic background of the patient or to a susceptible stage of cell development. These complex interrelations and the ethical ban on experiments in humans render it extremely difficult to prove the causative role for the virus.

Viruses may contribute to tumor development at various stages of the multistep carcinogenesis process and by different mechanisms. If viral activity is necessary, the virus should be found at some stage in every case in which the tumor occurs. Viral footprints do not, however, have to appear in cancer cells. Human immunodeficiency virus (HIV), for example, significantly increases the risk of development of Kaposi sarcomas and B-cell lymphomas, probably because of its suppressive effect on the immune system. For some herpesviruses and papillomaviruses, a 'hit and run' mechanism has been proposed, which implies virally induced irreversible damage at some point early in tumorigenesis, but no role later on in the maintenance of the malignant phenotype; the virus may therefore completely disappear from the cancer. Viruses may act as mutagens or, even more indirectly, by increasing the risk of mutations via induction of cell proliferation in the course of chronic inflammatory reactions. The etiologic significance of a virus is very difficult to prove in this case. Large-scale and long-term prospective epidemiological studies are the only way to define the risk of a given infection. As the virus may be present for short periods only, the infection is best monitored by the detection of specific antibodies. Previous studies focused on anticapsid antibodies, but with many DNA viruses the production of particles and oncogenic transformation appear to be mutually exclusive, so it might be more promising to screen for antibodies against early nonstructural viral proteins.

Following the classical concepts of virus-induced cell transformation, a tumor virus induces new genetic material into host cells by establishing a persistent infection. The expression of one or more viral oncogenes may then affect cell proliferation and/or differentiation. This can be tested *in vitro* by transformation assays which may result in cells that are tumorigenic in nude mice. If a virus acts in this way, one has to find viral genomes as well as virus-specific transcripts and oncogenic proteins in transformed cells and also in cancer cells if the viral functions are essential for maintaining the malignant phenotype. Tumor viruses may alternatively contribute to carcinogenesis by inserting viral transcription control elements in the vicinity of cellular proto-oncogenes. Viral DNA has to be detectable in these cases adjacent to relevant proto-oncogenes of cancer cells. A harmful integration is typically a very rare event among many random insertions, which is selected for by tumor growth *in vivo*. This mechanism cannot be mimicked by *in vitro* transformation assays.

The physical association of viral genes with tumor cells, in combination with data on oncogenic activity from cell culture or animal experiments, is usually regarded as a most convincing evidence for a role for a virus in human carcinogenesis; however, even better proof of the effective contribution of the virus is obtained from longitudinal epidemiological studies. Finally, the most convincing argument in favor of a necessary role for a tumor virus will be cancer prevention by intervention directed at the virus, such as specific vaccination.

Burkitt's Lymphoma

The malignant lymphoma that was recognized by Denis Burkitt in 1958 as a distinct disease entity in Africa was the first human neoplasm to be linked with a viral etiology. Burkitt's lymphoma (BL) is the most frequent type of childhood tumor found in some hot and humid lowland areas of Central and Eastern Africa, but sporadic cases of the disease, defined by the peculiar histopathology and chromosome translocations, occur throughout the world. Although, in the majority of cases, BL presents in younger children around 8 years of age as a unilateral swelling of the jaw, the disease is usually multifocal at diagnosis due to early metastasis; it characteristically involves liver, kidneys, ovaries or testes, lymphoid tissues in the gut, and endocrine or exocrine glands. In older children and young adults, mostly in the sporadic cases outside Africa, abdominal masses are the first sign of disease.

Lymphoid tumor cell lines derived from BL biopsies led to the discovery in 1964 by Epstein and colleagues of a new herpesvirus, termed Epstein–Barr virus (EBV). The cell lines usually contain EBV genomes as nonintegrated covalently closed circular double-stranded DNA (dsDNA) genomes of about 172 kb in high multiplicity; some lymphoblastoid cell lines carry the EBV genomes integrated into the cellular genomes. EBV is capable of immortalizing human B lymphocytes. The transformed cells express a viral nuclear antigen complex, termed EBNA, which consists of at least six proteins, and in addition latent membrane proteins (LMP). Genetic experiments identified EBNA-2 and LMP as the growth-transforming factors. BL-derived lymphoblastoid cell lines typically express EBNA-1, while, remarkably, the other EBNA proteins and LMP are not detectable. Some lymphoblastoid lines are in a semipermissive state; they produce mature herpesvirus particles spontaneously or can be induced to do so by substances such as the tumor-promoting phorbol ester, phorbol 12-myristate 13-acetate (PMA). BL lymphoma cells and lymphoblastoid tumor cell lines have the surface antigen markers of B lymphocytes; this correlates with a narrow host range of the virus; *in vitro* the virus selectively adsorbs and penetrates by binding of the virion envelope glycoprotein gp350/220 to the complement receptor 2 (CR2; CD21) of B lymphocytes or their precursors. In epithelial cell lines, transcripts encoding CD21 have been detected; however, expression of this receptor on primary epithelial cells remains to be demonstrated.

Indirect immunofluorescence testing with EBV-producing lymphoblastoid cell lines provided the basis for seroepidemiology. It showed that EBV is a ubiquitous virus that occurs in the majority of populations on a worldwide scale. Primary infection can lead to infectious mononucleosis or may remain inapparent without overt disease. BL typically follows early seroconversion during infancy; tumor-bearing children have high antibody titers against structural and early EBV proteins.

In spite of a general association between development of BL and the viral markers, the exact role of EBV in tumor pathogenesis has remained controversial. More than 90% of the tumors in areas of endemic BL contain EBV DNA and express EBNA, and the children have generally high titers of antibodies; however, in sporadic forms of BL that occur in other parts of the world the viral DNA and protein markers are present in only about 15–20%, and elevated antibody titers are not observed in the case of tumors devoid of viral markers. Thus, the presence of EBV persisting in certain compartments of B cells or their precursors may be a risk factor for the development of BL, but it cannot be the sole driving force for oncogenesis. So far, it is also difficult strictly to exclude the possibility that EBV is only a passenger of the tumor without contributing to its generation. Common denominators of all BL forms, endemic and sporadic, are certain chromosome translocations. Typically, the gene locus for the proto-oncogene c-*myc* (chromosome 8q29) is juxtaposed to the immunoglobulin heavy chain locus on the long arm of chromosome 14. The break points on the c-*myc* gene are located upstream of the promoter, in the first exon, or between the first and second exon of the proto-oncogene. Less frequently, c-*myc* is translocated to the immunoglobulin (chromosome 2p11) or (chromosome 22q11) light chain genes. It is generally believed that the translocations result in some form of c-*myc* deregulation, perhaps at the level of transcriptional control, mRNA processing or protein synthesis. A unifying concept to explain the role of EBV in BL proposes that the virus initiates the process of tumorigenesis through growth stimulation of a certain B-cell population. Polyclonal B-cell expansion, possibly favoured by malaria-induced impairment of T-cell functions, may enlarge the number of target cells for the necessary key event, chromosome translocation and deregulation of the proto-oncogene c-*myc*. An alternative may be the immortalization by EBV of a malaria-amplified pool of pre-existing c-*myc*-translocated B-cells. In both cases, early EBV infection and viral persistence would be an important risk factor for BL, primarily in its endemic forms.

EBV-Associated Lymphoproliferative Syndromes Other than BL

While primary infection with EBV usually remains without overt disease or manifests as benign infectious mononucleosis, rare cases develop into fatal lymphoproliferations with features of malignant B-cell lymphoma. About half of these cases occur in boys or male adolescents with an inherited defect in the immune system, termed X-linked lymphoproliferative syndrome (XLPS) or Duncan syndrome. The other cases are sporadic without a sex preponderance. Proliferating cells were shown to contain persisting EBV DNA and to express the viral latency genes EBNA and LMP. The infiltrating B-cell derivatives have been shown to be polyclonal in some cases; other processes appeared oligoclonal. The defects of the immune system leading to XLPS or fatal mononucleosis are not precisely known, as the children are not generally immunodeficient. Possibly it relates to functional impairment of natural killer (NK) cells, cytotoxic T cells or changes in the B cells that are the targets of EBV-induced growth stimulation. Notably, some of the patients do not have the normal antibody response to EBV antigens, particularly EBNA-1.

EBV sometimes induces fatal lymphoproliferative disease or lymphoma in globally immunodeficient individuals, either in cases of severe congenital immunodeficiencies or acquired immunosuppression in transplant recipients. Diffuse B-cell lymphomas, often localized in the central nervous system or other extranodular sites, are a frequent cause of morbidity and mortality in acquired immunodeficiency disease (AIDS). The tumors are often polyclonal initially, as they arise from several independent transformation events; they gradually evolve into an oligoclonal or even monoclonal proliferation. The tissues usually have the markers of persisting and actively transforming EBV, including EBNA and LMP expression. Similarly, the lymphomas of owl monkeys (*Aotus trivirgatus*) and cotton top marmosets (*Saguinus oedipus*) that are experimentally inoculated with EBV are considered to be immediate outgrowths of EBV-transformed B lymphoblasts. Presumably, deficiency in certain immune effector mechanisms, genetically determined or acquired, which are necessary to eliminate EBV-transformed B lymphoblasts from the body, leads to progressive lymphoproliferative diseases. On occasion it has been reported that human lymphomas with T-cell markers, such as nasal T-cell lymphomas, contain persisting EBV. A viral etiology of those tumors remains difficult to establish; the cell surface receptor for EBV on T cells is not yet known.

EBV genomes have been detected more recently in a large proportion (up to 60%) of cases of Hodgkin's disease. Distinct LMP-specific membrane and cytoplasmic staining has been found exclusively in Hodgkin and Reed–Sternberg cells of virus DNA-positive specimens, while EBNA-2 is not detected. This suggests a pattern of EBV gene expression different from that of B lymphoblastoid cells and BL. In view of the transforming potential of the LMP gene, it suggests a causal role of EBV in the case of Hodgkin's disease. Viral persistence and preferential expression of LMP has also been seen in some cases of CD30+ anaplastic large cell lymphoma, a heterogeneous group of high-grade malignant lymphomas at the borderline between Hodgkin's and non-Hodgkin's lymphomas. The role of EBV in angioimmunoblastic lymphoadenopathy remains to be determined.

Nasopharyngeal Carcinoma

Nasopharyngeal carcinomas (NPCs) are highly malignant neoplasms which mostly occur in adults between the ages of 20 and 50 years. Though the incidence is generally low in Europe and North

America, NPC is a frequent tumor in southern parts of China, in Tunisia, Central Africa and in the native population of Alaska. The prognosis is poor; most frequently, NPCs present with early metastasis into cervical lymph nodes and the skull. The association of EBV with NPC has been clearly established. Viral DNA is regularly found in all cases of poorly differentiated or lymphoepithelial NPC. Studies on the structure of the persisting episomal EBV genomes have indicated that the neoplastic epithelial cells contain a single clone of EBV in each case. Carcinoma cells consistently express EBNA-1 and, frequently, latent membrane proteins, while the EBNA-2 gene is not transcribed. There is a strong serological association between EBV and NPC. The sera of patients with NPC typically have high titers of immunoglobulin A (IgA) antibodies to structural viral components, latency proteins and replicative antigens. A similar association was found between EBV and several rare tumor forms that are also assumed to be derived from embryonic branchial cleft remnants. High IgA titers against EBV proteins and persisting viral DNA in the tumors have also been found in some forms of neoplasms from the parotid, thymus and lymphatic tissue of the oropharynx.

T-Cell Leukemia

Adult T-cell leukemia (ATL) was the first human disease to be causally linked to a retrovirus. ATL, first described as a frequent tumor form in southern regions of Japan, is a distinct disease entity that occurs in many other parts of the world, including Central Africa and the Caribbean basin. Epidemiology clearly demonstrated the association with human T-cell leukemia virus type 1 (HTLV-1). Serological surveys showed that antibodies against HTLV-1 were regularly found in leukemia patients, and frequently in their close contacts. Tumor cells mostly contain integrated proviral DNA; clonality of the tumor correlates with the monoclonal or oligoclonal integration pattern of the viral genomes. HTLV-1 can be detected by polymerase chain reaction (PCR) in peripheral lymphocytes of latently infected persons and ATL patients. If peripheral mononuclear blood cells are infected with HTLV-1 in cell culture, T cells are immortalized, resulting in continuous growth in suspension culture. The cell surface marker phenotype largely resembles the tumor cells which express high levels of IL-2Rα (α chain of the interleukin-2 receptor) and CD4. HTLV-1 has also been shown to be oncogenic in animal model systems.

ATL usually develops 30–50 years after perinatal infection with HTLV-1. The virus is most frequently transmitted by breast feeding and sexual contacts. The malignancy, arising after the long carrier phase, may be manifested as a lymphoma or acute leukemia, with high white blood cell count and a poor prognosis, usually being fatal within 6–8 months. Smoldering and chronic forms of ATL can convert into an acute course. Approximately 3% of the perinatally infected will develop ATL during their lifetime. Unlike retroviruses of other subgroups, HTLV-1 contains a 1.6 kb proviral genomic region coding for at least two regulatory polypeptides, the 40 kDa transcriptional transactivator Tax and the 27 kDa phosphoprotein Rex, which is required for the cytoplasmic targeting for structural protein mRNAs. Tax, a transactivator of the viral promoter and modulator of numerous cellular genes, appears to mediate the oncogenic effects of the virus; it induces polyclonal expansion of CD4+ T lymphocytes. The early virus-induced helper T-cell proliferation may precede a long period of tumor progression as growth becomes autonomous, turning independent of Tax expression.

HTLV-2, which frequently occurs in some tribes of native Americans, has been isolated repeatedly from the T-cell variant of hairy cell leukemia, but the etiology of T-cell malignancies by HTLV-2 has not been substantiated further until now. Like type 1, HTLV-2 is increasingly spread among intravenous drug abusers in European and American cities.

Genital Cancer

Clinical studies, and especially data from molecular biology, suggest that certain types of human papillomavirus (HPV) are of etiological importance for genital cancer. In developing countries, carcinoma of the cervix uteri is the most frequent type of female cancer. HPV DNA can be found in 80–90% of the tumors, and the early genes E6 and E7 are usually expressed. The most prevalent type in epidermoid carcinomas is HPV 16. HPV 18 may be preferentially associated with adenocarcinomas. Other types like HPV 31, 33, 35, 39, 45, 51, 52 or 56 have been detected in a few cases of squamous cell carcinoma each. HPV DNA was also demonstrated in the less prevalent carcinomas of the vulva, the vagina, the penis and the anus; HPV 16 is again the most frequent type, followed by HPV 18, HPV 6 and HPV 11. The significantly elevated prevalence of individual HPV types in cancers compared with the normal population led to the concept of HPVs with higher (HPV 16, 18, 45) and lower (HPV 6, 11) carcinogenic potential. This grouping is supported by first follow-up studies of the natural history of precancerous lesions associated with different HPVs and by differences in the *in vitro* transformation of keratinocytes.

HPV 16 and other members of the high-risk

papillomavirus group immortalize primary human keratinocytes and induce resistance to differentiation stimuli. Histological abnormalities can be observed in stratifying keratinocyte cultures that resemble those in precancerous, intraepithelial lesions *in vitro*. The cells are not tumorigenic in nude mice initially, but quickly change to an aneuploid karyotype, which is in keeping with frequently occurring abnormal mitoses in HPV 16-positive lesions. At higher passage level, malignant clones reproducibly arise, which indicates that HPV infection is sufficient to induce cancer cells in combination with additional spontaneous or virus-induced modifications. The viral genes E6 and E7 are required to trigger these effects. They encode proteins that are transactivators of transcription and are able to interact with the cellular proteins p53 and p105-RB (the retinoblastoma protein), respectively. The known cell-cycle regulating functions of these proteins are likely to be disturbed by this complex formation with the viral proteins. The E6 and E7 proteins of low-risk viruses display much lower affinities to the cellular proteins, in parallel with a lower or not detectable transforming potential *in vitro*.

Much attention has been paid to the possible role of viral DNA integration in tumor progression. HPV 18 DNA appears integrated into the cellular genome in almost all cervical cancers, and HPV 16 DNA in about two-thirds of the cases. This is in contrast with benign and premalignant lesions, where the viral DNA usually persists extrachromosomally. There is no evidence for a specific integration site, but HPV DNA has been repeatedly detected in the vicinity of the *myc* proto-oncogene in combination with an overexpression of the cellular gene.

The opening of the circular viral genome during integration frequently disrupts the regulator genes E1 and/or E2. Engineered mutants in these genes revealed increased transformation efficiency *in vitro*, so that naturally occurring inactivation may quantitatively enhance cell transformation.

In addition to the disruption of viral control mechanisms, there seems to be a failure of a cellular regulation of viral gene expression in malignant cells. The analysis of hybrids between HPV DNA-positive cervical cancer-derived cells and primary keratinocytes suggested that an inducible control system, possibly encoded by chromosome 11, can normally suppress viral transcription.

The persistence of viral DNA and the continual expression of transforming genes in advanced cancers suggest that HPV functions are also involved in the maintenance of the malignant phenotype. An experimental suppression of E6 and E7 expression inhibited the proliferation of HPV-positive cervical cancer cell lines and reduced the cloning efficiency in semisolid medium, thus indicating that the viral proteins are still modulating the growth of malignant cells.

The genital tract HPVs are also responsible for many HPV infections at extragenital mucosal sites such as the oral cavity and most notably the larynx. However, cancers arising in this field only rarely harbor HPV DNA. Case reports describe the presence of HPV 2, 6, 11, 16 or 30 in carcinomas of the tongue, the oral and nasal cavities, the larynx, the hypopharynx and the lung. The reason for the striking difference between the genital and aerodigestive tracts is not known. Either the etiology of oral and laryngeal cancers is unrelated to HPV, or the relevant HPV types are not yet characterized or the viral DNA is no longer necessary for cancer cells and is finally lost.

Skin Cancer

HPVs induce various proliferative skin lesions that are benign, like plantar, common and flat warts. An association between HPV and skin cancer becomes obvious in epidermodysplasia verruciformis (EV). EV patients are infected with a subgroup of HPVs, which induce characteristic persisting macular lesions disseminated over the body. Many EV patients develop squamous cell skin carcinomas, mainly at sun-exposed sites, which suggests a cocarcinogenic effect of ultraviolet light. The DNA of HPV 5 or 8 persists extrachromosomally in high copy number in more than 90% of the cancers. HPV14, 17, 20 or 47 were occasionally detected. The prevalence of specific HPVs is in striking contrast with the plurality of HPV in benign lesions and has been interpreted as reflecting a higher oncogenic potential of these types.

Oncogenes of EV-HPVs were mainly identified by their effects on rodent fibroblasts. The E6 gene induces altered morphology, reduced serum requirement, and anchorage-independent growth. In contrast with genital HPV, no complex formation could be detected between HPV8 E6 and the cellular p53 protein, which suggests different strategies of transformation. The HPV8 E2 gene, which encodes a transactivator of transcription, leads to reduced serum requirement and growth in soft agar. There is some indication of an increased transforming activity of E6 from HPV5, 8 and 47 when compared with E6 from related HPVs, which have not yet been detected in carcinomas.

A high prevalence of HPV DNA in squamous and basal cell carcinomas of the skin, particularly of immunosuppressed but also of immunocompetent patients, has most recently been demonstrated by highly sensitive PCRs. Evidence is accumulating for many novel HPV types related to EV HPVs and cutaneous types. Genital mucosal HPV types have also been found. That there is a strong association between genital HPV16 and squamous cell neoplasms from the finger is remarkable. Individual skin tumors were frequently noted to be infected by several HPVs. No single HPV type predominates in skin cancers of non-EV patients, so far as is known. The need for highly sensitive detection methods suggests that HPV DNA persists at very low concentrations in many skin cancers, perhaps at less than one genome copy per cancer cell. The relevance of these findings to the pathogenesis of cutaneous cancer remains to be determined. The possibilities discussed above for carcinomas of the aerodigestive tract are also valid for skin carcinomas.

Hepatocellular Carcinoma

Primary liver cancer is among the most common fatal malignancies of humans worldwide. An association with hepatitis B virus (HBV) from the hepadnavirus family was suggested by the geographical coincidence of a high incidence of hepatocellular carcinoma in southeast Asia and equatorial Africa with high rates of chronic HBV infections, generally contracted congenitally. Prospective studies demonstrated about a hundredfold increased risk of hepatoma among carriers of the HBV surface antigen (HBsAg). Integrated HBV DNA can be detected in a large proportion of the tumors from high-risk areas and in hepatoma-derived cell lines.

Liver cancer usually develops only after several decades of chronic HBV-induced hepatitis and may thus be triggered by accumulating genetic damage due to inflammation and continuous cell regeneration. A specific contribution of HBV might be expected from cis effects following integration of viral DNA, but except for a few case reports no consistent evidence has been obtained for the activation of particular proto-oncogenes. A transactivation of transcription may be more relevant; this can be achieved by the viral X protein, the large surface protein and a truncated preS$_2$/S protein. The viral preS$_2$/S gene, which normally encodes a surface protein, appears frequently disrupted in cancers as a consequence of DNA integration and then gives rise to the transactivator. All HBV transactivators exert pleiotropic effects via the protein kinase C/raf-controlled signal pathway, finally activating transcription factors such as AP-1 and NF-κB and proliferation. The analysis of viral integration patterns and functional assays suggest that at least one transactivator may function in most hepatomas. Multifocal nodular hyperplastic liver disease developed in mice transgenic for the HBV surface protein genes, and liver cancer arose in mice transgenic for the X gene. Mutations in the p53 tumor suppressor gene occur in about 30% of human hepatomas. They are observed more often in countries with dietary contamination by mutagenic aflatoxin and seem to be a late event in liver carcinogenesis. The complex formation between p53 and X protein as well as truncated preS$_2$/S may be relevant to p53 inactivation in patients with wild-type p53. The X protein was also shown to interact with elements of the DNA repair system, which may increase the mutation rate of p53.

HBV is the first human tumor virus against which vaccination programs have been initiated on a broad basis. First signs of a decrease in the incidence of hepatoma in populations vaccinated in the 1970s substantiate the viral role in cancer development.

More recently, seroepidemiological evidence was obtained for a correlation between hepatitis C virus (HCV) infections and hepatoma. Antibodies against HCV were detected in between 13% and over 80% of liver cancer patients around the world. Over 60% of acute hepatitis C becomes chronic and may progress to cirrhosis and hepatocellular carcinoma. Latency periods between primary infection and cancer are usually measured in decades but in some cases the intervals are rather short (5–10 years). The cumulative prevalence of hepatoma in cirrhotic HCV-infected patients is over 50%, indicating that HCV substantially increases the risk of hepatocellular carcinoma. HCV is related to flaviviruses and pestiviruses and is the first human tumor-related virus with an RNA genome and no DNA intermediate during replication. The role of the virus in carcinogenesis is not yet clear. Liver injury during chronic hepatitis may be responsible for malignant conversion but there is also some evidence that HCV is more directly involved. HCV appears to persist and replicate in hepatocytes during malignant transformation. The core protein has been shown to cooperate with the ras oncogene in transformation of primary rat embryo fibroblasts, to activate transcription of the c-myc proto-oncogene and to suppress the c-fos promoter. As regulation of cell death is now appreciated as an important factor in the pathogenesis of human malignancies, it is interesting to note that the HCV core protein can suppress cisplatin-mediated apoptosis in human cervical epithelial cells. Core gene variants that predominate in cancerous versus noncancerous lesions may point to a different oncogenic potential of various representatives of the HCV quasispecies. Experimental expression of the nonstructural protein NS3, a serine proteinase, leads to transformation of NIH3T3 cells and it has been speculated that NS3 may cleave and activate cellular proto-oncogene products.

Kaposi's Sarcoma

Kaposi's sarcoma (KS) was first described by Moriz Kaposi as 'multiple idiopathic pigmented sarcoma of the skin' in 1872. It is a multifocal, proliferative lesion of spindle-shaped cells with slit-like vascular spaces in skin and mucous membranes of the oral cavity, gastrointestinal tract and pleura. The tumor cells, termed KS spindle cells, are thought to be of endothelial origin. These tumor cells are likely not monoclonal in the early stages of KS. The 'classic' form of KS is a rare and often benign tumor of elderly males, mostly of Mediterranean or Jewish descent. Usually, the skin lesions of classic KS arise multifocally on the lower limbs and develop from patches to plaques and nodules over several years.

More aggressive, disseminated forms of KS have been described in Africa in the 1950s, and later in immunosuppressed organ transplant recipients. The etiology of this peculiar semimalignant neoplasia has always been an enigma, the favored hypothesis being a model where proliferation and transformation of endothelial cells are triggered in a paraendocrine manner by a host of proinflammatory cytokines and growth factors. Although this model is in agreement with some of the clinical features of this uncommon malignancy, it does not answer the question of what initiates the abnormal release of cytokines. An early hypothesis linked KS to infectious agents. The epidemiology of KS amongst patients with AIDS favored the latter hypothesis.

During the first decade of the AIDS epidemic, KS was at least 20 000 times more common in patients with AIDS than in the general population. Most notably, 20% of homosexual and bisexual patients developed KS, but only 1% of men with hemophilia. By employing the PCR-based representational difference analysis (RDA), Chang, Moore and colleagues searched for DNA sequences present in KS lesions but absent from uninvolved skin. This work resulted in the identification of DNA fragments of a novel human herpesvirus, now termed human herpesvirus 8 (HHV-8) or Kaposi's sarcoma-associated herpesvirus (KSHV). Numerous studies soon revealed that HHV-8 DNA is invariably found in all types of KS, where the majority of KS spindle cells are positive for HHV-8 DNA and transcripts. Searches in normal and diseased tissues other than KS showed that, at least in Northern Europe and the USA, HHV-8 DNA is infrequently detected in Caucasians. Only body cavity-based lymphomas (BCBL) and multifocal Castleman's disease, two rare B-lymphoproliferative disorders, were unequivocally HHV-8 DNA positive.

HHV-8 cell lines established from AIDS-associated cases of BCBL allowed for first studies of HHV-8 serology. In summary, the numerous studies available today clearly show that HHV-8 seropositivity closely reflects the risk of KS development. Antibodies against HHV-8 are usually detectable in 75–95% of KS patients but only in 1–5% of healthy blood donors in Northern Europe and the USA. Although the virus appears to be much more prevalent in Africa and Southern Europe, HHV-8 is closely linked to Kaposi's sarcoma. This is based both on seroepidemiology and DNA detection by PCR and *in situ* hybridization, suggesting a causal relationship between HHV-8 infection/reactivation and KS development.

Studies of HHV-8 genome structure and function also support the hypothesis of viral etiology. The complete genomic sequence revealed that HHV-8 belongs to the rhadinovirus subgroup of herpesviruses, whose best-characterized member is herpesvirus saimiri, an oncogenic virus of New World primates. The HHV-8 genome encodes an unusually high number of genes that have been captured from the host cell. Amongst them are several genes known to be involved in regulation of cell growth (D-cyclins) and apoptosis (bcl-2, v-Flip), signal transduction (IL-6, β-chemokines, IL8-receptor, interferon regulatory factor). Several HHV-8 genes have been found to have transforming potential in cell culture. Although further studies are required to substantiate the mechanism of oncogenesis by HHV-8, it becomes increasingly evident that HHV-8 is a causal factor for KS development.

Future Perspectives

Some two decades ago, only one human virus, EBV, was accepted as a candidate human tumor virus. Since then, the oncogenic potential of human papillomavirus, hepadnavirus and retrovirus has been clearly established. Now it has become evident that virus infections that may result in tumor formation are quite frequent. On a worldwide scale, more than 20% of all malignant tumor forms in females and about 8% of the tumors in males may be the late consequence of a previous virus infection. In most cases, long latency periods of many years or several decades elapse between primary infection by tumor viruses and first symptoms of cancer (**Table 1**). All human tumor viruses are widespread in the world population. They contribute to tumor disease, mainly by initiation of oncogenesis, but are not sufficient by themselves to cause a tumor. Thus, all human tumor viruses are important risk factors for cancer, but require additional events. This implies that mere proof of an infection with a tumor virus is of limited value for the management of patients and cancer prevention. Specific diagnostic tests have to be

Table 1 Latency periods for virus-associated tumors

Virus	Tumor	Latency period (years)
Hepatitis B virus	Hepatocellular carcinoma	30–50
Human T-cell leukemia virus type 1	T-cell leukemia	20–50
Human herpesvirus 8	Kaposi's sarcoma in immunosuppression	3–10
Human papillomavirus 5, 8	Squamous cell skin carcinoma of patients with epidermodysplasia verruciformis	5–15
Human papillomavirus 16, 18	Cervical cancer	5–25
Human papillomavirus 16, 18	Penile and vulval carcinoma	20–50
Epstein–Barr virus	Burkitt's lymphoma	3–12
Epstein–Barr virus	Nasopharyngeal carcinoma	30–40

Modified from zur Hausen H (1986) Intracellular surveillance of persisting viral infections. *Lancet* ii: 489.

designed which evaluate parameters of the viral infection more closely related to malignant conversion. Often the viruses cannot be traced unambiguously in the tumor; conventional virus isolation procedures usually remain unsuccessful: tumor tissues are usually not infectious. The neoplastic phenotype of HPV-positive genital carcinoma cells seems to be affected by viral functions, which raises the prospect of virus-specific pharmacological interference for adjuvant cancer therapy. In many cases, however, continuous viral expression is not detectable in malignant tumors. Primary infection and initial growth transformation apparently lead, through tumor progression, to a constitutive form of proliferation where viral gene products are not necessary for growth and the receptor molecules may no longer be functional. Thus, even in the longer term, antiviral gene therapy may not be successful for the treatment of the tumors, as they have become autonomous. Also in the distant future, the most efficient method for prophylaxis of virus-induced human tumors will probably be vaccination trials to prevent primary infection with the viruses.

See also: **Epstein-Barr virus (*Herpesviridae*): General features, Molecular biology; Hepadnaviruses (*Hepadnaviridae*): Avian hepatitis B virus, General features, Molecular biology; Hepatitis C virus (*Flaviviridae*); Human immunodeficiency viruses (*Retroviridae*): Molecular biology, Antiretroviral agents, General features; Human T-cell leukemia viruses (*Retroviridae*): HTLV-1, HTLV-2; Retroviral Oncogenes; Papillomaviruses – human (*Papovaviridae*): General features, Molecular biology; Transformation: Animal viruses.**

Further Reading

Chang Y, Cesarman E, Pessin MS *et al* (1994) Identification of herpesvirus-like DNA sequences in AIDS-associated Kaposi's sarcoma. *Science* 266: 1865.

Di Bisceglie AM (1995) Hepatitis C and hepatocellular carcinoma. *Semin. Liver Dis.* 15: 64.

IARC Working Group on the Evaluation of Carcinogenic Risks to Humans (1994) *Hepatitis viruses. IARC Monogr.* 59.

IARC Working Group on the Evaluation of Carcinogenic Risks to Humans (1995) *Human papillomaviruses. IARC Monogr.* 64.

Laimins LA (ed.) (1996) Viruses in human cancers. *Semin. Virol.* 7: 293.

Neipel F, Albrecht J and Fleckenstein B (1997) Cell-homologous genes in the Kaposi's sarcoma-associated rhadinovirus human herpesvirus 8: determinants of its pathogenicity? Minireview. *J. Virol.* 71: 4187

Pfister H (1996) The role of human papillomavirus in anogenital cancer. *Obstet. Gynecol. Clin. North Am.* 23: 579.

Pfister H and ter Schegget J (1997) Role of HPV in cutaneous premalignant and malignant tumors. *Clin. Dermatol.* 15: 335.

Rickinson AB (ed.) (1992) Viruses and human cancer. *Semin. Cancer Biol.* 3: 2049.

Smith MR and Greene WC (1991) Molecular biology of the type 1 human T-cell leukemia virus (HTLV-1) and adult T-cell leukemia. *J. Clin. Invest.* 87: 761.

Turkey Herpesvirus *see* Marek's Disease Virus (Herpesviridae)

TYMOVIRUSES

Adrian Gibbs, Research School of Biological Sciences, Australian National University, Canberra, Australia

Copyright © 1999 Academic Press

History and Distinguishing Features

Yellow mosaic and vein clearing diseases of several species of brassica found in the UK in the 1940s, were found to be caused by a stable sap and beetle-transmitted virus that was named turnip yellow mosaic virus (TYMV). Other similar viruses have been isolated since and found to form a clearly definable virus genus, which has been named *Tymovirus*, after the first found and type species. They have not been assigned to a family.

Around twenty tymoviruses are known. They infect dicotyledonous angiosperms, cause yellow mosaic diseases, are transmitted by beetles, but rarely by seed. They are readily transmitted experimentally by sap inoculation. Their virions are isometric and 25–30 nm in diameter. Their genomes are single molecules of single-stranded messenger-sense RNA about 6300 nucleotides long; 34–42% cytidylic acid. Their 5'-termini are capped, and most have a tRNA-like 3'-terminus. Their genomes replicate in small vesicles which form as invaginations of the outer membrane of chloroplasts.

Geographic Distribution

Tymoviruses have only been isolated from dicotyledonous plants, most of them wild. Most tymovirus species have natural and experimental host ranges restricted to one or a very few plant families and their geographic ranges are also mostly restricted. The species (and their normal geographic ranges) are Andean potato latent (the Andes), belladonna mottle (Europe), cacao yellow mosaic (Sierra Leone), calopogonium yellow mosaic (Malaysia), chayote mosaic (Central America) clitoria yellow vein (East Africa), desmodium yellow mosaic (USA), desmodium yellow mottle (Singapore), dulcamara mottle (UK), eggplant mosaic (Antilles), erysimum latent (Europe), kennedya yellow mosaic (Australia), melon rugose mosaic (Yemen), okra mosaic (Ivory Coast), ononis yellow mosaic (UK), passiflora yellow mosaic (Brazil), physalis mosaic (USA) (this virus was first called belladonna mottle virus-Iowa strain), plantago mottle (USA), scrophularia mottle (Germany), turnip yellow mosaic (Australia and Europe), voandezia necrotic mosaic (West Africa) and wild cucumber mosaic (USA) viruses, and also poinsettia mosaic virus (worldwide), which is a tentative tymovirus species.

Poinsettia mosaic virus has been carried internationally by the horticultural trade, and closely related, but distinct populations of turnip yellow mosaic virus have been found in Europe and Australia. However, every other tymovirus species seems to be confined to a single continent, and reports of wider distributions result from the use of serological tests, which do not adequately distinguish between tymovirus species. For example belladonna mottle virus was initially reported from both Europe and the USA, and clitoria yellow mosaic virus from both East Africa and Malaysia. However, in both instances, gene sequencing showed that the second record was not the same species; these are now known as physalis mosaic and calopogonium yellow mosaic viruses, respectively.

Host Ranges

Tymoviruses have been isolated from dicotyledonous plants; there is only one unconfirmed report of a tymovirus experimentally infecting a monocotyledonous plant. Most infect plants that use the C3 photosynthetic pathway, and only a very few C4 plants are susceptible. Individual tymoviruses have restricted natural host ranges and usually infect a few species from one family. Most have been isolated from wild plants, whereas species of all other genera/groups of plant viruses have mostly been isolated from crop plants. Most viruses that naturally infect wild plants cause few or no symptoms and do not affect growth, however tymoviruses cause bright yellow mosaic symptoms, and depress the growth of their wild natural hosts, but at least one such species, kennedya yellow mosaic virus, compensates for such damage by protecting its wild plant host against herbivores.

Tymoviruses have broader, but still restricted, experimental host ranges. They infect more species from the family of their natural hosts than from other families, and also a greater proportion of plant species from the same major division of the dicotyledons as their natural hosts than species from other divisions.

Molecular Biology

Virions

Tymoviral virions are isometric c.28 nm in diameter. Their shells are regular icosahedra of 180 subunits of a single protein species that cluster in fives or sixes in the surface of the virion shell to form the 32 morphological subunits, which can be seen in negatively stained virions. Purified virions sediment as two components. Those which sediment at 110–120S are nucleoprotein and each contains a single copy of the viral genome, which constitutes 35% of their mass. Some also contain a variable number of tRNA or virion protein mRNA molecules, and a variable number of polyamine molecules. The other virion component sediments at 50–55S and consists of the protein shell of the virion, and those of the solanaceous tymoviruses and ononis yellow mosaic virus also contain variable amounts of nongenomic RNA molecules.

Genome and encoded proteins

Tymoviral genomes are single molecules of about 6300 nucleotides of single-stranded RNA, and, when separated chemically from the virions, they are infectious. The genomes have a characteristic nucleotide composition; G 15–20%, A 17–24%, C 31–42% and U 20–29%. There are untranslated regions of the genome at both termini and between some open reading frames (ORFs) but these constitute only about 3% of the genome. They have a 5′-terminal m7GppppGp cap structure. Most tymovirus genomes also have a 3′-terminal sequence that can form a tRNA-like structure and that can be specifically valylated, but three tymoviruses, belladonna mottle, dulcamara mottle and erysimum latent, have a 3′-terminal sequence that can only form part of a tRNA-like structure, and dulcamara mottle has a 3′-terminal poly(A) sequence. All tymovirus genomes have three ORFs that are of similar size and arrangement in the genome. The largest is also the most conserved and spans most of the genome. It encodes a large replicase protein (RP: 1747–1874 residues, M_r 194 000–210 000) that has sequence motifs (NH_2- to -COOH-) characteristic of a N-methyltransferase, a papain-like protease, a helicase/nucleotide-binding fold and a replicase. Overlapping the 5′-terminal third of the RP, and always starting seven nucleotides to the 5′ side of the RP start codon, is an ORF that encodes an overlapping protein (OP) of variable length (440–750 residues, M_r 49 000–82 000) that is the least conserved of the proteins encoded by the virus. The OPs are very basic (pI 10.9–11.9), and may aid systemic spread of the virus in the plant. The third ORF, at the 3′ end of the genome, is of the virion protein (VP: 188–202 residues, M_r 19 600–21 500). The VP ORF is in different reading frames, relative to the RP/OP gene doublet, in different tymoviruses, and, in some, overlaps by a few nucleotides the 3′-terminal region of the RP ORF.

A region of about 50 nucleotides to the 5′ side of the start of the VP ORF, and hence in the 3′-terminal part of the RP ORF, is similar in all tymoviruses and two blocks of it are particularly conserved. One, which has been named the 'tymobox', is probably the VP mRNA promoter. It is 28–44 nucleotides from the start of the VP ORF and is 16 nucleotides in length. Eleven tymoviruses have tymoboxes with the same sequence (-GAGUCUGAAUUGCUUC-), there is a single nucleotide difference in three, and there are four differences in the tymobox of wild cucumber mosaic virus. Part of the tymobox sequence encodes the sequence, -ELL-, found near the C-terminus of all tymoviral RPs. The second conserved region occurs between the start of the VP ORF and the tymobox, seven or eight nucleotides from the latter. This is the translation initiation box -CAAU- (-CAAG- in one), and includes the 5′-terminal -AAU- found in the VP subgenomic mRNA of three tymoviruses.

The tymobox is useful as a genus-specific target for oligonucleotide probes and primers to isolate and sequence the VP gene of most tymoviruses.

Virion protein structure

The structure of the genome-containing virions of TYMV has been determined to a resolution of 0.32 nm. Each virion has a shell built from 180 identical VP molecules surrounding the folded genome. Each VP molecule is of 189 amino acid residues arranged as an elongated eight-stranded antiparallel β-barrel (jellyroll). The VP molecules are arranged in the shell as pentameric or hexameric clusters at the vertices of an icosahedron with deep furrows at the quasi-threefold axes; the outer radius of the shell is 15.9 nm from its center with the furrows at 12.1 nm. The C-termini of the VP molecules are external to the virion, and the N-termini are internal, and those grouped around the sixfold axes interact to form an annulus. During infection, histidine residues inside the VP may become deprotonated to aid disassembly. The genomic RNA also has some defined structure, possibly partial icosahedral symmetry, and there is a solvent-filled space of radius 2.5 nm at the center of the virion.

Only 73 of the amino acid residues of the VP are exposed at the surface of the virion, however not all are equally immunogenic or antigenic, indeed, despite being internal, the N-terminal peptide is a dominant immunogen. Thus the serological behavior of tymovirus virions is complex, involves only a small number of the amino acid residues of the VP, and may be an unsubtle indicator of tymovirus relationships.

Replication Strategy

Tymovirus genomes probably replicate in the vesicles

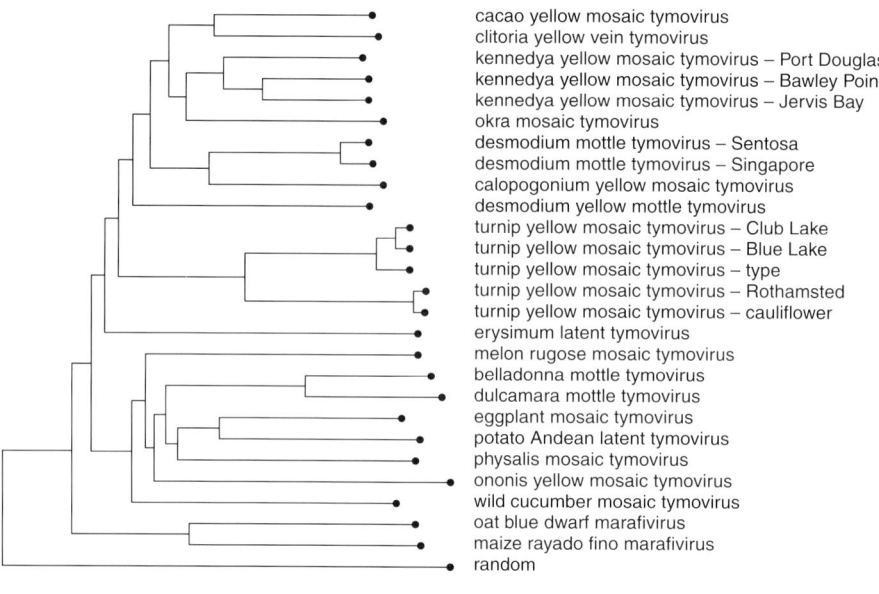

Figure 1 A neighbor-joining tree calculated from the percentage nucleotide differences (excluding gaps) between the virion protein genes of 24 tymovirus isolates and two marafiviruses aligned by the program CLUSTAL V (using default parameters). A random sequence was generated from the alignment by choosing randomly among the different nucleotides that occurred at each position in the alignment, and this was used as an outgroup. The bar represents a 20% nucleotide difference uncorrected for multiple changes.

that form in the margins of the chloroplasts of tymovirus-infected plants; these vesicles have been shown to contain the viral replicase complex and double-stranded RNA 'replicative intermediate' of the virus. It is probable that the OP and RP ORFs are translated directly from genomic RNA, but that of the VP from a subgenomic mRNA is transcribed from the negative genomic strand using the tymobox sequence as a promoter. Tymovirus proteins are produced by cytoplasmic ribosomes. The RP polyprotein is probably *cis*-hydrolyzed into its component parts by a viral protease in the central region of the RP; the first cut is between the helicase and replicase regions, and then the helicase and protease are separated.

Virions of the virus assemble at or near where the chloroplast vesicles connect with the cytoplasm. Virions and genome-free virion shells are found particularly around patches of vesicles, but also throughout the cytoplasm and all parts of infected plants. Virion shells may also accumulate in large numbers in nuclei.

Taxonomy and Evolution

Figure 1 shows a neighbor-joining tree calculated from the nucleotide sequence differences of the virion proteins of 24 tymoviruses. It can be seen that different isolates of each tymovirus species always cluster together, and that species fall into larger groupings that mostly correlate with the family of the plant from which they were isolated. The largest of the groups includes most of the tymoviruses isolated from legumes (**Fig. 1**), these form a sister group to the brassica-infecting tymoviruses, and the remaining major group includes all those isolated from solanaceous plants and cucurbits. The tymoviruses form a sister group to the marafiviruses. The replicase genes are known for seven tymoviruses and one marafivirus and their sequence relationships are totally congruent with those shown by the virion protein genes.

Tymoviruses are variable. Tymovirus isolates that infect the same range of plant species and cause closely similar symptoms are considered to be isolates of a single species. However, they may have virions that differ serologically and in their surface charge, and have genomes with sequence differences of up to 27% (turnip yellow mosaic virus). Some species have distinct subspecies, for example there are two subspecies of turnip yellow mosaic (the type and cauliflower subspecies), and three of kennedya yellow mosaic (the Port Douglas, Jervis Bay and Bawley Point subspecies).

The marafiviruses, which include oat blue dwarf (OBDV), maize rayado fino and Bermuda grass etched line viruses, form a 'sister' genus of the tymoviruses, and are closely related to them. All have particles of similar size and morphology, and the genome of OBDV has been found to be similar in size (6.509 kb), composition (42.8% C) and sequence to those of the tymoviruses; the complete replicase polyproteins of five tymoviruses differ from one another by up to 65% in sequence, whereas that of OBDV differs from the tymoviruses by 70%. The OBDV genome has a 'tymobox' sequence with 13/16 nucleotide identity to those of most tymoviruses and it encodes the same -ELL- motif. Marafiviruses differ from tymoviruses in several biological features. They mostly infect monocotyledonous plants (only OBDV is known to infect dicotyledons), they seem only to replicate in the phloem or in enations formed by hyperplasia of the procambium of the phloem, and their replication is not associated with chloroplasts or other cell organelles. They have leafhopper vectors and replicate in those vectors. Marafiviruses also differ significantly from tymoviruses in their molecular biology. Their genome does not encode an overlapping protein like that of the tymoviruses, and their virions have proteins of two sizes, that are mostly identical in sequence; the larger is produced by hydrolysis of the genomic transcript and the smaller is transcribed from a subgenomic mRNA, and lacks the N-terminal sequence of the larger protein.

The sequence motifs of the replicase protein (RP) of tymoviruses and marafiviruses also show clear similarities to those of the RPs of the capilloviruses, carlaviruses, closteroviruses and potexviruses, indicating that the RPs of all these viruses have a common ancestor; the RPs of the tymoviruses and OBDV differ from those of potato X and other potexviruses by 90–95% in sequence. The sequence motifs of the RPs also indicate that they may be very distantly related to the 'alpha-like viruses', which include alpha-, furo-, hordei-, rubi-, tobamo-, tobra- and tricornaviruses. Some of these viruses have isometric or bacilliform virions, which may have virion proteins that have a similar β-barrel (jellyroll) structure to those of the tymoviruses, and hence their VP genes may have a shared ancestor. However, all the viruses with filamentous or rod-shaped virions probably have four-stranded α-helix virion proteins encoded by genes unrelated to those encoding the jellyroll VPs. None of the viruses with replicase genes related to those of the tymoviruses has an overlapping (OP) gene, and hence the OP gene probably arose *de novo* in the 'proto-tymovirus'.

Epidemiology and Transmission

The known natural vectors of tymoviruses are all chrysomelid beetles (Halticidae and Galerucidae) except that of TYMV in Australia, which is a pill beetle (Byrrhidae). The vector beetles prefer feeding on plants that are tymovirus-infected rather than virus-free. A few tymoviruses are transmitted by the seed of a limited number of plant species, but not by their pollen. All may be transmitted by sap inoculation, but none by plant contact.

Pathogenicity and Symptoms

Tymoviruses cause yellow mosaics, vein-clearing and mottles. All plants infected with tymoviruses develop small characteristic vesicles within their chloroplasts attached to their outer membranes. These vesicles form as invaginations of the outer chloroplast membranes, and the bilayer membranes of those membranes and the vesicles are confluent.

Prevention and Control

Tymoviruses have mostly been found in uncultivated plants, and none is known to cause economically important diseases of crops.

See also: **Marafiviruses (Marafivirus); Potexviruses.**

Further Reading

Brunt A, Crabtree K, Dallwitz M, Gibbs A and Watson L (eds) (1996) *Viruses of Plants*. Oxon: CAB International.

Canady MA, Larson SB, Day J and McPherson A (1996) Crystal structure of turnip yellow mosaic virus. *Nature Struct. Biol.* 3: 771.

Gibbs A and Mackenzie AM (1998) Tymovirus isolation and genomic RNA extraction. In: Foster GD and Taylor SC (eds) *Plant Virology Protocols. Methods Mol. Biol.* 81: 219.

Hellendorn K, Michiels PJ, Buitenhuis R and Pleij CW (1996) Protonatable hairpins are conserved in the 5'-untranslated region of tymovirus RNAs. *Nucleic Acids Res.* 24: 4910–4917.

Hirth L and Givord L (1988) Tymoviruses. In: Koenig R (ed.) *The Viruses: the Plant Viruses 3*, p. 163. Plenum Press: New York and London.

Ty Elements   *see* **Retrotransposons of Fungi**

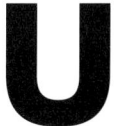

UMBRAVIRUSES

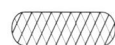

DJ Robinson and **AF Murant**, Scottish Crop Research Institute, Invergowrie, Dundee, UK

Copyright © 1999 Academic Press

History

Several of the viruses now placed in the genus *Umbravirus* have been known since the early days of plant virology but, because of their peculiar properties and the attendant difficulties in working with them, most have been little studied. The first to be described was tobacco mottle virus (TMoV), reported from Zimbabwe and Malawi by K. M. Smith in 1946. TMoV was shown to be mechanically transmissible but to depend on a helper virus that is not mechanically transmissible, tobacco vein distorting virus, for transmission by aphids in a persistent (circulative) manner. The two viruses together caused a disease in tobacco called 'rosette'. Several virus complexes with similar properties are now known and the dependent viruses in these complexes are placed together in the genus *Umbravirus*. The name was coined from Latin, *umbra*, meaning 'shade', 'shadow' and from English, *umbra*, 'a shadow', 'an uninvited guest accompanying an invited one'. All the helper viruses that have been identified are definitive or tentative members of the family *Luteoviridae*.

Most attention has been paid to umbraviruses associated with two diseases of major economic importance, carrot motley dwarf, which is damaging worldwide, and groundnut rosette, which is very serious and epidemic in Africa. The umbravirus carrot mottle virus (CMoV) was first described in 1964 from motley dwarf-diseased carrots in the UK. A similar but distinct umbravirus, called carrot mottle mimic virus (CMoMV), has recently been found in carrots in Australia. In both instances the helper virus is carrot red leaf luteovirus (CaRLV). In 1969, groundnut rosette virus (GRV) and its helper luteovirus, groundnut rosette assistor virus (GRAV), were recognized as causal agents of groundnut rosette disease, but it was not until 1988 that a satellite RNA of GRV was shown to be the main cause of the symptoms of rosette disease. Recently, pea enation mosaic virus (PEMV), a virus hitherto considered to have a bipartite genome and classified as the sole member of the genus *Enamovirus*, has been shown to be a complex of two viruses. PEMV-1, formerly PEMV RNA-1, is classified in the genus *Enamovirus*, family *Luteoviridae*, and PEMV-2, formerly PEMV RNA-2, is considered to be an umbravirus. The above-mentioned umbraviruses and others which are of lesser or unknown importance, are listed in **Table 1**, together with their helper viruses, where known, and their aphid vectors. The tentative members have either not been adequately characterized, or their putative helper virus has not been detected or identified.

Taxonomy and Classification

Umbraviruses have monopartite single-stranded RNA (ssRNA) genomes with a characteristic arrangement of open reading frames (ORFs) (**Fig. 1**). Amino acid sequence comparisons show that the putative RNA-dependent RNA polymerases encoded by the genomic RNA molecules of CMoMV, GRV and PEMV-2 belong to the so-called supergroup 2 of RNA polymerases, as do those of viruses in the genera *Carmovirus*, *Dianthovirus*, *Luteovirus*, *Machlomovirus*, *Necrovirus* and *Tombusvirus*. These enzymes are the only universally conserved proteins of positive-strand RNA viruses, and their affinities suggest that the genus *Umbravirus* might be considered to be in or close to the family *Tombusviridae*. Presently *Umbravirus* remains a genus unassigned to a family.

Virus Properties

In plants infected by umbraviruses unaccompanied by the helper virus, no particles of the kind associated with most plant viruses can be found by electron microscopy in leaf extracts, but infected leaves yield abundant infective ssRNA. However, the infectivity of CMoV and GRV in buffer extracts of leaves is surprisingly stable, surviving for about a day at room

Table 1 Umbraviruses, their helper luteoviruses and their main aphid vectors

Umbravirus	Helper luteovirus	Main aphid vector
Definitive Umbravirus species		
Bean yellow veinbanding virus (BYVBV)	Bean leaf roll virus (BLRV)	*Acyrthosiphon pisum*
	Pea enation mosaic virus-1 (PEMV-1)	
Carrot mottle virus (CMoV)	Carrot red leaf virus (CaRLV)	*Cavariella aegopodii*
Carrot mottle mimic virus (CMoMV)	Carrot red leaf virus (CaRLV)	*C. aegopodii*
Groundnut rosette virus (GRV)	Groundnut rosette assistor virus (GRAV)	*Aphis craccivora*
Lettuce speckles mottle virus (LSMV)	Beet western yellows virus (BWYV)	*Myzus persicae*
Pea enation mosaic virus-2 (PEMV-2)	PEMV-1	*Acyrthosiphon pisum*
Tobacco mottle virus (TMoV)	Tobacco vein distorting virus (TVDV)	*M. persicae*
Tentative Umbravirus species		
Sunflower crinkle virus (SCV)	Unknown	*Aphis gossypii*
(Sunflower rugose mosaic virus)		
Sunflower yellow blotch virus (SYBV)	Unknown	*Aphis gossypii*
(Sunflower yellow ringspot virus)		
Tobacco bushy-top virus (TBTV)	Unknown	*M. persicae*
Tobacco yellow vein virus (TYVV)	Tobacco yellow vein assistor virus (TYVAV)	*M. persicae*

temperature and for up to 15 days at 4–5°C. It is, however, very sensitive to treatment with organic solvents, and this suggests that the infective RNA is protected in lipid-containing structures. Vesicular structures about 50 nm in diameter occur in the cell vacuoles of CMoV-infected *Nicotiana clevelandii*, often associated with the tonoplast, and have also been found in partially purified preparations. Similar structures have been seen in plant cells infected with bean yellow veinbanding virus (BYVBV), lettuce speckles mottle virus (LSMV) and GRV. At first it was thought that these structures might be virus particles of a kind unusual among plant viruses but it now seems likely that they may be involved in virus replication and/or serve to protect the RNA. The present view is that umbraviruses do not form conventional virus particles but depend on the coat protein of the associated luteovirus for encapsidation and for transmission by the aphid vector of the helper.

Properties of the Genome

The genomes of umbraviruses consist of one linear segment of ssRNA. They are probably not polyadenylated at their 3′ends, but there is no information about structures at their 5′ends. The genomic RNA sequences of CMoMV, GRV and PEMV-2 comprise 4201, 4019 and 4253 nucleotides, respectively. Gel electrophoresis of double-stranded RNA (dsRNA) forms indicates that the genomes of other umbraviruses are of similar size.

The genomes of CMoMV, GRV and PEMV-2 each contain four ORFs (**Fig. 1**). A very short 5′noncoding region is followed by ORF 1, which codes for a potential product of M_r 31 000–37 000. ORF 2 overlaps ORF 1 in a different reading frame and could encode a product of M_r 64 000–65 000. The function of the ORF 1 product is unknown, but the potential ORF 2 product contains sequence motifs characteristic of viral RNA-dependent RNA polymerases. An untranslated region separates ORF 2 from the remaining two ORFs (3 and 4), which overlap one another almost completely in different reading frames. The putative products of these two ORFs are of M_r 26 000–29 000, and the ORF 4 product contains sequences typical of plant virus movement proteins. The ORF 3 products of CMoMV, GRV and PEMV-2 have 42–50% similarity to each other but no significant similarity to any other viral or nonviral proteins. The sequence of the predicted ORF 3 product therefore gives no clue to its possible function.

All three genomes lack genes for plausible coat proteins.

Replication

Strategy of replication of nucleic acid

Leaf tissue of plants infected with umbraviruses contains abundant dsRNA, including a prominent species of about 4.2–4.8 kbp corresponding in size to that expected for a double-stranded form of the genomic RNA. Replication of umbravirus RNA therefore presumably involves the ORF 2-encoded RNA-dependent RNA polymerase and a dsRNA

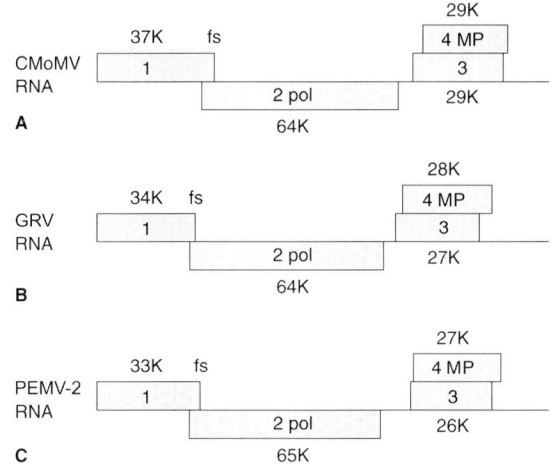

Figure 1 Diagram showing the arrangement of the ORFs in (**A**) CMoMV RNA, (**B**) GRV RNA and (**C**) PEMV-2 RNA. In each case the continuous horizontal line represents the RNA and the numbered blocks the correspondingly numbered ORFs. The M_r of the predicted translation product is shown adjacent to each ORF. ORFs that encode probable RNA-dependent RNA polymerases are marked 'pol', and those that encode probable cell-to-cell movement proteins are marked 'MP'. The positions of probable frameshift events are marked 'fs'. (Adapted from Taliansky M, Robinson DJ and Murant AF (1997) Complete nucleotide sequence and organization of the RNA genome of groundnut rosette umbravirus. *Journal of General Virology* **77**: 2335.)

intermediate, but no further details of the replication mechanism have been elucidated. A second prominent species of dsRNA, present in all plants infected with umbraviruses that have been examined, is of 1.1–1.5 kbp, and may be an intermediate in the synthesis of subgenomic RNA.

Characterization of translation

ORFs 1 and 2 are probably translated from genomic RNA as a single polypeptide of M_r 94 000–98 000 by a mechanism involving a −1 frameshift. ORF 2 does not have an appropriately positioned AUG initiation codon. Moreover, a 'shifty' heptanucleotide sequence is present just upstream of the ORF 1 termination codon and is flanked by sequences that could form stable stem–loop structures. These features are similar to ones associated with frameshifting sites in the genomes of several other plant and animal viruses.

The 1.1–1.5 kbp dsRNA found in umbravirus-infected plants is of the size expected for a subgenomic RNA for ORFs 3 and 4. For CMoMV, this dsRNA has been shown to include the sequences of ORFs 3 and 4, and the 3′ untranslated region. For GRV, corresponding ssRNA has been identified, which runs as two closely spaced bands in gel electrophoresis. Thus it is uncertain whether ORFs 3 and 4 are translated from the same subgenomic RNA species or two different ones.

Satellite RNA

Additional dsRNA species are associated with infection by some umbraviruses and, in the case of GRV, this dsRNA is known to represent a satellite RNA. GRV satellite RNA is found in all naturally occurring isolates of GRV, and is largely responsible for the symptoms of rosette disease in groundnut plants. Different variants of the satellite are responsible for different forms of the disease. Thus the agents of groundnut rosette disease comprise three components: the satellite RNA, GRV acting as a helper for replication of the satellite RNA, and GRAV acting as a helper for the encapsidation and aphid-transmission of GRV and its satellite RNA. Furthermore, for some reason that is not understood, the satellite RNA is also required for the GRAV-dependent aphid transmission of GRV, i.e. unlike most satellites, it is essential for the biological survival (though not the replication) of its helper virus. Most satellite RNA variants do not affect replication of the helper virus but at least one variant strongly downregulates GRV RNA synthesis.

Evolution

As mentioned above, umbraviruses have some affinities with viruses in the family *Tombusviridae* but whether they have lost or never had coat protein genes is idle speculation. Dependence of one virus on another for one or more gene functions is a fairly common feature among plant viruses. In most instances, the dependence of umbravirus on luteovirus is not reciprocated, but the PEMV complex appears to be a notable exception. Like other members of the family *Luteoviridae*, PEMV-1 lacks the ability to move outside the vascular system of infected plants but can 'borrow' the cell-to-cell movement function encoded by the umbravirus PEMV-2. It is thereby released from the confinement to the phloem that is typical of its family and as a result becomes transmissible by manual inoculation. Another member of the *Luteoviridae*, beet western yellows virus, has been reported to acquire limited manual transmissibility when in the presence of LSMV, and this may represent another example of the same phenomenon. The PEMV complex may perhaps illustrate the development of mutual interdependence that may have led to the evolution of multipartite genomes in other virus genera.

Serology

Because umbraviruses do not encode their own coat proteins but depend on their helper viruses for encapsidation, there is no information about serological relationships among umbraviruses.

Geographic Distribution

Carrot motley dwarf and pea enation mosaic diseases occur worldwide wherever their crop hosts are grown. However, it is unclear which of the viruses CMoV or CMoMV is associated with carrot motley dwarf disease in different parts of the world. Groundnut rosette disease occurs only in Africa, south of the Sahara. BYVBV is reported only from Europe, and LSMV only from California, USA. All other umbraviruses are reported only from Africa.

Host Range and Virus Propagation

Individual umbraviruses are confined in nature to one or a few host plant species. Their experimental host ranges are broader but still restricted. The host ranges of umbraviruses overlap, but do not necessarily coincide, with those of their helper viruses. The symptoms induced in infected plants are usually mottles or mosaics.

Experimentally, umbraviruses can be transmitted by manual inoculation, although sometimes with difficulty. They can be propagated in their natural hosts, but often an experimental host is more convenient. *Nicotiana benthamiana* and *N. clevelandii* have proved useful for propagation of CMoV, CMoMV, GRV and several other umbraviruses.

Transmission

In nature, umbraviruses are transmitted by aphids (**Table 1**), but only from plants that also contain a helper virus (**Table 1**). All helper viruses that have been characterized are definitive or tentative members of the family *Luteoviridae*. The mechanism of the dependent transmission is the encapsidation of the umbravirus RNA by the coat protein of the luteovirus. Transmission of the dependent umbravirus therefore occurs in the same persistent (circulative, nonpropagative) manner as that of the helper virus.

Epidemiology

Between crop growing seasons, umbraviruses must survive in plants that are also both hosts of the helper virus and feeding hosts of the vector. Sometimes the aphid vector too will survive on the same plants, but in cold winters in temperate climates, it may survive only in the form of eggs, and these may be laid on an alternate host that is not a host of the viruses. For example, the aphid *Cavariella aegopodii*, the vector of the CMoV/CaRLV complex, lays its eggs on willow (*Salix* spp.), which is not a host of either virus. The aphids produced on willow in the spring are therefore nonviruliferous and must re-acquire the virus complex from a perennial umbelliferous host such as *Anthriscus cerefolium* (cow parsley, Queen Anne's lace), or from overwintering carrot plants.

The components of the pea enation mosaic virus complex infect a wide range of leguminous plant species, of which the most important as overwintering hosts are probably *Medicago sativa* (alfalfa, lucerne) and *Vicia sativa* (common vetch). No nonleguminous natural hosts are known. The most important vector in nature is the pea aphid (*Acyrthosiphon pisum*).

Groundnuts, which originated in South America, are affected by rosette disease only in Africa south of the Sahara, and not in any other parts of the world to which they have been introduced. The causal viruses, GRV and GRAV, must therefore have come from wild plants indigenous to Africa. However, attempts to find an African plant species that is a host of both viruses have so far been unsuccessful. The viruses may now survive in overseasoning groundnut plants. Groundnut rosette is present in most seasons, but periodically becomes epidemic, causing devastating losses of great economic and social importance. The factors that determine the onset of epidemics are not understood, but are undoubtedly linked with the biology of the vector, *Aphis craccivora*.

Little is known about the ecology and epidemiology of other umbraviruses.

Pathology and Histopathology

Although all umbraviruses depend on a helper virus for transmission by vector insects, several of them are equally or more important than their helpers in the causation of disease symptoms. The umbravirus of greatest economic importance is GRV, which causes the most devastating virus disease of groundnut in Africa. However, in this case, as already mentioned, it is a GRV-dependent satellite RNA that is the actual cause of the symptoms.

Umbraviruses, even in the absence of their helper viruses, exhibit rapid systemic spread in plants. They infect cells throughout the leaf, though presumably the aphid-transmissible particles are restricted to the same tissues (in most instances the phloem) as the luteoviruses that provide their coat protein. In mesophyll cells infected with CMoV there is extensive development of cell wall outgrowths sheathing elongated plasmodesmatal tubules.

Prevention and Control

Vector Control

Preventing the spread of umbraviruses by controlling the aphid vector is rarely practical commercially, because severe disease outbreaks are erratic and difficult to predict. Also, especially in the case of GRV, which occurs mostly in the poorer African countries, use of insecticides may be too expensive. However, in many countries, carrot crops are sprayed intensively with insecticides, primarily for the prevention of carrot fly (*Psila rosae*) infestation, and this incidentally provides effective control of carrot motley dwarf disease.

Avoidance of Infection

For the avoidance of pea enation mosaic disease, it is sometimes recommended that pea or faba bean crops should be sited away from alfalfa or clover fields. In Africa, early planting and close spacing of groundnut are effective ways of avoiding rosette disease, because the flying aphid vector has difficulty in recognizing the crop once the plant cover is complete. This approach is also effective against tobacco rosette disease.

Host Plant Resistance

If resistant plant cultivars are available, this is undoubtedly the best approach. Resistance to GRV, inherited as a double recessive character, is found in some groundnut germplasm, and groundnut lines possessing this resistance have been developed, though they are often not preferred for commercial or cultural reasons.

See also: **Vector transmission of plant viruses; Luteovirus; Pea enation mosaic virus (*Luteoviridae*).**

Further Reading

Demler SA, de Zoeten GA, Adam G and Harris KF (1996) Pea enation mosaic enamovirus: properties and aphid transmission. In: Harrison BD and Murant AF (eds) *The Plant Viruses, Polyhedral Virions and Bipartite RNA Genomes*, vol. 5, p. 303. New York: Plenum Press.

Murant AF (1990) Recent research on the aetiology of groundnut rosette disease. *Ann. Rept. Scott. Crop Res. Inst. 1989* p. 138.

Murant AF (1993) Complexes of transmission-dependent and helper viruses. In: Matthews REF (ed.) *Diagnosis of Plant Virus Diseases*, p. 333. Boca Raton: CRC Press.

Ustilago Maydis Viruses   *see* Totiviruses

VACCINES AND IMMUNE RESPONSE

Gordon L Ada, Australian National University, Canberra, Australia

Copyright © 1999 Academic Press

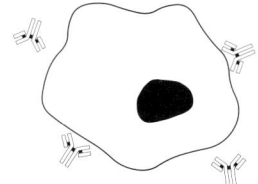

History

Any history of vaccination to control viral infections, however brief, begins with the story of smallpox and its final eradication. There were bicentenary celebrations in 1996 to celebrate the famous experiment of Edward Jenner in which he inoculated a boy, James Phipps, with cowpox material and demonstrated that he subsequently resisted a challenge with smallpox. Almost 100 years later, Louis Pasteur developed the rabies virus vaccine, and in 1935, an attenuated viral preparation to combat yellow fever was made and remains to this day a safe and effective vaccine. The first inactivated influenza virus vaccine became available in 1936. The production of these two vaccines was possible because of the newly developed technique of growing virus in the embryonated eggs of chickens.

However, the major event that accelerated viral vaccine development was the ability to grow many viruses in tissue culture. This began in the 1920s, but it was the studies by John Enders and colleagues in successfully growing polioviruses in cell culture which initiated an explosion of activity in this field. Jonas Salk produced the trivalent formalin-inactivated poliovirus vaccine and this was followed shortly afterwards by the oral live attenuated polio vaccines of Albert Sabin. Most viral vaccines in use today and those in clinical trials and probably close to registration (**Table 1**) are attenuated preparations.

A subunit preparation consisting of the surface glycoproteins of influenza virus, was subsequently made and is widely used because of its lower reactogenicity compared to whole virus. A new era of viral vaccine development was initiated when the hepatitis B surface antigen, originally isolated from infected blood, was prepared from DNA-transfected yeast cells for use as a vaccine.

Smallpox was declared eradicated in 1980, three years after the last case of endemic smallpox was detected, and nearly 14 years after the World Health Organization (WHO) had begun an intensified campaign to eradicate this disease. In 1985, the Pan American Health Organization (PAHO) initiated a program to eradicate indigenous wild-type polio from the Americas, and eradication was declared in 1994, three years after the last case was detected. WHO has declared the year 2000 as the target date for global eradication and there is a reasonable chance that this will be achieved. Following elimination of indigenous measles from some countries (e.g. Finland, the Caribbean Islands), PAHO has nominated the year 2000 as the date for eradication of this disease from the Americas.

Two Main Requirements of a Vaccine

The safety of a candidate vaccine has become of prime importance. Most of the vaccines listed in **Table 1** are very safe, but two in particular are less so. During the eradication campaign, most smallpox vaccines (vaccinia virus) had a level of side effects which made them unacceptable for current use. Safer preparations have since been made by the deletion of specific DNA sequences. Type 3 poliovirus in OPV can revert to virulence, and poliomyelitis occurs at the rate of about 3×10^6 doses of vaccine in recipients or their close contacts. Attenuated live vaccines may pose a risk to immunodeficient or -compromised people, but at least in the case of measles virus, even this is a very low risk.

The second requirement is efficacy, which is assessed as the ability to protect recipients from disease after a subsequent exposure to the wild-type infectious agent. Vaccine efficacy depends almost entirely on the nature and persistence of the induced immune response. Vaccines are usually given prophylactically and, as the time interval between vaccination and the subsequent exposure to challenge may be short (weeks) or long (years), efficacy depends on stimulation of the adaptive immune response, the

Table 1 Viral vaccines

Type	Infectious agents	
	Current vaccines	Products close to registration
Live, attenuated	Vaccinia	Cytomegalo
	Measles	Hepatitis A
	Yellow fever	Influenza
	Mumps	Dengue
	Polio (OPV)[a]	Parainfluenza
	Rota[a]	Japanese encephalitis
	Adeno[a]	
	Rubella	
	Varicella-Zoster	
Inactivated	Polio (IPV)	Hepatitis A
	Infuenza	
	Rabies	
	Japanese encephalitis	
Subunit	Hepatitis B	
	Influenza	
Combination	Measles, mumps, rubella (MMR)	

[a] Administered orally
OPV, Live polio virus; IPV, Inactivated polio virus.

lymphocytes, which have immunological memory. If a vaccine is used therapeutically, which may be deliberate or occur naturally if the vaccine is used in an endemic area, activated innate components may contribute to a protective effect. The efficacy of many vaccines may be predicted by the level of protective antibodies induced by vaccination, but where antigenic variation occurs, a high level of cell-mediated immune (CMI) responses may indicate a degree of protection.

Roles of antibodies

Specific antibody has three main roles: (1) to neutralize the infectivity of a virus; (2) to lyse infected cells which express viral antigens at the cell surface; and (3) to complex with viral debris from infected cells and help in its removal. Following vaccination, the continuing presence of specific antibody of increasing affinity which will bind to virus and prevent infection is regarded by vaccinologists as the most critical requirement of a vaccine. Many viruses naturally infect via a mucosal surface, and here, secretory immunoglobulin A (s.IgA) fulfills this role. In contrast, many vaccines are given parenterally, in which case, the IgM and IgG formed does not prevent the initial infection, but should prevent systemic spread, eg. polio and measles infection.

The mechanism of infectivity prevention by antibody varies between viruses, and even different immunoglobulin isotypes may have different effects. Viral replication may be prevented whether the antibody prevents virus adsorption to the cell, entry into the cell or expression of the viral genome.

Antiviral antibody may bind to antigens expressed on the infected cell plasma membrane and cause lysis – antibody-dependent cellular cytotoxicity (ADCC). Alternatively, lysis may be caused by certain antibody isotypes binding complement and the complex then binds to complement receptors on the infected cell surface. Antibody has been shown to clear some viral infections in T cell-deficient mice, eg. influenza and vaccinia virus infections. In contrast, antibody is inefficient at clearing ectromelia, lymphocytic choriomeningitis virus (LCMV) or Theiler's virus, which are natural pathogens of mice. However, in persistent infections such as LCMV in mice, antibody can prevent virus reaching sites such as the epidermis where CTLs are less effective.

Viral epitopes recognized by protective antibodies Generally, only one or a few antigens of a virus, those exposed to the medium, contain epitopes recognized by neutralizing antibodies. For the virus to survive extracellularly, it must be resistant to enzymes, particularly proteases, and this is usually achieved by having polymers of viral antigens – trimers (influenza hemagglutinin and human immunodeficiency virus envelope) or multimers (VP1 of polio) – so that the important epitopes are usually discontinuous sequences.

Roles of effector T cells

There are two classes of T cells – CD4+ (class II MHC-restricted) and CD8+ (class I MHC-restricted) – and two subclasses of each – CD4+Th1 and Th2, and CD8+Tc1 and Tc2. They are distinguished by their patterns of cytokine secretion. Because of similarities in these patterns, Th2 and Tc2 are called type 2 T cells, and Th1 and Tc1, type 1 T cells (*see also* **Immune Response, general features**). The main role of Th2 cells is 'helping' B cells make antibody. Th1 cells do this to a lesser extent, but in contrast to Th2 cells, they mediate delayed-type hypersensitivity reactions. From a vaccine development point of view, a major role of Tc1 is their ability to lyse virus-infected cells a long time before viral progeny is formed, so they are frequently called cytotoxic T cells (CTLs). **Table 2** lists some examples of viral infections in mice where there has been clearance or control of virus replication following transfer of specific CTLs.

Table 2 Examples of clearance or control of virus replication in infected mice following transfer of specific CD8+ cytotoxic T cells (CTLs, Tc1)

Orthomyxovirus (influenza virus)
Paramyxovirus (Sendai virus)
Poxvirus (vaccinia virus)
Pneumovirus (respiratory syncytial virus)
Arenavirus (lymphocytic choriomeningitis virus)
Alphaherpesvirus (herpes virus)
Betaherpesvirus (cytomegalovirus)

There are 'experiments of nature' which suggest a protective role for CTLs in infected people. In four situations where people were known to have been exposed to HIV but who were seronegative and virus could not be isolated, CTLs specific for known HIV CTL epitopes could be isolated from their blood.

Though cultured or cloned Th1 cells may also be cytotoxic, primary cells (without *in vitro* culture) are rarely so. Th (presumably Th1) cells have been shown to be protective in a herpes 2 virus infection – the zosteriform spread model. *In vitro*, CTL production is usually enhanced by the presence of TH1 cells, but *in vivo*, there are several examples where 'normal' levels of CTL activity were found following a viral infection in doctored mice lacking CD4+ T cells. However, it has also been shown that if the virus infection persists, CTL activity decreases over time compared to the situation in normal mice, which is similar to what occurs in many HIV-infected individuals when levels of CD4+ T cells greatly decrease and CTL activity disappears.

Sources and properties of T cell epitopes In contrast to the restricted number of viral antigens possessing epitopes recognized by neutralizing antibodies, potentially many viral antigens may contain T cell epitopes. They may be detected as follows.

1. Individual antigens are screened, sometimes using cells infected by a chimeric live vector.
2. A series of overlapping peptides is synthesized and each is tested for its ability to sensitize a target cell for lysis by CTLs.
3. Whereas peptides binding to class II MHC antigens vary considerably in length, averaging about 15 amino acids, those binding to class I MHC antigens are more homogeneous, the great majority being nonamers. The nonamers have a motif specific for MHC molecules of different allelic specificities, possessing two anchor positions that are critical for ligand binding. This has allowed protein sequences to be screened to find ligands potentially specific for different MHC antigens.
4. Peptide ligands can be 'stripped' from an infected cell and sequenced.

There were some general findings.

1. Where comprehensive studies have been made, e.g. influenza virus and HIV, the great majority of antigens possess potential CTL epitopes. With flaviviruses, the nonstructural proteins are the major source of CTL epitopes.
2. With both influenza and HIV, the internal antigens contain conserved sequence epitopes.
3. Not infrequently, one or a few epitopes may be dominant and these may be in a variable region or subject to mutation, both being potential mechanisms for the virus to escape immune control. A vaccine might need to include less dominant epitopes from conserved regions where mutations do not occur.
4. Even though a peptide will bind firmly to a MHC antigen of a given specificity, not all people with that allelic specificity but differing in the rest of the haplotype will respond to that peptide, because of crosstolerance with different self peptides.

Secondary Responses

Immunization/vaccination should achieve two major goals. The first is the continuing presence of high affinity specific antibody which will generally neutralize most (>95%) of the challenge virus. Probably, vaccines rarely if ever give 'sterilizing' immunity (100% prevention of infection). If sufficient virus escapes neutralization by pre-existing antibody to infect enough antigen presenting cells (APCs) the second effect is an enhanced CMI response, particularly CTLs. *In vitro*, limit dilution analyses show that following priming, there is an increase in the frequency of T cells of the particular specificity. However, these memory cells are also more easily activated than naive cells, and this may be a more important reason why a more rapid and greater CTL response is seen.

If the antigenic specificity (for neutralizing antibody) of the challenge virus differs grossly from that of the virus used for vaccination, as happens when antigenic shift occurs with influenza, or between different clades of HIV, the control and recovery from the challenge infection will depend very largely on an enhanced CMI response.

Table 3 Some factors favoring or obstructing the development of an effective viral vaccine

Favoring
1. Infection by wild-type agent induces immunity which clears the infection
2. Few important serotypes (DNA viruses); little or no antigenic drift (RNA viruses)
3. Antigens that are a source of protective B cell epitopes or important T cell epitopes are readily identified
4. The virus is not highly infectious
5. Infection is confined to one or few organs, e.g. the lung with influenza virus
6. There is readily available a relatively inexpensive animal model that mimics the human infectious process with onset of characteristic disease

Obstructing
7. Marked antigenic shift or drift
8. Viral DNA/cDNA integrates into the host cell genome; latency occurs
9. Virus infects a variety of cells distributed widely throughout the body
10. A latent infection may be transmitted by infected cells
11. Protective immunity does not occur after natural infection
    (a) infection persists due to suppression/evasion of CMI responses;
    (b) escape mutants (T and B cells) occur over time
12. Crucial cells of the immune system are infected or affected
13. Antibodies may enhance infection of susceptible cells
14. Lack of a suitable animal model

Protection Following Immunization by Different Routes

The area of mucosal surface in mammals is far greater than the area of skin, and many viruses infect via this route. The main sites of entry are oral, rectal, respiratory, urogenital and ocular. Following vaccination via a mucosal route such as the gut, the first line of defense is s.IgA, and the CMI responses originate from local lymphoid tissues such as the Peyer's patches. For example, OPV induces both a mucosal and systemic response whereas IPV induces only the latter which, however, is sufficient to prevent infection of the central nervous system and poliomyelitis. Measles vaccine is given parenterally; viremia occurs so that some virus reaches the respiratory tract and a mucosal, as well as sytemic response, occurs. There is still interest in administering this vaccine intranasally to achieve a stronger mucosal response which might also be less affected by maternally derived antibody.

There is a 'common mucosal system' so that an immune response induced say in the gut will cause traffic of immune cells to other mucosal sites. An example is the adenovirus vaccine. This is given orally but induces significant protection in the respiratory tract where the natural infection occurs. In contrast, using this approach, it seems to be more effective to administer antigen intranasally rather than orally to achieve immunity in the urogenital tract. For reasons that are not yet well understood, mucosal immunity tends to be shortlived.

Immunological Requirements of a Vaccine

1. Activation of APCs to facilitate antigen processing and enhancement of costimulator and cytokine production;
2. Stimulation of both T and B cells so that there is a high yield of memory cells;
3. Generation of type 1 and 2 T cells to several epitopes, preferably in conserved regions, to overcome the variation in the immune response in the population due to MHC polymorphism;
4. Persistence of antigen in its natural conformation on follicular dendritic cells (FDCs) in lymphoid tissues, where B memory cells are formed and recruited to form antibody-secreting cells (ASCs) so that antibody of high affinity is continually present.

Factors Affecting the Feasibility of Vaccine Development

Table 3 lists some of the factors which make it more straightforward to develop a vaccine against a virus, and these can be contrasted with those which tend to increase the difficulty. It can be readily seen that most of the latter points apply to HIV.

See also: **Immune response: General features, Cell mediated immune response; Persistent viral infection; Virus structure: Principles of virus structure.**

Further Reading

Ada GL and McElrath MJ (1996) Perspective. HIV-1 vaccine-induced cytotoxic T cell responses: potential role in vaccine efficacy. *AIDS Res. Hum. Retrov.* 13: 243.

Ada G and Ramsay A (1997) *Vaccines, Vaccination and the Immune Response*. Philadelphia: Lippincott–Raven.

Plotkin SA, Mortimer EA and Orenstein W (eds) (1998) *Vaccines*, 3rd edn. Philadelphia: WB Saunders.

Stratton KR, Howe CJ and Johnston RB (1994) *Adverse Events Associated with Childhood Vaccines: Evidence Bearing on Causality*. Washington, DC: Institute of Medicine, National Academy Press.

VACCINIA VIRUS (*POXVIRIDAE*)

Riccardo Wittek, Université de Lausanne, Lausanne, Switzerland

Copyright © 1999 Academic Press

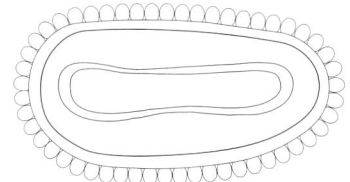

History

In 1980, the World Health Assembly announced that smallpox, once the most serious infectious disease of humankind, had been eradicated from all the countries of the world. Several factors were important in making the eradication campaign a unique success in the history of medicine. Among these was the active role played by WHO which organized the campaign and provided expertise in all relevant areas. Furthermore, variola virus, the agent of smallpox, had no animal reservoir and consequently, interrupting the chain of human-to-human transmission eliminated the virus. Finally, with vaccinia virus, an excellent vaccine for smallpox was available. The vaccine had a low production cost, could be freeze-dried and in this form was very heat stable obviating the need of a cold chain. In addition, the vaccine was easy to administer even by relatively untrained field workers and left a characteristic scar providing permanent evidence of vaccination which was important for WHO in assessing vaccination coverage.

It is not known when vaccinia virus was introduced as a smallpox vaccine. Edward Jenner, who was the first to demonstrate, at the end of the 18th century, that inoculation of a related poxvirus provided protection against challenge with variola virus, isolated his vaccine virus from a milkmaid infected with 'cowpox'. It is unclear what this virus was. Although, in modern times, vaccinia virus was occasionally isolated from skin lesions of infected cows, these cases were usually associated with contact with vaccinated humans and therefore, the cow does not seem to be the natural host of the virus. The origin of vaccinia virus thus remains a matter for speculation (see also: 'Evolution').

Taxonomy and Classification

Vaccinia virus is a member of the family *Poxviridae* which comprises a group of complex animal DNA viruses. The family is further subdivided into the two subfamilies, *Chordopoxvirinae* and *Entomopoxvirinae* whose representatives infect vertebrate and insect hosts, respectively. Within the subfamily, *Chordopoxvirinae* vaccinia virus belongs to the genus *Orthopoxvirus*.

Properties of the Virion

Poxviruses are among the largest and most complex viruses known. The particles have a typical brick-shape and measure about 300 × 250 nm. Two types of particles can be distinguished. Virions that are naturally released from the infected cells are surrounded by a Golgi-derived envelope. Virions that are released by experimental cell lysis lack this envelope, but are also infectious. Electron microscopy of negatively stained specimens reveals that the surface of nonenveloped particles is composed of tubular structures ('surface tubules'), which give the particles a characteristic appearance (**Fig. 1A**). However, more recent cryoelectron microscopy (**Fig. 1B**), which allows examination of hydrated virus particles, provided no evidence of surface tubules and it is conceivable that these structures represent a shrinkage artifact resulting from dehydration of particles prepared for electron microscopy by conventional procedures.

In thin sections of virions examined by conventional electron microscopy, the internal core structure can be visualized, which consists of an oval biconcave disk. The concavities of the core accommodate the two lateral bodies. Again, these structures are not seen by cryoelectron microscopy and their significance remains to be established. Cores prepared by treatment of virions with 2-mercaptoethanol and a nonionic detergent have a similar appearance both by conventional and cryoelectron microscopy (**Fig. 1C**).

Properties of the Genome

Vaccinia virions contain a large double-stranded DNA genome which has been entirely sequenced in the Copenhagen strain and shown to consist of 191 636 base pairs. Characteristic features of the molecules are the crosslinks that join the two DNA strands at both ends. The terminal 100 nucleotides or so consist of single-stranded loops. The genome is further characterized by the presence of long inverted terminal repeats of about 10 kbp. The terminal 3.5 kbp of these are mainly composed of a tandemly repeated 70 bp sequence.

Properties of the Proteins

The DNA sequence of the viral genome provides evidence for the presence of about 200 potential protein-coding sequences, but only relatively few proteins have been assigned a function. The majority of polypeptides with known or suspected functions are enzymes involved in nucleic acid metabolism. Examples are the subunits of RNA polymerase, enzymes involved in capping and polyadenylation of mRNA, DNA polymerase, thymidine and thymidylate kinase, DNA ligase and several more. Other proteins are structural components of the virion. Together with some enzymes, which are also packaged in the virus particle, the total number of virion polypeptides may be as high as 100. The envelope of extracellular virions contains at least six proteins, five of which are glycosylated. The 37 kDa major envelope antigen is acylated.

Physical Properties

The development of a stable smallpox vaccine was greatly facilitated by the fact that the infectivity of vaccinia virus is relatively unaffected by environmental conditions which inactivate most other viruses. This property, together with the large particle size, was also the reason why vaccinia virus was the first

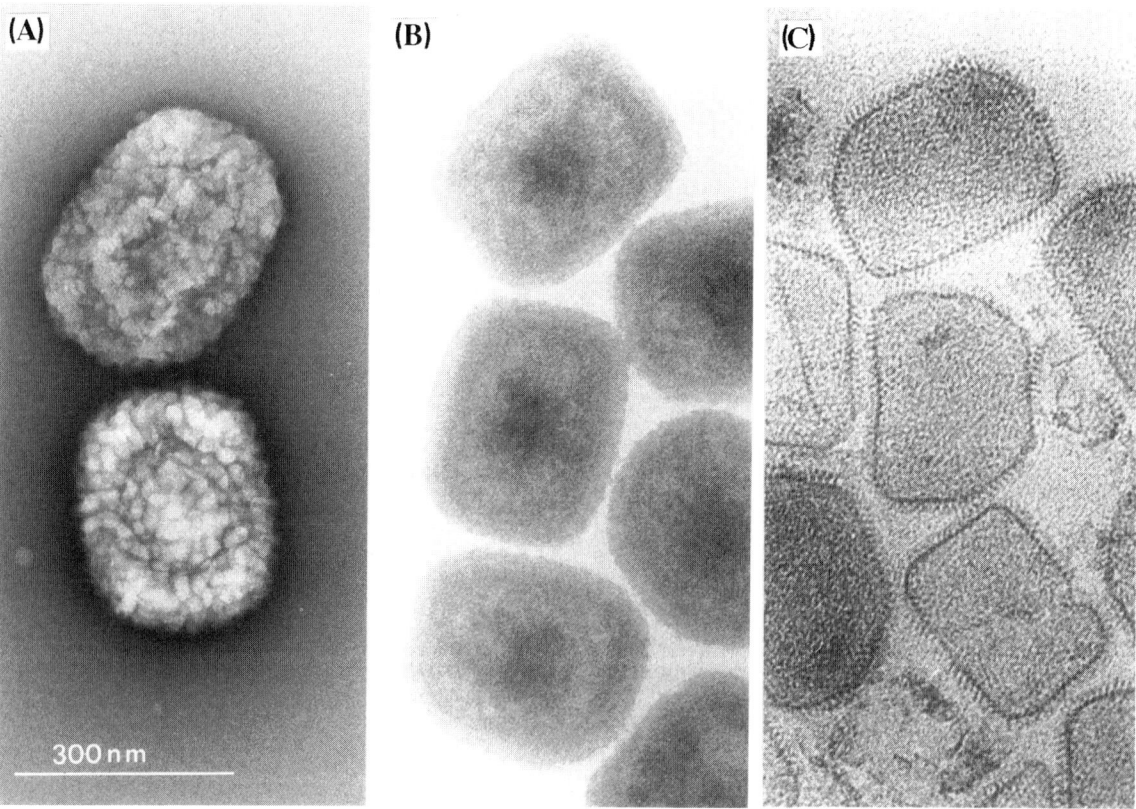

Figure 1 Structure of vaccinia virus including the viral core. (**A**) Conventional preparation of the virus by negative staining. (**B**) Vitrified sample observed by cryoelectron microscopy. The virus particles are in the native state and are floating in a thin layer of vitrified solution kept for observation at c. −160°C and are neither stained nor chemically fixed. (**C**) Core particles prepared as in (**B**). (Courtesy of M. Adrian and J. Dubochet.)

animal virus to be purified extensively. Heating at 55°C for 60 min, or at 50°C for 90 min completely destroys infectivity. Other methods for destroying infectivity were tested in attempts to produce an inactivated smallpox vaccine. Ultraviolet irradiation, formaldehyde treatment, photodynamic inactivation with methylene blue and gamma irradiation were all found to inactivate vaccinia virus, but some of these procedures also resulted in a loss of antigenicity.

Complete solubilization of vaccinia virus is achieved by heating at 100°C in the presence of sodium dodecylsulfate and reducing agents.

Strategy of Replication of Nucleic Acid

Poxviruses are unusual among DNA viruses in that their replication cycle takes place in the cytoplasm of the infected host cell. Upon penetration, the virus sheds its outer protein layers resulting in the release of the viral core containing the DNA and enzymes involved in the synthesis and modification of mRNA. A first burst of RNA synthesis occurs. Following expression of the early genes, the DNA is released from the core and replicated. This allows expression of the intermediate genes, the transcription of which requires a naked DNA template. After transcription of intermediate genes, late genes, many of which encode structural proteins, are expressed.

Replication of the genome occurs through synthesis of long concatemeric intermediates which are subsequently resolved into unit-length genomes. Concatemer resolution is a highly specific process and depends on a 20 bp element located adjacent to the hairpin loop in the mature DNA molecule. For a long time DNA replication itself was not believed to require specific origins of replication since any DNA transfected into vaccinia virus-infected cells is replicated to some extent. More recently, however, it was shown that optimal replication efficiency depends on 200 bp of sequences from the viral telomere.

Characterization of Transcription

Transcription of the different temporal classes of vaccinia virus genes requires specific promoters, which are short, a multisubunit RNA polymerase and stage-specific transcription factors.

Transcription of early genes depends on early promoter elements, which are about 30 bp long. An early transcription factor binds to these regulatory sequences. Termination of early transcription requires the virus-encoded capping enzyme and occurs about 50 bp downstream of a UUUUUNU signal in the nascent RNA chain. Early mRNAs are capped and polyadenylated and typically contain short 5' untranslated leader sequences.

Intermediate gene transcription requires the presence of the viral capping enzyme and two intermediate gene transcription factors which are able to activate intermediate gene transcription only after the DNA has been replicated. Interestingly, one of the intermediate gene transcription factors has also been purified from uninfected HeLa cells but not from nonpermissive cells. This finding challenges the dogma that exclusively virus-encoded proteins are used for transcription in vaccinia virus.

Late gene promoters also consist of about 30 bp and contain the highly conserved TAAAT motif in which transcription initiation occurs. Late mRNAs are heterogeneous in length, are polyadenylated and have a capped poly(A) leader sequence of about 35 Å residues. The leader is not encoded in the genome but is produced by stuttering of RNA polymerase in the TAAAT motif. In addition to RNA polymerase, four transcription factors are required for late gene transcription. Three of these are products of intermediate genes, the fourth is synthesized both before and after DNA replicaton.

Transcription in vaccinia virus is characterized by a cascade in which transcription of each temporal class of genes requires the presence of specific transcription factors which are made by the preceding temporal class of genes. Thus, early gene transcription factors are made late in infection, packaged in virions and used in the subsequent round of infection. Intermediate gene transcription factors are encoded by early genes, and late transcription factors by intermediate genes. The recent discovery of a cellular protein involved in intermediate gene transcription and the fact that one late gene transcription factor is made before and after DNA synthesis, requires some revision of the cascade model.

Characterization of Translation

Infection of cells by vaccinia virus results in rapid shut-off of host cell DNA, RNA and protein synthesis. Phosphorylation of ribosomal proteins and short polyadenylated viral RNAs has been implicated in the inhibition of cellular protein synthesis.

The preferential translation of temporal classes of mRNAs is probably a direct consequence of the half-life and abundance of mRNAs at a given time of infection.

Post-translational Processing

Several types of post-translational processing events occur in the maturation of viral proteins. The mature forms of three major core proteins and of the viral growth factor are generated by cleavage of higher-molecular-weight precursors. The envelope proteins, with the exception of the 37 kDa protein which is acylated, are all glycosylated. Finally, some viral proteins are phosphorylated or myristylated.

Assembly Site, Uptake, Release and Cytopathology

The penetration of cells by naked virions differs from that of enveloped particles. The strong temperature dependence of penetration of intracellular virions and its sensitivity to sodium fluoride and cytochalasin B indicate that the majority of such particles enter cells by endocytosis. In contrast, uptake of enveloped particles is relatively efficient at low temperature and insensitive to the above compounds suggesting that such particles penetrate by fusion of the viral envelope with the cell membrane. Intracellular and enveloped viruses appear to bind to different cellular receptors which have not yet been identified.

Since vaccinia virions are composed of a very large number of proteins, it is not surprising that virus assembly, which takes place in discrete cytoplasmic areas termed viral factories is a complex process which is still poorly understood and which requires several hours to be completed (**Fig. 2**).

For many years it was believed that formation of the intracellular naked virus (INV), now referred to as intracellular mature virus (IMV), involved a unique process of *de novo* membrane biogenesis mediated by viral enzymes, a concept which has been difficult for cell biologists to accept. Indeed, more recent data indicate that for the initial steps in morphogenesis vaccinia virus uses a membrane cisterna which is derived from the intermediate compartment between the endoplasmic reticulum (ER) and the Golgi stacks. The virus thus acquires two membranes simultaneously, the inner of which will become the core membrane and the outer of which will differentiate into the shell of the intracellular mature virus.

Morphogenesis results in the production of infectious virions containig two lipid membranes. A small fraction of these particles is further enveloped by two Golgi-derived membranes containing at least six viral antigens. Wrapped virions migrate along actin-containing microfilaments to the cell surface where the outer of the two membranes fuses with the plasma membrane. This results in the release of enveloped virions which are composed of the original naked particle enclosed in the inner Golgi membrane. This process of envelopment and release is relatively inefficient. Depending on virus strains and host cell, between 1% and 30% of the progeny is released as

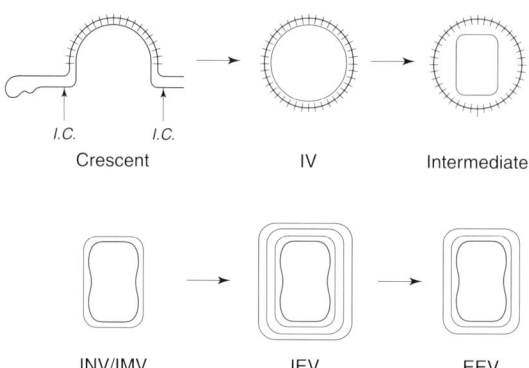

Figure 2 Model for vaccinia virus assembly. During the first envelopment step, a viral crescent is formed from cellular membranes derived from the intermediate compartment (*I.C.*, arrowheads). When the envelopment has been completed, an immature virus (IV) containing two tightly apposed membranes is formed. The morphologically distinct spicules of the crescents as well as the IV are indicated as lines in the outer membrane. These spicules become less visible as the virus matures. During the maturation of the virus particle, an intermediate form is seen in which two membranes become clearly visible; the inner one acquires the brick shape of the INV, while the outer membrane profile remains spherical. The next viral particle that is formed is the INV/IMV (intracellular naked virus or intracellular mature virus) where both membrane profiles are brick shaped. The INV becomes enwrapped by another cellular cisterna thereby forming the four-membraned intracellular enveloped virus (IEV). The IEV is believed to fuse with the plasma membrane, releasing the three-membraned extracellular enveloped virus (EEV) into the medium. Note that this model ignores the problem of how the DNA, which is found within the intermediate particle, enters the assembling virus. (Reproduced with permission of The Rockefeller University Press from Sodeik B, Doms RW, Ericsson M *et al* (1993) *J. Cell Biol.* 121: 521.)

enveloped particles. The majority of naked virions remain cell-associated even after cell death.

The current model of vaccinia virus biogenesis is represented schematically in **Fig. 2**.

Infection of cells in monolayer cultures induces several changes. Within a few hours after infection, the cells become rounded and retract from each other. Basophilic areas (=factories), which are the sites of virus replication, then appear in the cytoplasm. These areas develop into B-type inclusion bodies ('Guarneri bodies') which are distinct from the more prominent A-type inclusion bodies seen in cells infected with other orthopoxviruses. Infected cells die within about 15 h after infection.

Vaccinia Virus as a Eukaryotic Expression Vector

Foreign genetic information has been inserted into the vaccinia virus genome by homologous *in vivo* recombination. The standard procedure consists of fusing the foreign gene of interest to a vaccinia virus promoter and inserting the chimeric gene into the nonessential viral thymidine kinase gene contained in a recombinant plasmid. The resulting DNA is amplified and transfected into cells that have also been infected with wild-type virus. Upon viral DNA replication the thymidine kinase DNA sequences in the viral genome and recombinant plasmid undergo homologous recombination resulting in insertion of the foreign gene in the viral genome. Since this inactivates the viral thymidine kinase gene, recombinant virus can conveniently be selected on the basis of the thymidine kinase-negative phenotype.

Many alternative insertion sites into the viral genome and various selection procedures for isolating recombinant viruses have been described. It has also become possible to generate recombinant viruses by direct molecular cloning and packaging. Particularly high expression levels of foreign proteins have been obtained with the vaccinia virus/phage T7 hybrid system in which expression of the gene of interest is driven by the T7 promoter. T7 RNA polymerase is provided by a second recombinant virus used to co-infect cells. High expression levels of foreign proteins in this system requires cap-independent translation of the transcripts produced by T7 RNA polymerase. This has been achieved by fusing the target gene to sequences derived from the 5′ untranslated leader sequences of encephalomycarditis virus.

Recombinant vaccinia virus has become an invaluable tool to overexpress proteins of particular biological interest. Advantages of vaccinia virus compared to prokaryotic expression systems are the correct post translational processing and solubility of the proteins.

An exciting application of recombinant virus expressing antigens of other infectious agents is their use as live virus vaccines in human and veterinary medicine. Experimental animals immunized with recombinants expressing antigens of other pathogens produce neutralizing antibodies and a cell-mediated immune response and are protected against infection with the live pathogen. Advantages of such vaccines are the low production cost, stability, ease of administration, features that were major determinants for the success of the smallpox eradication program. The main argument against the introduction of recombinants is the residual virulence of vaccinia virus. Considerable effort has therefore been made to produce a safer vaccinia virus vector.

Geographic and Seasonal Distribution

Vaccinia virus is not associated with a naturally occurring disease in humans. The smallpox vaccine was extensively used worldwide but, after eradication of smallpox, vaccination was abandoned.

Rabbitpox virus, a highly virulent vaccinia virus strain, has caused outbreaks of a lethal pox disease in colonies of laboratory rabbits in Utrecht and New York. Several outbreaks of buffalopox occurred in Maharashtra state in India, where buffaloes are used for milk production. The disease is caused by an orthopoxvirus which is closely related to vaccinia virus, but different enough to justify classification as a subspecies of vaccinia virus.

Host Range and Virus Propagation

Vaccinia virus has a very broad host range and can infect most vertebrate animals. Mice and rabbits are the most commonly used experimental animals for studying the pathogenicity of virus mutants. The chorioallantoic membrane of developing chick embryos was widely used for virus propagation and for differentiating vaccinia virus from other poxviruses, but has been replaced by cultured cells. High virus titers can be obtained in most cell lines. Some of the most frequently used cells are HeLa cells, either grown in suspension or as monolayer cultures, mouse L cells, or CV-1 African green monkey kidney cells. Chinese hamster ovary (CHO) cells do not support virus multiplication. The gene that allows cowpox virus to replicate in CHO cells has been identified and inserted into the genome of recombinant vaccinia virus. The resulting virus can be propagated in CHO cells.

Genetics

The first vaccinia virus mutants were isolated on the chorioallantoic membrane of chick embryos where most strains normally produce red, hemorrhagic lesions (pocks). White pock lesions arise with a relatively high frequency and the viruses isolated from such pocks have been designated white pock mutants. Analysis of the genome of these mutants revealed large deletions near the termini of the DNA or more complex rearrangements involving both ends. In some white pock mutants, the deletions were also associated with an altered host range. A large number of temperature-sensitive and drug-resistant mutants have also been isolated. For many of these, the mutation was mapped in the genome by marker rescue experiments. Targeted insertional inactivation of particular genes has been widely used to study gene functions. Such knock-out mutants frequently display a small pock phenotype and/or are attenuated in experimental animals. These mutants also demonstrate that many genes are dispensable for virus replication in cultured cells but that their presence confers a selective advantage for virus propagation in the organism.

Evolution

Several hypotheses for the origin of vaccinia virus have been advanced, but none is entirely convincing. According to some of these, vaccinia virus was either derived from variola or cowpox virus, or is a hybrid between the two. Other authors propose that vaccinia virus is a 'fossil' and represents the maintenance in the laboratory of a virus of a domestic or wild animal that has otherwise become extinct. This view is supported by the fact that with the exception of buffalopox virus all vaccinia virus strains form a homogeneous group of viruses both with respect to biological properties and genome structure and are not more closely related to cowpox virus or variola virus than to other orthopoxvirus species. Therefore, the virus that was introduced by Jenner for smallpox vaccination and subsequently distributed worldwide, may indeed have been vaccinia virus.

At the genome level, differences between vaccinia virus strains are mainly due to variability in the terminal regions of the molecule, whereas the central part is highly conserved. Comparison of protein-coding regions between different strains typically show greater than 99% identity in amino acid sequences.

Buffalopox virus is also considered as a vaccinia virus strain and was probably derived from smallpox vaccine. The virus appears to have evolved more rapidly and has become a separate subspecies which is maintained in buffalo herds in certain parts of India.

Serologic Relationships and Variability

All orthopoxviruses show extensive serological cross-reactivity which is even more marked between individual vaccinia virus strains. Strains cannot, therefore, be distinguished by serological means. Restriction enzyme analysis of the viral genome has become the most reliable method for differentiating between vaccinia virus strains, and has largely replaced methods based on biological criteria such as pock morphology on the chorioallantoic membrane, or ceiling temperature.

Epidemiology

Vaccinia virus was occasionally spread from newly vaccinated humans to nonvaccinated individuals. This could lead to serious complications in cases where contraindications for vaccination of the unvaccinated contact existed. Transmission also occurred to domestic animals, such as cows and pigs and these animals in turn, represented a source of infection for humans. Buffalopox virus which probably also originated from vaccinia virus, was spread between animals by farmers. According to recent reports from India, buffalopox virus has acquired considerable pathogenicity for humans. Most outbreaks of rabbitpox in colonies of laboratory rabbits were caused by a vaccinia virus strain which was accidentally transmitted to the animals by laboratory workers. In some outbreaks, the source of infection was not traced.

Transmission and Tissue Tropism

The smallpox vaccine was usually introduced into the epidermis over the deltoid muscle. Jenner inoculated human subjects by a light scratch of the skin through a drop of vaccine and variations of this technique were used for a very long time. During the smallpox eradication campaign, other techniques for delivering vaccine were developed. Jet injectors were widely used in West Africa and Brazil. The major advance was the development of the bifurcated needle which could easily be used even by inexperienced vaccinators and which required no special maintenance.

Accidental transmission of vaccinia virus between humans or between humans and animals occurred by direct contact through minute skin lesions. In most outbreaks of rabbitpox, spread appeared to occur by the respiratory route; direct contact between animals was not necessary.

After smallpox vaccination of humans, virus replicated in the epidermis and remained confined to the site of inoculation. Spread to other parts of the body was only observed in the rare cases of complications. After infection of rabbits with rabbitpox virus by the respiratory route, virus spread through the body in a stepwise manner and replication occurred in various tissues.

Pathogenicity

The frequency of the rare, but serious complications of smallpox vaccination was related to the use of particular vaccinia virus strains. For instance, after the Bern strain, once in Austria, Switzerland and West Germany, was replaced by the Lister strain in 1971, the occurrence of complications of the central nervous system declined. Other strains with a good safety record are the New York City Board of Health strain and the Japanese LC16m8 strain. Since the residual virulence of vaccinia virus is the major obstacle for the introduction of recombinant virus as live vaccines against other pathogens, considerable effort is being made to make the virus a safer vector. Several nonessential genes have been deleted from the viral genome and in each case, the resulting mutant virus showed an attenuated phenotype in experimental animal models.

Rabbitpox virus is a highly virulent vaccinia virus strain for rabbits causing a rapidly lethal disease. Frequently death occurs before skin lesions have time to develop.

Clinical Features of Infection

After primary smallpox vaccination a papule developed in 3–5 days, rapidly became a vesicle and later became pustular, reaching its maximum size after 8–10 days. A scab then formed, which separated at 14–21 days leaving a typical vaccination scar. Vaccination produced a generalized infection with swelling and tenderness of the draining lymph nodes and mild fever. The vaccinees frequently felt miserable for a few days.

Apart from the 'normal' vaccination reactions, which were more intense than those seen with other human vaccines, a number of rare but serious complications occurred. These were of two kinds: those affecting the skin and those affecting the central nervous system. In the first group, progressive vaccinia was the least frequent, but most serious complication and was observed only in vaccinees with a deficient cell-mediated immune system. The clinical features of progressive vaccinia were a failure of the primary vaccination lesion to heal, appearance of lesions elsewhere on the body and progression of all lesions until the patient died. The fatality-rate was extremely high. Eczema vaccination was the second most serious skin affection and occurred among persons with eczema. This complication was characterized by the appearance of lesions on areas of the skin that were eczematous at the time or had previously been so. The fatality-rate was about 30%. Generalized vaccinia followed virus spread via the bloodstream. Lesions similar to the vaccination lesions appeared on many parts of the body. Generalized vaccinia had a good prognosis. Accidental infection occurred among laboratory workers in research facilities or vaccine production centers or in contacts of newly vaccinated persons and were most serious when they affected the eye. Complications affecting the central nervous system were encephalopathy, usually in children less than 2 years of age, and encephalomyelitis in older children and adults. These complications were of particular concern since they occurred in persons with no obvious contraindications for vaccination and had a high case-fatality rate.

Pathology and Histopathology

The pathology and histopathology of 'normal' skin lesions at various stages after smallpox vaccination were studied in biopsies. For more information, the reader is referred to the specialized literature which also deals with the pathology of the rare complications of vaccination.

Immune Response

Smallpox vaccination with vaccinia virus provided complete protection against smallpox for at least 5 years and some protection for over 30 years. Both humoral and cell-mediated immune responses were observed. Studies in mice indicated that cytotoxic T cells are more important for protection against mousepox than circulating antibodies. In humans, progressive vaccinia developed in patients with an impaired cell-mediated immune system, but normal humoral antibody responses, underlining the importance of cytotoxic T cells for limiting vaccinia virus spread and presumably also for providing protection against smallpox.

Evasion of the Host Immune Response

The recent discovery that poxviruses encode a whole arsenal of proteins whose functions are to counteract the host response to infection, has opened up a new field of exciting research. The list of such proteins includes a viral protein that blocks complement activation, thereby protecting intracellular virus from complement-mediated neutralization of infectivity. Other proteins target the host interferon response either by acting as soluble interferon receptors or by neutralizing the action of interferon-induced antiviral host proteins. Still other proteins interfere with the production of interleukin or compete for the binding of this cytokine to its cell surface receptor, or delay apoptosis. Some of these viral proteins exhibit unusual properties. For instance, in contrast to its cellular counterpart the virus-encoded secreted receptor for interleukin-1 binds only interleukin-1b but not interleukin-1a. The soluble viral interferon receptors on the other hand bind interferons from several different species. The study of these interesting viral proteins is expected to provide insight into the functions of host defense mechanisms which are particularly relevant for the control of infection by certain viruses.

Prevention and Control

After the eradication of smallpox, all countries have abandoned general, compulsory smallpox vaccination. Whether or not the staff in research institutes working with vaccinia virus should be vaccinated is a matter of controversy. Apart from the risk associated with smallpox vaccination, it will become increasingly more difficult in future to obtain vaccine and to find medical doctors proficient in the vaccination procedure.

Future Perspectives

Clearly, in future vaccinia virus vectors will continue to play an important role in basic and applied research. The future of vaccinia virus as a vaccine will depend on whether recombinant virus-expressing antigens of other pathogens will be accepted as live virus vaccines. The main argument against the introduction of such recombinants are the rare complications associated with the use of vaccinia virus as the smallpox vaccine. Considering the great potential of recombinant virus, the decision of whether or not to introduce such vaccines should only be made after a thorough risk–benefit evaluation and the development of safer vectors might influence the decision favorably.

See also: **Smallpox and monkeypox viruses (*Poxviridae*); Vaccines and immune response; Vectors: Animal viruses.**

Further Reading

Fenner F, Wittek R and Dumbell KR (1989) *The Orthopoxviruses*. New York: Academic Press.

Moss B (1996) Poxviridae: the viruses and their replication. In: Fields BN, Knipe DM, Howley PM *et al* (eds) *Fields Virology*, 3rd edn, p. 2637. Philadelphia: Lippincott-Raven.

Smith GL (1994) Virus strategies for evasion of the host response to infection. *Trends Microbiol.* 2: 81.

VARICELLA-ZOSTER VIRUS (*HERPESVIRIDAE*)

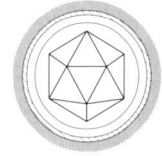

Contents
General Features
Molecular Biology

General Features

Jeffrey I Cohen and **Stephen E Straus**, Medical Virology Section, Laboratory of Clinical Investigation, National Institutes of Health, Bethesda, Maryland, USA

Copyright © 1999 Academic Press

History

Descriptions of vesicular rashes characteristic of chickenpox (varicella) date back to the ninth century. In 1875 Steiner showed that chickenpox was an infectious agent by transmitting the disease from chickenpox vesicle fluid to previously uninfected people. Shingles (zoster) has been recognized since ancient times. In 1909 Von Bokay suggested that chickenpox and shingles were related infections, an idea that was experimentally confirmed in the 1920s and 1930s when children inoculated with fluid from zoster vesicles were shown to contract chickenpox. By virtue of the remarkable dermatomal confinement of most zoster lesions, Garland suggested in 1943 that zoster was due to reactivation of varicella virus that had remained dormant or latent in sensory nerve ganglia.

The viral agents of varicella and zoster were first cultivated by Weller in 1952 and shown on morphologic, cytopathic and serologic criteria to be identical. In 1984 Straus and colleagues showed that viruses isolated during sequential episodes of chickenpox and zoster from the same patient had identical restriction endonuclease patterns, proving the concept of prolonged latent carriage of the virus. However, demonstration of latent virus within dorsal root ganglia awaited subsequent molecular studies using *in situ* hybridization and polymerase chain reaction (PCR) techniques.

Taxonomy and Classification

Varicella-zoster virus (VZV) is a member of the *Alphaherpesvirinae* subfamily, genus *Varicellovirus* of the family *Herpesviridae*. Other alphaherpesviruses that infect humans include herpes simplex viruses 1 and 2, and rarely cercopithicine herpesvirus (B virus). All of these agents exhibit relatively short replicative cycles, destroy the infected cell and establish latent infection in sensory ganglia.

Three subgroups of simian viruses cause severe varicella-like illnesses in nonhuman primates. These include the delta herpesvirus, Medical Lake macaque virus and chimpanzee herpesvirus. While these simian viruses are antigenically related to VZV, they are more homologous to each other than to VZV and are not known to infect humans.

Geographic and Seasonal Distribution

Varicella and zoster infections occur worldwide. Over 90% of varicella occurs during childhood in industrialized countries located in the temperate zone, but infection is commonly delayed until adulthood in tropical regions. Zoster may occur less frequently in tropical areas because of later acquisition of primary infection.

Varicella infection is epidemic each winter and spring, while zoster occurs throughout the year, without a seasonal preference.

Host Range and Virus Propagation

The reservoir for VZV is limited to humans. The virus inherently grows poorly in nonhuman animals or cell lines. Myers and colleagues, however, developed a guinea pig animal model of VZV infection by adapting the virus for growth in guinea pig embryo cells *in vitro*. Inoculation of animals results in a self-limited viremic infection and the emergence of both humoral and cellular immunity. Virus replicates initially in the nasopharynx and can be transmitted to other guinea pigs. Latent VZV DNA has been demonstrated in dorsal root and trigeminal ganglia. The same investigators extended their animal model to congenitally hairless Hartley guinea pigs with the advantage that some animals develop a papular erythematous rash. Rats and mice inoculated with VZV develop latent infection of dorsal root ganglia. Inoculation of VZV into fetal thymus and liver implants in SCID mice results in virus replication in T cells; inoculation of virus into subcutaneous fetal skin implants reproduces many of the histopathologic features of varicella.

An alternative, but less ideal animal model involves the common marmoset (*Callithrix jacchus*). VZV replicates in the lungs with a mild pneumonia and a subsequent humoral immune response. Inoculation of chimpanzees with VZV results in a transient rash containing viral DNA and evokes a modest humoral immune response. None of these animal models has, as yet, reproduced the disease pattern seen in humans, namely a vesicular rash and spontaneous reactivation from latency.

VZV is usually cultured in human fetal diploid lung cells in clinical laboratories. The virus has been cultivated in numerous other human cells including melanoma cells, primary human thyroid cells, astrocytes, Schwann cells and neurons, and can be grown in some simian cells including African green monkey kidney cells and Vero cells, and in guinea pig embryo fibroblasts.

VZV is extremely cell-associated. The titer of virus released into the cell culture supernatant is very low, and preparation of cell-free virus, by sonication or freeze-thawing cells, usually results in a marked drop in the viral titer. Therefore, virus propagation is usually performed by passage of infected cells on to uninfected cell monolayers. VZV is detected by its cytopathic effect, with refractile rounded cells that gradually detach from the monolayer, or by staining with fluorescein-labelled antibody.

Genetics

Several markers can be used to distinguish different strains of the virus. These include temperature sensitivity, plaque size, different effects on host cell lipid metabolism, antiviral sensitivity and restriction endonuclease cleavage patterns. The molecular basis for most of these strain differences are unknown, but viruses that are resistant to acyclovir are usually found to have mutations in their thymidine kinase gene. Other resistant strains have mutations in the DNA polymerase gene.

The entire genome of one prototypical laboratory strain of VZV consists of 124 884 bp. The identification of some viral genes was made by analogy to herpes simplex virus type 1 genes with similar sequences, and by genetic complementation studies in which cell lines expressing selected VZV proteins were used to support the growth of temperature-sensitive mutants of herpes simplex type 1 viruses. Recombinant VZV containing Epstein–Barr virus, hepatitis B virus or herpes simplex virus antigens have been constructed. Recently, a versatile cosmid transfection system has been developed that has allowed targeted deletion, insertion or mutagenesis of a number of individual viral genes products. For example, deletion of the VZV ORF10 gene, the homologue of the essential herpes simplex virus gene VP16, resulted in a virus that was unimpaired for growth *in vitro*.

Evolution

Comparison of the nucleotide and predicted amino acid sequences of VZV with herpes simplex virus types 1 and 2 indicates that these viruses originated from a common ancestor. They share similar gene arrangements and only five genes of VZV do not appear to have herpes simplex virus counterparts.

VZV is more distantly related to all other human herpesviruses, but many of the nonstructural proteins involved in viral replication have conserved elements and activities. Comparison of VZV, for example, with Epstein–Barr virus shows that the majority of VZV genes are homologous with Epstein–Barr virus. Three large blocks of genes are conserved, although rearranged within the two genomes.

Serologic Relationships and Variability

There is only one serotype of VZV. Antibodies detected by the complement fixation test and virus-specific IgM antibodies decline rapidly after convalescence from varicella. Other, more sensitive serologic tests recognize antibodies that persist for life, including immune adherence hemagglutination (IAHA), fluorescence antibody to membrane antigen (FAMA) and enzyme linked immunosorbent assay (ELISA). VZV-specific antibodies are boosted both by recrudescent infection (zoster) and by exposure to others with varicella.

Variability of VZV strains has been shown primarily by differences in restriction endonuclease patterns. Passage of individual strains *in vitro* eventually results in minor changes in restriction endonuclease patterns, predominantly through deletion or reiteration of small repeated elements scattered throughout the genome. Other than these sites, the genome sequence is remarkably stable. For example, the sequence of the thymidine kinase gene has been determined for several epidemiologically unrelated wild-type and acyclovir-resistant strains and found to possess >99% nucleotide and amino acid identity.

Epidemiology

Varicella may occur after exposure of susceptible persons to chickenpox or to herpes zoster. Over 95% of primary infections result in symptomatic chickenpox. Over 90% of individuals in temperate countries are infected with VZV before age 15.

Zoster is due to reactivation of VZV in patients who have previously had chickenpox; some of these patients may not recall the primary infection. Zoster is not clearly related to exposure to chickenpox or to other cases of zoster. About 10–20% of individuals ultimately develop herpes zoster; the risk of which rises steadily with age (**Fig. 1**). Severely immunocompromised patients, such as those with the acquired immune deficiency syndrome (AIDS), have a particularly high incidence of zoster. Recurrent zoster is uncommon; less than 4% of patients experience a second episode. Asymptomatic viremia has been detected in bone marrow transplant recipients and has been followed by recovery of cell-mediated immunity.

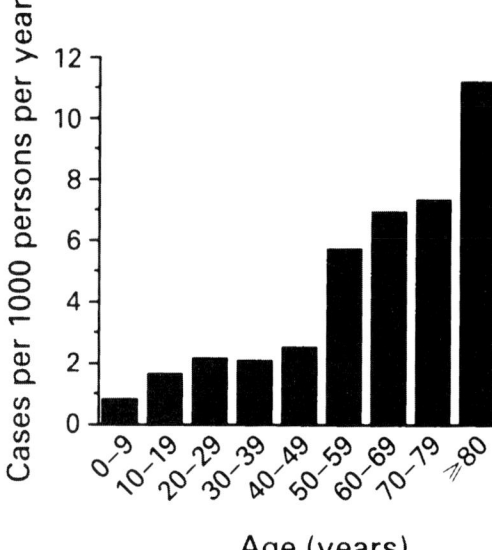

Figure 1 Incidence of herpes zoster per 1000 persons. (Reproduced with permission from Kost and Straus (1996).)

Transmission and Tissue Tropism

VZV is transmitted by the respiratory route. VZV has been detected by PCR in room air from patients with varicella or zoster. Intimate, rather than casual, contact is important for transmission. Chickenpox is highly contagious; about 60–90% of susceptible household contacts become infected. Herpes zoster is less contagious than chickenpox. Only 20–30% of susceptible contacts develop varicella. Patients with varicella are infectious from 2 days before the onset of the rash until all the lesions have crusted.

Primary infection with VZV results in viral replication in the upper respiratory tract and oropharynx, with lesions present on the respiratory mucosa. The infection subsequently spreads to the lymphatics and a mild viremia develops. Mononuclear cells are thought to support viral replication and convey the virus throughout the body. VZV DNA has been detected by PCR in the oropharynx, and virus has been cultured from the blood early during varicella. Further viral replication occurs in the reticuloendothelial system. A brisk secondary viremia results in spread to the periphery. Skin lesions begin with infection of the vascular endothelial cells and virus spreads to epithelial cells. At some time during the course of the infection the virus spreads to both

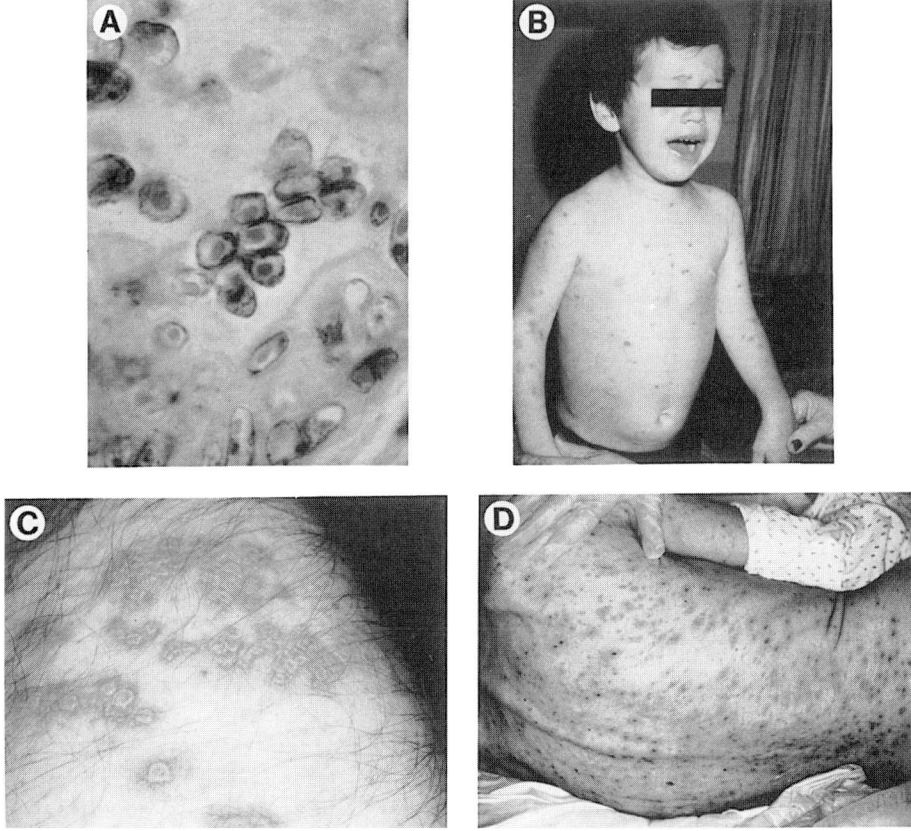

Figure 2 Histopathology and clinical findings of varicella-zoster virus infections. (**A**) Eosinophilic intranuclear inclusions from a skin biopsy in a patient with herpes zoster original magnification ×400. (**B**) Chickenpox in a child. (**C**) Localized zoster in an adult. (**D**) Disseminated zoster in a patient with chronic lymphocytic leukemia. (Reproduced with permission from Straus SE, Ostrove JM, Inchauspe G et al (1988) Varicella-zoster virus infections: biology, natural history, treatment, and prevention. *Ann. Intern. Med.* 108: 221–237.)

neurons and their surrounding satellite cells. During latency, VZV DNA can be detected in thoracic and trigeminal ganglia by PCR, but there are conflicting data regarding the cell types harboring the latent virus. Using *in situ* hybridization, VZV has been detected in neurons, in satellite cells, or in both cell types. During latency only about four of the 70 known viral genes remain expressed.

Zoster is due to reactivation of virus in the sensory ganglia. The factors leading to its reactivation are not known, but are associated with neural injury and cellular immune impairment. Reactivated virus spreads down the sensory nerve to the skin where the resulting vesicles are typically confined to a single dermatome. Viremia and subsequent cutaneous or visceral dissemination of lesions may occur in zoster, especially in immunocompromised patients.

Pathogenicity

Passage of wild-type VZV in cell culture by Takahashi in 1974 led to attenuation of the virus and changes in its temperature sensitivity and infectivity for certain cell lines. The resulting Oka vaccine strain has several differences in restriction endonuclease patterns from wild-type strains, but it is not known which of these differences contribute to attenuation.

Clinical Features of Infection

The incubation period for chickenpox is 2 weeks, with a range of 10–21 days. The disease begins with fever and malaise, followed by a generalized vesicular rash (**Fig. 2B**). Lesions tend to appear first on the head and trunk and then spread to the extremities. New lesions usually follow viremic waves for 3–5 days and, in the normal host, most lesions are crusted and healed by 2 weeks. Lesions in different stages coexist in an individual. The disease is usually self-limited in the normal host.

Complications of varicella are more common in neonates, in children with malnutrition, in immuno-compromised patients (e.g. malignancy or immunosuppressive therapy), in pregnant women, and in older adults. These complications include bacterial superinfection of the skin, pneumonia, hepatitis, encephalitis, thrombocytopenia and purpura fulminans. Reye syndrome occurs in rare children who take aspirin to treat varicella fevers. There are about 3–4 million cases of varicella each year in the USA, with about 100 deaths.

Zoster usually presents with pain and dysesthesias 1–4 days before the onset of the vesicular rash. The rash is usually painful and confined to a single dermatome (Fig. 2C), but may involve several adjacent dermatomes. Fever and malaise often accompany the rash. Vesicles are often pustular by day 4 and become crusted by day 10 in the normal host.

Postherpetic neuralgia, manifested by pain lasting for weeks to several years in the area of the initial rash, is the most common and disconcerting complication of zoster in the normal host. Less common complications include encephalitis, myelitis, the Ramsay Hunt syndrome (lesions in the ear canal, with auditory and facial nerve involvement), ophthalmoplegia, facial weakness and pneumonitis. Immunocompromised patients with zoster are more likely to develop disseminated disease with neurologic, ocular or visceral involvement (Fig. 2D). Patients with AIDS have a high frequency of zoster and may develop recurrent or chronic disease with verrucous, hyperkeratotic skin lesions.

Pathology and Histology

Varicella lesions are readily recognized in the skin and mucous membranes. However, similar lesions also occur in the mucosa of the respiratory and gastrointestinal tracts, liver, spleen and any tissue, and remain unrecognized except in severe cases. With severe disease there is inflammatory infiltration of the small vessels of most organs. Zoster causes inflammation and necrosis of the sensory ganglia and its nerves, and skin lesions which are histopathologically identical to those seen with varicella.

Cutaneous lesions due to VZV begin with infection of capillary endothelial cells, followed by direct spread to epidermal epithelial cells. The epidermis becomes edematous, with acantholysis and vesicle formation. Mononuclear cells infiltrate the small vessels of the dermis. Initially, vesicles contain clear fluid with cell-free virus, but later the vesicles become cloudy and contain neutrophils, macrophages, interferon and other cellular and humoral components of the inflammatory response pathways. Subsequently, the vesicles dry, leaving a crust that usually heals without scarring. Cells infected with VZV show eosinophilic intranuclear inclusions with multinucleate giant cell formation (Fig. 2A). These changes are not specific for VZV, as they are seen with herpes simplex and cytomegalovirus infections.

Immune Response

Infection with VZV elicits both a humoral and cellular immune response. The ability of VZV immune globulin (VZIG) to attenuate or prevent infection in exposed children (see Prevention and Control, below) indicates that virus-specific antibody is important in protection from primary infection. The presence of VZV-specific IgG does not correlate, however, with protection from zoster. Antibody to VZV is often present by the time the rash of varicella first appears. Virus-specific IgM, IgG and IgA are present within 5 days of symptomatic disease; however, only IgG persists for life. Antibodies to viral glycoproteins gE (gpI), gB (gpII), gH (gpIII) and the immediate early gene 62 product have been detected during acute infection, and the titers of antibodies to these proteins are boosted during recurrent infection. The mere presence of antibody to VZV glycoproteins in children with leukemia who had received live varicella vaccine was not adequate to prevent breakthrough varicella or zoster.

The cellular immune responses are thought to be more important in recovery from acute varicella infection and for prevention of, and recovery from, zoster. The level of cellular immunity correlates with disease severity during acute varicella. Cytotoxic T cells that lyse virus-infected cells are present by 2–3 days after the onset of the rash of varicella. Cell-mediated immunity, as measured by lymphocyte proliferative response, is directed against cells expressing glycoproteins gE, gB, gH, gI and gC (gpI–gpV, respectively), the immediate early genes 62 and 63, and presumably other gene products as well. Interferon is present in VZV vesicles.

Most varicella infections result in lifelong immunity to reinfection. Second episodes of varicella are rare; these individuals tend to have reduced humoral and cellular immunity to VZV at the time of the second infection. Zoster is associated with a reduction in cellular immunity to VZV that, in the normal host, is partially restored in response to this recurrent infection. Recurrent zoster is uncommon, except in severely immune deficient patients, such as those with AIDS.

Prevention and Control

Prevention of varicella can be achieved by restricting exposure or by resorting to either immunoglobulin prophylaxis or vaccination with live, attenuated virus. If given within 4 days of exposure to the virus,

VZIG prevents or attenuates varicella in seronegative persons. The preparation has no effect in modifying zoster. VZIG is recommended for individuals (1) with recent, close contact to patients with varicella or zoster, (2) who are susceptible to varicella, *and* (3) who fall in a high-risk category. The last group includes premature or certain newborn infants, pregnant women, and patients with congenital or acquired cellular immune deficiencies.

The live, attenuated varicella vaccine (Oka strain) was licensed in the USA in 1995 and is recommended for vaccination of all children and some susceptible adults. The vaccine protects normal children and adults, as well as children with malignancies, from clinical varicella. Most children develop adequate humoral and cellular immunity to varicella after a single dose of vaccine; additional doses enhance the degree of immunity and are recommended for adults. A rash may follow vaccination. It is usually mild, but can be severe if the vaccine is given to patients experiencing periods of profound cellular immune impairment. The live vaccine virus establishes neural latency and can reactivate. Thus, zoster has been reported in vaccinees, especially those who are immunocompromised, but the rate appears to be no higher than that following natural infection. Vaccination may be combined with VZIG for postexposure prophylaxis.

Patients with varicella or zoster should be isolated from susceptible persons until all lesions have crusted. This is particularly important for hospital workers and immune-deficient patients.

Acyclovir, vidarabine and leukocyte interferon have been used in the treatment of varicella and zoster in immunocompromised patients. Interferon proved to be an inadequate and impractical therapy. Vidarabine must be administered intravenously and is also less effective and more toxic than acyclovir. Acyclovir is the current treatment of choice for selected infections. It results in a shorter duration of symptoms and decreased visceral dissemination of varicella or zoster in the immunocompromised host. Acyclovir also prevents spread of trigeminal zoster to the eye and modestly shortens the duration of varicella and zoster symptoms in the normal host. Analogues of acyclovir, such as famciclovir and valaciclovir, result in higher levels of antiviral activity and have been licensed for oral therapy of zoster in the USA.

Acyclovir-resistant strains of VZV have been reported in patients with AIDS; these infections are best treated with foscarnet. Corticosteroids, when used early during zoster, reduce acute pain. Herpes zoster, particularly in elderly patients, may lead to prolonged and severe postherpetic neuralgia. Treatment of postherpetic neuralgia is difficult and often unsatisfactory, but many patients experience improvement with tricyclic antidepressant drugs like amitriptyline.

Future Perspectives

Widespread vaccination of children (both normal and immunocompromised) with the attenuated, live varicella vaccine should reduce the incidence and severity of varicella. The increase in humoral and cellular immunity after vaccination of elderly patients suggests that the vaccine might also reduce the frequency and severity of zoster and a large clinical trial is being planned to test this hypothesis. Because of the potential for the live vaccine to cause zoster, subunit vaccines (containing viral glycoproteins) may prove preferable.

See also: **Cytomegaloviruses (*Herpesviridae*): Animal cytomegaloviruses, General features (human), Molecular biology (human), Murine cytomegaloviruses; Herpes simplex viruses (*Herpesviridae*): General features, Molecular biology; Herpesviruses – baboon and chimpanzee (*Herpesviridae*); Immune response: Cell mediated immune response, General features.**

Further Reading

Arvin A, Moffat JF and Redman R (1996) Varicella-zoster virus: aspects of pathogenesis and host response to natural infection and varicella vaccine. *Adv. Virus Res.* 46: 263.

Cohen JI and Straus SE (1996) Varicella-zoster virus and its replication. In: Fields BN, Knipe DM, Howley PM *et al* (eds) *Fields Virology* 3rd edn, p. 2525. Philadelphia: Lippincott-Raven.

Ellis RW and White CJ (eds) (1996) The varicella-vaccine. *Infect. Dis. Clin. North Am.* 10: 457.

Kost RG and Straus SE (1996) Postherpetic neuralgia – pathogenesis, treatment, and prevention. *N Engl J Med* 335: 32.

Rentier B (ed.) (1995) Updated proceedings of the second international conference on the varicella-zoster virus. *Neurology* 45 (suppl. 8): S1.

Molecular Biology

William T Ruyechan and **John Hay**, Department of Microbiology, School of Medicine, State University of New York at Buffalo, Buffalo, New York, USA

Copyright © 1999 Academic Press

Properties of the Virion

The morphology of the varicella-zoster virus (VZV) virion is similar to that of other herpesviruses. The virion is 180–200 nm in diameter and is made up of four structurally distinct elements. The linear duplex viral DNA genome is packaged in a central 75 nm core, contained within an icosahedral nucleocapsid 100 nm in diameter, with 5:3:2 axial symmetry. The nucleocapsid is composed of 162 hexameric and pentameric capsomeres with central hollows wider on the outside than the inside. A proteinaceous tegument surrounds the nucleocapsid and is, in turn, surrounded by a lipid bilayer potentially derived from a number of cellular membranes, including the nuclear membrane and Golgi membranes. This lipid coat contains at least six virus-encoded glycoproteins which are visualized by electron microscopy as spikes or studs approximately 8 nm in length.

A minimum of 30 proteins ranging in size from ~ 250 to 17 kDa have been identified as components of the VZV virion. The capsid is composed primarily of the 155 kDa VZV major capsid protein which makes up the capsomeres. In addition, some 8–10 other polypeptides are also present in purified nucleocapsids based on sodium dodecyl sulfate-polyacrylamide gel electrophoresis (SDS–PAGE) analysis. Thus the capsid proteins and the glycoproteins account for somewhat less than half the virion proteins. The remainder are, by a process of elimination, contained in the tegument of the virus. Our knowledge of the VZV tegument proteins is incomplete. Recent work, however, has shown that two of the tegument components (the ORF10 protein and the IE62 protein) are the VZV homologues of the herpes simplex virus (HSV) alpha-*trans*-inducing factor (alpha-TIF) and the major immediate early transcriptional regulatory protein ICP4 (IE175). In addition, the products of VZV gene 47 (a protein kinase), gene 9 and the IE4 and IE63 proteins (both gene regulatory proteins) also appear to be present in the virion. The significance of the presence of these proteins is discussed in subsequent sections.

Properties of the Genome

The genome of VZV is a linear duplex DNA molecule with a bouyant density of 1.706 g cm^{-3} and an overall G + C content of 46%. The genome of VZV strain Dumas has been sequenced in its entirety and contains a total of 124 884 base pairs. The size and organization of VZV DNA indicated by this sequence are in good agreement with experimental data derived from a number of different strains over the last decade and it has been taken as the paradigm by workers in the field. The VZV genome is composed of two covalently joined segments designated L (long segment) and S (short segment) and is subdivided into four distinct domains based on sequence redundancy. These include a long unique region, U_L, ~ 105 kilobase pairs (kbp) in length and a short unique region, U_S, ~ 5.2 kbp in length, both of which are composed primarily, although not exclusively, of single-copy sequences. The U_L region is bounded by a short, 88.5 bp element (R_L) which is present in inverted orientation at the external (TR_L) and internal (IR_L) termini of the L segment. The S segment is also bounded by a set of inverted repeats termed TR_S and IR_S. These repeat elements, however, are much larger, being ~ 7.3 kbp in size. Both repeat elements are considerably higher in G+C content than the U_L and U_S segments with average values of 59% and 68% for R_S and R_L, respectively, as compared to $\sim 43\%$ for the single copy sequences.

The VZV genome exists as two predominant isomeric forms which result from inversion of the S segment. These two isomers, which have been designated P (prototype) and I_S (inverted S), are present in equimolar amounts and represent 90–95% of packaged VZV DNA. The remaining two isomeric possibilities, involving inversion of the L segment (I_L) and of both L and S (I_{LS}) with respect to the prototype, are also present but represent only 5–10% of the viral DNA. The four isomeric forms of VZV DNA are believed to result from general recombination during viral DNA synthesis. Why only two isomers predominate, as opposed to the four equally present in HSV is not clear, and this finding could indicate a preferential recognition of specific L-S joints by the VZV cleavage apparatus. Finally, a small and variable percentage of molecules (0.1–5.0%) can be isolated from virions as full-sized circular genomes. The origin of these molecules, the modes of their packaging and circularization, and the role they may play in the infectious cycle of the virus are unknown.

Properties of Viral Proteins

The VZV genome has been shown to contain at least 69 genes, three of which are diploid, encoding proteins that range in size from 8079 to 306 325 Da. Currently, approximately one-third of these proteins and/or their associated activities have been identified in VZV-infected cells. The functions of roughly another one-third have been inferred based on comparison of their genome location and predicted primary amino acid sequences with those of known HSV functions. Five of the open reading frames (ORFs) appear to be unique to VZV and one of these encodes a thymidylate synthetase activity. Not unexpectedly, several VZV proteins are not absolutely required for growth in cell culture; these include the products of ORFs 1, 8, 9A, 10, 13, 19, 36, 47 and 66. The VZV genes and their characteristics are given in **Table 1**.

Among the most extensively studied VZV protein species are the viral glycoproteins designated gB, gC, gE, gH, gI and gL (originally named gpII, gpV, gpI, gpIII, gpIV and gpVI). These glycoproteins are homologous to the HSV proteins of the same names, are incorporated into the lipid coat of the virion during maturation, and may appear on several cellular membranes in infected cells. Based on sequence homologies, there are likely to be several additional glycoprotein/membrane proteins that remain to be described. All of the known VZV glycoproteins appear to be heavily modified post-translationally.

Glycoprotein E (the most abundant VZV glycoprotein) and gI are believed to form an IgG Fc receptor and thus may have roles similar to that of their HSV counterparts. Glycoprotein B is assumed to be involved in viral attachment and fusion, whereas gH and gL form complexes that are transported to the cell surface, playing roles in cell fusion and cell-to-cell spread of VZV. Glycoprotein C varies considerably in size from strain to strain, has homology to the MHCII complex and may have a role in the pathogenesis of VZV in human tissue.

Homologues of all of the seven genes required for origin-dependent DNA synthesis in the HSV-1 system are present in the VZV genome. Of these seven predicted VZV gene products, only three have been characterized to any significant extent. These are the viral DNA polymerase, the major single-strand-binding protein and the origin-binding protein, that specifically recognizes DNA sequences at the VZV replication origin. The VZV DNA polymerase has been partially purified and is, like other herpesvirus enzymes, activated by monovalent cations with a peak activity at approximately 80 mM KCl. Finally, the VZV DNA polymerase is sensitive to phosphonoacetate and acyclovir, although to a lesser extent than the HSV-1 DNA polymerase. The VZV gene 29 single-stranded (ss) DNA binding protein is a major species in VZV-infected cells, contains a potential divalent metal binding site (zinc finger) and is present primarily in the nuclei of infected cells. The pattern observed is similar to the punctate and localized patchy staining seen with the HSV-1 major DNA-binding protein, suggesting a role in organization of proteins involved in DNA replication complexes, analogous to that of HSV ICP8. The remaining putative VZV origin-dependent replication genes (6, 16, 52 and 55) have not been examined in any detail.

VZV encodes proteins in ORFs 4, 61, 62 and 63 that are homologues of four of the five HSV immediate early genes. It is not yet clear that these are all 'immediate early' products in VZV, but three of them seem to be (IE4, IE62 and IE63); all are known to be involved in transactivation and transrepression of VZV transcription. VZV IE4 is homologous in genome location and, to a limited extent, in predicted amino acid sequence with the HSV U_L54 gene which encodes ICP27 (IE63). Based on transient expression assays, it is a potent transactivator of both homologous and heterologous promoters and can act synergistically with IE62 to enhance transcription. No evidence of a trans repressor activity has been identified, distinguishing IE4 from its HSV analogue, which acts both as a trans activator and a trans repressor. The ORF 61 product is phosphorylated and contains a RING finger domain, involved in metal binding and important for its functions. A similar region is found in the HSV-1 homologue (ICP0; IE110), a promiscuous trans activator of transcription. Used singly, the ORF 61 product can trans activate several VZV promoters and can further trans activate or repress the activating ability of both VZV IE4 and IE62; its activity appears to be cell type-specific. VZV IE62 is a phosphoprotein that both occurs in the virion tegument and will substantially enhance viral DNA infectivity. It is homologous to the HSV ICP4 (IE175) and is likely to be the major gene regulatory factor for VZV. It strongly trans activates VZV promoters of all kinetic classes through an N-terminal activation domain, reminiscent of a similar domain in HSV VP16. Thus, VZV IE62 may play some roles in VZV assigned to two proteins in HSV. IE62 is a sequence-specific DNA-binding protein, capable of regulating the activity of its own promoter. This promoter contains octamer-binding sites, as well as sites for CE/B and ATF binding. VZV IE63 is homologous to HSV ICP22 (IE68), and some evidence exists that it may, either singly, or in combination with IE62, play a role in VZV gene expression regulation. Also in the context of gene regulation, the ORF 10 tegument product (homologous to HSV VP16) is able to trans activate VZV promoters, but is much weaker than VP16 (or IE62).

Other VZV proteins that have been characterized include two protein kinases (from ORFs 47 and 66).

Table 1 Functions of VZV open reading frames

Gene	HSV	Mol. wt	Properties	Function
1		12103	phobic/C	Membrane[a]
2		25983		
3	UL55	19149		
4	UL54	51540	philic/N	(IE) Transcriptional regulator
5	UL53	38575	phobic	Glycoprotein K[a]
6	UL52	122541		DNA helicase/primase complex[a]
7	UL51	28245		
8	UL50	44816		dUTPase
9	UL49	32845	philic	Trafficking protein (cf. HSV VP22)
9A	UL49.5	9800		Membrane
10	UL48	46573		Tegument; transactivator
11	UL47	91825	philic/acidN	Tegument[a]
12	UL46	74269		
13		34531		Thymidylate synthetase
14	UL44	61350		Glycoprotein C
15	UL43	44522	phobic	Membrane?
16	UL42	46087		DNA polymerase accessory[a]
17	UL41	51365		Virion shut-off[a]
18	UL40	35395	acid	Ribonucleotide reductase (small)
19	UL39	86823		Ribonucleotide reductase (large)
20	UL38	53969		Capsid[a]
21	UL37	115774		Late/transcription regulation?[a]
22	UL36	306325		Tegument[a]
23	UL35	24416	phil/STQrich	Capsid[a]
24	UL34	30451	phobic/C	Phosphoprotein[a]
25	UL33	17460	philic/acidN	Virion[a]
26	UL32	65692		Virion?[a]
27	UL31	38234	philic/baseN	
28	UL30	134041		DNA polymerase
29	UL29	132133		Major ssDNA-binding protein
30	UL28	86968		Virion?[a]
31	UL27	98026		Glycoprotein B
32		15980	philic/acid	
33	UL26	66043		Protease/Capsid[a]
33.5	UL26.5	~34000		Assembly protein[a]
34	UL25	65182		Virion[a]
35	UL24	28973	basic	
36	UL23	37815		Pyrimidine deoxynucleoside kinase
37	UL22	93646		Glycoprotein H
38	UL21	60395		
39	UL20	27078	phobic	Membrane?[a]
40	UL19	154971		Major capsid
41	UL18	34387		Capsid[a]
42	UL15	82752		
45	ex1/2	(spliced)		
43	UL17	73905		
44	UL16	40243		
46	UL14	22544		
47	UL13	54347		Protein kinase
48	UL12	61268		Deoxyribonuclease
49	UL11	8907	philic	Virion[a]
50	UL10	48669	phobic	Glycoprotein M[a]

Table 1 Continued

Gene	HSV	Mol. wt	Properties	Function
51	UL9	94370		*ori*-binding protein
52	UL8	86343		DNA helicase/primase complex[a]
53	UL7	37417		
54	UL6	86776		Virion[a]
55	UL5	98844		DNA helicase/primase complex[a]
56	UL4	27166	S, T rich	
57		8079	philic/basic	
58	UL3	25093	philic/basic	
59	UL2	34375		Uracil-DNA glycosylase[a]
60	UL1	17616	acidic	Glycoprotein L
61	IE110	50913	philic	Transcriptional regulator
62	IE175	139989		(IE) Transcriptional regulator
63	US1	30494	philic/acid	(IE) Transcriptional regulator
64	US10	19868		Virion[a]
65	US9	11436	phobic	Tegument[a]
66	US3	43677		Protein kinase[a]
67	US7	39362		Glycoprotein I
68	US8	69953		Glycoprotein E

[a]Inferred from data with HSV.

The ORF 47 enzyme is found in the virion tegument, and can phosphorylate IE62, but not other VZV IE proteins. In addition, several enzymes of DNA metabolism are coded by VZV genes, including ribonucleotide reductase and thymidylate synthetase.

Physical Properties and Sensitivity to Environment

Due to the highly cell-associated nature of VZV and the relatively low yields of virus obtained from infected cells, very little work has been done on the physical properties and chemical composition of the virion. It is assumed that, based on its overall structural similiarity to other herpes virions, that the relative proportions of protein, nucleic acid and lipid are typical, as are the bouyant density and overall virion mass.

The VZV virion is highly sensitive to physical and chemical agents. The infectious particle is very labile, and cell-free virus preparations have very high particle:infectivity ratios. Virus from vesicle fluid appears to be more stable. VZV is temperature-sensitive and is inactivated rapidly and completely at 60°C and somewhat more slowly at lower temperatures. VZV is also sensitive to freezing, a property which contributes to difficulties in preparation and storage of high titer stocks. Quick freezing of the virus or infected cells and subsequent storage at −70°C, however, can result in less than 10% loss in titer. In contrast, the titer is rapidly lost on storage at −10°C.

Recent reports indicate that lyophilization of both infected cells and cell-free virus in the presence of sugar followed by storage at temperatures as high as −20°C results in complete titer preservation.

VZV is sensitive to pH, with loss of infectivity occurring below pH 6.2 and above pH 7.8. It is also sensitive to UV irradiation, to an extent similar to HSV-1 and HSV-2. VZV is susceptible to mechanical disruption, with 80–99% of infectivity lost after 2 min of sonication. This property may be responsible for some of the loss of infectivity seen on purification of the virus by ultracentrifugation, when a large number of damaged cell-free virions are observed in the electron microscope. HSV virions treated in the same manner are largely intact. A likely explanation for at least part of this VZV property is that virus particles may mature through lysosomal vesicles, allowing digestion of virion components by glycosidases and peptidases.

Replication of Nucleic Acid

The replication of VZV DNA has not been subject to extensive analysis, primarily due to the difficulty in obtaining sufficient numbers of synchronously infected cells. Consideration of the relative proportions of isomeric forms of the viral DNA and the frequency of novel junctions has led to the following model. On entry into the infected cell, the viral genome circularizes and undergoes a limited number of rounds of bidirectional replication. This initiates at the viral origin (ori) sequences (in the RS regions) consisting of an AT-rich palindrome and a CGTTCGCACTT sequence. During this phase, segment inversion may take place by intramolecular recombination between the inverted repeats. Replication, generating head-to-tail concatemers via a rolling circle mechanism, then accounts for the bulk of viral DNA synthesis. Finally, the newly synthesized DNA is cleaved into unit length molecules and packaged into preassembled capsids in the nucleus. The non-random proportions of isomeric DNA forms are postulated to result from a differential recognition of the normal and novel L-S joints by the viral cleavage system.

The full complement of viral and cellular proteins required for the complete replication of VZV DNA has not been identified. However, as indicated above and in **Table 1**, analogues of the seven genes required for origin-dependent replication of HSV have been identified in the VZV system and three of these have been partially characterized.

Characterization of Transcription

The enzyme responsible for transcription of VZV mRNAs is, presumably, the RNA polymerase II encoded by the host cell. As with other herpesviruses, no viral encoded RNA polymerase activity has been identified. Although 78 relatively abundant transcripts (reading from both strands) have actually been mapped to the VZV genome, as well as 33 less abundant and 29 large transcripts (6–11 kb), these numbers are underestimates of the true transcriptional capability of the genome.

Based on the extensive colinearity of the VZV and HSV genomes and the relatively high degree of functional homology predicted between VZV and HSV gene products, it is reasonable to assume that VZV transcription is regulated in the coordinated cascade scheme seen with other alphaherpesviruses. Direct experimental evidence for this scheme has been difficult to obtain due to the low titers of VZV obtained in cell culture. However, time course studies of protein synthesis have been carried out, which indicate that under conditions of near-synchronous infection, three major classes of VZV-specific proteins are apparent. They have been named immediate early (IE), early (E) and late (L) by analogy with HSV, and each temporal class contains proteins which are representative of such classes in other herpesvirus systems. For example, IE62 is synthesized in the IE phase, the gene 29 major DNA-binding protein is synthesized during the E phase, and the major capsid protein is synthesized at peak levels during the L phase of protein synthesis. Despite these similarities, though, VZV transcription is often different from that of HSV-1. For example, the VZV ORF 10 protein, corresponding to the HSV VP16 (virion trans activator) lacks the acidic carboxy-terminal region which is responsible for the trans inducing activity of that protein. VZV has apparently evolved a separate strategy for the efficient initial transcription of its immediate early genes, probably involving IE62.

Other general features of VZV transcription are apparent from studies of transcription from specific genes. As of this writing, detailed transcript mapping has been carried out on relatively few VZV genes. One finding from these studies is that VZV may use atypical *cis*-acting transcriptional control elements. For example, several consensus TATA box elements may be present upstream of transcriptional start sites but are not used, whereas nonconventional AT-rich regions function to initiate transcription. Similarly, transactivation of VZV promoters often occurs using unusual upstream sequences. Analysis of the 3′ ends of VZV genes also reveals differences in the utilization of *cis*-acting polyadenylation sites. Canonical polyadenylation signals for transcripts are often ignored and atypical sequences are utilized preferentially, although GU-rich elements (as in HSV) are usually present. Generally, multiple transcripts are often derived from one gene sequence, but there is no documented evidence for splicing. Indeed, in some VZV genes with spliced mRNAs in their HSV counterparts, there is no spliced VZV mRNA; it is predicted from the genome sequence that ORFs 42/45 will be spliced, however.

Characterization of Translation

Little is known about the details of translation in VZV-infected cells. It is assumed that mRNAs are translated in a fashion similar to that seen in HSV-infected cells and that translation occurs both on free and membrane-bound polyribosomes. Following translation, the majority of viral proteins are efficiently transported to the nucleus where they carry out their roles in viral replication.

Post-translational Processing

Thus far, the most extensively studied post-translationally processed VZV proteins are the glycoproteins. All are N-linked glycosylated and the majority show additional modifications including O-linked glycosylation, sulfation and phosphorylation. For example, VZV gE contains both O-linked and N-linked glycans, and is heavily sulfated and phosphorylated, with phosphorylation occurring at the level of both the polypeptide chain and glycosyl residues. The phosphorylated amino acids are serine

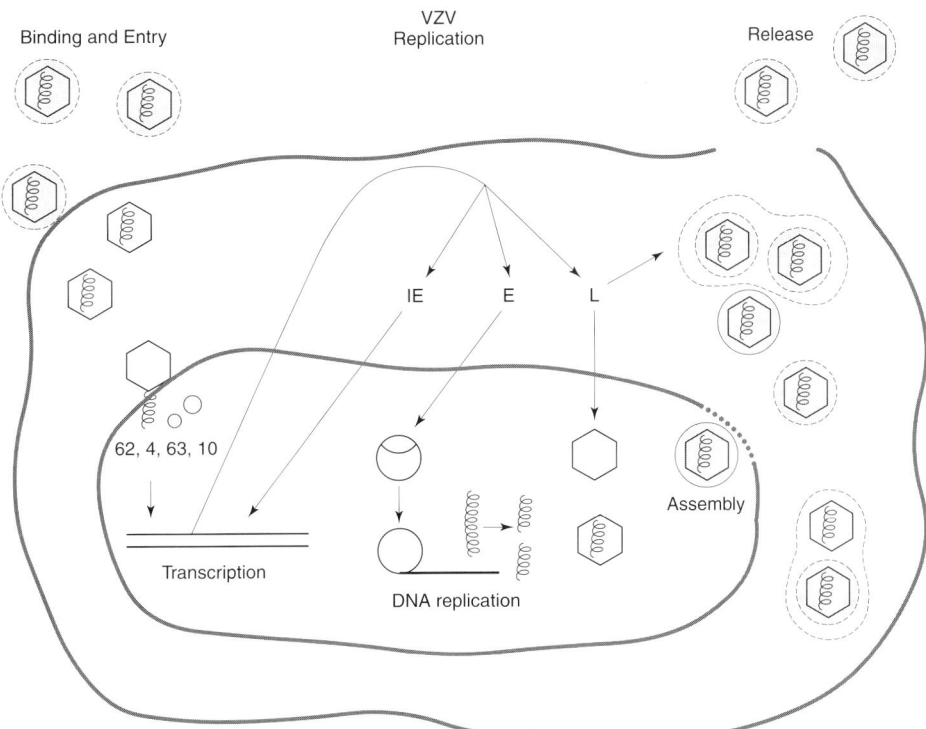

Figure 1 Schematic diagram of the proposed infectious cycle of VZV during lytic infection. Infection is initiated by binding of the virus to the plasma membrane of susceptible cells followed by fusion of the viral envelope and entry of the virus. Following uncoating, the viral DNA, along with tegument components, enters the nucleus where three temporal classes of proteins (IE, E and L) are produced. Transcription of IE mRNA may be enhanced by the IE62 protein which is carried into the cell as a major tegument component. DNA synthesis takes place during the E phase possibly utilizing both bidirectional and rolling circle mechanisms. During the L phase, progeny DNA are packaged into preformed capsids, in the nucleus. These may be enveloped by budding through the nuclear membrane. Enveloped particles acquire a second envelope by budding into cytoplasmic vesicles, which may fuse with lysosomal vesicle. Nucleocapsids may also cross the nuclear membrane and become enveloped in large cytoplasmic vesicles. The membranes surrounding all of these vesicles may ultimately fuse with the plasma membrane, resulting in release of the virus. In cell culture, much of this released virus may have damaged envelope structures.

and threonine but not tyrosine, and the enzymes involved are probably cellular casein kinases I and II. The enzyme responsible for the phosphorylation of the complex oligosaccharides has not been identified, nor has a specific role for the phosphorylated or sulfated residues.

Other viral proteins are modified, particularly by phosphorylation, including IE62 and the ORF 61 protein. IE62 has a predicted molecular weight of 140 kDa, but migrates at approximately 175 kDa on SDS–PAGE, showing evidence of differently phosphorylated forms. The functional significance of the phosphorylation of VZV proteins is unknown.

Assembly Site Uptake, Release, Cytopathology

Models for assembly and release of VZV virions are derived both from extensive, well-established electron microscopic studies and from analyses of VZV glycoprotein biosynthesis and trafficking in infected cells, but no consensus exists (**Fig. 1**). Fully assembled capsids containing unit length genomes comprising all four possible isomeric forms appear to be released from the nucleus, either naked, or having acquired a lipid envelope from the nuclear lamella. In the former case, nucleocapsids acquire their envelope by budding into large cytoplasmic vesicles into which viral glycoproteins have been inserted (via the Golgi), and are released from the cell through reverse endocytosis. In the latter case, vesicles with enveloped particles fuse with lysosomes, in which degradation of virions may take place. The involvement of lysosomes in this case is proposed to rest on their mannose-6-phosphate receptors binding this sugar on the surface of VZV particles. This apparently will not occur in the human host, since the cells in the superficial layers of the skin lack lysosomal vesicles. Perhaps this is also why vesicle fluid virus tends to have a higher and more stable titer.

In tissue culture, cells infected with VZV initially show increased refractility followed by rounding and swelling. Multinucleated cells are common, although the extent of syncytium formation is less than that seen with HSV strains of syncytial plaque morphology. Eventually, the infected cells detach from the support surface, producing readily discernible plaques. The nuclei of infected cells are larger than those of uninfected cells with marginally located chromatin and peripherally located nucleoli. Eosinophilic proteinaceous intranuclear inclusion bodies are present which occupy the sites of viral DNA replication. The nature and function of these inclusion bodies are unknown. Chromosomal aberrations and chromosome and chromatid breakage have also been observed.

Subjects for Further Investigation

A variety of interesting and fundamental questions remain to be answered concerning this important human herpesvirus. One of these is the cellular location and nature of latent VZV infection. Several early reports indicated that the sites of latency were neuronal cells within the dorsal root ganglia but later studies pointed to satellite cells surrounding the neuron. This has led to a model for reactivation of latency in which virus reactivating in satellite cells or neurons lytically infects the neuron resulting in cell destruction. This model is consistent both with the normally singular recrudescence of the virus, and with neuronal damage and postzoster neuralgia associated with reactivation of VZV. Another important feature of VZV latency is the state of expression from the viral genome. Unlike HSV, which appears to produce only a single transcript in the latent state known as the latency associated transcript (LAT), several messages are expressed in cells latently infected with VZV, corresponding to IE4, IE62, IE63, ORF 21 and ORF 29. Assuming translation of these mRNAs in latently infected cells, four of these 'latency proteins' have gene regulatory capacity, and may serve to control the latent state.

A second question involves the factors delineating VZV pathogenesis. Currently there are two obvious areas for investigation. The first involves the identification and understanding of both the *cis*- and *trans*-acting factors involved in the regulation of expression of VZV genes. Why, for example, has the virus evolved to use noncanonical transcription start and stop sites? Which specific viral polypeptides are involved in recognition of such sequences and how many cellular factors are involved? The roles of the known transcriptional regulatory proteins (IE4, IE62, IE63, ORF 61 and ORF 10) will have to be evaluated *in vivo*, in order to define their true roles during productive infection in the human host. Such an approach could also lead to the identification of host cell factors which influence the control of VZV expression. A second set of proteins for which we have only vague functional ideas are the glycoproteins. Some obvious questions are: why does VZV have fewer glycoproteins than HSV and how does this affect its pathogenesis? And do the VZV glycoproteins modulate tissue tropism of VZV?

These questions are all germane to the fact that an effective live attenuated vaccine strain (Oka) has been developed and is in widespread use in children in the industrialized world. However, the specific molecular nature of its attenuation is unknown. In recent studies in a SCID-hu model for VZV infection, it has been demonstrated that the Oka vaccine virus grows well in T-lymphocytes but not in skin cells, consistent with its antigenicity, as well as its relative inability to cause the typical varicella rash. In analogous experiments, VZV lacking gC has been shown to replicate poorly in skin cells, suggesting that this glycoprotein is a virulence factor for the virus. Now that we have a good animal model, as well as a reliable method for construction of viral mutants, we can anticipate substantial new data on VZV replication, both *in vivo* and *in vitro*.

See also: **Herpes simplex viruses (*Herpesviridae*): General features, Molecular biology; Latency; Persistent viral infection.**

Further Reading

Arvin AM (1996) Varicella zoster virus. In: Fields BN, Knipe DM, Howley PM *et al* (eds) *Fields' Virology*. Philadelphia: Lippincott-Raven.

Arvin AM and Gershon AA (1996) Live attenuated varicella vaccine. *Annu. Rev. Microbiol.* 50: 59.

Cohen JI (1996) Varicella zoster virus. The virus. *Inf. Dis. Clin. North Am.* 10: 457.

Cohen JI and Straus SE (1996) Varicella zoster virus and its replication. In: Fields BN, Knipe DM, Howley PM *et al* (eds) *Fields Virology*. Philadelphia: Lippincott-Raven.

Hay J and Ruyechan WT (1994) Varicella zoster virus – a different kind of herpesvirus latency? *Semin. Virol.* 5: 241.

Variola Virus   *see* Smallpox and Monkeypox Viruses

VECTORS

Contents
Animal Viruses
Plant Viruses

Animal Viruses

Geoffrey Kitchingman and **J Victor Garcia**, Department of Virology and Molecular Biology, St. Jude Children's Research Hospital, Memphis, Tennessee, USA

Copyright © 1999 Academic Press

Introduction

Researchers have exploited knowledge of the structure of viral genomes to insert DNA from foreign sources (transgenes) for over 20 years. Vectors, as such recombinant molecules are known, were initially generated from the genomes of the smaller DNA viruses (papovavirus and papillomavirus families). Knowledge of the genome structure of the larger DNA viruses (adenovirus, herpesvirus, poxvirus and baculovirus) and RNA viruses has expanded the numbers and types of backbones available for generating vectors. Each virus family, and vector backbone, has its own set of advantages and disadvantages that identify the types of operations for which they can optimally be used. Scientists have used these vector systems: (1) to study gene regulation; (2) in mRNA processing; (3) to achieve high-level expression of biologically active proteins; (4) to address questions of the structure–function relationship of specific polypeptides; (5) to investigate the immunobiology of specific pathogens; (6) to develop recombinant vaccine candidates and serodiagnostic reagents; and (7) to understand and treat cancer and genetic diseases in the clinic.

The salient features of many, but not all, RNA and DNA virus-based vectors will be discussed here. Not included are some of the vectors used infrequently, including the original vectors derived from papova- and papillomaviruses.

Adeno-associated Virus Vectors

Adeno-associated viruses (AAV) belong to the family *Parvoviridae*, genus *Dependovirus*. As indicated in their name, these viruses are replication defective and depend on other viruses for factors required for replication. In the laboratory, the factors are generally supplied by adenovirus or herpesvirus co-infection.

The AAV vector genome consists of a single-stranded DNA of 4.7 kb, with 150 bp palindromic sequences or inverted terminal repeat sequences (ITRs) at both ends. These two ITRs are all that is needed for packaging and integration into the host genome. AAV vectors can be constructed with up to 5 kb of exogenous DNA between the two ITRs. The transgene inserted between the ITRs must have its own promoter, as these sequences do not function as promoters. During infection, a low percentage of the viral genomes will integrate into the host chromosome. Wild-type AAV has a propensity to integrate at a specific site in human chromosome 19, but the currently available AAV vectors have lost this property and integrate randomly into the genome of the target cell.

A number of systems have been developed for using the AAV DNA backbone as a vector for gene transfer, with varying degrees of success. Despite the relatively simple genomic structure of AAV, vector systems require three components: one that supplies the AAV capsid proteins, the transgene containing vector and the helper virus. The need for helper virus results in contamination of vector preparations with helper virus particles or with denatured viral proteins, even after extensive purification and heat inactivation of vector stocks. This contamination is undesirable for the implementation of AAV vectors in clinical applications. Identification of the adenovirus genes required for complementation of AAV has allowed the development of new schemes that use a non-replicating adenovirus genomic plasmid as a helper. When co-transfected with the AAV vector and the AAV helper construct, vector preparations free of replication-competent adenovirus and wild-type AAV can be produced at relatively high titers. However, this system is based on transient transfection of cell lines, which would make large-scale clinical implementation of protocols using AAV vectors difficult. Efforts to develop stable cell lines for the production of AAV vectors are still at an early stage, but their availability is likely to facilitate evaluation of this potentially useful vector system.

AAV vectors are being developed almost exclusively as vehicles for gene transfer and gene therapy in a clinical setting. Several features of AAV make it attractive for these uses. The virus is nonpathogenic

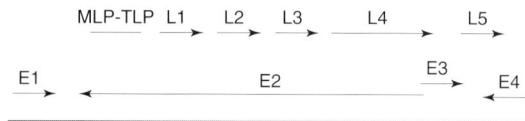

Figure 1 Adenovirus transcription map. Early (E) and late (L) transcription units are represented by solid lines relative to the 36 kb adenovirus genome. Arrowheads indicate direction of transcription. Each transcription unit gives rise to families of mRNAs derived by differential splicing events. The late mRNAs are generated by differential splicing and polyadenylation site utilization and all are initiated from the major late promoter (MLP) and contain the tripartite leader (TPL).

and has a broad host range and tissue tropism. A major advantage is its ability to infect nondividing cells, and its potential for targeted integration. In preclinical model systems the levels and duration of transgene expression have varied, so it is not entirely certain that therapeutic levels of expression can be achieved. Transduced cells do not elicit a cytotoxic T cell response, a common occurrence when using adenovirus vectors. Phase I clinical trials are underway to evaluate toxicity in humans.

Adenovirus Vectors

The human adenovirus (Ad) family consists of at least 49 members that have been classified into six subgroups based on a variety of biological and molecular characteristics. Two members of the subgroup C adenoviruses, Ad2 and Ad5, form the backbone for the majority of Ad vectors in use today. The viral genome is divided into five early and five late gene regions, with each region coding for a multiplicity of mRNAs and proteins (**Fig. 1**). All coding regions are by and large essential, with the exception of the early region 3 (E3), which is not necessary for growth in tissue culture. The viral genome is approximately 36 kb in length, and studies have shown that up to 105% of the viral genome can be packaged. High titer virus vector preparations are relatively easy to prepare and consequently they have found many uses, including the expression of large amounts of transgenes, in vaccine development, and especially in the area of gene therapy. Some of the types of adenovirus vectors used to date are discussed below.

There are two basic methods for inserting foreign genes (transgenes) into adenovirus vectors, methods that are also used for the larger DNA viruses. The first is through homologous recombination, which can be carried out in tissue culture cells, bacteria or yeast. The gene of interest is inserted into a shuttle vector containing about 2–4 kb of the viral genome, and it is co-transfected with DNA representing (at minimum) the remainder of the viral genome into the cells of choice. Recombinants can be selected by analyzing individual plaques, or by including marker genes in the shuttle plasmid that allow visual selection. The second method of construction of adenovirus vectors involves cloning of the whole genome in bacterial plasmids. An advantage of this method is that most of the characterization can be performed on the plasmid, and all plaques arising from transfection into human cells should contain the transgene. The maximal length of the transgene is directly dependent on the number of viral genes deleted. Most vectors are based on E1A- and E1B-deleted backbones, and can hold transgenes of up to 4 kb. Deletion of the nonessential E3 region brings the packaging capacity to about 7 kb, and deletion of additional early region genes further increases the packaging capacity. Every essential gene deleted has to be complemented, and cell lines expressing various complements of these genes are available. The promoter used to drive transgene expression will dictate the relative level of expression, and transgenes with and without introns are expressed equally well. With the exception of hematopoietic cells, adenovirus vectors efficiently infect most cell types.

Adenovirus vectors do not integrate, so expression of transgenes is limited to the time the vector DNA is maintained episomally in the cell. The viral episome is stable in cells, so when terminally differentiated cells are infected, the viral genome will last for essentially the life of the cell. *In vivo*, adenovirus causes significant immune responses, which is also true for adenovirus vectors, so this is potentially a limiting factor for their use in animals or humans.

Adenovirus, especially the attenuated virus produced when E1A and E1B are deleted, is generally innocuous for immunocompetent adults, and vaccines for a variety of human viruses are under development using Ad vectors for transgene delivery. Virus genes inserted into Ad vectors for vaccine development include genes from hepatitis B, human immunodeficiency virus (HIV), herpes simplex virus and pseudorabies, but to date no vaccine has come into common use. Humoral responses were elicited with the hepatitis B/Ad recombinant in chimpanzees, but they only partially protected against hepatitis B challenge. Other methods of gene delivery, including other viruses and direct injection of DNA, are finding their way into clinical trials, and it is likely that few adenovirus vectors will be used for vaccine development.

Adenovirus vectors have been used in numerous clinical trials to deliver therapeutic and/or toxic compound to cells. Use of Ad vectors for delivery of therapeutic proteins has generally not been successful. The extent to which adults are already armed against adenovirus infections was underestimated in these trials. There are a number of physical and immunological barriers to adenovirus infection that diminish the duration and extent of transgene expression. These include: (1) physical barriers to infection; (2) virus removal from the blood through unknown mechanisms; and (3) the presence of a memory immune response to the virus. The initial failures with the subgroup C backbone-based Ad vectors has led to the development of a variety of vectors based on backbones from other subgroups to which the majority of the population has not been exposed. Vectors lacking all viral genes have also been developed, but have not yet been put to use in the clinic.

Adenovirus vectors that are potentially selectively toxic to tumor cells are now in clinical trials. Adenovirus mutants that replicate only in cells lacking p53 are being tested in clinical trials for their ability to specifically kill tumor cells (in combination with chemotherapy). Vectors carrying tumor suppressor genes such as p53 and Rb are being tested in numerous clinical trials for their efficacy in halting tumor growth. Vectors that carry transgenes for enzymes that convert prodrugs to their active forms are being developed. The transgene is expressed under the control of a promoter that is either tumor or tissue specific. Ad vectors with altered tropisms are being developed to target tumors or specific tissues. One problem with many of these approaches is that the virus is large and does not readily diffuse from the site of injection, and therefore killing can be quite localized. Thus, adenovirus vector-mediated therapy of cancer is likely to be an additional tool for the oncologist, to be worked into a regimen of more traditional chemotherapy and radiotherapy.

Adenovirus vectors are being developed for use in nonmalignant disease therapy. A vector containing the gene encoding vascular endothelial growth factor is being used to try to help ischemic hearts grow new blood vessels. Other vectors are being used to try to prevent the closure of blood vessels newly opened in angioplasty.

Adenovirus vectors are finding their way into many niches in medicine, but it is safe to say that researchers are still learning how to use the virus most effectively.

Poxvirus-based Vector Systems

Poxviruses are widespread in nature and tend to have a limited host range. They are large DNA viruses, with genomes of about 190 kb in length. They differ from other DNA viruses in that they replicate solely in the cytoplasm of cells. This requires the virus to encode nearly all of the enzymes involved in replication of the virus, many of which are found in the virus particle and enter a cell with the virus. Poxvirus particles can package DNA at least 25 kb larger than the wild-type genome, and deletion of nonessential genes can significantly increase the size of foreign DNA that can be inserted into the vector. Poxvirus vectors grow well in cells of the native host, and the virus can readily be purified to high titers. Vectors based on human, animal and avian poxviruses have been developed, each with a particular set of advantages for a given application.

Poxvirus DNA is not infectious because of the requirement for virus particle-associated enzymes, and the generation of recombinants requires the use of infectious virus. The favored technique is based on marker rescue, originally developed to map mutants in the viral genome. The technique is similar to the homologous recombination method used with adenovirus vectors, but cells are first infected with a virus whose genome is to be altered and then transfected with a plasmid containing the transgene between viral sequences normally contiguous in the genome. The relative level of homologous recombination is low, about 0.1%, so efficient selection methods have been developed. These include inactivating the viral thymidine kinase gene by insertion of the foreign gene within it, and the insertion of genes encoding visual marker proteins in the rescuing plasmid. Because poxvirus vectors replicate in the cytoplasm and use poxvirus-encoded enzymes, transgenes must be placed under the control of poxvirus promoters for expression (some exceptions are discussed below). There are three classes of poxvirus promoters, early, intermediate and late, and the timing and level of expression of any transgene can be regulated by the choice of promoter. Proteins produced in poxvirus expression systems are processed and transported normally, so relatively high levels of production of normal protein are possible in permissive and nonpermissive cell lines.

Vaccinia virus is the favored vector for a variety of applications. Many different variations on the straight transgene-containing vector have been developed. Systems are available for expression of proteins from recombinant plasmids introduced into vaccinia virus-infected cells. This type of transient expression system affords much higher levels of transgene expression than conventional transfection systems. Inducible expression systems based upon the bacteriophage T7 and T3 RNA polymerase promoter and the *Escherichia coli* lac operator–repressor systems have been developed. The RNA polymerase can either be constitutively expressed in the cell line, or be brought in by a co-infecting virus. The gene to be expressed, under the control of the T3 or T7 promoter elements, is introduced into the cells either as an expression plasmid or as part of a vaccinia virus vector. These approaches allow for controlled expression, which is especially important when the protein product is cytotoxic.

Poxvirus expression systems have been used to express hundreds of proteins of biological and medical importance. The practical application of vaccinia virus vaccine candidates has been demonstrated in both the veterinary and human fields. Vaccinia was used successfully as a vaccine for the eradication of smallpox. Other examples of its use include vaccinia virus recombinants to protect raccoons against rabies, a capripoxvirus vector to protect cattle against rinderpest, a swinepox vector to protect pigs against pseudorabies, and fowlpox vectors to protect chickens against influenza virus, Newcastle disease virus and infectious bursal virus. Clinical trials with a vaccinia-based HIV-1(IIIB) *env* recombinant have been initiated in the USA. Results from these studies clearly demonstrated the ability of this recombinant to prime an immunological response in the recipients, although the response was suboptimal in some individuals. A vaccinia virus-based vector expressing the Epstein–Barr virus membrane glycoprotein has been used in China with some success in preventing natural infection.

New vectors have recently been developed that address some of the safety concerns of the original vectors. A strain of vaccinia virus with 18 genes implicated in the virulence and host range of the virus deleted has been developed. Another vector, based on a canarypoxvirus, replicates only in avian species. When this vector is introduced into nonavian cells, the transgene is expressed. Preliminary studies demonstrate that both are effective in generating high levels of transgene expression, and that in a vaccine setting they can both induce protective immunity. A canarypoxvirus-based vector expressing the rabies G glycoprotein has been assessed in phase I clinical trials in Europe and the USA, with encouraging results. In addition, vectors expressing the human cell surface protein CD80 are in clinical trials. This protein is involved in T cell recognition of target cells, so its expression in tumor cells potentially enhances the ability of the immune system to recognize cancer cells. This tumor vaccine approach is expanding, as poxvirus vectors encoding a variety of tumor antigens are currently undergoing preclinical testing. Given the large capacity of the vectors, genes encoding both tumor antigens and immune system recognition enhancing molecules could be inserted into a single virus.

Poxvirus vector-based systems have demonstrated their utility for expression of foreign genes for study in tissue culture, for use as a vaccine vehicle in both animals and humans, and they are beginning to be used for treating cancer. Because of the wide variety of available vectors, and the safety features that have been built into them, poxvirus vectors will increasingly become the vector of choice for a variety of applications.

Baculovirus Expression Vectors

Baculoviruses are pathogenic insect viruses that have been investigated for possible use as biological control agents for insect pests. Recently, these viruses have proven useful in the development of helper-independent vectors for overexpression of foreign genes in eucaryotic cells. Baculoviruses contain a double-stranded DNA genome of around 130 kb, and the DNA is infectious. The main attraction of this system is the ability to produce very large quantities of transgene protein, but until recently the system was limited to insect cells. Recent developments have considerably expanded the potential of the baculovirus vector system for use in mammalian cells.

Baculovirus vectors are generally produced by homologous recombination between a shuttle vector and a wild-type genome, using the viral polyhedrin gene as the recombination target. Shuttle vectors often contain the transgene of interest plus a selectable marker gene, although inactivation of the polyhedrin gene through transgene insertion gives rise to plaques that can be differentiated from those of wild-type virus. The polyhedrin gene of baculoviruses such as *Autographa californica* nuclear polyhedrosis virus (AcMNPV) is expressed at very late times of infection and produces a protein that surrounds the mature virus particle to form an occlusion body in insect larvae. Polyhedrin protein expression in infected tissue culture cells can continue for days following initial infection and often amounts to 50% of the total cell protein. The polyhedrin protein is not essential for replication of the virus in tissue culture, and transgenes placed under the control of its promoter can be expressed to levels approaching that of the polyhedrin itself. The virus has a rod-shaped capsid and has a large capacity for packaging foreign DNA. Baculoviruses do not productively infect vertebrate cells, but modifications to the system have allowed transgene expression in a variety of mammalian cell lines, further expanding the potential of the vector system.

Baculovirus vectors have found their greatest use in the production of large quantities of protein for purification. While insect cells can post-translationally modify proteins correctly, there were concerns that they could not process high-mannose glycans like mammalian cells. However, recent reports on human plasminogen expressed in insect cells show that the enzymes necessary for processing high-mannose glycans can be activated with glycan processing identical to that found in the human-expressed protein. These are important considerations if baculovirus-expressed products are to have the same biological and immunological properties as that of the native protein. Baculovirus-expressed protein was used in the first human clinical trials for an acquired immune deficiency syndrome (AIDS) vaccine, using an HIV-1 (IIIB) *env* gene product purified from insect cells. Its general utility for production of purified proteins for clinical use remains to be demonstrated.

Herpesvirus Vectors

Two herpesviruses are emerging as alternatives for the development of gene transfer vectors: herpes simplex virus (HSV) and Epstein–Barr virus (EBV). HSV has a genome of approximately 155 kb in length, which is maintained as a concatemerized circular or linear episome in infected cells. It efficiently infects cells, including nondividing cells, from a wide variety of organisms, and is able to establish a persistent infection. Its genome can accommodate large amounts of foreign DNA, and a number of vector systems have been developed. The EBV-based systems have not been developed as extensively and currently employ replication-defective EBV strains. Unlike HSV, EBV vectors have a very limited tropism and their possible usefulness remains to be explored. The main difficulty using these two systems is the need for almost complete virus genomes that are very complex and large in size, making manipulations exceedingly difficult. The eventual usefulness of these systems will be dictated by further simplifications that render them more manageable in the laboratory and that facilitate vector production.

Helper-dependent and -independent systems have been developed for preclinical evaluation. The helper-independent systems have basically the complete viral genome with one or more transgenes substituted for nonessential viral genes. These vectors are rendered defective for growth by deletion of essential genes, permitting their growth only on complementing cell lines. So far these vectors have met with limited success in model systems because of leakiness in the system, which leads to cytotoxicity and cell death. The requirements for maintenance of gene expression during the latent state in neuronal cell types are also currently unknown, so prolonged transgene expression has been difficult to obtain. The second type of HSV vector is the helper-dependent system. The vectors contain only the sequences required for replication and packaging, but all the other functions must be supplied in *trans* from a helper virus. While such systems are capable of producing high-titer amplicon-containing virus, they are almost invariably contaminated with large quantities of the helper virus. Recent improvements in the amplicon system have allowed the generation of relatively high-titer amplicon preparations with much lower levels of contamination with helper virus. These systems hold promise for use in clinical situations, especially in gene transfer to neuronal cells, but further development of the system is required.

Retrovirus Vectors

Retroviruses are ubiquitous in nature and have a relatively simple RNA genome of around 9 kb in length. By reverse transcription, the RNA genome becomes a double-stranded DNA that integrates into the host chromosome and is stably transmitted to progeny cells. Specific aspects of the life cycle of retroviruses and their relatively simple genome have facilitated their development into gene transfer vectors. Most of the vectors currently used for basic science and for clinical applications are based on murine leukemia viruses. Because of the high efficiency with which retroviral vectors can transduce a variety of cell types from many different species, they have become a method of choice for gene transfer experiments.

Retrovirus vectors can be produced by either transient transfection of cells, or by the generation of stable producer cell lines. In both cases, the transcription units for the packaging functions for the virus particle and that for the transgene are on separate genetic elements. The packaging proteins are provided in *trans*, either by a co-transfected second plasmid that encodes the proteins needed for particle formation, reverse transcription and integration of the vector (transient production), or by a packaging cell line that contains these genes integrated into the chromosome (**Fig. 2**). Separation of the *trans* functions into several plasmids is important to minimize the chance that a wild-type replication competent virus may be generated by a recombination event. Packaging cell lines are able to generate large numbers of virus particles without a genome. These particles are empty because the packaging construct does not contain the information needed for specific incorporation of RNA into the virus particle. This is an important aspect of the system because it prevents the transmission of genomic information encoding virus proteins. The vector plasmid contains all of the *cis*

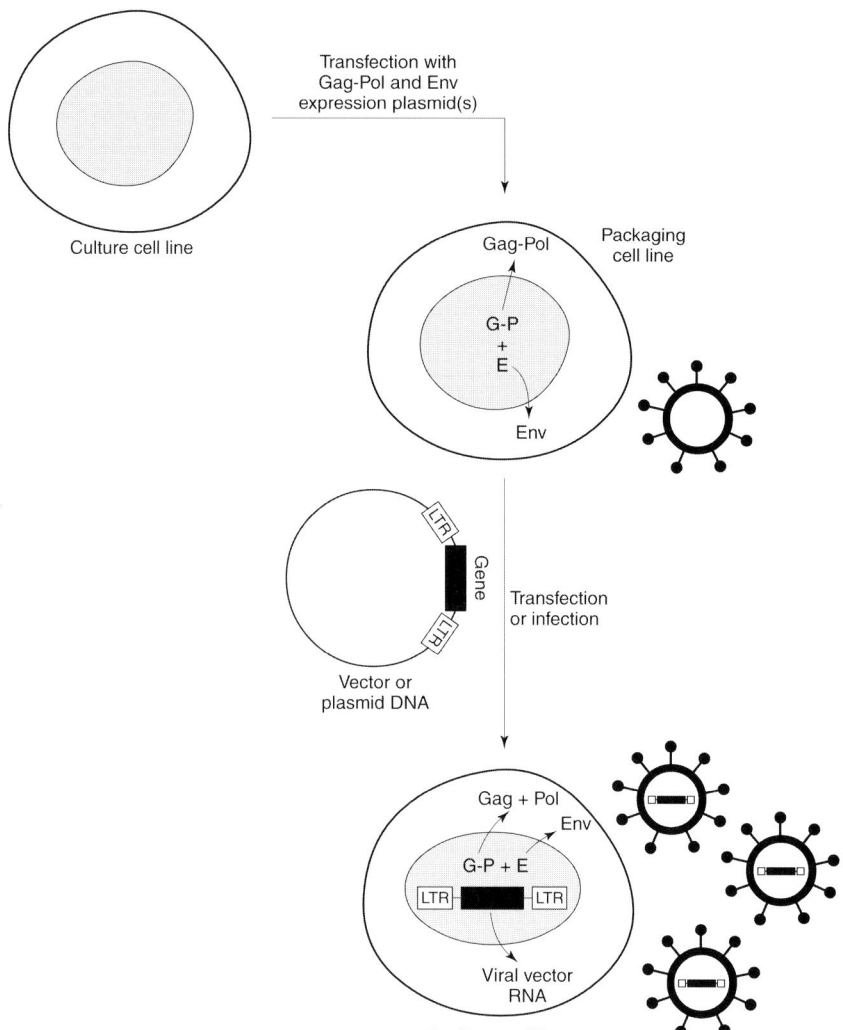

Figure 2 Construction of a retrovirus packaging cell line. Plasmids encoding the Gag-Pol polyprotein are transfected into cells. Clones expressing high levels of 'empty' virus particles in the supernatant are identified. An envelope expression construct is then transfected into the Gag-Pol-expressing clone and clones expressing high levels of both Gag-Pol and Env are identified. Finally, a retrovirus vector is introduced into the Gag-Pol-Env cell line and clones producing the highest levels of transducing particles are identified. Once cloned, these producer cell lines are stable and can be expanded to produce large amounts of vector for clinical or basic science experimentation. LTR, long terminal repeat.

elements necessary for transcription and polyadenylation of the transgene, and for reverse transcription and encapsidation (packaging) of the vector RNA. Once the vector that contains the packaging signal is introduced into the packaging cell, or cotransfected with a plasmid containing the genes for the packaging functions, particles are generated that contain the vector genome. The vector-containing particles are infectious and can introduce new genetic information into the genome of a target cell.

Producer cell lines can be made that express different envelope proteins, cell surface glycoproteins (*env*) needed for attachment and penetration into the target cell. By using *env* proteins from different retroviruses, the species specificity and tissue tropism of the vector can be altered. Recently, retrovirus vectors that use the vesicular stomatitis virus G protein in place of *env* have been produced. In addition to having a broad host range and tissue specificity, such vectors can be concentrated by centrifugation, which is not possible with *env*-containing vectors. Expression of the transgene in vectors can be under the control of the viral long terminal repeat promoter, or of an exogenous promoter such as the cytomegalovirus or SV40 early promoters. It is possible to express multiple genes under the control of a single promoter through the introduction of an element termed an internal ribosome entry site, which can be derived from an RNA virus such as encephalomyocarditis virus. Because retrovirus vectors can be made free of wild-type virus, there is no expression of virus proteins in the transduced cell. Therefore, retrovirus vector-transduced cells do not induce virus-specific immune responses.

Advantages of the retrovirus gene transfer system include stable integration of the vector into the genome of target cells, the wide tropism of the available vectors, the relative ease of vector production, and the large number of vector and producer cell lines available for both basic research and clinical applications. Some disadvantages include: (1) integration of the vector into the genome of the host is random, which can potentially lead to gene mutation; (2) a limited packaging capacity; and (3) an inability to transduce nondiving cells. This last limitation has been resolved by using lentiviruses, such as HIV, instead of murine leukemia viruses to derive the packaging components and packaging cell lines. Lentivirus-based vectors have shown significant promise in early evaluations. Undoubtedly, lentivirus-based vectors are likely to complement the existing battery of vectors and possibly expand the usefulness of this system to nondividing targets such as liver, brain and the hematopoietic stem cell.

RNA Virus Vector Systems

Researchers are investigating the potential of RNA genome-containing viral vectors, such as poliovirus, alphaviruses, influenza virus and vesicular stomatitis virus (VSV). These viruses have the potential advantage of not having a DNA phase in their replication cycle, which provides a measure of safety for their use in humans. Negative-strand viruses such as influenza and VSV do not undergo measurable rates of homologous RNA recombination, which contributes to the stability and safety of these vectors. Expression of foreign proteins has now been shown for vectors derived from influenza, rabies, VSV, respiratory syncytial virus, SV5 and Sendai virus. The foreign proteins include antigens derived from other viruses, bacteria and parasites, and in general have represented attempts to derive vaccines for agents for which no adequate vaccine currently exists. The vectors produced thus far have coded for a single antigen, and we can expect that in the near future vectors encoding multiple antigens will become available. While the larger DNA viruses such as adenovirus, herpesvirus and the poxviruses code for proteins capable of downmodulating the immune response, no such proteins have been found in RNA viruses. Some of the RNA viruses have been shown to be excellent inducers of both cellular and humoral immune responses in humans.

Poliovirus, a positive-strand RNA virus, has been used to express a number of foreign genes. Poliovirus vectors expressing epitopes derived from hepatitis A virus, rhinovirus 14, human papillomavirus 16, foot-and-mouth disease virus and HIV have been produced. A poliovirus–HIV chimera has been shown to elicit anti-HIV antibodies in rabbits. Furthermore, this antiserum neutralized a wide range of American and African HIV-1 isolates. The major disadvantage of polio, relative to the negative-strand RNA virus vector systems, is that the systems that have been developed thus far have a limited capacity for foreign sequences.

Alphavirus (Sindbis virus and Semliki Forest virus)-based vector systems have also been introduced. The value of such systems is derived from the ability to use these vectors in a wide range of mammalian cells, as a plasmid, or a recombinant progeny virus. Noncytopathic Sindbis virus replicons that replicate in BHK cells and express large amounts of foreign protein have been produced. These vector systems are bipartite, contain a selectable marker for selection, and are capable of expressing the transgene protein at high levels for prolonged periods of time. They do not contain a complete complement of viral genes and thus no infectious particles can be produced. The vectors are probably minimally immunogenic for the parent viral components, as there is little of the parental viral RNA in the vector and structural proteins are not produced. Because of all of these features, the latest generation of alphavirus vectors have a number of safety advantages over some of the DNA virus-based vector systems, and could see applications soon not only in terms of vaccine development but also in the gene therapy arena. Since they replicate in the cytoplasm, and get distributed into the dividing cells without affecting the chromosomal make-up, many safety concerns could be satisfied. Use in the latter area is likely to be limited initially to the introduction of vectors into cells that can be grown in culture for periods of time to permit selection.

For vaccines, cytolytic virus vectors that stimulate an immune response to the virus infection may be useful in stimulating a response against a heterologous protein. Derivatives of Venezuelan equine encephalitis virus that show a self-limiting replication *in vivo* have been used to generate a protective immunity against influenza virus in animals.

Future Perspectives

Viral vectors have changed the way science is done, from the expression of single proteins in cells, to the generation of new vaccines and to the implementation of new therapeutic strategies for the cure of genetic diseases and the treatment of cancer and other diseases. The variety of viral vectors continues to grow, and much is being learned about the advantages and disadvantages of each type. Practical application in the future will be based on extensive knowledge gained of the structures of viral genomes, their replication strategies and the response of immune systems to infection by such vectors. Such practical application will turn these causes of diseases into tools for curing disease.

See also: **Adenoviruses (*Adenoviridae*): Animal viruses, General features, Malignant transformation and oncology, Molecular biology; Baculoviruses (*Baculoviridae*): Granuloviruses, Nucleopolyhedrovirus; Herpes simplex viruses (*Herpesviridae*): General features, Molecular biology; Epstein-Barr virus (*Herpesviridae*): General features, Molecular biology; Human immunodeficiency viruses (*Retroviridae*): Molecular biology, Anti-retroviral agents, General features; Polioviruses (*Picornaviridae*): General features, Molecular biology; Papillomaviruses – human (*Papovaviridae*): General features, Molecular biology; Vaccinia virus (*Poxviridae*); Vesicular stomatitus viruses (*Rhabdoviridae*).**

Further Reading

Ertl HC and Xiang Z (1996) Novel vaccine approaches. *J. Immunol.* 156: 3579.

Moss B (1996) Genetically engineered poxviruses for recombinant gene expression, vaccination, and safety. *Proc. Natl Acad. Sci. USA* 93: 11341.

Garoff H and Li KJ (1998) Recent advances in gene expression using alphavirus vectors. *Curr. Opin. Biotechnol.* 9: 464.

Matsushita T, Elliger S, Elliger C et al (1998) Adeno-associated virus vectors can be efficiently produced without helper virus. *Gene Ther.* 5: 938.

Palese P (1998) RNA virus vectors: where are we and where do we need to go? (Commentary) *Proc. Natl Acad. Sci. USA* 95: 12750.

Paoletti E (1996) Applications of pox virus vectors to vaccination: an update. *Proc. Natl Acad. Sci. USA* 93: 11349.

Robbins PD and Ghivizzani SC (1998) Viral vectors for gene therapy. *Pharmacol. Ther.* 80: 35.

Rolph MS and Ramshaw IA (1997) Recombinant viruses as vaccines and immunological tools. *Curr. Opin. Immunol.* 9: 517.

Stavropoulos TA (1998) An enhanced packaging system for helper-dependent herpes simplex virus vectors. *J. Virol.* 72: 7137.

Plant Viruses

Thomas Hohn, Friedrich Miescher Institute, Basel, Switzerland

Rob Goldbach, Agricultural University, Wageningen, The Netherlands

Copyright © 1999 Academic Press

Introduction

Virus vectors have become useful tools for introducing genes into a variety of organisms. The first successful virus vectors were derivatives of the bacteriophage λ, with the help of which the first homologous and heterologous gene libraries were established in *Escherichia coli*. Likewise, a number of animal viruses were used to introduce foreign genes into animal cells where they replicated and were expressed. The two most important types are based on the double-stranded (ds)DNA papovaviruses, e.g. bovine papillomavirus, and those based on retroviruses. While papovavirus vectors replicate as circular dsDNA, retroviral vectors mediate the incorporation of the passenger gene into the host chromatin. All of the cases mentioned above lead to relative stability of the passenger gene in the transfected cell, since their replication as dsDNA involves a proofreading mechanism.

Neither true dsDNA viruses nor viruses mediating DNA integration have yet been found amongst the large variety of plant viruses. Accordingly, experiments with plant virus vectors are based on single-stranded (ss)DNA viruses, pararetroviruses and RNA viruses; replication in all these cases can lead to genome rearrangements, because single-strand intermediates are involved on which proofreading mechanisms do not apply and where template switching could occur. If the design and use of the virus vector interferes with viral replication, expression or other vital functions, the passenger gene will be removed from the vector population within a few generations. The passenger gene will in any case be finally eliminated unless it provides some selective advantage. This instability can be also looked upon as a benefit, since it provides biological containment: hybrid plant virus derivatives released purposely or accidentally into the environment are unlikely to maintain a nonselective gene. Stable transformation of plants, on the other hand, can be achieved either with the help of *Agrobacterium*-derived vectors, which mediate integration of passenger DNA into the plant chromatin, or by direct gene transfer.

Another peculiarity of plant viruses is their mechanism of spreading within the host tissue. Spreading usually makes use of the plasmodesmata (cytoplasmic connections between individual cells) which are thought to become modified to allow passage of viral nucleic acid or particles. Since plant cells in culture lack these connections, their infection with viruses or viral genomes usually depends upon artificial methods, such as electroporation or polyethylene glycol (PEG) treatment, and further spread will not occur. In contrast, animal viruses have developed methods to both leave and enter cells, e.g. by exo- and endocytosis, and are, therefore, able to spread through host cell cultures after the initial infection.

Inoculation of Plants with Virus and Vectors

Many plant viruses, irrespective of whether their genome consists of DNA or RNA, can be inoculated mechanically on to plant leaves using an abrasive. In these cases, naked nucleic acid or manipulated derivatives can also usually be used as an inoculum. A further method is agroinoculation, which was first developed with CaMV (see **Table 1** for definitions of virus abbreviations) and potato spindle tuber viroid and makes use of the DNA-transfer machinery of *Agrobacterium tumefaciens*, the cause of crown gall disease in a number of dicotyledons. Using this method, multimers, or at least 'one-and-a-bit-mers', of the virus genome are cloned between the T-DNA borders of the *Agrobacterium tumefaciens* Ti-plasmid and this manipulated T-DNA is introduced into the plant upon bacterial infection. Once in the plant cell, probably in the nucleus, the viral genome can escape either by recombination or by the direct production of monomeric replicative intermediates, such as the CaMV 35S pregenomic RNA.

Table 1 Plant virus names and their abbreviations

Virus	Abbreviation	Group
African cassava mosaic[a]	ACMV	Bipartite gemini
Cassava latent[a]	CLV	
Alfalfa mosaic	AlMV	–
Beet curly top	BCTV	Monopartite gemini
Brome mosaic	BMV	Bromo
Beet necrotic yellow vein	BNYVV	Furo
Barley stripe mosaic	BSMV	Hordei
Barley yellow dwarf	BYDV	Luteo
Beet western yellows	BWYV	Luteo
Cauliflower mosaic	CaMV	Caulimo
Cowpea chlorotic mottle	CCMV	Bromo
Cucumber mosaic	CMV	Cucumo
Cucumber necrosis	CNV	Tombus
Cowpea mosaic	CPMV	Como
Cymbidium ringspot	CyRSV	Tombus
Digitaria streak	DSV	Monopartite gemini
Maize streak	MSV	Monopartite gemini
Odontoglossum ringspot	ORSV	Tobamo
Pea early browning	PEBV	Tobra
Plum pox	PPV	Poty
Potato X	PVX	Potex
Red clover necrotic mosaic	RCNMV	Diantho
Rice tungro bacilliform	RTBV	Badna
Tomato bushy stunt	TBSV	Tombus
Turnip crinkle	TCV	Carmo
Tomato golden mosaic	TGMV	Bipartite gemini
Tobacco mosaic	TMV	Tobamo
Tobacco rattle	TRV	Tobra
Tobacco vein mottling	TVMV	Poty
Turnip yellow mosaic	TYMV	Tymo
White clover mosaic	WClMV	Potex
Wheat dwarf	WDV	Monopartite gemini

[a] The same virus.

Certain viruses and their nucleic acids are not infectious on mechanical inoculation. This group contains many viruses that are restricted to the phloem tissue, being directly introduced there by their insect vectors. Among these are many viruses that have members of the *Gramineae* as hosts, plants that are also not susceptible to crown gall disease. It was thus surprising that maize plants could be infected with MSV by agroinoculation. This success indicated that *Gramineae* are also susceptible to T-DNA transfer, and opened a route to the introduction of a number of different viruses that could not enter by other artificial means, e.g. WDV into wheat and RTBV into rice.

Pararetrovirus Vectors

Pararetroviruses, like retroviruses, use both the host nucleus and the cytoplasm for replication. In the nucleus, viral DNA is transcribed into terminally redundant RNA, in the cytoplasm the RNA is reverse transcribed into DNA, which is transported either directly or via new infections into the nucleus. Pararetrovirus DNA accumulates (but does not replicate) in the form of supercoiled circles, while retrovirus DNA is inserted in a terminally redundant form into the host chromatin. Plant pararetroviruses exist as two groups, the icosahedral caulimoviruses and the bacilliform badnaviruses. The genomes of these viruses are all around 8000 bp in length.

So far, only CaMV, a caulimovirus from this group, has been used as a vector. The seven open reading frames (ORFs) of this virus are arranged densely packed on the pregenomic 35S RNA, and it is thought that all but one of the ORFs are translated from this polycistronic messenger. Infection can be achieved in the laboratory by mechanical inoculation with virus particles or virus DNA and thus ORF 2, which codes for an aphid transmission factor, becomes dispensable. In view of this, an ORF-2-replacement vector was constructed and used to clone, express and spread systemically payloads through turnips. By this means, the ORFs for bacterial dihydrofolate reductase (DHFR; 240 bp), the Chinese hamster metallothionein (200 bp), human αD interferon (500 bp), and BNYVV ORF N (171 bp) were cloned, spread systemically and expressed in plants.

From these successful and other unsuccessful experiments, it was learned that sequences introduced into the CaMV genome are frequently lost, probably as a result of illegal template switching of the nascent minus or plus DNA strands as well as negative selection against the inserted DNA sequence. These recombination events could be minimized by avoiding homologies at the insertion site, and selection for the deletions could be minimized by avoiding whatever might interfere with the virus life cycle as follows:

1. The total size of the genome should not, or should only slightly, exceed the original viral genome length of 8000 bp. About 700 bp can be capitalized by deletion of ORF 2, as mentioned above, and ORF 7, which is also dispensable for virus growth. Allowing for overpackaging of 300 bp, a payload of about 1000 bp seems to be the upper limit. CaMV vectors to clone a larger payload might be developed from artificial bipartite CaMV genomes, which together contain all essential functions and lack recombination targets.
2. The tightly packed ORF organization should be maintained, probably because of the unusual CaMV translation mechanism. Experience has shown that noncoding sequences between CaMV and passenger ORFs diminish vector stability.
3. Inserted sequences should not interfere with CaMV gene expression and replication. For instance, the insertion of an RNA polyadenylation signal would interfere with the production of pregenomic RNA, insertion of a new promoter might occlude the original CaMV promoters and an intron would not survive the transcription/reverse transcription cycle for very long.
4. Sequences leading to gene products that interfere with virus replication either directly or by affecting the host cell must be avoided.

CaMV and its derived vectors do not proliferate efficiently in cell culture; while DNA replicative intermediates can be found in infected protoplasts, mature virus particles are absent or rare. This might be explained by developmental control of genome replication versus translation. Both processes depend on the same 35S RNA, and one can assume a control mechanism that switches between these two functions. In protoplasts and the derived cell cultures, the switch is apparently set to genome replication and particle formation is inhibited.

It is also likely that other plant pararetroviruses can be developed as gene vectors, collectively covering a large host range. This would also include the *Gramineae* if, e.g. RTBV is considered. Since this virus has a bacilliform capsid, overpackaging might be less of a problem.

Geminivirus Vectors

Geminiviruses (**Table 2**) contain 2.5–3 kb of circular ssDNA. They are characterized by twinned (geminate) icosahedral particles. Geminiviruses of dicotyledonous plants are usually, but not always, bipartite

Table 2 Geminivirus vectors

Virus	Partite	Target	Host	Payload
TGMV	Bi-	Plants	Nicotiana tabacum	CAT, GUS, NPT-II
ACMV	Bi-	Plants	Nicotiana benthamiana	CAT
MSV	Mono-	Protoplasts	Zea mays	NPT-II, GUS, DSI
WDV	Mono-	Protoplasts	Triticum monococcum	NPT-II, CAT, βGAL

and transmitted by white flies; geminiviruses of monocotyledonous plants are monopartite and transmitted by leafhoppers. Usually, component 'A' of the bipartite geminiviruses is sufficient for replication in single cells, while component B is required for systemic spread and needs component A for replication. With respect to their bidirectional expression strategy, geminiviruses resemble the animal polyomaviruses and simian virus 40 (SV40). Their intranuclear dsDNA forms contain two non-coding regions, one harboring the clockwise and counter-clockwise promoters and the other containing the two polyadenylators. Transcription in one direction (in consensus clockwise) produces RNAs coding for structural proteins, and transcription in the other direction gives RNAs required for DNA replication.

The coat proteins of geminiviruses are dispensable for genome replication but are required for insect transmission, and in the case of the monopartite viruses are also required for virus spread within the plant. Accordingly, mutants in the coat protein gene of bipartite geminiviruses can still replicate in single cells and spread through the host plant. Coat protein mutants of monopartite geminiviruses do not spread.

Geminivirus coat protein replacement vectors have been introduced into plants by either mechanical means or agroinoculation. Vectors based on component A DNA of bipartite geminiviruses can spread if component B is provided either as a transgene or as a co-inoculum. However, when transgenes of these vectors are used or transient expression in protoplasts or leaf disks is studied, component B is not required. Monopartite geminivirus vectors are so far restricted to transient expression experiments in localized patches of plant tissue disks, seed-derived embryos or cell cultures.

The following additional observations have been made.

1. In addition to the coat protein gene, the small ORF of unknown function located further upstream can also be replaced by the payload. Deletion or replacement mutants of the counter-clockwise coding regions, however, are defective in replication.

2. Systemically spreading vectors are unstable if they are either smaller or larger than wild-type virus; rearrangements occur which restore the original size. The reason for this size dependence in the absence of packaging is not known. Non-spreading vectors, on the other hand, can exceed normal genome size by up to 4 kb, for instance when they harbor the long β-glucuronidase (GUS) or neomycin phosphotransferase (NPT) II coding regions.

3. Geminivirus vectors also tolerate the insertion of additional promoters, e.g. the CaMV 35S promoter, which leads to a large increase in payload expression without affecting replication.

4. An E. coli replicon can also be incorporated into monopartite geminivirus genomes, creating shuttle vectors that replicate and express a payload gene in both bacteria and protoplasts of Gramineae.

RNA Viruses as Gene Vectors

Infectivity of cloned cDNA

To develop RNA viruses as gene vectors, it is essential that infectious RNA can be generated from cloned cDNA copies. This has been achieved for a growing number of plus-strand RNA viruses (but not minus-strand viruses) using four different approaches.

1. With a cDNA clone directly. Only limited results have been reported so far (excluding the viroids), namely for A1MV RNA3 and TMV RNA; in both cases, the cDNAs gave rise to virus at a very low level. The infectivity found here is probably due to transcription from unidentified promoters.

2. As cDNA fused to the CaMV 35S promoter. This results in more efficient production of progeny virus, as reported for BMV and BNYVV RNA 3 and RNA4.

3. By agroinoculation. This has been achieved for BWYV, a luteovirus, using a cDNA clone provided with a ribozyme sequence to enable in vivo run-off transcription.

4. As in vitro run-off transcripts, from linearized full-length cDNA clones, using phage SP6, T7, T3 or E.

coli RNA polymerase, in combination with their respective promoters. This is by far the most frequent approach, and infectious transcripts have been synthesized for more than 20 different RNA viruses belonging to 15 distinct taxonomic groups (**Table 3**). It is essential for infectivity that the transcripts are not only of full length but also (almost) identical to the natural viral RNAs. Some problems may arise here since most promoters extend into the transcribed region, resulting in transcripts that start with extra nonviral nucleotides. In general, it has been found that nonviral residues at the 3' end are better tolerated than extra nucleotides at the 5' end, which mostly lead to a significant drop in infectivity.

The best results have been obtained with *in vitro* transcription systems using SP6, T3 or T7 promoters and the corresponding specific polymerases. These systems are highly efficient (up to 20 μg of transcript from 1 μg of template) and can be designed to yield almost authentic termini. However, if the first viral nucleotide is not *a priori* a G residue, one extra G residue must be tolerated at the 5' end. It should be noted that, in most cases studied, the extra nonviral nucleotides were deleted in progeny RNAs. In cases of virus with capped genomic RNAs, the addition of a cap structure at the 5' end of the transcripts often enhances infectivity. For BSMV RNAs capping seems to be an absolute requirement. There is an additional complication with viruses belonging to the 'picornalike superfamily', e.g. the como-, nepo- and potyviruses. The genomic RNAs of these viruses possess a protein (denoted VPg) covalently linked to the 5' end. Nevertheless, both capped and uncapped *in vitro* transcripts have been shown to be infectious.

Insertion and expression of foreign genes

Cloned full-length copies from which infectivity can be recovered by following one of the approaches discussed above provide a good starting point for constructing replicons that can be used as gene vectors (**Table 3**). Of course, insertion of foreign sequences should not interfere with any viral function or process (e.g. RNA replication, subgenomic mRNA synthesis, translation, encapsidation) required for (helper-independent) infectivity.

With respect to noncoding sequences, the terminal sequences should at least be retained for replication, while for some viral RNAs (e.g. BMV RNA3) internal noncoding sequences also appear to contain obligatory *cis*-acting replication signals.

With respect to the introduction of payloads into coding sequences ('replacement' vectors), the following points can be made.

Table 3 Plant viral cDNAs reported to generate infectious *in vitro* transcripts

Group	Virus
Alfalfa mosaic	AlMV (RNA3)
Bromo	BMV, CCMV (RNA1–3)
Carmo	TCV
Como	CPMV (RNA1–2)
Cucumo	CMV (RNA1–3)
Diantho	RCNMV (RNA1–2)
Furo	BNYVV (RNA1–4)
Hordei	BSMV (RNA α, β, γ)
Luteo	BYDV, BWYV
Potex	PVX, WClMV
Poty	PPV, TVMV
Tobamo	TMV
Tobra	PEBV, TRV (RNA1–2)
Tombus	CNV, CYRSV, TBSV
Tymo	TYMV

Genes encoding proteins involved in RNA replication

All plant RNA viruses so far studied possess one or more cistrons encoding replication proteins (e.g. putative helicase, viral polymerase). It is obvious that any manipulation of these genes will lead to non-replicating transcripts unless the functions can be provided in *trans*. This is feasible, e.g. by transformation of host plants with functional copies of the affected genes (transgenic tobacco plants expressing the RNA1 and RNA2 products of AlMV are able to support RNA3 replication) or by co-inoculation with helper virus (smaller TMV RNA-derived replicons co-replicate and spread systemically with TMV helper virus). In both cases, however, the viral vector has lost its truly independent character.

The movement protein gene(s)

A considerable number of plant RNA viruses encode a so-called 'movement protein' which is actively involved in cell-to-cell spread of the viral genome (e.g. tobamoviruses) or viral particle (e.g. comoviruses) through plasmodesmata. Its coding sequence should be retained if systemic spread of the viral vector is desired. This is true for TMV for the 30 kD protein, for BMV for the RNA3-encoded 32 kD protein and for CPMV for the M-RNA-encoded 58 kD/48 kD protein pair. For expression in protoplast systems or cultured cell suspensions, the movement protein cistron can be omitted and the site exploited.

Table 4 Heterologous gene expression from plant RNA viral genomes

Group	Virus	Insertion site	Gene	Expression system
Bromo	BMV	Coat protein gene	CAT	Protoplasts
Furo	BNYVV	25 kD gene (RNA3)	GUS	Inoculated leaf
Hordei	BSMV	βb gene (RNAβ)	LUC	Protoplasts
Tobamo	TMV	Coat protein gene	CAT	Inoculated leaf
		Coat protein gene	ENK	Protoplasts
		Extra site[a]	NPT-II	Whole plant
		Extra site[a]	DHFR	Whole plant

[a] From inserted ORSV coat protein promoter.

The coat protein gene(s)

The viral coat protein gene can, in some instances, be manipulated in order to express foreign sequences, though it always leads to lower fitness in terms of systemic spread. Although for some viruses the coat protein is dispensable for cell-to-cell movement (e.g. TMV), this structural protein cannot be omitted for long-distance transport of the inoculated vector (via the vascular system) throughout the whole plant. Therefore, replacement of coat protein genes by reporter genes (e.g. CAT, **Table 4**) always leads to naked, infectious RNA which is confined to the inoculated leaf. Such replacement vectors can, however, be efficiently expressed in protoplast systems (**Table 4**). The problem of limited spread has recently been circumvented for TMV by creating a viral vector (TB2) which contained a duplicated subgenomic promoter of the coat protein gene, enabling the expression of both the coat protein and the payload gene (NPT II, DHFR). It was found that the duplicated promoter should be cloned from a different tobamovirus with enough sequence divergency (i.e. ORSV) to avoid removal by homologous recombination.

Miscellaneous genes

Further genes with potential for exploitation as vectors exist in some viruses. Their function has usually not been resolved, although some of them have been shown to be dispensable for both viral RNA replication and systemic spread. For example, in the quadripartite RNA virus BNYVV, both RNA3 (specifying a 25 kD protein) and RNA-4 (specifying a 31 kD protein) have been shown to be dispensable and are in fact lost after serial mechanical inoculation. Large internal parts of both these RNAs can be deleted without affecting replication. Insertions of the bacterial GUS gene in a deletion-containing RNA3 cDNA has been shown to give rise to detectable GUS activity in the inoculated leaf (**Table 3**) and amplification of the transcript. A further example of successful replacement, this time with BSMV, is insertion of the firefly luciferase (LUC) coding sequence into the βb gene (located on β-RNA and encoding a 58 kD protein with a helicase motif), which resulted in infectious virus expressing high-level luciferase activity in both tobacco and maize protoplasts. However, luciferase activity was not detected in extracts of whole plants inoculated with BSMV RNAs α, β or the LUC-gene-containing RNA, which is consistent with the replaced βb protein being essential for multiplication in whole plants.

Independent versus 'disarmed' vectors

From the previous paragraph, it is clear that viral RNA vectors able to replicate and spread independently through whole plants should contain all cis- and trans-acting factors involved in RNA replication, encapsidation and spread. Two approaches have been shown to be successful for the development of such helper-independent vectors, i.e. the insertion of a ('recombination-proof') extra promoter, as shown for TMV, and the replacement of non- or less essential genes (e.g. BNYVV 25 kD gene).

As an alternative, 'disarmed' viral vectors could be constructed for foreign gene expression in plants, which lack one or more essential functions and are able to multiply only in target plants transformed with the required gene(s). The properly constructed transgenic plant which is required provides a bonus in the form of control over the spread of field-released genetically engineered virus. This approach is indeed feasible, as shown by the replication of engineered AlMV RNA3 molecules in tobacco plants transformed with the AlMV replicase genes, and the complementation of spread-deficient TMV strains in transgenic plants expressing the TMV 30 kD movement protein.

Plant Viruses as Vectors for Studying DNA and RNA Rearrangements

Virus vectors have also been used for purposes other than expression of a payload ORF.

Splicing

Cloning of introns in virus vectors allows precise measurement of the efficiency and accuracy of splicing in monocotyledons and dicotyledons. The precise excision of an intron introduced into a CaMV vector verified the intron and was a proof for reverse transcription of CaMV.

Recombination

Experiments can be designed which make use of essentially nonviable virus hybrids which become viable upon specific genome rearrangements. The most obvious examples, already mentioned in the course of discussing agroinoculation, are given by 'one-and-a-bit-mer' of manipulated caulimo- and geminivirus genomes which release viable virus upon recombination. If the redundant portions of these constructs are derived from different viral strains, questions can be answered concerning the recombination mechanism, the presence of recombination hot spots, the degree of homology required, etc. Escape of pregenomic virus RNA by transcription was observed if the promoter/polyadenylator region of CaMV constituted the terminal redundancy. If transgenic *Brassica napus* plants were produced containing CaMV one-and-a-bit-mers arranged such that CaMV could not escape by simple transcription, true recombination events could be scored by appearance of viral symptoms. Sequence analysis of recombinant molecules suggested that mismatch repair was linked to the recombination process. Intermolecular recombination could also be studied, i.e. between transgenic CaMV ORF 4 and supertransfected complementary virus sequences.

Infectious transcripts from cloned RNA viruses have been very useful for studying RNA recombination, e.g. in bromoviruses, and for analyzing and understanding the *cis*- and *trans*-acting factors in RNA replication.

Agrobacterium T-DNA transfer

A CaMV-based system was used to analyze independent *Agrobacterium* transfer DNA (T-DNA) transfer events. The complete T-DNA without the border sequences was replaced by the virus genome such that a viable replicon could be produced by circularization upon transfection of plants. Analysis of this replicon revealed rather conserved right border remnants, while sequences remaining at the left border were more variable. The presence of small direct repeats between some of the joined ends showed that linear T-DNA had been transported to the plant.

Transposition

Using WDV and MSV vectors that contained the maize transposable element *Ac* or its defective *Ds* derivatives, excision of the transposable element could be studied in protoplasts and whole maize plants. Excision of the *Ds* element was dependent on the presence of *Ac*. The junction sequences left on the viral genomes after excision revealed the typical footprints.

Conclusions

Based on the limited and (sometimes) rather preliminary results obtained so far, it may be concluded that plant viruses can be engineered into gene vectors able to express desired genes. Systems are described that allow expression in single plant cells; others allow replication, expression and spread through the plant, either independently or as 'disarmed vectors' in the presence of a helper virus, or within a transgenic host carrying the missing functions.

The advantages of the viral vector transfection systems are ease of handling, the short time periods required to obtain results and the replication of the vectors to high copy numbers which can result in expression levels much higher than in transgenic plants.

Because of the lack of any proofreading mechanism and the large number of replication cycles (even in a single cell), one might imagine that payload genes in RNA virus and pararetrovirus vectors would rapidly accumulate point mutations, leading to inactivation of these nonessential inserts. The (limited) experimental data obtained so far, however, indicate that at least for the duration of a single protoplast batch or plant infection, functional proteins can be obtained in desirable amounts. It is not excluded that viral vectors eventually lose their capacity to encode a functional protein upon serial passage, although this would merely provide an advantage in view of biological containment.

A second issue of concern is the risk of recombination involving viral vectors. Indeed, it has now been well documented that viral genomes, including those of RNA viruses, are frequently the subject of recombinational events. One obvious mechanism for recombination in all classes of plant viral vectors relies on template switches of the nascent DNA and RNA strands. On the one hand, nonviral inserts in viral vectors might become lost by recombination because of the lack of selective pressure; the consequences seem only to be beneficial with respect to biological containment, since viral vectors will not survive for long in nature. On the other hand, new functional viral genomes may arise from recombinational events involving (disarmed) RNA vectors, co-infecting (helper-) viruses and transgenes, which could lead to undesired spread of pathogens. Although so far no evidence has been obtained for such events, it is clear that critical risk-assessment analyses should be performed prior to possible release of viral vectors in agricultural practice.

See also: **Bromoviruses (*Bromoviridae*); Geminiviruses (*Geminiviridae*).**

Further Reading

Ahlquist P and Pacha RF (1991) Gene amplification and expression by RNA viruses and potential for further application to plant gene transfer. *Physiol. Plant.* 79: 163.

Bakkeren G *et al.* (1989) Recovery of *Agrobacterium tumefaciens* T-DNA molecules in whole plants early after transfection. *Cell* 57: 847.

Beachy RN, Fitcher JH, Hein MB (1996) Use of plant viruses for delivery of vaccine epitopes. *Annals of The New York Academy of Sciences* 792: 43–9.

Brisson N and Hohn T (1988) Plant virus vectors: CaMV. In: Weissbach A and Weissbach H (eds) *Methods for Plant Molecular Biology*, p. 437. San Diego: Academic Press.

Donson J *et al.* (1991) Systemic expression of a bacterial gene by a tobacco mosaic virus-based vector. *Proc. Natl Acad. Sci. U.S.A.* 88: 7204.

Gray SM (1996) Plant virus proteins involved in natural vector transmission. *Trends in Microbiology* 4: 259–64.

Hohn B *et al.* (1987) Plant DNA viruses as gene vectors. *CIBA Found.* 133: 185.

Joshi L, Joshi V and Ow DW (1991) BSMV genome mediated expression of a foreign gene in dicot and monocot plant cells. *EMBO J.* 9: 2663.

Matzeit V *et al.* (1991) Wheat dwarf virus vectors replicate and express foreign genes in cells of monocotyledonous plants. *Plant Cell* 3: 247.

Mushegian AR, Shepherd RJ (1995) Genetic elements of plant viruses as tools for genetic engineering. *Microbiological Reviews* 59: 548–78.

[This article is reproduced from the 1st edn (1994).]

VECTOR TRANSMISSION OF PLANT VIRUSES

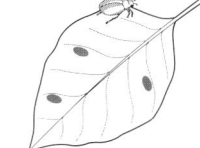

Stewart M Gray, USDA, ARS and Department of Plant Pathology, Cornell University, Ithaca, New York, USA

D'Ann Rochon, Agriculture and Agri-Food Canada, Pacific Agri-Food Research Centre, Summerland, British Columbia, Canada

Copyright © 1999 Academic Press

Introduction

It has been nearly 100 years since a leafhopper was confirmed as the vector of rice dwarf virus. Several hundred plant viruses have since been identified, a majority of which are dependent upon a vector for transmission between, and inoculation into, plant hosts. The plant viruses have evolved many interesting and biologically complex associations with their vectors, which include arthropods, nematodes and fungi. Although there is a great deal known about the general biology of most virus–vector interactions, we are only beginning to understand the molecular and cellular mechanisms that regulate the transmission processes and determine the efficiency of transmission.

General Mechanisms of Virus Transmission by Arthropods and Nematodes

In the early years viruses were said to be either mechanically transmitted or biologically transmitted by their vectors. Biological transmission was the specific association of a virus with a particular arthropod species or genus and the virus replicated in the vector. Mechanical transmission referred to the nonspecific transmission of viruses, usually by multiple vector species. The viruses did not replicate in the vector and transmission was thought to occur by the simple contamination of vector mouthparts. Most plant viruses do not replicate in their vectors, but it was quickly realized the transmission process involved more than just contaminated mouthparts.

The early work on plant virus–vector associations was related to timing events, e.g. acquisition and inoculation periods, retention periods and latent periods (the time between ingestion of the virus and the ability of the vector to inoculate a healthy host). Therefore, the terminology evolved to describe time events. Nonpersistent viruses are not retained by the vector for more than a few hours. Semipersistent viruses are retained for days or possibly weeks. Nonpersistent and semipersistent viruses are acquired and inoculated within seconds or minutes, and do not require a latent period, nor do they replicate in the vector. Persistent viruses are retained for the life of the vector. These viruses require longer acquisition and inoculation times (hours to days), and latent periods of one day to several weeks.

As additional data were generated on the mechanisms of transmission, other variations of the terminology evolved. The nonpersistent and semipersistent viruses were found to associate specifically with the epicuticle that lines the stylets (mouthparts) or foregut, respectively, of their arthropod and nematode vectors and were often referred to as stylet-borne or foregut-borne viruses.

All of the above terms were developed for use with aphid and leafhopper vectors and are applicable to many plant viruses. However, as additional arthropod, nematode and fungal vectors were discovered and their associations with viruses were studied, terminology problems arose, especially with regard to fungal vectors.

In recent times the terms circulative and noncirculative have been widely used. Circulative refers to the requirements that the virus be actively transported across cell membranes and internalized by the vector. These viruses, which would include the persistent viruses, can be further divided into propagative viruses, which replicate in their arthropod vector in addition to their plant hosts, and nonpropagative viruses which only replicate in their plant hosts. Noncirculative viruses do not cross vector cell membranes and are carried externally either on the vector surface or on the cuticle lining of the vector's mouthparts or foregut. These would include both the nonpersistent and semipersistent viruses.

The noncirculative and circulative classification is simple and can be used for all plant viruses that require a vector for optimal existence in nature. There is of course some loss of definition and categorization, but subgrouping, such as nonpersistent and semipersistent, can be added if they pertain to a particular vector taxa. There would, of course, be the paradoxical virus–vector associations that may not easily fit into the proposed scheme. For example, beetle-transmitted viruses and the myirid bug-transmitted velvet tobacco mottle virus may utilize both circulative and noncirculative transmission mechanisms. Additionally, these terms have not been adapted for use with viruses transmitted by fungal vectors (see below).

Vector Feeding Mechanics and Behavior

Plant viruses are incapable of penetrating the plant cell wall and require a wound to gain entrance. However, the cell they enter must be viable so the virus can replicate and translate movement proteins that enable it to move to neighboring unwounded cells. A majority of arthropod and nematode vectors of plant viruses have piercing–sucking mouthparts which are ideal for inoculating plant viruses into plant cells. The hollow needle-like mouthparts can penetrate the plant cell wall by mechanical force and with the help of salivary and gut enzymes. The cell membrane is easily breached by mechanical force, making the cell contents available as food. The most significant feature of this type of feeding is that it does not irreparably damage the plant cell.

The general feeding behavior of many arthropod and nematode vectors also aids in the inoculation process. The acceptance or rejection of a plant host is accomplished by a series of brief probes into multiple epidermal cells. These 'taste-tests' are sufficient to inoculate the noncirculative, nonpersistent viruses. This type of transmission mechanism does not require the plant to be a host of the vector for the virus to establish an infection. Accordingly, most of the noncirculative, nonpersistent plant viruses are transmitted by numerous species within one vector taxon. For example, individual potyviruses are transmitted by numerous aphid species, but are not transmitted by whiteflies or leafhoppers.

If the brief feeding probes indicate the plant is an acceptable host or food source then the vector is likely to initiate prolonged feeding. This may occur in numerous epidermal or mesophyll cells, or more often the insect will seek out its preferred feeding site, the carbohydrate-rich phloem sap. Prolonged feeding allows for the inoculation of the semipersistent, noncirculative viruses as well as the circulative viruses. The transmission strategy of these viruses is to associate with one, or at most a few, vector species for the life of the vector. The virus and the vector share overlapping host ranges and this ensures the virus will be delivered to a new host when the vector moves to a new host.

There are insect vectors (mainly beetles) of plant viruses that have chewing mouthparts and a more indiscriminate feeding behavior than the piercing–sucking insects and nematodes. Inoculation by beetles was, until recently, considered to be a mechanical process; virus contaminating the mouthparts was deposited into the wound, or virus in the gut was regurgitated as the beetle fed. The process is now known to be extremely specific and biologically complex. Viruses are inoculated into a gross wound resulting from the chewing action of the beetle because the virus can rapidly translocate in xylem elements away from the site of inoculation and infect cells away from the feeding site. Several viruses that are not transmitted by beetles can be acquired and are present in the hemolymph and gut regurgitant that is deposited into and around the feeding sites. The nontransmissible virus is apparently inactivated at the wound site or unable to gain entrance to a functional plant cell capable of sustaining a virus infection.

The transmission of plant viruses has been found to be extremely complex even in situations where initially it may have appeared to be a simple, nonspecific mechanical inoculation. The details of many of these molecular and cellular mechanisms regulating the transmission of plant viruses are described in subsequent sections.

Noncirculative Transmission

The noncirculative method of transmission is not widely associated with animal virus transmission, but it is the method of choice for a majority of plant viruses (**Table 1**). The noncirculative viruses are transmitted by arthropod and nematode vectors and can be further subdivided into nonpersistent and semipersistent categories. Semipersistent viruses tend to be associated with the cuticle lining the foregut of the vector (**Fig. 1**) and are retained for several days or weeks (months or years in some). Transmission efficiency increases as the acquisition feeding time increases, which suggests that virus is stably bound and accumulates until binding sites are saturated. In contrast, the nonpersistent viruses are retained only for a few hours and are easily lost during feeding probes. Furthermore, transmission efficiency rapidly decreases as acquisition feeding time increases. This suggests that bound virus is easily dislodged during prolonged feeding and subsequently ingested virus cannot associate with sites along the stylets.

There are two current theories for the mechanics of noncirculative, nonpersistent transmission. The ingestion–egestion model suggests that transmissible virus adheres to the cuticle at the stylet tips or further inside the mouthparts or foregut during ingestion of plant material. Bound virus is subsequently released during periods of regurgitation and salivation. The ingestion–salivation model acknowledges that virus can bind at multiple sites along the anterior alimentary canal, but the transmitted virus is limited to that which is bound to the proximal tip of the maxillary stylet where the food and salivary canals are fused. Virus is released by the act of salivation rather than by regurgitation (**Fig. 1**).

The most complete understanding of the mechanisms of noncirculative virus transmission comes from work on the aphid-transmitted potyviruses and caulimoviruses, both of which are nonpersistent and require a nonstructural, virus-coded protein referred to as a helper component, or aphid transmission factor to be transmitted (**Table 1**). Although there are several hypotheses for the role of helper in virus–vector interactions, one is emerging as the most plausible. The 'bridge' hypothesis suggests that the helper acts to mediate the attachment of virus to the cuticle lining of the vector mouthparts. Purified virus is not transmissible, but if aphids are given access to a solution containing helper prior to or along with purified virus then transmission can occur. Ultrastructural and immunolabeling evidence indicates that potyvirus fed to aphids along with helper becomes embedded in a matrix material bound to the cuticle, and helper protein is a component of the matrix. If aphids are fed on virus without helper, the matrix material is absent and virus is not retained.

The potyvirus coat protein contains a DAG amino acid motif located near the N-terminus. Mutations within this domain or adjacent to this domain abolish transmission and also prevent accumulation of virus in the stylets. Additionally, all of the potyvirus helper factors studied to date contain two characteristic amino acid motifs, a KITC box and a PTK box. Mutations in or adjacent to these motifs render the virus nontransmissible by the natural vector. A specific mutation of the KITC sequence to EITC abolished transmission, but did not affect the *in vitro* binding of virus to the helper. Furthermore, the virus was not observed on the stylets when acquired with the EITC-mutant helper, but was observed when acquired along with wild-type helper. These data indicate that the KITC box functions in aphid–helper interactions rather than helper–virus interactions. In contrast, mutations in the PTK box abolished helper–virus interactions *in vitro*; therefore this domain may play a role in attachment of the virus to the helper. Alternatively, mutations in the PTK box may prevent dimerization of the helper, which is the active configuration of the helper protein.

Analysis of the cauliflower mosaic caulimovirus (CaMV) helper provides further evidence of the bridge hypothesis. The CaMV helper accumulates in paracrystals in the cytoplasm of infected plant cells

Table 1 Mechanism of transmission and the principal vectors of plant virus families

Virus taxa	Number of members[a]	Principal vector taxa[b]	Transmission mechanism[c]	Helper required[d]
Caulimovirus	17	Aphids	NC-NP	Yes
Fabavirus	2	Aphids	NC-NP	No
Potyvirus	186	Aphids	NC-NP	Yes
Carlavirus	55	Aphids	NC-NP	No
Cucumovirus	3	Aphids	NC-NP	No
Alfamovirus	1	Aphids	NC-NP	No
Machlomovirus	1	Thrips/beetle	NC-NP	No
Macluravirus	2	Aphids	NC-NP	No
Potexvirus	55	Aphids (7/10), mites (2/10),	NC-NP	No
Badnavirus	16	Mealybugs (3/6), leafhopper (1/6)	NC-SP	No
Closterovirus	25	Aphids (10/19), whiteflies (6/19), mealybugs (2/19)	NC-SP	No*
Nepovirus	39	Nematodes	NC-SP	No*
Sequivirus	2	Aphids	NC-SP	No
Tobravirus	4	Nematodes	NC-SP	No
Trichovirus	6	Aphids (1/3), mealybugs (1/3), mites (1/3)	NC-SP	No
Waikavirus	3	Aphids (1/3), leafhopper (2/3)	NC-SP	No
Necrovirus	3	Fungi	*in vitro*	No
Tombusvirus	12	Fungi (1/12)	*in vitro*	No
Varicosavirus	4	Fungi	*in vitro*	No
Enamovirus	1	Aphids	C-Npr	No
Geminivirus				
Bigeminivirus	41	Whiteflies	C-Npr	No*
Hybrigeminivirus	2	Treehoppers	C-Npr	No
Monogeminivirus	11	Leafhoppers	C-Npr	No
Luteovirus	27	Aphids	C-Npr	No
Nanavirus	5	Aphids	C-Npr	No
Umbravirus	10	Aphids	C-Npr	Yes
Bromovirus	6	Beetles	C-Npr*	No
Carmovirus	22	Beetles (3/10)	C-Npr*	No
Comovirus	14	Beetles	C-Npr*	No
Sobemovirus	17	Beetles (6/8)	C-Npr*	No
Tymovirus	21	Beetles	C-Npr*	No
Rymovirus	7	Mites	?	No
Bymovirus	6	Fungi	*in vivo*	No
Furovirus	12	Fungi	*in vivo*	No
Bunyaviridae				
Tospovirus	5	Thrips	C-Pr	No
Marafivirus	3	Leafhopper	C-Pr	No
Reoviridae				
Phytoreovirus	5	Leafhopper	C-Pr	No
Fijivirus	6	Planthopper	C-Pr	No
Oryzavirus	2	Planthopper	C-Pr	No
Rhabdoviridae				
Phytorhabdovirus	32	Aphid (1/3), leafhopper (1/3), planthopper (1/3)	C-Pr	No
Cytorhabdovirus	17	Aphid (3/7), planthopper (4/7)	C-Pr	No
Nucleorhabdovirus	38	Aphid (7/17), leafhopper (4/17), planthopper (6/17)	C-Pr	No
Tenuivirus	10	Planthopper	C-Pr	No

[a] The number of members of each group was obtained from Brunt AA *et al* (1996) *Viruses of Plants*. Cambridge: CAB International.
[b] Indicates the vector taxa that is commonly associated with the transmission of the members of the virus group. In cases where multiple vector taxa have been reported to vector members of the virus group, the number of viruses vectored by that insect

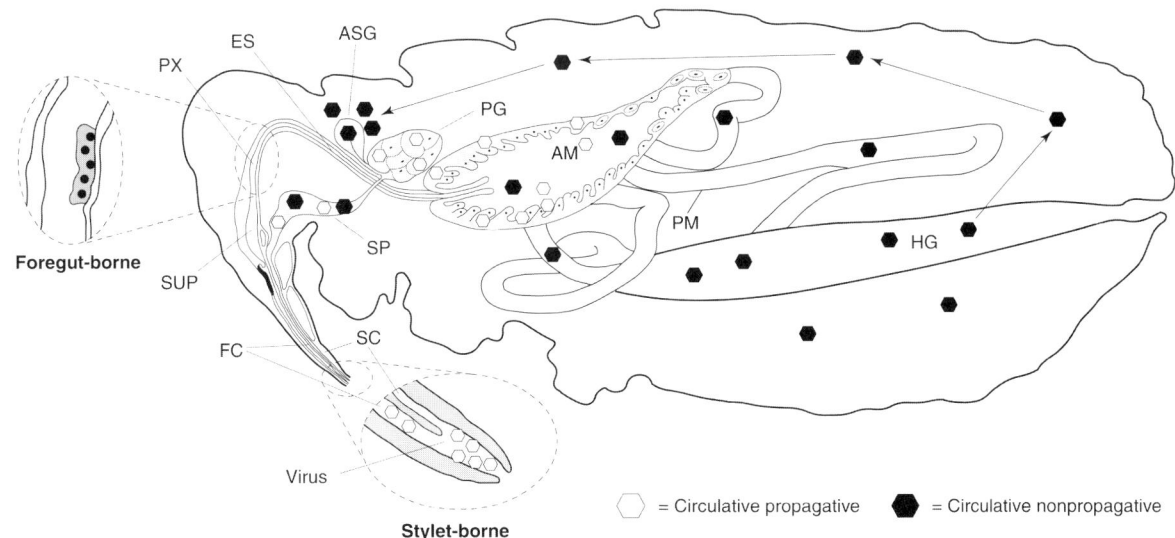

Figure 1 Mechanisms of transmission of plant viruses by arthropods with piercing–sucking mouthparts. The general anatomy of the alimentary system and the salivary system is shown; the areas relevant to virus transmission are labeled. One inset shows a detailed view of the distal end of the mouthparts where the food canal (FC) and salivary canal (SC) empty into a common space. The current model of transmission of stylet-borne (nonpersistent, noncirculative) viruses suggests that transmissible virus is retained at the distal tip of the stylets and then released by salivary secretions as the insect salivates during feeding. A second inset shows a detailed view of foregut-borne (semipersistent, noncirculative) viruses attached to the cuticle lining of the foregut, a region that would include the sucking pump (SUP), pharynx (PX) and esophagus (ES). Note the virus is embedded in a matrix material attached to the cuticle. The origin or composition of the matrix material is unknown. The circulative nonpropagative viruses will pass through the foregut into the anterior midgut (AM), posterior midgut (PM) and then into the hindgut (HG). They do not infect the gut cells but are transported through the posterior midgut or hindgut cells and released into the hemocele (body cavity). Current information indicates these viruses specifically associate with the accessory salivary glands (ASG) and are transported across the ASG cells and then released into the salivary canal (SC). The circulative propagative viruses will infect the midgut cells and subsequently infect other tissues. These viruses ultimately associate with the principal salivary glands (PG) and possibly ASG prior to their release into the SC. SP, salivary pump.

from which active helper can be solubilized. Mutations in the C-terminal domain of the CaMV helper abolish helper–virus binding *in vitro* and aphid transmission. Mutations in the N-terminus also abolish aphid transmission, but the helper retains its ability to bind to virions *in vitro*. These results suggest the C-terminus of the helper protein binds to virus particles, while the N-terminus of the helper protein is free to bind to sites in the aphid and bridge the indirect association of the virus particles to the insect cuticle.

Not all viruses transmitted in a noncirculative manner require a helper protein or helper virus (**Table 1**). Purified alfamoviruses, carlaviruses and cucumoviruses can be transmitted by aphids without helpers. Studies with cucumber mosaic cucumovirus have shown that transmission is regulated solely by the capsid protein. It is not known if these viruses are retained in similar locations in the vector.

The mechanisms of semipersistent transmission are not well studied. They may share some attributes with nonpersistent transmission but differences in sites of virus binding to the vector and times of retention indicate major differences in release of virus, if not in mechanisms of binding. There are few experimental data to explain how virus particles bound to the epicuticle substrate are released. The N-terminus of the potyvirus coat protein which binds the helper protein is often proteolytically cleaved *in vitro* without any deleterious effect on its infectivity.

---

taxa/the number of viruses tested for transmission is given. Information obtained from Brunt AA *et al* (1996) *Viruses of Plants*. Cambridge: CAB International.
[c] NC-NP, noncirculative, nonpersistent; NC-SP, noncirculative, nonpersistent; C-Npr, circulative, nonpropagative; C-Npr*, viruses transmitted by beetles do circulate in the insect hemolymph, but may also use a noncirculative mechanism of transmission as well; C-Pr, circulative, propagative. All mechanisms are defined in the text.
[d] Virus require a virus-encoded nonstructural helper protein or a helper virus for transmission; * indicates that there is some information that suggests a helper may be required for the transmission of some members of these virus families.

Similarly, the C-terminus of the nematode-transmitted tobacco rattle tobravirus can be cleaved from the particle without adversely affecting the virus. It is possible that proteases in the vector saliva or regurgitated gut secretions can act to cut the virus particle loose. Conformation differences in virus–helper–vector combinations and/or exposure to different enzymes and ionic conditions, depending on the site of retention, may account for differences between nonpersistent and semipersistent viruses and also for the differences in the specificity or transmission efficiency of vectors for the same virus.

Circulative Transmission

The mechanism of circulative transmission requires the virus to be internalized by the arthropod vector; there are no known circulative nematode transmitted plant viruses (**Table 1**). As previously mentioned, the circulative viruses are further divided into two subgroups: propagative viruses, those which replicate in their arthropod vectors (similar to the arboviruses); and the nonpropagative viruses.

Circulative, nonpropagative transmission

This type of transmission has been best studied with the luteoviruses and pea enation mosaic enamovirus (PEMV). The members of the luteovirus group and PEMV are each efficiently transmitted by one or, at most, a few aphid species. All the viruses share a common circulative pathway (**Fig. 1**) and biology within their aphid vectors. Ultrastructural studies have shown that ingested virus is not degraded or inactivated in the gut. Acquisition of virus into the aphid hemocele (body cavity) occurs either through the posterior midgut or hindgut epithelial cells by endocytosis. Virus is transported through the cell cytoplasm in vesicles that ultimately fuse with the basal plasmalemma, releasing particles into the space between the membrane and the basal lamina. Virus apparently moves rapidly across the basal lamina and into the hemocele. In most virus isolate–aphid species combinations, virus is acquired into the hemocele regardless if the aphid is a vector of that particular virus isolate. The gut does not appear to be a major barrier to luteovirus acquisition, although the process is specific for luteoviruses. Morphologically similar viruses can accumulate in the gut, but are not acquired into the hemocele.

Virus in the hemocele must pass through the salivary gland cells via an endocytosis pathway to be released by the vector into the plant. The salivary glands in aphids consist of two principal glands and two accessory salivary glands (ASG). Luteoviruses and PEMV associate exclusively with the ASG and more specifically with the anterior portion of these four celled glands. The ASG may function as an excretory organ in aphids and it is possible that luteoviruses have evolved to take advantage of specific excretory pathways to access the salivary ducts. An inability of luteovirus isolates to penetrate the ASG of nonvector aphids has long been known to contribute to the vector specificity. Recently it was shown that both the basal lamina and the basal plasmalemma function as independent barriers to transmission in different luteovirus isolate–aphid species combinations.

Studies of multiple luteovirus isolates in multiple nonvector aphid species has shown that the hindgut barrier or either of the two ASG associated barriers can function as the primary barrier of transmission for the same virus in different aphid species or in the same aphid for different virus isolates. This indicates that different membrane attachment sites (receptors) and/or different virus attachment protein domains are used at each transmission barrier by different virus isolate–aphid species combinations. Receptors on the aphid cell membranes have not been identified. However, the luteovirus and PEMV encoded proteins involved in aphid transmission have been studied and both virus groups share some structural features. The virus capsid contains a predominant coat protein ($c.$ 22–24 kDa) and a minor amount of a larger protein translated via a readthrough of the coat protein stop codon. The full-length luteovirus coat protein readthrough is $c.$ 72–74 kDa, but the C-terminal half of the 50 kDa readthrough domain is proteolytically processed to yield a 55–58 kDa coat protein readthrough commonly associated with purified virus preparations. It is not known if this type of processing actually occurs *in vivo*, but the C-terminal readthrough domain is not required for aphid transmission. The PEMV capsid also contains a coat protein readthrough, but the protein is inherently shorter than the luteovirus counterpart and does not undergo further processing.

The readthrough protein is not required for particle assembly or plant infection, and although particles containing only the 22–24 kDa coat protein are not aphid transmissible, ingested particles are found in the hemolymph. These results indicate that the coat protein regulates the uptake of the virus through the hindgut, and suggest the N-terminal portion of the readthrough domain regulates the virus–ASG associations. When luteovirus coat protein genes were expressed in insect cells using a baculovirus expression vector, virus-like particles (VLPs) were assembled. The readthrough-minus VLPs were purified and either fed to aphids through a Parafilm membrane or injected directly into the hemocele.

Ultrastructural examination of the aphids revealed the ingested particles were acquired through the gut into the hemocele, but, surprisingly, VLPs were observed in the accessory salivary gland cells and in the salivary ducts. These results are consistent with earlier studies showing that readthrough was not required for acquisition through the gut, but contrasted with the hypothesis that readthrough regulated the transport of virus through the accessory salivary gland. What then is the function of the readthrough domain, if any, in the aphid transmission process?

Aphids harbor endosymbiotic bacteria of the genus *Buchnera* in specialized cells located in the abdomen, called mycetocytes. Neither the aphid nor the bacteria are able to survive and reproduce without the other. All of the benefits that the bacteria provide for the aphid are unknown, but they are likely to provide essential amino acids the aphid is unable to synthesize. In addition, the bacteria produce copious amounts of a chaperonin protein named symbionin, a homologue of the *Escherichia coli* GroEL chaperonin protein.

Six luteoviruses and the related PEMV were all shown to bind specifically, but differentially, to *E. coli* GroEL and symbionin homologues from vector and nonvector aphids *in vitro*. The binding capacity was not correlated with transmission efficiency of the aphid, suggesting that if symbionin plays a role in transmission it does not play a role in vector specificity. A mutational analysis indicated the N-terminal portion of the readthrough domain contained the determinants for symbionin binding. Finally, virions that did not contain readthrough protein and did not bind symbionin *in vitro* were less persistent in the aphid hemolymph than wild-type virus. These studies provide convincing data that symbionin can interact specifically with luteoviruses and PEMV *in vitro* and may slow the degradation of virus in hemolymph. The mechanisms of degradation of virus in the hemolymph are unknown, nor is it known whether the attachment of symbionin to the virus protects the virus from targeting by the aphid immune system; alternatively, it may facilitate virus movement into the accessory salivary gland.

The coat protein readthrough appears to be a requirement for vector transmission of luteovirus and PEMV, but not for all circulative, nonpropagative viruses. Geminiviruses are single-stranded circular DNA viruses that have been divided into three taxonomic groups or genera (**Table 1**). The viruses within the monogeminivirus and hybrigeminivirus genera are each transmitted by a different species of leafhopper or treehopper. Viruses within the bigeminivirus genera are all transmitted by whiteflies.

Geminiviruses have been observed in the gut epithelial cells and associated with salivary glands of whitefly vectors. They are assumed to follow a similar circulative route through the whitefly as the aphid transmitted luteoviruses, although no detailed ultrastructural studies have been published. Several lines of evidence suggest that the transmission mechanisms used by the geminiviruses differ from that of the luteoviruses.

The geminivirus coat protein has been shown to be the sole determinant of transmission of some whitefly-borne viruses, a property that was recently mapped to the N-terminus of the coat protein of abutilon mosaic bigeminivirus. The coat protein was also shown to be the sole determinant of whether a geminivirus was transmitted by a whitefly or a leafhopper. However, the coat protein does not solely determine the transmission phenotype of all geminiviruses. A genomic analysis of tomato golden mosaic bigeminivirus indicated that, although the coat protein was required for acquisition of the virus, both genomic components were required for transmission. DNA B was essential for the accumulation of virus in the whitefly, while DNA A was required for the successful inoculation of plants by viruliferous insects. It is not understood if either or both genomic sequences are directly influencing virus–insect interactions or plant–virus interactions that may indirectly influence transmission efficiency.

Studies of geminivirus titer over time in whiteflies have not been able to show conclusively an increase that would suggest virus replication, but the viral DNA does persist in the insect longer than its infectivity would suggest. No replicative forms of the viral DNA have been detected within the insect, which also argues against the replication of virus in the insect. However, squash leaf curl virus was observed in several whitefly tissues and the presence of virus was associated with cytopathological abnormalities in some tissues. Furthermore, the presence of the virus in the insect can have detrimental effects on the biology and reproduction of the vector. Both of these observations would suggest virus replication. Additionally, tomato yellow leaf curl virus was recently reported to be transmitted transovarially in its whitefly vector. This type of vertical transmission usually indicates the virus is replicating in the vector, but geminiviruses may have evolved a mechanism to cross the transovarial transmission barriers without replicating in that tissue, or perhaps there is some low level amount of infection of reproductive tissues. No cytopathological effects, deleterious reproductive effects or transovarial transmission have been documented for aphids fed on luteovirus-infected plants.

Circulative, propagative viruses

The plant-infecting viruses within this classification (**Table 1**) are those most closely related to the animal-infecting arboviruses. Indeed three of the five taxonomic groups considered here have animal infecting members: rhabdoviruses, reoviruses and bunyaviruses. The plant viruses within these groups could be considered as plant-infecting arboviruses or phytoarboviruses.

The phytoarboviruses, with few notable exceptions such as the tomato spotted wilt tospovirus, are not economically important and have not been intensively studied. Their genomes tend to be relatively large and complex and they have remained recalcitrant to many of the modern molecular biology techniques. In addition, it has been difficult to generate sufficient numbers of stable mutants with phenotypes related to vector transmission. These are problems that have also plagued arbovirus research but, on the other hand, arbovirus research has benefited tremendously from the establishment of cultured vector cell lines and the ability to conduct detailed genetic studies on vector populations. Both of these research strategies have been difficult to develop and apply to the insect vectors of the phytoarboviruses.

Similar to the circulative, nonpropagative viruses, the individual phytoarboviruses tend to be transmitted by only one or a limited number of closely related vector species. Furthermore, many of the individuals within a population of any given vector species are not able to transmit the virus, although many can support virus replication. Consequently much of the research on transmission has investigated the movement of virus in vectors and the mechanisms of vector specificity. The general pathway through the arthropod is similar for all these viruses (**Fig. 1**). Virus is imbibed along with the plant sap and attaches to and infects midgut cells, usually reaching high titers in these tissues. Virus is released into the hemocele and secondarily infects other tissues, including reproductive tissues from which the virus can spread vertically to offspring. Horizontal transmission to other plant or animal hosts occurs following infection of salivary tissues and subsequently release of infectious virus from the glands in the salivary secretions that are injected into the host during feeding.

Vector competence (ability to transmit) is determined not only by the ability of the virus to replicate in the various tissues of the vector, but also by the ability of the virus to successfully enter and exit the tissues. The cellular barriers to transmission have been extensively studied and include a midgut infection barrier, which was first demonstrated for eastern equine encephalomyelitis alphavirus and has subsequently been demonstrated for other animal- and plant-infecting viruses. An active midgut infection barrier will effectively render the arthropod immune to the virus. Other barriers allow infection of the arthropod, but virus is not transmitted. A midgut escape barrier has been demonstrated for tomato spotted wilt tospovirus (*Bunyaviradae*) in the adult stage of the thrip vector. Virus can infect and replicate in midgut cells of both larval and adult thrips, but virus can only disseminate from larval midgut cells into other thrip tissues, therefore it must be acquired by the larval thrips to be transmitted. Wound tumor reovirus and sowthistle yellow vein rhabdovirus, both phytoarboviruses, are able to invade and replicate in several tissues of their leafhopper or aphid vectors, respectively. However, in nontransmitting individuals the viruses were not associated with the salivary glands. This suggests the existence of a salivary gland infection barrier, but does not rule out the possibility that the virus is not able to survive in the hemolymph or hemolymph-associated cells that would come in contact with the salivary glands. A salivary gland escape barrier has also been demonstrated for some arboviruses in their mosquito vectors, but has not been demonstrated for any phytoarbovirus. Similar to the situation described earlier for the circulative, nonpropagative luteoviruses, the specific barrier may differ for any combination of virus and vector and no generalities seem to be applicable.

The molecular and physiological basis for virus–vector interactions at these various barriers that regulate transmission are not well understood, but it is clear that genetic elements of the vector ultimately decide if a particular species or individual within a species of arthropod is able to vector a particular virus strain. Environmental or abiotic factors also play a role in determining virus–vector interactions, but in general these factors seem to influence the efficiency of the interaction rather than to determine the ability of the interaction to take place.

Virus transmission by vectors is not controlled solely by the vector: the virus also contributes to the overall process. Limited progress has been made in understanding the phytoarbovirus genes and gene products that influence vector transmission. A lack of stable cell lines from insect vector species and a difficulty in developing stable mutants with a transmission-deficient phenotype have contributed to the slow progress, but recently cell lines have been established for leafhopper vectors of reoviruses as well as for thrip vectors of tomato spotted wilt tospovirus.

Despite an absence of vector cell lines, progress on the identification of virus genes whose function is related to transmission has been made by studying virus associations with whole insects. The animal-infecting La Cross bunyavirus glycoproteins have long been implicated in vector transmission and recently it was shown that the tomato spotted wilt bunyavirus glycoproteins interact with two different thrip proteins, one of which was associated with midgut tissues. The tissue association of the other was not determined. The glycoproteins are likely involved with cell attachment and virus entry.

Studies on whole, virus-infected insects have also identified differences in virus RNA and protein accumulation between the plant and insect hosts. A nonstructural protein of maize stripe tenuivirus and rice grassy stunt tenuivirus accumulates in maize and rice, but not in the leafhopper vector. The function of the nonstructural protein is unknown. Perhaps it serves as a plant virus movement protein or aids in the initial uptake of virus by the vector, but would not subsequently be needed to be produced by the vector. In contrast to the aforementioned studies, the RNAs encoding the two maize stripe virus glycoproteins are abundant in both insect and plant host cells, and all serologically detectable rice dwarf reovirus proteins are present in both insect and plant hosts. Similar findings of no qualitative differences in viral RNAs or proteins have been reported for the alphaviruses. However, there were differences in the post-translational processing of the viral proteins between the mosquito and vertebrate hosts.

Another major problem in understanding phytoarbovirus–vector interactions has been in developing or identifying stable mutants that have altered vector transmission phenotypes. The viruses have all remained recalcitrant to many of the modern molecular biology techniques. Infectious DNA clones have not yet been produced and therefore a directed mutational strategy is not possible, nor is a reverse genetic approach to identifying gene function. A limited number of transmission mutants have been obtained by repeated mechanical inoculation of plant hosts without going through the insect host. A strain of the rice dwarf reovirus maintained for 12 years in vegetatively propagated rice plants had lost the P2 outer capsid protein due to a point mutation that introduced a termination codon in the open reading frame. The P2-minus virus was able to infect plants, but was unable to infect the leafhopper vector and be transmitted to plants.

Vegetative propagation of wound tumor reovirus-infected plants also resulted in leafhopper transmission-defective virus isolates. This was later found to result from the generation of defective RNAs of four of the 12 genomic sequences. These defective viruses were not able to infect the leafhopper vector cells, but were able to maintain a near wild-type infection of the plant host. Presumably all of the virus functions necessary to infect the plant host were contained on the eight remaining genomic segments, whereas one or more of the four defective segments provided for, as of yet, undefined functions specific for infection of the insect host. The data that have been generated thus far point to the conclusion that outer capsid proteins of the phytoarboviruses are, as would be predicted, involved in the infection of insect cells, i.e. attachment proteins. These would not be necessary for plant hosts because of the cell wall, which must be breached by totally different mechanisms than the cell membrane of insect hosts.

There is very limited reference to the continued serial passage of phytoarboviruses in their insect vector. Sowthistle yellow vein rhabdovirus was mechanically passaged by injecting virus into the hemocele of aphid vectors. Continuous serial passage did give rise to virus isolates that were difficult to transmit to plants and also more pathogenic to the vector. The reasons for the low probability of transmission was not determined and may have been a deficiency in systemic plant infection or an inability to move through all the transmission barriers in the aphid. With the advances in technologies that now allow further characterization of such mutants, there should be advances in our understanding of virus–vector interactions despite the difficulties with vector cell cultures and a lack of infectious clones of the viruses.

Viruses with Fungal Vectors

The terminologies and concepts described in the previous sections were all developed for multicellular organisms that feed on plant tissues. These are not easily adapted to virus transmission by fungal vectors. Although the fungi are multicellular, the vector is the unicellular zoospore. Furthermore, the acquisition of virus by the fungus does not involve feeding and ingestion comparable to the arthropod or nematode vectors discussed previously. Therefore, different terminology has been applied to the transmission of viruses by fungi.

Properties of Fungal Vectors

The fungally transmitted viruses belong to at least seven plant virus genera contained within at least four families (**Table 1**). The fungi known to be involved in vector transmission are zoosporic obligate parasites of plant roots and include two species of Chytridiomycetes (*Olpidium bornovanus* (formerly *O. radicale*) and *O. brassicae*) and three species of Plasmodiophoromycetes (*Polymyxa graminis, P. be-*

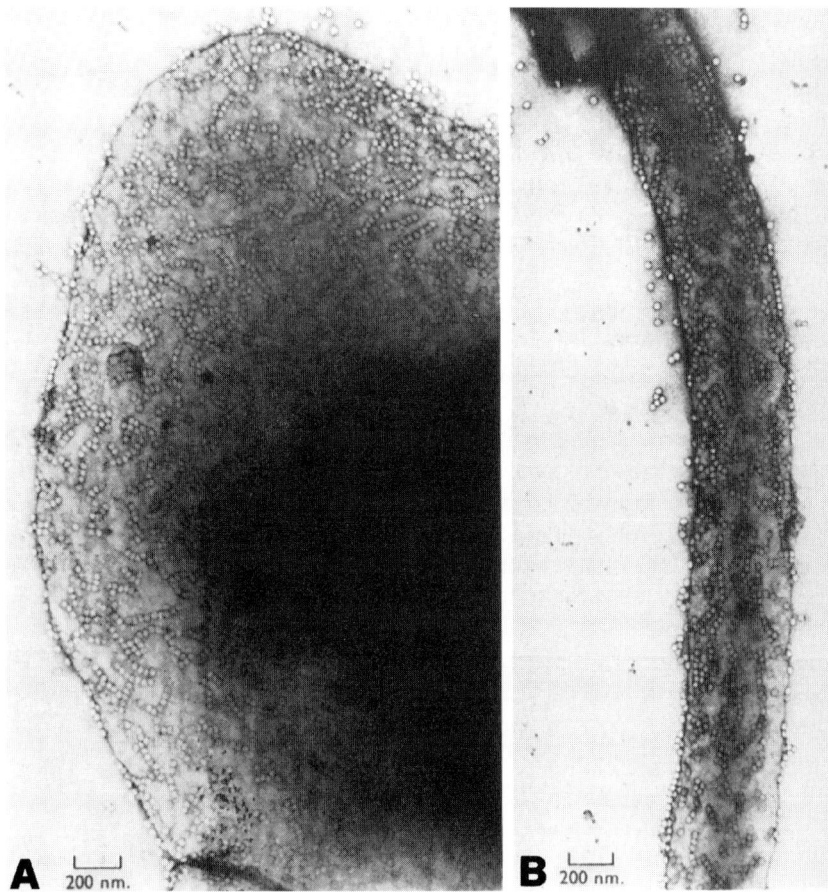

Figure 2 Electron micrograph showing binding of tobacco necrosis virus particles to the plasmalemma of the body (**A**) and to the axonemal sheath of the flagellum (**B**) of *Olpidium brassicae* zoospores. (Reprinted with permission from Temmink JHM, Campbell RM and Smith PR (1970) Specificity and site of *in vitro* acquisition of tobacco necrosis virus by zoospores of *Olpidium brassicae*. *J. Gen. Virol.* 9: 201–213.)

tae and *Spongospora subterannea*). The genera *Polymyxa* and *Olpidium* apparently cause little or no direct damage to crops but the viruses they vector can cause significant disease.

Most of the viruses vectored by *Olpidium* species are members of the family *Tombusviridae* and, as such, are small, spherical viruses containing single-stranded RNA genomes. Exceptions to this are the 'varicosaviruses' which are double-stranded RNA viruses with rod-shaped virus particles. Viruses with plasmodiophorid vectors are rod shaped and usually contain segmented single-stranded RNA genomes.

Olpidium spp. have zoospores which are uniflagellate, whereas *Polymyxa* and *Spongospora* spp. have biflagellate, heterokont zoospores. The developmental stages of these fungi are similar. Resting spores (or cystosori in the Plasmodiophoromycetes) produced in plant roots are released into the soil when roots decay. The resting spores germinate and produce motile zoospores which swim to roots and encyst when they encounter epidermal cells. Encystment involves withdrawal of the flagellum, attachment to root cell walls, and secretion of a thin cyst wall. The protoplasm of the zoospore is then released into the host cell and divides into a multinucleated plasmodium, which then develops into a sporangium. The sporangium liberates secondary zoospores, which are either released into the soil to infect other root cells, or which infect adjacent root cells. Vegetative sporangia produce the thick-walled resting spores. These are essential for survival of the fungus in the absence of a host and also permit survival of virus for extended lengths of time (>20 years for viruses transmitted in the *in vivo* fashion, see below).

Fungal Transmission Mechanisms

Two types of fungal–vector relationships are recognized: *in vitro* and *in vivo*. They are distinguished by the method of acquisition of the virus by the fungus and the location of the virus relative to the fungal resting spore (internal or external). In *in vitro* transmission the virus is carried externally on the zoospores (**Fig. 2**) and virus is not found within resting spores. In *in vivo* transmission, virus is acquired during growth of the fungus in a virus-infected plant and is found within resting spores. The location of a virus particle relative to a resting spore can be determined by treating resting spores with strong chemicals that are known to inactivate virus exposed to them (e.g. 20% Na_3PO_4 or 5 mol l^{-1} HCl). A virus carried internally will remain transmissible following treatment, whereas a virus on the surface will not. Alternatively, mixing virus with zoospores obtained from virus-free plants in solution and then inoculating roots with the suspension can result in infection by *in vitro* transmitted viruses, but viruses transmitted *in vivo* will not be acquired by the zoospores in solution and cannot infect plants inoculated with the suspension. *Olpidium* spp. are the only vectors identified that transmit virus *in vitro*, whereas *in vivo* transmission occurs with *Olpidium* spp., *Polymyxa* and *Spongospora* vectors. There is no evidence for replication of fungally transmitted viruses in their vectors.

In vitro transmission

The mechanism of *in vitro* transmission has been best described using tobacco necrosis necrovirus (TNV) and its vector *O. brassicae,* but was also later demonstrated for cucumber necrosis tombusvirus (CNV) and *O. bornovanus*. The virus is adsorbed on to the surface of the zoospore (**Fig. 2**) as it moves through the soil following independent release of the fungus and virus into the soil. The source of zoospores can either be from vegetative sporangia or from resting spores. The source of virus can be from infected root material obtained during the growing season or from other decaying plant parts after the crop is harvested. The acquisition time is short, in the range of 5–15 min, and the virus is very stably adsorbed to the plasmalemma of the body and the axonemal sheath of the zoospore. Electron microscopy studies have shown that adsorption is very specific: TNV binds *O. brassicae* zoospores but not *O. bornovanus* zoospores; CNV binds *O. bornovanus* zoospores but not *O. brassicae* zoospores. In addition, there is intraspecific variation in transmission efficiency. Different *O. brassicae* isolates vary in their ability to transmit TNV and three categories of vector efficiency could be identified: efficient vectors, inefficient vectors and nonvectors. Virus is not absorbed on to zoospores of a nonvector isolate and inefficient vector isolates adsorb fewer particles than zoospores of efficient vectors. The ability or inability of particles to bind zoospores appears to play a major role in the specificity of transmission.

The manner in which bound virus enters a root cell following zoospore encystment has not been extensively studied. It has been suggested that virions enter the zoospore protoplasm as the flagellum is retracted during encystment. Virus then enters a root cell when the zoospore protoplasm is discharged.

The molecular basis of *in vitro* transmission is also not well understood. Work with CNV and its fungal vector *O. bornovanus* has shown that virus particles are required for transmission. Further work in which the coat protein (CP) gene of CNV was exchanged with that of the nontransmissible tomato bushy stunt virus showed that the CNV CP contains transmission-specificity determinants. Transmission-defective CNV mutants have been isolated by repeated mechanical passaging. The transmission deficiencies were found to be due to either a deleted CP gene, the inability to express CP or an altered CP. One characterized mutant contained a single amino acid substitution in the CP shell domain which decreased transmissibility to less than 20% that of wild-type virus without affecting particle stability, virus accumulation or infectivity. This mutant also showed a decreased ability to bind zoospores in an *in vitro* binding assay, providing further evidence that binding plays a critical role in the transmission process. In addition, binding of CNV to *O. bornovanus* zoospores has been found to be saturable, specific and pH dependent. These studies suggest that a specific zoospore receptor may be involved in mediating viral attachment.

In vivo transmission

Viruses such as beet necrotic yellow vein furovirus (BNYVV) and barley yellow mosaic bymovirus (BaYMV) are transmitted by the *in vivo* mechanism and have been visualized within zoospores and resting spores of their fungal vectors. The virus must be acquired by the fungus within an infected host plant, but the timing and mechanisms of acquisition are unknown. A majority of the research has focused on roles of virus-encoded proteins in the transmission process.

Similar to the luteoviruses described earlier, the furovirus capsid contains a predominant coat protein and lesser amounts of a coat protein readthrough. Repeated mechanical passage of BNYVV and soil-borne wheat mosaic furovirus (SBWMV) results in transmission-defective mutants, a trait that is associated with the accumulation of deletion mutations in the readthrough domain. These results suggest that the readthrough domain contains sequences which can promote interactions between particles and fungus. Deletion analysis, along with alanine scanning mutagenesis, has identified a KTER amino acid motif near the C-terminus of the BNYVV readthrough as being important for the fungus transmission process. A similar sequence (KTEIR) is found in the readthrough domain of SBWMV.

Bymoviruses do not translate a coat protein readthrough. The repeated mechanical transfer of a BaYMV strain resulted in the loss of fungus transmission and a spontaneous approximate 1 kb deletion in RNA2. The deleted region is from a protein which is associated with crystalline inclusion bodies in infected tissue. Alignments of portions of the protein products of RNA2 of two bymoviruses and the readthrough portion of several furovirus capsids has revealed that certain amino acid combinations (ER or QR) are found consistently in all the viruses. These amino acids occur on the outside of the protein and therefore may be available for interaction with the fungus vector. In addition, certain conserved regions are absent in nontransmissible deletion mutants. These studies suggest that bymoviruses and furoviruses encode similar proteins for facilitating their transmission.

See also: **Luteovirus; Geminiviruses (*Geminiviridae*); Potyviruses (*Potyviridae*); Plant pararetroviruses (*Caulimoviridae*): Caulimoviruses: general features, Caulimoviruses: molecular biology; Tospoviruses (*Bunyaviridae*).**

Further Reading

Adams MJ (1991) Transmission of plant viruses by fungi. *Ann. Appl. Biol.* 118: 479.

Ammar ED (1994) Propagative transmission of plant and animal viruses by insects: factors affecting vector specificity and competence. In: Harris KF (ed.) *Advances in Disease Vector Research*, vol. 10, p. 289. New York: Springer-Verlag.

Brown DJF, Robertson WM and Trudgill DL (1995) Transmission of viruses by plant nematodes. *Annu. Rev. Phytopathol.* 33: 223.

Campbell RN (1996) Fungal transmission of plant viruses. *Annu. Rev. Phytopathol.* 34: 87.

Gergerich RC and Scott HA (1991) Determinants in the specificity of virus transmission by leaf-feeding beetles. In: Harris KF (ed.) *Advances in Disease Vector Research*, vol. 8, p. 1. New York: Springer-Verlag.

Gildow FE (1999) Luteovirus transmission and mechanisms regulating vector-specificity. In: *Luteoviridea*. Wallingford: CAB International.

Pirone TP and Blanc S (1996) Helper-dependent vector transmission of plant viruses. *Ann. Rev. Phytopathol.* 34: 227.

Venezuelan Equine Encephalitis Virus see Equine Encephalitis Viruses

---

Vesicular Exanthema Virus see Caliciviruses

VESICULAR STOMATITIS VIRUSES (*RHABDOVIRIDAE*)

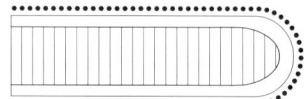

Luis L Rodriguez, Plum Island Animal Disease Center, Agricultural Research Service, United States Department of Agriculture, Greenport, New York, USA

Stuart T Nichol, Special Pathogens Branch, Division of Viral and Rickettsial Diseases, National Center for Infectious Diseases, Centers for Disease Control and Prevention, Atlanta, Georgia, USA

Copyright © 1999 Academic Press

History

Vesicular stomatitis viruses (VSVs) are rhabdoviruses which infect a wide range of wild and domestic animals, and several groups of insects. VSVs are best known as the cause of vesicular stomatitis (VS), a disease characterized by vesicular lesions in the mouth, tongue, udder teats and hoof coronary bands of cattle, horses and pigs. Clinical disease occurs every year in farming areas from northern South America to

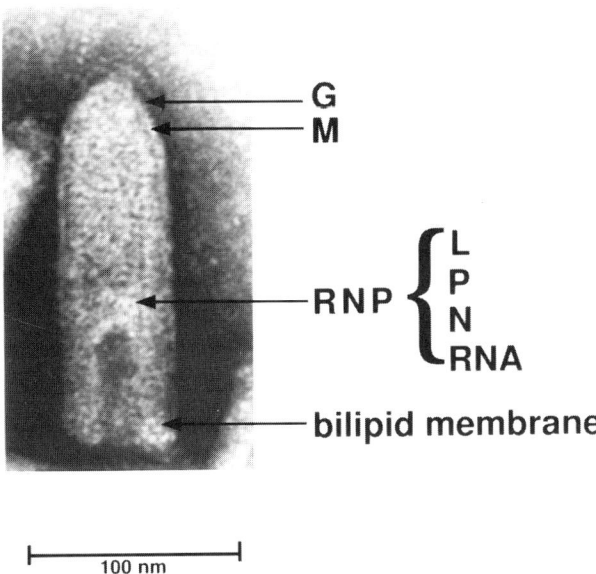

Figure 1 Electron micrograph of VSV-IN. Location of virion components is indicated. RNP is ribonucleoprotein.

southern Mexico where VSVs seem to have a stable natural cycle and are considered endemic. Humans living in these areas are often infected, and consequently develop flu-like symptoms. Early records of disease compatible with VS such as 'sore tongue' in pigs and 'hoof loss' in horses date back to the early 1800s in the Southeastern US and Central America. In 1862, a vesicular and febrile illness compatible with VS affected thousands of army horses in the US during the Civil War. The first large epizootic of VS to be described in detail occurred in 1916 in the US. The contagious, febrile and vesicular disease spread rapidly from Colorado to the East Coast, affecting large numbers of horses and mules and to a lesser extent cattle. Large epizootics have continued to occur in the US, on an approximately 10 year cycle, mostly in south western states.

Taxonomy and Classification

VSVs are classified in the order *Mononegavirales* (non-segmented-negative-sense RNA viruses), family *Rhabdoviridae*, genus *Vesiculovirus*. All rhabdoviruses share a characteristic bullet- or rod-shaped morphology and basic biochemical properties (**Fig. 1**). VSVs are grouped together on the basis of antigenic crossreactivity and genetic and biochemical relatedness. Two main serotypes, Indiana (IN) and New Jersey (NJ), have been defined based on cross-neutralization properties. The prototype strain of the IN serotype (VSV-IN1) was isolated in 1925 from an outbreak in cattle in Richmond, Indiana. A year later, the prototype virus strain of the NJ serotype (VSV-NJ) was isolated from cattle in New Jersey. Other VSVs serologically related to but distinct from VSV-IN1 have been found. Cocal virus, a virus isolated from mites in 1961 in Trinidad became the prototype strain of the VSV-IN type 2 (VSV-IN2). Another IN-related virus was isolated in 1964 from a mule in Alagoas, Brazil and became the prototype strain of VSV-IN type 3 (VSV-IN3). Many viruses serologically related to VSVs have been found, such as, Calchaqui in Argentina, Maraba and Carajas in Brazil, all isolated from insects, and Piry isolated from an opossum in Brazil.

Properties of the Virion

VSV particles are rod-shaped (hence the name rhabdo, from the Greek for rod) enveloped viruses of approximate dimensions 70 × 180 nm (**Fig. 1**). The virion core consists of a helical ribonucleoprotein (RNP) structure containing the RNA genome. The protein components of RNP cores consist of nucleocapsid (N) protein, the polymerase-associated phosphoprotein (P) and the large (L) polymerase protein. Based on studies using electron microscopy it has been estimated that there are 1258, 466 and 50 molecules of N, P and L, respectively, in each virion core of VSV-IN1. The matrix (M) protein is closely associated with the core structure, and provides structural support to the bullet-shaped helical RNP. The RNP is enveloped by a bilipid membrane derived from the host cell. Embedded in the membrane is the surface glycoprotein (G). The majority of the G molecule protrudes to the exterior of the viral particle and the short cytoplasmic tail contacts the underlying M protein.

Physical Properties

VS virions consist of approximately 74% protein, 20% lipid, 3% RNA and 3% carbohydrate. Infectivity is unstable at pH 3, but relatively stable in the pH range 5–10. It is rapidly inactivated at 56°C and by UV and X-ray irradiation. Infectivity is also sensitive to lipid solvents, detergents, formalin and various disinfectants such as bleach.

Properties of the Genome

The single-stranded non-segmented negative-sense RNA genome of VSV is approximately 11 kb in length. These linear RNA molecules possess 5′-phosphate and 3′-hydroxyl groups, and lack 5′ cap or 3′ poly(A) tail structures. The termini exhibit limited self-complementarity which may be involved in the circularization of the genome. The naked RNA

Table 1 Properties of proteins of vesicular stomatitis virus (NJ serotype)[a]

Protein	Biochemical characteristics	Localization and function(s)
Nucleocapsid (N)	422 aa; pI 5.8–6.3; 47–48 kDa	Encapsidates RNA to form nucleocapsid, essential component of transcription–replication complex
Phosphoprotein (P)	274 aa; acidic pI 4.2–4.3; 30–31 kDa; phosphorylated	Part of viral polymerase complex, mediates binding of L to nucleocapsid cores
Large (L)	2109 aa; basic pI 8.6–8.8; 241–242 kDa	Nucleocapsid, multifunctional enzyme, protein kinase, polymerase, capping, methylation and poly(A) addition
Matrix (M)	229 aa; highly basic pI 9.9; 26–27 kDa, phosphorylated	Forms scaffolding of nucleocapsids, promotes virus assembly, regulates genome transcription, inhibits host-cell gene expression, most abundant virion protein
Glycoprotein (G)	517 aa; 57–58 kDa class I membrane protein, N-glycosylated at 2 Asp residues	Major protein on viral envelope, attaches to cell receptor(s), mediates membrane fusion at low pH, induces cell toxicity, target of virus-neutralizing antibodies
C and C'	Coded in second ORF of P gene, 55 and 65 aa respectively, highly basic, arginine-rich	Nonstructural with unknown function

[a] Similar properties have been reported for VSV-IN1 proteins. aa, amino acids.

is not infectious. The nucleotide sequences of the complete genomes of VSV-IN1 and VSV-NJ have been determined. Furthermore, infectious virus has been recovered from plasmids containing the full-length genome of VSV-IN1. This has allowed extensive studies on the genome structure, transcription and replication strategies of VSV (see replication section).

Properties of the Proteins

VSV-NJ and VSV-IN1 code for seven proteins; five structural proteins (N, P, M, G, L) are coded in separate nonoverlapping open reading frames (ORFs) whereas two small highly basic nonstructural proteins (C and C') are coded in a second ORF within the P gene. The following details relate to VSV-NJ proteins unless otherwise stated (for details see **Table 1**). The N protein encapsidates the viral RNA, it is an essential component of actively transcribing or replicating viral cores and functions in close association with the P protein. The P protein is a highly phosphorylated protein associated with viral polymerase activity. It mediates the binding of the L protein to the nucleocapsid core and facilitates access of the polymerase to the RNA template during transcription and replication. Phosphorylation of P protein seems to be necessary for optimal transcriptase activity of the RNP complex. C and C' are nonstructural proteins of which the exact role in the life cycle of VSV is not clear. Engineered viruses that do not express C proteins are indistinguishable from wild-type virus in protein synthesis, virus production and host-protein synthesis shut off in tissue culture cells. The large L protein is a multifunctional enzyme required in only catalytic amounts and probably performs most of the polymerase-associated functions of the virus such as RNA synthesis, capping, methylation and poly(A) addition. It also has protein kinase activity which preferentially phosphorylates serine residues on the P protein. The matrix protein (M) is the most abundant protein of virions. M binds specifically to G protein monomers and promotes their trimerization, it also associates with the cellular lipid bilayer through the C-terminal domain to promote the condensation of viral RNP cores into tightly coiled helical structures that are subsequently enveloped and released as virions. The M protein, in tight association with RNPs, inhibits genome transcription and may play an important role in the correct regulation of viral genome transcription.

The G protein is a typical class I membrane-associated glycoprotein, with the N-terminal 90% of the molecule projecting from the surface of the virion or infected cell, a hydrophobic transmembrane domain anchoring the protein in the membrane, and a C-terminal 28-amino acid cytoplasmic domain projecting to the interior of the virion or infected cells. The G protein forms trimers that constitute the approximately 400 spikes on the virion envelope. The G protein plays a major role in attachment, penetration of VSV into susceptible cells and budding of virions from infected cells. It is the major target of VSV-specific neutralizing antibodies and is capable of inducing cell membrane fusion at low pH.

Replication Cycle

Unless otherwise stated, the following description of viral replication (**Fig. 2**) is that of VSV-IN1, although

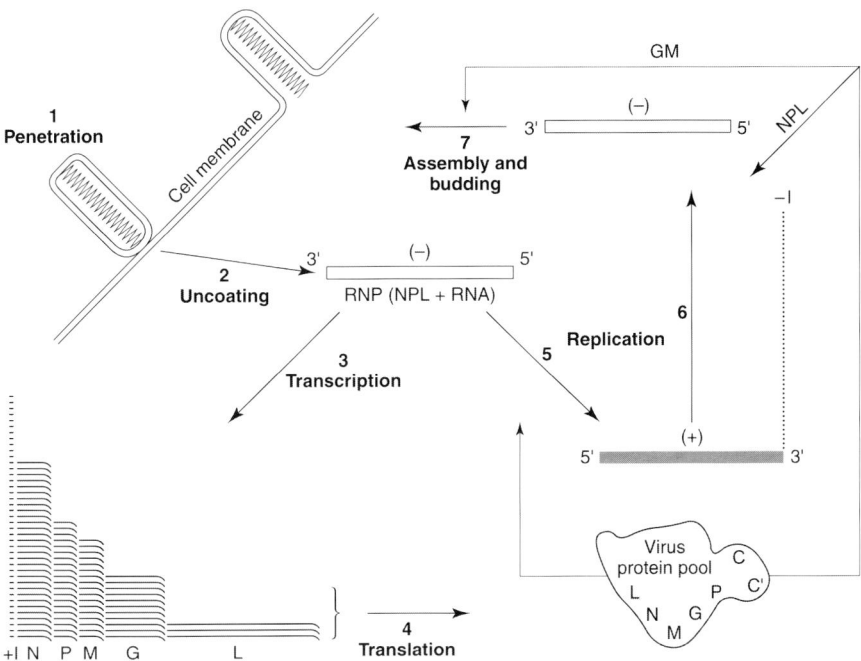

Figure 2 Model of VSV replication cycle. The major steps in the replication cycle of VSV are shown in diagram form. Open bars represent viral negative-sense RNA and closed bars represent viral positive-sense RNA. Refer to the text for discussion of steps 1–7.

it is likely to be representative of events occurring with the other VSVs. The infection cycle starts when the VSV G protein interacts with receptors on the host cell surface (such as phosphatidylserine). The virion penetrates by receptor-mediated endocytosis (**Fig. 2**, step 1). Once inside the cell, the G protein mediates the fusion of the cell and viral membranes under the low-pH conditions in the endosomes (**Fig. 2**, step 2). The viral ribonucleoprotein or nucleocapsid is released in the cytoplasm and the negative-sense viral RNA is transcribed by the virion-associated polymerase complex to produce six viral transcripts (**Fig. 2,** step 3). Active transcribing complexes consist of the template, made up of the RNA genome in tight association with the N protein, together with the polymerase, consisting of the phosphoprotein (P) and large (L) protein. The polymerase complex starts transcribing at a single entry site at the 3′ end of the genome and transcribes each gene in decreasing amounts as it moves away from the entry site. Therefore, the gene order provides an efficient way of regulating gene expression, where proteins necessary in larger amounts are located near the 3′ end and are transcribed in larger amounts and those needed in smaller amounts are located towards the 5′ end and are transcribed less frequently (i.e. 3′ N>P>M>G>L 5′). The complex initiates transcription by completing a 47-nucleotide transcript termed the leader RNA which is an exact copy of the genome 3′ end. This is followed by an untranscribed junctional sequence AAA (AAAA in VSV-NJ). The leader transcript which is neither capped nor polyadenylated, is transported to the nucleus where it inhibits host cell transcription. The leader transcript is followed by the N mRNA, which is capped during synthesis by the virion polymerase complex. At the end of the N gene, and indeed of all five viral genes, is the sequence 5′-AGUUUUUUUCAUA-3′ which signals the termination and polyadenylation of the mRNA. The mRNA poly(A) tract is probably synthesized by the viral polymerase slipping or chattering on the 7 U stretch. In an essentially identical manner, the polymerase completes the sequential synthesis of the remaining four mRNAs. Translation of the mRNAs is coupled to the transcription process and the protein amounts reflect the relative abundance of each mRNA (**Fig. 2**, step 4). Subsequently, after translation of viral proteins has occurred, a switch is made to synthesis of full-length positive-sense copies of the genome (**Fig. 2**, step 5). The switch mechanism is not fully understood but it requires protein synthesis and perhaps the participation of host cell factors. The critical step is the readthrough of the first junction encountered by the polymerase, i.e. the leader-N gene junction. The polymerase must be altered so as to no longer recognize the termination signal at this junction and continue down the full length of the genome. The simplest model fitting most of the experimental data proposes that rising levels of encapsidation of the nascent positive-strand leader RNAs by N protein reaches a threshold whereby it prevents the polymerase complex from recognizing the termination signals. Once full-length positive-strand synthesis occurs, production of the virus negative-sense RNA genomes necessary for packaging into released virions commences (**Fig. 2**, step 6). A negative-sense leader RNA which represents a 46-nucleotide copy of the 3' end of the positive-sense template can be found in infected cells. Its function is not known but it is probably synthesized in a manner similar to the positive sense leader RNA, i.e. in the presence of limiting levels of N protein the nascent negative-sense RNA synthesis terminates after the leader RNA transcript. In the presence of optimal levels of N protein the efficient encapsidation of the nascent strand pushes the polymerase through the termination signal and allows the polymerase complex to complete the synthesis of the entire negative-sense RNA genome. Such a proposed mechanism is attractive as it closely couples the production of virion RNA with the availability of viral proteins necessary for virion production.

The five viral mRNAs are transcribed in the cytoplasm of infected cells and their translation is directly coupled to the transcription process. Four of the viral mRNAs, N, P, M and L, are translated on free polysomes in a manner essentially analogous to cellular mRNAs. The G mRNA is translated on membrane-bound polysomes, the N-terminus of the newly emerging G protein has a 16 amino acid hydrophobic signal peptide which targets the protein to the rough endoplasmic reticulum (ER). The signal peptide is cleaved in the lumen of the ER. The protein is glycosylated as it is transported through the Golgi complex and is eventually expressed on the cell surface membrane in a trimeric form.

Assembly and Release

The glycoprotein forms patches on the surface of the infected cells. The M protein appears to form a bridge between the G protein membrane patches and virion RNP cores and promotes the tight condensation of the cores and their assembly into mature virion particles. These are then released by budding from the surface of the cell (**Fig. 2**, step 7). Considerable virus release occurs prior to the eventual disruption and death of the host cell. VSVs are generally highly cytopathic causing rapid cell death (in less than 12 h in some cases) in susceptible cells. Both M and G proteins and the viral inhibition of cell macromolecular synthesis have been shown to be involved in the cytotoxicity and death of infected cells.

Growth in Tissue Culture

The growth of VSVs is supported by a large number of vertebrate and insect tissue culture cells. VSV grows to high titers (8–9 $\log_{10}$) and produces dramatic cytopathic effect (CPE) in vertebrate cells such as cell lines and primary cultures of hamster, bovine and primate origin. In contrast, CPE is less obvious or absent and titers are lower in insect cells including several cell lines from mosquitoes (*Aedes albopictus* and *Aedes aegypti*).

Geographic and Seasonal Distribution

VSVs have been isolated almost exclusively from New World mammals and insects. Disease epizootics have been reported as far north as Canada, and as far south as Argentina. According to the intervals between outbreaks of clinical disease, there are areas of high, moderate or low VS activity with intervals of less than 1 year, 2–10 years or more than 10 years, respectively (**Fig. 3**). VSV-NJ infections are the most common, and have the widest distribution, with isolations as far north as Canada and as far south as Peru. VSV-IN1 has a similar wide geographical distribution but is less frequently encountered. VSV-IN2 (Cocal) viral infections have been detected in Trinidad, Brazil and

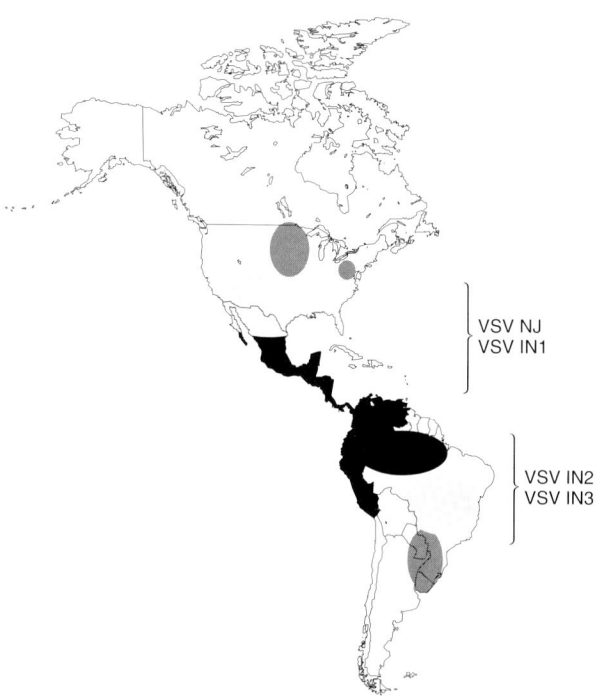

Figure 3 Geographical distribution of VSV serotypes. Areas are shaded according to the approximate interval between outbreaks of clinical vesicular stomatitis: □, never reported; ▨, > 10 years; ▨, 2–10 years; ■, 1 year.

Argentina. The last reported outbreaks caused by VSV-IN 2 date back to 1979 in Brazil. VSV-IN3 (Alagoas) is the main cause of VS outbreaks in Brazil. VS outbreaks often follow natural features of the land (e.g. spreading throughout river valley systems rather than along road systems or trucking routes) and tend to have a marked seasonality. In temperate regions, they begin in the late spring, peak in the late summer and cease with the first frosts of late fall/early winter. In more tropical regions, the epizootics frequently appear at the cessation of rainy seasons. In both regions, the seasons of high VSV activity tend to correlate with high insect population levels.

There are only two reports of suspected VS epizootics outside of the New World. The first was an apparent VS outbreak in horses and mules in Transvaal, South Africa in the late nineteenth century. The second was a VS outbreak in France during World War I which was initiated by a shipment of infected US army horses. There is no evidence of VSV activity persisting for prolonged periods in either of these continents. VS is a mandatory reportable disease in most countries, either because of it being exotic in those countries or for the similarity of its clinical signs to those caused by foot-and-mouth disease virus, a virus exotic or under eradication in most parts of the world.

Natural History

VSVs seem to infect a wide range of hosts in endemic areas, with evidence of viral infections in wild small mammals such as: cotton rats (*Sigmodon* spp.), rice rats (*Oryzomis* spp.) and field mice (*Peromyscus* spp. and *Reithrodontomys* spp.); arboreal mammals such as bats (many species) and howler monkeys (*Alloata palliatta*); and large wild mammals such as white tail deer (*Odocoileus virginianus*) and feral swine (*Sus scrofa*). Infections of wild animals seem to be asymptomatic. Insects are also infected by VSVs, with isolations reported from sand flies (*Lutzomyia* spp.), black flies (*Simulium* spp.), midges (*Culicoides* spp.), mosquitoes (*Culex* spp., *Aedes* spp.), eye gnats (*Hippelates* spp.), mites (*Gigantolaelaps* spp.) and domestic flies (*Musca domestica*). No disease symptoms are observed in insects and their importance in the maintenance and transmission of VS disease is unclear. However, the ability of VSVs to replicate and be transovarially transmitted in sand flies and black flies and the seasonal appearance of clinical disease, suggests a role for these insects in the natural cycle of VSV. Since transovarial transmission of VSV in insects is inefficient it has been proposed that natural reservoirs, in which the virus induces high titers in the blood, are necessary for hematophagous insects to maintain the virus in nature. However, to date such wild or domestic natural reservoir(s) remain elusive.

One of the best documented VSV endemic foci is on Ossabaw Island, a barrier island off the coast of Georgia in southeastern US. On this island, the local feral swine population is infected every year by VSV-NJ. Several lines of evidence indicate that the sand fly (*Lutzomyia shannoni*) is the vector responsible for VSV-NJ transmission to feral swine. First, *L. shannoni* is the only species of sand fly on the island. Second, VSV-NJ has been isolated not only from hematophagous females but also from nonhematophagous male sand flies which indicates that transovarial transmission must have occurred in these flies. Third, the population peak of sand flies on the island precedes by about a month the peak in seroconversion rates of sentinel pigs, and fourth, it was found that the virus is transmitted most often to sentinel pigs in those habitats of the island where the sand flies are abundant, such as maritime live oak forests. However, the reservoir that feeds this apparent insect–swine cycle in Ossabaw remains unknown, since neither deer nor feral swine from the island were capable of producing detectable viremias after experimental inoculation with the local strain of VSV-NJ. Other studies in well-documented endemic areas in Costa Rica have shown that the presence of clinical VS in dairy cattle is associated with the presence of forested areas near the affected farms, where wild animals including rodents, primates and bats have high antibody prevalence to VSV, and also where sand flies and black flies are present. The role of these wild animals and insects in the natural cycle of VSV is to be determined.

Evolution

RNA-dependent RNA-polymerase of VSVs has an estimated error rate of $1-4 \times 10^{-4}$ substitutions per base incorporated. As a consequence of this high error rate, every time the genome is replicated new variants arise producing a heterogeneous virus progeny referred to as a 'quasispecies'. VSV uses this genetic variability to adapt and persist in its natural niche. Despite the high mutation rate of VSV *in vitro*, naturally occurring VSVs show a clear pattern of genetic stability (**Fig. 4**). There is good correlation between viral phylogeny and the location of virus isolation, indicating that many lineages and sublineages are maintained in infection foci of limited geographical distribution (**Fig. 4**). There is no correlation between lineages and host species, i.e. there is not a distinct VSV of any particular host species. Viruses isolated from mammals and insects in the same endemic area usually have identical se-

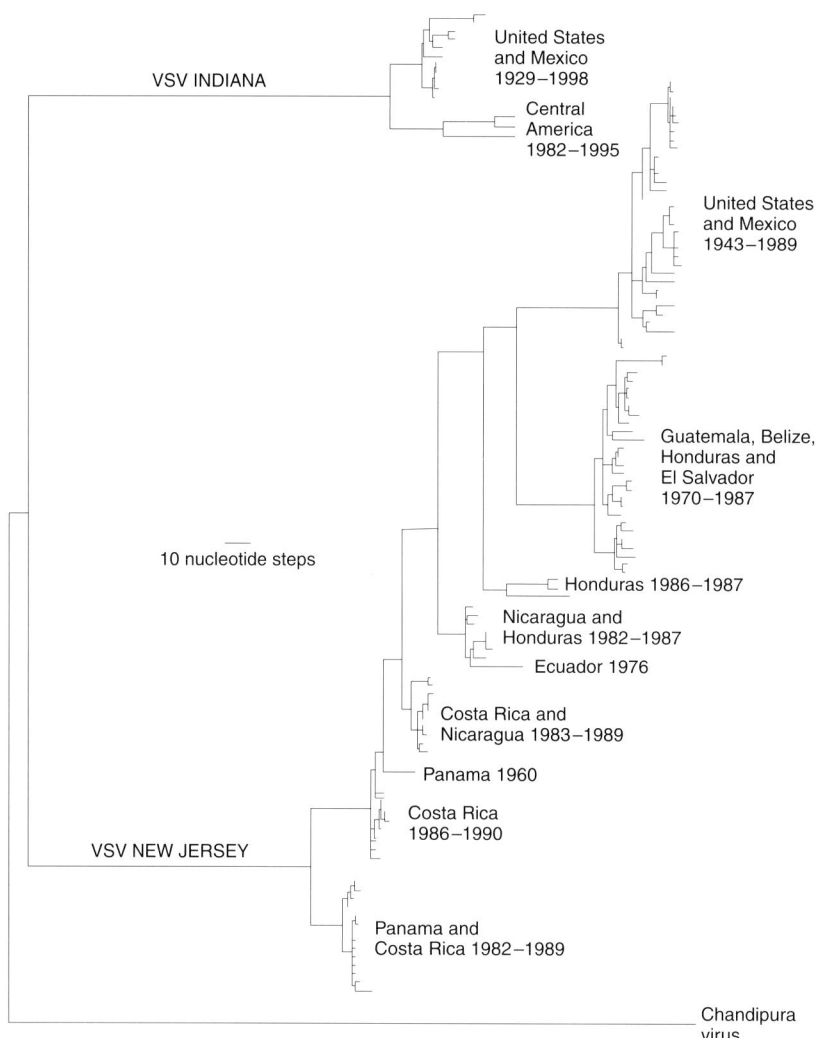

Figure 4 Evolutionary tree topology for VSV-NJ and VSV-IN1 from North and Central America, obtained by maximum parsimony analysis of partial phosphoprotein sequences from 122 VSV isolates. Genetic distance is proportional to the length of horizontal lines. Vertical distances are for graphic display only.

quence, furthermore, viruses isolated in these areas 30 years apart are more closely related than viruses from the same year but from different areas. The absence of a molecular clock contrasts with the evolutionary pattern of other RNA viruses such as human influenza A viruses which show a clear relationship between year of isolation and position within a phylogenetic tree. The evolutionary pattern of influenza virus A is driven mainly by the immune response of the infected hosts, where new antigenic variants capable of escaping the immune response have a selective advantage. In contrast, sequence analysis of VSVs causing clinical disease in Central and North America suggest that ecological factors rather than immune selection are the major forces driving VSV evolution (**Fig. 4**). For instance, viruses originating less than 25 km apart but from different ecological zones had different sequences, whereas viruses originating over 800 km apart but from areas of similar ecological characteristics had identical sequences. The ancestral origin of the VSVs is currently unclear. A relatively conserved gene order and limited sequence similarity with other nonsegmented negative-strand RNA animal viruses suggest a common, albeit very ancient, ancestor.

Serological Relationships and Variability

All VSVs share common N protein epitopes which are group specific and are usually detected by complement fixation assay. The two major VSV serotypes, IN and NJ, have been defined by crossneutralization assays using antibodies to the surface glycoprotein (G). Limited antigenic variation has been observed among natural virus isolates of VSV-NJ. Greater antigenic diversity is seen among VSV-IN with at least three distinct types identified. Antisera raised to virus of one IN type will neutralize virus of another type but to a lesser degree. Although some antigenic variation can be found, there is no evidence of distinct antigenic drift of VSVs in nature (see Evolution section).

Epidemiology

The epidemiological characteristics of VS outbreaks depend to a large extent on whether the outbreak occurs in an endemic or a nonendemic area. Endemic areas are located in tropical and subtropical areas of the Americas where the interval between clinical outbreaks is less than one year. An epidemiologic study carried out in an endemic area of dairy production in Costa Rica reported clinical cases starting in November, peaking in December and January and continuing until March (the dry season in this area begins in November and continues through May). Most clinical cases occurred in adult lactating cattle (average age 5.4 years) and were caused by VSV-NJ (90%) and to a lesser extent IN 1 (10%). The majority of the adult population, including those that became clinically ill, had significant titers of neutralizing antibodies to VSV-NJ (93%) and VSV-IN1 (25%). Interestingly, there was no evidence for genetic drift in the viral glycoprotein gene in viruses recovered from these cases, despite the fact that clinically affected animals had high titers of neutralizing antibodies prior to clinical disease. In these endemic areas many animals, particularly young animals (less than 2 years) become seropositive to VSV during periods of clinical activity without showing any signs of clinical disease.

VSV causes periodic large-scale disease epizootics of cattle, horses and swine in non-endemic areas with peaks of activity approximately every 10 years. Clinical cases appear in many premises in a short period of time, generally during the summer months, and the disease disappears with the first frosts. However, in 1982–83 a large outbreak of VSV-NJ in western US persisted well into the winter months. After the 1982/83 outbreaks, VS has occurred in Southwestern US in 1995, 1997 and 1998. All cases in 1995 were caused by VSV-NJ, however, during the 1997 and 1998 outbreaks, VSV-IN1 was the major cause of clinical cases. Interestingly, this was the first report of VSV-IN1 in the US since 1966. It is not known what the sources of VSVs are for the US outbreaks. Nucleotide sequencing of virus isolates from US in 1982/83 showed that these viruses were very close to each other, they differed greatly from viruses from the only documented endemic focus in the US in Ossabaw Island, Georgia, but were related to VS strains circulating in Mexico during the same years. VSV-IN type 2 and type 3 cause outbreaks mainly in South America. Little is known regarding the epidemiology of these two virus types.

Transmission and Tissue Tropism

There is little information regarding transmission and tissue tropism of VSVs. Presumably domestic animals are infected by bites from insect vectors. Viral activity is most obvious in cattle, horses and pigs because of their clinical signs. However, it is likely that these animals play little or no role in the maintenance and transmission of the virus in nature, since infected animals do not show detectable viremias. There is no virus shedding in milk, feces or urine. Fluid from vesicular lesions contains large amounts of infectious virus ($>10^{10}$ PFU ml^{-1}) which can serve as a source for mechanical transmission from animal to animal. However, attempts to reproduce animal-to-animal transmission of VSV have met with only occasional success. Experimental data would suggest that the epidermal layer probably needs to be broken or abraded for successful direct viral transmission. Several lines of evidence suggest that VSVs are insect viruses and the infection of animals may be incidental. Tissue tropism of VSVs in insects has not been studied extensively, although the midgut and fat body have been shown to be major sites of VSV-NJ viral replication in sand flies. Serological surveys of humans in areas enzootic for VSVs suggest that human infection can be relatively common. Numerous cases of infection of laboratory workers, veterinarians and animal handlers have been reported. These are usually associated with viral entry through breaks in the skin or exposure to high virus titer aerosols such as infected animals sneezing in the faces of susceptible individuals. Human to human transmission has never been reported.

Tissue tropism of the virus in naturally infected animals is poorly understood. It seems likely that the majority of viral replication is found close to the site of entry of the virus and remains relatively localized. However, cases in which lesions appear in multiple sites (hoof, mouth and teats) in the same animal might suggest that generalization occurs through blood circulation. The localized nature of the vesicular lesions in the mouth (tongue, gum, lips), coronary band of the hoof and the skin of the teats or prepuce, suggest a tropism to tissues in these areas. It has been shown that the virus replicates in the *stratum spinosum* layer of the skin. However, the physiological basis of this tropism remains unknown.

Pathogenicity

The majority of VSV natural infections of domestic animals appear to be asymptomatic, as seroconversion in the absence of obvious clinical symptoms is frequently observed. Data from epidemiologic studies have showed that physiological state (e.g. lactation, pregnancy, age) are significant risk factors for clinical VS, suggesting that host, rather than viral factors likely determine the clinical outcome of infections. However, tissue-culture-grown virus appears to quickly lose the ability to produce clinical disease when reintroduced into animals. This might be related to loss in fitness of the viral quasi-species by repeated passage in tissue culture (see Evolution section).

Clinical Features of Infection

VS disease in cattle, horses and swine is characterized by the appearance of vesicular lesions on the mouth (tongue, lips, gums), teats, or hoof coronary band epithelium layer approximately 2–4 days after inoculation of the virus. Animals rarely exhibit lesions at more than one site, but when it happens it is usually in serologically naive animals introduced to endemic areas or infected during large epizootics. Depression, lameness, fever and excessive salivation are often seen before vesicles are detected. Alterations in hepatic enzyme levels suggest that VSV infection may also affect the liver in cattle and humans. In dairy cattle, milk production virtually ceases and weight loss can be as much as 300 pounds (140 kg) in beef cattle. This is especially true if mouth lesions become too sore for animals to eat, or they become too lame to get to food and water. Mastitis is a common consequence of the infection due to milk retention (caused by pain during milking) and secondary infections. In severe cases the udder can be lost to gangrenous mastitis. In most cases healing of lesions occurs within 7–10 days. Human VSV infections are characterized by an influenza-like illness after 24–48 h incubation. The majority of cases develop a biphasic fever accompanied by malaise, myalgia, headache, photophobia and chills. Vesicles appear on the tongue, oral and pharyngeal mucosa, lips or nose in a minority of cases. There is one report of VSV causing severe encephalitis in a child.

Pathology and Histopathology

The main lesions associated with clinical VSV infections are the vesicles that can appear in the tongue, the mouth, the hoof coronary bands or on the skin of the teat or prepuce. Vesicles begin as small blanched areas, the epithelium separates from the basal layer and forms a vesicle filled with clear-yellowish fluid. Vesicles rupture easily leaving a red surface which usually heals in 1–2 weeks if they are kept free of secondary bacterial infections. Necropsy reports of infected animals are rare since VSV does not cause mortality. No gross lesions of internal organs have been reported in experimentally infected animals. Histopathological examination of vesicular lesions reveals that lesions develop in the *stratum germinativum* where intercellular edema is observed. Cells become necrotic later which results in the separation of the epithelial layers above the *stratum basale* and accumulation of vesicular fluid.

Immune Response

Little is known about the immune response to VSV in domestic animals or wild natural hosts. However, VSV has been used extensively to study the immune response to viruses in laboratory animals, particularly mice. There are three major components in the immune response to VSV: the nonspecific immunity (interferon and nitric oxide); humoral immunity (antibodies); and cellular immunity (T cells). Interferon seems to play a role in survival of laboratory mice inoculated with VSV. Naturally occurring VSV strains differ in their capacity to induce interferon *in vitro*; in general VSV-NJ strains induce higher interferon responses than VSV-IN1. However, there is no clear correlation between interferon induction capacity of VSV strains and their pathogenesis *in vivo*. Neutralizing antibodies directed against VSV glycoprotein play an important role in protection of laboratory animals against VSV. The exact mechanism of protection is not clear, since virus–antibody complexes are still capable of binding to susceptible cells but do not initiate infection. The majority of cattle, horses and pigs living in endemic areas have neutralizing antibodies to VSV. However, it seems that the presence of neutralizing antibodies is not sufficient to prevent clinical disease in these animals. This may be explained by the majority of viral replication being localized in the epithelium.

Experiments in cattle and swine have demonstrated proliferative responses of peripheral blood mononuclear (PBM) cells to VSV antigens which could be detected at 3 weeks postinoculation in swine or postvaccination in cattle. In both cases, these responses could still be detected 6 months later. However, the role of the cellular immune response in protection against VSV is questionable since laboratory animals devoid of direct and indirect cytotoxicity, but capable of humoral response, survive VSV infections.

Prevention and Control of VSVs

The first step in controlling VS is rapid detection of clinical cases. Differential diagnosis particularly to distinguish VS from foot-and-mouth-disease is important. Diagnostic methods currently used include complement fixation, fluorescent antibody and isolation in cell culture. Other detection methods include antigen-capture ELISA and reverse-transcriptase-polymerase chain reaction (RT-PCR). Epithelium or vesicular fluid from fresh lesions are ideal samples for submission. In premises affected with VS in non-endemic areas, quarantine is usually established to avoid further spread of the disease. Within the affected premises, control measures include insect control and cleaning and disinfection with bleach of feed and water troughs, milking equipment and any utensils that could transfer the virus between animals. Since it has been suggested that scarification plays a role in virus entry, rough hay or overgrown pastures should be avoided.

Several inactivated vaccines containing both serotypes NJ and IN1 have been used in South and Central America. Although their effectiveness has not been rigorously tested, a recent report indicates that an oil-based bivalent vaccine decreased the incidence of clinical disease by as much as 25-fold among vaccinated cattle in endemic areas of Colombia. Other vaccine approaches including subunit vaccines and Vaccinia vectors containing G protein have had limited success in laboratory trials using domestic animals and have not been tested in the field. International control of VS is by means of import/export control on the movement of animals with significant neutralizing antibody titers to VSVs.

Future Perspectives

Despite significant efforts made during the last 30 years, many of the questions about the natural cycle of VSV remain unanswered. There is compelling evidence indicating that VSVs are transmitted to domestic animals by blood-sucking insects. However, despite the testing of many species of wild and domestic mammals, none has been found capable of producing the sustained viremias necessary to be a source of virus for insects. The genetic stability of VSV in endemic areas and the specific ecological characteristics associated with different VSV genotypes, indicate that there could be different natural cycles of VSV under different ecological conditions. The fact that VSV activity can be traced to very specific ecological conditions and even to specific forest types in endemic areas, should be taken into consideration in designing future studies on the natural cycle of VSV.

The ability to obtain infectious VSV-IN from cDNA clones has opened a new chapter in VSV research, since by using reverse genetics it is now possible to dissect the role that individual genes and genome sequences play in the life cycle of VSV, both within the cell and also within the animal and insect hosts. The availability of VSV cDNA clones has also made possible the inclusion of foreign genes in the VSV genome, which are expressed and incorporated in the virion along with other viral structural proteins, providing the potential to use VSV as a vector for vaccine delivery. One of the most interesting applications of this technology is the incorporation of the human immunodeficiency virus 1 (HIV-1) cell receptor CD4 and coreceptor CXCR4 in the VSV virion. This virus is unable to infect normal cells but infects and kills those expressing HIV-1 membrane fusion protein on their surface, making it a 'guided' killer for HIV-1-infected cells only.

See also: **Rabies virus (*Rhabdoviridae*); Rabies-like viruses (*Rhabdoviridae*).**

Further Reading

Banerjee AK and Barik S (1992) Gene expression of vesicular stomatitis virus genome RNA. *Virology* 188: 417.

Dietzschold B, Rupprecht CE, Zhen FF and Koprowski H (1996) In: Fields BN, Knipe DM, Howley PM *et al* (eds) *Fields Virology* 3rd edn, p. 1137. Philadelphia: Lippincott-Raven.

Wagner RR and Rose JK (1996) In: Fields BN Knipe DM, Howley PM *et al* (eds) *Fields Virology* 3rd edn, p. 1121. Philadelphia: Lippincott-Raven.

VIRAL MEMBRANES

John Lenard, Department of Physiology and Biophysics, Robert Wood Johnson Medical School, University of Medicine and Dentistry of New Jersey, Piscataway, USA

Copyright © 1999 Academic Press

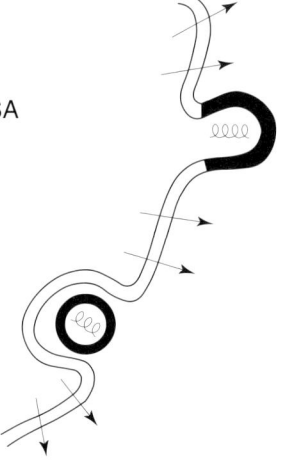

Introduction

Viruses of many kinds possess lipids as integral components of their structure. Lipid-containing, or enveloped, viruses include *Corona-*, *Orthymyxo-*, *Paramyxo-*, *Bunya-*, *Rhabdo-*, *Toga-*, *Retro-*, *Herpes-*, *Baculo-* and *Poxviridae*. Despite the great diversity of these viruses in regard to structure, replicative strategy, host range and pathogenicity, the function of the lipid is the same in all of them: to form a membrane surrounding the encapsidated viral genome. In all these viruses the lipids form a continuous bilayer that functions as a permeability barrier protecting the viral nucleocapsid from the external milieu. Embedded in the bilayer are numerous copies of a limited number (usually one or two) of virally encoded transmembrane proteins that are required for virus entry into a host cell. These proteins must mediate two essential functions: attachment of the virion to the cell surface; and fusion of the viral envelope with a cell membrane.

The membrane is acquired during viral assembly within an infected cell. Membrane acquisition generally occurs by budding of the viral nucleocapsid through a particular cellular membrane, which is characteristic for each enveloped virus. Many of the viruses mentioned above bud through the plasma membrane. However, bunyaviruses bud through the Golgi apparatus, coronaviruses take their membranes chiefly from the endoplasmic reticulum and herpesviruses bud from the nuclear membrane. Poxviruses, which are among the largest and most complex animal viruses, are unique in not acquiring membrane by simple budding. They acquire several membranes through a series of interactions with different elements of the intracellular membrane transport system.

Viruses that lack lipids often possess capsids or shells consisting only of viral protein. These structures perform the same functions as viral membranes, i.e. protection of the genome, attachment to a suitable host cell and facilitation of its entry into the host cell. Increasingly, the actions of these proteins are being shown to resemble those of the glycoproteins of enveloped viruses.

Viral Bilayer

Knowledge of the structure of viral membrane bilayers has come chiefly from the study of a few viruses that are easily grown in large quantities in the laboratory, namely the orthomyxo-, paramyxo-, rhabdo- and togaviruses. In these, the bilayer arrangement of the lipids has been directly demonstrated using physical methods, and the lipid composition of various viruses grown under different conditions has been described in detail. Since all of these viruses acquire their bilayer by budding through the host cell's plasma membrane, the viral membrane contains the lipids present there. Wide variations of lipid composition are tolerated, and most of the lipids display the properties characteristic of lipids in a bilayer, not those of protein-bound lipids. The precise content of each individual phospholipid or glycolipid in a viral membrane does not always reflect the bulk composition of the host cell membrane from which it was derived, however. This difference may arise from interactions of lipids with the viral membrane proteins, or from inhomogeneity in the host cell membrane.

Intact virions are impermeant to proteases and other enzymes. Indeed, virions can swell and shrink in response to changes in osmolarity, showing that the viral membrane is impermeant to small molecules and ions as well as large proteins. This property indicates that the viral membrane consists of an intact bilayer, completely surrounding the encapsidated viral genome. It is generally assumed that intact bilayers are characteristic of all enveloped viruses, and not just for those few for which this property has actually been demonstrated.

Viral Membrane Proteins

The proteins of viral membranes, like those of other membranes, may be classified as either integral or peripheral. Integral proteins are those that span the membrane one or more times, and thus cannot be solubilized without disrupting the bilayer, e.g. with detergents. Peripheral proteins do not cross the membrane, and can be removed from it and solubilized by treatment with aqueous salts or chaotropic agents, which do not destroy the bilayer.

Integral membrane proteins of enveloped viruses generally span the membrane only once; an exception is the E1 protein of coronavirus, which spans the membrane three times. Each membrane-spanning, or transmembrane, or anchoring, domain is a sequence of 18–27 predominantly hydrophobic amino acid residues. Transmembrane sequences are inherently insoluble in water, so that integral membrane proteins require the presence of detergents to be soluble. In the absence of detergents or lipids, membrane proteins tend to aggregate as rosettes, with the transmembrane sequences clustered together at the center of the rosette, in order to minimize contact with water. Viral membrane proteins can be reinserted into lipid bilayers of defined composition by mixing detergent-solubilized proteins and lipids together, then removing the detergent by dialysis or centrifugation. These reconstituted viral membranes often possess biological activity.

As much as 90% of the polypeptide chain of a viral membrane protein may be external to the bilayer, where it is accessible to degradation by added proteases. In some favorable cases, nearly the entire external domain can be recovered intact and correctly folded after limited proteolysis, facilitating crystallization and structural analysis. The best example is the influenza virus HA protein. The external portions of viral membrane proteins generally possess oligosaccharide side chains, identical to those of cellular proteins in attachment position and structure. Often, they also possess disulfide bonds. These post-translational modifications reflect the viral proteins' synthesis at, assembly within and translocation through, the cell's rough endoplasmic reticulum (see Membrane Synthesis below).

Peripheral proteins are attached to the viral membrane by a combination of electrostatic and hydrophobic interactions. Although they may penetrate the bilayer to some extent, they do not cross it as the integral proteins do. Viral peripheral proteins include the M1 protein of influenza, the M proteins of paramyxo- and rhabdoviruses, and the MA proteins of retroviruses.

Attachment of Viruses to Host Cells

The first step in infection, attachment of the virus to the outer surface of the host cell, is performed by the membranes of enveloped viruses. Each virus recognizes a unique feature of its host cell membrane. Thus, the nearly total specificity of human immunodeficiency virus (HIV)-1 for cells expressing CD4 protein is conferred by the affinity of the viral envelope protein gp120 for this cell surface 'receptor'. Other enveloped viruses bind to different specific cell surface proteins to initiate infection. An emerging generalization is that, even when viruses bind to true cell surface receptors that normally initiate complex intracellular responses such as phosphorylation cascades, these responses are not essential for viral infectivity. The virus is simply using a characteristic surface landmark to identify and attach to its appropriate host cell.

Orthomyxo- and paramyxoviruses have a broader receptor specificity than was discussed above. Their hemagglutinin (HA and HN, respectively) glycoproteins bind to sialic acid residues attached to various cell surface proteins and lipids. Sialic acids are bound to the host cell membrane through several different kinds of glycosidic linkages, and different virus strains show some preference for sialic acid residues in particular linkages. The most nonspecific of the enveloped viruses may be the rhabdoviruses, represented by vesicular stomatitis virus (VSV) and rabies, which bind indiscriminately to clusters of negative charges, whether created by lipids, proteins or oligosaccharides. This nonspecific binding property helps to account for the extremely broad host range of these viruses.

Viral Fusion

Before viral transcription and replication can commence, the viral genome must cross the barriers presented by both the viral envelope and the cell membrane. Fusion of the viral membrane with a cellular membrane accomplishes this, introducing the viral genome into the host cell cytoplasm. Fusion, like cell attachment, is a property conferred upon each virus by one (or perhaps, in some cases, more) envelope glycoprotein. In most well-studied cases (notably the orthomyxo-, paramyxo-, rhabdo- and togaviruses) fusion does not require the participation of cell proteins, as virions and reconstituted viral

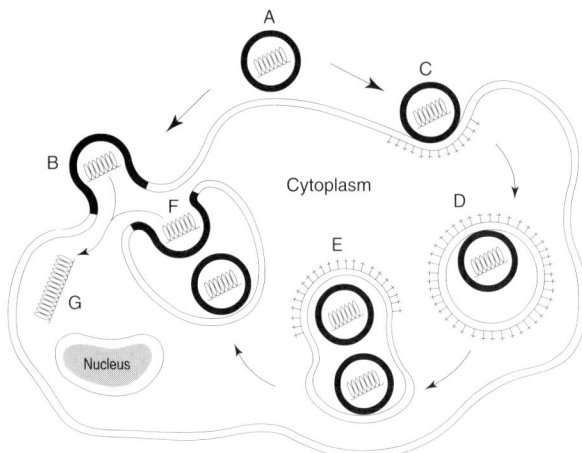

Figure 1 The two major pathways for cellular penetration and uncoating of enveloped viruses. Uncoating begins with attachment of the virion to the cell surface (A), through the binding of an integral viral membrane protein to a 'receptor' on the cell surface, which may be a specific cell protein, an oligosaccharide or a patch of charged lipids. Attachment is followed by fusion, mediated by a viral protein which may or may not be of the same type as the attachment protein. If the viral fusion protein is active at neutral pH, fusion can occur directly with the plasma membrane (B). Alternatively, if fusion requires an acidic pH, the virion must first be endocytosed via the coated pit–coated vesicle pathway (C,D). The viral fusion protein is activated in the acidic endosomes (E,F). Both pathways result in the introduction of the viral nucleocapsid, containing the viral genome, into the cytoplasm (G). For viruses that undergo transcription and replication in the nucleus (such as orthomyxoviruses and most DNA viruses), uncoating is followed by transport of the nucleocapsid through the nuclear pores into the nucleus by unrelated processes.

membranes (often called 'virosomes') fuse readily with protein-free liposomes and planar lipid bilayers.

The fusion proteins of the paramyxoviruses differ from those of the orthomyxo-, rhabdo- and togaviruses in regard to the pH at which they act. While the former are active at neutral pH, the latter require a more acidic environment, usually below pH 6, for fusion. This difference has profound consequences, as it reflects two distinctly different modes of viral entry (**Fig. 1**). The paramyxoviruses, and others capable of fusing at neutral pH, can fuse with the cells' plasma membranes under normal conditions, i.e. at the neutral pH of extracellular fluid or culture medium (**Fig. 1B,G**). Those viruses that fuse only at acidic pH, on the other hand, must first be internalized from the cell surface into specialized vacuoles, the endosomes. Although this process brings the virus inside the cell, the viral genome is still separated from the cell cytoplasm by the same two membranes as before. The endosomes are acidic, however, which activates the viral fusion protein and allows fusion between the viral and endosomal membranes (**Fig. 1C–G**). The pH dependence of viral fusion activity, which is conveniently measured as virus-induced hemolysis, or by a variety of direct fusion assays, serves to distinguish between viruses that enter the cell by the two distinct routes shown in **Fig. 1**.

The two different routes of cell entry shown in **Fig. 1** are differentially inhibitable by specific compounds. A variety of membrane-permeant or 'lysosomotropic' amines (notably chloroquine, ammonia and methylamine, but also including a variety of local anesthetics, tranquilizers and other commonly used pharmaceuticals) possess the property of being able to diffuse across membranes only in their unprotonated, uncharged form. The protonated, charged form of these compounds thus accumulates in acidic compartments such as the endosomes, raising the endosomal pH and preventing the activation of acid-dependent viral fusion proteins. Lysosomotropic amines generally have no effect on the entry of those enveloped viruses that fuse at neutral pH.

Viral fusion proteins are generally glycoproteins which possess a single transmembrane domain, and which assemble into multimers, usually homotrimers. In the last few years considerable progress has been made in understanding the molecular events that occur during viral fusion. Fusion mediated by the influenza fusion protein, HA, has been the most thoroughly studied and is the best understood, since the three-dimensional structure of its proteolytically derived extracellular portion has been determined by x-ray crystallography. The fusion-competent form of HA arises from proteolytic cleavage of an inactive precursor, HA0, to yield HA1 and HA2. The single transmembrane domain is in HA2, to which HA1 is attached by disulfide bonds. HA1 is primarily concerned with cell attachment, while HA2 chiefly mediates the fusion reaction, which relies on three structural features of the molecule:

1. *The fusion peptide*, situated at the N-terminus of HA2. This hydrophobic sequence was recognized early as a conserved feature between influenza and paramyxovirus fusion proteins. Its release from constraint by the proteolytic cleavage that creates HA2 is an essential element in the proteolytic activation of HA.

2. *The three-stranded coiled-coil* that comprises the stem of the HA trimer at neutral pH. The low pH-mediated activation of HA for fusion consists of a rearrangement and extension of this coiled-coil. This repositions the fusion peptide, from a sequestered location close to the viral membrane to an exposed position at the extreme end of the newly elongated coil. This enables the fusion

peptide to contact and penetrate the target membrane (**Fig. 2**).

3. *The transmembrane domain of HA2.* An essential role of this domain was demonstrated through the use of a mutant from which it had been deleted. When the entire external portion of HA was anchored through a lipid only into the outer leaflet of the membrane bilayer, it was no longer capable of mediating fusion. However, it could still catalyze half the reaction, or hemifusion, a process in which only the outer leaflets of the two membrane bilayers become mixed.

Using influenza HA protein as the model, viral fusion may be considered to occur in a series of discrete steps following virus-receptor binding (**Fig. 3**):

1. *Activation of the fusion protein* by conformational rearrangement. For influenza HA this is induced by acid, and consists of the extension of the coiled-coil stalk and exposure of the fusion peptide (**Fig. 2**). For fusion proteins that act at neutral pH, other activation processes operate. Some paramyxovirus fusion proteins (named F) may be activated by interaction with a partner viral protein, the cell attachment protein HN. For the HIV-1 fusion protein, activation is thought to occur by interaction with one of several chemokine receptors present on the surface of host cells (part of step 1, **Fig. 3**).
2. *Penetration of the fusion peptide* into the target bilayer, thus linking the viral bilayer with the target bilayer (step 1, **Fig. 3**).
3. *Relocation of the extended coiled coil stem* so as to bring the two linked membranes into close apposition (part of step 3, **Fig. 3**).
4. *Hemifusion* between the outer leaflets of the viral membrane and the target membrane. This may be mediated by the fusion peptide. Hemifusion is initiated by formation of a *stalk*, a lipid structure of very high negative curvature that provides continuity between the two outer leaflets. Mixing of outer leaflet lipids, but not those of the inner leaflet, characterizes hemifusion (step 3, **Fig. 3**).
5. *Formation of fusion pores.* The transition from the structure present in the hemifused state (the *hemifusion diaphragm*, a small area consisting of a single bilayer composed of the inner leaflets of the two reacting membranes; **Fig. 3**) to the fusion pore is energetically favorable. This transition requires participation of the transmembrane domain of the viral fusion protein (step 4, **Fig. 3**).
6. *Enlargement of the fusion pore.* Initially, fusion pores allow only flickering electrical contact between the aqueous compartments. The pore eventually widens out to permit transfer of the viral genome or other large molecules, thus completing the fusion process (step 5, **Fig. 3**).

It should be noted that the mechanism by which the viral fusion protein catalyzes (3)–(6) above is not yet understood. The major recognized fusion intermediates – the stalk, the hemifusion diaphragm and the fusion pore – are predominantly lipidic in nature, and have been defined in pure lipid systems. None the less, it has been estimated that HA-mediated fusion requires the concerted action of at least three HA trimers (step 2, **Fig. 3**). It seems likely that all viral fusion reactions proceed through a very similar series of steps. A more detailed understanding of the mechanisms of viral fusion would be of fundamental importance, and might also suggest new avenues for antiviral therapeutic intervention.

Membrane Synthesis

Viruses in general make maximal use of mechanisms already in place in the infected cell to perform their functions. Hence, viral protein synthesis is carried out on host cell ribosomes. Synthesis of viral membrane proteins occurs on membrane-bound ribosomes, from

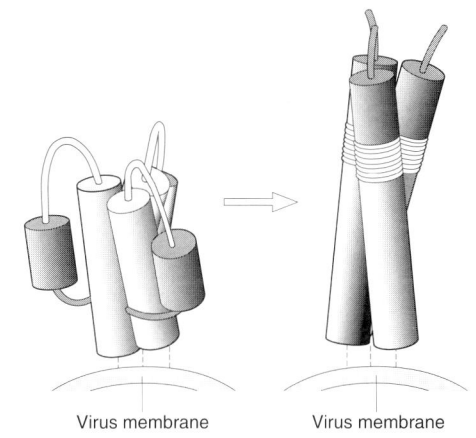

Figure 2 How influenza HA protein is activated for fusion by low pH. *Left:* A simplified representation of the trimeric structure of HA2 at neutral pH, as revealed by x-ray crystallography. Cylinders represent α helices; the light colored cylinders interact to form a three-stranded coiled-coil stem. The 'fusion peptide', which extends from the short, dark cylinders, is sequestered close to the viral membrane. *Right:* Upon exposure to low pH (e.g. inside an endosome), the previously unordered region shown in white becomes helical and extends the coiled-coils, which are still further extended by incorporation of the darkly colored region as shown. This repositions the fusion peptide to the end of the coiled-coils, enabling it to insert into a target membrane. (Modified with permission from Carr CM and Kim PS (1993) *Cell* 73: 823–832.)

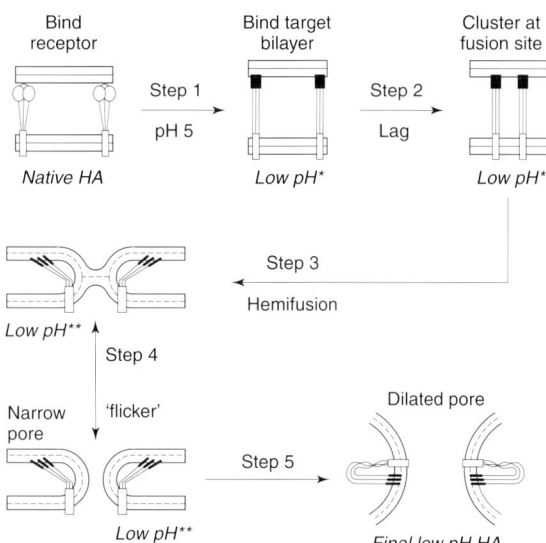

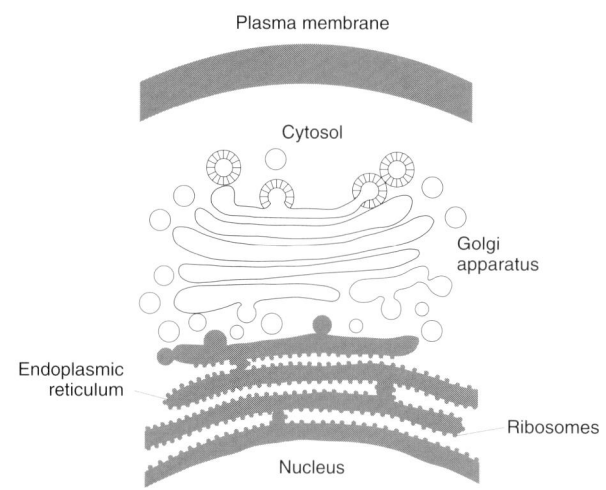

Figure 3 Sequence of events during HA-mediated virus fusion. See text for details. (Reproduced with permission from Hernandez et al (1996).) 'Low pH*' and 'Low pH**' are successive low pH-mediated conformations postulated by Hernandez et al (1996) to mediate the successive fusion events.

Figure 4 Endoplasmic reticulum–Golgi–plasma membrane system of a cell. All viral and cellular integral membrane proteins are synthesized by ribosomes bound to the endoplasmic reticulum membrane. Proteins destined for the plasma membrane then undergo vesicular transport to the nearest lamella of the Golgi apparatus (the 'cis' face). A series of sequential vesicular transport steps then carries these proteins through the Golgi to the 'trans' face and out to the plasma membrane. In polarized cells, further sorting steps target the viral protein to the apical or basolateral plasma membrane. Assembly and budding of different enveloped viruses occurs at characteristic points within this membrane system.

which they are inserted, always in the correct orientation, into the endoplasmic reticulum membrane. There they are glycosylated and assembled into multimeric form. The influenza HA protein, for example, is assembled into the trimers that form the 'spikes' seen in electron micrographs of the surface of influenza virions. The viral glycoproteins may then be further processed through the Golgi and on to the plasma membrane (**Fig. 4**). In fact, the membrane proteins of VSV, influenza, and several other enveloped viruses have provided valuable tools for the study of these transport processes. This is because many of these viruses possess only one major membrane protein, which is expressed in infected cells at very high levels. Further, host cell protein synthesis is inhibited by both VSV and influenza infection, so large amounts of a single membrane protein are produced and correctly processed in infected cells.

Viral proteins are targeted to specific cellular locations by the same mechanisms that cells use for their own membrane proteins. Viral proteins, in fact, are widely used in the study of these targeting mechanisms. Newly synthesized VSV G protein, for example, is targeted to the basolateral plasma membranes of polarized cells. Newly synthesized influenza HA protein, on the other hand, is delivered to the apical plasma membranes of the same polarized cells. Similarly, the retention of coronavirus glycoproteins by the endoplasmic reticulum, and of bunyavirus glycoproteins by the Golgi, are thought to reflect the operation of the same cellular mechanisms that retain resident cellular proteins in these organelles. The localization of viral membrane proteins is of particular importance, as it determines the location of viral assembly and budding.

As described above, the lipids of the viral membrane are taken from the host cell membrane during budding. No new lipids are specifically synthesized in response to viral infection, and viruses seem to tolerate wide variations in their lipid composition. Alterations in cellular lipid metabolism have been reported to result from some viral infections in cultured cells, but these are most likely secondary to other cytopathic effects; there is no indication that they play an important role in the progress of the infection.

Virus Assembly

The budding process consists of the wrapping of a specific piece of membrane around the previously assembled nucleocapsid, which contains the viral genome. The process is shown diagrammatically in **Fig. 5**. The specificity of the process is remarkable in

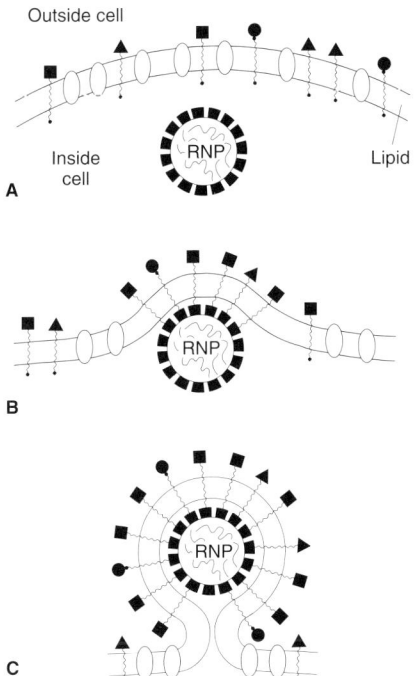

Figure 5 One kind of virus budding. Viral glycoproteins, inserted into the cellular membrane at the endoplasmic reticulum (**Fig. 4**), associate with the assembled viral nucleocapsid. The direct association pictured here is characteristic of togaviruses. For other viruses, possessing helical nucleocapsids, the association is mediated by a peripheral membrane protein. Cellular membrane proteins are excluded from the envelope of the mature virion. This may occur during assembly, as pictured, or by prior formation of a viral membrane patch, before the nucleocapsid arrives at the membrane.

that the completed viral envelope contains viral proteins and host cell lipids almost exclusively, with host cell membrane proteins being almost completely excluded.

Viruses can bud anywhere in the endoplasmic reticulum–Golgi–plasma membrane pathway shown in **Fig. 4**. While the parmyxo-, orthomyxo-, rhabdo- and togaviruses (and many others) generally bud from the plasma membrane, they have also been shown to bud intracellularly under certain conditions. Other viruses normally bud intracellularly, from the endoplasmic reticulum or Golgi apparatus, e.g. coronaviruses and bunyaviruses, respectively. In these cases the nucleocapsid, assembled in the cytoplasm, buds into the lumen of the appropriate organelle. The assembled virus is often seen inside vesicles in electron micrographs, producing a double-shelled appearance. Eventually, the newly formed virion may be secreted out of the cell through the normal secretory pathway, although this does not always occur efficiently.

In many cases viral assembly occurs at the plasma membrane. Some retroviruses assemble there, while others do not; this has provided a classical basis for distinguishing between different types of retroviruses. In orthomyxo-, paramyxo- and rhabdoviruses, budding is mediated by a peripheral membrane protein (called M). Surprisingly, this protein does not interact specifically with the corresponding viral membrane glycoproteins; in fact, successful budding has been observed in the complete absence of viral glycoproteins. This lack of specificity has made possible the creation of pseudotype viruses, possessing the encapsidated genome of one virus and the membrane glycoproteins of another. Since the membrane proteins determine host range and host cell specificity (see above), pseudotypes have proven useful in redirecting specific viral genomes to alternate host cells.

In contrast, togaviruses, which lack any M protein, possess an icosahedral nucleocapsid, which interacts directly with the viral membrane protein. Completed virions contain an equal number of nucleocapsid and membrane protein molecules. Both are in a similar geometric arrangement, so in this case specific interaction between the two proteins appears likely.

See also: **Human immunodeficiency viruses (*Retroviridae*): Molecular biology, Anti-retroviral agents, General features; Influenza viruses (*Orthomyxoviridae*): General features, Molecular biology, Structure of antigens; Pathogenesis: Animal viruses; Replication of viruses; Sendai virus (*Paramyxoviridae*); Virus structure: Atomic structure, Principles of virus structure; Viral receptors.**

Further Reading

Hernandez LD, Hoffman LR, Wolfsberg TG and White JM (1996) Virus–cell and cell–cell fusion. *Ann. Rev. Cell Dev. Biol.* 12: 627.

Lenard J (1996) Negative-strand virus M and retrovirus MA proteins: all in a family? *Virology* 216: 289.

Lodish H, Baltimore D, Berk A *et al* (1995) Synthesis of plasma membrane, secretory and lysosomal proteins. In: *Molecular Cell Biology* 3rd edn, p. 669. New York: Freeman.

VIRAL RECEPTORS

Horacio U Saragovi, **Gordon J Sauvé** and **Mark I Greene**, University of Pennsylvania School of Medicine, Philadelphia, Pennsylvania, USA

Copyright © 1999 Academic Press

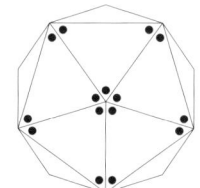

Introduction

Virus–host interactions are complex processes that span binding to cells, entry, dissemination and finally lytic or persistent infection. The first step, binding to host molecules that serve as viral receptors, is critical in all subsequent events. However, host cell alterations can occur in the virtual absence of entry and infection. These effects are due to viral binding to the cellular receptor and the activation of second messenger systems linked to the receptor.

Several viruses reportedly exploit cellular molecules for binding (see **Table 1**). Two interesting examples are the human immunodeficiency virus (HIV) and the vaccinia virus. HIV gp120 appears to bind to two distinct molecules, CD4 in T cells and galactosylceramide in brain. No homologies have been reported between gp120 and Class II major histocompatibility complex (MHC) molecules which are the biological ligand of CD4. Furthermore, it seems that the sites of CD4–Class II interaction are distinct from sites of CD4–gp120 interaction. This example emphasizes the evolution of the gp120 molecule as an effective binding agent for two completely different receptors. In contrast, the vaccinia VGF protein appears to bind to the epidermal growth factor (EGF) receptor. Vaccinia virus VGF is partially homologous to EGF which may explain its binding to EGF receptors. Therefore, some viruses may mimic the biological ligand of the cellular receptor.

Viruses have been proven to be invaluable tools in the molecular dissection of cellular processes and immune regulation. We have been studying the cellular receptor for reovirus type 3 and the role of this receptor in growth and development. Reoviruses provide an excellent model for the study of viral binding which includes biological effects. Furthermore, the as yet unknown structure of the reovirus receptor and its putative biological ligand provides an interesting system in which receptor biological function can be analyzed. In the following section we describe the role of reovirus type 3 cellular receptor in growth and differentiation of a variety of tissue types. New findings also point to the development of novel vaccines and drugs to treat viral infections.

The Reovirus Type 3 Cellular Receptor (Reo3R)

Reo3R was initially analyzed by Fields and colleagues when mammalian lymphocytes and neurons were recognized to express a molecule utilized by the reovirus as its attachment site. Initially, cellular tropism by reovirus type 3 was linked to the expression of the viral hemagglutinin (HA) encoded by the $\sigma 1$ viral gene. Later, receptor-ligand assays using murine cells and labeled virus demonstrated that reovirus type 3 binds to lymphoid cells and fibroblasts with similar affinity. In contrast, reovirus type 1 or a recombinant construct of reovirus type 3 expressing type 1 HA was found to bind to fibroblast L cells but did not bind to lymphocytes (**Table 2**). The viral HA determines both the serotype specificity and the ability of reovirus to bind to cells. Thus, the HA type 1 (HA1) and HA type 3 (HA3) appear to recognize and bind to different and nonoverlapping structures on cell surfaces. These cell surface molecules bound by viral HA are exploited as cellular receptors for reovirus.

Table 1 Cell surface molecules that serve as viral receptors

Virus	Putative receptor
Vaccinia	EGF receptor
Sendai	Gangliosides
Epstein–Barr	C3d receptor
Lactic dehydrogenase	Ia and Fc receptors
Rabies	Acetylcholine receptors
Rhinovirus	ICAM-I adhesion molecules
HIV (in T cells)	CD4
HIV (in brain)	Galactosylceramide

Abbreviations: EGF, epidermal growth factor; HIV, human immunodeficiency virus.

Table 2 Binding affinity of *Reoviridae* to murine cell lines

Cell type	K_d for reovirus type 3 (nM)	K_d for reovirus type 1 (nM)
R1.1 thymoma	0.6	Not detected
Fibroblast cells	0.8	0.4

The R1.1 murine thymoma cells express $\sim 50\,000$ Reo3R molecules per cell and the murine L fibroblasts express $\sim 100\,000$ Reo3R molecules per cell.

Table 3 Sequence comparison of MAb 87.92.6 variable heavy (V_H) and light (V_L) chains with HA3

87.92.6 V_H	43	Q	G	L	E	W	I	G	R	I	D	P	A	N	G		56
Reovirus HA3	317	Q	S	M	–	W	I	G	I	V	S	**Y**	**S**	**G**	**S**	**G**	**L**	N	332
87.92.6 V_L	39	K	P	G	K	T	N	K	L	L	I	**Y**	**S**	**G**	**S**	**T**	**L**	Q	55
									I				Reo3R binding				I	

Amino acid sequence similarity of the reovirus type 3 σ1 protein and MAb 87.92.6 light chain CDR2 is shown using the single-letter code. Amino acid numbers of the proteins are shown, and the regions within HA3 and V_L required for Reo3R binding are indicated. Bold letters indicate amino acid homology between viral protein and mAb.

To analyze Reo3R in detail, we obtained a murine monoclonal antibody (MAb) directed against the receptor. The anti-Reo3R MAb 87.92.6 was raised against MAb 9BG5 which binds and neutralizes HA3. Thus, the interactions of MAb 9BG5 with MAb 87.92.6 or HA3, and the interactions of HA3 and MAb 87.92.6 with the cellular receptor, can be studied. An important feature of this model is that binding to Reo3R is accomplished by a structure that is shared by MAb 87.92.6, the HA3 and their analogues. It has been demonstrated that the light chain variable region (V_L) of MAb 87.92.6 (specifically the complementarity determining region 2; CDR2) bears the internal image of HA3 (**Table 3**), emphasizing the relevance of structural domains in binding to Reo3R. Conversely, it has been hypothesized that Reo3R may bear the internal image of MAb 9BG5. Work in progress towards the molecular cloning of Reo3R cDNA will answer this question.

Given the primary sequence and structural similarity between HA3 and MAb 87.92.6, it is not surprising that the MAb prevents reovirus type 3 attachment to cells and primes mice to develop humoral or cellular immunity to the virus. Most importantly, binding of MAb 87.92.6 or its peptide analogues to Reo3R elicits receptor-mediated biological effects identical to those elicited by binding of inactivated virus to cells. Functional effects include the inhibition of mitogen-induced proliferation of T cells, maturation of oligodendrocytes and demyelination of neurons. Peptide analogues derived from V_L amino acids 45–55, as well as a synthetic nonaminoacid-based β-loop structure which mimics this region, also bind to Reo3R and elicit functional responses, indicating that receptor ligation generates the biological effects. Thus the technology developed using the Reo3R system might lead to the development of new drugs to modulate immune responses and affect neural development.

Effects mediated upon Reo3R binding are so profound and significant that an important role for the cellular receptor is suggested, resulting in an increased interest in understanding the cognate function of this surface molecule. Unlike other viral receptors the biological functions of which are known (e.g. CD4 is the HIV receptor and its biological ligands are Class II MHC gene products), it is not known whether Reo3R is also a true receptor with a true ligand. We will discuss evidence addressing this question in the next section.

Functional Studies of Reo3R

Reoviral infection takes place primarily in the gut epithelium, and can be spread to neutral tissue by an as yet unclear mechanism. The uncoupling of viral entry and replication processes is emphasized by the fact that, while productive infection occurs in the epithelium, latent chronic infection can take place in lymphoid cells. Obviously Reo3R must be expressed on epithelial, neural and lymphoid tissues for viral binding, and studies with MAb 87.92.6 have determined that the viral receptor is the same for these three cell types. However, the varied effects manifested upon receptor ligation suggest that expression of Reo3R has different repercussions for different tissues. Therefore, in order better to understand the function of Reo3R, we have studied its expression and the functional consequences of receptor engagement with the use of anti-Reo3R MAb 87.92.6.

Lymphoid cells

Most (80%) freshly isolated murine splenic B cells express Reo3R. In contrast, only a small proportion (5–15%) of resting splenic T cells and thymocytes express Reo3R. Interestingly, activation of T cells with concanavalinA (ConA) mitogen induces expression of Reo3R to detectable levels after 24h and optimally after 36h. Therefore, Reo3R is constitutively expressed in splenic B cells, but is inducible in T-cells, suggesting that differential regulation of transcription or translation occurs. The kinetics of expression in T cells parallel those of other inducible T-cell activation markers such as interleukin 2 (IL-2) receptor p55 (α) subunit and transferrin receptor, suggesting that Reo3R plays an important role in cellular immunity. After expression of Reo3R has been induced in T cells, binding by inactivated virus,

MAb 87.92.6, peptides derived for the MAb V_L domain or synthetic compounds that mimic these structures to the cell surface leads to a dramatic inhibition of proliferation even in the presence of the powerful stimulator ConA.

Litle is known about the mechanism of inhibition, but it does not involve cell death. Alternative possibilities include (i) blocking of an as yet unidentified biological ligand to the receptor or (ii) induction of receptor-mediated inhibitory signals. An exciting recent development has been the demonstration that inhibitory effects require ligation of Reo3R at the cell surface. In contrast to the negative growth regulation induced by Reo3R extracellular ligation, intracellular ligation has no effect on T cell proliferation. The data, however, do not clarify which of the possible mechanisms for inhibition may be operational.

Central nervous system (CNS)

The CNS is an important target of reovirus type 3 infection. Mature oligodendrocytes and both type 1 and 2 astrocytes, but not glial progenitor cells, express Reo3R. Surface Reo3R appears at an early stage of development prior to expression of myelin basic protein (MBP).

The effects of MAb 87.92.6 and its peptides in neural tissue have been tested *in vitro* and *in vivo*. In both systems neural tissue biology is altered and demyelination is induced, suggesting that Reo3R normally plays an important role in oligodendrocyte differentiation. Thus, it may be possible to create analogues of MAb 87.92.6 that stimulate myelin synthesis *in vivo* leading to the development of new drugs to modulate immune responses and affect neural development. A recent advance in this area has shown that synthetic analogues of MAb 87.92.6 bind Reo3R and induce functional effects, emphasizing the usefulness of viruses in analyzing receptor biology.

Future studies will reveal the structure and function of Reo3R, define the true physiological ligand(s) and provide insights into the signal transducing pathways by which this receptor exerts its important effects.

See also: **Cell structure and function in virus infections; Human immunodeficiency viruses (*Retroviridae*): General features; Pathogenesis: Animal viruses; Reoviruses (*Reoviridae*): General features; Replication of viruses; Virus–host cell interactions.**

Further Reading

Cohen JA *et al* (1989) In: Sercarz E (ed.) *Antigenic Determinants and Immune Regulation*, vol 46, p. 126. Basel: Karger.

Holmes KV, Tresnan DB and Zelus BD (1997) Virus-receptor interactions in the enteric tract. Virus-receptor interactions. *Adv. Exp. Med. Biol.* 412: 125.

Miller AD (1996) Cell-surface receptors for retroviruses and implications for gene transfer. *Proc. Natl Acad. Sci. USA* 93(21): 11407.

Moore JP, Trkola A and Dragic T (1997) Co-receptors for HIV-1 entry. *Curr. Opin. Immunol.* 9(4): 551.

Norkin LC (1995) Virus receptors: implications for pathogenesis and the design of antiviral agents. *Clin. Microbiol. Rev.* 8(2): 293.

Williams WV *et al* (1990) *Trends Biotechnol.* 8: 256.

[This article is reproduced from the 1st edn (1994).]

VIROIDS

Robert A Owens, Molecular Plant Pathology Laboratory, Beltsville Agricultural Research Center, Beltsville, Maryland, USA

Copyright © 1999 Academic Press

Introduction

Viroids are the smallest known agents of infectious disease – small (246–375 nucleotides), highly structured, circular, single-stranded RNAs which lack both a protein capsid and detectable messenger RNA activity. Whereas viruses have been described as 'obligate parasites of the cell's translational system' and supply some or most of the genetic information required for their replication, viroids can be regarded as 'obligate parasites of the cell's transcriptional machinery'. Thus far, viroids are known to infect only plants.

History

While scientific investigation of plant diseases now known to be caused by plant viruses did not begin until the late nineteenth century, the earliest written records of plant viral disease date to the eighth century AD. The first viroid disease to be studied by plant pathologists was potato spindle tuber disease. In 1923, its infectious nature and ability to spread in the field led Schultz and Folsom to group potato spindle tuber disease with several other 'degeneration diseases' of potatoes. These maladies, long attributed to senility, 'reversion', or loss of vigor caused by prolonged asexual reproduction, are now known to be caused by infection with conventional RNA viruses. Nearly 50 years were to elapse between the first published descriptions of potato spindle tuber disease and Diener's 1971 demonstration of the fundamental differences between the structure and properties of its causal agent, potato spindle tuber viroid (PSTVd), and those of conventional plant viruses.

Growers and plant pathologists are unlikely to have simply overlooked diseases with symptoms as severe as those of chrysanthemum stunt or cucumber pale fruit, two other viroid diseases first reported after World War II. Thus, certain aspects of modern agricultural practice seem to have favored the appearance of viroid diseases in the twentieth century. Large-scale monoculture of genetically identical crops and the commercial propagation/distribution of many cultivars are two comparatively modern developments which can facilitate the development of serious disease problems following the chance transfer of viroids from wild hosts to cultivated plants.

Genome Structure

Efforts to understand how viroids replicate and cause disease without the assistance of any viroid-encoded polypeptides have prompted detailed analysis of their structure. Viroids possess rather unusual properties for single-stranded RNAs (e.g. a pronounced resistance to digestion by ribonuclease and a highly cooperative thermal denaturation profile), leading to an early realization that they might have an unusual higher-order structure. Their small size also made viroids tempting objects for detailed structural investigation.

To date, the complete sequences of more than 20 distinct viroid species plus a large number of sequence variants have been determined (**Table 1**). All known viroids are single-stranded circular RNAs which contain 246–399 unmodified nucleotides and lack any unusual 2,′5′-phosphodiester bonds or 2′-phosphate moieties. Electron microscopy, optical melting and other physicochemical studies, and theoretical calculations of their lowest free-energy secondary structure all indicate that PSTVd and related viroids assume a highly base-paired, rod-like conformation *in vitro* (**Fig. 1**). Pairwise sequence comparisons of PSTVd with several related viroids suggest that the series of short double helices and small internal loops which comprise this so-called 'native' structure are organized into five domains whose boundaries are defined by sharp changes in sequence similarity.

As implied by its name, the 'conserved central domain' is the most highly conserved viroid domain and is believed to contain the site where multimeric viroid RNAs are cleaved and ligated to form circular progeny. The 'pathogenicity domain' contains one or more structural elements which modulate symptom expression, and the relatively small 'variable domain' exhibits the greatest sequence variability between otherwise closely-related viroids. The two 'terminal domains' appear to play an important role in viroid replication and evolution. Although these five domains were first identified in members of the PSTVd viroid group, ASSVd and related viroids also contain a similar domain arrangement. (See **Table 1** for explanation of abbreviations.) Certain viroids such as *Columnea* latent viroid appear to be 'mosaic molecules' formed by exchange of domains between two or more viroids infecting the same cell. Individual plants of the *Coleus blumei* cultivar 'Ruhm von Luxemburg' may contain as many as three viroid species, one of which (i.e. CbVd 2) represents a fusion product of the right half of CbVd 1 and the left half of CbVd 3. RNA rearrangement/recombination can also occur within individual domains, thereby leading, in the case of CCCVd, to duplication of the right terminal domain plus part of the variable domain, as disease progresses. The presence of domains in ASBVd and other ribozyme-containing viroids remains uncertain pending identification of additional group members.

Much less is currently known about viroid tertiary structure, especially *in vivo* where these molecules accumulate as ribonucleoprotein particles. Although the extended, rod-like nature of the 'native' structure might suggest that viroids lack significant tertiary structure, the ability of UV irradiation to crosslink certain nucleotides within the conserved central domain of PSTVd provided the first definitive evidence for such tertiary interactions. Similar UV-sensitive structural elements have also been discovered in a number of other RNAs, including 5S ribosomal RNA, adenovirus VAI RNA, and the viroid-like domain of the hepatitis delta virus genome. Studies of the spontaneous self-cleavage of various ASBVd-related RNAs as well as the nuclease-dependent conversion of multimeric PSTVd RNAs into monomers have provided additional evidence for the functional importance of viroid tertiary structure.

Classification

Viroids of known sequence have recently been assigned to one of two taxonomic families based upon differences in the structural and functional properties of their genomes (**Table 1**). Members of the *Pospiviroidae* (type member, potato spindle tuber viroid) have a rod-like secondary structure that contains five structural–functional domains. Two members of the *Avsunviroidae* (type member, avocado sunblotch viroid), in contrast, appear to adopt a branched conformation, and multimeric RNAs of all three known family members undergo spontaneous self-cleavage *in vitro*. Groups of independently replicating sequence variants that show >90% sequence homology in pairwise comparisons have been arbitrarily defined as viroid species.

Phylogenetic evidence for an evolutionary link between viroids and other viroid-like subviral RNAs has been presented by Elena *et al* (**Fig. 2**). Among several subviral RNAs possibly related to viroids is carnation small viroid-like RNA, a 275 nt circular molecule with self-cleaving hammerhead structures in both its plus and minus strands. This novel retroviroid-like element shares certain features with both viroids and a small RNA transcript from newt.

Host Range and Transmission

All viroids are mechanically transmissible, and most are naturally transmitted from plant to plant by humans and their tools. Nevertheless, individual viroids vary greatly in their ability to infect and replicate in different plant species. PSTVd can replicate in about 160 primarily solanaceous hosts, while only two members of the Lauraceae are known

Table 1 Viroids of known nucleotide sequence (1998)

Family[a]	Genus[a]	Name	Abbreviation	Nucleotides[b]
Pospiviroidae	Pospiviroid	Chrysanthemum stunt	CSVd	354–356
		Citrus exocortis	CEVd	368–375 (463)
		Columnea latent	CLVd	370–373
		Iresine	IrVd	370
		Mexican papita	MPVd	359–360
		Potato spindle tuber	PSTVd	358–361 (341)
		Tomato apical stunt	TASVd	360–363
		Tomato planta macho	TPMVd	360
	Cocadviroid	Citrus viroid IV	CVd-IV	284
		Coconut cadang-cadang	CCCVd	246–247 (287–301)
		Coconut tinangaja	CTiVd	254
		Hop latent	HLVd	256
	Hostuviroid	Hop stunt[c]	HSVd	294–303
	Apscaviroid	Apple dimple fruit	ADFVd	306
		Apple scar skin[d]	ASSVd	329–334
		Australian grapevine	AGVd	369
		Citrus bent leaf	CBLVd	315, 318
		Citrus viroid III	CVd-III	294, 297
		Grapevine yellow speckle 1	GYSVd 1	336–388
		Grapevine yellow speckle 2	GYSVd 2	363
		Pear blister canker	PBCVd	315
	Coleviroid	*Coleus blumei* 1	CbVd 1	248–251
		Coleus blumei 2	CbVd 2	301
		Coleus blumei 3	CbVd 3	361–364
Avsunviroidae	Avsunviroid	Avocado sunblotch	ASBVd	246–251
	Pelamoviroid	Chrysanthemum chlorotic mottle	CChMVd	398, 399
		Peach latent mosaic	PLMVd	336–337

[a] Classification follows scheme proposed by Flores *et al* (see Seventh Report of the International Committee on Taxonomy of Viruses). The nucleotide sequences of apple fruit crinkle, burdock stunt, eggplant latent, *Nicotiana glutinosa* stunt, pigeon pea mosaic mottle and tomato bunchy top viroids are currently unknown; thus, these viroids have not been assigned to specific genera.
[b] Sizes of variants containing insertions or deletions arising *in vivo* are shown in parentheses.
[c] Includes cucumber pale fruit, citrus cachexia, peach dapple and plum dapple viroids.
[d] Includes pear rusty skin and dapple apple viroids.
[e] Formerly named grapevine viroid 1B.

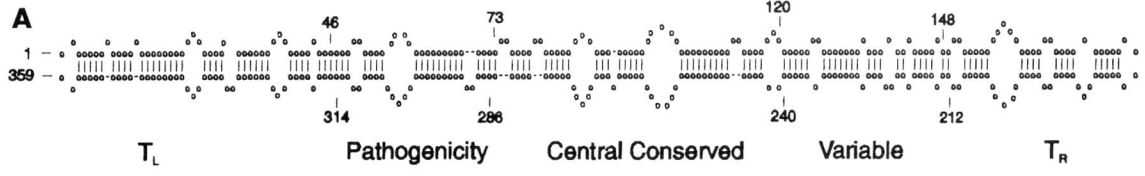

Potato spindle tuber viroid

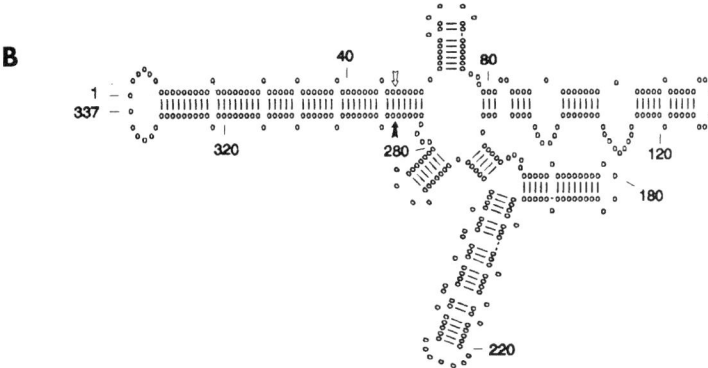

Peach latent mosaic viroid

Figure 1 Secondary structures of potato spindle tuber and peach latent mosaic viroids. (**A**) A rod-like secondary structure for PSTVd is supported by a variety of physical studies as well as chemical and enzymatic mapping data. Boundaries of the terminal-left (T_L), pathogenicity, central conserved, variable and terminal-right (T_R) domains are indicated by vertical lines. (**B**) Proposed lowest-free-energy structure of PLMVd. Predicted self-cleavage sites in the plus and minus strands are indicated by filled and open arrows, respectively. (Redrawn from Hernandez and Flores (1991) *Proc. Natl. Acad. Sci. USA* 89: 3711.)

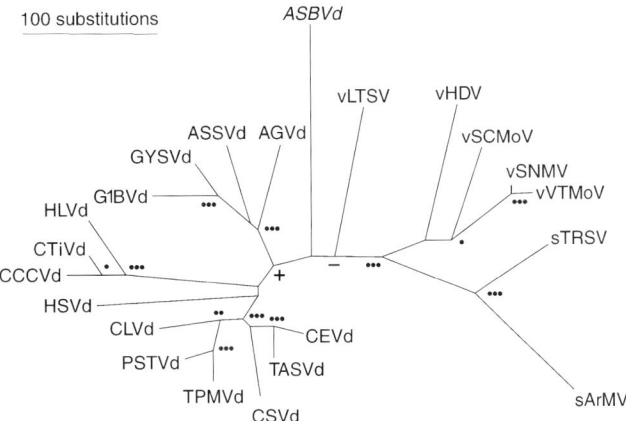

Figure 2 Consensus phylogenetic tree containing 22 viroids, viroid-like satellite RNAs and the viroid-like domain of hepatitis delta virus RNA. ASBVd has been taken as outgroup. •••, Group monophyletic in all 1000 bootstrap replicates; ••, monophyletic in more than 99%; •, in more than 95%; +, in more than 90%; and −, in more than 80% of all replicates. From ASBVd to the left of the figure groups are considered as being within the viroid family, and from ASBVd to the right (including the viroid-like domain of HDV RNA) as within the satellite family. For example, satellite tobacco ringspot virus (sTRSV) and satellite *Arabis* mosaic virus (sArMV) (satellite family) or CCCVd, CTiVd and HLVd (viroid family) conformed to two well-defined monophyletic groups in all bootstrap replicates. G1BVd, grapevine viroid 1B; LTSV, Lucerne transient streak virus; ScMoV, subterranean clover mottle virus; SNMV, *Solanum nodiflorum* mosaic virus; VTMoV, velvet tobacco mottle virus. Other abbreviations as in **Table 1**. (From Elena SF *et al* (1991) *Proc. Natl. Acad. Sci. USA* 88: 5631, with permission.)

to support ASBVd replication. HSVd has a particularly wide host range which includes several herbaceous species as well as woody perennials (e.g. grapes, citrus and various *Prunus* spp.). Many natural hosts of viroids are either vegetatively propagated crops, such as potato and chrysanthemum, or those that are subjected to repeated grafting or pruning operations. PSTVd, ASBVd and CbVd can all be vertically transmitted through pollen and/or true seed, but the significance of this mode of transmission in the natural spread of disease is unclear. PSTVd can be encapsidated by potato leafroll luteovirus (PLRV) as well as velvet tobacco mottle sobemovirus, and epidemiological surveys suggest that PLRV can facilitate viroid spread under field conditions.

Commonly used techniques for the experimental transmission of viroids include the standard leaf abrasion methods developed for use with conventional viruses, various 'razor slashing' methods in which phloem tissue in the stem or petiole is inoculated via cuts made with a razor blade previously dipped into the inoculum, and, in the case of CCCVd, high-pressure injection into folded apical leaves. PSTVd and HSVd have also been experimentally transmitted by 'Agroinoculation', a technique in which a modified *Agrobacterium tumefaciens* Ti plasmid is used to introduce full-length viroid cDNA into the potential host cell. In both cases, Agro-inoculation was able to overcome a marked host resistance to mechanical inoculation. Identification of the molecular mechanism(s) which determine host range remains an important research goal.

Symptomatology

Viroids and conventional plant viruses induce a very similar range of macroscopic symptoms (and presumably metabolic changes) in their hosts. Symptom expression is usually optimal at the same relatively high temperatures that promote viroid replication (i.e. 30–33°C). Prominent among metabolic changes are dramatic alterations in growth regulator levels. Stunting and leaf epinasty (a downward curling of the leaf lamina resulting from unbalanced growth within the various cell layers) are often considered the classic symptoms of viroid infection, and other commonly observed symptoms include vein clearing, veinal discoloration or necrosis, and the appearance of localized chlorotic/necrotic spots or mottling in the foliage. Viroid infections only rarely kill the host (**Figs 3** and **4**).

Viroid infections are also accompanied by a number of cytopathic effects – various chloroplast and cell wall abnormalities, the formation of membranous structures (so-called 'plasmalemmasomes' or 'paramural bodies') in the cytoplasm, and the accumulation of electron-dense deposits in both chloroplasts and cytoplasm. A combination of subcellular fractionation and *in situ* hybridization studies has shown that the plus and minus strands of PSTVd and related viroids both accumulate in the nucleolus. Precise partitioning between the nucleoplasm and nucleolus remains to be established, but this nucleolar localization may have important implications for replication and pathogenicity. ASBVd, in contrast, appears to be associated with chloroplast thalykoid membranes rather than the nucleoli of infected cells, thereby raisng the possibility that a host-encoded enzyme other than RNA polymerase II may be responsible for its replication (see below).

Geographic Distribution

Viroids such as PSTVd, HSVd, CEVd and ASBVd are widely distributed throughout the world, while others have never been detected outside the areas where they were first reported. Several factors may contribute to this variation in distribution pattern. Among the crops most affected by viroid diseases are a number of valuable woody perennials such as grapes, citrus, various pome and stone fruits, and hops. Propagation and distribution of improved cultivars is becoming increasingly commercialized, with the result that many are now grown worldwide. The international exchange of plant germplasm has also continued to increase at a rapid rate. In both instances, the large number of latent (asymptomatic) hosts facilitates viroid spread. Also, several newly-discovered viroids affect either tropical or subtropical crops. The combination of the generally high temperature optimum for viroid replication and an increased interest in diseases affecting tropical crops is likely to cause a continued shift in the known geographic distribution of viroid diseases.

Epidemiology and Control

While many viroids were first detected in ornamental or crop plants, most viroid diseases are thought to be the result of their chance transfer from endemically-infected wild species to susceptible cultivars. Several lines of circumstantial evidence are consistent with this hypothesis:

- The experimental host ranges of several viroids include many wild species, and these wild species often tolerate viroid replication without the appearance of recognizable disease symptoms.
- Although coevolution of host and pathogen is often accompanied by appearance of gene-for-gene ver-

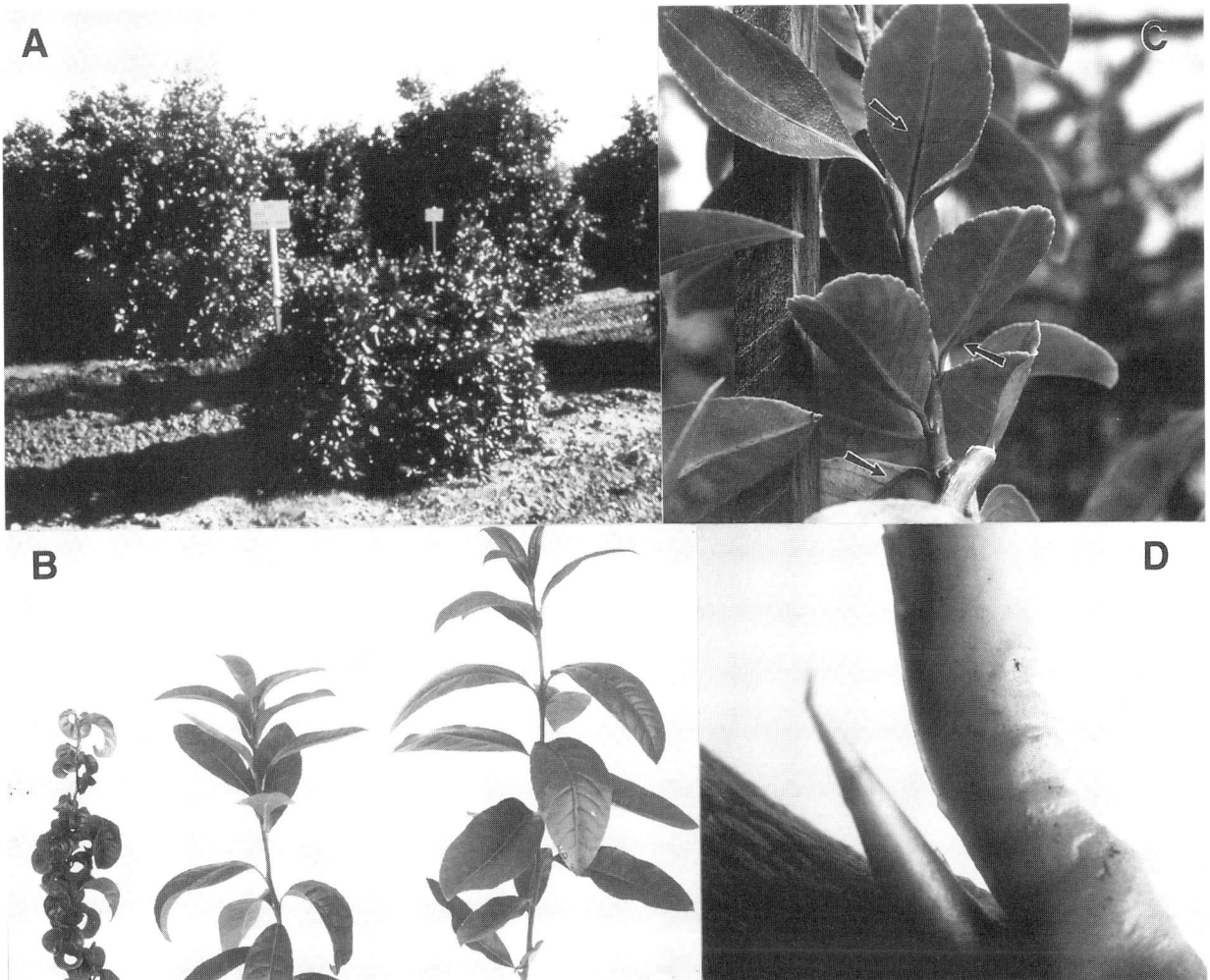

Figure 3 Characteristic symptoms of viroid infection in citrus. (**A**) Dwarfing of sweet orange induced by citrus viroid(s). Note the difference in height between the infected tree (foreground) and uninfected trees. (**B**) Leaf epinasty in 'Etrog' citron induced by severe (left) and mild (center) isolates of citrus exocortis viroid. The plant on the right is an uninfected control. (**C, D**) Additional symptoms of viroid infection in 'Etrog' citron: Midvein and petiole browning (arrows) and petiole wrinkling induced by citrus viroid III. (Photographs courtesy of S.M. Garnsey and L. Levy.)

tical resistance, no useful sources of resistance to PSTVd has been identified in the cultivated potato.
- Viroids and/or viroid-related RNAs closely related to TPMVd and CCCVd have been detected in weeds and other wild vegetation growing near fields containing viroid-infected plants.

Viroid diseases may also arise by transfer between cultivated crop species. Studies conducted in the People's Republic of China have shown that pears provide a latent reservoir for ASSVd; likewise, while there is no obvious correlation between disease status and the presence of HSVd in grapes, this viroid is known to cause severe disease in hops. In both instances, the two crops are often grown in close proximity.

All viroid diseases pose a potential threat to agriculture, and several are of considerable economic importance. Coconut cadang-cadang has killed over 30 million palms in the Philippines since it was first recognized in the early 1930s, and estimates of the resulting loss in copra production are in the range of US $80–100 per tree (1987 estimate). Ready transmission of PSTVd by vegetative propagation, foliar contact and true seed or pollen poses a potentially serious threat to potato production, germplasm collections and breeding programs. For many plant viruses, the preferred method of prevention involves incorporation of genetic resistance into the genomes of commercially desirable cultivars. Unfortunately, no useful sources of natural resistance to viroid disease are known, and thermotherapy and/or mer-

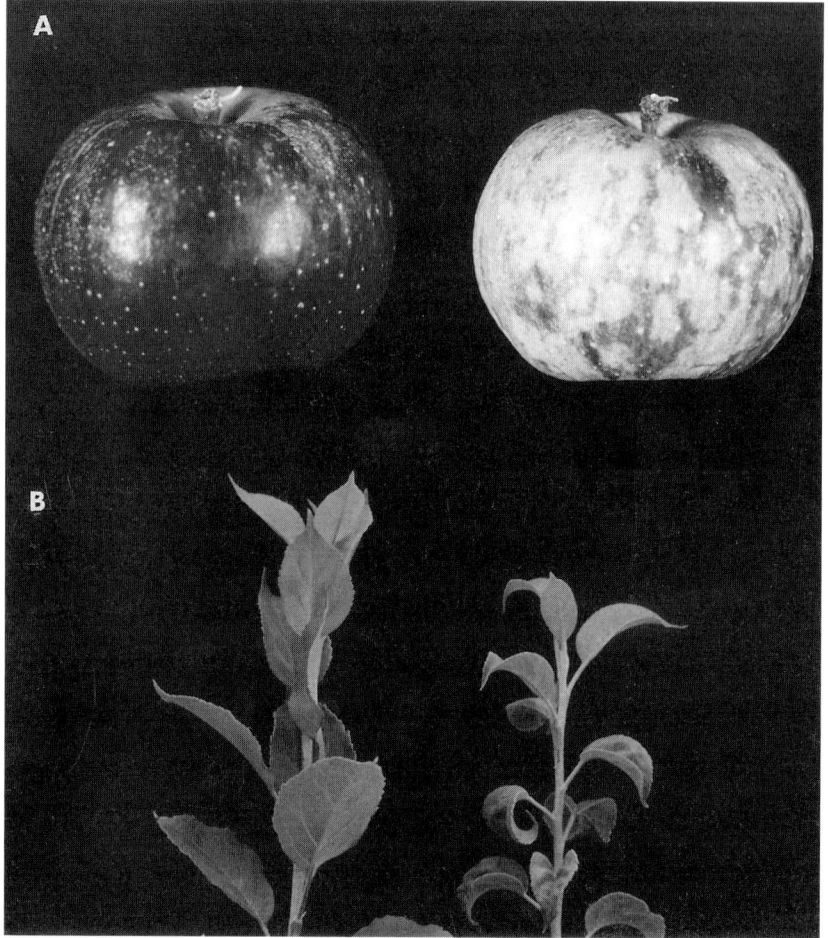

Figure 4 Characteristic symptoms of viroid infection in apple. (**A**) Normal (left) and dappled (right) fruit from 5-year-old orchard-grown 'Lord Lambourne' trees. The tree producing dappled fruit was infected with apple scar skin viroid. (**B**) Leaf epinasty induced by apple scar skin viroid in the variety 'Stark's Earliest'. The plant on the left is an uninfected control. (Photographs courtesy of E.V. Podleckis.)

istem culture protocols have not been widely adopted. Thus, suitable diagnostic tests for the rapid, specific and reliable detection of viroids continue to play a prominent role in disease control efforts.

Tests based upon their unique physical or chemical properties have largely supplanted biological assays for viroid detection. Problems associated with viroid bioassays include the often extended period of time required for completion (weeks to months) and difficulties in detecting mild or latent strains of the pathogen. Several rapid (1–2 day) protocols involving two-dimensional or bidirectional polyacrylamide gel electrophoresis have been developed which take advantage of the circular nature of viroids. Using these protocols, subnanogram amounts of viroid can be unambiguously detected without the use of radioactive isotopes, but neither bioassay nor electrophoretic assays are well suited for the routine analysis of large numbers of samples. Because viroids lack a protein capsid, antibody-based diagnostic techniques are not applicable.

In recent years, diagnostic procedures based upon nucleic acid hybridization or the polymerase chain reaction have become widely used. The simplest methods involve the hybridization of a highly radioactive viroid-complementary DNA or RNA probe to viroid samples that have been bound to a solid support, followed by autoradiographic detection of the resulting DNA–RNA or RNA–RNA hybrids. Such conventional 'dot blot' assays can detect picogram amounts of viroids using clarified plant sap rather than purified nucleic acid as the viroid source, but sample preparation is often a significant stumbling block. Polymerase chain reaction-based protocols are finding increasing acceptance in those cases where either this level of sensitivity is inadequate or a number of closely-related viroids are present in the same sample.

Molecular Biology

Although apparently devoid of messenger RNA activity, viroids replicate autonomously and induce disease in a wide variety of plant species. The many gaps in our present understanding of the biological properties of these unusual molecules have been aptly summarized by Diener as a series of questions:

- What molecular signals do viroids possess (and cellular RNAs evidently lack) that induce certain host enzyme(s) to accept them as templates for the synthesis of complementary RNA molecules?
- What are the molecular mechanisms responsible for viroid replication? Are these mechanisms also operative in uninfected cells? If so, what are their functions?
- How do viroids induce disease? In the absence of viroid-specified proteins, disease must arise from direct interaction(s) of viroids (or their complementary RNA molecules) with as yet unidentified host cell constituents.
- What are the molecular determinants of viroid host range? Are viroids restricted to higher plants, or do they have counterparts in animals?
- How did viroids originate?

Over the past several years, considerable information has accumulated concerning the molecular biology of viroid replication, pathogenesis and host range determination. The precise nature of the molecular signals involved nevertheless remains elusive.

Replication

Viroid replication is believed to proceed via a 'rolling circle' mechanism involving the synthesis of a minus-strand RNA template. A variety of multimeric plus- and minus-strand viroid RNAs have been detected by nucleic acid hybridization. ASBVd replication appears to utilize a symmetric replication cycle in which the multimeric minus strand is first cleaved to unit-length molecules and circularized before serving as template for the synthesis of multimeric ASBV plus strands. PSTVd and related viroids appear to utilize an asymmetric cycle in which the multimeric minus strand is directly copied into a multimeric plus-strand precursor.

A variety of host-encoded enzymes have been implicated in different aspects of viroid replication. Low concentrations of α-amanitin specifically inhibit the synthesis of both PSTVd plus and minus strands in nuclei isolated from infected tomato, strongly suggesting the involvement of RNA-dependent RNA polymerase II in the replication of PSTVd and related viroids. Localization of both the mature viroid and the replicative intermediates within the nucleolus would seem to argue against the involvement of RNA polymerase II in their synthesis, but this contradiction may be more apparent than real. One or more host-encoded nuclease activities appear to be required for the specific cleavage of multimeric PSTVd plus strands, while both plus- and minus-strand ASBVd RNAs transcribed *in vitro* undergo a spontaneous self-cleavage to form linear monomers. The final step in viroid replication is the ligation of linear monomers to form mature circular progeny. Plant cells are known to contain RNA ligase activities which can act upon the 5'-hydroxyl and 2',3'-cyclic phosphate termini formed during either cleavage pathway, and ribonuclease T1 is able to generate circular RNA molecules from PSTVd-specific RNA transcripts by cleavage and intramolecular ligation *in vitro*.

During replication, the rod-like native structure of PSTVd and related viroids must rearrange to assume one or more as-yet-undefined alternative conformations. How a viroid 'switches' between these different conformations remains to be determined. As shown in **Fig. 5**, there is compelling biochemical and molecular genetic evidence for the ability of dimeric ASBVd minus-strand RNA to undergo spontaneous *in vitro* cleavage via two different (but related) structures. The preferred pathway for enzymatic processing of longer-than-unit-length PSTVd plus-strand RNAs seems to involve a cleavage site formed by rearrangement of the conserved central domain, but other less efficient sites can also be used *in vivo*.

Pathogenicity

Both viroid cDNAs and their RNA transcripts are infectious when inoculated on to susceptible plants, a fact which provides a unique opportunity to relate sequence (and hence structural) variation to pathogenicity. Infectivity studies with chimeras constructed by exchanging the pathogenicity domains of naturally occurring mild and severe strains of CEVd have clearly shown that the pathogenicity domain contains important determinants of symptom expression. Sequence variation within the variable domain of CEVd also influenced viroid titer in infected plants. Application of a similar experimental strategy to TASVd revealed the presence of a third pathogenicity determinant located in the left terminal loop.

The ability of novel viroid chimeras to replicate and move normally from cell-to-cell implies certain basic similarities between their structures *in vitro* and *in vivo* but provides no information about the nature of the molecular interactions responsible for symptom development. Viroid infections are accompanied by quantitative changes in a variety of host-encoded

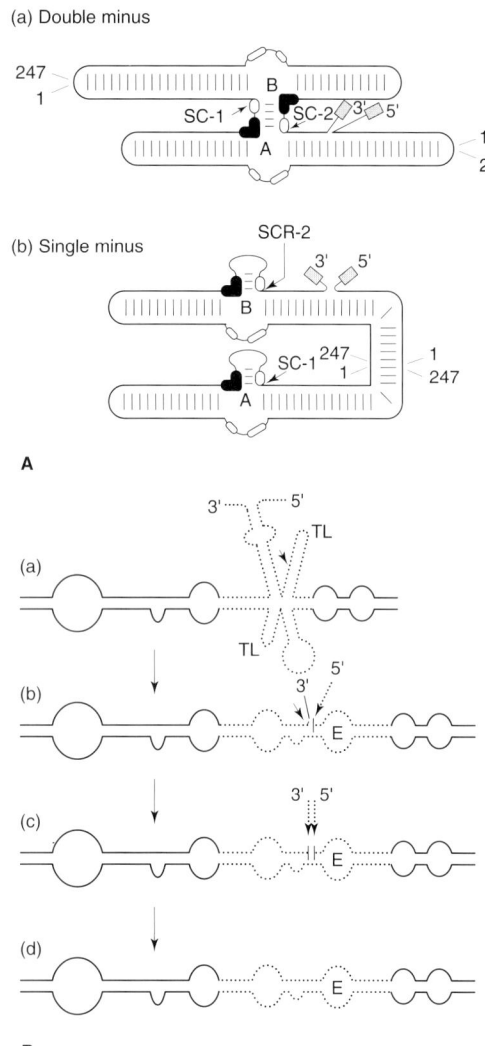

Figure 5 Cleavage of multimeric viroid RNAs requires rearrangement of the native structure. (**A**) A dimeric minus ASBVd RNA transcribed *in vitro* from a *Bst*NI dimeric cDNA clone can fold to produce a structure containing either a double- (**a**) or single- (**b**) hammerhead. Self-cleavage sites, labeled SC-1 and SC-2, are indicated by arrows; stippled boxes, vector sequences at 5′ and 3′ ends; closed boxes, conserved GAAAC sequences labeled A and B; open boxes, remaining conserved nucleotides. Base-pairing is represented by lines between RNA strands. (From Davies C *et al* (1991) *Nucl. Acids Res.* 19: 1893, with permission.) (**B**) Processing of a longer-than-unit-length plus PSTVd RNA transcript in a potato nuclear extract. The central conserved region of the substrate for the first cleavage reaction (**a**) contains a tetraloop (denoted TL). (**b**) After dissociation of the 5′ segment from the cleavage site, the new 5′ end refolds and is stabilized by formation of a UV-sensitive loop E, while the 3′ end partially base-pairs with the lower strand. Single-stranded nucleotides at the 3′ end are then cleaved between positions 95 and 96 (**c**), and ligation of the 5′ and 3′ termini (**d**) results in formation of mature circular progeny. (From Baumstark T *et al* (1997) *EMBO J.* 16: 599, with permission.)

proteins. Certain of these proteins may be 'pathogenesis-related' proteins whose synthesis or activation is part of a general host reaction to both biotic and abiotic stresses; others, such as a 140 kDa protein whose accumulation requires the presence of a replicating low molecular weight viroid or viral satellite RNA, may be more specific. In tobacco, PSTVd infection results in the preferential phosphorylation of a host-encoded 68 kDa protein that is immunologically related to an interferon-inducible, double-stranded RNA-dependent mammalian protein kinase of similar size. Diener and coworkers have presented evidence for the differential activation of the human kinase by PSTVd strains of varying pathogenicity. Although major differences have been reported in the overall three-dimensional conformations of the pathogenicity domain from a series of PSTVd strains, precise cause and effect relationships for the role of protein kinase(s) in viroid pathogenicity remain to be established.

Host range

Perhaps as a result of its involvement in the cleavage/ligation of multimeric plus-strand progeny RNA, a variety of evidence indicates that the central conserved region of PSTVd and related viroids also plays an important role in determining host range. For example, a severe isolate of PSTVd known as KF 440-2 replicates very poorly in tobacco, but a single nucleotide substitution in the so-called 'loop E' portion of the central conserved region results in a dramatic increase in the rate of replication and systemic movement. The biological properties of Columnea latent viroid also suggest that this domain contains one or more host range determinants. As described above, CLVd appears to be a natural mosaic of sequences present in other viroids; phylogenetic analysis (**Fig. 2**) suggests that it can be considered to be a PSTVd-related viroid whose conserved central domain has been replaced by that of HSVd. Like HSVd (but unlike other PSTVd-related viroids), CLVd is able to replicate and cause disease in cucumber.

Origin and Evolution

As discussed by Matthews, available evidence suggests three possible origins for viruses: (1) descent from molecules present in a prebiotic RNA world; (2) descent from normal host RNAs; and (3) degeneration from simple obligate cellular parasites. Present-day plant viruses form four clusters (i.e. single-stranded positive-sense RNA viruses (three superfamilies); plant reoviruses, rhabdoviruses and bunyaviruses; caulimoviruses; and geminiviruses) and the existence of these clusters may reflect their different origins. Much of the early speculation about viroid origin involved their possible origin as 'escaped introns' (i.e. descent from normal host RNAs). More recently, however, viroids have been proposed to represent 'living fossils' of a precellular RNA world that assumed an intracellular mode of existence sometime after the evolution of cellular organisms.

According to Diener, the chief proponent of this view, the inherent stability of viroids and viroid-like RNAs which arises from their small size and circularity would have enhanced the probability of their survival in primitive, error-prone RNA self-replicating systems and assured their complete replication without the need for initiation or termination signals. Most viroids (but not satellite RNAs or random sequences of the same base composition) also display structural periodicities with repeat units of 12, 60 or 80 nucleotides. The high error rate of prebiotic replication systems would be expected to have favored the evolution of polyploid genomes, and the mechanism of viroid replication (i.e. rolling-circle transcription of a circular template) provides an effective means of genome duplication.

Viroids and viroid-like satellite RNAs all possess efficient mechanisms for the precise cleavage of their oligomeric replication intermediates to form monomeric progeny. As discussed earlier, PSTVd and related viroids appear to require proteinaceous host factor(s) for cleavage, but others (the self-cleaving viroids and viroid-like satellite RNAs) function as self-cleaving RNA enzymes far smaller and simpler than those derived from introns. Thus, ASBVd and the other self-cleaving viroids may represent an evolutionary link between viroids and satellite RNAs. No viroid is known to code for protein, a fact that is consistent with the possibility that viroids are phylogenetically older than introns. It is conceivable that introns may be 'captured' viroids, rather than viroids 'escaped' introns.

See also: **Hepatitis Delta virus; Diagnostic techniques: Detection of viral antigens, nucleic acids and specific antibodies; Epidemiology of viral diseases; Pathogenesis: Plant viruses; Plant resistance to viruses: Natural resistance; Satellite RNAs and Satellite viruses; Ribozymes.**

Further Reading

Diener TO (1979) *Viroids and Viroid Diseases*. New York: Wiley Interscience.

Diener TO (ed.) (1987) *The Viroids*. New York: Plenum Press.

Flores R, Di Serio F and Hernàndez C (1997) Viroids: the noncoding genomes. *Semin.Virol.* 8: 65.

Matthews REF (1991) *Plant Virology*, 3rd edn. New York: Academic Press.

Semancik JS (ed.) (1987) *Viroids and Viroid-Like Pathogens*. Boca Raton: CRC Press.

Symons RH (ed.) (1990) Viroids and related pathogenic RNAs. *Semin. Virol.* 1: 75.

VIRUS SPECIES

Marc HV Van Regenmortel, UPR 9021 IBMC CNRS, Strasbourg, France

Copyright © 1999 Academic Press

Introduction

The question of what is a virus species is part of the general problem of how the diversified world of viruses should be organized to achieve a coherent scheme of distinct and easily recognizable viral entities. Virus taxonomy suffers from a bad image among virologists, the subject often being equated with arcane debates about proposed names for newly discovered viruses or theoretical discussions about possible phylogenetic relationships of little relevance to practising virologists. This is unfortunate since virus classification and the demarcation of virus species are subjects of fundamental importance for clarifying the nature and identity of the objects studied by virologists and for allowing virology to develop into a mature scientific discipline.

The first internationally organized attempt to introduce some order in the bewildering variety of viruses took place at the International Congress of Microbiology held in Moscow in 1966. A committee was created, later called the International Committee on Taxonomy of Viruses (ICTV) which was given the task of developing a single, universal taxonomic scheme for all the viruses infecting animals (vertebrates, invertebrates and protozoa), plants (higher plants and algae), bacteria, fungi and archaea. Since 1971 the ICTV, operating on behalf of the world community of virologists, has produced six reports describing the current state of virus taxonomy; a seventh one is due for publication in 1999. The current system of virus classification uses the classical hierarchical levels of order, family, genus and species. At present 184 genera have been recognized and of these, 161 are classified in 54 families.

Although the species is the most fundamental unit in all biological classifications, it took many years before an internationally agreed definition of virus species applicable to all viruses became generally accepted and was ratified by the ICTV. The virologists who study viruses that infect plants had been particularly reluctant to admit that the species concept could be used in virology. Some of these virologists argued that the only legitimate definition of species was that of *biological species*, used for sexually reproducing organisms but which is clearly not applicable to entities such as viruses that replicate by clonal means. However, a great variety of species concepts exists and some of them may be applicable to viruses. Unfortunately, there is no general agreement among biologists on what counts as a good species concept. Before outlining the concept of virus species, it will be helpful, therefore, to define a few terms and to analyze some of the key concepts used in biological classification.

What is a Virus?

A virus is an elementary biosystem that possesses some of the properties of living systems such as having a genome and being able to adapt to changing environments. However, viruses cannot capture and store free energy and they are not functionally active outside their host cells. Although viruses are pathogens, they should not be equated with pathogenic microorganisms.

A virus has both *intrinsic properties* (e.g. its size) and *relational properties* (e.g. its host), the second type of property existing only by virtue of a relation with other objects. These properties are either *resultant properties* already possessed by the components of the virus (e.g. the mass of the virion equals the sum of the mass of its parts) or *emergent properties* that are only possessed by the system as a whole and are not present in its constituent parts (e.g. the viral replication cycle or the viral ecological niche). It should be stressed that only cells and multicellular systems possess the emergent property of being alive and that this property is not present in subcellular components or individual molecules. A virus becomes part of a living system only after its genome has been integrated in the host cell and viral replication is made possible through the metabolic activity of the cell. Viruses are thus not organisms and they lead only a kind of borrowed life.

It is also important to clearly distinguish between the entity called a virus and a single, discrete virus particle or virion. The virion possesses intrinsic biochemical and structural properties which, incidentally, include as one of the phenotypic characters the composition and sequence of the viral genome (although this is generally called the genotype). A virus, on the other hand, possesses in addition a number of relational and emergent properties that become actualized, for instance during the viral replication cycle, i.e. when the virus forms an integrated whole with its host cell. A virus can thus not be reduced to the physical constituents and chemical composition of a virion and it is necessary to include in its description the functional activity it possesses inside its host, as well as a variety of other biotic interactions. Furthermore, the hereditary material of a particular virus cannot be described in terms of the unique genomic sequence present in a single virion. The genome of a virus is not a single molecular species but must be viewed as a dynamic population consisting of the thousands of viral mutants that are always present in a given viral clone. This population, which is the target of selection, is referred to as a viral quasi-species (see below).

Classes, Fuzzy Sets and Species

One of the difficulties in defining species is that the term is used in many different ways which unfortunately are not always clearly distinguished. For instance, the term species is often used to designate groups of real organisms studied by taxonomists, in which case it refers to concrete objects, i.e. material things that are located in time and space. One popular taxonomic theory views species as concrete individuals in the sense that they correspond to historical entities related by common descent. The thesis that species should be regarded as individuals instead of classes has led to vigorous debate, but this has not solved the species problem in biology.

Classes

A second meaning of the term species is that of a class, i.e. a conceptual construct or abstraction that does not exist on its own in the absence of someone conceiving of the idea. Properties and classes are related abstract entities. Whatever is said about a thing is seen as ascribing a property to it, and the thing thereby becomes a member of a particular class. If a virus has a positive-strand RNA genome, it

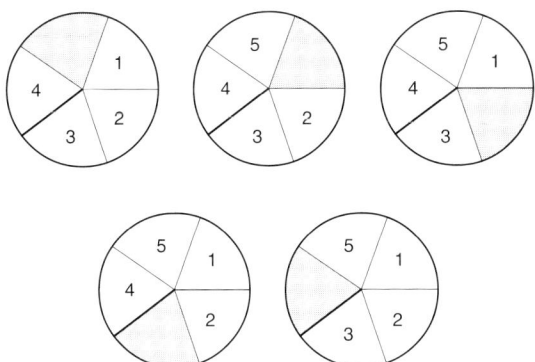

Figure 1 Five members of a polythetic class characterized by five properties, 1–5. Each member possesses several of these properties, but no single property is present in all the members of the class. The missing property in each case is represented by the hatched sector.

becomes automatically a member of the class of positive-strand RNA viruses. Such a class is called a universal class because it is defined by a single property, or a combination of properties, necessarily present in all the members of the class.

A biological classification is a conceptual construction made up of classes with a hierarchical structure, the ranks being the species, genus, family, order and phylum. It must be emphasized that the classes or taxonomic categories used for building up a classification are conceptual constructions that do not correspond to groups of real organisms with a spatiotemporal location. It is thus impossible for a biologist ever to encounter an abstract genus or species when handling organisms. It is odd that many biologists who readily accept that genera, families or orders are conceptual constructions of the mind, i.e. abstractions, insist that species have a real existence in space and time and are not abstract classes. It seems that species are more readily perceived as populations of real organisms rather than as abstractions. On the other hand, higher ranks such as genera and families, are more easily accepted as universal classes defined by one or more properties present in every member of the class. One problem with the species class is that its members, i.e. living organisms, undergo continuous developmental and evolutionary changes in time, and are therefore always endowed with intrinsic variability. This seems to contradict the notion that such organisms could belong to a universal class, seen as immutable and timeless. It also seems problematic to speak of the origin of species if one conceives of them as abstract concepts with neither beginning nor end in time. However, these difficulties disappear when species are viewed, not as classical, universal classes, but as polythetic classes, the members of which share only a certain number of characteristic attributes which can change with time. Whereas a traditional class is defined by the necessary presence of at least one property in all its members, the members of a polythetic class need not have a single defining property in common (**Fig. 1**). When species are viewed as polythetic classes, it is possible to accommodate individuals that lack one or other character normally considered typical for the species. The concept of polythetic species is thus particularly suited for dealing with replicating biological entities endowed with intrinsic variability and undergoing continual evolutionary changes. When viewed in this way, species correspond to fuzzy sets with hazy boundaries, and it is not possible to draw sharp boundaries between them as is done with classical sets and universal classes.

Fuzzy sets

The use of vagueness or fuzziness as a descriptor of reality has a long history in Western philosophy. Vagueness stems from a continuum with innumerable steps and is exemplified in the well-known sorites paradox of the heap described by Greek philosophers. This paradox arises because it is impossible to say how many grains of sand can be removed from a heap before it stops being a heap. This implies that the concept of heap cannot be defined in a precise manner. In a similar way, fuzzy sets have no sharp boundaries, and since the set is defined by a vague predicate, membership of a fuzzy set is not an all-or-nothing matter. This means that the law of excluded middle of classical logic (a swan is either white or nonwhite) does not apply, as in some cases it may not be possible to ascertain if an object is a member of the set or not. Handling fuzzy sets, therefore, falls outside the scope of classical, bivalent logic. In a biological classification, it may sometimes be necessary to allocate an organism to a particular species purely as a matter of convention or convenience rather than logical necessity.

Science is based on empirical observations, the precision of which is always limited. Scientific evidence, therefore, can never be assigned the absolute truth value possessed by certain types of statement in formal logic that lack factual reference. Scientific knowledge always remains approximate and incomplete and it would be counterproductive to look for certainty and for absolutely precise boundaries where none exist. When fuzziness is accepted as an unavoidable ingredient of species taxa, spurious problems of definition disappear and it becomes possible to describe species in terms of continuums devoid of artificial sharp edges. In a similar way, colors can be distinguished conceptually in spite of the continuous nature of the spectrum of electromagnetic waves, and mountain peaks are given names although there are no sharp boundaries in geological rock formations.

Species

The traditional view of species is that they correspond to groups of similar organisms that can breed among themselves and produce fertile offspring. Mayr's classical definition of biological species states that 'species are groups of interbreeding natural populations that are reproductively isolated from other such species'. This definition has been criticized because if defines species as a population instead of a class; furthermore it applies only to organisms that reproduce sexually and it ignores the phenomenon of interspecies hybridization that is widespread in the plant kingdom. Since groups of plants lie on a continuum from completely interfertile to completely reproductively isolated, the criterion of infertility for demarcating species is very often inapplicable and the choice of what constitutes a significant breeding discontinuity is rather arbitrary. In order to make it applicable to asexual organisms, Mayr subsequently modified his definition and stated that 'a species is a reproductive community of populations, reproductively isolated from others, that occupies a specific niche in nature'.

As biologists became increasingly committed to evolutionary theory, several authors introduced the notion of evolutionary species corresponding to a time-slice in an evolving lineage. By including in the definition the idea of ancestry and descent, the concept of species acquired an internal cohesion which was absent when species were defined on a morphological or phenetic basis, i.e. only in terms of similarity. However, the evolutionary species concept remains a highly theoretical one as it gives no indication of how individual time-slices of evolving lineages segregate into separate species. Transition from one species to another during evolution occurs within an uninterrupted chain of replicating nucleic acid molecules and ancestral-descendant organisms and there are no criteria for deciding how far back in time a species can be traced. It is thus as difficult to demarcate boundaries in time in order to identify evolutionary species as it is to define clear-cut breeding discontinuities for identifying biological species.

For most practical purposes, biologists today still tend to distinguish between different species on a phenetic or morphological basis. As noted before, the genomic sequence of an organism is also a phenotypic trait and it seems that the overall degree of phenotypic difference observed between organisms, which also includes genomic divergence, is roughly proportional to the amount of evolutionary distance from a common ancestor. This is the reason why phenetic species defined only in terms of overall similarity are often very similar to the species defined as lineages of ancestral-descendant populations.

What is a Virus Species?

The rationale for using the species concept in viral taxonomy is that viruses are biological entities and not simply chemicals. Viruses possess genes, replicate, evolve and are adapted to particular biotic habitats and ecological niches. Like all biological entities that possess the ability to replicate and reproduce themselves, viruses are endowed with an intrinsic variability derived from the error-prone process of nucleic acid replication. Whereas the molecules of a compound studied by a chemist are all identical, the virus particles in a clone always include thousands of mutants which constitute a so-called quasi-species population. This built-in variability allows any biological system to become adapted through selection and in the end guarantees its survival.

In 1981, the ICTV proposed the following definition of virus species: 'A virus species is a concept that will normally be represented by a cluster of strains from a variety of sources, or a population of strains from a particular source, which have in common a set of correlating stable properties that separate the cluster from other clusters of strains.' This definition does not explain what a strain is and it proposes grouping viruses purely on a phenetic basis without considering the cohesive forces present in ancestral-descendant populations. In 1989, the author proposed a definition of virus species which took into account that a species is a polythetic class, the members of which are united by relational properties of descent and by occupation of a particular biotic niche. In 1991, the ICTV endorsed this definition, which states that: 'A virus species is a polythetic class of viruses constituting a replicating lineage and occupying a particular ecological niche.'

Virus species as polythetic class

As shown in **Fig. 1**, there is no single attribute in a polythetic class that can be used to indicate that a virus qualifies as a member of a particular species. A polythetic class consists of members that have several properties in common, although there is no single defining property which is present in all the members of a particular species and absent in the members of other species. A single discriminating character, for instance a particular host reaction or a certain degree of genome sequence dissimilarity, cannot be used as an absolute criterion for differentiating two species within the same genus. Attempts to use a single discriminating character for distinguishing species would fail because of the inherent variability of members of the species, and furthermore it would contradict the notion that species are not universal classes definable by a single property. The situation is different with higher taxa, such as genera and families, which are universal classes and consist of members that share one or more defining properties that are both necessary and sufficient for class membership. As far as virus species are concerned, it is always a combination of statistically covariant properties that provides the rationale for deciding that a particular virus should be considered a member of a species.

Virus species as a replicating lineage

This part of the definition acknowledges that a virus species, in addition to being a polythetic class, is made up of members that represent an evolving lineage. The membership of a virus species varies over time but all its members share descent from a common ancestor. It should be noted that shared descent is a property that also links different species and different genera.

The genomic plasticity inherent in any viral replicating lineage leads to continual phenotypic variation that makes the virus species a polythetic rather than a universal class. It should be stressed that a single criterion, such as the degree of genome sequence divergence or the potential for genetic reassortment, cannot serve as a criterion for species demarcation. Classifying viral genomes should not be confused with classifying viruses. Genome comparisons cannot by themselves justify taxonomic placements that would disregard the biotic and phenotypic properties which are the main reason why virologists want to classify viruses.

Ecological niche occupancy

The ecological niche refers to biotic properties of members of a virus species, such as host range, tissue tropism, virulence, pathogenesis, host responses, vectors and habitat. The ecological niche does not simply refer to a location in three-dimensional space but is a functional concept based on relational properties of the virus. The niche is not a property of the environment but a property of the virus and there can therefore be no vacant or empty niches but only unoccupied habitats or geographical spaces. In the absence of the virus, its ecological niche property is also absent and the notion of a vacant niche is thus meaningless. A niche provides the needs that must be met for the virus to replicate and to survive and it is restricted to the relations that have a positive biological advantage for the virus.

Taxonomic Polythetic Species Versus Molecular Quasi-species

As mentioned above, the genome of a virus cannot be defined by a unique sequence corresponding to a so-called wild type but consists of a distribution of mutant sequences, each one differing in one or a few nucleotide positions from the consensus sequence of the clone. This consensus sequence, identified by sequencing a clone, may give the impression of a stable, unique structure, although it corresponds in fact to the average of a large number of different individual sequences. Since RNA viruses have genomes that replicate in the absence of repair mechanisms, they evolve very rapidly, with a mutation frequency per nucleotide site in the genome of 10^{-3}–10^{-5}. The genome of an RNA virus therefore consists of a master sequence corresponding to the most fit genome sequence under a given environment, together with thousands of competing mutants. Such a population is usually referred to as a quasi-species, a somewhat unfortunate term as it may seem to imply that the virus corresponds to some sort of imperfect species, as opposed to a 'true' or genuine species that would possess a single, invariant genome sequence. Such idealized species, of course, do not exist. The term quasi-species was introduced by Eigen and his colleagues to describe self-replicating RNA molecules which, because of mutation, do not consist of a unique molecular species. In this context, the term species refers to a purely chemical entity, i.e. a species of molecule, and not to the taxonomic concept of virus species as a variable biological entity. Whereas all the members of a chemical species are identical molecules, the members of a virus species are not. Taxonomic species are thus automatically quasi-species in the molecular sense.

Virus Species Demarcation

Although the acceptance of a definition of virus species by the international virological community was an important step for establishing a unified virus classification system based on the traditional taxonomic categories, it should be stressed that such a definition is of little use for deciding if a particular virus isolate is a member of a certain species or not. The reason for this is that definitions apply only to abstract concepts such as the notion of species taken as a category or class used in classification. Individual viruses located in time and space cannot be 'defined'

Table 1 Characters that would demarcate virus isolates as distinct species in the families *Potyviridae* and *Geminiviridae* (Van Regenmortel et al, 1997).

Character	Potyviridae	Geminiviridae
Genome features	—	Different numbers of genome components
	—	Different organization of genes in the genome
	—	No transcomplementation of gene products
	—	No pseudorecombination between components
Genome sequence	< *c.* 85% identical over whole sequence	< *c.* 90% identical in coat protein sequence
	< *c.* 75% identical in 3′ noncoding region	—
Protein features	Different polyprotein cleavage sites	—
	Virions react differently with key antibodies	Virions react differently with key antibodies
	< *c.* 90% identical in coat protein sequence	< *c.* 90% identical in coat protein sequence
Transmission	Different vector species	Different vector species
	Different seed transmissibility	—
Effects in infected tissue	Different inclusion body morphology	—
	No crossprotection effects	—
	—	Different tissue tropism
Host range	Different in key species	Different in key species

but can only be identified by means of so-called diagnostic properties. The difference between definition and identification can be clarified by the following analogy. It is possible to define the concept of a human family in terms of an ancestral-descendant population comprising parents, grandparents, children, siblings, etc., but such a definition of the family concept would be of no help whatsoever for recognizing the members of the Smith family who have gathered for the annual school concert and for distinguishing them from members of the Brown family. What is required is a set of characters and diagnostic properties that can be used for identifying individual members of a family or species. It is thus necessary to reach an agreement about which diagnostic properties are most useful for identifying the members of a virus species.

The identification of a virus isolate is a comparative process based on a number of different characters that will indicate the extent of relationship of the isolate with members of an established species. Since species are polythetic, the comparison must involve several characters rather than the presence or absence of a single key feature. For species diagnosis it is of course essential not to use characters that are present in all the members of a genus or family, as these obviously will not permit species demarcation within the group. Characters such as virion morphology, genome organization, method of replication and the number and size of structural and nonstructural viral proteins are family- or genus-defining properties that are of little value for identifying individual species. The following characters are useful for discriminating between virus species within the same genus:

- genome sequence relatedness,
- natural host range,
- cell and tissue tropism,
- pathogenicity and cytopathology,
- mode of transmission,
- physicochemical properties,
- antigenic properties.

A list of characters that have been used to decide if two virus isolates belonging to the plant virus families *Potyviridae* or *Geminiviridae* are different species or not are listed in **Table 1**. Some criteria are the same for the two families, others are qualitatively the same but quantitatively different and some criteria do not apply to viruses in both families. No one criterion has an absolute supremacy over others; some are more informative and discriminatory than others, but it is the sum total of the information that is gathered which allows reliable species demarcation. Once different species have been established on this basis in the classification scheme, it may be sufficient to check for the presence of a few characters in a particular isolate to be able to allocate it to a particular species.

In each genus, one species for which considerable knowledge is available is designated as the type species. However, this designation does not imply that the properties of the type species are most typical and representative of the properties of all species in the genus.

See also: **Diagnostic techniques: Detection of viral antigens, nucleic acids and specific antibodies, Isolation and identification by culture and microscopy; Lysogeny and prophage; Phage ecology, evolution and speciation; Phage taxonomy and classification; Quasispecies; Recombination of viruses; Taxonomy and classification – general; Taxonomy of viruses (Quantitive).**

Further Reading

Claridge MF, Dawah HA and Wilson MR (eds) (1997) *Species. The Units of Biodiversity.* London: Chapman & Hall.

Gibbs A, Calisher CH and Garcia-Arenal F (eds) (1995) *Molecular Basis of Virus Evolution.* Cambridge: Cambridge University Press.

Mayo MA and Pringle CR (1998) Virus taxonomy 1997. *J. Gen. Virol.* 79: 649.

Murphy FA, Fauquet CM, Bishop DHL *et al* (eds) (1995) *Virus Taxonomy.* Sixth Report of the International Committee on Taxonomy of Viruses. Vienna: Springer.

Van Regenmortel MHV (1990) Virus species, a much overlooked but essential concept in virus classification. *Intervirology* 31: 241.

Van Regenmortel MHV, Bishop DHL, Fauquet CM *et al* (1997) Guidelines to the demarcation of virus species. *Arch. Virol.* 142: 1505.

VIRUS STRUCTURE

Contents
Atomic structure
Principles of virus structure

Atomic Structure

Ming Luo, Center for Macromolecular Crystallography, The University of Alabama, Birmingham, Alabama, USA

Copyright © 1999 Academic Press

Architecture of Viruses

Viruses have two essential components: protein and nucleic acid. A closed capsid may be formed by one type or a few types of proteins to encapsidate the nucleic acid genome. The protein capsid can have a helical (filamentous virus) or icosahedral (spherical virus) symmetry. The symmetry allows a small protein unit to assemble into a large particle. The helical symmetry is described by the diameter d, the pitch P, and the number of subunits per turn. There are as many capsid proteins as necessary for completely covering the nucleic acid genome. The icosahedral symmetry is defined by six fivefold axes, ten threefold axes, and 15 twofold axes. A number T, called the *triangulation number*, indicates how many quasisymmetrical subunit interactions there are within one asymmetrical region of the icosahedron. There are a total of $60T$ copies of proteins in one icosahedral capsid. In some viruses, there is a membrane envelope wrapped around the protein–nucleic acid core. There are proteins on the surface of the envelope.

Methods of Structure Determination

X-ray diffraction is the common technique used for studying the atomic structure of proteins and nucleic acids. When X-rays strike electrons of the atoms in a stationary specimen, a diffraction pattern of different intensities is generated and recorded. By analysis of the diffraction pattern and the intensities, a three-dimensional electron density map (EDM) can be calculated by Fourier transformation. A three-dimensional chemical structure could be built based on the interpretation of the EDM. Two types of X-ray diffraction experiments are useful for virus structure studies: fiber diffraction (for filamentous viruses) and crystallography (for spherical viruses and globular viral proteins).

Atomic Structure of Helical Viruses

The disc of the tobacco mosaic virus (TMV) coat protein has been crystallized and its atomic structure resolved by X-ray crystallography. The intact TMV structure containing the nucleic acid could only be determined by X-ray fiber diffraction experiments, as could that of Pf2 phage. The coat proteins of TMV and Pf2 contain mainly α-helices and the nucleic acid interacts with the coat protein with one base (Pf2) or three bases (TMV) per protein unit. The axis of the coat protein helix coincides with that of the nucleic acid. The coat proteins of TMV have many aggregation forms, depending on pH or ionic strength. The TMV RNA is inserted into the coat protein helix in the growing virus particle. The coat protein of Pf2 was added one by one to the DNA helix emerging from the membrane.

Atomic Structure of Spherical Viruses

Spherical viruses without a membrane envelope form large single crystals under proper conditions. Their atomic structure can be determined by X-ray crystallography with the aid of supercomputers and synchrotron X-ray sources. Since 1978, numerous atomic structures of viruses have been reported. These include the plant RNA viruses tomato bushy stunt virus (TBSV), southern bean mosaic virus (SBMV), satellite tobacco necrosis virus (STNV), bean pot mottle virus (BPMV), and cow pea mosaic virus (CPMV); the animal RNA viruses human rhinovirus, poliovirus, black beetle virus (BBV), Mengo virus, foot-and-mouth disease virus (FMDV), Theiler's murine encephalomyelitis virus (TMEV), coxsackievirus, and tetravirus; and the animal DNA viruses canine parvovirus (CPV), simian virus 40 (SV40), bluetongue virus and adenovirus hexon; as well as the bacteriophages MS2 and ϕx174.

Most capsid proteins of these viruses contain an antiparallel, eightstranded β-barrel folding motif. The motif has a wedge-shaped block with four β-strands (BIDG) on one side and another four (CHEF) on the other. There are also two conserved α-helices (A and B), one is between βC and βD, the other between βE and βF. In animal viruses, there are large loops inserted in between the β-strands. These loops form the surface features of individual viruses. The wedge shape is best suited to making a concealed icosahedral shell.

A virus capsid may contain multiple copies of the β-barrel fold with the same amino acid sequence (such as $T = 3$ TBSV or $T = 1$ CPV) or with different amino acid sequences (such as pseudo $T = 3$ rhinovirus). In some cases there are two β-barrel folds in a single polypeptide (such as CPMV and adenovirus hexon). Capsid proteins of spherical viruses can have other motifs such as plane β-sheet in MS2 and α-helices in bluetongue virus.

Atomic Structure of Viral Proteins

There are many functional viral proteins that do not have any symmetrical quaternary structure in virus particles. Therefore, their atomic structure has to be studied by crystallizing isolated proteins. Crystal structures have been determined for the hemagglutinin (HA) and the neuraminidase (NA) of enveloped influenza virus, and the protease and reverse transcriptase of human immunodeficiency virus (HIV) and other retrovirus, matrix and capsid proteins (influenza virus and HIV/SIV), a fragment of the HIV glycoprotein gp41, the protease of picornaviruses, the protease and the thymidine kinase of herpesvirus, the protease of hepatitis C virus, the receptor binding domain of adenovirus fiber and the envelope glycoprotein of tick-borne encephalitis virus.

The HA has two domains in the subunit and the functional molecule is a trimer. The domain extending from the membrane contains α-helices and β-sheets. This domain forms the base interacting with the membrane envelope. The distal domain has an eight-stranded β-barrel fold similar to that seen in the spherical viruses. This domain bears the binding site for sialic acid, the receptor for influenza virus on the cell surface. The membrane fusion peptide at the N terminus of HA_2 is located in the membrane-interacting domain.

The NA is a tetrametric molecule and its subunit contains six sheets of four β-strands each. The six β-sheets are arranged like the blades of a propeller. The enzymatic site is at a hydrophobic depression in the center of the β-sheets. The antibody recognition site has been defined on the external surface near the enzymatic site by the atomic structure of the NA complexed with Fab fragments.

The HIV protease is an aspartic acid protease with two β-sheets in each subunit. The enzyme has to dimerize before it becomes active. This activation mechanism has an important role in HIV assembly. The virus assembly complex attached to the membrane will not proceed during maturation until all the necessary components are present to initiate dimerization of the protease.

The matrix protein of influenza virus contains at least two α-helix domains and works as a dimer in the virion. The N-terminal domain has a hydrophobic surface which can bind membrane, while the middle domain has a positively charged surface that interacts with the RNA. This bifunctional protein can simultaneously bind membrane and RNA. The matrix protein and the capsid protein of HIV have similar folds as the matrix protein of influenza virus when compared with each domain. In HIV, the two proteins are initially covalently linked, as are the two domains in the matrix protein of influenza virus. After being cleaved during maturation, the matrix protein remains bound to membrane and the capsid protein binds to the RNA nucleocomplex.

Nucleic Acid–Protein Interaction

The viral nucleic acid genome is always packaged inside the protein capsid. Usually the structure of the nucleic acid cannot be observed in a single crystal X-ray diffraction experiment because of the random orientation of the icosahedral particles in the crystal. However, in rare cases, the nucleic acid might assume icosahedral symmetry by interacting with the protein capsid. Fragments of the complete genome make the same conformation, although with different nucleotide sequences, at locations related by icosahedral symmetry. Such structures have been seen in BPMV (RNA virus) and CPV (DNA virus). The bases are stacked either as in A-type RNA helix (BPMV) or to form a coiled conformation to fit the interactions with the protein capsid. These viruses readily form empty virus particles and have a hydrophobic pocket on the interior surface of the capsid. The nucleic acid generally interacts nonspecifically with the protein.

Evolution

The highly conserved β-barrel motif of the viral capsid protein indicates that many viruses must have evolved from a single origin. The unique three-dimensional structure of this motif is required for capsid assembly and it is generally conserved over a longer period of time than the amino acid sequence. The superposition of the capsid proteins from different viruses can be used to estimate the branch point in the evolutionary tree for each virus group. The structural alignment not only relates plant viruses to animal viruses, RNA viruses to DNA viruses, but also viruses to other proteins like concanavalin A, which has a similar fold and competes with poliovirus for its cellular receptor. The evolutionary relationship of these viruses is supported by amino acid sequence alignment of more conserved viral proteins, such as the viral RNA polymerase. The structural similarities of the matrix and capsid proteins, as well as the surface glycoproteins of influenza virus and HIV, further support the idea of a common evolutionary origin among enveloped viruses.

Assembly

The icosahedral capsid is assembled from smaller units made of several protein subunits. In small animal RNA viruses, a protomeric unit is first formed with one copy of each polypeptide after translation. The termini of the subunits are intertwined with each other to hold the subunits together in the protomer. The protomers are then associated as pentamers, which in turn form the complete icosahedral virion while encapsidating the viral RNA. In $T = 3$ or $T = 1$ plant RNA viruses, the pentamers are formed by dimers of the capsid proteins. In adenovirus and SV40, the capsid proteins form hexon units (three polypeptides, each has two β-barrels) or pentamers before they assemble into an icosahedral shell. The assembly of enveloped viruses like influenza virus is directed by the matrix protein, which initiates the assembly at the cellular membrane.

Host Receptor Recognition Site

Animal viruses have to recognize a specific host cellular receptor for entry during infection. Host receptor binding is the initial step in the viral life cycle and could be an effective target for preventing viral infection. Based on the atomic structure of animal viruses, it was found that the receptor recognition site is located in an area surrounded by hypervariable regions of the antigenic sites. Usually the area is in a depression (called the 'canyon') on the viral surface that is protected from recognition by host antibodies. This structural feature is present in rhinovirus, and the active site of influenza virus NA. The receptor-binding site on influenza virus HA does not have a deep depression, but it is surrounded by antigenic sites.

Antigenic Sites

Antibodies are the first line of defense by the immune system against a viral infection. The epitopes combined with the neutralizing antibodies are mapped on a few isolated locations on the surface of viral proteins. The structure of the influenza virus NA complexed with Fab fragments showed that the antibody makes contact with an area about 6 nm^2 and the epitope spans four discontinuous polypeptides. Therefore, an effective vaccine usually needs to include a complete viral protein or a large fragment. The binding of the antibodies does not change the structure of the antigen. The exact mechanism by which antibodies neutralize antigens is still unclear.

Antiviral Agents

Viral infectious diseases can be cured if an agent can be administered to stop viral infection. Such agents have been synthesized and shown to bind to the capsid of rhinovirus in the crystal structure. The compounds were inserted into the hydrophobic pocket within the β-barrel of the major capsid protein VP1. Binding of the compounds stops uncoating of the virion and the receptor binding, which results in the failure of release of the viral RNA into the cytoplasm. These compounds inhibit infections of several other RNA viruses and may be effective against other viruses after modification, as the β-barrel structure exists in many viruses.

The most successful antiviral drugs are the HIV protease inhibitors, which are developed based on the atomic structure of the protease. Through interactive cycles of computer modeling, chemical synthesis and structural studies of the protein–inhibitor complexes, a panel of clinically effective drugs has been brought to the market and shown benefits to patients. Inhibitors of influenza virus NA are also under development by the same method.

For an illustration of protein crystallography used to determine protein structure, see **Color Plate 30**.

See also: **Virus structure: Principles of virus structure; Viral receptors; Influenza viruses (*Orthomyxoviridae*): General features, Molecular biology, Structure of antigens.**

Further Reading

Fields BN, Knipe DM, Howley PM *et al* (eds) (1996) *Fields Virology*, 3rd edn, pp 59–99. Philadelphia: Lippincott-Raven.

Jones I and Stuart D (1996) Journey to the core of HIV. *Nat. Struct. Biol.* 3: 818.

Rossmann MG and Johnson JE (1989) Icosahedral RNA virus structure. *Annu. Rev. Biochem.* 58: 533.

Principles of Virus Structure

John E Johnson and **Jeffrey A Speir**, Department of Molecular Biology, The Scripps Research Institute, La Jolla, California, USA

Copyright © 1999 Academic Press

Introduction

The virion is a nucleoprotein particle designed to move the viral genome between susceptible cells of a host and between susceptible hosts. An important limitation on the size of the viral genome is its container, the protein capsid. The virion has a variety of functions during the virus life cycle (**Table 1**); however, the principles dictating its architecture result from the need to provide a container of maximum size with a minimum amount of genetic information. The universal strategy evolved for the packaging of viral nucleic acid requires multiple copies of one or more protein subunit types arranged symmetrically about the genome. The assembly of these subunits into nucleoprotein particles is, in many cases, a spontaneous process that results in a minimum free energy structure under intracellular conditions. The two broad classes of symmetric virions are helical rods and spherical particles.

The nucleoprotein helix can, in principle, package a genome of any size. Extensive studies of tobacco mosaic virus (TMV) show that protein subunits will continue to add to the extending rod as long as there is exposed RNA. Protein transitions required to form the TMV helix from various aggregates of subunits are now understood at the atomic level. It is clear that subunits forming the helix display significant polymorphism in the course of assembly; however,

Table 1 Functions of the virus capsid in simple RNA viruses

Assembly	Subunits must assemble to form a protective shell for the RNA
Package	Subunits must specifically package the viral RNA
Infection	The capsid may actively participate in virus infection processes.
Binding to receptors	Binding to receptors and mediating cell entry (animal)
Transport	Virion transport within the host (plant)
Mutation	Capsid protein mutation to avoid the immune system
Replication	Some capsid proteins function as a primer for viral RNA replication

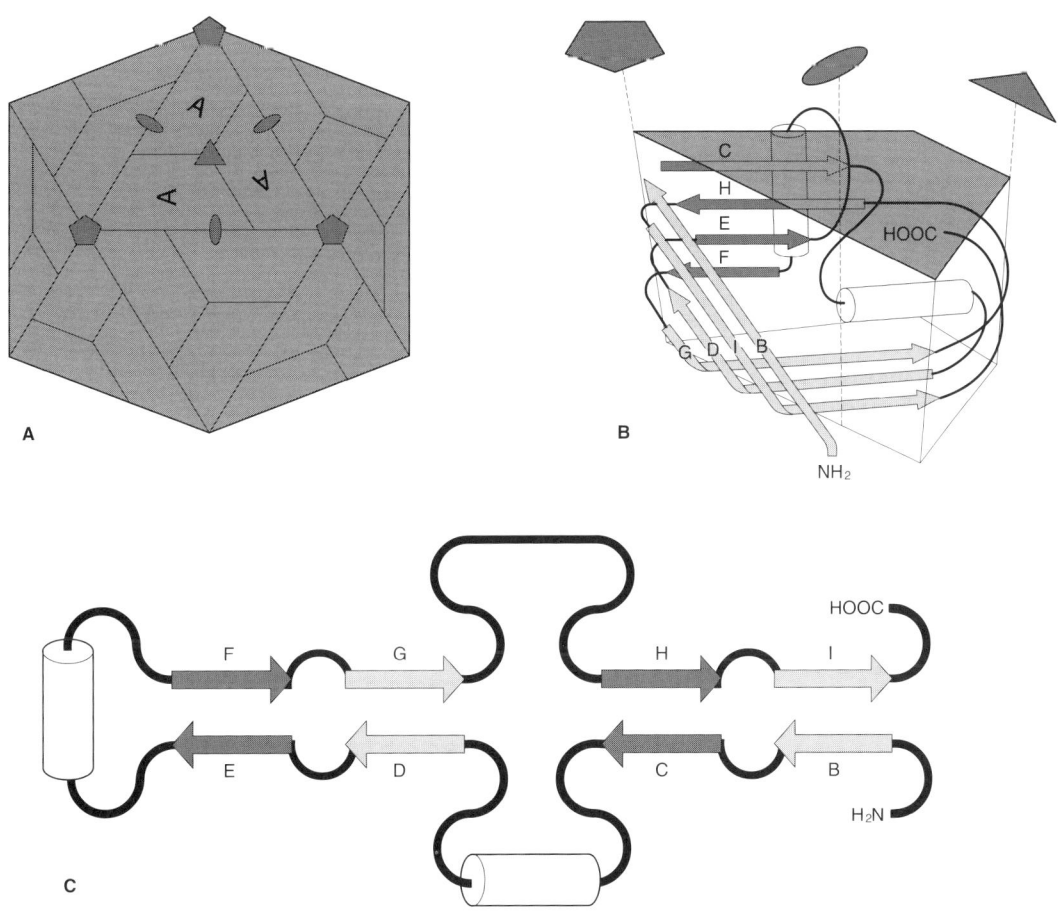

Figure 1 (**A**) The icosahedral capsid contains 60 identical copies of the protein subunit (blue) labeled A. These are related by fivefold (yellow pentagons at vertices), threefold (yellow triangles in faces) and twofold (yellow ellipses at edges) symmetry elements. For a given sized subunit this point group symmetry generates the largest possible assembly (60 subunits) in which every protein lies in an identical environment. (**B**) A schematic representation of the subunit building block found in many RNA and some DNA viral structures. Such subunits have complementary interfacial surfaces which, when they repeatedly interact, lead to the symmetry of the icosahedron. The tertiary structure of the subunit is an eight-stranded β-barrel with the topology of the jellyroll (see (**C**), β-strand and helix coloring is identical to (**B**). Subunit sizes generally range between 20 and 40 kDa with variation among different viruses occurring at the N-and C-termini and in the size of insertions between strands of the β-sheet. These insertions generally do not occur at the narrow end of the wedge (B–C, H–I, D–E and F–G turns). (**C**) The topology of viral β-barrel showing the connections between strands of the sheets (represented by yellow or red arrows) and positions of the insertions between strands. The green cylinders represent helices that are usually conserved. The C–D, E–F and G–H loops often contain large insertions. (**For color references see Color Plate 31.**)

excluding the two ends of the rod, all subunits are in identical environments in the mature helical virion. This is the ideal protein context for a minimum free energy structure. In spite of these packaging and structural attributes the helical virion must be deficient in functional requirements that are common for animal viruses because they are found only among plant and bacterial viruses. Even among plant viruses only seven of the 25 recognized groups are helical. The large majority of all viruses are roughly spherical in shape.

The architectural principles for constructing a 'spherical' virus were first articulated by Crick and Watson in 1956. They suggested that identical subunits were probably distributed with the symmetry of Platonic polyhedra (the tetrahedron, 12 equivalent positions; the octahedron, 24 equivalent positions; or the icosahedron, 60 equivalent positions). Subunits distributed with the symmetry of the icosahedron (**Fig. 1A**) provide the maximum sized particle in which all copies of a subunit will lie in identical positions. The repeated interaction of chemically complementary surfaces at the subunit interfaces leads naturally to such a symmetric particle. The 'instructions' required for assembly are contained in the tertiary structure of the subunit (**Fig. 1B, C**). The actual assembly of the protein capsids is a remarkably accurate process. The use of subunits for the construction of organized complexes places strict control on the process and will naturally eliminate defective units. The reversible formation of noncovalent bonds between properly folded subunits leads naturally to error free assembly and a minimum free energy structure.

Crystallographic studies of more than 40 unique viruses have demonstrated that there are a limited number of folds utilized in forming viral capsids. **Figure 2** shows schematically the folds of subunits from viruses infecting vertebrates, insects and bacteria. By far the most common fold is the eight-stranded antiparallel β sandwich shown schematically in **Fig. 1B**. Other folds include one that is closely similar to the protease enzyme chymotrypsin.

Early ideas explaining spherical virus architecture were extended on the basis of physical studies of small spherical RNA plant viruses. The large yields and ease of preparation made them ideal subjects for investigations requiring substantial quantities of material. Protein subunits forming virus capsids of this type are usually 20–40 kDa. An example of a virus consistent with the Crick and Watson hypothesis is satellite tobacco necrosis virus (STNV) which is formed from 60 identical 25 kDa subunits. The particle outer radius is 80 Å and the radius of the internal cavity is 60 Å, providing a volume of 9×10^5 Å^3 for packaging RNA. A single hydrated ribonucleotide in a virion will occupy on average roughly 600 to 700 Å^3. The STNV volume is adequate to package a genome of only 1200–1300 nucleotides. STNV is a satellite virus and the packaged genome codes for only the coat protein. Proteins required for RNA replication are supplied by the 'helper virus', tobacco necrosis virus. Most simple ribovirus genomes contain coding capacity for at least two proteins, roughly 1200 nucleotides for the capsid protein and 2500 nucleotides for a RNA-directed RNA polymerase. The inner radius required to package a minimal genome is 90 Å. Consistent with this requirement were experimental studies showing that the vast majority of simple spherical viruses had outer radii of at least 125 Å which corresponds to inner radii of roughly 100 Å. Such particles had to be formed from more than 60 subunits, yet X-ray diffraction patterns of crystalline tomato bushy stunt virus (TBSV) and turnip yellow mosaic virus (TYMV) were consistent with icosahedral symmetry. Although a number of investigators developed hypotheses explaining the apparent inconsistent observations, in 1962 Caspar and Klug derived a general method for the construction of icosahedral capsids that contained multiples of 60 subunits. The method for systematically enumerating all possible quasi-equivalent structures was similar to that used by Buckminster Fuller in constructing geodesic domes. The quasi-equivalent theory of Caspar and Klug has explained the distribution of morphological units (features identifiable at low resolution by electron microscopy often corresponding to hexamer, pentamer, trimer or dimer aggregate of the subunits) on all structures observed to date, but the results from high resolution crystallographic studies have shown some remarkable inconsistencies with the microscopic principles upon which the theory is based.

Quasi-equivalence is best visualized graphically. Formally, subunits forming quasi-equivalent structures must be capable of assembling into both hexamers (which are conceptually viewed as planar) and pentamers (which are convex because one subunit has been removed from the planar hexamer and yet similar (quasi-equivalent) contacts are maintained). If subunits assembled as all hexamers, the result would be a sheet of hexamers and a closed shell could not form (**Fig. 3A**). The rules of quasi-equivalence described a systematic procedure for inserting pentamers into the hexagonal net in such a way as to form a closed shell with exact icosahedral symmetry. **Figure 3** illustrates this principle and the selection rules for inserting pentamers. **Figure 4** illustrates how the morphogenesis of such an assembly may occur using the crystallographic structure of cowpea chlorotic mottle virus (CCMV) as inspiration. CCMV, although solved only recently, was the first virus structure that agreed in detail with the predictions of Caspar and Klug.

The quasi-equivalence theory has been universally successful in describing surface morphology of spherical viruses observed in the electron microscope and, prior to the first high resolution crystallographic structure of a virus, it was assumed that the underlying assumptions of Caspar and Klug were essentially correct. The structure of TBSV determined at 2.9 Å resolution revealed an unexpected variation from the concept of quasi-equivalence which was defined as 'any small nonrandom variation in a regular bonding pattern that leads to a more stable structure than does strictly equivalent bonding'. Unlike CCMV, the structure of TBSV showed that differences occurring between pentamer interactions and hexamer interactions were not small variations in bonding patterns, but almost totally different bonding patterns. **Figure 5A** shows diagrammatically the subunit interactions in the shell of TBSV, southern bean mosaic virus (SBMV), BBV and TCV. These high resolution structures revealed that the mathematical concept of quasi-equivalence predicted surface lattices with high fidelity, but *not* for the reasons expected. Bonding contacts between quasi-threefold related subunits are maintained with little deviation

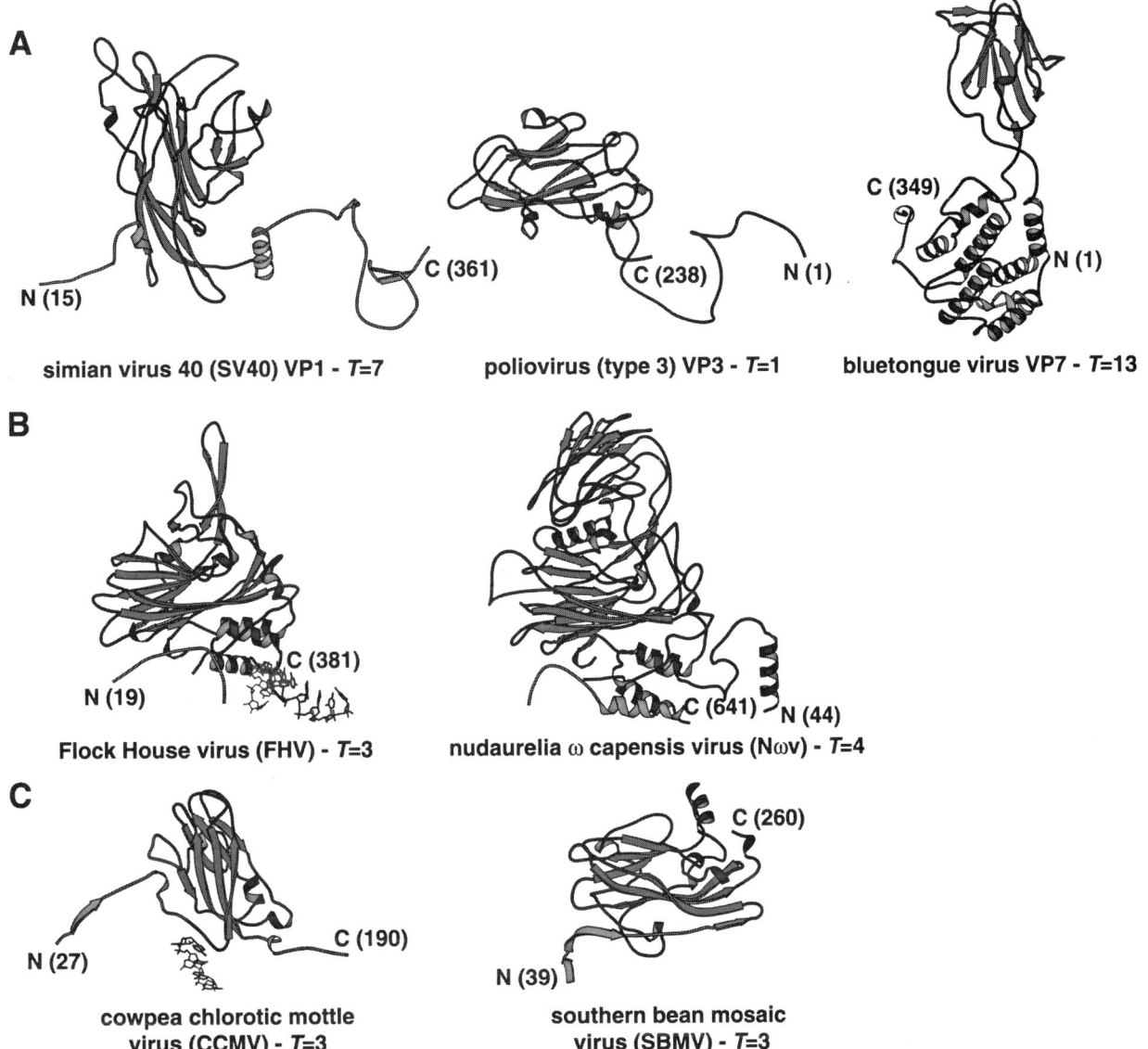

Figure 2 Structure of (**A**) vertebrate, (**B**) insect and (**C**) plant virus protein subunits that assemble into icosahedral shells. The name of the virus appears below the corresponding protein subunit along with the capsid triangulation number T (explained in **Fig. 3**). The N- and C-termini are labeled with the residue numbers in brackets. Many virus subunit structures determined to near atomic resolution have the β-barrel fold and/or insertions with nearly all β-secondary structure (colored red, see **Fig. 1B, C**). Multiple copies (from 180 to 780) of the single subunit shown for each virus, except for that of poliovirus, form the entire icosahedral protein shell. Assembly of icosahedral virus particles with more than 60 subunits (e.g. see **Fig. 1A**) requires quasi-symmetric interactions (nonidentical interactions between neighboring identical subunits, discussed in detail later in this chapter, see **Figs 3** and **4**) often involving subtle to extensive differences in structure at the subunit N- and C-termini. The subunit regions involved in quasi-symmetric interactions critical to virion structure and assembly are colored green (only a single variation is shown for each virus). The 'switch' in structure between identical subunits is a response to differences in the local chemical environment, defined the number of subunits forming the icosahedral shell, in order to maintain similar bonding between neighboring subunits. The structural variations include the presence or absence of highly ordered RNA structure (green stick models) in FHV and CCMV. Poliovirus utilizes multiple copies of two additional subunits highly similar to VP3 to form a complete virion. Thus, there is no quasi-symmetry in poliovirus (note the absence of any green highlights) since neighboring subunits are different proteins. (**For color references see Color Plate 32.**)

from exact symmetry, while quasi-twofold contacts and icosahedral twofold contacts (which are predicted to be very similar) are quite different. The hexamer quasi-symmetry is better described as a trimer of dimers in the TBSV and related structures. Unlike the conceptual model and the CCMV capsid

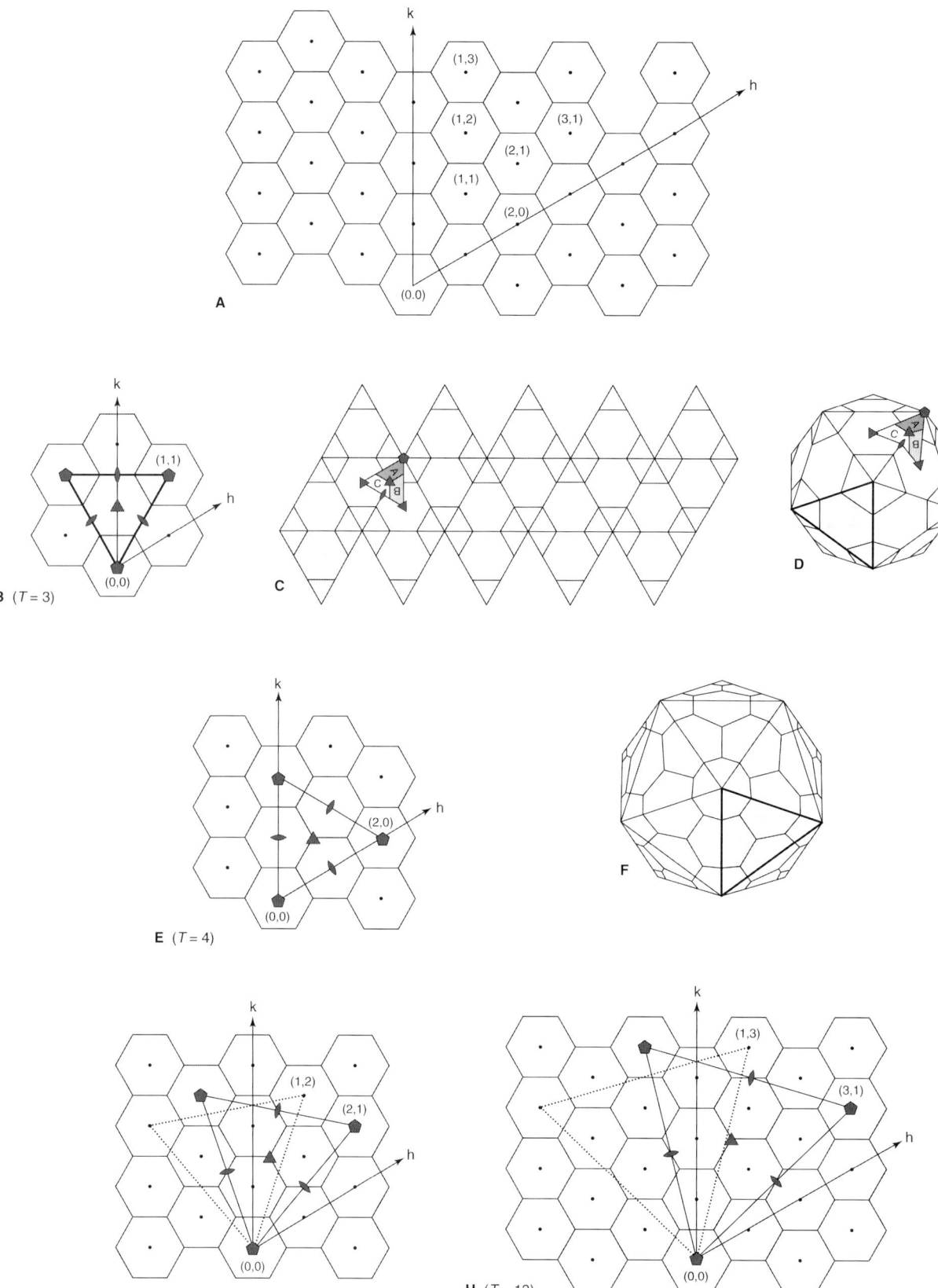

(**Fig. 5B**), the particle curvature in TBSV results from both pentamers and hexamers.

The high resolution $T = 3$ structures showed that the overall features of the quasi-equivalent theory were correct, but that the underlying concepts of quasi-equivalent bonding had to be revised. The first low (22.5 Å) resolution structure of a $T = 7$ virus required an even greater conceptual adjustment to the underlying principles of quasi-equivalence. Rayment, Baker and Caspar reported, in 1982, that the polyomavirus capsid contained 72 capsomeres, as previously reported from electron microscopy studies, but that all the capsomeres were pentamers of protein subunits even though they were located at hexavalent lattice points. The $T = 7$ surface lattice predicts 12 pentamers and 60 hexamers, thus the prediction of the number and position of the morphological units is correct, but the fine structure of the morphological units is incorrect. Although the result was highly controversial when first reported, additional electron microscopy studies and the 3.5 Å resolution X-ray structure of polyomavirus have fully confirmed the all-pentamer structure. This result clearly shows the limits of theory in predicting virus structure and indicates that further understanding of capsid structure will come only from experimental studies. The structure of the polyomavirus and its relatives illustrates an important concept when considering surface lattice formation. The important feature is not the symmetry of the morphological unit positioned on the hexamer sites, but only its ability to accommodate six neighbors (it is a hexavalent position). Normally this is accomplished by morphological units with sixfold symmetry, but here, rather acrobatic molecular switching has permitted a pentamer of subunits to accommodate six neighbors. Although the all-pentamer capsid has been observed for the $T = 7$ structure of papillomaviruses, cauli-

---

Figure 3 Geometric principles for generating icosahedral quasi-equivalent surface lattices. These four constructions show the relation between icosahedral symmetry axes and quasi-equivalent symmetry axes. The latter are symmetry elements that hold only in a local environment. (**A**) It is assumed in quasi-equivalence theory that hexamers and pentamers can be interchanged at a particular position in the surface lattice. Hexamers are initially considered planar (an array of hexamers forms a flat sheet as shown) and pentamers are considered convex, introducing curvature in the sheet of hexamers when they are inserted. Inserting 12 pentamers at appropriate positions in the hexamer net generates the closed icosahedral shell, composed of hexamers and pentamers. The positions at which hexamers are replaced by pentamers are defined by the indices **h** and **k** measured along the labeled axes. The values of (**h, k**) used in the following examples are labeled. To construct a model of a particular quasi-equivalent lattice, one face of an icosahedron (equilateral triangles colored orange in (**B–F**) is generated in the hexagonal net. The origin (0,0) is replaced with a pentamer, and the (**h,k**) hexamer is replaced by a pentamer. The third replaced hexamer is identified by threefold symmetry (i.e. complete the equilateral triangle). Each quasi-equivalent lattice is identified by a number $T = \mathbf{h}^2 + \mathbf{hk} + \mathbf{k}^2$ where **h** and **k** are the indices used above. T indicates the number of quasi-equivalent units in the icosahedral asymmetric unit (a hexamer contains six units and a pentamer contains five units). For the purpose of these constructions it is convenient to choose the icosahedral asymmetric unit as one-third of an icosahedral face defined by the triangle connecting a threefold axis to two adjacent fivefold axes. Other asymmetric units can be chosen such as the triangle connecting two adjacent threefold axes and an adjacent fivefold axis (see (**C**) and **Fig. 5**). The total number of units in the particle is $60T$, given the symmetry of the icosahedron. The number of pentamers must be 12 and the number of hexamers is $(60T - 60)/6 = 10(T - 1)$. (**B**) One face of the icosahedron for a $T = 3$ surface lattice is identified by the orange triangle with the bold outline (this corresponds to a face of the icosahedron in **Fig. 1A**). The yellow symmetry labels are the same as those defined in **Fig. 1**. The hexamer replaced has coordinates **h** = 1, **k** = 1. The icosahedral asymmetric unit is one-third of this face and it contains three quasi-equivalent units (two units from the hexamer coincident with the threefold axis and one unit from the pentamer). (**C**) Arranging 20 identical faces of the icosahedron as shown can generate the three-dimensional model of the quasi-equivalent lattice. Three quasiequivalent units labeled A (blue), B (red) and C (green) are shown. These correspond to the three quasi-equivalent units defined in **Figs 4** and **5** rather than the alternative definition used in (**A**) and (**B**). (**D**) The folded icosahedron is shown with hexamers and pentamers outlined. The orange face represents the triangle originally generated from the hexagonal net. The $T = 3$ surface lattice represented in this construction has the appearance of a soccer ball. The trapezoids labeled A, B and C identify quasi-equivalent units in one icosahedral asymmetric unit of the rhombic tri-icontahedron discussed in **Fig. 5**. (**E**) An example of a $T = 4$ icosahedral face (**h** = 2, **k** = 0). In this case the hexamers are coincident with icosahedral twofold axes. (**F**) A folded $T = 4$ icosahedron with the orange face corresponding to the face outlined in the hexagonal net. Note that folding the lattice has required that the hexamers have the curvature of the icosahedral edges. (**G**) A single icosahedral face generated from the hexagonal net for a $T = 7$ lattice. Note that there are two different $T = 7$ lattices (**h** = 2, **k** = 1 in bold outline; and **h** = 1, **k** = 2 in dashed outline). These lattices are the mirror images of each other. To fully define such a lattice, the arrangement of hexamers and pentamers must be established as well as the enantiomorph of the lattice. (**H**) A single icosahedral face for a $T = 13$ lattice is shown. The two enantiomorphs of the quasi-equivalent lattice (**h** = 3, **k** = 1 – bold; and **h** = 1, **k** = 3 – dashed) are outlined. The procedure for generating quasi-equivalent models described here does not exactly correspond to the one described by Caspar and Klug (1962). Caspar and Klug distinguish between different icosadeltahedra by a number $P = \mathbf{h}^2 + \mathbf{hk} + \mathbf{k}^2$ where **h** and **k** are integers that contain no common factors but 1. The deltahedra are triangulated to different degrees described by an integer f that can take on any value. In their definition $T = Pf^2$. The description in this figure has no restrictions on common factors between h and k, thus $T = \mathbf{h}^2 + \mathbf{hk} + \mathbf{k}^2$ for all positive integers. The final models are identical to those described by Caspar and Klug. (**For color references see Color Plate 33.**)

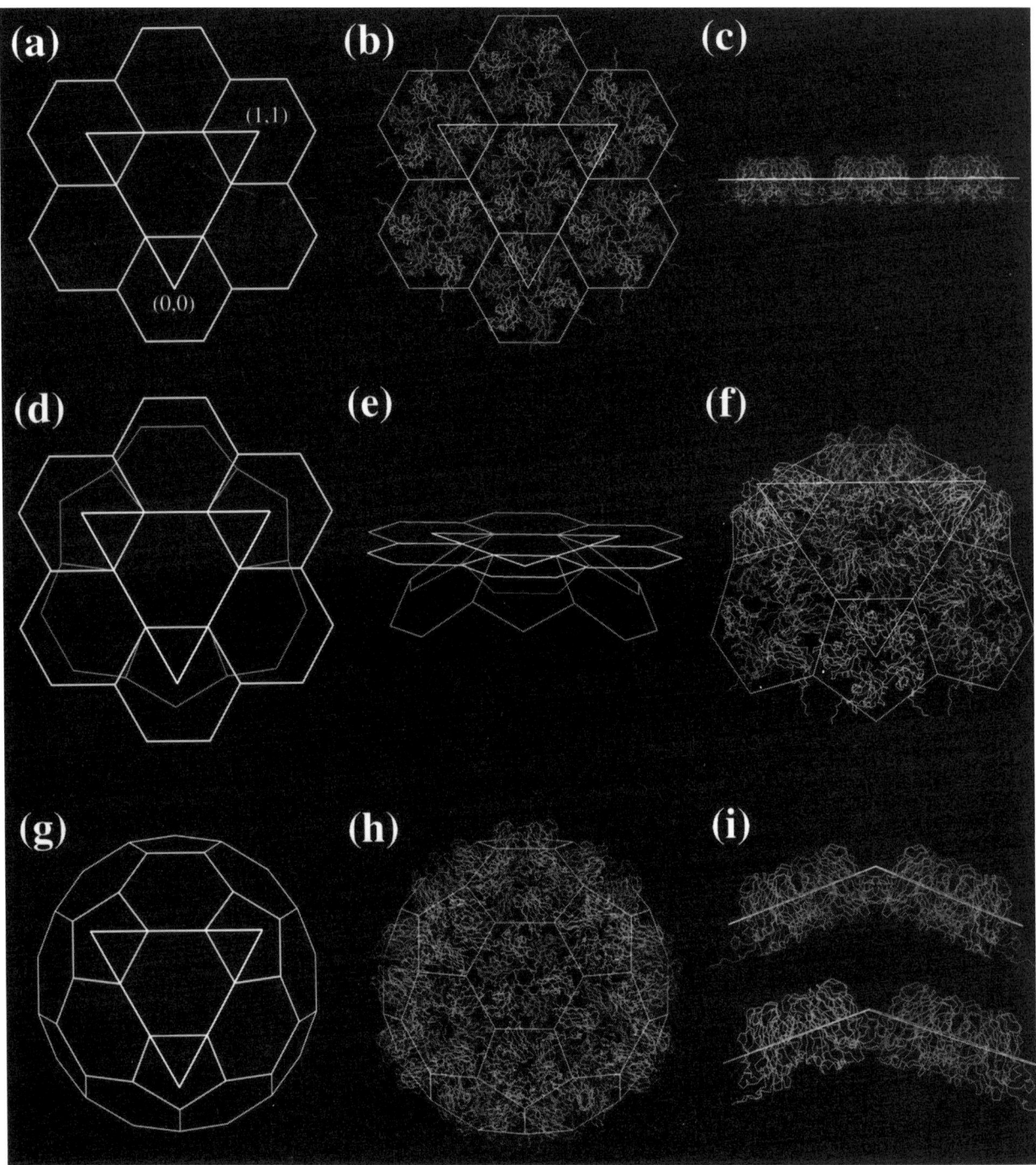

Figure 4 Molecular graphics construction of a $T = 3$ quasi-equivalent icosahedron. (**a**) Hexagonal sheet overlaid with the triangular coordinates (white) for a theoretical $T = 3$ quasi-equivalent icosahedron (**h** = 1, **k** = 1, see **Fig. 3B**). The sheet has true sixfold rotational symmetry about axes passing through the hexamer centers, which are normal to the sheet. (**b**) Copies of the hexamer coordinates from the CCMV X-ray structure (colored by asymmetric unit position, see **Fig. 5**) can be positioned in the sheet by simple translations. (**c**) A side view of the modeled sheet demonstrates its planarity. (**d**) Hexamers at the corners of the white (**h** = 1, **k** = 1) triangle become pentamers. The planar sheet (yellow model) takes on curvature to maintain contacts between the polygons (green model). (**e**) The magnitude of the pentamer-induced curvature is displayed in the side view of the partial polyhedron. (**f**) Coordinates of the CCMV X-ray structure fit this construction without any manipulation. (**g**) A completed $T = 3$ icosahedral model. The 12 pentamers generate curvature that closes the structure. This cage (a truncated icosahedron) accurately describes the geometric morphology of CCMV (**h**) which is composed of modular, planar pentamers (12) and hexamers (20). Angular pentamer–hexamer and hexamer–hexamer interfaces (**i**) stabilize curvature in the absence of convex pentamers used to construct the soccer ball of **Fig. 3D** (see also **Fig. 5**). (**For color references see Color Plate 34.**)

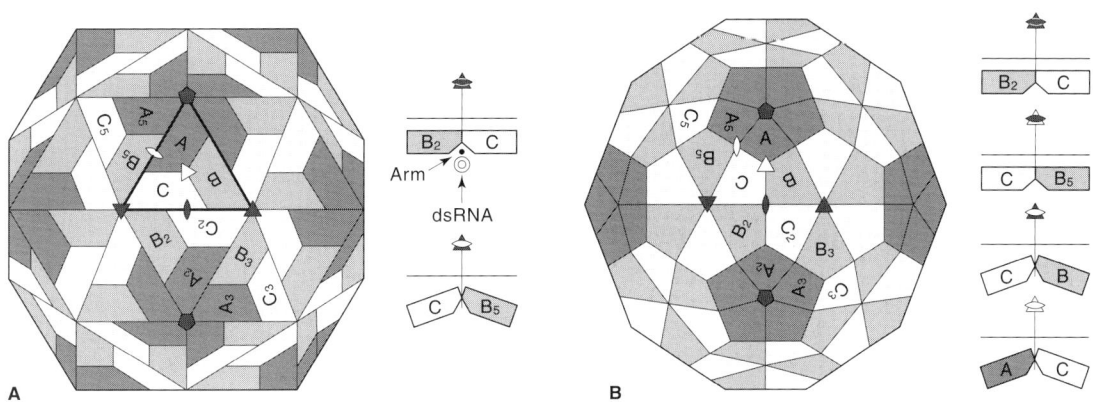

Figure 5 Although quasi-equivalence theory can predict, on geometrical principles, the organization of hexamers and pentamers in a viral capsid, the detailed arrangement of subunits can only be established empirically. High-resolution X-ray structures of $T = 3$ plant and insect viruses show that the particles are organized like the icosahedral rhombic tri-icontahedron or truncated icosahedron (**Fig. 4**). A convenient definition of the icosahedral asymmetric unit for both geometrical shapes is the wedge defined by icosahedral threefold axes left and right of the particle center and an icosahedral fivefold axis at the top. The icosahedral asymmetric unit contains three subunits labeled A (blue), B (red) and C (green) (see **Fig. 3C, D**). The asymmetric unit polygons represent chemically identical protein subunits that occupy slightly different geometrical (chemical) environments as indicated by differences in their coloring. Polygons with subscripts are related to A, B, and C by icosahedral symmetry (i.e. A to A_5 by fivefold rotation). The shapes of the $T = 3$ soccer ball model in **Fig. 3D**, truncated icosahedron in **Fig. 4** and rhombic tri-icontahedron are all different; however, the quasi-symmetric axes are in the same positions relative to the icosahedral symmetry axes for all three models. Quasi-threefold and quasi-twofold axes are represented by the white symbols. The quasi-sixfold axes are coincident with the icosahedral threefold axes in $T = 3$ particles as shown in **Figs 3B–D** and **4**. (**A**) The rhombic tri-icontahedron is constructed by placing rhombic faces perpendicular to icosahedral twofold symmetry axes (yellow ellipse). Thus, the A, B and C polygons are coplanar within each asymmetric unit. The shape of the subunit in $T = 3$ plant and insect viruses is nearly identical to the shape of the subunit in the $T = 1$ virus and they pack in a very similar fashion. The $T = 1$ subunits in one face (**Fig. 1A**) are related by an icosahedral threefold axis, while the $T = 3$ subunits in one face are related by a quasi-threefold axis. The dihedral angle between subunits C and B_5 (juxtaposed across quasi-twofold axes) is 144° and is referred to as a bent contact (bottom right image), while the dihedral angle between subunits C and B_2 (juxtaposed across icosahedral twofold axes) is 180° and is referred to as a flat contact (top right image). Two dramatically different contacts between subunits with identical amino acid sequences are generated by the insertion of an extra polypeptide from the N-terminal portion of the C subunit into the groove formed at the flat contact. This polypeptide is called an 'arm'. The flat contact can also be upheld by insertion of nucleic acid structure into the same groove. The N-terminal arms of the A and B subunits are disordered, and nucleic acid structure has not been observed in the groove across the quasi-twofold axis; thus, C and B_5 are in direct contact as in, for example, the X-ray structure of FHV. (**B**) A truncated icosahedron achieves curvature at different interfaces compared to the rhombic tri-icontahedron. Interactions between B_2–C and between C–B_5 polygons are both defined by 180° dihedral angles (side view at top right) whereas bends similar in magnitude occur within the asymmetric unit at the B–C and C–A polygon interfaces (138° and 142°, respectively; side view at bottom right). This creates the planar pentamer and hexamer morphological units characteristic of the truncated icosahedron and the CCMV X-ray structure (**Fig. 4h**). (**For color references see Color Plate 35.**)

flower mosaic virus appears to have the hexamer/pentamer distribution predicted by quasi-equivalent theory, as do the $T = 7$ capsids of the λ-like bacteriophage, HK97. A substantial number of complex virus structures have been determined by cryoelectronmicroscopy and the surface lattices agree well with the predictions of quasi-equivalence. Thus there is considerable confidence in the lattice assignments, but the capsomere and therefore number of subunits must be carefully confirmed.

A number of viral capsids are constructed with pseudo $T = 3$ symmetry. These structures contain β-barrel subunits (**Fig. 1B**) in the quasi-equivalent environments formed in $T = 3$ structures, but each of the three β-barrels in the asymmetric unit has a unique amino acid sequence. Rather than 180 identical subunits, the $P = 3$ particles contain 60 copies each of three different subunits (**Fig. 6**). These structures do not require quasi-equivalent bonding because each unique interface will have different amino acids interacting, rather than the same subunits forming different contacts. The animal picornaviruses have capsids of this type. Animal virus capsids undergo rapid mutation to avoid recognition by the circulating immune system. Capsids composed of three subunit types could mutate in one subunit without affecting the other two. This would be less likely to affect assembly or other functions of the particle in $P = 3$ shells than it would in $T = 3$ shells. At least one plant virus group displays $P = 3$ shells,

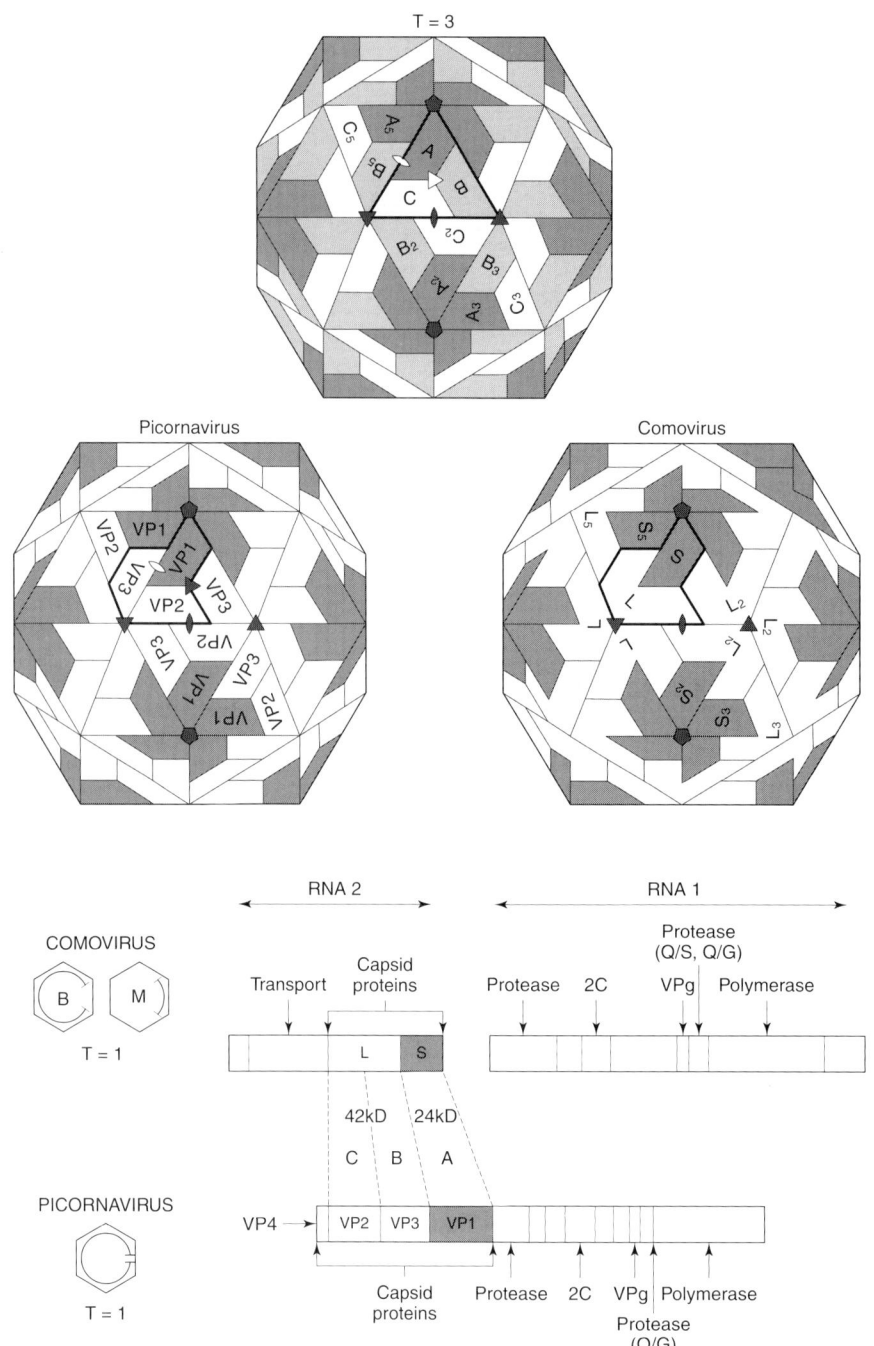

Figure 6 A comparison of $T = 3$, picornavirus and comovirus capsids. In each case, one trapezoid represents a β-barrel and the icosahedral asymmetric units are outlined in bold. The icosahedral asymmetric unit of the $T = 3$ shell contains three identical subunits labeled A, B and C (see **Fig. 5**). The asymmetric unit of the picornavirus capsid contains three β-barrels, but each has a characteristic amino acid sequence labeled VP1, VP2 and VP3. The comovirus capsid is similar to the picornavirus capsid except that two of the β-barrels (corresponding to the green VP2 and VP3 units) are covalently linked to form a single polypeptide, the large protein subunit (L), while the small protein subunit (S) corresponds to VP1 (note the similar color shading). The individual subunits of the comovirus and picornavirus capsids are in identical geometrical (chemical) environments (e.g. VP1 and S are always pentamers) making these $T = 1$ capsids. Comoviruses and picornaviruses have a similar gene order, and the nonstructural 2C and polymerase genes display significant sequence homology. The relationship between the capsid subunit positions in these viruses and their location in the genes is indicated by color coding and the labels A, B and C in the gene diagram. (**For color references see Color Plate 36.**)

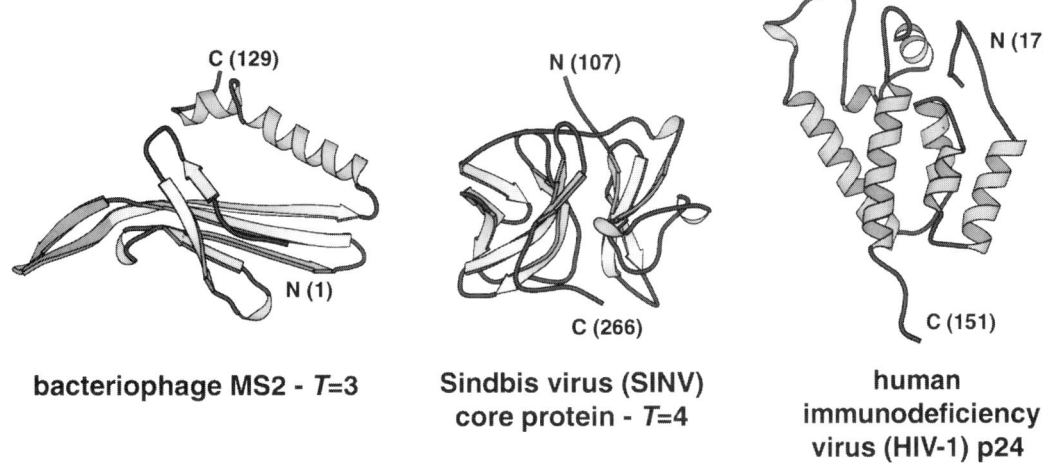

Figure 7 Viral capsid subunits having a fold other than the β-barrel. The MS2 and SINV subunits assemble into icosahedral shells with the T numbers shown. The SINV core is further surrounded by a lipid bilayer and glycoprotein spikes to form the complete virus particle. HIV-1 p24 does not form a capsid with icosahedral symmetry. Together with other products from Gag protein cleavage by the viral protease, p24 forms a conical core structure that encloses the HIV nucleocapsid protein–RNA complex.

the comoviruses. An interesting variation occurs in these capsids when compared with the picornaviruses. Two of the domains forming the shell are contained in a single polypeptide chain. This phenomenon is readily understood in the context of the synthesis of the subunits in picornaviruses and comoviruses. In both cases the proteins are synthesized as a polyprotein that is subsequently cleaved into functional proteins by a virally encoded protease. Clearly one of the cleavage sites in picornaviruses is missing in the comoviruses, resulting in these two domains being still a 'polyprotein'.

Other icosahedral shells containing more than one type of protein subunit have been investigated by high resolution electron microscopy and X-ray crystallography.

Subunit Tertiary Structure

The dominant tertiary fold observed in high resolution X-ray structures determined to date is the eight-stranded β-barrel illustrated in **Fig. 1B**. This fold has been observed in a wide range of viruses. The wedge shape is ideally suited to form pentamers and hexamers, as it does in $T = 3$ virus and $P = 3$ viruses. In other viruses, however, the wedge is not found in this favorable geometric environment. Canine parvovirus, the phage ϕX174, the DNA tumor virus SV40 and adenovirus hexons have the β-barrel fold, but its geometrical environment in each of these viruses is very different from that observed in the $T = 3$ and $P = 3$ viruses.

In all cases the residues in the β-barrel form most of the contiguous shell, while insertions between strands of the barrel project outward. In some cases these insertions can be up to 100 residues or more, creating additional domains of the protein. Extensions at the N-terminus are generally on the interior of the shell, and in many plant and some animal viruses this portion will be extremely basic. These regions are generally not visible in X-ray structures because they are assuming different structures and do not obey icosahedral symmetry. Extensions at the C-terminus are generally external. In the case of TBSV and TCV an entire protruding domain is created by the 90 residues following the polypeptide that forms the contiguous shell (**Fig. 2**).

Although infrequent, other tertiary structures have been seen in viral capsid subunits (**Fig. 7**). The RNA phage MS2 was found to have an entirely different fold than the β-barrels observed in other $T = 3$ structures. What is more, like CCMV, the quaternary structure of MS2 is more closely related to the quasi-equivalence of subunit interactions originally envisioned by Caspar and Klug. The difference between quasi and icosahedral twofold axes are extremely small and the difference in contacts at the pentamers and hexamers seems to be regulated by a loop between two strands that is extended at hexamer axes and folded down at pentamer contacts.

Another tertiary structure found is in the core protein of Sindbis virus. In this case subunits were purified and crystallized because the intact nucleoprotein core was not stable enough to crystallize. The fold found was that of chymotrypsin. It was previously known that this subunit functions as an enzyme because it cuts itself out of a polyprotein after synthesis. Generally the structure has shorter loops than found in chymotrypsin, but the topology and active site are conserved. The C-terminal tryptophane, where the cleavage occurs, is still in the active site of the subunit. These subunits form $T = 4$ shells with the viral RNA. In this case a protein fold with a totally different function has been adapted to form shells. The N-terminal region of this protein (residues 1–100) is composed predominately of basic residues and is not visible in the crystal structure.

The principles of virus structure discussed reflect the level of current understanding for a few relatively simple virus systems. More than 40 unique virus structures have been determined at moderate to high resolution (35 nm or higher) by X-ray crystallography and coordinates are available for these capsids in the Brookhaven Protein Data Bank. This structural information has allowed an understanding of virus assembly and disassembly at the chemical level and this has led to the rational design of antiviral agents that effect particle stability. Approximately 30 virus structures, many with dimensions greater than 80 nm, have been determined at moderate resolution (~ 2 nm) with cryo-electron microscopy and image reconstruction and these structures have revealed organizational principles of exceptional complexity. The large icosahedral viruses extend the principles of quasiequivalence to multisubunit capsid types, but it remains a unifying theme over a remarkable range of virus particle size.

Complex Virus Structures

Many viruses are composed of complex particles with specific functions associated with different structural elements. Complex bacteriophages, for example, have been a subject of study for decades, and the details of their morphogenesis and low resolution structure have been determined. A variety of viruses contain multiple copies of different subunits in their capsids, and the structural roles of each subunit type are still being determined. In most cases these particles are too large to be analyzed by crystallography, but some have been successfully examined by high resolution electron microscopy. Many viruses of medical importance are enveloped by a membrane that contains functionally important proteins. Usually a quasi-symmetric nucleoprotein particle assembles in the cytoplasm and the membrane and associated proteins are acquired when the particle buds through the plasma membrane of the host cell. In the paramyxoviruses, two proteins in the membrane (neuraminidase and hemagglutinin) have been purified, crystallized and analyzed at high resolution. There are a number of examples in which envelopes have been removed and nucleoprotein cores have been analyzed by cryoelectronmicroscopy and image analysis. Their structures display a variety of T numbers, and they are not significantly different from nonenveloped protein capsids. The largest structure ever determined by crystallography is the core of the nonenveloped, double-stranded RNA bluetongue virus that is delivered to the cytoplasm of infected cells. The particle is over 600 Å in diameter, has a $T = 13$ outer capsid and an inner capsid with $T = 1$ symmetry formed of 120 copies of the same gene product. The subunit that forms the outer $T = 13$ shell is shown in **Fig. 2**.

The continued rapid development of single crystal X-ray diffraction, cryo-electron microscopy and associated image processing techniques virtually guarantees rapid progress in understanding the structure and function of large complex viruses. These complex structures will certainly provide insights for broader biological mechanisms as well.

See also: **Virus structure: Atomic structure; Comoviruses (*Comoviridae*); Human immunodeficiency viruses (*Retroviridae*): Molecular biology, Antiretroviral agents, General features; Picornaviruses – insect (*Picornaviridae*); Polioviruses (*Picornaviridae*): General features, Molecular biology; Sindbis and Semliki Forest viruses (*Togaviridae*); Single-stranded RNA phages (*Leviviridae*).**

Further Reading

Caspar DLD (1980) Movement and self-control in protein assemblies. Quasi-equivalence revisited. *Biophys. J.* 32: 103.

Caspar DLD and Klug A (1962) Physical principles in the construction of regular viruses. *Cold Spring Harbor Symp. Quant. Biol.* 27: 1.

Grimes J, Burroughs J, Gouet P *et al* (1998) The atomic structure of the bluetongue virus core. *Nature* 395: 470.

Johnson JE (1996) Functional implications of protein–protein interactions in icosahedral viruses. *Proc. Natl Acad. Sci. USA* 93: 27.

Johnson J and Speir J (1997) Quasi-equivalent viruses: a paradigm for protein assemblies. *J. Mol. Biol.* 269: 665.

VIRUS–HOST CELL INTERACTIONS

Patricia Whitaker-Dowling and **Julius S Youngner**, University of Pittsburgh School of Medicine, Pittsburgh, Pennsylvania, USA

Copyright © 1999 Academic Press

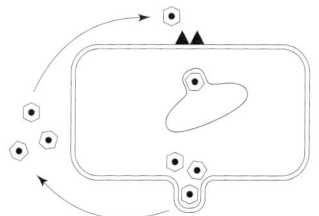

Introduction

The topic of virus–host cell interactions spans all of virology and provides some of the most important insights into this field. Since viruses are intracellular parasites, they rely on their host cells for the energy, macromolecular synthesis machinery and the work benches for genome replication and particle assembly. Because of this dependence, viruses have evolved a myriad of mechanisms for exploiting normal host cell functions. Often this exploitation is associated with damage to the host cell which may be one of the major factors in the pathology and disease caused by viruses. The material in this entry is confined to model systems of virus–host cell interactions that involve the infection by animal viruses of cells in culture.

The past few decades have witnessed a dramatic expansion of our knowledge of animal viruses. These advances have provided a detailed understanding of the structure and composition of the viral genome and the virus particle as well as insight into the replication strategies used by viruses and the regulation of viral gene expression during infection. Development of an understanding of the virus growth cycle has proved easier than a clear comprehension of the interaction of the virus with the host cell. Owing to the complexity of the cell, many of the effects of virus infection on the host occur by mechanisms yet to be determined.

Types of Virus Infections

When a virus infects a cell, the outcomes that may occur can be grouped into several general categories which are determined by the particular virus involved, as well as by the type of cell and its functional state. Productive infections result in the formation of progeny virus and usually cause the destruction of the host cell. In some cases the host cells are not all destroyed, leading to persistent infections in which the surviving cells multiply and continue to produce progeny viruses. When persistent infections occur in which the viral genome is present but no infectious virus is produced, these infections are referred to as latent infections. In such infections some level of viral gene expression is usually detectable although virions are not produced. When genetic information of the virus is integrated as DNA into the host cell genome or is carried as episomal DNA, transforming infections may take place. Such infections can cause an oncogenic alteration of the growth properties of the cell. Abortive infections occur when viruses infect cells that are nonpermissive or only partially permissive. In this instance, the virus is able to enter the cell but because some step essential for viral replication is absent, the replication cycle does not go to completion and no progeny are produced. Such abortive infections may or may not cause cell death.

A few examples follow which demonstrate that different outcomes of infection are dependent on the particular virus and host cell involved, as well as on the state of the host cell. For example, influenza A virus causes a productive, cytolytic infection of a line of canine kidney cells (MDCK). However, when the same virus infects the L cell line of mouse fibroblasts an abortive infection occurs because of a block at the level of virion RNA replication. The same mouse L cell line supports a productive, cytolytic infection by vesicular stomatitis virus (VSV). However, if the L cells are pretreated with interferon, the functional state of the cells is altered; the VSV replication cycle is blocked at the level of protein synthesis and an abortive infection results. When VSV infects insect cell lines derived from *Aedes* or *Drosophila*, productive noncytolytic infections occur. Continuous passage of the insect cell lines reveals that they have become persistently infected and continuously produce infective virus without any signs of cytopathology. Adeno-associated virus (AAV), a parvovirus, is capable of a productive or a latent infection depending upon whether or not the host cells are co-infected with a helper virus such as adenovirus. In some host cells, AAV can cause a latent infection by integrating its DNA into the host cell genome.

There are instances in which infection with a second unrelated virus can dramatically alter the type of infection produced by certain viruses. As mentioned in the preceding paragraph, adeno-associated viruses are capable of productive, cytolytic infections only in cells co-infected with adenovirus. Human adeno-viruses can multiply in monkey cells only in the presence of SV40, a simian papovavirus that supplies a helper function that permits translation of adenovirus mRNAs. In rabbit corneal cells, co-infection with vaccinia or some other poxviruses can convert nonproductive infections with VSV into cytolytic infections.

Effects of Virus Infection on the Host Cell

Effects on host cell morphology and viability

The most readily recognized effects of viruses on host cells are those that involve morphologic changes or cell death. Enders defined viral cytopathogenicity as 'the capacity to induce any demonstrable departure from the normal either in the morphological or functional properties of cells'. The space available for this entry precludes a comprehensive survey of all the cytopathic effects induced by infection with the various families of animal viruses. However, one of the most striking observations that emerges from an overview of the effects of viruses on host cells is how little is known of the mechanisms by which viruses induce cytopathology. The production of cytopathic effects has been observed with most families of viruses and in many cases the viral gene(s) involved or implicated in these morphological changes has been defined. However, in most cases the mechanisms responsible for cell destruction have not been identified. It is fair to say that one of the most fundamental questions of virology, namely, how viruses kill cells, remains for the most part unanswered.

Effects on host cell macromolecular synthesis

Many of the investigations of the effect of virus infection on the host cell have centered on virus-induced alterations of host cell macromolecular synthesis. While these studies are important to an understanding of the viral growth cycle and have yielded significant insights into the control of host cell gene expression, there is no direct evidence that inhibition at this level is the direct cause of visible cytopathology or cell death. In fact, treatment of host cells with drugs such as actinomycin D and cycloheximide, which inhibit nucleic acid and protein synthesis, does not mimic the morphological changes produced by virus infection. Nevertheless, viruses do employ a variety of strategies to affect the host cell at the level of gene expression.

Effects on host cell DNA and RNA synthesis A variety of DNA and RNA viruses are capable of affecting gene expression by directly altering the host cell genome. For example, the host cell DNA is degraded after infection with poxviruses. Herpes-, picorna- and reoviruses cause a displacement of the cellular chromatin, while an inhibition of host DNA synthesis has been reported following infection with herpes-, pox-, adeno-, picorna-, reo-, alpha- and rhabdoviruses. This inhibition of host DNA synthesis may be a direct effect of a virus factor in the nucleus or a secondary consequence of the inhibition of host cell protein synthesis.

Viral products can directly affect the activity of cellular RNA polymerases and cause an inhibition of host RNA synthesis. Such an inhibition has been seen with VSV and polioviruses. In the case of VSV, both a small viral-encoded RNA molecule (leader RNA) and a viral protein (the matrix M protein) have been implicated in the inhibition of the cellular polymerases at the level of RNA synthesis initiation. Another mechanism to inhibit host RNA synthesis is employed by polioviruses. These agents encode a protease that is capable of cleaving transcription factors required by host RNA polymerases II and III. Reo- and alphaviruses also block host RNA synthesis but the mechanism of this inhibition is not known. Synthesis is not the only level at which viruses can affect host mRNA. Infection with herpes- and poxviruses increases the rate of host mRNA degradation. A unique effect on host cell mRNA is produced by influenza viruses. These agents cleave the cap structure and the first 10–13 nucleotides from the 5′ ends of newly synthesized host mRNAs, and utilize this oligomer as a primer for viral mRNA synthesis. Another mechanism that affects host RNA is seen with adenoviruses; in this instance, infection inhibits the transport of host mRNA out of the nucleus.

Effects on host cell protein synthesis Although much effort has been directed at understanding the effect of virus infection on host protein synthesis, it is unlikely that an inhibition of host protein synthesis is required for successful virus replication. Many viruses, such as paramyxo-, papova- and retroviruses do not normally inhibit host protein synthesis during their replication. Furthermore, mutant viruses that are defective in their ability to shut down host protein synthesis are not necessarily defective for virus growth. In fact, VSV mutants selected during a persistent infection have a reduced ability to inhibit the host's translational machinery; nevertheless, these mutants grow to higher titer during a lytic growth cycle than the parental wild-type virus. With several virus families, infection causes a selective inhibition of the translation of host cell mRNA. Such viruses include picorna-, pox-, herpes-, adeno-, rhabdo-, reo- and orthomyxoviruses. In many cases this inhibition is accompanied by a decrease in the overall rate of protein synthesis in the infected cell. It is likely that this overall inhibition occurs at the level of initiation of protein synthesis since, where it has been examined, the average size of the polysomes in the infected cells is reduced.

The most clearly defined case of virus-induced damage to the translational machinery of the host cell is the effect of poliovirus on one of the translation initiation factors. Following infection with poliovirus, the cap binding complex responsible for recognition of the capped 5′ end of cellular mRNA is inactivated by a proteolytic cleavage of the p220 component of the complex. It has been speculated that the destruction of the p220 protein confers a selective advantage on the translation of poliovirus messages which are uncapped. Infection with poliovirus also causes the release of host mRNA from the cytoskeleton.

Virus-mediated inactivation of other initiation factors for protein synthesis has also been reported. Translational extracts prepared from VSV-infected cells are deficient in eucaryotic initiation factor 2 (eIF-2) activity in one report and eIF-3 in another, while infection with reoviruses impairs the function of eIF-2. It has recently been shown that vaccinia virus, a poxvirus, encodes a small protein which has significant homology to the α subunit of eIF-2. This protein may function as a replacement initiation factor since there is evidence that it may be important in making the virus resistant to inhibition by interferon.

Another viral strategy to inhibit host protein synthesis involves a direct competition of viral and host RNAs. VSV and reoviruses compete successfully with the host for the translational machinery through sheer abundance of viral transcripts. Mengovirus, a picornavirus, produces mRNA which initiates translation more efficiently than the bulk of the host message and, in addition, synthesizes a factor that causes an overall inhibition of protein synthesis in infected cells.

It has been suggested that selective translation of viral mRNA may also occur following changes in intracellular ion concentrations during infection. Increased plasma membrane permeability is a common cytopathic effect of virus infection which can alter the intracellular levels of sodium and potassium ions. Under conditions that cause increased intracellular sodium ion concentrations, the translation of viral mRNAs may be unimpaired while the translation of host mRNAs is severely reduced. Such a differential effect on virus and host protein synthesis has been reported for cells infected with poliovirus, encephalomyocarditis virus, VSV, reovirus and Sindbis virus. In the case of Sindbis virus, the shutdown of host protein synthesis following infection has been correlated temporally with an increase in permeability of the plasma membrane.

Effects on host cell membranes and cytoskeleton

In addition to altering membrane permeability, virus infection can cause other changes in the membranes of the host cell. Insertion of viral proteins into the plasma membrane can induce syncytia formation by fusing infected cells with neighboring uninfected cells. This fusion can be induced either from without by input virions or from within by newly synthesized viral fusion protein made during infection. The ability to fuse cells, which is characteristic of the paramyxovirus family, is also seen with herpes-, flavi-, lenti-, pox- and coronaviruses. Flaviviruses can also affect internal membranes by causing the proliferation of the rough endoplasmic reticulum, a site associated with the assembly of viral particles. Reo-, picorna- and alphavirus infections frequently produce a significant increase in vesicle formation in the cytoplasm.

Cytolytic virus infections generally cause a progressive loss of integrity of the lysosomal membranes. Two phases of damage are recognized. In the first phase, which in some cases is reversible, the lysosomes become permeable to small molecules and are able to concentrate dyes such as neutral red. Visible evidence of this phenomenon is seen with a mutant strain of Newcastle disease virus, a paramyxovirus, which produces red plaques when assayed using an agar overlay containing neutral red. Concentration of this vital stain in lysosomes can also be detected in cells infected with certain strains of influenza A virus. In this instance a ring of darkly staining cells surrounds a clear area of unstained dead cells. In the second phase of lysosomal damage the membrane becomes so permeable that lysosomal enzymes are released into the cytoplasm. As a rule, this release occurs late in the replicative cycle. The release of lysosomal enzymes into the cytoplasm has been described for a wide variety of viruses such as picorna-, pox-, herpes-, orthomyxo-, paramyxo-, corona-, adeno- and papovaviruses. The mechanism responsible for this type of virus-induced cytopathology and the role it plays in cell death have not been clearly defined.

One of the most common signs of virus-induced cytopathology is cell rounding, a morphological change which has been correlated with alterations in the cytoskeleton. Disruption of one or more of the elements of the cytoskeleton has been described after infection with several viruses. Early gene products of herpes, vaccinia and SV40 viruses produce a disassembly of the actin-containing microfilaments, while infection with polio- and reoviruses causes an alteration and reorganization of the virimentin-containing intermediate filaments of the cytoskeleton. Microtubules, another element of the cytoskeleton, are depolymerized following infection with herpes simplex virus 1 (HSV-1), canine distemper virus and frog virus-3. It has been reported that infection with VSV causes a sequential disassembly of all three filament components of the cytoskeleton. The mechanisms by which virus infections disrupt the cytoskeleton are not known and it is not clear whether these morphologic changes are a direct effect of some virus product or a secondary consequence of some other aspect of virus-induced cytopathology. It is interesting to note that in normal cells polyribosomes are closely associated with the cytoskeleton, and on the basis of this association it is possible to speculate that some of the effects of virus infection on the host translational apparatus may be caused by virus-induced changes in the integrity of the cytoskeleton.

Viruses also use the structural elements of the cytoskeleton as the work benches for virion assembly and for transport of viral products within the cell. Examples of this function of the cytoskeleton include adenoviruses which appear to use the microtubules for movement within the infected cell; Newcastle disease virus, the viral products of which are associated with actin filaments; and reoviruses which produce inclusion bodies found in association with microtubules and are the site of viral RNA synthesis and virion assembly. It has also been suggested that, in VSV infections, assembly of nucleocapsids occurs in close association with the cytoskeleton.

Inclusion bodies

Another commonly recognized form of virus-induced alteration of the infected host cell is the formation of intracellular masses called inclusion bodies. It should be noted that at the beginning of this century the discovery of a characteristic cytoplasmic inclusion, the Negri body, in cells infected with rabies virus provided an effective diagnostic test for this disease. Depending upon the virus, these intracellular masses may consist of either virions or unassembled viral products. Inclusion bodies may occur in the cytoplasm, as in cells infected with pox-, paramyxo-, orthomyo-, reo-, rubella or rabies viruses, or may be found in the nucleus in cells infected with adeno- and herpesviruses.

Transformation of host cells

In addition to producing various forms of cell destruction, some families of animal viruses are capable of inducing cell transformation. In most cases, transformation is associated with integration of the viral genome into the host cell DNA or maintenance of viral DNA in an episomal state. Only one family of RNA viruses, the retroviruses, is capable of transforming cells. This family of viruses induces transformation through the action of a variety of oncogenes that are cellular in origin and that are not part of or necessary to the virus replicative cycle. There are several families of DNA viruses that are the cause of or are associated with tumor induction in animals and cell transformation in cultured cells. These include polyoma-, adeno-, herpes-, papilloma-, hepadna- and poxviruses. In contrast to the RNA viruses, the genes of DNA viruses responsible for transformation are viral in origin and required for virus replication.

Is It Murder or Suicide?

It is clear from the information reviewed above that the mechanisms responsible for cell death following virus infection have not been clearly defined. Perhaps the reason it has been so difficult to explain how viruses kill cells is that they do not do this directly. An alternative to a direct cell killing is the induction by viruses of a suicide function in infected cells. It would be advantageous for a cell, as part of a metazoan, to induce an apoptosis-like function in response to viral infection rather than to continue on as a factory producing a constant stream of progeny virus. Some recent evidence has appeared that lends support to this possibility. The cytopathic effect of human immunodeficiency virus (HIV) infection has been associated with apoptosis; and in another report, a noncytopathic latent infection of B cells with Epstein–Barr virus (EBV) has been associated with an inhibition of the apoptosis function. In this connection, it is interesting to note that latent infection with EBV blocks the killing of B cells by VSV with little or no effect on the replicative ability of this RNA virus. These observations provide some basis for suggesting that virus-associated cell killing may involve the induction of apoptosis or some other suicide function in the infected cell.

Resistance of Cells to Virus Infection

The major determining factor of the susceptibility of a cell to a particular virus is the ability of the viral attachment proteins to recognize and interact with specific receptors on the cell surface. In many cases, cells are resistant to infection by a particular virus simply because of the lack of appropriate surface receptors. A dramatic example of this type of resistance is seen when chicken fibroblast cells, which lack specific receptor molecules on their plasma membranes, are exposed to poliovirus. Infection does not take place because the viruses cannot adsorb to the cell membrane. However, the avian cells are fully able to support the growth of poliovirus if transfected with the virion RNA rather than infected with intact virions. In addition to cell surface viral receptors, the host range of some viruses can be determined by other factors such as host cell transcriptional regulators. There is evidence that suggests that viruses from the herpes-, polyoma-, retro- and hepadnavirus families can replicate only in cells that express the appropriate factors that permit recognition of the viral enhancers.

Although viruses have an adaptive advantage in terms of genetic plasticity, cells are not totally powerless to mount a defensive response to viral infection. The best characterized defense that cells have evolved for protection against viral infection is the interferon system. The interferon family of proteins that is produced in response to viral infection promotes the development of an antiviral state through the induction of a second group of proteins. Two of these proteins, the 2'-5' A synthetase and the protein kinase, have been well characterized and evidence has accumulated that demonstrates their role in the development of the interferon-mediated antiviral state. Perhaps the best evidence to suggest that these proteins are actually involved in the interferon-induced antiviral state comes from the fact that several families of viruses have evolved factors that are capable of blocking the activity of the 2'-5' A synthetase (herpes- and poxviruses) and the protein kinase (herpes-, pox-, adeno-, reo- and orthomyxoviruses).

Viruses as Tools for Probing the Host Cell

Many of the crucial discoveries concerning cellular processes were offshoots of investigations into the replication cycle of viruses or derived from the use of viruses as model systems. This is particularly true for understanding the mechanisms involved in gene expression. It is apparent that all viruses must use the host cell translational apparatus for the synthesis of viral proteins and that many DNA viruses depend on the host transcriptional and DNA replication machinery as well. Consequently, investigation of the intricacies of viral gene expression has led to the discovery of nearly all identified host factors involved in host genome replication, RNA splicing, enhancer sequences, the scanning model for the initiation of protein synthesis, the use of translational frameshifting for gene expression, and the manner in which proteins are targeted within the cell. This list, which is far from exhaustive, will surely be expanded in the future.

It would be difficult to overestimate the impact of the study of tumor viruses on our understanding of the mechanisms involved in transformation and the nature of the cancer cell. In spite of the fact that most naturally occurring cancers of humans and animals are not caused by viruses, investigation of transforming viruses, and retroviruses in particular, has led to an understanding of the major mechanisms and cellular genes responsible for transformation. A detailed review of this subject can be found elsewhere in this volume.

See also: **Cell structure and function in virus infections; Enteroviruses (*Picornaviridae*): Human enteroviruses (serotypes 68–71); Host genetic resistance; Influenza viruses (*Orthomyxoviridae*): General features; Interferons: Therapy of aids and cancer; Pathogenesis: Animal viruses; Persistent viral infection; Polioviruses (*Picornaviridae*): General features; Replication of viruses.**

Further Reading

Frankel-Conrat H and Wagner RR (eds) (1984) *Comprehensive Virology*, Vol. 19, *Viral Cytopathology*. New York: Plenum Press.

Knipe DM (1990) Virus–host cell interactions. In Fields BN *et al.* (eds) *Virology*, 2nd edn, p. 1091. New York: Raven Press.

Norkin LC (1995) Virus receptors: implications for pathogenesis and the design of antiviral agents. *Clin. Microbiol. Rev.* 8(2): 293.

[This article is reproduced from the 1st edn (1994).]

VISNA-MAEDI VIRUSES (*RETROVIRIDAE*)

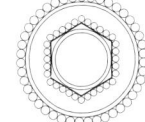

Opendra Narayan, Johns Hopkins University School of Medicine, Baltimore, Maryland, USA

Copyright © 1999 Academic Press

History

Visna and maedi are Icelandic terms for two sheep diseases characterized by wasting paralysis and progressive labored breathing respectively. These diseases broke out in epizootic proportions among Icelandic sheep following introduction of European sheep into the local flocks. The newly introduced

Karakul rams had gone through a long pre-importation quarantine period and had come from flocks with no history of the type of disease that broke out in Iceland. These animals were intended to provide a new gene pool for native Icelandic animals which had been maintained in isolation on the island for several centuries. The new diseases spread rapidly among the Icelandic sheep, involving as many as 50% of the animals in some flocks. Maedi was the predominant disease with visna occurring mainly as a complication. The disease complex was finally eradicated from the islands during the 1960s by slaughter of all sheep on the farms that had affected animals. The farms were then restocked with sheep from other parts of the island that had had no contact with the foreign sheep or local sheep with the disease syndromes. Virus obtained from sick animals was the origin of the prototype visna-maedi virus. In 1974, a virus genetically and serologically related to visna-maedi virus was obtained from goats affected with arthritis and encephalitis in Washington State. This virus was named caprine arthritis encephalitis virus (CAEV).

Clinical and Pathological Criteria

Clinical signs of visna are gradual weight loss and gradual weakening of the hind legs followed by ataxia. These signs progress slowly during a period of months to cachexia and paralysis of the hindlimbs. Rarely, forelimbs are also involved in the paralytic syndrome. Signs of maedi are characterized by weight loss, labored breathing, a dry cough and inability to keep up with the rest of the flock. Both of these diseases occur in adult animals, 2–3 years old, and the disease syndromes last 6–8 months. Arthritis synovitis also occurs in some sheep and is the hallmark of the infection in goats. Similar to visna-maedi, this disease appears in adult life of the animals. Clinically, signs of swelling of the carpal joints ('knees') appear first and this progresses to arthritis and eventual lameness. The encephalitis in goats is confined to kids and becomes apparent a few weeks after birth. This progresses to paralysis and eventually death. In all cases, the animals have normal blood counts. They do not develop fever and all have normal appetites. They do not succumb to opportunistic infections.

Pathology

Histologically, all of the lesions in sheep and goats are characterized by infiltration and proliferation of mononuclear cells consisting of macrophages, B lymphocytes and T lymphocytes in the affected tissues. In the brain, this inflammation is accompanied by demyelination and necrotizing changes in the neural parenchyma. In the lungs, these mononuclear cells infiltrate into the interalveolar interstitial areas of the lung causing consolidation of the organ and physical obliteration of the alveoli. The arthritis consists of thickening and infiltration of mononuclear cells into the synovial lining of the joint and accumulation of large amounts of synovial fluid. This is followed later by degeneration and calcification of the articular facets of the joint and eventually degeneration in the bone. Massive lymphadenopathy accompanies these organ-specific diseases.

There are only a few reports of visna from other parts of the world but pulmonary lesions in sheep similar to maedi had been described previously in the USA and subsequently in several other countries except Australia and New Zealand. In the Netherlands the disease was called Zwoegerziekte, in South Africa, Graaf Reinet, in France, La Bouhite, in the USA, Montana lung disease and/or progressive pneumonia, etc. This provides a clear indication at the pathological level that visna-maedi viruses are present in sheep throughout the world. Modern diagnostic procedures have confirmed this, but unlike the experience in Iceland, the disease in most sheep populations occurs mainly sporadically and usually only in adult animals. The caprine disease complex has also been reported in most of the industrialized countries of the world, including New Zealand and Australia. The infection is rare in most underdeveloped countries where herds are small and isolated.

Host Range and Epizootiology

Visna-maedi virus replicates best in sheep and CAEV in goats. However, reciprocal infection has been documented. Further, some strains of ovine virus such as those found in the USA are biologically more similar to CAEV than Icelandic visna-maedi virus. These viruses are infectious for other small ruminant animal species. Such cross-over infections have been documented in zoos. The viruses are spread mainly by colostrum, milk and respiratory exudates. Under field conditions, viral transmission from mother to offspring is very efficient but localized unless the milk is used for feeding other animals. Virus is also disseminated by poor management practices and this has led to local epizootics. A high rate of transmission occurs in poorly ventilated barns during winter months and this is exacerbated further during intercurrent respiratory infections (caused by other agents) that cause increased production of respiratory exudates. Minimal spread occurs during summer months while animals are on pasture. Infected macrophages in colostrum milk and respiratory exudates are a source of the infection. Intercurrent mastitis causes increased numbers of infected macrophages in the milk and this increases the efficiency of transmission. The major mechanism of dissemination of CAEV has been the dairy husbandry practice by which all kids were fed pooled milk. This guaranteed infection in all kids when only a single infected lactating female may have been present in the herd.

Taxonomy and Classification

By the early 1960s, Icelandic investigators had established that the visna-maedi syndrome was caused by a new virus which replicated productively in stationary ovine cell cultures and caused acute cytopathic effects characterized by fusion of the cells into multinucleated giant cells. Paradoxically, sheep inoculated with the virus at that time remained clinically well for several months. Onset of clinical disease occurred insidiously and progressed slowly but inexorably, leading to death. These findings led to the definition of the viruses as 'slow viruses', the forerunner of the present term, lentiviruses. CAEV had similar biological properties. Some 10 years after the discovery of reverse transcriptase in retroviruses by Temin and Baltimore, the ovine and caprine viruses were both shown to be retroviruses. As lenti-retroviruses, these new agents were distinct from the oncogenic retroviruses which require dividing cells for replication and the oncogenic and transforming properties of which are associated with defective helper virus-dependent replication. The viruses also differ from spuma retroviruses which are not associated with disease. This new ungulate lentivirus, visna, was shown to share similar genetic and biological properties with the lentiviruses of horses, cattle, cats, macaques and humans. Its genome has approximately 9.5 kb of nucleotide sequences and its reverse transcriptase enzyme requires Mg^{2+} instead of Mn^{2+} to catalyze transcription of viral RNA to DNA. In addition to the long terminal repeat (LTR)-gag-pol-env-LTR arrangement of the proviral DNA of retroviruses, visna virus and other lentiviruses also have open reading frames that encode regulatory genes important for replication of the virus. *Tat* and *rev* are examples of these genes.

Variability

The lentiviruses of sheep are genetically and biologically highly heterogeneous. The high mutation rate of the virus has been attributed in part to mistake-prone reverse transcription of viral RNA to DNA. The high mutation rate may be more apparent than real, however, because many mutations in the *env* gene of the virus are viable and viruses with distinct biological properties can be selected by various host systems. Mutant viruses with slow and fast replication rates have been selected by various tissues. Virus-neutralizing antibodies select for neutralization-escape variants (antigenic drift viruses) and macrophages in various tissues such as the brain, lung, synovium and mammary glands select for specific viral phenotypes that replicate optimally in these tissues.

Immune Responses

The envelope proteins of the lentivirus elicit biological responses of greatest importance in the infection. Neutralization epitopes in the envelope consist of either linear peptides or conformational structures and induce antibodies that inhibit replication of the virus. Other epitopes in the viral envelope induce antibodies that bind viral particles but do not neutralize infectivity. These antibodies thus bind to viral particles and enhance entry into target macrophages by Fc receptor-mediated endocytosis. Such antibodies comprise the so-called enhancing antibodies. Cytotoxic CD8 T lymphocytes are also induced by the virus. While these cells, along with neutralizing antibodies, probably lower the virus load *in vivo*, they are incapable of curing the infection, because the virus usually persists for the lifetime of the animal. Part of the failure of the immune responses to eliminate the virus may be due to the integrated unexpressed viral genome in precursor cells in the animal.

Cell Biology and Pathogenesis

The main cell type that supports visna replication *in vivo* is the macrophage-lineage cell, and virus-laden macrophages can be found in all tissues with lesions such as the encephalitic brain, the pneumonic lung, the arthritic joint and mastitic mammary gland. Intense viral replication in local macrophage populations along with local overproduction of cytokines lead to worsening of the inflammatory lesion and more viral replication. Hence, the progressive nature of the lesion and the disease. In animals with organ-specific disease, there is also a high level of infection in precursor cells in bone marrow and in dendritic cells in the blood. In subclinically infected animals that do not have organ-specific lesions, the virus is found at a low rate in the bone marrow and in rare cells in blood but not in tissues. Factors causing the upregulation of viral replication in specific macrophages in tissues have not yet been identified. Studies on viral replication in monocytes (immature macrophages) and in mature macrophages have shown that the viral life cycle is incomplete in the monocytes and mature viral particle formation occurs only in the mature macrophages. The linkage between the life cycle of the virus to that of the cell is probably due in part to the requirement for DNA binding proteins c-Fos and c-Jun (present only in mature cells) to activate viral transcription in the virus LTR. The LTR of the proviral DNA has AP-1 and AP-4 sites which specifically interact with these proteins in mature cells and result in increased transcription of viral RNA. Linkage of the viral life cycle to the physiology of the macrophage as the cell begins its life cycle in the bone marrow and ends in the tissues has relevance in both the disease state in the animals and the mechanism of transmission of the virus in body fluids to other animals.

Prevention and Control

The most effective mechanism for control of lentiviruses in sheep and goats has been the prevention of infection. This has been achieved by removal of infected animals and their young from flocks, prevention of consumption of colostrum and correction of management practices that facilitate enhancement of the spread of virus in respiratory exudates and milk. The sexual route is not a major mechanism for transmission of these viruses. Lentivirus proteins are poor at inducing protective immunity, and such mechanisms have not been investigated thoroughly.

Future Perspectives

These viruses are agricultural pathogens with effects that are in general too subtle to grasp the attention of regulatory agencies. They provide excellent models of human immunodeficiency virus (HIV) infection since they represent an example of natural lentivirus infection in which the host usually wins the battle. More studies in the future may be directed to investigations on mechanisms by which these hosts keep their viruses in check and mechanisms by which virulent strains of these viruses cause disease.

See also: **Bovine immunodeficiency virus (*Retroviridae*); Feline immunodeficiency virus (*Retroviridae*); Human immunodeficiency viruses (*Retroviridae*): Molecular biology; Pathogenesis: Animal viruses; Simian immunodeficiency viruses (*Retroviridae*).**

Further Reading

Clements JE, Hu L, Lindstrom L, Powell A, Rexroad C and Zink MC (1996) Molecular studies of visna virus gene expression: analysis of envelope gene expression in transgenic sheep. *AIDS Research & Human Retroviruses* 12: 42–3.

Haase AT (1988) Pathogenesis of lentivirus infections. *Nature (London)* 322: 130.

Narayan O and Clements JE (1989) Biology and pathogenesis of lentiviruses. *J. Gen. Virol.* 70: 1617.

Narayan O and Cork LC (1985) Lentiviral diseases of sheep and goats: chronic pneumonia, leukoencephalomyelitis and arthritis. *Rev. Infect. Dis.* 7: 89.

Pepin M, Vitu C, Russo P, Mornex JF and Peterhans E (1998) Maedi-visna virus infection in sheep: a review. *Veterinary Research* 29: 341–67.

[This article is reproduced from the 1st edn (1994).]

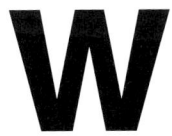

WAIKAVIRUSES (*SEQUIVIRIDAE*)

Donald T. Gordon, The Ohio State University, Wooster, Ohio, USA

Copyright © 1999 Academic Press

History

Maize chlorotic dwarf was first recognized in the early 1960s in the southeastern USA. Initially, the disease was thought to be incited by the maize dwarf mosaic potyvirus, and in the late 1960s by the Ohio corn stunt agent (CSA-OH). The maize chlorotic dwarf virus (MCDV) was initially characterized in 1972. MCDV and CSA-OH were subsequently shown to be identical. MCDV infections were also frequently associated with symptoms of another similar disease, the Mississippi corn stunt.

Tungro, Philippine for 'degenerated growth', was similarly first recognized in the early 1960s. It was observed at the International Rice Research Institute (IRRI) in the Philippines. The disease was known by other names in countries of South and Southeast Asia and as early as 1859 in Indonesia. Initially, spherical or isometric particles, 30 nm in diameter, were associated with the tungro disease and the virus was named rice tungro virus (RTV). Later, small bacilliform virus particles were also associated with the disease and both spherical and bacilliform particles were observed frequently in rice (*Oryza sativa*) plants expressing tungro symptoms. The virus with the isometric particles was renamed rice tungro spherical virus (RTSV), and the second virus rice tungro bacilliform virus (RTBV). RTSV is also named rice tungro waikavirus. The rice waika disease was discovered in 1971 in southwestern Japan. Initially, the disease was known as the 'waisei' or stunting phenomenon in Japanese. In 1973, the disease became known as 'rice waika' (stunting) and the virus was named the rice waika virus (RWV). RWV is confined to Japan.

Anthriscus yellows virus (AYV) was first isolated in 1968 from *Anthriscus sylvestris*. AYV is the least agriculturally important of the waikaviruses and has been the least studied. Interest in AYV comes from its role as a helper virus in the transmission of parsnip yellow fleck *sequivirus* (PYFV). In the following sections, where nothing is known for AYV reference to the virus is omitted.

Taxonomy and Classification

The genus *Waikavirus* was approved in 1995 by the International Committee on Taxonomy of Viruses (ICTV). Previously, the genus was referred to as the maize chlorotic dwarf virus group by the ICTV (1993). Species of the *Waikavirus* include the RTSV, which is the type species, MCDV, RWV and AYV. The genus is classified in the family *Sequiviridae*. The latter is not classified at upper taxonomic levels of class and order.

The waikaviruses are differentiated from the sequiviruses, the other genus of the *Sequiviridae*, by genome organization and size with the genome of PYFV, the *Sequivirus* type species, being smaller, about 10 kb in length, and lacking a 3' poly(A) tract. The amino acid sequences of the conserved motifs of the waikavirus polyprotein most closely resemble those of the *Comoviridae* and *Picornaviridae*, and the genome organization that of the *Picornaviridae*. The waikaviruses belong to the picornavirus superfamily.

Geographic and Seasonal Distribution

The geographical distributions of MCDV and RTSV are the western and eastern hemispheres, respectively, where they occur in temperate and subtropical regions. MCDV occurs in 18 states in the southeastern quadrant of the USA, from the east coast to eastern Texas and north to southern Missouri and the Ohio river valley and in Pennsylvania and Arizona and Mexico. MCDV occurrences are delimited by the overlapping distributions of Johnson grass (*Sorghum halepense*), the overwintering host, and the principal vector, *Graminella nigrifrons*.

Tungro, and presumably RTSV, occurs in the Philippines, Malaysia, Indonesia, Thailand, India, Bangladesh, China, Nepal, Pakistan, Sri Lanka and

Vietnam and RWV in Japan. AYV occurs in Scotland and possibly England and other northern European countries where the transmission-dependent PYFV occurs.

During the growing season, MCDV occurs in maize (*Zea mays*) and a few crop and weed grass species. Over winter, when maize is not present, the virus survives in perennial grass species, most notably in the rhizomes of Johnson grass. For RTSV seasonal occurrence is principally in rice, during the growing season, and rice stubble, ratoons and volunteer plants between rice crops. RTSV infects various weed grass species. When long rice-free periods occur between rice plantings, the virus may occur primarily in weed hosts. RWV occurs in rice and in several wild rice species during the growing season. Between seasons the virus survives in rice ratoons and in the roots of rice stubble.

Host Range and Virus Propagation

Hosts of MCDV, RTSV and RWV are species within the *Poaceae*. The principal cultivated host of MCDV is maize, in which economic yield loss occurs. Several other cultivated species including sorghum (*Sorghum bicolor*) are susceptible but no important disease caused by MCDV has been recorded for these species. The principal natural host is Johnson grass, a perennial grass species and the overwintering host of MCDV. Other perennial and grass hosts are known but have no known role in the epidemiology of the virus. Maize is the principal propagation host.

Rice is the principal host of RTSV. In addition to cultivated rice, wild rice, weed grasses and other crop plants are alternate hosts of the tungro viruses. Hosts of RWV include rice and wild rice species. Rice is the propagation host of RTSV and RWV.

Hosts of AYV are *Anthriscus sylvestris* (anthriscus), *A. cerefolium* (chervil) and *Corandrum sativium* (coriander). Coriander is the preferred propagation host.

Genetics

The genomes of MCDV and RTSV contain a large single component, single-stranded (ss), linear, positive-sense, 3′ polyadenylated RNA consisting of one major open reading frame (ORF) which encodes a large polyprotein. The latter is presumably cleaved by a self-encoded protease(s) to yield individual functional proteins, the total number of which is unknown. Further, it is not known whether the 5′ end of the genome has a 7-methylguanosine or a VPg, although a VPg is probable. The sizes of the sequenced genomes are 11 786 nt (MCDV-OH), 11 813 nt (MCDV-TN) and 12 433 nt (RTSV-PH1). The genomes of other RTSV isolates may be 253 nt shorter. The 5′ untranslated leader sequence ranges in length from 435 to 514 nt and is followed by a large ORF which encodes a polyprotein of 3342–3473 amino acids. The 5′ leader contains extensive secondary structure and multiple AUG triplets before the large ORF internal initiation AUG. Immediately downstream of the noncoding 5′ leader is P1, a putative polypeptide of c. 78 kDa or 644 amino acids in length. Downstream of the putative P1 protein are the encoding sequences of the capsid proteins CP2, CP3 and CP1 of MCDV or CP1, CP2 and CP3 of RTSV. Electrophoretically estimated M_rs for CP1 (MCDV) and CP3 (RTSV), which are equivalent, are 30–35 kDa; CP2 (MCDV)/CP1 (RTSV), 22.5–27.1 kDa; and CP3 (MCDV)/CP2 (RTSV), 18–24.5 kDa. The three CPs of each virus are immunologically distinct. Polyprotein sequences downstream of the structural proteins contain domains characteristic of proteins with nucleoside triphosphate (NTP) binding, picornaviral serine-like 3C protease and RNA-dependent RNA polymerase (RdRP) domains. A serine-like proteinase, with similarity to the cysteine proteinase of cowpea mosaic *comovirus*, appears to be involved in the cleavage of the individual proteins from the polyprotein. The C-terminal portion of the RTSV polyprotein is processed into a penultimate 35 kDa protease and a C-terminal 68 kDa RdRP. The protein(s) between the C-terminus of CP3 and the C-terminal protease and RdRP has not been identified but contains the NTP-binding domain. The 3′ terminal noncoding region (NCR) sequence ranges from 956 to 1240 nt in length, which is unusually long for a plant virus genome and is a distinctive characteristic of the waikavirus genome. A small ORF (ORF 1) occurs in the 5′ NCR of MCDV-TN and another (ORF 3) in the 3′ NCR. Two small ORFs (ORF 2 and 3) occur in 3′ NCR of RTSV. Subgenomic RNAs but not proteins have been detected for the RTSV small ORFs, whereas neither have been detected for MCDV-TN.

The AYV genome is a single species of RNA with an electrophoretically estimated 10 600 ± 70 nt. Virions contain four electrophoretic CP species of M_rs 35.0, 28.4, 24.3 and 22.3 kDa, respectively.

Evolution

Waikaviruses appear to have an evolutionary relationship with the plant and animal picornaviruses. Waikaviruses resemble the animal picornaviruses in having: (1) a large polyadenylated unsegmented (+)-sense ssRNA genome with a 3′ poly(A) tract; (2) an isometric virion containing three similarly sized CPs;

Table 1 Predicted amino acid sequence identities between portions and the entire polyprotein of MCDV-TN and of other waikaviruses, a sequivirus and plant and animal picornaviruses

Virus	CP1	CP2	CP3	NTP-binding	Proteinase	Replicase	Entire polyprotein
MCDV OH or T	60	71	68	86	76	80	60
RTSV	35	41	45	69	38	65	37
PYFV	23	18	24	37	19	41	22
Cowpea mosaic *comovirus*[a]	—	—	—	32	—	33	—
Tomato black ring *nepovirus*[a]	—	—	—	—	—	30	—
Hepatitis A virus[b]	—	—	—	31	—	24	—
Polio virus[b]	—	—	—	24	—	—	—

[a] A plant picornavirus.
[b] An animal picornavirus.
Reproduced from Reddick BB, Habera LF and Law MD (1997) Nucleotide sequence and taxonomy of maize chlorotic dwarf virus within the family Sequiviridae. *J. Gen. Virol.* 78:1165–1174, with permission of the senior author and the journal.

(3) location of the CP encoding sequences upstream of the putative genome replication proteins; (4) polyprotein expression; and (5) a polyprotein processing involving a 3C-type virus-encoded protease. Preliminary comparisons of the waikavirus sequences, principally the amino acid sequences of the CP2, NTP-binding region and replicase, with those of the plant and animal picornaviruses support an evolutionary relationship. The greater similarity of the genome organization of the waikaviruses with that of the animal picornaviruses suggests a closer evolutionary relationship between the waikaviruses and the animal picornaviruses than between the latter and the other plant picornaviruses of the *Comoviridae* and *Potyviridae*. This greater similarity suggests that the waikaviruses may be more closely related to the ancestral virus of the plant picornaviruses that may have evolved from the animal picornaviruses.

Serologic Relationships and Variability

MCDV strains include the severe, white stripe (WS), type (T) or Ohio (OH), and M1. MCDV-M1 differs from MCDV-T in that its CP2 and CP3 are slightly larger. Also full, partially full and empty virus particles occur *in situ* and *in vitro* for M1, whereas for T and WS mainly full particles occur. Also, the CP1s of M1 and T show no serological relationship, whereas T and WS are serologically indistinguishable. Infection of maize by individual strains causes only mild symptoms, with M1 causing the mildest symptoms, whereas co-infection by T and M1 incites severe symptoms. MCDV-M1 and MCDV-T show a 54% sequence similarity for a corresponding region of 839 nt at the 3' end of their genomes. Based on predicted amino acid sequences of the polyprotein, MCDV-TN has a sequence identity of 60% to MCDV-OH. It is less closely related to other picornaviruses (**Table 1**).

The waikaviruses share many characteristics with the animal picornaviruses (see Evolution). Differences include the putative P1 protein, which is larger than the leader (L) proteins of the two *Picornaviridae* genera with L proteins and which is absent for the remaining three genera. Also, MCDV and RTSV lack a CP equivalent to the *Picornaviridae* VP4.

Like MCDV, some RTSV isolates show symptomatological differences. A virulent RTSV strain from the Philippines, Vt6, readily infects rice cultivar TKM6, which is highly resistant to the IRRI strain A. RTSV isolates from India also show differences in virulence on TKM6. RTSV isolates from Thailand, Malaysia and India are serologically indistinguishable from the Philippines isolate when tested with antisera to the individual CPs of the latter. However, CP3 of the Indian RTSV isolate has a slightly higher electrophoretic mobility, which allows it to be differentiated from Southeast Asian isolates. Nucleotide and predicted amino acid sequences of part of the CP1 gene also show that Indian and Bangladeshi RTSV isolates are different from the Philippine and Malaysian isolates, suggesting the existence of two strain groups. Isolates from Thailand and Nepal may be mixtures of the two groups.

RTSV isolates also show variability in their sequences and organization in the 3' terminus downstream of the large ORF. Significant sequence differences exist in ORF 2 of isolates from the Philippines (RTSV-PH-2), Thailand and India compared to ORF 2 of RTSV-PH-1. Also, a repeating nucleotide sequence in the 3' NCR of RTSV-PH-1 is absent in the sequences of the other isolates. Because RTSV causes indistinct symptoms on many rice varieties and antisera to the virion or individual CPs do not differentiate isolates, sequence analysis will be required to differentiate additional RTSV variants.

In Japan two strains of RWV occur: the common or C strain and a more virulent strain S. Since RWV or RTSV assists in the transmission of RTBV by the leafhopper *Nephotettix virescens* and symptoms incited by RWV in combination with RTBV are similar to those of the tungro virus complex (RTBV + RTSV), RWV is believed to be identical or closely related to RTSV.

Epidemiology

The epidemiology of the waikaviruses depends principally on virus and vector sources for early infections. MCDV survives winters in the USA in the rhizomes of infected Johnson grass. Its principal leafhopper vector, *G. nigrifrons*, is one of the most common leafhopper species in the eastern half of the USA and frequently the most abundant leafhopper on maize. In the southern USA, *G. nigrifrons* overwinters as adults and eggs on winter grasses, grains and grazing crops which allow survival in the absence of maize. Most of these overwintering hosts are not virus hosts. In the northern USA, where winter temperatures are probably too low for leafhopper survival, *G. nigrifrons* may be introduced at the beginning of each growing season by migration from the southern overwintering areas. *G. nigrifrons* presumably acquires MCDV from virus-infected Johnson grass early in the season and initiates the disease anew in seedling maize.

Outbreaks of tungro are unpredictable and appear suddenly over large areas, frequently followed by disease disappearance in the next season. Virus sources for these outbreaks include infected rice stubble and volunteer rice ratoons, which may act as vector sources as well, especially in asynchronously planted areas. Weed grasses generally are relatively poor virus sources. Rice nursery beds may also serve as a virus source. In single-crop areas with a long rice-free period, virus may be introduced by long distance migration of viruliferous leafhoppers from virus endemic areas and locally by leafhoppers from infected weeds in and near rice plantings. *N. virescens*, the dominant and most efficient vector, is monophagous and prefers rice, whereas the relatively inefficient *N. nigropictus* prefers weeds. In areas of overlapping rice plantings, *N. virescens* may be of greater importance in virus spread and survival, whereas in single-cropping areas, *N. nigropictus* may be important in transmitting the virus among weed hosts in fallow fields.

The primary source of RWV for leafhopper acquisition is infected rice plants, rice stubble and spring ratoons. Winter host plants of *N. cincticeps*, the principal vector, are restricted to several grass species that are not virus hosts. Since rice plants do not survive over winter in most areas of Japan where RWV occurs owing to cold temperatures, migration of *N. virescens* from the disease-free islands, where it overwinters, to the areas of virus occurrence and then to areas where the virus does not overwinter may perpetuate RWV in the latter.

Transmission and Tissue Tropism

The waikaviruses are obligately vector transmitted in nature. The principal vectors of MCDV, RTSV and RWV are the leafhopper species *G. nigrifrons*, *N. virescens* and *N. cincticeps*, respectively. AYV is transmitted by the aphid *Cavariella aegopodii*. These vectors acquire and inoculate the viruses following a 10–15 min to 2 h acquisition access period and a 2 min to 2 h inoculation access period, respectively, and usually lose inoculativity within up to 4 days following acquisition and always following a molt. Preacquisition starvation has no effect on transmission efficiency and there is no detectable latent period in vectors. The viruses are not transovarially transmitted in their vectors. Leafhopper nymphal instars as well as adults transmit the viruses with similar efficiencies. The virus–vector relationship is semipersistent and transmission presumably involves a virus-encoded helper component (HC) protein.

RTSV is required for transmission of RTBV, which occurs only when the leafhopper has previously or simultaneously fed on RTSV-infected plants from which it acquires the putative RTSV HC. RTSV can be transmitted independently. AYV also acts as a helper virus for the transmission of PYFV, presumably by providing an HC for the transmission of PYFV.

Vectors acquire the viruses while ingesting from phloem cells and retain the viruses at sites on the lining of the vector's foregut. The particles are surrounded by a lightly or densely staining matrix, which in turn is embedded in a lightly staining material (M material) overlying the lining of the foregut. The matrix presumably allows virus retention within the vector for transmission. The viruses are released from these sites to infect phloem cells when the vectors extravasate during subsequent phloem feeding. The viruses are mainly phloem limited in infected plants and presumably move cell-to-cell via plasmodesmata.

Pathogenicity

Maize chlorotic dwarf and rice tungro are incited by

co-infections of MCDV and RTSV plus other viruses, respectively. For maize chlorotic dwarf, the severe symptoms are caused by synergistic co-infections of MCDV-T and MCDV-M1, which individually cause mild symptoms. However, not all field occurrences of the disease involve co-infections by isolates of the two viruses, making the disease etiology problematic.

Rice tungro is caused by co-infections of RTSV and RTBV. RTBV alone causes symptoms of moderate stunting and dark green and transitory yellow-orange discoloration of leaves, whereas RTSV alone causes no conspicuous symptoms. RWV occurs alone unassociated with RTBV.

AYV may occur alone or with PYFV.

Clinical Features and Infection

The principal symptoms incited by MCDV on susceptible maize are a reduction in plant height, chlorotic clearing or banding of tertiary veins and red or yellow discoloration of upper leaves. Symptoms of plant stunting or dwarfing and red or yellow leaf discoloration are often associated with infections of maize by the corn stunt spiroplasma or maize bushy stunt phytoplasma. MCDV infections can be differentiated from infections by the latter two pathogens by the diagnostic chlorotic vein clearing or banding of tertiary veins.

RTSV incites almost no symptoms and infected plants appear green with only mild stunting. Moderately resistant cultivars may exhibit recovery from tungro symptoms incited by RTSV plus RTBV, whereas stunting and leaf discoloration persist on susceptible cultivars. Tungro symptoms may show similarity to feeding damage caused by N. virescens, vector of both viruses, and symptoms caused by leafhopper feeding may be mistaken for those caused by the viruses and vice versa. Both the tungro virus (RTSV plus RTBV) and N. virescens cause foliar discoloration (orange or reddish-brown), reduction in tiller numbers, plant stunting and plant death when large numbers of leafhoppers feed on rice plants during tillering. Plants recover from leafhopper- but not virus-caused stunting.

RWV causes stunting and yellowing of leaves, but symptoms are less severe than those of RTSV plus RTBV. Leaf discoloration ranges from green to yellow and is transitory, not appearing on subsequently emerging leaves. Stunting symptoms persist.

AYV is associated with no conspicuous symptoms for infections of *Anthriscus sylvestris*, its principal host, but causes stunting and reddish purple leaf discoloration on *A. cerefolium*.

Pathology and Histopathology

Waikaviruses, which have 30 nm diameter isometric particles, are mostly phloem-limited in sieve tubes, companion cells and phloem parenchyma and cause distinctive inclusions detected by both light and electron microscopy. For MCDV, these inclusions include electron-dense granular and fibrous, fibriform or striated sheet inclusions. The former resemble the currant-bun inclusions of AYV and the viroplasms of RTSV and RWV. The fibrous inclusions are unique to MCDV infections. For the M1 and WS strains of MCDV, accumulations of virus-like particles occur within the dense granular inclusions, whereas with type strain isolates most of these inclusions contain no or very few virus-like particles. Individual virus-like particles are rarely found in the surrounding cytoplasm. In maize leaf cells infected with the WS isolate, the chloroplasts are deformed; and in stunted plants doubly infected with MCDV-T and MCDV-M1, some phloem cells degenerate. Histological changes include plugging of xylem but not phloem, reduced thickness of the leaf cuticular layer, and reduction of the diameter of the sieve elements in the rachis.

In RTSV-infected cells, inclusions include amorphous X bodies and lattice or tubular structures as well as viroplasms. Viroplasms are not membrane bound and appear as masses of electron-dense bodies. Virus particles are mostly scattered in the cytoplasm or vacuoles. Small vesicles, containing fibers and occasionally RTSV particles, are found in the cytoplasm, usually along the cell wall. RWV particles present in vacuoles are often in crystalline arrays. Phloem necrosis is observed with RWV infection. AYV-infected chervil petioles show phloem cells containing clusters of isometric virus-like particles embedded in amorphous densely staining material.

Prevention and Control

The recommended control for MCDV, RTSV and RWV is the cultivation of virus-resistant or -tolerant cultivars. For MCDV, no maize hybrids are immune and only a few are highly resistant. Other means of MCDV control include early planting, herbicide eradication of Johnson grass, and leafhopper vector control using the systemic insecticide carbofuran. Of these, widespread Johnson grass eradication and vector control are effective but problematic, being costly and potentially harmful to the environment. Cultivation of resistant or tolerant hybrids in combination with Johnson grass eradication and early planting is sufficient to limit yield loss due to the virus.

While RTSV causes only mild to inconspicuous

symptoms and presumably little or no yield loss, its control is important because of its role in RTBV transmission by the leafhopper vector and in inciting the severe symptoms of tungro when co-infecting with RTBV. While control of tungro is possible by use of vector resistance, the latter has been short-lived due to its breakdown after a few seasons. Resistance in rice is available for RTSV, but not for RTBV, and can provide an effective control of tungro in large fields, as plants infected with RTBV do not serve as sources for secondary spread of the virus in the absence of RTSV. However, RTSV resistance may be ineffective in small plots where high numbers of viruliferous vectors migrate from neighboring fields. Other means of tungro control include: (1) eradication of rice stubble and volunteer seedlings; (2) early transplanting; (3) large scale synchronous rice planting followed by a sustained fallow period; and (4) application of insecticides, especially carbofuran, for vector control. Control of RWV involves use of insecticides and cultivation of resistant varieties.

Future Perspectives

To complete knowledge of the waikavirus genome organization and protein functions, determination of the function(s) and the numbers and sizes of proteins is needed for the following portions of the polyprotein: the putative P1 protein downstream of the 5′ leader sequence and the sequences downstream of the structural proteins which contain an NTP-binding domain. Information is also needed on whether an RTSV-like C-terminal protease and RdRP are also present in the C-terminus of the MCDV polyprotein. Also, it is not known whether the cysteine-like C-terminal protease alone cleaves the viral polyproteins to release all the functional proteins. Functions are also unknown for the unusually long 5′- and 3′-terminal NCR and the small ORFs of the terminal NCRs of several waikavirus genomes. The designations of the three CPs (CP1, CP2 and CP3) need to be uniform among the waikaviruses. Finally, the relationship of the encapsidated small RNAs, found in slower sedimenting particles of some waikaviruses, to their associated viruses is unresolved.

Among the unresolved taxonomic questions is the relationship between MCDV-OH and MCDV-TN, which seem sufficiently distinct based on sequence identities to consider them as distinct waikaviruses. MCDV-M1 may also be a distinct species, but the similarity of its sequence to that of MCDV-TN is unknown. Also, nucleotide sequence information for the RWV genome would resolve its relationship with RTSV.

Other matters concerning the waikaviruses in need of demonstration are the HC protein, the role of MCDV-OH and -M1 in inciting the severe symptoms of maize chlorotic dwarf, and biological differences among waikavirus isolates differentiated by sequence and sometimes serological characteristics.

Finally, several characteristics of AYV raise the question of whether it is properly classified as a waikavirus. These characteristics are its apparent smaller genome, the presence of four rather than three CP species, an aphid rather than a leafhopper vector, and a dicot rather than monocot host range. The sequence of the AYV genome is needed to resolve this question.

See also: **Sequiviruses (*Sequiviridae*); Plant virus disease – economic aspects; Pathogenesis: Plant viruses.**

Further Reading

Anjaneyulu A, Satapathy MK and Shukla VD (1995) *Rice Tungro*. Lebanon, NH: Science Publishers, Inc.

CAB International (1999) Maize chlorotic dwarf waikavirus [original text by D. T. Gordon]. In: *Crop Protection Compendium*. Wallingford, UK: CAB International.

Hull R (1996) Molecular biology of rice tungro viruses. *Ann. Rev. Phytopathol.* 34: 275.

Thole V and Hull R (1998) Rice tungro spherical virus polyprotein processing: identification of a virus-encoded protease and mutational analysis of putative cleavage sites. *Virology* 247: 106.

Wesselbron Virus   *see* **Encephalitis Viruses**

West Nile Encephalitis Virus   *see* **Encephalitis Viruses**

Western Equine Encephalitis Virus   *see* **Equine Encephalitis Viruses**

YABAPOX AND TANAPOX VIRUSES (*POXVIRIDAE*)

HA Rouhandeh, Torrey Pines Cancer/Aids Research Institute, San Diego, California, USA

Copyright © 1999 Academic Press

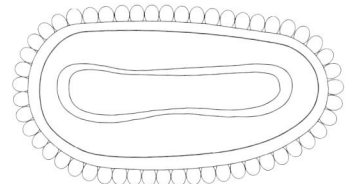

History

The disease produced by Yabapox virus is characterized by formation of tumors that regress slowly. The disease was first observed in 1958 in captive Rhesus monkeys housed in open pens in Yaba, Nigeria. At first the disease was confined to Asian monkeys and one baboon. Later one species of African monkey (*Cercopithecus aethiops tantalus*) became infected with the virus. In 1969 a spontaneous outbreak of the disease occurred in monkeys housed in Roswell Park Memorial Institute in Buffalo, New York. Infection of a laboratory worker reported in 1963 showed the virus to be pathogenic for humans.

The disease produced by Tanapox virus is characterized by a mild febrile illness in humans with one or two pock-like lesions developing on the upper part of the body. Two outbreaks occurred in 1957 and 1962 among the indigenous population living in the Tana River Valley in Kenya. In 1966 outbreaks occurred in monkey colonies in the USA and in humans having contact with the animals. Although Tanapox virus was first isolated from humans during an outbreak of the disease, it, like Yabapox virus, primarily causes a disease of macaque monkeys.

Taxonomy and Classification

The International Committee for Taxonomy of Viruses (ICTV) has proposed a classification of *Yatapoxviruses* as the genus name for Yabapox virus and Tanapox virus (as well as Yabavirus-like disease) within the *Poxviridae*.

Evolution

Both Tanapox and Yabapox viruses have been identified within the last 40 years. As far as is known, both viruses originated in monkeys. Human infections of Tanapox are believed to have originated from monkeys through the mosquito as a vector.

Properties of the Virion

Yabapox virus measures 250–280 µm in the long axis. The surface consists of thread-like structures which are randomly formed around the viral particle. Both Yabapox and Tanapox viruses are symmetrical and dumbbell-shaped; both contain a core with lateral bodies in the concavities and a double lipoprotein bilayer envelope comparable to other poxviruses.

Properties of the Genome

Yabapox and Tanapox viruses contain linear double-stranded DNA; the number of segments of 3′ terminal poly(A) tracts present or absent is presently unknown for these viruses. The size of both DNAs is estimated to be approximately 145 kbp with a molecular mass of 119×10^3 kD. The G+C content is $32.5 \pm 0.5\%$.

Properties of Virus Proteins

Tanapox virus contains approximately 55 proteins ranging in size from about 200 to 11 kDa. Yabapox virus contains approximately 44 proteins of which 21 are core-associated, ranging in molecular mass from 220 to 10 kDa. Four enzymatic activities have been identified with purified Yaba virions: DNase with pH optimum at 5.0; DNase with pH optimum at 7.8; RNA polymerase; and nucleotide phosphohydrolase.

Physical Properties

Yabapox viral DNA has a density of 1.6905 g ml^{-1} in CsCl and its T_m value in 0.015 M citrate in saline is 82.3°C.

Replication of Yabapox Virus

Nucleic acid

Viral DNA is detected 3 h after infection. At 6 h postinfection 7–10S RNA is detected which increases in amount after 12 h. At 24 h after infection, 14–15S RNA as well as 7–10S RNA is detected. The first and largest peak of mRNA synthesis occurs between 11 and 12 h postinfection and a second slightly smaller peak occurs between 21 and 23 h after infection. Late in the infection cycle, viral DNA is present in the host cell nucleus.

Protein synthesis

Yabapox viral proteins are synthesized at different times after infection and can be grouped into two classes, early and late. Early proteins are synthesized before the onset of viral DNA replication (3 h postinfection). Some of the proteins in this group are structural and continue to be synthesized in the presence of DNA inhibitor. Late viral proteins are detected at 6 h postinfection and continue to increase in number during the infection period. Viral infection does not inhibit host protein synthesis.

Virus synthesis

Yabapox virus is synthesized in the cytoplasm. At 35°C, the minimum length of replicative cycle is 35 h; however, maximum virus yields are not obtained until 75 h postinfection. Synthesis of at least two viral structural antigens occurs in the presence of the DNA inhibitor, cytosine arabinofuranoside, indicating potential transcription and translation of these antigens from parental DNA. The first progeny DNA is completed after 20 h postinfection, but is not detected in infectious form until 35 h postinfection. The maximum rate of progeny DNA synthesis occurs between 20 and 30 h postinfection. Viral DNA synthesis continues until 45–50 h after infection.

Morphogenesis

Within 3 h postinfection, the adsorption and phagocytosis of Yabapox virus particles by the cells can be seen by electron microscopy. This is followed by the disruption of the phagocytic vacuole membrane, with the release of viral DNA into the cytoplasm. At 24 h postinfection, large cytoplasmic inclusions termed 'factories' are observed. A typical factory contains a large number of viral particles, particulate glycogen, DNA-containing electron dense material, and small membranous spherical structures (40 nm in diameter) designated as 'micelles'.

Transformation

Various cell lines of monkey kidney cells have been transformed with UV-irradiated Yabapox virus. Two different cloned restriction enzyme fragments can also transform CV-1 monkey kidney cells. Transformed cells do not produce virus but exhibit biological characteristics typical of transformed cells. These include increased saturation density, reduced serum requirements for growth, and ability to grow in soft agar. The morphological alterations of transformed cells are similar to Yabapox virus-induced tumor cells and are characterized by loss of contact inhibition, multinucleated cells, and cytoplasmic lipid droplets. Southern blot hybridization showed that sequences homologous to low molecular weight viral DNA (5.1, 4.8 and 3.9 kbp) are present in transformed cells. Virus-specific antigens detected by immunofluorescence assays are found in the cytoplasm of transformed cells. Four virus-specific proteins, with molecular masses of 160, 140, 108 and 74 kD, are contained in transformed cells immunoprecipitated with sera from tumor-bearing monkeys.

Serological Relationships and Variability

Serologically Tanapox and Yabapox viruses show minimal to moderate cross-reactivity. The presence of type-common and type-specific antigens has been demonstrated. Yabapox viral infection fully protects primates against Tanapox virus challenges. In monkeys infected with Tanapox virus then challenged with Yabapox virus, symptoms were delayed in developing, and histiocytomas were smaller.

Complement fixing (CF) and complement fixing inhibiting (CFI) antibodies were demonstrated in the clinical and convalescent stages, respectively, of Rhesus monkeys infected with either Tanapox or Yabapox viruses. The persistence of CF antibody in monkeys infected with Tanapox virus is from 10 to 12 weeks; in monkeys infected with Yabapox virus CF antibody persists up to 35 weeks postinfection.

Epidemiology

The epidemiology of Tanapox virus is believed to be a reservoir of monkeys in the wild in Kenya from which the natives of the Tana River Valley are occasionally infected as a result of mosquito transmission of the virus. An outbreak occurred in monkey colonies in California, Oregon and Texas in 1965 and 1966 and spread to men in contact with the housed diseased animals. Tanapox of man is essentially a zoonosis. Yabapox is believed to be epidemic in scope in African and Asian monkeys. Infection in man occurs only through injection of the virus.

Transmission and Tissue Tropism

Yabapox and Tanapox viruses are both believed to be transmitted by insect vectors. Yabapox virus transforms fibrocytes of the dermis and subcutaneous cells to pleomorphic polygonal cells. The histiocyte gives rise to the tumor. In monkeys inoculated with Yabapox virus, histiocytes migrate into the infected area by 48 h postinoculation. After 3–5 days, the histiocytes undergo striking morphologic alterations and proliferate rapidly, leading to tumor formation. Intravenous inoculation results in many tumors in the heart, lungs, muscles and subcutaneous tissues of susceptible monkeys.

Tanapox viral infection is histiologically distinct from Yabapox. It affects the epidermis almost exclusively, resulting in hypertrophy and thickening of the epithelial layers of the skin with swelling and ballooning of the deeper epithelial cells; there is little cellular infiltration into the underlying dermis.

Pathogenicity

Because of the lack of studies on the prevalence of either Yabapox or Tanapox disease in the population of monkeys in the wild, little is know about pathogenicity. However, both viruses are of low pathogenicity in housed monkey populations. Pathogenicity from monkeys to humans is probably nonexistent in the case of both viruses in that each depends upon a vector or artificial means of transmission.

Clinical Features of Infection

In humans, Tanapox starts with a short febrile illness lasting 3–4 days and sometimes a severe headache, backache and pronounced prostration also occur. During the course of the febrile illness, one or two pock-like lesions appear on the upper part of the body, usually on the upper arm, face, neck and trunk. The lesion resembles a modified smallpox lesion in a vaccinated individual, except there is no pustulation in the Tanapox lesion. The illness is nonfatal and of short duration.

In monkeys, Yabapox is characterized by tumors on the hairless areas of the face, on the palms and interdigital areas and on the mucosal surfaces of the nostrils, sinuses, lips and palate. The benign tumors develop 5 days after inoculation, grow to 25–45 mm in diameter and project up to 25 mm in diameter. Tumor growth proceeds steadily, reaching a maximum in 6 weeks, after which regression occurs and is completed by 12 weeks postinoculation.

Pathology and Histopathology

In Yabapox infection tumor cells which develop are characterized by the appearance of multinucleated cells, cytoplasmic granulation, nuclear enlargement, nucleolar hypertrophy and the formulation of numerous lipid vacuoles in the cytoplasm. Granular inclusions in the cytoplasm stain positively for DNA with acridine orange.

Tanapox virus infection is characterized by hypertrophy and thickening of the epithelial layers with swelling and ballooning of the deeper epithelial cells, which show vacuolation of cell nuclei and eosinophilic cytoplasmic inclusions.

Immune Response

In Yabapox, circulating neutralizing antibody is ineffective in preventing growth of established tumors. Immunity to superinfection is present when tumors are present or regressing, but after total regression of tumors, re-infection results in new tumor formation.

In Tanapox infection immunity persists in monkeys for at least nine months following healing of the skin lesions.

Prevention and Control

Prevention of Tanapox in the human population is thought to be controllable by controlling the mosquito population and avoidance of mosquito-infested areas where the disease is epidemic in monkeys. Control of both diseases in housed monkeys has been accomplished by control of insects and by strict isolation of infected animals.

Future Perspectives

The control of Tanapox in the human population presents a serious problem because of the highly isolated and rare epidemiology of the disease and its non-serious nature. More studies of wild monkey populations where the disease is epidemic are needed in order to determine for certain how the disease is spread. If both diseases are spread by mosquitoes as postulated, complete control is unlikely to be achieved.

See also: **Smallpox and monkeypox viruses (*Poxviridae*); Zoonoses.**

Further Reading

Amano H, Ueda Y and Miyamura T (1995) Identification and characterization of the thymidine kinase gene of Yaba virus. *J. Gen. Virol.* 76 (Pt 5): 1109.

Knight C *et al*. (1989) Studies on Tanapox virus. *Virology* 172: 116.

Rouhandeh H (1988) Yaba virus. In: Darai G (ed.) *Virus Diseases in Laboratory and Captive Animals*. Boston: Martinus Nijhoff Publishers.

[This article is reproduced from the 1st edn (1994).]

YEAST RNA VIRUSES (*TOTIVIRIDAE*)

Lionel Benard, **Herman Edskes**, **Juan Carlos Ribas** and **Reed B Wickner**, Laboratory of Biochemistry and Genetics, National Institutes of Health, Bethesda, Maryland, USA

Copyright © 1999 Academic Press

History

Some strains of the yeast *Saccharomyces cerevisiae* secrete a protein toxin that kills other strains, but to which the secreting strain is itself immune. Toxin production ability is inherited as a non-mendelian trait. This finding (in 1963) by Makower and Bevan led to the discovery of viral particles containing various double-stranded RNAs (dsRNAs), one of which, called M, was correlated with the killer phenomenon. Studies of this area have taken two directions, one concerned with the virology of the system, and the other with the processing, secretion and action of the toxin and the mechanism of immunity.

Classification

Yeast RNA viruses belong to the genus *Totivirus* of the *Totiviridae* family. Other genera in the family are *Giardiavirus* and *Leishmaniavirus*.

Yeast RNA Replicons

Four completely distinct RNA to RNA replication systems have been found in various strains of *S. cerevisiae*: L-A and its satellites (including M), L-BC, 20S RNA and 23S RNA. The L-A and L-BC systems are encapsidated, whereas the 20S and 23S RNAs apparently replicate naked in the cells (**Table 1**). None of the viruses are known to have a natural extracellular infectious cycle, although they can be introduced into spheroplasts along with transforming DNA plasmids. All are efficiently transmitted from cell to cell by the cytoplasmic mixing that occurs on mating. Perhaps because mating is a very frequent event for yeasts in nature, these viruses are widespread and most strains have more than one. The best studied is the L-A virus (**Fig. 1**) and its satellite viruses, M_1, M_2, M_3 and M_{28}, encoding different killer toxins and immunity functions. Defective interfering deletion mutants of L-A and M_1 have been described. Yeast strains also contain at least four families of retroviruses. Recently, brome mosaic virus and flockhouse virus have been found able to replicate in yeast, a result that promises further

Table 1 RNA replicons in *Saccharomyces cerevisiae*

	kb	Proteins encoded	Comments
dsRNA viruses			
L-A	4.6	76 kDa major coat protein = Gag 170 kDa Gag-Pol fusion protein	Single segment ribosomal frameshifting no 5′ cap or 3′ poly(A) Gag has decapping activity
M_1, M_2, M_{28},...	1.0–1.8	Preprotoxin-immunity protein	Satellites of L-A
L-BC	4.6	78 kDa major coat protein = Cap 175 kDa Cap-Pol fusion protein	
ssRNA replicons			
20S RNA	2.8	90 kDa RNA-dependent RNA polymerase	W dsRNA is RF; circular form seen
23S RNA	3.2	RNA-dependent RNA polymerase	T dsRNA is RF supported by cDNA clones for segs. 1 and 2
Brome mosaic V. segment 3		*URA3*	

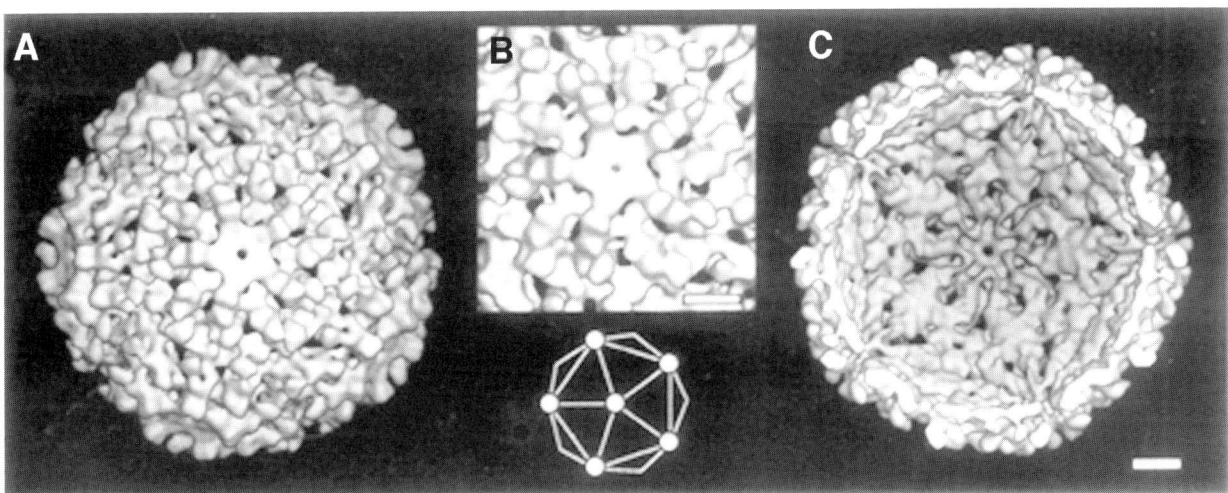

Figure 1 Cryo-electron microscopic reconstruction of L-A viral particles shows them to have icosahedral symmetry with a T=1 triangulation number. Each particle is composed of 120 Gag molecules, 60 pairs of Gag molecules with the members of a pair in two different environments. The outer (**A**, **B**) and inner (**C**) surfaces are shown at 20 Å resolution. Scale bar, 50 Å. (Reproduced with permission from Steven AC, Trus BL, Booy FP et al (1997) The making and breaking of symmetry in virus capsid assembly: glimpses of capsid biology from cryoelectron microscopy. *FASEB J.* 11: 733.)

widening of the scope of application of yeast studies to virology. Yeast RNA replicons are summarized in **Table 1**.

L-A Replication Cycle

L-A is a dsRNA virus that has a single 4.6 kb segment, and viral particles contain a single molecule of L-A dsRNA. The viral particles have a 76 kDa major coat protein (Gag) and a minor 170 kDa protein (Gag-Pol) whose N-terminal portion is a Gag monomer and whose C-terminal portion binds ssRNA and is the RNA polymerase. A conservative transcriptase activity of the particles produces viral plus-strands and extrudes them from the particles. The plus ssRNA is translated to form viral particle proteins (see below) and is also the species packaged to form new viral particles. These particles then make the minus-strand on the plus-strand template to form L-A dsRNA-containing particles and complete the cycle (**Fig. 2**).

Satellite viruses of L-A, such as M_1, use the L-A-encoded coat proteins. Again, a single viral plus-strand is packaged to form new particles, but after replication and transcription, the new transcripts often remain inside the viral particle where a second (or more) dsRNA molecule is formed by a second replication event. This is called 'headful replication' to distinguish it from the 'headful packaging' phenomena seen in many bacteriophages. In the case of L-A and its satellites, a single viral plus-strand is packaged and then it replicates inside the particle until the head is full. Then all new transcripts are extruded from the particle.

The *cis* signals responsible for packaging and replication have been defined on L-A (**Fig. 3**) and M_1. The packaging proteins recognize a stem–loop structure located about 400 nucleotides from the 3' end of either L-A or M_1. The sequence of the stem is not important, only that it is a stem, but an A residue that protrudes on the 5' side of the stem is critical, as is the loop sequence. The replication reaction requires that the template has both an internal site that largely overlaps with the packaging site (and may be identical to it) and a specific 3'-terminal sequence and structure.

The packaging of viral (+) strands involves recognition of the packaging site by residues 67–213 of the Pol domain of the Gag-Pol fusion protein. There are two copies of the fusion protein per particle.

L-A Expression: Ribosomal Frameshifting in a dsRNA Virus

L-A plus-strands encode the 76 kDa viral major coat protein (called Gag in analogy with retroviruses) and a 170 kDa Gag-Pol fusion protein, formed, as in the case of retroviruses, by a −1 ribosomal frameshift (**Fig. 3**). The structure responsible for the frameshifting is a slippery site, GGGUUUA, followed by an RNA pseudoknot, both located in the region of overlap of the *gag* and *pol* open reading frames. The efficiency of frameshifting appears to be critical for viral propagation, suggesting that the balance of Gag and Gag-Pol fusion proteins may be important in the assembly process. Since no eukaryotic cellular gene is known to use −1 ribosomal frameshifting as part of its expression strategy, these results suggest that drugs affecting this process may be useful for antiviral therapy.

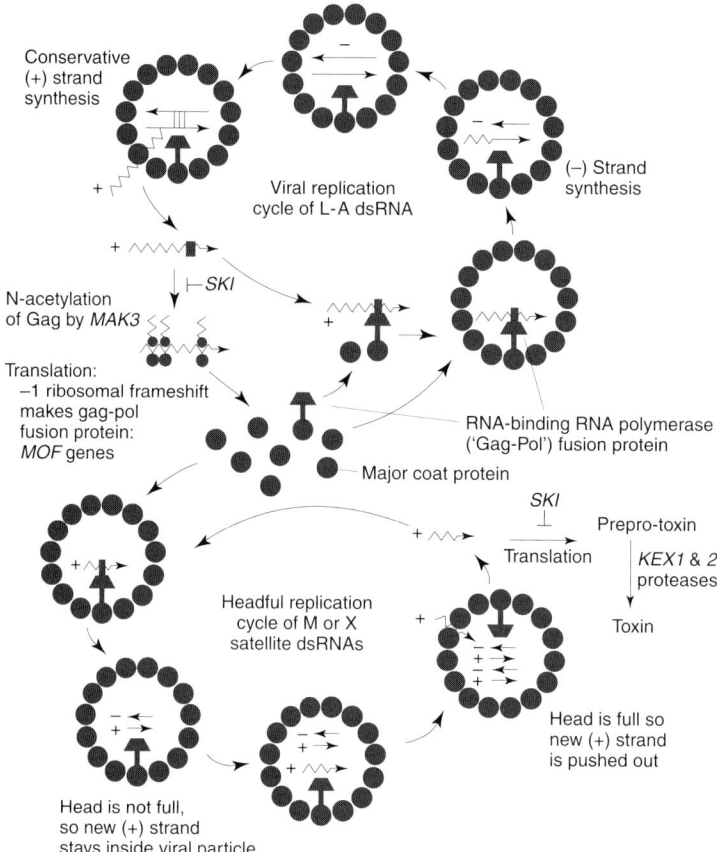

Figure 2 Replication cycles of L-A and its satellites.

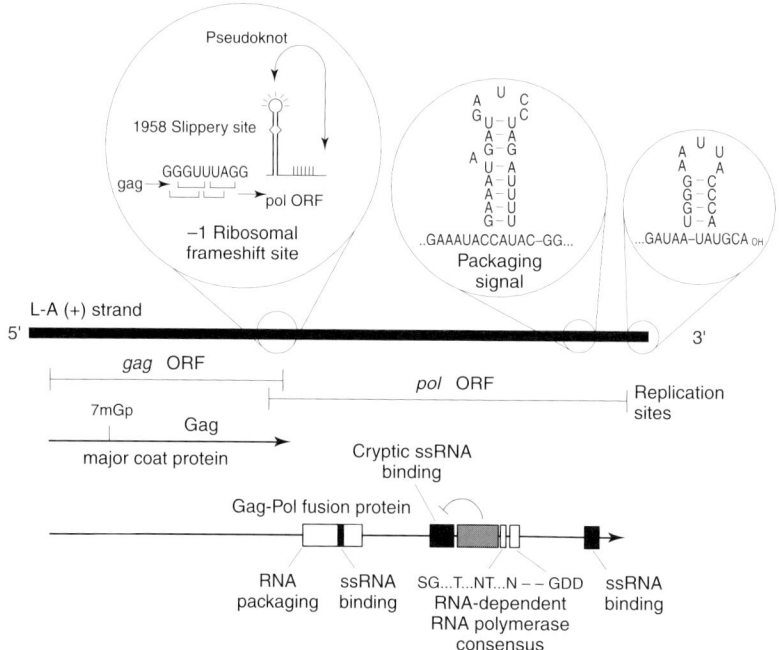

Figure 3 Expression of L-A-encoded information. The two L-A ORFs encode a chimeric RNA polymerase-RNA binding protein with a major coat protein domain. ORF 1 (Gag) is the major coat protein, whereas ORF 2 (Pol) encodes a region with the consensus sequence patterns for the RNA-dependent RNA polymerases of plus ssRNA viruses and dsRNA viruses. Pol also has three ssRNA binding domains, the N-terminal one of which is necessary for packaging viral (+) strands.

Table 2 Chromosomal genes affecting yeast RNA viruses

Gene(s)	Encodes	RNA affected	Mechanism
MAK3	N-Acetyltransferase	L-A, M	Viral assembly
MAK1, 7, 8, 11, 16, 18, 27, ...	60S ribosomal subunit proteins and assembly factors	L-A, M	Expression of viral poly(A)-mRNA
SKI1/XRN1	5'-exoribonuclease	L-A, M	Viral mRNA stability
SKI2, 3, 8	System blocking translation of nonpoly(A) mRNA	L-A, M, L-BC, 20S	Blocks viral translation
SKI6	3'-exoribonuclease required for 60S ribosomal subunit assembly	L-A, M	Blocks viral translation
porin, NUC1	Mitochondrial functions	L-A	?
CLO1	?	L-BC	?

The structure of the Gag-Pol fusion protein suggested a packaging mechanism for L-A in which the Pol part of the fusion protein captures a viral (+) strand and the Gag part primes polymerization of the coat by association with Gag molecules. This results in the natural packaging of one viral (+) strand per particle.

Why do L-A, retroviruses and a number of plus single-stranded (ss) RNA viruses use ribosomal frameshifting and readthrough of termination codons to make Gag-Pol and other fusion proteins? dsRNA viruses, plus ssRNA viruses and retroviruses all use their plus-strands as mRNA, as the form of the genome that is packaged to make new particles and as a template for replication. If they were to use splicing or RNA editing for the purpose of fusing open reading frames, they would be generating mutants unless the spliced out region contained a site essential for packaging or replicating the genome. Retroviruses often splice, but they remove the packaging site in so doing so that the spliced mRNAs will not be packaged. Insofar as is known, plus ssRNA viruses and dsRNA viruses do not splice, perhaps for this reason. Minus ssRNA viruses do splice and edit their RNAs.

Host Functions

Over 40 chromosomal genes affecting the propagation and expression of the L-A or M dsRNA genomes in yeast have been defined and a single gene is needed for L-BC (Table 2). Chromosomal (host) mutants that lose the M_1 genome are generally called *mak* mutants (for maintenance of killer). Among the 30 genes of this type are three, MAK3, MAK10 and MAK31, which are necessary for the propagation of L-A. MAK3 is now known to encode an N-acetyltransferase responsible for acetylating the N-terminus of the major coat protein (Gag) encoded by L-A. This acetylation appears to be necessary for the assembly of viral particles. This parallels the N-terminal myristylation necessary for proper assembly of poliovirus and proper localization of retrovirus Gag protein assembly.

Over 20 *MAK* genes encode proteins of the 60S ribosomal subunit or other factors necessary for 60S ribosomal subunit assembly. Deficiency of 60S subunits leads to loss or decreased copy number of L-A and M dsRNAs. The mechanism of this effect may be due to inefficient translation of the viral mRNA, which lacks 3' poly(A). It has been suggested that the mRNA 3' poly(A) structure facilitates the joining of the 60S subunit to the 40S subunit waiting at the initiator AUG. A deficiency of 60S subunits should therefore adversely affect translation of nonpoly(A) mRNAs (e.g. viral mRNA) more than the poly(A)$^+$ cellular mRNA.

Mutations of any of seven genes, called *SKI* genes (for superkiller, the phenotype of the mutants), result in elevated copy number of L-A, M, L-BC and 20S RNA (23S RNA has not been tested). SKI1 (= XRN1) encodes a 5'-exoribonuclease specific for uncapped RNAs (such as viral (+) strands) and known to be the major enzyme degrading cellular mRNAs. The L-A Gag protein can decap cellular mRNAs, probably as a means to distract the SKI1 exoribonuclease from degrading viral mRNAs by providing other substrates to engage its attention.

Mutations in SKI2, 3, 6 or 8 result in derepressed translation of mRNAs lacking a 3'-poly(A) structure. It has been suggested that they act by affecting 60S ribosome biogenesis, but so far only *ski6* mutants have been proven to have altered 60S subunits. Ski3p is also known to be a nuclear protein, and Ski2p is highly homologous to a mammalian nucleolar protein. In strains carrying M dsRNA, *ski* mutants are cold-sensitive, temperature-sensitive or unable to grow at any temperature, depending on the presence of other nonchromosomal factors. The SKI system acts on L-A, M, L-BC and 20S RNA (see below), to lower their copy numbers in the cell.

A distinct system, affecting only L-A, is defined by mutations in the mitochondrial outer membrane porin and the major mitochondrial nuclease (*NUC1*). Growth on nonfermentable carbon sources is also known to elevate the copy number of L-A, indicating that a complex relationship exists between these viruses and mitochondrial functions.

Killer Toxin Processing and Mammalian Prohormone Processing

The killer toxin is encoded by M_1 as a precursor protein which apparently gives immunity to cells carrying M_1. The toxin has two subunits which, in close analogy to insulin, are processed from the preproprotein by removal of a signal sequence and a peptide between the subunits (**Fig. 4**). This analogy with mammalian prohormone processing is more than superficial. The *kex1* and *kex2* mutations were originally isolated based on their inability to secrete K_1 killer toxin and the yeast α mating pheromone. The *KEX2* product was then found to be a protease cleaving specifically C-terminal pairs of basic residues, and *KEX1* is another protease that removes the two basic residues. This is just like the processing of insulin, pro-opiomelanocortin and other mammalian hormones. Indeed, using sequence information from *KEX2* or functional complementation of *kex2* mutants, several mammalian protease genes have been isolated which are candidates for the physiological prohormone processing enzymes. Moreover, the yeast *KEX2* gene can substitute for the mammalian proteases in processing prohormones.

Toxin Action

The K_1 killer toxin must bind first to (1 → 6) β-D-glucan, a major structural component of yeast cell walls. The K_{28} toxin binds first to cell wall mannans. However, since spheroplasts remain sensitive to these toxins, there must be a receptor further downstream in the process. The K_1 toxin acts by creating proton pores in the membrane.

20S RNA Replicon and T and W dsRNA

20S RNA was discovered in 1971 as a species whose synthesis is induced when cells are transferred to the media that are used to induce meiosis and sporulation in yeast (potassium acetate medium). Subsequent studies showed that some strains were unable to produce 20S RNA under these conditions, and that there was no role for 20S RNA in sporulation. Thus, some strains that could sporulate made no 20S RNA and some that could not sporulate could make 20S RNA. It was also shown that the ability to induce 20S RNA synthesis was inherited as a non-mendelian factor.

Recently, most of 20S RNA has been cloned and

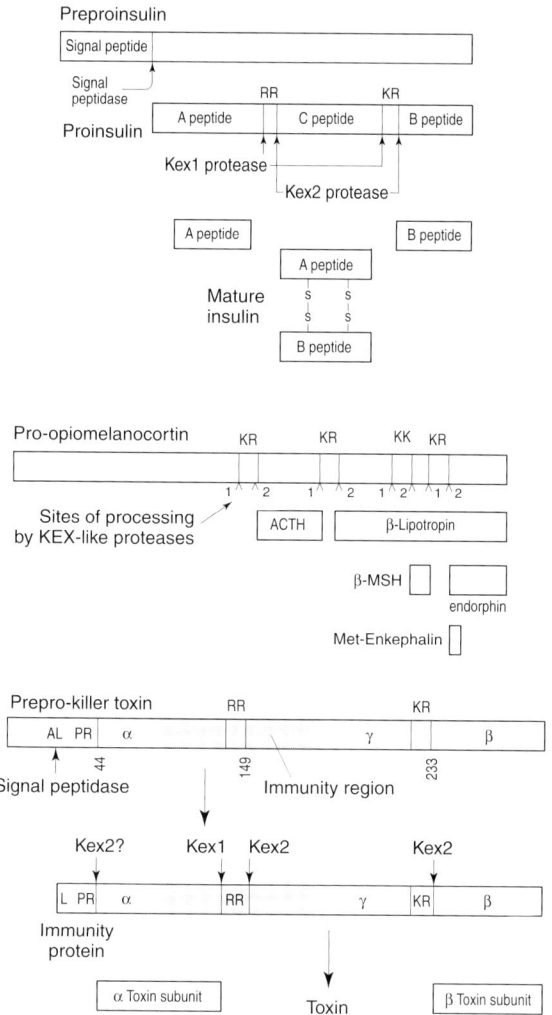

Figure 4 Preprotoxin processing resembles mammalian hormone processing. The two subunits of both insulin and killer toxin are cleaved out of their precursor hormones by Kex-like proteases. These enzymes were first discovered in the killer system and this led to their discovery in mammalian cells.

sequenced. 20S RNA is not encoded by any cellular DNA (chromosomal or otherwise). It replicates via an RNA to RNA mechanism. Electron microscopy of 20S RNA coated with T4 gene 32 protein and cross-linked with glutaraldehyde showed mostly circles, and dimer length molecules of both plus and minus polarity have also been detected *in vivo*, consistent with a rolling circle mode of replication. However, the inability to clone all the way around the 20S RNA circle suggests that either there is unusual structure at the uncloneable site, or a fundamentally linear molecule whose ends are held together by some structure. A linear structure is also indicated by biochemical experiments. At this time the structure of 20S RNA remains unclear.

Two low copy number dsRNAs, called T and W,

were described in 1984. Neither was homologous to cellular DNAs and the copy number of both was induced by growth at elevated temperatures. W was recently cloned and sequenced and was found to be identical to 20S RNA. Indeed, 20S RNA copy number is also induced at high temperature. Since the copy number of 20S RNA is always 10-fold or more that of W, W may be viewed as a replicative form of 20S RNA. Their sequence shows a single long open reading frame encoding a protein of about 90 kDa with some homology to the RNA-dependent RNA polymerases of plus-strand RNA viruses. T dsRNA encodes a similar putative RNA-dependent RNA polymerase. These proteins are found in extracts specifically associated with their respective templates, and the 20S RNA polymerase activity has actually been demonstrated *in vitro*.

Applications

Since killer strains kill nonkiller strains when cocultivated, brewing strains have been modified to include a killer virus so that strains present in the grapes (barley, hops, etc.) will not spoil the brewing process. This application is in use today. Vectors based on the toxin secretion signals have also been developed.

Future Perspectives

The ease with which yeast is manipulated genetically and the high yields of L-A virus that can be easily obtained from engineered strains have made possible extensive characterization of the genetics of this virus and its satellites and their relationship with their host. The *in vitro* replication, packaging and transcription systems were the first developed among the dsRNA viruses of eukaryotes, and few such systems have been developed for any RNA viruses. It is likely that the mechanisms found for L-A will not be unique to this system. Among the important problems to be solved are (1) development of an RNA transfection system so that the L-A virus may be used as a vector, (2) further pursuit of the mechanisms of transcription, replication and packaging and application of this information to viruses of higher systems, (3) further elucidation of the mechanisms by which the *SKI* genes control virus propagation, (4) further understanding of the role of host genes that the virus uses for its propagation, and (5) study of the role of various host components in ribosomal frameshifting and search for pharmacologic agents affecting this process – a new approach to antivirals.

The 20S RNA system (and the related T dsRNA system) have only begun to be studied. The question of the nature of the circularity of 20S RNA and the mechanism by which its propagation is controlled, including the massive 10 000-fold amplification on acetate medium, are of great interest. If it is a true circle of RNA, it is likely to self-cleave and self-ligate as do related viroid systems.

See also: **Partitiviruses – fungal (*Partitiviridae*); Prions: Yeast and Fungi; Retroviruses – type D (*Retroviridae*); Totiviruses (*Totiviridae*): General features,** *Ustilago maydis* **viruses; Vectors: Animal viruses, Plant viruses; Viroids.**

Further Reading

Bussey H (1991) K1 killer toxin, a pore-forming protein from yeast. *Mol. Microbiol.* 5: 2339.

Esteban R, Rodriguez-Cousino N and Esteban LM (1993) Genomic organization of T and W, a new family of double-stranded RNAs from *Saccharomyces cerevisiae*. *Prog. Nucl. Acid Res.* 46: 155.

Steiner DF, Smeekens SP, Ohagi S and Chan SJ (1992) The new enzymology of precursor processing endoproteases. *J. Biol. Chem.* 267: 23435.

Wickner RB (1996) Double-stranded RNA viruses of yeast. *Microbiol Rev* 60: 250.

Wickner RB (1996) Viruses of yeasts, fungi and parasitic microorganisms. In: Fields BN, Knipe DM, Howley PM, *et al* (eds) *Fields Virology*, 3rd edn. Philadelphia: Lippincott–Raven.

YELLOW FEVER VIRUS (*FLAVIVIRIDAE*)

Thomas P Monath, OraVax Inc., Cambridge, Massachusetts, USA

Copyright © 1999 Academic Press

History

Yellow fever was first described as a disease entity in 1648 in Mexico. The origins of the disease are in doubt, but the susceptibility of New World – but not African – monkey species to lethal infection (suggesting contact with the virus in relatively recent times) indicates an African origin of the virus. Whether or not yellow fever in its enzootic form (transmitted between monkeys and sylvan mosquito species) predated the Spanish Conquest in tropical America, it was the slave trade that led to the introduction from Africa of the domestic mosquito vector, Aedes aegypti and the emergence of epidemic (urban) yellow fever. Yellow fever was one of the great scourges of mankind during the eighteenth and nineteenth centuries, with epidemics affecting coastal cities in the Americas, Europe and West Africa. The mode of spread of the disease was the subject of great debate. Mosquito transmission was suggested as early as 1848, was emphasized by the Cuban physician, Carlos Finlay in 1881, and finally was proven by Walter Reed and his colleagues in 1900. Reed et al also demonstrated that yellow fever was a filterable 'virus', although the etiology of the disease remained in dispute until isolation of the virus in 1927. In the decade that followed, quantitative virological and serological methods were established, allowing precise diagnostic, epidemiological and pathogenesis studies as well as the development and evaluation of live, attenuated vaccines.

Taxonomy and Classification

Yellow fever virus is the prototype member of the family *Flaviviridae*, genus *Flavivirus*, and the virus after which the family and genus were named (*flavus*, Lat. yellow). The genus consists of at least 68 viruses grouped on the basis of shared antigenic determinants and physicochemical properties (see below). The relatively specific neutralization test using polyclonal antisera has been used to distinguish at least eight antigenic complexes to which closely-related flaviviruses are assigned. Neutralization epitopes of yellow fever virus are sufficiently different from other flaviviruses to preclude assignment to a complex.

Properties of the Virion

Virions are spherical, 40–50 nm in diameter, and have short surface projections. The nucleocapsid has icosahedral symmetry, contains the RNA genome and a single core protein, and is surrounded by a lipid bilayer envelope. Approximately 66% of the virion is composed of protein, 12% carbohydrate and 17% lipid. Viral infectivity is rapidly inactivated by heat (56°C for 30 min), ultraviolet radiation and lipid detergents.

Morphogenesis of yellow fever virus occurs at intracellular (endoplasmic reticular, ER) membranes. Mature virions accumulate in these membranes, are transported to the cell surface, and released by exocytosis. Budding of virions into the lumen of the ER is rarely observed and may be an extremely rapid event.

In secretory cells (such as the mosquito salivary gland and a variety of exocrine and endocrine glands infected in mammals), virion assembly occurs in concert with host cell secretory components and virions are released in secretory granules. Flavivirus infection often proceeds without markedly disturbing host cell function or macromolecular synthesis.

Properties of the Genome

The viral genome is composed of a single linear strand of infectious (positive polarity) RNA, 10 862 nucleotides in length, with a mass of 3750 kDa. The 5' terminus has a type 1 cap, and the 3' terminus is not polyadenylated. The GC content is 49.7%. The viral genome contains a single long open reading frame 10 233 nucleotides in length, encoding 11 viral proteins (**Fig. 1**). The remainder of the genome comprises short 5' (118 nucleotides) and 3' (511 nucleotides) noncoding regions. Nucleotide conservation is seen between the 5' terminus of the plus strand and the 3' terminus of the minus strand, serving as common recognition sequences for the viral polymerase. The 3' terminus forms a stable hairpin loop involved in binding to the capsid protein.

Viral Proteins

The three virion structural proteins are encoded by the 5' one-fourth of the genome, in the sequence C (capsid), prM (precursor to the mature membrane (M) protein) and E (envelope) (**Fig. 1**). The remainder of the open reading frame encodes eight nonstructural proteins, in the order illustrated. Translation begins at the 5' terminus of the viral genome, and the individual proteins are produced after translation by a series of enzymatic cleavages. The C protein (12–14 kDa) interacts with RNA in the virion nucleocapsid; its hydrophobic C terminus anchors nucleocapsids to ER membranes, and provides signal sequence for prM. The prM glycoprotein (18–19 kDa), present intracellularly, is cleaved by a furin-like protease at the time of virus maturation to form M in the extracellular virion. The M protein spans the viral membrane, and has exposed antigenic domains that may play a minor role in the induction of protective immunity. However, the E glycoprotein (53–54 kDa) is the major surface structure and subserves many biological functions, including cell attachment, hemagglutination and neutralization. Important to these functions is the three-dimensional configuration of E protein, determined by disulfide bonding. Epitopes with strain-specific, type-specific and flavivirus group-reactive specificities are present in the E glycoprotein. As is the case for similar proteins, the C

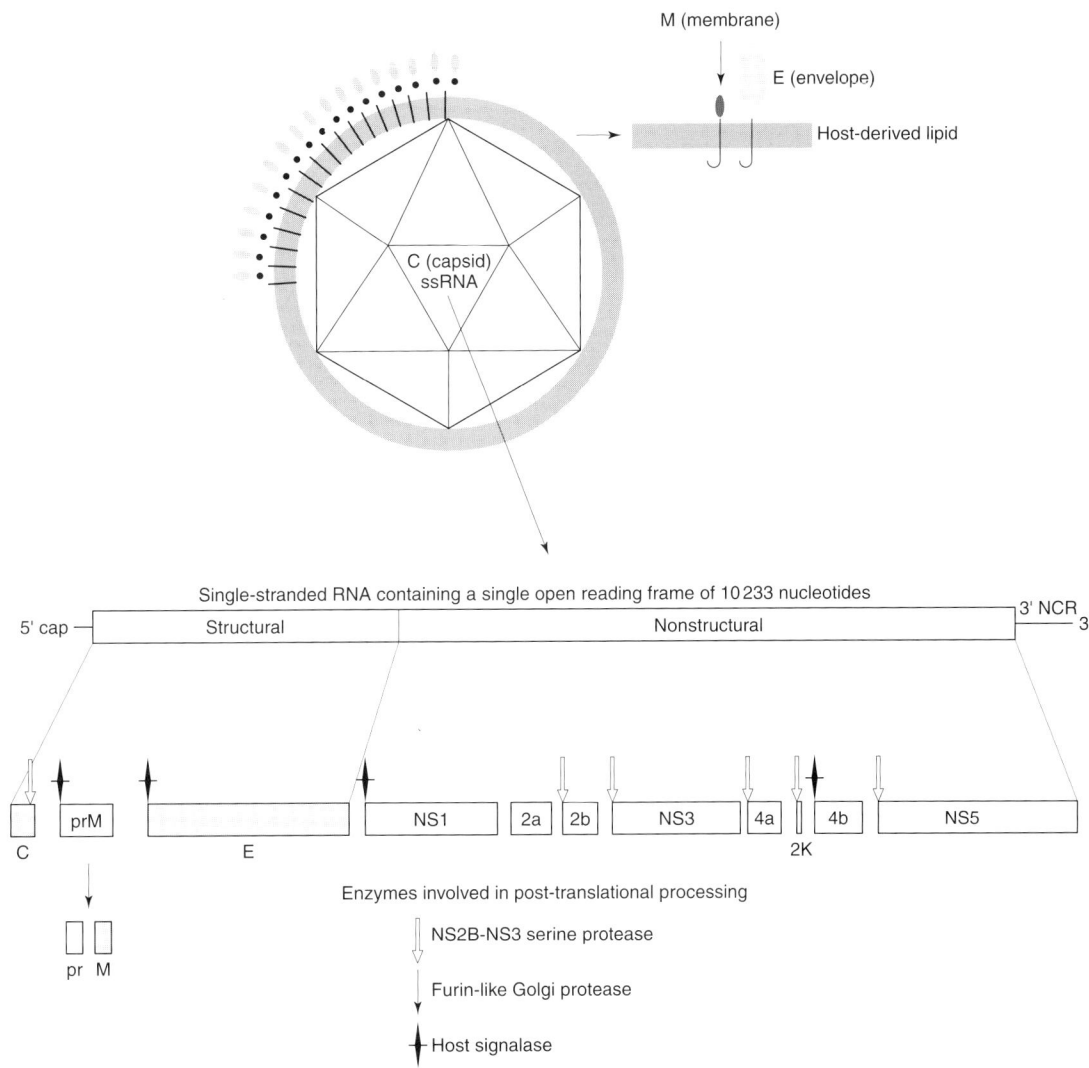

Figure 1 Yellow fever (flavivirus) virion and genome, showing the structural and nonstructural protein coding regions. The genome is characterized by type 1 5′ cap structure, followed by a short noncoding region and a long open reading frame of over 10 000 nucleotides encoding the structural (C-prM-E) and nonstructural (NS1–NS5) proteins. The genome lacks a 3′ poly(A) tail.

terminus contains hydrophobic sequences forming the protein anchor in the lipid membrane. The crystallographic structure of the E glycoprotein reveals a head-to-tail dimer composed of a 170 Å long rod anchored to the membrane at its basal end, with its long axis parallel to the virion surface. The C-terminus resembles an immunoglobulin constant domain and is connected by a flexible region to the central part of the molecule (domain I) with up-and-down topology having eight antiparallel β strands and containing the N-terminus. Two long loops (domain II) extending laterally are responsible for dimerization. A conserved stretch of 14 amino acids at the tip of one of the domain II loops constitutes the fusion domain responsible for internalization of nucleocapsids from endosomes into the cytoplasm of the infected cell. Domain III contains ligands involved in binding cell receptors. Neutralization determinants are conformational, and are scattered on the outer surface of all three flavivirus structural domains. The nonstructural NS1 glycoprotein is found both within infected cells and extracellularly (as circulating antigen with complement-fixing properties). Expressed on the cell surface, NS1 is a target for antibodies involved in clearance of virus infection. The highly conserved NS3 protein (68–70 kDa) has helicase, protease and RNA triphosphatase functions. NS5 (103–105 kDa) is the RNA polymerase. The functions of NS2A, NS2B, NS4A and NS4B are not clear.

Replication

After gaining entry to the cell, genomic, plus-strand RNA is translated and RNA replication proceeds by

Table 1 Amino acid differences between Asibi virus and attenuated 17D vaccines

Nucleotide	Gene	Amino acid	Asibi	17D-204 and 17DD vaccines
854	M	36	Leu	Phe
1127	E	52	Gly	Arg
1482		170	Ala	Val
1491		173	Thr	Ile
1572		200	Lys	Thr
1870		299	Met	Ile
1887		305	Ser	Phe
2112		380	Thr	Arg
2193		407	Ala	Val
3371	NS1	307	Ile	Val
3860	NS2a	118	Met	Val
4007		167	Thr	Ala
4022		172	Thr	Ala
4056		183	Ser	Phe
4505	NS2b	109	Ile	Leu
6023	NS3	485	Asp	Asn
6876	NS4a	146	Val	Ala
7171	NS4b	95	Ile	Met
10142	NS5	836	Glu	Lys
10338		900	Pro	Leu
10367	(3′NCR)		U	C
10418			U	C
10800			G	A
10847			A	C

synthesis of complementary minus strands. New plus strands are transcribed from genome-length minus-strand templates. Duplex RNA molecules (replicative forms) are thus formed in the infected cell. New genome-length plus strands serve as mRNAs for translation of structural and nonstructural proteins, as templates for transcription of new minus strands for replication, and as genomes for inclusion into nucleocapsids for production of mature virus particles.

Variation and Evolution

Nucleotide sequence analysis of the E gene revealed that yellow fever virus evolved early in the lineage of mosquito-borne flaviviruses, approximately 3000 years ago.

Yellow fever virus is distantly related to other flaviviruses by serologic tests and in terms of homology in RNA sequences. Strains of yellow fever virus from different geographic regions can be distinguished by RNA fingerprinting and are presently classified into three genotypes, one from West Africa, one from Central and East Africa, and one from South America. A high degree of homology has been noted between strains belonging to one topotype.

Molecular Basis of Virulence

The genomes of the attenuated 17D and the French neurotropic vaccines and their wild-type parents, Asibi and the French viscerotropic virus have been compared. The 17D and Asibi viruses differ at 20 amino acids, and four nucleotides in the 3′ noncoding region (**Table 1**). Because of the functional importance of the E protein in attachment and entry to cells, one or more of the seven amino acid differences that separate Asibi and the vaccine strains are likely to play a role in attenuation. The role of the E glycoprotein in neurovirulence of flaviviruses has been established by studies in which the E gene of a nonneurovirulent virus has been replaced by the corresponding gene of a virulent virus, resulting in a conversion to neurovirulent phenotype. Four of the seven amino acid differences in the E gene are nonconservative ($52^{Gly \rightarrow Arg}$; $200^{Lys \rightarrow Thr}$; $305^{Ser \rightarrow Phe}$; and $380^{Thr \rightarrow Arg}$). At least three wild yellow fever virus strains with different passage histories or geographic origins are identical at these codons, suggesting that the mutations in 17D vaccine are in part responsible for attenuation. Residues 52 and 200 are located at the base of domain II, where mutations might affect acid-dependent conformational change in the endosome required for entry. The conservative change at position $173^{Thr \to Ile}$ corresponds to a site in tick-borne encephalitis virus at which a neutralization escape mutant had reduced neuroinvasiveness in mice. Residue 173 encodes an epitope recognized by wild-type specific monoclonal antibody and reversion at this site is correlated with the neurovirulence phenotype of a plaque variant recovered from a 17D vaccine. The nonconservative changes at E-305 and E-380 are located in domain III, which contains the determinants involved in tropism and cell attachment. Residue 305 is located on the outer surface of domain III and residue 380 is located in a highly conserved region in mosquito-borne flaviviruses implicated in cell receptor interactions. Sequence analysis of virus recovered from the brain of a 3-year-old child in the USA, who died of encephalitis following 17D immunization, revealed a mutation near the E-305 residue (at $303^{Glu \to Lys}$); the mutant had increased neurovirulence for mice and monkeys. Other studies emphasize the multigenic nature of virulence and suggest that one or more of the 10 amino acid changes in the nonstructural proteins or the changes in the 3' noncoding region of the virus may contribute to the attenuation of 17D vaccine.

Little is known about the molecular basis of viscerotropism (the ability of wild-type yellow fever virus to replicate and damage nonneural tissue, particularly the liver), or the mutations responsible for loss of this trait in 17D vaccine. Sequence comparison of the French viscerotropic strain with that of the French neurotropic vaccine (FNV) revealed 77 (0.7%) nucleotide and 35 (1%) amino acid changes scattered throughout the genome, with the highest frequency of mutations in the C, M, E, NS2a, 2K and NS4b proteins. The large number of differences and lack of biological data on the role of these mutations preclude speculations on the genetic basis of viscerotropism. Sequence comparison of FNV with 17D vaccines (which also have attenuated viscerotropism) revealed only two shared differences from the parental and other wild-type yellow fever viruses. These common differences, which evolved during the development of vaccine strains by completely distinct processes, were at positions in the M protein ($35^{Leu \to Phe}$) and NS4b ($95^{Ile \to Met}$). It is unclear whether these mutations are involved in loss of viscerotropism.

Host Range and Virus Propagation

A highly conserved region in domain III of the E glycoprotein incorporates an RGD motif and is the probable site of virus–cell attachment. Cell membrane receptors also remain to be elucidated. Because of the broad host range of the flaviviruses, cell receptors may be molecules with conserved structure across the chordate and arthropod phyla. Yellow fever and other flaviviruses enter cells by typical receptor-mediated endocytosis.

Yellow fever virus replicates and produces cytopathic effects and plaque formation in a wide variety of cell cultures, including: primary chick and duck embryo cells; continuous porcine, hamster, rabbit and monkey kidney cell lines; and cells of human origin (e.g. HeLa, KB, Chang liver, SW-13 cells). The virus replicates in Fc-receptor bearing macrophages and macrophage cell lines, and replication is enhanced by antibody. Mosquito cell lines, especially *Ae. pseudoscutellaris* (AP-61) cells, are highly susceptible and are often used for primary isolation or efficient laboratory propagation of virus.

The most sensitive method for virus isolation and assay is the intrathoracic inoculation of mosquitoes, such as *Toxorhynchites* spp. or *Ae. aegypti*. Infected mosquitoes show no signs of illness, and the presence of virus must be demonstrated by immunofluorescence or subpassage to a susceptible host. Infant mice succumb within 6–8 days to encephalitis; at about 8 days of age, mice become resistant to lethal infection by the peripheral route, while remaining susceptible to intracerebral challenge. After parenteral virus infection, a number of subhuman primate species develop fatal hepatitis resembling the human disease. The only nonprimate species that develops lethal hepatitis in response to yellow fever infection is the European hedgehog, *Erinaceus europaeus*. Antibodies have been found in a wide variety of wild vertebrates collected in the field. Wild animals have also been experimentally infected with yellow fever virus, including rodents, bats and marsupials. With the possible exception of opossums in South America, the data do not support a role for nonprimate species in transmission cycles.

Geographic and Seasonal Distribution

Yellow fever virus presently occurs in tropical areas of South America and Africa. *Ae. aegypti*-infested regions of North and Central America, the Caribbean and southern Europe were intermittently invaded by the disease until the early part of this century and are still considered at risk, should the virus be introduced. Despite the prevalence of *Ae. aegypti* in tropical Asia, yellow fever has never reached that continent, possibly because transmission in Africa and South America occurs in relatively inaccessible areas and because crossprotection is afforded by immunity to dengue

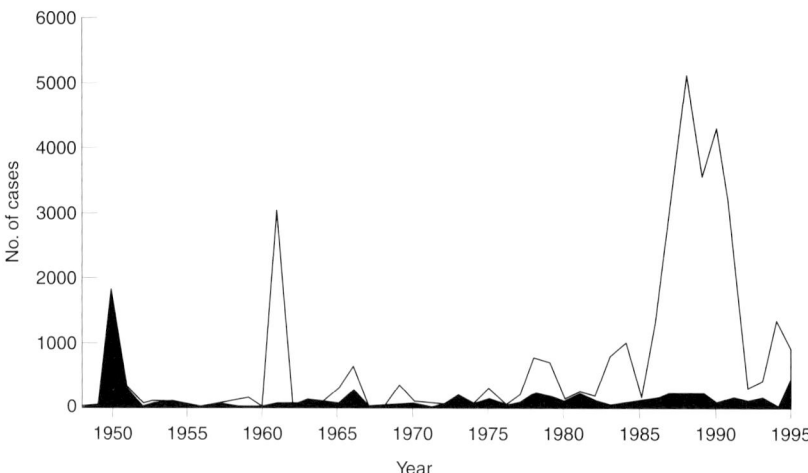

Figure 2 Officially reported incidence of yellow fever cases in South America (■) and Africa (□). The recent upsurge in incidence is due to a series of severe epidemics in Nigeria. Official reports greatly underestimate the true morbidity due to this disease.

viruses; dengue immunity is nearly universal in many parts of Asia. Asian populations of *Ae. aegypti* are relatively inefficient vectors; thus, vector competence may also provide a partial barrier to the spread of yellow fever in Asia.

The breeding of many mosquito species engaged in yellow fever transmission occurs in tree-holes and is highly dependent on rainfall. Transmission waxes during the tropical rainy season and wanes or ceases during the dry season. Breeding of the domestic mosquito, *Ae. aegypti*, occurs in manmade containers used for water storage and is thus less influenced by seasonal rainfall; where this species becomes involved in virus transmission, outbreaks may occur during the dry season.

Disease Incidence

Official notifications underestimate the true incidence of the disease by 10- to 250-fold. The number of cases officially reported annually from South America and Africa is shown in **Fig. 2**, and their geographic distribution in **Fig. 3**. The incidence in Africa has increased dramatically in recent years, due principally to a series of epidemics in Nigeria. Some epidemics in Nigeria and elsewhere in Africa have been very large, involving 100 000 or more cases, with case-fatality rates of over 20%.

Epidemiology and Transmission

Yellow fever virus is present in the blood of infected, susceptible hosts (humans and subhuman primates) for several days, during which mosquito vectors taking a blood-meal may become infected. The virus undergoes sequential replication in the midgut epithelium, body and salivary glands of the mosquito, a temperature-dependent process that takes a week or more to complete – the so-called extrinsic incubation period – before the vector is capable of transmitting virus by refeeding on a second host.

Two cycles of transmission are distinguished by the hosts and vectors involved. The urban cycle involves humans as the viremic host and *Ae. aegypti* mosquitoes, breeding in manmade containers. The forest cycle involves virus transmission between subhuman primates and tree-hole breeding mosquito vectors. The rate of transmission of yellow fever virus in the forest cycle can vary greatly, depending on the density of vectors and the available population of immunologically susceptible monkeys. In South America, some primate species succumb to fatal disease, and die-offs of these animals may provide a clue to yellow fever activity; in Africa, monkeys generally develop subclinical infections. Humans exposed in the forest to infected tree-hole mosquitoes may acquire yellow fever. In South America, this form (so-called jungle yellow fever) accounts for all cases in the last 50 years. Jungle yellow fever strikes mainly young adult males engaged in timbering and agricultural pursuits in the Amazon and Orinoco river basins. The principal mosquito vectors are species of the genus *Haemagogus*. The disappearance in the early 1940s of urban yellow fever, once a major endemic and epidemic disease in South American towns and cities, was attributed to successful programs to control the domestic vector, *Ae. aegypti*. However, in the last 10–15 years, *Ae. aegypti* has reinvaded much of the territory in South America from which it had formerly been eliminated, raising the spectre of urban epidemics in the future. Although

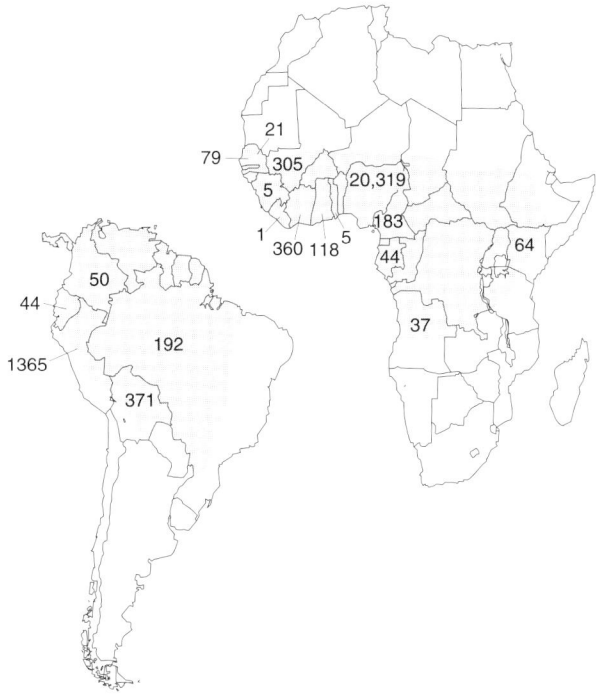

Figure 3 Geographic distribution of yellow fever cases, 1985–1996.

vaccine-induced immunity provides a degree of protection against such outbreaks, the level of coverage is presently incomplete.

The epidemiology of yellow fever in Africa is more complex than in the New World. The virus is present in a vast area of tropical Africa. Sporadic cases of jungle yellow fever occur in the rainforest zone, where the virus is maintained in a cycle involving monkeys and *Ae. africanus* mosquitoes, but such cases are rarely recognized because of inadequate surveillance. Unlike South America, tree-hole breeding *Aedes* spp. are also involved in epidemic transmission. Amplification of the virus transmission cycle occurs in moist savanna and forest-savanna transition zones, where the density of tree-hole *Aedes* reaches high levels during the rainy season. In these circumstances, humans are frequently infected. In urban areas or areas of low rainfall, where water storage practices favor breeding of domestic *Ae. aegypti*, this vector may be involved in epidemic spread, with humans serving as the viremic host.

Clinical Features

Subclinical or abortive infections occur more frequently than full-blown yellow fever. In its classical form, the disease begins suddenly, 3–6 days after the bite of an infected mosquito, with fever, headache, low back pain, muscle aches, loss of appetite and nausea. This period of infection is clinically non-specific, and corresponds to the viremic phase when the patient is infectious for feeding mosquitoes. It may be followed by a brief period of remission, during which signs and symptoms abate. The patient then becomes increasingly ill, entering the period of intoxication, with reappearance of fever, vomiting, dehydration, abdominal pain, and the appearance of jaundice, protein in the urine, signs of renal failure, and hemorrhages, most notably the vomiting of blood. Virus is no longer present in the blood. Approximately 20 to 50% of patients who progress to this stage die between the 7th and 10th day after onset, with deepening renal and hepatic failure, shock, delirium and convulsions.

Pathology and Pathogenesis

In humans, pathologic changes in the liver include swelling and necrosis of hepatocytes in the midzone of the liver lobule, with sparing of cells in the portal area and surrounding the central veins. Viral antigen and RNA are demonstrable by immunocytochemistry and nucleic acid hybridization in cells undergoing these pathologic changes, and cytopathology is mediated by direct viral injury. Hepatocytes may undergo apoptosis. Inflammatory changes are absent or minimal, and patients with hepatitis who recover do not develop residual scarring or cirrhosis. The kidneys show acute tubular necrosis, probably the result of reduced perfusion of blood rather than direct viral injury. Focal degeneration of muscle cells may be present in the heart. Spleen and lymph nodes show necrosis of B cell areas. The brain shows edema and petechial hemorrhages, but viral invasion and encephalitis are very rare events. Hemorrhage results principally from decreased synthesis of clotting factors by the liver. The mediators of hypotension and shock remain to be elucidated.

The pathogenesis of yellow fever has been studied in subhuman primates and mice, but our level of understanding is at the descriptive rather than the mechanistic level. Susceptible monkeys develop an illness similar to humans. Initial sites of virus replication have not been clearly defined, but probably include lymphatic tissue draining the site of virus inoculation. Viremia follows, with infection of the liver. Early virus replication occurs in fixed macrophages (Kupffer cells) in the liver, which undergo necrosis. The virus then invades hepatocytes, which develop accelerated cytopathologic changes during the 24 hours before death. Yellow fever virus demonstrates both viscerotropism (infection of liver, lymphoid and other visceral tissues) and neurotropism (infection and inflammation of the brain). In primates, viscerotropic infection is the rule; animals inoculated intracerebrally replicate virus in brain tissue and develop histopathologic evidence of encephalitis, but die of hepatitis. In contrast, mice develop brain infection without evidence of hepatitis.

Immune Response

Antibodies of both IgM and IgG subclass measurable by binding assays (immunofluorescence, ELISA), hemagglutination inhibition and neutralization appear 5–7 days after onset of illness (8–14 days after infection). IgM antibodies tend to wane to low or undetectable levels between 6 and 12 months after infection, although, in one study IgM neutralizing antibodies were still detectable several years after yellow fever immunization. Complement-fixing antibodies appear in the second week after infection, wane between 3–6 months later, provide a reliable indicator of recent wild-type yellow fever infection, and are rarely demonstrable after yellow fever vaccination. IgG neutralizing antibodies persist for at least 35 years, probably for life, and provide solid protection against reinfection. Antibodies to heterologous flaviviruses, such as Zika, dengue and Wesselsbron viruses, provide partial crossprotection against yellow fever. Complement-dependent antibody-mediated cytolysis of cells with exposed NS1 protein sequences may play a role in virus clearance and recovery, as well as in protection in the previously-immunized host. Little is known about cell-mediated responses in yellow fever. Limited studies in mice suggest that nonspecific resistance is mediated by interferon, NK cells and macrophages, and that cytotoxic T cells are important in clearance of yellow fever infection.

Prevention and Control

The control of domestic Ae. aegypti mosquitoes is an important measure, but has proven difficult to sustain. The most effective approach to prevention is immunization of the human population in endemic areas. Yellow fever 17D is a live, attenuated vaccine produced in embryonated eggs. Over 300 million people have been immunized with this inexpensive product, which has proven safe and highly effective. Recent efforts have focused on the production of a new vaccine derived from a full-length cDNA clone that generates infectious transcripts. By this approach it may ultimately be possible to produce chimeric vaccines with heterologous cassette genes incorporated into the 17D yellow fever vaccine backbone.

See also: **Dengue viruses (Flaviviridae); Pathogenesis: Animal viruses; Replication of viruses; Zoonoses.**

Further Reading

Barrett ADT (1997) Yellow fever vaccine. Biologicals 25: 17.

Chambers TJ, Hahn CS, Galler R and Rice CM (1990) Flavivirus genome organization, expression, and replication. Annu. Rec. Microbiol. 44: 649.

Chang GJ, Cropp CB, Kinney RM, Trent DW and Gubler DJ (1995) Nucleotide sequence variation of the envelope protein gene identifies two distinct genotypes of yellow fever virus. J. Virol. 69: 5773.

Monath TP (1986) Pathobiology of the flaviviruses. In: Schlesinger S and Schlesinger MJ (eds) The Togaviridae and Flaviviridae, p. 375. New York: Plenum Press.

Monath TP (1987) Yellow fever: a medically neglected disease. Rec. Infect. Dis. 9: 165.

Monath TP (ed.) (1989) Yellow fever. In: The Arboviruses: Epidemiology and Ecology, vol. V, p. 139. Boca Raton: CRC Press.

Monath TP (1991) Yellow fever: Victor, Victoria? Am. J. Trop. Med. Hyg. 45: 1.

Rice CM, Lenches EM, Eddy SR et al (1985) Nucleotide sequence of yellow fever virus: implications for flavivirus gene expression and evolution. Science 229: 726.

Robertson SE, Hull BP, Tomori O et al (1996) Yellow fever: a decade of reemergence (reprinted). JAMA 276: 1157.

Zanotto PM, Gould EA, Gao GF et al (1996) Population dynamics of flaviviruses revealed by molecular phylogenies. Proc. Natl Acad. Sci. USA 93: 548.

ZOONOSES

Thomas M Yuill, Institute for Environmental Studies, University of Wisconsin, Madison, Wisconsin, USA

Copyright © 1999 Academic Press

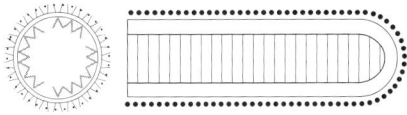

Introduction

Zoonoses are diseases transmissible from vertebrate animals, other than humans, to people. Hundreds of viruses in a wide range of families are zoonotic. Mammals, birds, reptiles and probably amphibians are reservoir or amplifier hosts for these viral zoonoses. Frequently, these viruses cause little or no overt disease in their nonhuman vertebrate hosts. Some zoonotic viruses have very limited host ranges, others may infect a wide range of vertebrates. Human infection may vary from unapparent to fatal disease. Some viral zoonoses have been recognized since ancient times, others have become public health problems recently. Both new and old viral zoonoses are especially important in emerging and re-emerging virus diseases.

Transmission

Transmission of zoonotic viruses may occur by a variety of routes. Rabies is transmitted by *direct contact* through the bite of an infected animal. *Indirect contact* transmission of other zoonoses occurs by ingestion of contaminated food and water, as is the case with the hantaviral and arenaviral hemorrhagic fevers. *Nosocomial* arenavirus and filovirus infections have been problems in hospitals caring for patients where isolation has not been adequate. *Aerosol transmission* of Venezuelan equine encephalitis virus has occasionally been a problem in the laboratory, where virus-bearing microdroplets have been widely circulated, with many resulting human cases. *Vertical (in utero)* transmission of arenaviruses results in persistent virus infection in the offspring. A large number of viral zoonoses throughout the world are *vector-* or *arthropod-borne*.

Some Common Zoonotic Viruses Around the World

Viral zoonotic diseases occur on every continent except, perhaps, Antarctica. Some are found around the world, in a variety of ecological settings. Others are found only in very limited ecologic and geographic foci. The panorama of viral zoonotic diseases is constantly changing. Although hundreds of viruses have been shown to infect both humans and animals, the importance of many of these viruses, as agents of either human or animal disease, has not yet been established. Some of the more important viral zoonoses will be discussed briefly.

Rabies virus

Rabies is one of the oldest reported zoonoses. Rabies virus infection causes nervous system disease that ends in death. Animals can become infected without nervous system involvement or disease, develop antibodies, and survive, but play no role in transmission. Classical rabies is found all around the world except in Antarctica, Britain, the Hawaiian Islands, Australia and New Zealand. Transmission occurs by the bite of an infected mammal that has virus in its saliva. Aerosol (droplet) transmission to humans has been reported, although rarely. Dogs and cats are the main reservoirs, especially in the tropical developing countries where more than 99% of all human deaths due to rabies occur. In the industrialized countries, wild mammals are the main reservoirs and the species involved vary from region to region. Translocation of rabid wild animals by hunting groups has been a cause of rabies spread in the USA. The principal species are: in North America, skunks, raccoons and foxes; in Europe, foxes; and in the Caribbean, mongooses. Bats in all enzootic regions harbor rabies, with vampire bats especially important in the Neotropics. Rabies virus is classified in the *Lyssavirus* genus of the family *Rhabdoviridae*. Genetic relationships between rabies isolates from different species and geographic areas have been established by genomic sequence analysis. Rabies-related viruses have been found in bats in Australia (Australian bat lyssavirus) and Britain and other European countries

(European bat lyssaviruses). Still more distantly-related lyssaviruses, some zoonotic, are found in Africa. Diagnosis is based on characteristic altered behavior of infected mammals, confirmed by isolation of virus or demonstration of intracellular antigen by immunofluorescence or of virus genomic sequences by nested reverse transcription–polymerase chain reaction (RT-PCR) confirmed by Southern blot hybridization. Postexposure treatment is accomplished by thorough washing of the bite wound, administration of hyperimmune serum or globulin, and administration of antirabies vaccine (prepared in human diploid cells, purified chick embryos or purified Vero cells). Dogs and cats in enzootic areas should be vaccinated. Other domestic animals and humans at high risk should be also vaccinated. Vaccination campaigns of free-ranging red fox populations in Europe and raccoons and coyotes in the USA have been carried out by oral administration of recombinant vaccinia-vectored vaccines in bait.

Hantavirus hemorrhagic fevers and pulmonary syndrome viruses

Hantaviruses are a newly-recognized complex of public health importance. These viruses belong to the *Hantavirus* genus of the *Bunyaviridae* family. Hantaan virus causes Korean hemorrhagic fever, and occurs in east Asia, especially in Korea, China and eastern Russia. Closely related rodent-associated hantaviruses cause milder hemorrhagic fever with renal syndrome in humans and have been reported from Scandinavia, Europe and Russia (Puumala virus), The Balkans (Dobrava-Belgrade virus), Russia and Asia as well as port areas around the world (Seoul virus). The similarity of many *Rattus* spp.-associated viruses globally suggests that movement of rats through commercial shipping has spread the virus as well. Seoul virus has been found in laboratory rats, with transmission to personnel there. Direct transmission of these viruses among rodents or from rodents to humans may occur by bite. A group of hantaviruses have been newly recognized with the appearance of highly fatal hantavirus pulmonary syndrome (HPS) in humans. As of June, 1998, 183 cases of HPS from 29 states and 24 cases from three Canadian provinces have been reported. Western hemisphere rodent-maintained hantaviruses that cause HPS include Sin Nombre (Alaska, across Canada, the USA except the southeast, south to central Mexico), New York (eastern USA, Canada and Mexico), Black Creek Canal (eastern Canada, USA; northern South America), Bayou (south central and southeast USA), Andes (southern South America) and Laguna Negra from a vesper mouse (southern South America). Lechiguanas and Oran viruses have also been associated with HPS cases in Argentina. There is evidence of direct human-to-human transmission of Andes virus. Several other rodent hantaviruses newly discovered in Europe, Asia and the Americas have not been associated with human disease. Hantaviruses are harbored by wild rodents which often live in close association with humans. Virus is shed in urine and other excreta. Outbreaks of HPS have been associated with ecological changes and invasion of human habitations by expanding rodent populations. Diagnosis has been complicated by the lack of efficient and sensitive isolation and serological methods, which explains why these 'new' viruses have only recently been isolated and characterized. Cell cultures, immunofluorescence or RT-PCR are used to isolate or detect virus, or to test for antibody. Because some of these agents are highly pathogenic to humans, work with them must be carried out in facilities that provide a high degree of biocontainment. Rodent control and avoidance of exposure to rodent excreta, especially in dust, are the only methods available currently for prevention of transmission to humans.

Arenavirus hemorrhagic fever viruses

Arenavirus hemorrhagic fever (HF) viruses, like the hantaviruses, are rodent associated, and can also cause severe disease in humans. Lymphocytic choriomeningitis (LCM) virus, the first arenavirus isolated, came from a person with encephalitis residing in the USA. Junin virus occurs in Argentina, Machupo virus in Bolivia, Guanarito virus in Venezuela, Sabia virus in Brazil and Lassa virus in West Africa. A complex of related arenaviruses that do not cause human disease occur in the Americas and Africa. These pathogenic arenaviruses establish persistent infection in their rodent hosts, and virus is shed in urine, infecting humans who live in close contact with these contaminated environments. Transmission may occur when people are in contact with blood or fresh carcasses of infected rodents. Lassa fever is also transmitted in rural hospitals to other people in contact with blood from viremic patients. Diagnosis is accomplished by virus isolation in cell culture, but detection of virus may require use of specific antibody and immunofluorescent or enzyme labeling. These techniques, as well as cDNA hybridization probes, are also used to detect viral products in tissues of infected humans or rodents. Diagnosis may also be established serologically by a diagnostic rise of specific IgG, or detection of IgM antibodies. Except for LCM virus, isolation of HF viruses pathogenic for humans requires the use of biosafety level 4 facilities. Serological tests such as ELISA can be done reliably with inactivated antigen at a lower level of biosafety. Control of these diseases is attempted mainly by reduction of rodent populations, as was done successfully with Bolivian HF, and by avoidance of dust containing rodent excreta. Prevention of human disease by vaccination is possible. A live attenuated vaccine has been developed for Argentine HF, and a vaccinia-vectored vaccine has been developed for Lassa fever. Ribivirin is effective for treating arenavirus infection if administered early in the course of infection.

Yellow fever virus

Yellow fever (YF), first recognized clinically in the Neotropics in the sixteenth century, periodically ravaged human populations in the Americas, Europe and Africa until as recently as the beginning of the twentieth century. Infection causes hemorrhagic disease with severe liver damage and death in up to half of the most acute cases. Presently, the virus is maintained enzootically in Africa and the tropical Americas in primates and arboreal mosquitoes. Humans or primates transport the virus from its sylvan cycle in forested areas to rural or urban areas, where other vector mosquitoes transmit it. YF may be a public health time bomb: there has been an alarming increase in human cases in West Africa in recent years, and, for the first time in history, in Kenya in 1992–1993. Although the number of 'jungle' YF cases in the American tropics has not increased as dramatically, re-establishment of the major urban vector, *Aedes aegypti*, and the recent appearance and spread of a potential YF mosquito vector, the Asian tiger mosquito (*Ae. albopictus*), in the hemisphere is a cause for serious concern. The risk of introduction of YF into cities is real. There have been recent instances of individuals infected acutely with sylvan yellow fever traveling to four South American urban centers infested with *Ae. aegypti*, but, fortunately, without subsequent transmission. YF virus is a flavivirus in the *Togaviridae* family. Diagnosis is by virus isolation in cell culture or in inoculated mosquitoes, detection of circulating antigens, demonstration of a significant raise in specific YF virus antibodies, or by observing viral inclusion bodies or antigen in tissues taken at postmortem examination. Insecticide spraying and elimination of breeding sites in homes can be used for vector control in epidemic situations. Disease can be prevented in humans by vaccination. Unfortunately, many countries have not been able to maintain an adequate level of immunity in populations in areas of risk and have to resort to emergency immunization programs when cases are detected. Because cases often occur in remote areas, it is difficult for many national health services to provide adequate vaccination coverage quickly in the face of YF outbreaks.

West Nile virus

West Nile (WN) virus, a close relative of Japanese encephalitis virus, occurs from India and Pakistan westward through the Middle East and into Africa, and northward into Europe and the republics of the former USSR. Mild infection to acute febrile disease with rash, and occasional encephalitis (mainly in the elderly), is produced in humans. *Culex* spp. are the main vectors, and birds are the vertebrate hosts. Diagnosis is by virus isolation and serological means. Unlike the related flavivirus encephalitides, WN virus can be isolated from the blood of human patients relatively commonly.

Chikungunya virus

Chikungunya (CHIK) virus has been responsible for acute febrile disease with rash and severe arthralgia in people in Africa and Asia. The epidemiology in Africa is similar to yellow fever; CHIK virus is maintained in sylvan or savanna cycles involving wild primates and arboreal *Aedes* mosquitoes. In both Africa and Asia, the virus also has an urban cycle involving humans and *Ae. aegypti* mosquitoes. Two outbreaks in Thailand in 1995 also involved *Ae. albopictus* mosquitoes. Virus can be recovered frequently from the blood of acute phase patients. The virus is an alphavirus of the *Togaviridae* family. The virus can be isolated in mammalian or mosquito cell cultures, although suckling mouse and mosquito inoculation are also sensitive systems. The virus has been transmitted to laboratory workers in the laboratory via aerosols created during virus isolation and passage. Serologic tests (neutralizing antibody or IgM capture ELISA test) are useful for diagnosis. Control of the sylvan and savanna enzootic cycles is not feasible. The urban cycle can be controlled by reduction of *Ae. aegypti* breeding sites and adult populations. No vaccine is available.

Sindbis virus

Sindbis (SIN) virus is one of the most widely distributed arthropod-borne viruses in the world, being found in Africa, Europe, Asia and Australia. Disease in humans is usually mild, and is characterized by acute fever, with arthralgia and rash. SIN virus is maintained in wild bird populations, with transmission by *Culex* spp. mosquitoes. In Africa and the Middle East, WN is often found in the same ecosystems where WN virus is being transmitted. The virus is an alphavirus of the *Togaviridae*. Phylogenetic analysis indicates that there is one major genetic cluster of western SIN virus strains in Africa and another in Australia and Asia. There is evidence of some geographic mixing western strains of SIN virus that suggests long-distance transport via migrating birds. Diagnosis is accomplished by virus isolation, demonstration of virus genomic sequences by RT-PCR or by serological means. There is no vaccine available. Since many of the mosquito vectors breed in extensive rice fields, large-scale control would be expensive.

Crimean–Congo hemorrhagic fever virus

Crimean–Congo hemorrhagic fever (CCHF) virus is very widely distributed, and is found from eastern Europe and the Crimean, eastward through the Middle East to western China, and southward through Africa to South Africa. CCHF is characterized by severe hemorrhagic fever with hepatitis, with case mortality of 10–50%. Asymptomatic infections also occur. Maintenance of CCHF virus involves horizontal transmission from *Hyalomma* ticks to mammals, and vertical transmission in ticks through the eggs. Immature ticks feed on small mammals, and the adult ticks feed on cattle and other large mammals. *Hyalomma* ticks have also been found on birds migrating between Europe and Africa – a mechanism for long-distance dispersal of the virus. Recent human CCHF cases in workers handling livestock and their products in Saudi Arabia and the United Arab Emirates have been attributed to importation of infected cattle and their ticks from Somalia and the Sudan. Diagnosis is by virus isolation, demonstration of viral nucleic acid sequences by RT-PCR, *in situ* hybridization or immunohistochemistry or by serological techniques. There are no vaccine or tick control measures available.

Sandfly fever viruses

Sandfly fever (Sicilian, Naples and Toscana) viruses are endemic in the Mediterranean area (southern Europe, North Africa and Southwest Asia). They cause acute febrile disease in humans, with occasional aseptic meningitis. In central Italy, Toscana virus caused one-third of previously undiagnosed cases of aseptic meningitis. The viruses are members of the *Phlebovirus* genus of the *Bunyaviridae*. They are transovarially and horizontally transmitted by phlebotomine sandflies. Wild mammals are presumed reservoirs.

Viruses Occurring in the Americas

Encephalitis viruses

Venezuelan equine encephalitis (VEE) has been a major public and animal health problem in tropical and subtropical areas of the Americas. VEE virus is made up of a closely related complex of subtypes with several varieties, which have differing epidemiologies, geographic distributions and disease importance. The epizootic/epidemic (VEE IAB and IC) virus variants are of greatest concern. In equine animals, the virus causes acute encephalitis, and case fatality may approach 80%. Survivors may have serious neurological deficits. Although the case fatality rate in humans is low (less than 1%), the large numbers of acutely infected people that occur during an epidemic may completely overwhelm the local health care system. VEE IAB and IC viruses are maintained in northern South America, where they have periodically swept through Venezuela and Colombia in epidemic waves, with occasional extension into Ecuador and massively through Central America into Mexico and South Texas. Epidemic spread depends on the availability of susceptible equine populations (the amplifying host) and abundant mosquito vectors of several species. Although the interepidemic maintenance systems remain undefined, there is some recent evidence that the epidemic form may be enzootic in Central America, causing sporadic cases in equine animals there. There is other evidence that the epizootic strains may arise by mutation of subtype ID enzootic virus. The enzootic strains are maintained in limited foci involving rodents and *Culex* (*Melanconion*) spp. mosquitoes from Florida to Argentina. With the exception of subtype IE, which caused epizootics in horses in 1993 in Chiapas and in 1996 in Oaxaca State, Mexico, these virus strains do not cause disease in equine animals, but can cause acute febrile illness in humans. The VEE complex viruses are in the *Alphavirus* genus of the *Togaviridae*. Diagnosis is usually done by antibody detection (IgG or IgM ELISA test) because virus isolation from clinical cases is difficult (except from the blood of early febrile cases in infected herds of equine animals), although RT-PCR may detect viral genomic sequences. Viruses are subtyped with monoclonal antibodies in plaque-reduction neutralization or ELISA tests. There is an effective live, attenuated vaccine for both human and equine use. Because the maintenance of equine herd immunity is costly, most animal health agencies do not carry out ongoing, intensive vaccination campaigns. Thus, the risk of reoccurrence of explosive outbreaks remains.

Eastern (EEE) and western (WEE) equine encephalitis viruses occur in epidemic form in North America, but have also been found in Central and South America. Generally, EEE is maintained in eastern North America but has caused scattered epizootics and cases in the Caribbean, and in Central and South America. EEE virus can be divided into a North

American–Caribbean clade, an Amazon Basin clade, and a Trinidad, Venezuela, Guyana, Ecuador and Argentina clade. WEE occurs in western and prairie states and provinces and along the west coast. WEE has caused sporadic cases of encephalitis in equine animals, but not humans, in Argentina and Uruguay. Both involve wild birds and mosquito vectors, with spillover into equine populations and humans, causing clinical encephalitis and death. Central nervous sequelae may occur among survivors. Diagnosis is by isolation of the virus in mice or cell cultures, by demonstration of viral RNA by RT-PCR or of viral antigen by capture ELISA. Isolation from brain tissue of clinical encephalitis cases is difficult. Demonstration of IgG antibody by a variety of tests, or IgM antibody by capture ELISA, is of diagnostic value. Effective vaccines are available commercially for equine animals, and experimental vaccines are used for laboratory personnel. Effective mosquito abatement to control vector populations has been carried out in the West for many years. Insecticide application is used for vector control in epidemic situations.

St Louis encephalitis (SLE) virus occurs from Canada to Argentina and causes sporadic but extensive epidemics in the USA, with most epidemics occurring in the west, down the Ohio and Mississippi valleys into Texas, and in Florida. Wild passerine birds are amplifying hosts in North America, but in the Southeastern USA and the Neotropics mammals may play an epidemiologic role in virus maintenance and transmission. SLE virus is transmitted by *Culex* spp. mosquitoes in the USA. SLE virus is a flavivirus of the *Togaviridae*, and is closely related to Japanese encephalitis virus. RNA oligonucleotide fingerprint patterns indicate that the virus varies by geographic region. In humans, SLE is characterized by febrile disease, with subsequent encephalitis or aseptic meningitis, and strikes older people more often than the young. Diagnosis is accomplished by virus isolation, demonstration of viral genomic sequences by RT-PCR or antigens by ELISA capture. Serological diagnosis is made by demonstration of rising titer of IgG by standard techniques, or presence of specific IgM by ELISA tests. Since no vaccine is available, SLE prevention and control relies on surveillance, vector control and screening of dwelling windows and doors.

Powassan (POW) virus is a North American member of the flavivirus tick-borne encephalitis complex. Although POW virus is widely distributed across the USA and Canada, and westward into far eastern Russia, disease (febrile, with encephalitis) has only been detected in the eastern states and provinces of North America. The transmission cycle involves small mammals and *Ixodes* ticks.

La Crosse (LAC) and other California serogroup encephalitides are human pathogens in North America. LAC encephalitis is the most common arthropod-borne virus disease in this region, affecting mainly preschool-aged children. It is endemic in the Upper Midwest, but occasional cases occur elsewhere. Although fatality is uncommon, the disease is severe enough to cause prolonged hospitalization. LAC virus is maintained transovarially in treehole breeding *Ae. triseriatus* mosquitoes with horizontal transmission to small forest mammal reservoirs and to humans. The other California group viruses affecting people have similar epidemiologies, but do not cause disease as commonly. California encephalitis virus was isolated in California, and has occasionally caused human disease there. Snowshoe hare (SSH) virus occurs in the Northern USA and across Canada, and has caused human encephalitis in the eastern provinces. Jamestown Canyon (JC) virus is widely distributed across the USA, and has been shown to cause human disease, mainly in adults in the Midwest, and to infect deer. Like LAC virus, these other viruses have the same close epidemiological relationship with their *Aedes* vectors. These viruses are members of the California serogroup of the *Bunyavirus* genus of the *Bunyaviridae* family. SSH virus is an antigenic variant of LAC virus. Oligonucleotide analysis has shown differences in LAC viruses from the eastern and the western parts of its geographic range in the Midwest. Diagnosis is nearly always by serological means, with demonstration of an antibody rise during illness. There are no vaccines for the LAC group viruses. LAC has been controlled in a few places by eliminating vector breeding sites through filling treeholes and removing discarded rubber tires.

Colorado tick fever virus

Colorado tick fever (CTF) is endemic in sagebrush–pine–juniper habitats of the higher elevations (over 1200 meters) in the mountains of the western states and provinces of North America. Although seldom fatal, CTF can cause serious disease in humans, with prolonged convalescence. CTF may present as hemorrhagic or central nervous system disease, and is most severe in preadolescent children. Males are infected over twice as frequently as are females. The virus is transmitted by and overwinters in *Dermacentor andersoni*. Wild rodents are the vertebrate hosts, and develop a prolonged viremia. CTF virus is classified in the *Coltivirus* genus of the family *Reoviridae* and is serologically related to Eyach virus from Germany. Diagnosis is by virus isolation from erythrocytes, or demonstration of CTF viral antigen by immunofluorescence, during the long viremia.

Serologic diagnosis may be problematic because antibodies develop late in the course of infection. Avoidance of tick bites is the main preventive measure available, but control of rodents and the ticks that inhabit their burrows can be applied in foci of virus maintenance in the field.

Vesicular stomatitis virus

Vesicular stomatitis (VS) virus is of major economic concern as a cause of acute, febrile vesicular disease in cattle, mainly in Central and northern South America and in the USA. Both of the major serotypes, VS-Indiana and VS-New Jersey, cause influenza-like illness in humans and are an occupational hazard to people handling cattle. The VS viruses comprise a complex of related serotypes and subtypes in the Americas, with related vesiculoviruses (*Rhabdoviridae* family) viruses in Africa and Asia. Many of these viruses are transmitted horizontally and transovarially by phlebotomine sandflies, with evidence for infection of wild rodents and other small mammals. However, the role of these mammals in the epidemiology of VS viruses is unclear because they do not develop viremia. Thus, the host and vector transmission cycles of VS viruses in the Americas are not well understood. Diagnosis is established by isolation of the virus in cell cultures, demonstration of antigen in vesicular fluid or tissues of infected animals, or demonstration of specific RNA sequences by RT-PCR. Serological diagnosis may be complicated by lack of specificity of tests and by normal fluctuations of antibody titers. The experimental vaccines developed for use in domestic animals have not yet been commercialized.

Other Neotropical viruses

Oropouche virus, a Simbu serogroup bunyavirus, causes epidemics, occasionally severe, of acute febrile disease with arthralgia and occasional aseptic meningitis in humans in the Brazilian and Peruvian Amazon as well as Panama. During rainy season epidemics, the virus is transmitted by *Culicoides paraensis* biting midges. Enzootic maintenance cycles are believed to involve forest mammals and arboreal mosquitoes.

Mayaro (MAY) virus occurs epidemically in the Brazilian and Bolivian Amazon Basin, and has also been associated with human disease in Surinam and Trinidad. In humans, the acute, nonfatal, febrile disease with rash is clinically similar to CHIK, an alphavirus to which it is antigenically and taxonomically related. MAY virus appears to be maintained in nature in a cycle similar to that of yellow fever, with arboreal mosquito vectors and primate hosts, but also involving other mammals and birds.

Rocio virus was first isolated from fatal human encephalitis cases during an explosive outbreak of acute febrile disease in coastal Sao Paulo State, Brazil in 1975, after which time sporadic outbreaks have continued. This virus is an ungrouped flavivirus in the *Togaviridae*, and is serologically related to Murray Valley encephalitis virus from Australia. The epidemiology is unclear but probably involves wild birds, and several mosquito species are suspected vectors.

Viruses Occurring in Europe

Tahyna (TAH) virus is widely distributed in Europe, and has been reported in Africa. TAH virus produces an influenza-like febrile disease, with occasional central nervous system involvement. The virus is a bunyavirus of the California serogroup, in the *Bunyaviridae*. Like La Crosse virus, small forest mammals are TAH virus reservoirs, and the virus is horizontally and transovarially transmitted by *Aedes* mosquitoes. There are no effective control measures.

Omsk hemorrhagic fever occurs in a localized area of western Siberia. Disease can be severe, with up to 3% case fatality, and sequelae are common. This virus is a member of the tick-borne encephalitis (TBE) complex of the flaviviruses. The virus is epizootic in wild muskrats, which had been introduced into the area, and is associated with ixodid ticks. Muskrat handlers are at highest risk of infection. Water voles and other rodents are also vertebrate hosts of the virus. TBE virus vaccine is used in high-risk individuals to provide protection.

Central European tick-borne encephalitis (CETBE) virus is also a member of the TBE complex of flaviviruses. Because recreation in wooded areas has increased in recent years, CETBE has become the most frequent arthropod-borne disease in Europe. The virus occurs in deciduous forests in western Europe from the Mediterranean countries, westward to France, and northward to the Scandinavian countries. It is maintained in a transmission cycle involving small mammals and *Ixodes* spp. ticks. Human infection also occurs through the consumption of unpasteurized milk from infected cows. Infection can be prevented by an inactivated vaccine and avoidance of tick bites.

Cowpox virus is an orthopoxvirus in the *Poxviridae*. It has a wide host range. Domestic cats are the most important source of human infection, transmitting the virus from wild rodent reservoirs to people. In addition to cattle, this virus has produced severe, generalized infections in a variety of incidental animal hosts in zoos and circuses, including elephants and large cats, which may die. Humans develop typical poxvirus lesions (vesicle and pustule formation), usually on the hands. Laboratory diagnosis (characterization of isolated virus) is required to differentiate cowpox from other nodule-forming zoonotic poxviruses such as orf virus, bovine papular stomatitis virus and pseudopoxvirus, which are worldwide in distribution.

Viruses Occurring in Africa

Rift Valley fever virus

Rift Valley fever (RVF) is among the most serious arbovirus infections in Africa today. Repeated RVF epidemics in sub-Saharan Africa cause serious disease in small ruminant animals and humans. RVF disease has expanded its historical geographic range in the livestock-raising areas of eastern and southern Africa over the past 25 years, causing a massive epidemic in Egypt in 1977–1978, appearing in epidemic form along the Mauritania–Senegal border 10 years later and in Madagascar in 1990–1991. Cattle, sheep and humans are affected. Abortion storms with febrile disease and bloody diarrhea occur in ruminant animals, and mortality may be heavy in young stock. Most infected humans develop febrile disease, with prolonged convalescence. A few individuals develop more severe disease, with liver necrosis, hemorrhagic pneumonia, meningoencephalitis and retinitis with vision loss. The human case fatality rate is less than 1%. RVF virus is in the *Phlebovirus* genus of the *Bunyaviridae*. In sub-Saharan Africa, RVF virus is closely tied to its *Aedes* mosquito vectors. RVF vectors transmit the virus transovarially and horizontally. The virus persists in mosquito eggs laid around seasonally flooded pools and depressions called 'dambos'. When the rains come and dambos flood, the eggs hatch and infected mosquitoes emerge and begin transmission. The vertebrate reservoir hosts of RVF virus are unknown. Agricultural development projects in Africa must take into account that creation of larval habitats (artificial dambos) may lead to epidemics of RVF, as happened in West Africa. Diagnosis depends on virus isolation and serologic testing. Field and laboratory workers need to exercise caution to avoid becoming infected by exposure to the virus during postmortem examination of animals or processing materials in the laboratory. A high level of biosecurity is required. Both live attenuated and inactivated vaccines are available for animals, but the unpredictability of scattered, sporadic RVF outbreaks across sub-Saharan Africa is a major obstacle for implementation of extensive, cost-effective vaccination programs. An inactivated vaccine is available for laboratory and field workers at high risk of infection.

Marburg and Ebola viruses

The reappearance of epidemic Ebola disease in Kikwit, Democratic Republic of the Congo (formerly Zaire) in 1995 and Makokou, Gabon in 1996 again focused international attention on this hemorrhagic disease. Marburg and Ebola viruses have sporadically caused severe hemorrhagic fever in humans. Marburg virus, although of African origin, first appeared in laboratory workers in Germany who had handled cell cultures originating from African primates. Later, epidemics of severe hemorrhagic fever occurred in the Sudan and in Zaire, and Ebola virus was isolated. These viruses produce hemorrhagic shock syndrome and visceral organ necrosis, and have the highest case fatality rate (30–90%) of the hemorrhagic fevers. These viruses, with their bizarre filamentous, pleomorphic morphology, belong to the *Filoviridae* family. They are presumed to be zoonotic, but their hosts in nature and mechanisms of transmission in the field have not been determined. Most of the Makokou, Gabon patients had very recently butchered chimpanzees. A variant of Ebola virus has been isolated from chimpanzees from Côte D'Ivoire, but since wild primates suffer severe disease, they are unlikely to be maintenance reservoirs. Nosocomial transmission of Marburg and Ebola viruses has occurred frequently; a high level of patient isolation and biosafety containment are essential to avoid hospital- and laboratory-acquired infection. An outbreak of simian hemorrhagic disease, caused by a Marburg/Ebola-like filovirus, occurred in a primate-holding facility, but without evidence of related human disease among animal care personnel. The virus can be detected by electron microscopic examination of tissue or isolation of the virus in cell culture. Serologic diagnosis is accomplished by means of indirect immunofluorescence or ELISA test, with antigen specificity confirmed by western blot. No vaccines or control measures are available.

Monkeypox virus

The largest epidemic of human monkeypox ever documented occurred in the Katako-Kombe area of the Democratic Republic of the Congo (formerly Zaire) in 1996–1997, with over 500 people becoming ill and five deaths. Primary monkey-to-human transmission occurred, as did subsequent secondary human-to-human spread. Human monkeypox is a severe, smallpox-like illness. Monkeypox belongs to the *Orthopoxvirus* genus of the *Poxviridae*. The virus is enzootic in wild primates and squirrels in the rainforests of West and Central Africa. Vaccinia is protective against infection, but its use has been discontinued with the eradication of smallpox. A new drug, cidofovir, has been reported to be effective in preventing overt disease and death in monkeys infected experimentally.

O'nyong-nyong virus

O'nyong-nyong virus disease initially occurred in 1959 in Uganda and spread to Kenya, Tanzania, Malawi and Senegal, infecting 2 million people. O'nyong-nyong virus is considered a subtype of Chikungunya virus, and is widespread in eastern sub-Saharan Africa. The disease it produces and its epidemiology are similar to CHIK, with *Anopheles* spp. as the main mosquito vector. Igbo Ora virus is also antigenically related to CHIK virus, and has been isolated from humans in West Africa.

Semliki Forest virus

Semliki Forest (SF) virus caused an extensive epidemic of human disease in Bangui, Central African Republic, in 1987. SF virus is an alphavirus in the *Togaviridae*. It occurs across East, Central and West Africa, and has been isolated from various mosquitoes and from wild birds. Antibodies have been also found in wild mammals. The SF virus maintenance cycle probably involves *Ae. africanus* mosquitoes and vervet monkeys.

Orungo virus

Orungo (ORU) virus caused mild epidemic disease (fever, nausea, headache and rash) in Nigeria. The virus occurs in a band across Africa from Uganda to Sierra Leone. It is an orbivirus in the *Reoviridae*. ORU is probably mosquito transmitted, but the species that transmit it in nature are not known. Although the vertebrate reservoir hosts are unknown, wild primates have antibody and are suspected to be involved in virus maintenance.

Viruses Occurring in Asia

Kyasanur Forest disease (KFD) was first recognized in India in 1957, when an acute hemorrhagic disease appeared in wild monkeys and people frequenting forested areas. KFD has been slowly spreading in India. KFD virus is a member of the tick-borne encephalitis complex of flaviviruses. The basic virus maintenance cycle involves forest mammals (primates, rodents, bats and insectivores) and ixodid ticks, mainly *Haemaphysalis spinigera*. The virus can be isolated in mice and cell cultures, including tick cells. An inactivated vaccine provides some protection to people at risk of infection.

Japanese encephalitis virus

Japanese encephalitis (JE) is found in a broad area from far eastern Russia, northeastern Asia through China and Southeast Asia to Papua New Guinea and the Torres Strait Islands of Australia and westward into India. One of the world's arthropod-borne encephalitides, JE causes the greatest number of clinical human cases – thousands annually – predominantly in children. It produces encephalitis in humans and horses, and acute febrile disease with abortion in swine, an amplifying host. Herons and egrets are wildlife amplifying hosts. The virus is transmitted by *Culex* spp. mosquitoes. The overwintering mechanism in temperate Asia is unknown. JE virus is a member of a complex of four related flaviviruses in the *Togaviridae* family. RNA oligonucleotide analysis indicates that there are differences in JE virus isolates from different vertebrate species, and between strains from different geographic areas. Diagnosis is by means of virus isolation or demonstration of JE virus genomic sequences by RT-PCR, IgG antibody rise, or of specific IgM in acute sera. Prevention of disease is mainly through vaccination of humans, horses and swine. A bivalent vaccine is used that incorporates the two recognized antigenic variants. Insecticides and integrated pest control measures that include natural compounds (*Bacillus thurengiensis* toxins), larvicidal fish, and larval habitat modification have been successfully used in China. Use of pyrethroid-impregnated bed netting can also prevent transmission.

Viruses Occurring in Australia

Murray Valley encephalitis virus

Murray Valley encephalitis (MVE) occurs primarily in southeastern Australia, with cases appearing occasionally in other parts of the country and in Papua New Guinea. Febrile disease leads to encephalitis and, in severe cases, death. Neurologic sequelae are common in survivors. Children are predominantly affected. Large water birds are the main vertebrate amplifying hosts, but mammals are also reservoirs. The virus is transmitted mainly by *Culex annulirostris* mosquitoes. It is maintained in northern Australia and New Guinea and is believed to be introduced into southern Australia in years of high rainfall. MVE virus is a flavivirus of the *Togaviridae* and is closely related to Japanese encephalitis. RNA sequencing indicates that the Australian strains of MVE virus are similar to, but different from Papua New Guinea isolates. Like JE, MVE diagnosis depends on virus isolation and serological testing. No vaccine is available. Control is achieved through application of larvicides.

Ross River virus

Ross River (RR) virus has caused annual epidemics of febrile disease with polyarthritis and rash in tropical and temperate eastern Australia. Within the past two decades, RR virus has spread through several Pacific islands in epidemic form and appears to have become endemic in New Caledonia. Convalescence can be long. RR virus is an alphavirus of the *Togaviridae* family. The enzootic maintenance cycles of RR virus in Australia are not well defined, but wild and domestic mammals appear to be the reservoir hosts, and the principal mosquito vectors are salt marsh *Aedes* spp. and freshwater *Culex* spp. In the Pacific Islands, the virus was probably transmitted from person to person by *Aedes* mosquitoes.

Kunjin virus

Kunjin virus has caused scattered cases of fever, myalgia and polyarthralgia across Australia and in clusters in central Queensland and northern Western Australia. Kunjin virus is a flavivirus of the *Togaviridae*, and is related to WN and MVE viruses. The virus is believed to be maintained in wild bird–*Cx annulirostris* transmission cycles similar to MVE virus.

Burmah Forest virus

Burmah Forest virus causes subclinical and clinical infections in humans, including fever, myalgia, polyarthalgia and rash. It is an alphavirus in the *Togaviridae*. The virus appears to be endemic in eastern Australia, and its mosquito vectors and vertebrate hosts have not been established.

Control

Control of zoonotic virus diseases is accomplished by breaking the cycle of transmission. This is usually achieved by eliminating or immunizing vertebrate hosts, and reducing vector populations. Reduction of reservoir host populations is usually not accomplished because it is too expensive, not environmentally safe, and not technically or logistically feasible. However, there have been some notable exceptions. Bolivian hemorrhagic fever, caused by Machupo virus, was controlled by reduction of its rodent hosts through intensive rodenticiding. The principal vampire bat reservoir of rabies, *Desmodus rotundus*, is being controlled by the application of warfarin-type anticoagulants, either directly to the bats themselves or to the cattle upon which they feed (with no harm to the cattle). Control programs like these have to be continuous to be effective. Their reduction or discontinuation results in host population recovery through reproduction and immigration, which may result in re-emergence of disease sweeping through the increasing, susceptible cohort.

Immunization of hosts is both promising and discouraging. After decades of research, safe and effective rabies vaccines are being used for immunization of humans, domesticated animals and some wildlife species. The human diploid cell vaccine is extremely effective, free of adverse effects and widely available but at a cost too high for use in many developing countries. Safe, effective animal vaccines of cell culture origin are on the market. After some initial public resistance, raccoon populations in the eastern USA and wild foxes in Europe are being successfully immunized by means of an oral, vaccinia-vectored recombinant vaccine. This experience illustrates the need for public understanding, in order to counteract fear of the unknown – in this case, field use of a genetically engineered virus. Other vectored rabies vaccines are under development for control of mongoose-transmitted rabies in the Caribbean. Vaccines will not be developed for many zoonotic viral diseases that affect relatively few people and are of very limited concern geographically. With limited markets for new vaccines, there is no economic incentive to justify the several millions of dollars for the research and testing required for licensure and commercialization of these products.

Vector control is another promising but difficult area of zoonoses reduction or elimination. Insecticide application has become more problematic because both vectors themselves, as well as public opinion, have become more resistant to their use. Integrated pest management techniques, well developed for the control of many crop insects, along with the use of natural pesticides such as *Bacillus thurengiensis* toxin, offers promise for the effective, environmentally safe control of dipterous vectors. Control of tick vectors is likely to remain a problem for some time to come.

Emerging and Reemerging Zoonoses

Ecological change

Human disturbance has become a feature of nearly every part of the planet. All too often these disturbances create habitats that favor increases in populations of key hosts and vectors, with subsequent increased transmission of viral zoonoses. Nowhere are ecological changes happening more rapidly and profoundly than in the world's tropics. Conversion of tropical forests to agricultural ecosystems simplifies diverse ecosystems and provides either native or introduced host or vector species the conditions necessary to become more abundant, and sustain intensified virus transmission in areas where people live and work. In Africa, recent yellow fever epidemics have been increasing dramatically in agricultural areas. Some agricultural irrigation development projects have created extensive vector breeding habitats, with an increase in mosquito-transmitted disease. The extensive dams constructed in Senegal were followed by epidemics of Rift Valley fever, with numerous cases of disease in humans and small ruminant animals. The public health consequences of development projects must never be overlooked.

Global climate change will also bring ecological changes and shifts of human populations that will affect the occurrence of viral zoonoses. Although experts debate the geography, severity and rapidity of the oncoming greenhouse effect, there is general consensus that changes in the global climate will happen with unprecedented speed. With those changes will come alterations in the geography of natural and agricultural ecosystems, with corresponding changes in the distribution of zoonotic diseases and the intensity of their transmission. It is clear that El Niño–southern oscillation phenomena have increased rainfall, with resulting increases in rodent populations and occurrence of hantavirus pulmonary syndrome in the Southwestern USA, and increased breeding sites for mosquito vectors of Rift Valley fever virus in Africa. While it is not possible to predict accurately what the world will be like in 100 years, nor what zoonotic diseases are likely to be most troublesome, it is certain that things will be different, and constant surveillance will be essential to avoid serious problems or deal promptly and effectively with the ones that arise.

Movement of zoonotic viruses can result from the displacement of infected animals, contaminated animal products and virus-carrying arthropod vectors. It is clear that illegal translocation of wild raccoons for hunting purposes, with inadvertent movement of rabies-infected animals, was responsible for initiating the recent rabies epizootic in the Middle Atlantic states. Pets, sport, laboratory and agricultural animals are moving around the world as never before. Although international and national regulations have been established to prevent movement of infected individuals, it is not possible to test for all possible zoonotic viruses, and prevent them from crossing international boundaries. Moreover, significant numbers of animals of high commercial value move illegally. Psittacine and other exotic birds worth hundreds to thousands of dollars each cross illegally into the USA, despite intensive government efforts to halt this smuggling. The importation of highly virulent Newcastle disease (ND) virus has been occasionally linked to smuggled birds. The costly ND outbreak (more than $50 million to control) in southern California in the early 1970s was linked to the importation of an infected pet bird from Asia. Subsequently, highly lethal ND virus has been found in smuggled parrots. Although not a serious infection in humans, ND is highly transmissible and can be extremely lethal in poultry and costly to that industry.

Zoonotic viruses may be transported by movement of arthropod vectors, too. Just as the yellow fever mosquito, *Ae. aegypti*, moved around the world in water casks aboard sailing vessels, mosquitoes are transported around the world in international commerce. Ships still transport mosquito vectors. The Asian tiger mosquito, *Ae. albopictus*, has become established in the Western Hemisphere after multiple introductions in eggs deposited in used tires. This mosquito is capable of transmitting yellow fever, Venezuelan equine encephalitis, Jamestown Canyon (JC) and La Crosse (LAC) encephalitis viruses. It remains to be seen if this highly competitive exotic vector, with its peridomestic habits, will carry yellow fever virus from its jungle cycle to the urban, human amplified cycle in the American tropics, increase the numbers of La Crosse encephalitis cases in south temperate or subtropical areas of the USA, or facilitate emergence of LACV × JCV recombinants. Perhaps of greater concern, modern transport aircraft have been shown to move vector mosquitoes internationally. Nature can move vectors as well. For example, windblown biting insects, such as culicoid midges, have been shown to account for the spread of some arthropod-borne virus diseases of animals, in some cases over long distances. There is no reason to believe that vectors of human diseases cannot move similarly.

Human activity alters animal populations, contact between wild and domestic animals, and human–animal interactions, changing the occurrence of zoonotic diseases and the risk of infection to humans. For example, emergence of new influenza strains is related to the interaction of populations of people, pigs and aquatic birds. It is hypothesized that the emergence of the new H5N1 influenza strain in Hong Kong in 1997 was the result of a chain of events resulting in transmission from migrating shorebirds to ducks, to chickens, and finally to humans. Fortunately, this pathogenic strain was not easily transmitted from human to human, or a serious pandemic could have resulted.

Social change

Increasing human populations place great demands on the public health and other government services, especially in developing countries where needs for zoonosis diagnosis, control and prevention are greatest and resources are most limited. Some preventive measures could be implemented by the people who live in the affected areas themselves, and at minimal cost, if they knew why and how they needed to do it. Public education and information is essential for control and prevention of zoonotic diseases; however, it takes more than civic action to deal with them. Delivery of public education, disease surveillance and diagnosis and the technical materials and logistical support for control or preventive programs depend on national or international scientific and financial support. Because serious zoonotic viral diseases, such as rabies, yellow fever, Venezuelan equine encephalitis and the hemorrhagic fevers, know nothing of international boundaries, international technical cooperation and financial support are imperative.

See also: ***Bunyaviridae***: **General features; Replication; Diagnostic techniques: Detection of viral antigens, nucleic acids and specific antibodies; Isolation and identification by culture and microscopy; Encephalitis viruses (*Flaviviridae*):** Encephalitis viruses and related viruses causing hemorrhagic disease; Tick-borne encephalitis and Wesselsbron viruses; Hantaviruses (*Bunyaviridae*); Lassa, Junin, Machupo and Guanarito viruses (*Arenaviridae*); Rhabdoviruses (*Rhabdoviridae*): Plant rhabdoviruses; Ungrouped mammalian, bird and fish rhabdoviruses; Emerging and re-emerging virus diseases; Marburg and Ebola viruses (*Filoviridae*).

Further Reading

Beran GW and Steele JH (eds) (1994) *Handbook of Zoonoses*, Section B, Viral, 2nd edn. Boca Raton: CRC Press.

Fenner FJ, Gibbs EPJ, Murphy FA *et al* (eds) (1987) *Veterinary Virology*. San Diego: Academic Press.

Fields BN, Knipe DM and Howley PM (eds) (1990) *Virology*, 2nd edn. New York: Raven Press.

Hubbert WT, McCulloch WF and Schnurrenberg PR (eds) (1975) *Diseases Transmitted from Animals to Man* 6th edn. Springfield IL: CC Thomas.

Hugh-Jones M, Hubbert WT and Hagstad HV (1995) *Zoonoses: Recognition, Control and Prevention*. Ames: Iowa State University Press.

Monath TP (ed.) (1988–1989). *The Arboviruses: Epidemiology and Ecology*, vols I–V. Boca Raton: CRC Press.

APPENDIX

This appendix lists the updated ICTV virus name index published in the 1999 Seventh ICTV Report.[1] It lists all virus names, with nomenclature based on the ICTV code of 1999. Because of differences in publication schedules, some virus names in *Encyclopedia* entries may differ form those listed in the Appendix. While not all viruses listed are addressed by the *Encyclopedia*, the list provides a ready reference source for all viruses, from the most recognized to the most obscure.

Species names are in italics; names not in italics indicate synonym, strain, serotype, genotype, and clade or isolate names. Abbreviation virus names are enclosed in parenthesis. The family name is also indicated for each virus name.

10924 virus, *Arenaviridae*
12056 virus, *Arenaviridae*
1324Cg/79 virus, *Bunyaviridae*
3076 virus, *Arenaviridae*
3099 virus, *Arenaviridae*
3739 virus, *Arenaviridae*
63U-11 virus, (63UV), *Bunyaviridae*
75V 2374 virus, (V2374V), *Bunyaviridae*
75V 2621 virus, (V2621V), *Bunyaviridae*
78V 2441 virus, (V2441V), *Bunyaviridae*

AA288-77 virus, *Arenaviridae*
Abadina virus, (ABAV), *Reoviridae*
Abelson murine leukemia virus, (AbMLV), *Retroviridae*
Above Maiden virus, *Reoviridae*
Abras virus, (ABRV), *Bunyaviridae*
Abraxas grossulariata cypovirus 8, (AgCPV-8), *Reoviridae*
Abu Hammad virus, (AHV), *Bunyaviridae*
Abu Mina virus, (ABMV), *Bunyaviridae*
Abutilon mosaic virus, (AbMV), *Geminiviridae*
Abutilon yellows virus, (AbYV), *Closteroviridae*
Acado virus, (ACDV), *Reoviridae*
Acalypha yellow mosaic virus, (AYMV), *Geminiviridae*
Acara virus, (ACAV), *Bunyaviridae*
Acciptrid herpesvirus 1, (AcHV-1), *Herpesviridae*
Acetobacter phage pKG-2, (pKG-2), *Myoviridae*
Acetobacter phage pKG-3, (pKG-3), *Myoviridae*
Acherontia atropas virus, (AaV), *Tetraviridae*
Acheta domestica densovirus, (AdDNV), *Parvoviridae*
Acholeplasma phage 0c1r, (0c1r), *Inoviridae*
Acholeplasma phage 10tur, (10tur), *Inoviridae*
Acholeplasma phage L2, (L2), *Plasmaviridae*
Acholeplasma phage M1, (M1), *Plasmaviridae*
Acholeplasma phage MV-G51, (G51), *Inoviridae*
Acholeplasma phage MV-L1, (L1), *Inoviridae*
Acholeplasma phage MV-L51, (L51), *Inoviridae*
Acholeplasma phage O1, (O1), *Plasmaviridae*
Acholeplasma phage v1, (v1), *Plasmaviridae*
Acholeplasma phage v2, (v2), *Plasmaviridae*
Acholeplasma phage v4, (v4), *Plasmaviridae*
Acholeplasma phage v5, (v5), *Plasmaviridae*
Acholeplasma phage v7, (v7), *Plasmaviridae*
Acid-stable equine picornaviruses, (EqPV), *Picornaviridae*
Acinetobacter phage 133, (133), *Myoviridae*
Acinetobacter phage 205, (205), *Leviviridae*
Acinetobacter phage 531, (531), *Siphoviridae*
Acinetobacter phage A10/45, (A10/45), *Myoviridae*
Acinetobacter phage A3/2, (A3/2), *Myoviridae*
Acinetobacter phage A36, (A36), *Podoviridae*
Acinetobacter phage BS46, (BS46), *Myoviridae*
Acinetobacter phage E13, (E13), *Siphoviridae*
Acinetobacter phage E14, (E14), *Myoviridae*
Acinetobacter phage E4, (E4), *Myoviridae*
Acinetobacter phage E5, (E5), *Myoviridae*

---

[1] van Regenmortel *et al.* (1999) *Virus Taxonomy Seventh ICTV Report*. Academic Press, London, UK.

Acipenserid herpesvirus 1, (AciHV-1), *Herpesviridae*
Acipenserid herpesvirus 2, (AciHV-2), *Herpesviridae*
Acrobasis zelleri entomopoxvirus 'L', (AZEV), *Poxviridae*
Actias selene cypovirus 4, (AsCPV-4), *Reoviridae*
Actinomycetes phage 108/016, (108/016), *Myoviridae*
Actinomycetes phage 119, (119), *Siphoviridae*
Actinomycetes phage A1-Dat, (A1-Dat), *Siphoviridae*
Actinomycetes phage Bir, (Bir), *Siphoviridae*
Actinomycetes phage M_1, (M_1), *Siphoviridae*
Actinomycetes phage MSP8, (MSP8), *Siphoviridae*
Actinomycetes phage P-a-1, (P-a-1), *Siphoviridae*
Actinomycetes phage R_1, (R_1), *Siphoviridae*
Actinomycetes phage R_2, (R_2), *Siphoviridae*
Actinomycetes phage SK1, (SK1), *Myoviridae*
Actinomycetes phage SV2, (SV2), *Siphoviridae*
Actinomycetes phage VP5, (VP5), *Siphoviridae*
Actinomycetes phage ΦC, (ΦC), *Siphoviridae*
Actinomycetes phage φ115-A, (φ115-A), *Siphoviridae*
Actinomycetes phage φ150A, (φ150A), *Siphoviridae*
Actinomycetes phage φ31C, (φ31C), *Siphoviridae*
Actinomycetes phage φUW21, (φUW21), *Siphoviridae*
Acute bee paralysis virus, (ABPV), Unassigned
Acyrthosiphon pisum virus, (APV), Unassigned
Adelaide River virus, (ARV), *Rhabdoviridae*
Adeno-associated virus 1, (AAV-1), *Parvoviridae*
Adeno-associated virus 2, (AAV-2), *Parvoviridae*
Adeno-associated virus 3, (AAV-3), *Parvoviridae*
Adeno-associated virus 4, (AAV-4), *Parvoviridae*
Adeno-associated virus 5, (AAV-5), *Parvoviridae*
Adeno-associated virus 6, (AAV-6), *Parvoviridae*
Aedes aegypti densovirus, (AaDNV), *Parvoviridae*
Aedes aegypti entomopoxvirus, (AAEV), *Poxviridae*
Aedes albopictus densovirus, (AlDNV), *Parvoviridae*
Aedes pseudoscutellaris densovirus, (ApDNV), *Parvoviridae*
Aedes sollicitans NPV, (AesoNPV), *Baculoviridae*
Aedes taeniorhynchus iridescent virus, *Iridoviridae*
Aeromonas phage 1, (1), *Myoviridae*
Aeromonas phage 25, (25), *Myoviridae*
Aeromonas phage 29, (29), *Myoviridae*
Aeromonas phage 31, (31), *Myoviridae*
Aeromonas phage 37, (37), *Myoviridae*
Aeromonas phage 40R, (40R), *Myoviridae*
Aeromonas phage 40RR2.8t, (40RR2.8t), *Myoviridae*
Aeromonas phage 43, (43), *Myoviridae*
Aeromonas phage 51, (51), *Myoviridae*
Aeromonas phage 59.1, (59.1), *Myoviridae*
Aeromonas phage 65, (65), *Myoviridae*
Aeromonas phage Aa-1, (Aa-1), *Podoviridae*
Aeromonas phage Aeh1, (Aeh1), *Myoviridae*
Aeromonas phage Aeh2, (Aeh2), *Myoviridae*
African cassava mosaic virus, (ACMV), *Geminiviridae*
African green monkey cytomegalovirus, *Herpesviridae*
African green monkey EBV-like virus, *Herpesviridae*
African green monkey polyomavirus, (AGMPyV), *Polyomaviridae*
African horse sickness virus 1 to 9, (AHSV-1 to 9), *Reoviridae*
African horse sickness virus, (AHSV), *Reoviridae*
African swine fever virus, (ASFV), *Asfarviridae*
AG80-663 virus, (AG80V), *Togaviridae*
AG83-1746 virus, (AG1746V), *Bunyaviridae*
AG83-497 virus, (AG497V), *Bunyaviridae*
Agaricus bisporus virus 1, (ABV-1), Unassigned
Agaricus bisporus virus 4, (AbV-4), *Partitiviridae*
Ageratum yellow vein virus, (AYVV), *Geminiviridae*
Aglais urticae cypovirus 2, (AuCPV-2), *Reoviridae*
Aglais urticae cypovirus 6, (AuCPV-6), *Reoviridae*
Aglaonema bacilliform virus, (ABV), *Caulimoviridae*
Agraulis vanillae cypovirus 2, (AvaCPV-2), *Reoviridae*
Agraulis vanillae densovirus, (AvDNV), *Parvoviridae*
Agraulis vanillae virus, (AvV), *Tetraviridae*
Agrobacterium phage PIIBNV6, (PIIBNV6), *Myoviridae*
Agrobacterium phage PS8, (PS8), *Siphoviridae*
Agrobacterium phage PT11, (PT11), *Siphoviridae*
Agrobacterium phage Ψ, (Ψ), *Siphoviridae*
Agrochola helvola cypovirus 6, (AhCPV-6), *Reoviridae*
Agrochola lychnidis cypovirus 6, (AlCPV-6), *Reoviridae*
Agropyron mosaic virus, (AgMV), *Potyviridae*
Agrotis segetum cypovirus 9, (AsCPV-9), *Reoviridae*
Aguacate virus, (AGUV), *Bunyaviridae*
Ahlum waterborne virus, (AWBV), *Tombusviridae*
Aichi virus, (AiV), *Picornaviridae*
Aino virus, (AINOV), *Bunyaviridae*
Akabane virus, (AKAV), *Bunyaviridae*
AKR (endogenous), murine leukemia virus, (AKRMLV), *Retroviridae*
Alajuela virus, (ALJV), *Bunyaviridae*
Alcaligenes phage 8764, (8764), *Siphoviridae*
Alcaligenes phage A5/A6, (A5/A6), *Siphoviridae*
Alcaligenes phage A6, (A6), *Myoviridae*
Alcelaphine herpesvirus 1, (AlHV-1), *Herpesviridae*
Alcelaphine herpesvirus 2, (AlHV-2), *Herpesviridae*
Alenquer virus, (ALEV), *Bunyaviridae*
Aleutian disease virus, *Parvoviridae*
Aleutian mink disease virus, (AMDV), *Parvoviridae*
Alfalfa cryptic virus 1, (ACV-1), *Partitiviridae*
Alfalfa cryptic virus 2, (ACV-2), *Partitiviridae*
Alfalfa latent virus, *Carlavirus*
Alfalfa mosaic virus, (AMV), *Bromoviridae*
Alfuy virus, (ALFV), *Flaviviridae*

Alligatorweed stunting virus, (AWSV), *Closteroviridae*
Allomyces arbuscula virus, (AAV), Unassigned
Almeirim virus, (ALMV), *Reoviridae*
Almpiwar virus, (ALMV), *Rhabdoviridae*
Alpinia mosaic virus, (AlpMV), *Potyviridae*
Alstroemeria carlavirus, *Carlavirus*
Alstroemeria mosaic virus, (AlMV), *Potyviridae*
Alstroemeria streak virus, (AlStV), *Potyviridae*
Altamira virus, (ALTV), *Reoviridae*
Alternanthera mosaic virus, (AltMV), *Potexvirus*
Alteromonas phage PM2, (PM2), *Corticoviridae*
Althea rosea enation virus, (AREV), *Geminiviridae*
Amapari virus, (AMAV), *Arenaviridae*
Amaranthus leaf mottle virus, (AmLMV), *Potyviridae*
Amazon lily mosaic virus, (ALiMV), *Potyviridae*
Ambystoma tigrinum stebbensi virus, (ATV), *Iridoviridae*
American ground squirrel cytomegalovirus, *Herpesviridae*
American hop latent virus, (AHLV), *Carlavirus*
American oyster reovirus 13p2V, (13p2V), *Reoviridae*
American plum line pattern virus, (APLPV), *Bromoviridae*
Amsacta moorei entomopoxvirus 'L', (AMEV), *Poxviridae*
Amyelosis chronic stunt virus, (ACSV), *Caliciviridae*
AN 20410 virus, *Arenaviridae*
AN 21366 virus, *Arenaviridae*
Anagrapha falcifera NPV, (AnfaMNPV), *Baculoviridae*
Anagyris vein yellowing virus, *Tymovirus*
Anaitis plagiata cypovirus 3, (ApCPV-3), *Reoviridae*
Anaitis plagiata cypovirus 6, (ApCPV-6), *Reoviridae*
Ananindeua virus, (ANUV), *Bunyaviridae*
Anatid herpesvirus 1, (AnHV-1), *Herpesviridae*
Andasibe virus, (ANDV), *Reoviridae*
Andean potato latent virus, (APLV), *Tymovirus*
Andean potato mottle virus, (APMoV), *Comoviridae*
Andes virus, (ANDV), *Bunyaviridae*
Aneilema virus, (AneV), *Potyviridae*
Angel fish reovirus, (AFRV), *Reoviridae*
Anguillid herpesvirus 1, (AngHV-1), *Herpesviridae*
Anhanga virus, (ANHV), *Bunyaviridae*
Anhembi virus, (AMBV), *Bunyaviridae*
Anomala cuprea entomopoxvirus, (ACEV), *Poxviridae*
Anopheles A virus, (ANAV), *Bunyaviridae*
Anopheles B virus, (ANBV), *Bunyaviridae*
Antequera virus, (ANTV), *Bunyaviridae*
Antheraea eucalypti virus (AeV) *Tetraviridae*
Antheraea mylitta cypovirus 4, (AmCPV-4), *Reoviridae*
Antheraea pernyi cypovirus 4, (ApCPV-4), *Reoviridae*

Anthoxanthum latent blanching virus, (ALBV), *Hordeivirus*
Anthoxanthum mosaic virus, (AntMV), *Potyviridae*
Anthriscus latent virus, (AntLV), *Carlavirus*
Anthriscus yellows virus, (AYV), *Sequiviridae*
Anti xanthomista cypovirus 6, (AxCPV-6), *Reoviridae*
Anticarsia gemmatalis iridescent virus, (AGIV), *Iridoviridae*
Anticarsia gemmatalis MNPV, (AgMNPV), *Baculoviridae*
Aotine herpesvirus 1, (AoHV-1), *Herpesviridae*
Aotine herpesvirus 3, (AoHV-3), *Herpesviridae*
Apanteles crassicornis bracovirus, (AcBV), *Polydnaviridae*
Apanteles fumiferanae bracovirus, (AfBV), *Polydnaviridae*
Apeu virus, (APEUV), *Bunyaviridae*
Aphid lethal paralysis virus, (ALPV), Unassigned
Aphodius tasmaniae entomopoxvirus, (ATEV), *Poxviridae*
Apis iridescent virus, *Iridoviridae*
Apoi virus, (APOIV), *Flaviviridae*
Aporophyla lutulenta cypovirus 10, (AlCPV-10), *Reoviridae*
Apple chlorotic leaf spot virus, (ACLSV), *Trichovirus*
Apple dimple fruit viroid, (ADFVd), *Pospiviroidae*
Apple fruit crinkle viroid, (AFCVd), *Avsunviroidae*
Apple mosaic virus, (ApMV), *Bromoviridae*
Apple scar skin viroid, (ASSVd), *Pospiviroidae*
Apple stem grooving virus, (ASGV), *Capillovirus*
Apple stem pitting virus, (ASPV), *Foveavirus*
Aquareovirus A, (ARV-A), *Reoviridae*
Aquareovirus B, (ARV-B), *Reoviridae*
Aquareovirus C, (ARV-C), *Reoviridae*
Aquareovirus D, (ARV-D), *Reoviridae*
Aquareovirus E, (ARV-E), *Reoviridae*
Aquareovirus F, (ARV-F), *Reoviridae*
Aquilegia necrotic mosaic virus, (ANMV), *Caulimoviridae*
Aquilegia virus, (AqV), *Potyviridae*
Arabidopsis thaliana Ta1 virus, (AthTa1V), *Pseudoviridae*
Arabis mosaic virus large satellite RNA, Satellite
Arabis mosaic virus small satellite RNA, Satellite
Arabis mosaic virus, (ArMV), *Comoviridae*
Araguari virus, (ARAV), Unassigned
Aransas Bay virus, (ABV), *Bunyaviridae*
Araujia mosaic virus, (ArjMV), *Potyviridae*
Arbia virus, (ARBV), *Bunyaviridae*
Arboledas virus, (ADSV), *Bunyaviridae*
Arbroath virus, (ABRV), *Reoviridae*
Arctia caja cypovirus 2, (AcCPV-2), *Reoviridae*
Arctia caja cypovirus 3, (AcCPV-3), *Reoviridae*
Arctia villica cypovirus 2, (AviCPV-2), *Reoviridae*

Arctic squirrel hepatitis virus, (ASHV), *Hepadnaviridae*
Argentine turtle herpesvirus, *Herpesviridae*
Arkansas bee virus, (ABV), Unassigned
Arkonam virus, *Reoviridae*
Armadillidium vulgare iridescent virus, *Iridoviridae*
Armstrong virus, *Arenaviridae*
Aroa virus, (AROAV), *Flaviviridae*
Arphia conspersa entomopoxvirus 'O', (ACOEV), *Poxviridae*
Arracacha latent virus, (ALV), *Carlavirus*
Arracacha virus A, (AVA), *Comoviridae*
Arracacha virus B, (AVB), *Comoviridae*
Arracacha virus Y, (AVY), *Potyviridae*
Artichoke Aegean ringspot virus, (AARSV), *Comoviridae*
Artichoke curly dwarf virus, (ACDV), *Potexvirus*
Artichoke Italian latent virus, (AILV), *Comoviridae*
Artichoke latent virus M, (ArLVM), *Carlavirus*
Artichoke latent virus S, (ArLVS), *Carlavirus*
Artichoke latent virus, (ArLV), *Potyviridae*
Artichoke mottled crinkle virus, (AMCV), *Tombusviridae*
Artichoke vein banding virus, (AVBV), *Comoviridae*
Artichoke yellow ringspot virus, (AYRSV), *Comoviridae*
Artogeia rapae granulovirus, (ArGV), *Baculoviridae*
Aruac virus, (ARUV), *Rhabdoviridae*
Arumowot virus, (AMTV), *Bunyaviridae*
Ascogaster argentifrons bracovirus, (AaBV), *Polydnaviridae*
Ascogaster quadridentata bracovirus, (AqBV), *Polydnaviridae*
Asinine herpesvirus 1, *Herpesviridae*
Asinine herpesvirus 2, *Herpesviridae*
Asinine herpesvirus 3, *Herpesviridae*
Asparagus virus 1, (AV-1), *Potyviridae*
Asparagus virus 2, (AV-2), *Bromoviridae*
Asparagus virus 3, (AV-3), *Potexvirus*
Aspergillus foetidus virus F, (AFV-F), Unassigned
Aspergillus foetidus virus S, (AFV-S), *Totiviridae*
Aspergillus niger virus S, (AnV-S), *Totiviridae*
Aspergillus ochraceous virus, (AoV), *Partitiviridae*
Asystasia gangetica mottle virus, (AGMoV), *Potyviridae*
Asystasia golden mosaic virus, (AGMV), *Geminiviridae*
Ateline herpesvirus 1, (AtHV-1), *Herpesviridae*
Ateline herpesvirus 2, (AtHV-2), *Herpesviridae*
Ateline herpesvirus 3, (AtHV-3), *Herpesviridae*
Atkinsonella hypxylon virus, (AhV), *Partitiviridae*
Atlantic salmon reovirus ASV, (ASRV), *Reoviridae*
Atlantic salmon reovirus HBR, (HBRV), *Reoviridae*
Atlantic salmon reovirus TSV, (TSRV), *Reoviridae*
Atropa belladonna virus, (AtBV), *Rhabdoviridae*

Aucuba bacilliform virus, (AuBV), *Caulimoviridae*
Aura virus, (AURAV), *Togaviridae*
Australian bat lyssavirus, (ABLV), *Rhabdoviridae*
Australian grapevine viroid, (AGVd), *Pospiviroidae*
Autographa californica MNPV, (AcMNPV), *Baculoviridae*
Autographa gamma cypovirus 12, (AgCPV-12), *Reoviridae*
Auzduk disease virus, *Poxviridae*
AV 9310135 virus, *Arenaviridae*
Avalon virus, (AVAV), *Bunyaviridae*
Avian adeno-associated virus, (AAAV), *Parvoviridae*
Avian carcinoma Mill Hill virus 2, (ACMHV-2), *Retroviridae*
Avian encephalomyelitis-like virus, (AEV), *Picornaviridae*
Avian entero-like virus 2 to 4, (AELV-2 to 4), *Picornaviridae*
Avian leukosis virus - HPRS103, (ALV-J), *Retroviridae*
Avian leukosis virus - RSA, (ALV-A), *Retroviridae*
Avian leukosis virus, (ALV), *Retroviridae*
Avian myeloblastosis virus, (AMV), *Retroviridae*
Avian myelocytomatosis virus 29, (AMCV-29), *Retroviridae*
Avian nephritis virus 1 to 3, (ANV-1 to 3), *Picornaviridae*
Avian orthoreovirus 176, (ARV-176), *Reoviridae*
Avian orthoreovirus S1133, (ARV-S1133), *Reoviridae*
Avian orthoreovirus SK138a, (ARV-138), *Reoviridae*
Avian orthoreovirus, (ARV), *Reoviridae*
Avian parainfluenza virus 1, (APMV-1), *Paramyxoviridae*
Avian paramyxovirus 2 (Yucaipa), (APMV-2), *Paramyxoviridae*
Avian paramyxovirus 3, (APMV-3), *Paramyxoviridae*
Avian paramyxovirus 4, (APMV-4), *Paramyxoviridae*
Avian paramyxovirus 5 (Kunitachi), (APMV-5), *Paramyxoviridae*
Avian paramyxovirus 6, (APMV-6), *Paramyxoviridae*
Avian paramyxovirus 7, (APMV-7), *Paramyxoviridae*
Avian paramyxovirus 8, (APMV-8), *Paramyxoviridae*
Avian paramyxovirus 9, (APMV-9), *Paramyxoviridae*
Avian pneumovirus, *Paramyxoviridae*
Avian sarcoma virus CT10, (ASV-CT10), *Retroviridae*
Avocado sunblotch viroid, (ASBVd), *Avsunviroidae*
Azotobacter phage A12, (A12), *Podoviridae*
Azuki bean mosaic virus, *Potyviridae*

B19 virus, (B19V), *Parvoviridae*
Babahoya virus, (BABV), *Bunyaviridae*
Babanki virus, *Togaviridae*
Baboon herpesvirus, *Herpesviridae*

Baboon orthoreovirus, (BRV), *Reoviridae*
Baboon polyomavirus 2, (PPyV), *Polyomaviridae*
Bacillus phage 1A, (1A), *Siphoviridae*
Bacillus phage 2C, (2C), *Myoviridae*
Bacillus phage AP50, (AP50), *Tectiviridae*
Bacillus phage AR1, (AR1), *Myoviridae*
Bacillus phage AR13, (AR13), *Podoviridae*
Bacillus phage B103, (B103), *Podoviridae*
Bacillus phage B1715V1, (B1715V1), *Siphoviridae*
Bacillus phage Bace-11, (Bace-11), *Myoviridae*
Bacillus phage BLE, (BLE), *Siphoviridae*
Bacillus phage CP-54, (CP-54), *Myoviridae*
Bacillus phage G, (G), *Myoviridae*
Bacillus phage GA-1, (GA-1), *Podoviridae*
Bacillus phage GS1, (GS1), *Myoviridae*
Bacillus phage I9, (I9), *Myoviridae*
Bacillus phage II, (II), *Siphoviridae*
Bacillus phage IPy-1, (IPy-1), *Siphoviridae*
Bacillus phage M2, (M2), *Podoviridae*
Bacillus phage mor1, (mor1), *Siphoviridae*
Bacillus phage MP13, (MP13), *Myoviridae*
Bacillus phage MP15, (MP15), *Siphoviridae*
Bacillus phage MY2, (MY2), *Podoviridae*
Bacillus phage Nf, (Nf), *Podoviridae*
Bacillus phage NLP-1, (NLP-1), *Myoviridae*
Bacillus phage PBP1, (PBP1), *Siphoviridae*
Bacillus phage PBS1, (PBS1), *Myoviridae*
Bacillus phage PZA, (PZA), *Podoviridae*
Bacillus phage PZE, (PZE), *Podoviridae*
Bacillus phage SF5, (SF5), *Podoviridae*
Bacillus phage SN45, (SN45), *Siphoviridae*
Bacillus phage SP01, (SP01), *Myoviridae*
Bacillus phage SP10, (SP10), *Myoviridae*
Bacillus phage SP15, (SP15), *Myoviridae*
Bacillus phage SP3, (SP3), *Myoviridae*
Bacillus phage SP5, (SP5), *Myoviridae*
Bacillus phage SP50, (SP50), *Myoviridae*
Bacillus phage SP8, (SP8), *Myoviridae*
Bacillus phage SP82, (SP82), *Myoviridae*
Bacillus phage SPP1, (SPP1), *Siphoviridae*
Bacillus phage Spy-2, (Spy-2), *Myoviridae*
Bacillus phage Spy-3, (Spy-3), *Myoviridae*
Bacillus phage SPβ, (SPβ), *Siphoviridae*
Bacillus phage SST, (SST), *Myoviridae*
Bacillus phage SW, (SW), *Myoviridae*
Bacillus phage Tb10, (Tb10), *Siphoviridae*
Bacillus phage TP-15, (TP15), *Siphoviridae*
Bacillus phage type F, (type F), *Siphoviridae*
Bacillus phage α, (α), *Siphoviridae*
Bacillus phage φ105, (φ105), *Siphoviridae*
Bacillus phage φ15, (φ15), *Podoviridae*
Bacillus phage φ25, (φ25), *Myoviridae*
Bacillus phage φ29, (φ29), *Podoviridae*
Bacillus phage φBa1, (φBa1), *Podoviridae*
Bacillus phage φe, (φe), *Myoviridae*

Bacillus phage φNS11, (φNS11), *Tectiviridae*
Bagaza virus, (BAGV), *Flaviviridae*
Bahia Grande virus, (BGV), *Rhabdoviridae*
Bahig virus, (BAHV), *Bunyaviridae*
Bajra streak virus, (BaSV), *Geminiviridae*
Bakau virus, (BAKV), *Bunyaviridae*
Bakel virus, (BAKV), *Bunyaviridae*
Baku virus, (BAKUV), *Reoviridae*
Bald eagle herpesvirus, *Herpesviridae*
Bamboo mosaic virus satellite RNA, Satellite
Bamboo mosaic virus, (BaMV), *Potexvirus*
Banana bract mosaic virus, (BBrMV), *Potyviridae*
Banana bunchy top virus, (BBTV), *Nanovirus*
Banana streak virus, (BSV), *Caulimoviridae*
Banded krait herpesvirus, *Herpesviridae*
Bandia virus, (BDAV), *Bunyaviridae*
Bangoran virus, (BGNV), *Rhabdoviridae*
Bangui virus, (BGIV), *Bunyaviridae*
Banna virus (China), (BAV-Ch), *Reoviridae*
Banna virus (China-HN131), (BAV-HN131V), *Reoviridae*
Banna virus (China-HN191), (BAV-HN191V), *Reoviridae*
Banna virus (China-HN295), (BAV-HN295V), *Reoviridae*
Banna virus (China-HN59), (BAV-HN59V), *Reoviridae*
Banna virus (Indonesia-6423), (BAV-In6423), *Reoviridae*
Banna virus (Indonesia-6969), (BAV-In6969), *Reoviridae*
Banna virus (Indonesia-7043), (BAV-In7043), *Reoviridae*
Banna virus, (BAV), *Reoviridae*
Banzi virus, (BANV), *Flaviviridae*
Barfin flounder nervous necrosis virus, (BFNNV), *Nodaviridae*
Barley mild mosaic virus, (BaMMV), *Potyviridae*
Barley stripe mosaic virus, (BSMV), *Hordeivirus*
Barley virus B1, (BarV-B1), *Potexvirus*
Barley yellow dwarf virus – GPV, (BYDV-GPV), *Luteoviridae*
Barley yellow dwarf virus – MAV, (BYDV-MAV), *Luteoviridae*
Barley yellow dwarf virus – PAV, (BYDV-PAV), *Luteoviridae*
Barley yellow dwarf virus – RGV, *Luteoviridae*
Barley yellow dwarf virus – RMV, (BYDV-RMV), *Luteoviridae*
Barley yellow dwarf virus – SGV, (BYDV-SGV), *Luteoviridae*
Barley yellow dwarf virus satellite RNA, Satellite
Barley yellow mosaic virus, (BaYMV), *Potyviridae*
Barley yellow striate mosaic virus, (BYSMV), *Rhabdoviridae*

Barmah Forest virus, (BFV), *Togaviridae*
Barramundi virus-1, (BaV), *Picornaviridae*
Barranqueras virus, (BQSV), *Bunyaviridae*
Barur virus, (BARV), *Rhabdoviridae*
Bashkiria Cg18-20 virus, *Bunyaviridae*
Batai virus, (BATV), *Bunyaviridae*
Batama virus, (BMAV), *Bunyaviridae*
Batken virus, *Orthomyxoviridae*
Batu Cave virus, (BCV), *Flaviviridae*
Bauline virus, (BAUV), *Reoviridae*
Bayou virus, (BAYV), *Bunyaviridae*
Bdellovibrio phage MAC 1, (MAC-1), *Microviridae*
Bdellovibrio phage MAC 1', (MAC-1'), *Microviridae*
Bdellovibrio phage MAC 2, (MAC-2), *Microviridae*
Bdellovibrio phage MAC 4, (MAC-4), *Microviridae*
Bdellovibrio phage MAC 4', (MAC-4'), *Microviridae*
Bdellovibrio phage MAC 5, (MAC-5), *Microviridae*
Bdellovibrio phage MAC 7, (MAC-7), *Microviridae*
Beak and feather disease virus, (BFDV), *Circoviridae*
BeAn 157575 virus, (BeAnV-157575), *Rhabdoviridae*
BeAn 277 virus, (GMAV), *Bunyaviridae*
BeAn 293022 virus, *Arenaviridae*
BeAn 47693 virus, (BUJV), *Bunyaviridae*
BeAn 70563 virus, *Arenaviridae*
BeAn 8582 virus, (CAPV), *Bunyaviridae*
Bean angular mosaic virus, *Carlavirus*
Bean calico mosaic virus, (BCaMV), *Geminiviridae*
Bean common mosaic necrosis virus, (BCMNV), *Potyviridae*
Bean common mosaic virus, (BCMV), *Potyviridae*
Bean dwarf mosaic virus, (BDMV), *Geminiviridae*
Bean golden mosaic virus – Brazil, (BGMV-Br), *Geminiviridae*
Bean golden mosaic virus – Dom. Rep., (BGMV-DR), *Geminiviridae*
Bean golden mosaic virus – Guatemala, (BGMV-Gua), *Geminiviridae*
Bean golden mosaic virus – Puerto Rico, (BGMV-PR), *Geminiviridae*
Bean leafroll virus, (BLRV), *Luteoviridae*
Bean mild mosaic virus, (BMMV), *Tombusviridae*
Bean pod mottle virus, (BPMV), *Comoviridae*
Bean rugose mosaic virus, (BRMV), *Comoviridae*
Bean yellow dwarf virus, (BeYDV), *Geminiviridae*
Bean yellow mosaic virus, (BYMV), *Potyviridae*
Bean yellow vein-banding virus, (BYVBV), *Umbravirus*
BeAr 328208 virus, (BAV), *Bunyaviridae*
Bearded iris mosaic virus, *Potyviridae*
Bebaru virus, (BEBV), *Togaviridae*
Bee iridescent virus, *Iridoviridae*
Bee virus X, (BXV), Unassigned
Bee virus Y, (BYV), Unassigned
Beet cryptic virus 1, (BCV-1), *Partitiviridae*
Beet cryptic virus 2, (BCV-2), *Partitiviridae*

Beet cryptic virus 3, (BCV-3), *Partitiviridae*
Beet curly top virus Iran/CFH, (BCTV-CFH), *Geminiviridae*
Beet curly top virus Worland, (BCTV-Wor), *Geminiviridae*
Beet curly top virus, (BCTV), *Geminiviridae*
Beet leaf curl virus, (BLCV), *Rhabdoviridae*
Beet mild yellowing virus, (BMYV), *Luteoviridae*
Beet mosaic virus, (BtMV), *Potyviridae*
Beet necrotic yellow vein virus satellite - like RNA5, Satellite
Beet necrotic yellow vein virus, (BNYVV), *Benyvirus*
Beet pseudoyellows virus, (BPYV), *Closteroviridae*
Beet ringspot virus satellite RNA, Satellite
Beet ringspot virus, (BRSV), *Comoviridae*
Beet soil-borne mosaic virus, (BSBMV), *Benyvirus*
Beet soil-borne virus, (BSBV), *Pomovirus*
Beet virus Q, (BVQ), *Pomovirus*
Beet western yellows virus, (BWYV), *Luteoviridae*
Beet yellow stunt virus, (BYSV), *Closteroviridae*
Beet yellows virus, (BYV), *Closteroviridae*
BeH 2251 virus, (CDUV), *Bunyaviridae*
Belem virus, (BLMV), *Bunyaviridae*
Belladonna mottle virus, (BeMV), *Tymovirus*
Belmont virus, (BELV), *Bunyaviridae*
Beltera virus, (BELTV), *Bunyaviridae*
Benevides virus, (BENV), *Bunyaviridae*
Benfica virus, (BENV), *Bunyaviridae*
Berkeley bee virus, (BBV), Unassigned
Bermejo virus, *Bunyaviridae*
Bermuda grass etched-line virus, (BELV), *Marafivirus*
Berrimah virus, (BRMV), *Rhabdoviridae*
Bertioga virus, (BERV), *Bunyaviridae*
Bhanja virus, (BHAV), *Bunyaviridae*
Bhendi yellow vein mosaic virus, (BYVMV), *Geminiviridae*
Bidens mosaic virus, (BiMV), *Potyviridae*
Bidens mottle virus, (BiMoV), *Potyviridae*
Biken-1 virus, *Bunyaviridae*
Bimbo virus, (BBOV), *Rhabdoviridae*
Bimiti virus, (BIMV), *Bunyaviridae*
Birao virus, (BIRV), *Bunyaviridae*
Biston betularia cypovirus 6, (BbCPV-6), *Reoviridae*
Bivens Arm virus, (BAV), *Rhabdoviridae*
BK polyomavirus, (BKPyV), *Polyomaviridae*
Black beetle iridescent virus, *Iridoviridae*
Black beetle virus, (BBV), *Nodaviridae*
Black Creek Canal virus, (BCCV), *Bunyaviridae*
Black footed penguin herpesvirus, *Herpesviridae*
Black queen cell virus, (BQCV), Unassigned
Black raspberry necrosis virus, (BRNV), Unassigned
Black stork herpesvirus, *Herpesviridae*
Blackcurrant reversion associated virus, (BRAV), *Comoviridae*
Blackeye cowpea mosaic virus, *Potyviridae*

Blackgram mottle virus, (BMoV), *Tombusviridae*
Bloodland Lake virus, (BLLV), *Bunyaviridae*
Blue crab virus, (BCV), *Rhabdoviridae*
Blue River virus, *Bunyaviridae*
Blueberry leaf mottle virus, (BLMoV), *Comoviridae*
Blueberry mosaic viroid-like RNA, (BluMVd-RNA), *Avsunviroidae*
Blueberry red ringspot virus, (BRRV), *Caulimoviridae*
Blueberry scorch virus, (BlScV), *Carlavirus*
Blueberry shock virus, (BlShV), *Bromoviridae*
Blueberry shoestring virus, (BSSV), *Sobemovirus*
Bluetongue virus 1 to 24, (BTV-1 to 24), *Reoviridae*
Bluetongue virus, (BTV), *Reoviridae*
B-lymphotropic polyomavirus, (LPyV), *Polyomaviridae*
Boa herpesvirus, *Herpesviridae*
Bobaya virus, (BOBV), *Bunyaviridae*
Bobia virus, (BIAV), *Bunyaviridae*
Bobwhite quail herpesvirus, *Herpesviridae*
Bohle iridovirus, (BIV), *Iridoviridae*
Boid herpesvirus 1, (BoiHV-1), *Herpesviridae*
Boletus virus X, (BolVX), *Potexvirus*
Boloria dia cypovirus 2, (BdCPV-2), *Reoviridae*
Bombyx mori cypovirus 1, (BmCPV-1), *Reoviridae*
Bombyx mori densovirus, (BmDNV), *Parvoviridae*
Bombyx mori mag virus, (BmoMagV), *Metaviridae*
Bombyx mori NPV, (BmNPV), *Baculoviridae*
Boolarra virus, (BoV), *Nodaviridae*
Boraceia virus, (BORV), *Bunyaviridae*
Border disease virus BD31, *Flaviviridae*
Border disease virus X818, *Flaviviridae*
Border disease virus, (BDV), *Flaviviridae*
Borna disease virus, (BDV), *Bornaviridae*
Botambi virus, (BOTV), *Bunyaviridae*
Boteke virus, (BTKV), *Rhabdoviridae*
Bouboui virus, (BOUV), *Flaviviridae*
Bovine adeno-associated virus, (BAAV), *Parvoviridae*
Bovine adenovirus 1, (BAdV-1), *Adenoviridae*
Bovine adenovirus 10, (BAdV-10), *Adenoviridae*
Bovine adenovirus 2, (BAdV-2), *Adenoviridae*
Bovine adenovirus 3, (BAdV-3), *Adenoviridae*
Bovine adenovirus 4 to 8, (BAdV-4 to 8), *Adenoviridae*
Bovine adenovirus 9, (BAdV-9), *Adenoviridae*
Bovine adenovirus A, (BAdV-A), *Adenoviridae*
Bovine adenovirus B, (BAdV-B), *Adenoviridae*
Bovine adenovirus C, (BAdV-C), *Adenoviridae*
Bovine astrovirus 1, (BAstV-1), *Astroviridae*
Bovine astrovirus 2, (BAstV-2), *Astroviridae*
Bovine astrovirus, (BAstV), *Astroviridae*
Bovine calicivirus, (VESV/Bos-1), *Caliciviridae*
Bovine encephalitis virus, *Herpesviridae*
Bovine enteric calicivirus, (BoCV), *Caliciviridae*
Bovine enterovirus 1, (BEV-1), *Picornaviridae*
Bovine enterovirus 2, (BEV-2), *Picornaviridae*
Bovine enterovirus, (BEV), *Picornaviridae*
Bovine ephemeral fever virus, (BEFV), *Rhabdoviridae*
Bovine foamy virus, (BFV), *Retroviridae*
Bovine herpesvirus 1, (BoHV-1), *Herpesviridae*
Bovine herpesvirus 2, (BoHV-2), *Herpesviridae*
Bovine herpesvirus 4, (BoHV-4), *Herpesviridae*
Bovine herpesvirus 5, (BoHV-5), *Herpesviridae*
Bovine immunodeficiency virus, (BIV), *Retroviridae*
Bovine leukemia virus, (BLV), *Retroviridae*
Bovine mamillitis virus, *Herpesviridae*
Bovine papillomavirus 1 to 4, (BPV-1 to 4), *Papillomaviridae*
Bovine papillomavirus, (BPV), *Papillomaviridae*
Bovine papular stomatitis virus, (BPSV), *Poxviridae*
Bovine parainfluenza virus 3, (BPIV-3), *Paramyxoviridae*
Bovine parvovirus, (BPV), *Parvoviridae*
Bovine polyomavirus, (BPyV), *Polyomaviridae*
Bovine respiratory syncytial virus, (BRSV), *Paramyxoviridae*
Bovine rhinovirus 1, (BRV-1), *Picornaviridae*
Bovine rhinovirus 2, (BRV-2), *Picornaviridae*
Bovine rhinovirus 3, (BRV-3), *Picornaviridae*
Bovine viral diarrhea virus 1 CP7, *Flaviviridae*
Bovine viral diarrhea virus 1 NADL, *Flaviviridae*
Bovine viral diarrhea virus 1 Osloss, *Flaviviridae*
Bovine viral diarrhea virus 1 SD-1, *Flaviviridae*
Bovine viral diarrhea virus 1, (BVDV-1), *Flaviviridae*
Bovine viral diarrhea virus 2 C413, *Flaviviridae*
Bovine viral diarrhea virus 2 strain 890, *Flaviviridae*
Bovine viral diarrhea virus 2, (BVDV-2), *Flaviviridae*
Box turtle virus 3, (TV3), *Iridoviridae*
Bozo virus, (BOZOV), *Bunyaviridae*
Brachypodium yellow streak virus, (BYSV), Unassigned
Bramble yellow mosaic virus, (BrmYMV), *Potyviridae*
Brazilian wheat spike virus, (BWSpV), *Tenuivirus*
Broad bean mottle virus, (BBMV), *Bromoviridae*
Broad bean necrosis virus, (BBNV), *Pomovirus*
Broad bean stain virus, (BBSV), *Comoviridae*
Broad bean true mosaic virus, (BBTMV), *Comoviridae*
Broad bean wilt virus 1, (BBWV-1), *Comoviridae*
Broad bean wilt virus 2, (BBWV-2), *Comoviridae*
Broadhaven virus, (BRDV), *Reoviridae*
Broccoli necrotic yellows virus, (BNYV), *Rhabdoviridae*
Brome mosaic virus, (BMV), *Bromoviridae*
Brome streak virus, (BStV), *Potyviridae*
Bromus striate mosaic virus, (BrSMV), *Geminiviridae*
Brucella phage Tb, (Tb), *Podoviridae*
Bruconha virus, (BRUV), *Bunyaviridae*
Bryonia mottle virus, (BryMoV), *Potyviridae*

BT 4971 virus, (PATV), *Bunyaviridae*
Bubaline herpesvirus 1, (BuHV-1), *Herpesviridae*
Budgerigar fledgling polyomavirus, (BFPyV),
  Polyomaviridae
Buenaventura virus, (BUEV), *Bunyaviridae*
Buffalopox virus, (BPXV), *Poxviridae*
Buggy Creek virus, *Togaviridae*
Bujaru virus, (BUJV), *Bunyaviridae*
Bukalasa bat virus, (BBV), *Flaviviridae*
Bunyamwera virus, (BUNV), *Bunyaviridae*
Bunyip creek virus, (BCV), *Reoviridae*
Burdock stunt viroid, (BuSVd), *Avsunviroidae*
Burdock yellows virus, (BuYV), *Closteroviridae*
Bushbush virus, (BSBV), *Bunyaviridae*
Bussuquara virus, (BSQV), *Flaviviridae*
Buthus occitanus reovirus, (BoRV), *Reoviridae*
Butterbur mosaic virus, (ButMV), *Carlavirus*
Buttonwillow virus, (BUTV), *Bunyaviridae*
B-virus; Herpesvirus simiae, *Herpesviridae*
Bwamba virus, (BWAV), *Bunyaviridae*

Cabassou virus, (CABV), *Togaviridae*
Cacao swollen shoot virus, (CSSV), *Caulimoviridae*
Cacao virus, (CACV), *Bunyaviridae*
Cacao yellow mosaic virus, (CYMV), *Tymovirus*
Cache Valley virus, (CVV), *Bunyaviridae*
Cacipacore virus, (CPCV), *Flaviviridae*
Cactus virus 2, (CV-2), *Carlavirus*
Cactus virus X, (CVX), *Potexvirus*
Caddo Canyon virus, (CDCV), *Bunyaviridae*
Caenorhabditis elegans Cer1 virus, (CelCer1V),
  Metaviridae
Caimito virus, (CAIV), *Bunyaviridae*
Calanthe mild mosaic virus, (CalMMV), *Potyviridae*
Calchaqui virus, (CQIV), *Rhabdoviridae*
California encephalitis virus, (CEV), *Bunyaviridae*
California harbor seal poxvirus, (SPV), *Poxviridae*
California hare coltivirus, (CTFV-Ca), *Reoviridae*
Callimorpha quadripuntata virus, (CqV),
  Tetraviridae
Callistephus chinensis chlorosis virus, (CCCV),
  Rhabdoviridae
Calliteara pudibunda virus, (CpV), *Tetraviridae*
Callitrichine herpesvirus 1, (CalHV-1), *Herpesviridae*
Callitrichine herpesvirus 2, (CalHV-2), *Herpesviridae*
Calopogonium yellow vein virus, (CalYVV),
  Tymovirus
Camel contagious ecthyma virus, *Poxviridae*
Camellia yellow mottle virus, (CYMoV),
  Varicosavirus
Camelpox virus, (CMLV), *Poxviridae*
Campoletis aprilis ichnovirus, (CaIV), *Polydnaviridae*
Campoletis flavicincta ichnovirus, (CfIV),
  Polydnaviridae

Campoletis sonorensis ichnovirus, (CsIV),
  Polydnaviridae
Campoletis sp. ichnovirus, (CspIV), *Polydnaviridae*
Camptochironomus tentans entomopoxvirus,
  (CTEV), *Poxviridae*
Cananeia virus, (CNAV), *Bunyaviridae*
Canary reed mosaic virus, (CRMV), *Potyviridae*
Canarypox virus, (CNPV), *Poxviridae*
Canavalia maritima mosaic virus, (CnMMV),
  Potyviridae
Canid herpesvirus 1, (CaHV-1), *Herpesviridae*
Caninde virus, (CANV), *Reoviridae*
Canine adeno-associated virus, (CAAV),
  Parvoviridae
Canine adenovirus 1, (CAdV-1), *Adenoviridae*
Canine adenovirus 2, (CAdV-2), *Adenoviridae*
Canine adenovirus, (CAdV), *Adenoviridae*
Canine calicivirus, (CaCV), *Caliciviridae*
Canine distemper virus, (CDV), *Paramyxoviridae*
Canine herpesvirus, *Herpesviridae*
Canine minute virus, (CMV), *Parvoviridae*
Canine oral papillomavirus, (COPV),
  Papillomaviridae
Canine parvovirus, (CPV), *Parvoviridae*
Canna yellow mottle virus, (CaYMV),
  Caulimoviridae
Cano Delgadito virus, (CADV), *Bunyaviridae*
Cape Wrath virus, (CWV), *Reoviridae*
Caper latent virus, (CapLV), *Carlavirus*
Capim virus, (CAPV), *Bunyaviridae*
Caprine adenovirus, (GAdV), *Adenoviridae*
Caprine arthritis encephalitis virus, (CAEV),
  Retroviridae
Caprine herpesvirus 1, (CpHV-1), *Herpesviridae*
Capuchin herpesvirus AL-5, *Herpesviridae*
Capuchin herpesvirus AP-18, *Herpesviridae*
Carajas virus, (CJSV), *Rhabdoviridae*
Caraparu virus, (CARV), *Bunyaviridae*
Caraway latent virus, (CawLV), *Carlavirus*
Carcinus mediterraneus W2 virus, (CcRV-W2),
  Reoviridae
Cardamine chlorotic fleck virus, (CCFV),
  Tombusviridae
Cardamine latent virus, (CaLV), *Carlavirus*
Cardamom mosaic virus, (CdMV), *Potyviridae*
Cardiochiles nigriceps bracovirus, (CnBV),
  Polydnaviridae
Carey Island virus, (CIV), *Flaviviridae*
Carnation bacilliform virus, (CBV), *Rhabdoviridae*
Carnation cryptic virus 1, (CCV-1), *Partitiviridae*
Carnation cryptic virus 2, (CCV-2), *Partitiviridae*
Carnation etched ring virus, (CERV), *Caulimoviridae*
Carnation Italian ringspot virus, (CIRV),
  Tombusviridae
Carnation latent virus, (CLV), *Carlavirus*

Carnation mottle virus, (CarMV), *Tombusviridae*
Carnation necrotic fleck virus, (CNFV), *Closteroviridae*
Carnation ringspot virus, (CRSV), *Tombusviridae*
Carnation vein mottle virus, (CVMoV), *Potyviridae*
Carnation yellow stripe virus, (CYSV), *Tombusviridae*
Carp pox herpesvirus, *Herpesviridae*
Carrot latent virus, (CtLV), *Rhabdoviridae*
Carrot mosaic virus, (CtMV), *Potyviridae*
Carrot mottle mimic virus, (CMoMV), *Umbravirus*
Carrot mottle virus, (CMoV), *Umbravirus*
Carrot red leaf virus, (CtRLV), *Luteoviridae*
Carrot temperate virus 1, (CTeV-1), *Partitiviridae*
Carrot temperate virus 2, (CTeV-2), *Partitiviridae*
Carrot temperate virus 3, (CTeV-3), *Partitiviridae*
Carrot temperate virus 4, (CTeV-4), *Partitiviridae*
Carrot thin leaf virus, (CTLV), *Potyviridae*
Carrot yellow leaf virus, (CYLV), *Closteroviridae*
Casinaria arjuna ichnovirus, (CarIV), *Polydnaviridae*
Casinaria forcipata ichnovirus, (CfoIV), *Polydnaviridae*
Casinaria infesta ichnovirus, (CiIV), *Polydnaviridae*
Casinaria sp. ichnovirus, (CaspIV), *Polydnaviridae*
Casphalia extranea densovirus, (CeDNV), *Parvoviridae*
Cassava American latent virus, (CsALV), *Comoviridae*
Cassava common mosaic virus, (CsCMV), *Potexvirus*
Cassava green mottle virus, (CsGMV), *Comoviridae*
Cassava Ivorian bacilliform virus, (CsIBV), Unassigned
Cassava symptomless virus, (CsSLV), *Rhabdoviridae*
Cassava vein mosaic virus, (CsVMV), *Caulimoviridae*
Cassava virus C, (CsVC), *Ourmiavirus*
Cassava virus X, (CsVX), *Potexvirus*
Cassia mild mosaic virus, (CasMMV), *Carlavirus*
Cassia yellow blotch virus, (CYBV), *Bromoviridae*
Cassia yellow spot virus, (CasYSV), *Potyviridae*
Catu virus, (CATUV), *Bunyaviridae*
Cauliflower mosaic virus, (CaMV), *Caulimoviridae*
Caulobacter phage φCb12r, (φCB12r), *Leviviridae*
Caulobacter phage φCb2, (φCb2), *Leviviridae*
Caulobacter phage φCb23r, (φCb23r), *Leviviridae*
Caulobacter phage φCb4, (φCb4), *Leviviridae*
Caulobacter phage φCb5, (φCb5), *Leviviridae*
Caulobacter phage φCb8r, (φCb8r), *Leviviridae*
Caulobacter phage φCb9, (φCb9), *Leviviridae*
Caulobacter phage φCP18, (φCP18), *Leviviridae*
Caulobacter phage φCP2, (φCP2), *Leviviridae*
Caulobacter phage φCr14, (φCr14), *Leviviridae*
Caulobacter phage φCr28, (φCr28), *Leviviridae*
Caulobacter phage φCr24, (φCr24), *Myoviridae*
Berne virus, (BEV), *Coronviridae*

Bovine coronavirus, (BCoV), *Coronviridae*
Bovine torovirus, (BoTV), *Coronviridae*
Breda virus, (BRV), *Coronviridae*
Canine coronavirus, (CCoV), *Coronviridae*
Caulobacter phage φCd1, (φCd1), *Podoviridae*
Caviid herpesvirus 1, (CavHV-1), *Herpesviridae*
Caviid herpesvirus 2, (CavHV-2), *Herpesviridae*
Caviid herpesvirus 3, (CavHV-3), *Herpesviridae*
CbaAr 426 virus, (CAV), *Bunyaviridae*
Cebine herpesvirus 1, (CbHV-1), *Herpesviridae*
Cebine herpesvirus 2, (CbHV-2), *Herpesviridae*
Celery mosaic virus, (CeMV), *Potyviridae*
Celery yellow mosaic virus, (CeYMV), *Potyviridae*
Cell fusing agent virus, (CFAV), *Flaviviridae*
Centrosema mosaic virus, (CenMV), *Potexvirus*
Ceratitis capitata reovirus, *Reoviridae*
Ceratitis I virus, (CIV), *Reoviridae*
Ceratitis V virus, (CVV), Unassigned
Ceratobium mosaic virus, (CerMV), *Potyviridae*
Cercopithecine herpesvirus 1, (CeHV-1), *Herpesviridae*
Cercopithecine herpesvirus 10, (CeHV-10), *Herpesviridae*
Cercopithecine herpesvirus 12, (CeHV-12), *Herpesviridae*
Cercopithecine herpesvirus 13, (CeHV-13), *Herpesviridae*
Cercopithecine herpesvirus 14, (CeHV-14), *Herpesviridae*
Cercopithecine herpesvirus 15, (CeHV-15), *Herpesviridae*
Cercopithecine herpesvirus 16, (CeHV-16), *Herpesviridae*
Cercopithecine herpesvirus 17, (CeHV-17), *Herpesviridae*
Cercopithecine herpesvirus 2, (CeHV-2), *Herpesviridae*
Cercopithecine herpesvirus 3, (CeHV-3), *Herpesviridae*
Cercopithecine herpesvirus 4, (CeHV-4), *Herpesviridae*
Cercopithecine herpesvirus 5, (CeHV-5), *Herpesviridae*
Cercopithecine herpesvirus 8, (CeHV-8), *Herpesviridae*
Cercopithecine herpesvirus 9, (CeHV-9), *Herpesviridae*
Cercopithecine herpesvirus SA8, *Herpesviridae*
Cereal chlorotic mottle virus, (CCMoV), *Rhabdoviridae*
Cereal yellow dwarf – RPV satellite virus, Satellite
Cereal yellow dwarf virus – rpv, (CYDV-RPV), *Luteoviridae*
Cervid herpesvirus 1, (CvHV-1), *Herpesviridae*
Cervid herpesvirus 2, (CvHV-2), *Herpesviridae*

Cestrum yellow leaf curling virus, (CmYLCV), *Caulimoviridae*
Cetacean calicivirus, (VESV/Tur-1), *Caliciviridae*
Cetacean morbillivirus virus, (CeMV), *Paramyxoviridae*
CEV BFS-283, (CEV), *Bunyaviridae*
Chaco virus, (CHOV), *Rhabdoviridae*
Chagres virus, *Bunyaviridae*
Chamois contagious ecthyma virus, *Poxviridae*
Chandipura virus, (CHPV), *Rhabdoviridae*
Chandiru virus, (CDUV), *Bunyaviridae*
Changuinola virus, (CGLV), *Reoviridae*
Changuinola virus, (CGLV), *Reoviridae*
Channel catfish reovirus, (CRV), *Reoviridae*
Channel catfish virus, *Herpesviridae*
Chara australis virus, (CAV), Unassigned
Chara corallina virus, Unassigned
Charleville virus, (CHVV), *Rhabdoviridae*
Chayote mosaic virus, (ChMV), *Tymovirus*
Chelonid herpesvirus 1, (ChHV-1), *Herpesviridae*
Chelonid herpesvirus 2, (ChHV-2), *Herpesviridae*
Chelonid herpesvirus 3, (ChHV-3), *Herpesviridae*
Chelonid herpesvirus 4, (ChHV-4), *Herpesviridae*
Chelonus altitudinis bracovirus, (CalBV), *Polydnaviridae*
Chelonus blackburni bracovirus, (CbBV), *Polydnaviridae*
Chelonus inanitus bracovirus, (CinaBV), *Polydnaviridae*
Chelonus insularis bracovirus, (CinsBV), *Polydnaviridae*
Chelonus nr. curvimaculatus bracovirus, (CcBV), *Polydnaviridae*
Chelonus texanus bracovirus, (CtBV), *Polydnaviridae*
Chenopodium necrosis virus, (ChNV), *Tombusviridae*
Chenuda virus, (CNUV), *Reoviridae*
Chenuda virus, (CNUV), *Reoviridae*
Cherry green ring mottle virus, (CGRMV), *Foveavirus*
Cherry leaf roll virus, (CLRV), *Comoviridae*
Cherry rasp leaf virus, (CRLV), *Comoviridae*
Cherry rosette virus, (CRV), *Comoviridae*
Cherry virus A, (CVA), *Capillovirus*
Chick syncytial virus, (CSV), *Retroviridae*
Chicken anemia virus, (CAV), *Circoviridae*
Chicken parvovirus, (ChPV), *Parvoviridae*
Chicken rotavirus 555, (AvRV-G/555), *Reoviridae*
Chicken rotavirus A4, (AvRV-F/A4), *Reoviridae*
Chicken rotavirus 132, (AvRV-D/132), *Reoviridae*
Chickpea bushy dwarf virus, (CpBDV), *Potyviridae*
Chickpea chlorotic dwarf virus, (CpCDV), *Geminiviridae*
Chickpea filiform virus, (CpFV), *Potyviridae*
Chickpea stunt disease associated virus, (CpSDaV), *Luteoviridae*
Chicory yellow blotch virus, (ChYBV), *Carlavirus*
Chicory yellow mottle virus large satellite RNA, Satellite
Chicory yellow mottle virus satellite RNA, Satellite
Chicory yellow mottle virus, (ChYMV), *Comoviridae*
Chikungunya virus, (CHIKV), *Togaviridae*
Chilibre virus VP-118D, (CHIV), *Bunyaviridae*
Chilibre virus, (CHIV), *Bunyaviridae*
Chilli veinal mottle virus, (ChiVMV), *Potyviridae*
Chilo iridescent virus, *Iridoviridae*
Chim virus, (CHIMV), *Bunyaviridae*
Chimpanzee adenovirus C2, (ChAdV-C2), *Adenoviridae*
Chimpanzee adenovirus strain Y34, (ChAdV-Y34), *Adenoviridae*
Chimpanzee foamy virus human isolate, (CFV/Hu), *Retroviridae*
Chimpanzee foamy virus, (CFV), *Retroviridae*
Chinese rape mosaic virus, *Tobamovirus*
Chinese yam necrotic mosaic virus, (ChYNMV), *Carlavirus*
Chino del tomate virus, (CdTV), *Geminiviridae*
Chinook salmon reovirus B, (GRCV), *Reoviridae*
Chinook salmon reovirus DRC, (DRCRV), *Reoviridae*
Chinook salmon reovirus ICR, (ICRV), *Reoviridae*
Chinook salmon reovirus LBS, (LBSV), *Reoviridae*
Chinook salmon reovirus YRC, (YRCV), *Reoviridae*
Chironomus attenuatus entomopoxvirus, (CAEV), *Poxviridae*
Chironomus luridus entomopoxvirus, (CLEV), *Poxviridae*
Chironomus plumosus entomopoxvirus, (CPEV), *Poxviridae*
Chlamydia phage 1, (Ch-1), *Microviridae*
Chloris striate mosaic virus, (CSMV), *Geminiviridae*
Chobar Gorge virus, (CGV), *Reoviridae*
Chobar Gorge virus, (CGV), *Reoviridae*
Choristoneura biennis entomopoxvirus 'L', (CBEV), *Poxviridae*
Choristoneura conflicta entomopoxvirus 'L', (CCEV), *Poxviridae*
Choristoneura diversuma entomopoxvirus 'L', (CDEV), *Poxviridae*
Choristoneura fumiferana cypovirus 7, (CfCPV-7), *Reoviridae*
Choristoneura fumiferana entomopoxvirus 'L', (CFEV), *Poxviridae*
Choristoneura fumiferana MNPV, (CfMNPV), *Baculoviridae*
Chorizagrotis auxiliars entomopoxvirus 'L', (CXEV), *Poxviridae*
Chronic bee paralysis virus, (CBPV), Unassigned

Chronic bee-paralysis satellite virus, Satellite
Chrysanthemum aspermy virus, *Bromoviridae*
Chrysanthemum chlorotic mottle viroid, (CChMVd), *Avsunviroidae*
Chrysanthemum frutescens virus, (CFV), *Rhabdoviridae*
Chrysanthemum stem necrosis virus, (CSNV), *Bunyaviridae*
Chrysanthemum stunt viroid, (CSVd), *Pospiviroidae*
Chrysanthemum vein chlorosis virus, (CVCV), *Rhabdoviridae*
Chrysanthemum virus B, (CVB), *Carlavirus*
Chub reovirus, (CHRV), *Reoviridae*
Chum salmon reovirus CSV, (CSRV), *Reoviridae*
Chum salmon reovirus F, (PSRV), *Reoviridae*
Chysochromulina brevifilum virus PW1, (CbV-PW1), *Phycodnaviridae*
Chysochromulina brevifilum virus PW3, (CbV-PW3), *Phycodnaviridae*
Ciconiid herpesvirus 1, (CiHV-1), *Herpesviridae*
Cimex lactularius reovirus, (ClRV), *Reoviridae*
Citrus bent leaf viroid, (CBLVd), *Pospiviroidae*
Citrus cachexia viroid, *Pospiviroidae*
Citrus exocortis viroid, (CEVd), *Pospiviroidae*
Citrus III viroid, (CVd-III), *Pospiviroidae*
Citrus IV viroid, (CVd-IV), *Pospiviroidae*
Citrus leaf rugose virus, (CiLRV), *Bromoviridae*
Citrus leprosis virus, (CiLV), *Rhabdoviridae*
Citrus mosaic virus, (CMBV), *Caulimoviridae*
Citrus psorosis virus, (CPsV), *Ophiovirus*
Citrus tatter leaf virus, *Capillovirus*
Citrus tristeza virus, (CTV), *Closteroviridae*
Citrus variegation virus, (CVV), *Bromoviridae*
Cladosporium fulvum T-1 virus, (CfuT1V), *Metaviridae*
Classical swine fever virus Alfort/187, *Flaviviridae*
Classical swine fever virus Alfort-Tübingen, *Flaviviridae*
Classical swine fever virus Brescia, *Flaviviridae*
Classical swine fever virus C strain, *Flaviviridae*
Classical swine fever virus, (CSFV), *Flaviviridae*
Clitoria yellow mosaic virus, (CtYMV), *Potyviridae*
Clitoria yellow vein virus, (CYVV), *Tymovirus*
Clo Mor virus, (CMV), *Bunyaviridae*
Clostridium phage CEβ, (CEβ), *Myoviridae*
Clostridium phage F1, (F1), *Siphoviridae*
Clostridium phage HM2, (HM2), *Podoviridae*
Clostridium phage HM3, (HM3), *Myoviridae*
Clostridium phage HM7, (HM7), *Siphoviridae*
Cloudy wing virus, (CWV), Unassigned
Clover enation virus, (ClEV), *Rhabdoviridae*
Clover yellow mosaic virus, (ClYMV), *Potexvirus*
Clover yellow vein virus, (ClYVV), *Potyviridae*
Clover yellows virus, (CYV), *Closteroviridae*
CoAr 1071 virus, (CA1071V), *Bunyaviridae*

CoAr 3624 virus, (CA3624V), *Bunyaviridae*
CoAr 3627 virus, (CA3627V), *Bunyaviridae*
Coastal Plains virus, (CPV), *Rhabdoviridae*
Cocal virus, (COCV), *Rhabdoviridae*
Cockatoo entero-like virus, (CELV), *Picornaviridae*
Cocksfoot mild mosaic virus, (CMMV), *Sobemovirus*
Cocksfoot mottle virus, (CoMV), *Sobemovirus*
Cocksfoot streak virus, (CSV), *Potyviridae*
Cocoa necrosis virus, (CoNV), *Comoviridae*
Coconut cadang-cadang viroid, (CCCVd), *Pospiviroidae*
Coconut foliar decay virus, (CFDV), *Nanovirus*
Coconut tinangaja viroid, (CTiVd), *Pospiviroidae*
Coffee ringspot virus, (CoRSV), *Rhabdoviridae*
Coho salmon reovirus CSR, (CSRV), *Reoviridae*
Coho salmon reovirus ELC, (ELCV), *Reoviridae*
Coho salmon reovirus SCS, (SCSV), *Reoviridae*
ColAn 57389 virus, (CA57389V), *Bunyaviridae*
Cole latent virus, (CoLV), *Carlavirus*
Coleus blumei viroid 1, (CbVd-1), *Pospiviroidae*
Coleus blumei viroid 2, (CbVd-2), *Pospiviroidae*
Coleus blumei viroid 3, (CbVd-3), *Pospiviroidae*
Colletotrichum lindemuthianum virus, (CLV), Unassigned
Colocasia bobone disease virus, (CBDV), *Rhabdoviridae*
Colombian datura virus, (CDV), *Potyviridae*
Colony B North virus, *Reoviridae*
Colony virus, (COYV), *Reoviridae*
Colorado tick fever virus, (CTFV), *Reoviridae*
Columbia SK virus, *Picornaviridae*
Columbid herpesvirus 1, (CoHV-1), *Herpesviridae*
Columnea latent viroid, (CLVd), *Pospiviroidae*
Commelina mosaic virus, (ComMV), *Potyviridae*
Commelina virus X, (ComVX), *Potexvirus*
Commelina yellow mottle virus, (ComYMV), *Caulimoviridae*
Connecticut virus, (CNTV), *Rhabdoviridae*
Convict Creek 107 virus, *Bunyaviridae*
Convict Creek 74 virus, *Bunyaviridae*
Corfou virus, (CFUV), *Bunyaviridae*
Coriander feathery red vein virus, (CFRVV), *Rhabdoviridae*
Cormorant herpesvirus, *Herpesviridae*
Corriparta virus, (CORV), *Reoviridae*
Corriparta virus, (CORV), *Reoviridae*
Coryneform phage A19, (A19), *Myoviridae*
Coryneforms phage 7/26, (7/26), *Podoviridae*
Coryneforms phage AN25S-1, (AN25S-1), *Podoviridae*
Coryneforms phage Arp, (Arp), *Siphoviridae*
Coryneforms phage BL3, (BL3), *Siphoviridae*
Coryneforms phage CONX, (CONX), *Siphoviridae*
Coryneforms phage MT, (MT), *Siphoviridae*
Coryneforms phage α, (α), *Siphoviridae*

Coryneforms phage β, (β), *Siphoviridae*
Coryneforms phage φA8010, (φA8010), *Siphoviridae*
Costelytra zealandica iridescent virus, *Iridoviridae*
Cote d'Ivoire Ebola virus, (CIEBOV), *Filoviridae*
Cotesia congregata bracovirus, (CcBV), *Polydnaviridae*
Cotesia flavipes bracovirus, (CfBV), *Polydnaviridae*
Cotesia glomerata bracovirus, (CgBV), *Polydnaviridae*
Cotesia hyphantriae bracovirus, (ChBV), *Polydnaviridae*
Cotesia kariyai bracovirus, (CkBV), *Polydnaviridae*
Cotesia marginiventris bracovirus, (CmaBV), *Polydnaviridae*
Cotesia melanoscela bracovirus, (CmeBV), *Polydnaviridae*
Cotesia rubecula bracovirus, (CrBV), *Polydnaviridae*
Cotesia schaeferi bracovirus, (CsBV), *Polydnaviridae*
Cotia virus, (CPV), *Poxviridae*
Cotton leaf crumple virus, (CLCrV), *Geminiviridae*
Cotton leaf curl virus - Pakistan 1, (CLCuV-Pk1), *Geminiviridae*
Cotton leaf curl virus - Pakistan 2, (CLCuV-Pk2), *Geminiviridae*
Cottontail rabbit herpesvirus, *Herpesviridae*
Cottontail rabbit papillomavirus, (CRPV), *Papillomaviridae*
Cow parsnip mosaic virus, (CPaMV), *Rhabdoviridae*
Cowbone Ridge virus, (CRV), *Flaviviridae*
Cowpea aphid-borne mosaic virus, (CABMV), *Potyviridae*
Cowpea chlorotic mottle virus, (CCMV), *Bromoviridae*
Cowpea golden mosaic virus, (CPGMV), *Geminiviridae*
Cowpea green vein banding virus, (CGVBV), *Potyviridae*
Cowpea mild mottle virus, (CPMMV), *Carlavirus*
Cowpea mosaic virus, (CPMV), *Comoviridae*
Cowpea mottle virus, (CPMoV), *Tombusviridae*
Cowpea rugose mosaic virus, (CPRMV), *Potyviridae*
Cowpea severe mosaic virus, (CPSMV), *Comoviridae*
Cowpox virus, (CPXV), *Poxviridae*
Crane herpesvirus, *Herpesviridae*
Cricetid herpesvirus, (CrHV-1), *Herpesviridae*
Cricket paralysis virus, (CrPV), "CrPV-like viruses"
Crimean-Congo hemorrhagic fever virus, *Bunyaviridae*
Crimson clover latent virus, (CCLV), *Comoviridae*
Crinum mosaic virus, (CriMV), *Potyviridae*
Croatian clover virus, (CroCV), *Potyviridae*
Crocus tomasinianus virus, *Potyviridae*
Croton yellow vein mosaic virus, (CYVMV), *Geminiviridae*
Crowpox virus, (CRPV), *Poxviridae*

Cryphonectria hypovirus 1-EP713, (CHV1-EP713), *Hypoviridae*
Cryphonectria hypovirus 1-EP747, (CHV1-EP747), *Hypoviridae*
Cryphonectria hypovirus 2-NB58, (CHV2-NB58), *Hypoviridae*
Cryphonectria hypovirus 3-GH2, (CHV3-GH2), *Hypoviridae*
Cryphonectria hypovirus 4-SR2, (CHV4-SR2), *Hypoviridae*
Cryphonectria parasitica mitovirus 1-NB631, (CpMV1-NB631), *Narnaviridae*
CSIRO village virus, (CVGV), *Reoviridae*
Cucumber chlorotic spot virus, (CCSV), *Closteroviridae*
Cucumber cryptic virus, (CuCV), *Partitiviridae*
Cucumber green mottle mosaic virus, (CGMMV), *Tobamovirus*
Cucumber leaf spot virus, (CLSV), *Tombusviridae*
Cucumber mosaic virus satellite RNA, Satellite
Cucumber mosaic virus, (CMV), *Bromoviridae*
Cucumber necrosis virus, (CuNV), *Tombusviridae*
Cucumber pale fruit viroid, *Pospiviroidae*
Cucumber soil-borne virus, (CuSBV), *Tombusviridae*
Cucurbit aphid-borne yellows virus, (CABYV), *Luteoviridae*
Cucurbit yellow stunting disorder virus, (CYSDV), *Closteroviridae*
CUMC-B11 virus, *Bunyaviridae*
Cyanobacteria phage A-4(L), (A-4(L)), *Podoviridae*
Cyanobacteria phage AC-1, (AC-1), *Podoviridae*
Cyanobacteria phage AS-1, (AS-1), *Myoviridae*
Cyanobacteria phage LPP-1, (LPP-1), *Podoviridae*
Cyanobacteria phage N1, (N1), *Myoviridae*
Cyanobacteria phage S-2L, (S-2L), *Siphoviridae*
Cyanobacteria phage S-4L, (S-4L), *Siphoviridae*
Cyanobacteria phage S-6(L), (S-6(L)), *Myoviridae*
Cyanobacteria phage SM-1, (SM-1), *Podoviridae*
Cycas necrotic stunt virus, (CNSV), *Comoviridae*
Cydia pomonella granulovirus, (CpGV), *Baculoviridae*
Cymbidium mosaic virus, (CymMV), *Potexvirus*
Cymbidium ringspot virus satellite RNA, Satellite
Cymbidium ringspot virus, (CymRSV), *Tombusviridae*
Cynara virus, (CraV), *Rhabdoviridae*
Cynodon mosaic virus, (CynMV), *Carlavirus*
Cynosurus mottle virus, (CnMoV), *Sobemovirus*
Cypovirus 1, (CPV-1), *Reoviridae*
Cypovirus 10, (CPV-10), *Reoviridae*
Cypovirus 11, (CPV-11), *Reoviridae*
Cypovirus 12, (CPV-12), *Reoviridae*
Cypovirus 13, (CPV-13), *Reoviridae*
Cypovirus 14, (CPV-14), *Reoviridae*
Cypovirus 2, (CPV-2), *Reoviridae*

Cypovirus 3, (CPV-3), *Reoviridae*
Cypovirus 4, (CPV-4), *Reoviridae*
Cypovirus 5, (CPV-5), *Reoviridae*
Cypovirus 6, (CPV-6), *Reoviridae*
Cypovirus 7, (CPV-7), *Reoviridae*
Cypovirus 8, (CPV-8), *Reoviridae*
Cypovirus 9, (CPV-9), *Reoviridae*
Cyprinid herpesvirus 1, (CyHV-1), *Herpesviridae*
Cyprinid herpesvirus 2, (CyHV-2), *Herpesviridae*
Cypripedium calceolus virus, (CypCV), *Potyviridae*

Dab lymphocystis disease virus, *Iridoviridae*
Dabakala virus, (DABV), *Bunyaviridae*
Dacus oleae reovirus, (DoRV), *Reoviridae*
D'Aguilar virus, (DAGV), *Reoviridae*
Dahlia mosaic virus, (DMV), *Caulimoviridae*
Dak AN B 188d virus, *Arenaviridae*
Dakar bat virus, (DBV), *Flaviviridae*
DakArK 7292 virus, (DAKV-7292), *Rhabdoviridae*
Danaus plexippus cypovirus 3, (DpCPV-3), *Reoviridae*
Dandelion latent virus, (DaLV), *Carlavirus*
Dandelion yellow mosaic virus, (DaYMV), *Sequiviridae*
Daphne virus S, (DVS), *Carlavirus*
Daphne virus X, (DVX), *Potexvirus*
Daphne virus Y, (DVY), *Potyviridae*
Dapple apple viroid, *Pospiviroidae*
Darna trima virus, (DtV), *Tetraviridae*
Dasheen mosaic virus, (DsMV), *Potyviridae*
Dasychira pudibunda cypovirus 2, (DpCPV-2), *Reoviridae*
Dasychira pudibunda virus, (DpV), *Tetraviridae*
Datura distortion mosaic virus, (DDMV), *Potyviridae*
Datura mosaic virus, (DTMV), *Potyviridae*
Datura necrosis virus, (DNV), *Potyviridae*
Datura shoestring virus, (DSSV), *Potyviridae*
Datura virus 437, (DV-437), *Potyviridae*
Datura yellow vein virus, (DYVV), *Rhabdoviridae*
Deer fibroma virus, *Papillomaviridae*
Deer papillomavirus, (DPV), *Papillomaviridae*
Deformed wing virus, (DWV), Unassigned
Demodema boranensis entomopoxvirus, (DBEV), *Poxviridae*
Dendrobium leaf streak virus, (DLSV), *Rhabdoviridae*
Dendrobium mosaic virus, *Potyviridae*
Dendrobium vein necrosis virus, (DVNV), *Closteroviridae*
Dendrolimus spectabilis cypovirus 1, (DsCPV-1), *Reoviridae*
Dengue virus type 1, (DENV-1), *Flaviviridae*
Dengue virus type 2, (DENV-2), *Flaviviridae*

Dengue virus type 3, (DENV-3), *Flaviviridae*
Dengue virus type 4, (DENV-4), *Flaviviridae*
Dengue virus, (DENV), *Flaviviridae*
Dera Ghazi Khan virus, (DGKV), *Bunyaviridae*
Dermolepida albohirtum entomopoxvirus, (DAEV), *Poxviridae*
Desert Shield virus, (DSV-395), *Caliciviridae*
Desmodium mosaic virus, (DesMV), *Potyviridae*
Desmodium yellow mottle virus, (DYMoV), *Tymovirus*
Desulfurolobus virus DAFV, (DAFV), *Lipothrixiviridae*
Dhori virus, (DHOV), *Orthomyxoviridae*
Diadegma acronyctae ichnovirus, (DaIV), *Polydnaviridae*
Diadegma interruptum ichnovirus, (DiIV), *Polydnaviridae*
Diadegma terebrans ichnovirus, (DtIV), *Polydnaviridae*
Diadromus pulchellus ascovirus 1a, (DpAV-1a), *Ascoviridae*
Diadromus pulchellus reovirus, (DpRV), *Reoviridae*
Diatraea saccharalis densovirus, (DsDNV), *Parvoviridae*
Dicentrarchus labrax encephalitis virus, (DlEV), *Nodaviridae*
Digitaria streak virus, (DSV), *Geminiviridae*
Digitaria striate mosaic virus, (DiSMV), *Geminiviridae*
Digitaria striate virus, (DiSV), *Rhabdoviridae*
Diodea vein chlorosis virus, (DVCV), *Closteroviridae*
Diolcogaster facetosa bracovirus, (DfBV), *Polydnaviridae*
Dioscorea alata ring mottle virus, *Potyviridae*
Dioscorea bacilliform virus, (DBV), *Caulimoviridae*
Dioscorea green banding virus, *Potyviridae*
Dioscorea latent virus, (DLV), *Potexvirus*
Dioscorea trifida virus, (DTV), *Potyviridae*
Dipladenia mosaic virus, (DipMV), *Potyviridae*
Diplocarpon rosae virus, (DrV), *Partitiviridae*
Dobrava-Belgrade virus, (DOBV), *Bunyaviridae*
Dock mottling mosaic virus, (DMMV), *Potyviridae*
Doctor fish virus, (DFV), *Iridoviridae*
Dolichos yellow mosaic virus, (DoYMV), *Geminiviridae*
Dolphin poxvirus, (DOV), *Poxviridae*
Dorcopsis wallaby herpesvirus, *Herpesviridae*
Douglas virus, (DOUV), *Bunyaviridae*
Drosophila ananassae Tom virus, (DanTomV), *Metaviridae*
Drosophila C virus, (DCV), "CrPV-like viruses"
Drosophila F virus, (DFV), *Reoviridae*
Drosophila line virus, (DLV), *Nodaviridae*
Drosophila melanogaster 176 virus, (Dme176V), *Metaviridae*

Drosophila melanogaster 1731 virus, (Dme1731V), *Pseudoviridae*
Drosophila melanogaster 297 virus, (Dme297V), *Metaviridae*
Drosophila melanogaster 412 virus, (Dme412V), *Metaviridae*
Drosophila melanogaster copia virus, (DmeCopV), *Pseudoviridae*
Drosophila melanogaster gypsy virus, (DmeGypV), *Metaviridae*
Drosophila melanogaster mdg1 virus, (DmeMdg1V), *Metaviridae*
Drosophila melanogaster mdg4 virus, (DmeMdg4V), *Metaviridae*
Drosophila melanogaster micropia virus, (DmeMicV), *Metaviridae*
Drosophila P virus, (DPV), Unassigned
Drosophila S virus, (DSV), *Reoviridae*
Drosophila virilis Ulysses virus, (DviUllV), *Metaviridae*
Drosophila X virus, (DXV), *Birnaviridae*
Drosophilia A virus, (DAV), Unassigned
Duck adenovirus 2, (DAdV-2), *Adenoviridae*
Duck adenovirus, (DAdV), *Adenoviridae*
Duck astrovirus 1, (DAstV-1), *Astroviridae*
Duck astrovirus, (DAstV), *Astroviridae*
Duck hepatitis B virus, (DHBV), *Hepadnaviridae*
Duck hepatitis virus 1, (DHV-1), *Picornaviridae*
Duck hepatitis virus 3, (DHV-3), *Picornaviridae*
Duck plague herpesvirus, *Herpesviridae*
Dugbe virus, (DUGV), *Bunyaviridae*
Dulcamara mottle virus, (DuMV), *Tymovirus*
Dulcamara virus A, (DuVA), *Carlavirus*
Dulcamara virus B, (DuVB), *Carlavirus*
Dusona sp. ichnovirus, (DspIV), *Polydnaviridae*
Duvenhage virus, (DUVV), *Rhabdoviridae*

East African cassava mosaic virus, (EACMV), *Geminiviridae*
Eastern equine encephalitis virus, (EEEV), *Togaviridae*
Echinochloa hoja blanca virus, (EHBV), *Tenuivirus*
Echinochloa ragged stunt virus, (ERSV), *Reoviridae*
Eclipta yellow vein virus, (EYVV), *Geminiviridae*
Ectocarpus fasciculatus virus a, (EfV-a), *Phycodnaviridae*
Ectocarpus siliculosus virus 1, (EsV-1), *Phycodnaviridae*
Ectocarpus siliculosus virus a, (EsV-a), *Phycodnaviridae*
Ectromelia virus, (ECTV), *Poxviridae*
Edge Hill virus, (EHV), *Flaviviridae*
Edmonston virus, *Paramyxoviridae*
EDS virus, *Adenoviridae*

Eel virus American, (EVA), *Rhabdoviridae*
Eel virus B12, (EEV-B12), *Rhabdoviridae*
Eel virus C26, (EEV-C26), *Rhabdoviridae*
EgAN 1825-61 virus, (EGAV), *Bunyaviridae*
Egg drop syndrome virus, (DAdV-1), *Adenoviridae*
Eggplant green mosaic virus, (EGMV), *Potyviridae*
Eggplant latent viroid, (ELVd), *Avsunviroidae*
Eggplant mild mottle virus, (EMMV), *Carlavirus*
Eggplant mosaic virus, (EMV), *Tymovirus*
Eggplant mottled crinkle virus, (EMCV), *Tombusviridae*
Eggplant mottled dwarf virus, (EMDV), *Rhabdoviridae*
Eggplant severe mottle virus, (ESMoV), *Potyviridae*
Eggplant virus, *Carlavirus*
Eggplant yellow mosaic virus, (EYMV), *Geminiviridae*
Egtved virus, *Rhabdoviridae*
Egypt bee virus, (EBV), Unassigned
El Moro Canyon virus, (ELMCV), *Bunyaviridae*
Elapid herpesvirus 1, (EpHV-1), *Herpesviridae*
Elderberry latent virus, (ElLV), *Tombusviridae*
Elderberry symptomless virus, (ESLV), *Carlavirus*
Elderberry virus A, *Carlavirus*
Elephant loxodontol herpesvirus, *Herpesviridae*
Elephantid herpesvirus 1, (ElHV-1), *Herpesviridae*
Ellidaey virus, (ELLV), *Reoviridae*
Elm mottle virus, (EMoV), *Bromoviridae*
Embu virus, (ERV), *Poxviridae*
Encephalomyocarditis virus, (EMCV), *Picornaviridae*
Endive necrotic mosaic virus, (ENMV), *Potyviridae*
Enseada virus, (ENSV), *Bunyaviridae*
Entamoeba virus, (ENTV), *Rhabdoviridae*
Entebbe bat virus, (ENTV), *Flaviviridae*
Enterobacteria phage φK, (φK), *Microviridae*
Enterobacteria phage μ2, (μ2), *Leviviridae*
Enterobacteria phage 01, (01), *Myoviridae*
Enterobacteria phage 1, (1), *Myoviridae*
Enterobacteria phage 102, (102), *Siphoviridae*
Enterobacteria phage 103, (103), *Siphoviridae*
Enterobacteria phage 11F, (11F), *Myoviridae*
Enterobacteria phage 121, (121), *Myoviridae*
Enterobacteria phage 150, (150), *Siphoviridae*
Enterobacteria phage 16-19, (16-19), *Myoviridae*
Enterobacteria phage 168, (168), *Siphoviridae*
Enterobacteria phage 174, (174), *Siphoviridae*
Enterobacteria phage 186, (186), *Myoviridae*
Enterobacteria phage 1φ1, (1φ1), *Microviridae*
Enterobacteria phage 1φ3, (1φ3), *Microviridae*
Enterobacteria phage 1φ7, (1φ7), *Microviridae*
Enterobacteria phage 1φ9, (1φ9), *Microviridae*
Enterobacteria phage 299, (299), *Myoviridae*
Enterobacteria phage 2D/13, (2D/13), *Microviridae*
Enterobacteria phage 3, (3), *Myoviridae*
Enterobacteria phage 3T+, (3T+), *Myoviridae*

Enterobacteria phage 50, (50), *Myoviridae*
Enterobacteria phage 5845, (5845), *Myoviridae*
Enterobacteria phage 66F, (66F), *Myoviridae*
Enterobacteria phage 7-11, (7-11), *Podoviridae*
Enterobacteria phage 7480b, (7480b), *Podoviridae*
Enterobacteria phage 8893, (8893), *Myoviridae*
Enterobacteria phage 9/0, (9/0), *Myoviridae*
Enterobacteria phage 9266, (9266), *Myoviridae*
Enterobacteria phage AE2, (AE2), *Inoviridae*
Enterobacteria phage B6, (B6), *Leviviridae*
Enterobacteria phage B7, (B7), *Leviviridae*
Enterobacteria phage BA14, (Ba14), *Podoviridae*
Enterobacteria phage BE/1, (BE/1), *Microviridae*
Enterobacteria phage Beccles, (Beccles), *Myoviridae*
Enterobacteria phage BF23, (BF23), *Siphoviridae*
Enterobacteria phage BZ13, (BZ13), *Leviviridae*
Enterobacteria phage C-1, (C-1), *Leviviridae*
Enterobacteria phage C16, (C16), *Myoviridae*
Enterobacteria phage C-2, (C-2), *Inoviridae*
Enterobacteria phage C2, (C2), *Leviviridae*
Enterobacteria phage D108, (D108), *Myoviridae*
Enterobacteria phage D20, (D20), *Siphoviridae*
Enterobacteria phage D2A, (D2A), *Myoviridae*
Enterobacteria phage D6, (D6), *Myoviridae*
Enterobacteria phage D8, (D8), *Myoviridae*
Enterobacteria phage DdVI, (DdVI), *Myoviridae*
Enterobacteria phage dφ3, (dφ3), *Microviridae*
Enterobacteria phage dφ4, (dφ4), *Microviridae*
Enterobacteria phage dφ5, (dφ5), *Microviridae*
Enterobacteria phage Ec9, (Ec9), *Inoviridae*
Enterobacteria phage Esc-7-11, (Esc-7-11), *Podoviridae*
Enterobacteria phage f1, (f1), *Inoviridae*
Enterobacteria phage F10, (F10), *Myoviridae*
Enterobacteria phage f2, (f2), *Leviviridae*
Enterobacteria phage F7, (F7), *Myoviridae*
Enterobacteria phage FC3-9, (FC3-9), *Myoviridae*
Enterobacteria phage fcan, (fcan), *Leviviridae*
Enterobacteria phage fd, (fd), *Inoviridae*
Enterobacteria phage FI, (FI), *Leviviridae*
Enterobacteria phage Folac, (Folac), *Leviviridae*
Enterobacteria phage fr, (fr), *Leviviridae*
Enterobacteria phage Fsα, (Fsα), *Myoviridae*
Enterobacteria phage G13, (G13), *Microviridae*
Enterobacteria phage G14, (G14), *Microviridae*
Enterobacteria phage G4, (G4), *Microviridae*
Enterobacteria phage G6, (G6), *Microviridae*
Enterobacteria phage GA, (GA), *Leviviridae*
Enterobacteria phage H, (H), *Podoviridae*
Enterobacteria phage H-19J, (H-19J), *Siphoviridae*
Enterobacteria phage Hi, (Hi), *Siphoviridae*
Enterobacteria phage HK022, (HK022), *Siphoviridae*
Enterobacteria phage HK97, (HK97), *Siphoviridae*
Enterobacteria phage HR, (HR), *Inoviridae*
Enterobacteria phage I$_2$-2, (I$_2$-2), *Inoviridae*
Enterobacteria phage ID2, (ID2), *Leviviridae*
Enterobacteria phage If1, (If1), *Inoviridae*
Enterobacteria phage IKe, (IKe), *Inoviridae*
Enterobacteria phage IV, (IV), *Podoviridae*
Enterobacteria phage Iα, (Iα), *Leviviridae*
Enterobacteria phage j2, (j2), *Myoviridae*
Enterobacteria phage Jersey, (Jersey), *Siphoviridae*
Enterobacteria phage JP34, (JP34), *Leviviridae*
Enterobacteria phage JP501, (JP501), *Leviviridae*
Enterobacteria phage K11, (K11), *Podoviridae*
Enterobacteria phage Kl3, (Kl3), *Myoviridae*
Enterobacteria phage Kl9, (Kl9), *Myoviridae*
Enterobacteria phage KU1, (KU1), *Leviviridae*
Enterobacteria phage L, (L), *Podoviridae*
Enterobacteria phage L17, (L17), *Tectiviridae*
Enterobacteria phage LP7, (LP7), *Podoviridae*
Enterobacteria phage M, (M), *Leviviridae*
Enterobacteria phage M11, (M11), *Leviviridae*
Enterobacteria phage M12, (M12), *Leviviridae*
Enterobacteria phage M13, (M13, Ff), *Inoviridae*
Enterobacteria phage M20, (M20), *Microviridae*
Enterobacteria phage Mg40, (Mg40), *Podoviridae*
Enterobacteria phage MS2, (MS2), *Leviviridae*
Enterobacteria phage Mu, (Mu), *Myoviridae*
Enterobacteria phage Mu-1, (Mu-1), *Myoviridae*
Enterobacteria phage MX1, (MX1), *Leviviridae*
Enterobacteria phage N4, (N4), *Podoviridae*
Enterobacteria phage NL95, (NL95), *Leviviridae*
Enterobacteria phage P1, (P1), *Myoviridae*
Enterobacteria phage P1D, (P1D), *Myoviridae*
Enterobacteria phage P2, (P2), *Myoviridae*
Enterobacteria phage P22, (P22), *Podoviridae*
Enterobacteria phage P7, (P7), *Myoviridae*
Enterobacteria phage PA-2, (PA-2), *Siphoviridae*
Enterobacteria phage PB, (PB), *Siphoviridae*
Enterobacteria phage pilHα, (pilHα), *Leviviridae*
Enterobacteria phage Pk2, (Pk2), *Myoviridae*
Enterobacteria phage PR3, (PR3), *Tectiviridae*
Enterobacteria phage PR4, (PR4), *Tectiviridae*
Enterobacteria phage PR5, (PR5), *Tectiviridae*
Enterobacteria phage PR64FS, (PR64FS), *Inoviridae*
Enterobacteria phage PR772, (PR772), *Tectiviridae*
Enterobacteria phage PRD1, (PRD1), *Tectiviridae*
Enterobacteria phage PSA78, (PSA78), *Podoviridae*
Enterobacteria phage PST, (PST), *Myoviridae*
Enterobacteria phage PTB, (PTB), *Podoviridae*
Enterobacteria phage Qβ, (Qβ), *Leviviridae*
Enterobacteria phage R, (R), *Podoviridae*
Enterobacteria phage R17, (R17), *Leviviridae*
Enterobacteria phage R23, (R23), *Leviviridae*
Enterobacteria phage R34, (R34), *Leviviridae*
Enterobacteria phage RB42, (RB42), *Myoviridae*
Enterobacteria phage RB43, (RB43), *Myoviridae*
Enterobacteria phage RB49, (RB49), *Myoviridae*
Enterobacteria phage RB69, (RB69), *Myoviridae*

Enterobacteria phage S13, (S13), *Microviridae*
Enterobacteria phage San 2, (San2), *Siphoviridae*
Enterobacteria phage sd, (sd), *Podoviridae*
Enterobacteria phage SF, (SF), *Inoviridae*
Enterobacteria phage Sf6, (Sf6), *Podoviridae*
Enterobacteria phage SKII, (SKII), *Myoviridae*
Enterobacteria phage SKV, (SKV), *Myoviridae*
Enterobacteria phage SKX, (SKX), *Myoviridae*
Enterobacteria phage SMB, (SMB), *Myoviridae*
Enterobacteria phage SMP2, (SMP2), *Myoviridae*
Enterobacteria phage SP, (SP), *Leviviridae*
Enterobacteria phage SP6, (SP6), *Podoviridae*
Enterobacteria phage ST, (ST), *Leviviridae*
Enterobacteria phage St-1, (St-1), *Microviridae*
Enterobacteria phage SV14, (SV14), *Myoviridae*
Enterobacteria phage SV3, (SV3), *Myoviridae*
Enterobacteria phage T1, (T1), *Siphoviridae*
Enterobacteria phage T2, (T2), *Myoviridae*
Enterobacteria phage T3, (T3), *Podoviridae*
Enterobacteria phage T4, (T4), *Myoviridae*
Enterobacteria phage T5, (T5), *Siphoviridae*
Enterobacteria phage T6, (T6), *Myoviridae*
Enterobacteria phage T7, (T7), *Podoviridae*
Enterobacteria phage tf-1, (tf-1), *Inoviridae*
Enterobacteria phage TH1, (TH1), *Leviviridae*
Enterobacteria phage TW18, (TW18), *Leviviridae*
Enterobacteria phage TW28, (TW28), *Leviviridae*
Enterobacteria phage U3, (U3), *Microviridae*
Enterobacteria phage UC-1, (UC-1), *Siphoviridae*
Enterobacteria phage ViI, (ViI), *Myoviridae*
Enterobacteria phage ViII, (ViII), *Siphoviridae*
Enterobacteria phage VK, (VK), *Leviviridae*
Enterobacteria phage W31, (W31), *Podoviridae*
Enterobacteria phage WA/1, (WA/1), *Microviridae*
Enterobacteria phage WF/1, (WF/1), *Microviridae*
Enterobacteria phage WPK, (WPK), *Podoviridae*
Enterobacteria phage WW/1, (WW/1), *Microviridae*
Enterobacteria phage Wϕ, (Wϕ), *Myoviridae*
Enterobacteria phage X, (X), *Inoviridae*
Enterobacteria phage X-2, (X-2), *Inoviridae*
Enterobacteria phage Y, (Y), *Podoviridae*
Enterobacteria phage ZG/1, (ZG/1), *Leviviridae*
Enterobacteria phage ZG/3A, (ZG/3A), *Siphoviridae*
Enterobacteria phage ZIK/1, (ZIK/1), *Leviviridae*
Enterobacteria phage ZJ/1, (ZJ/1), *Leviviridae*
Enterobacteria phage ZJ/2, (ZJ/2), *Inoviridae*
Enterobacteria phage ZL/3, (ZL/3), *Leviviridae*
Enterobacteria phage ZS/3, (ZS/3), *Leviviridae*
Enterobacteria phage ΦD328, (ΦD328), *Siphoviridae*
Enterobacteria phage Ω8, (Ω8), *Podoviridae*
Enterobacteria phage α1, (α1), *Myoviridae*
Enterobacteria phage α10, (α10), *Microviridae*
Enterobacteria phage α15, (α15), *Leviviridae*
Enterobacteria phage α3, (α3), *Microviridae*
Enterobacteria phage β, (β), *Leviviridae*

Enterobacteria phage β4, (β4), *Siphoviridae*
Enterobacteria phage χ, (χ), *Siphoviridae*
Enterobacteria phage δ1, (δ1), *Microviridae*
Enterobacteria phage δ6, (δ6), *Microviridae*
Enterobacteria phage δA, (δA), *Inoviridae*
Enterobacteria phage ϕ80, (ϕ80), *Siphoviridae*
Enterobacteria phage ϕ92, (ϕ92), *Myoviridae*
Enterobacteria phage ϕA, (ϕA), *Microviridae*
Enterobacteria phage ϕR, (ϕR), *Microviridae*
Enterobacteria phage ϕW39, (ϕW39), *Myoviridae*
Enterobacteria phage ϕX174, (ϕX174), *Microviridae*
Enterobacteria phage ϕ1.2, (ϕ1.2), *Podoviridae*
Enterobacteria phage $\phi\gamma$, ($\phi\gamma$), *Siphoviridae*
Enterobacteria phage η8, (η8), *Microviridae*
Enterobacteria phage; λ, (λ), *Siphoviridae*
Enterobacteria phage μ, (μ), *Myoviridae*
Enterobacteria phage τ, (τ), *Leviviridae*
Enterobacteria phage ζ3, (ζ3), *Microviridae*
Enterobacteria phage ϕI, (ϕI), *Podoviridae*
Enterobacteria phage ϕII, (ϕII), *Podoviridae*
Enterobacteria phage ϕye03, (ϕye03), *Podoviridae*
Enterobacterial phage ViIII, (ViIII), *Podoviridae*
Enytus montanus ichnovirus, (EmIV), *Polydnaviridae*
Epirus cherry virus, (EpCV), *Ourmiavirus*
Epizootic haematopoietic necrosis virus, (EHNV), *Iridoviridae*
Epizootic hemorrhagic disease virus 1 to 8, (EHDV-1 to 8), *Reoviridae*
Epizootic hemorrhagic disease virus, (EHDV), *Reoviridae*
Epstein-Barr virus, *Herpesviridae*
Equid herpesvirus 1, (EHV-1), *Herpesviridae*
Equid herpesvirus 2, (EHV-2), *Herpesviridae*
Equid herpesvirus 3, (EHV-3), *Herpesviridae*
Equid herpesvirus 4, (EHV-4), *Herpesviridae*
Equid herpesvirus 5, (EHV-5), *Herpesviridae*
Equid herpesvirus 6, (EHV-6), *Herpesviridae*
Equid herpesvirus 7, (EHV-7), *Herpesviridae*
Equid herpesvirus 8, (EHV-8), *Herpesviridae*
Equid herpesvirus 9, (EHV-9), *Herpesviridae*
Equine abortion virus, *Herpesviridae*
Equine adeno-associated virus, (EAAV), *Parvoviridae*
Equine adenovirus 1, (EAdV-1), *Adenoviridae*
Equine adenovirus 2, (EAdV-2), *Adenoviridae*
Equine adenovirus A, (EAdV-A), *Adenoviridae*
Equine adenovirus B, (EAdV-B), *Adenoviridae*
Equine arteritis virus, (EAV), *Arteriviridae*
Equine coital exanthema virus, *Herpesviridae*
Equine encephalosis virus 1 to 7, (EEV-1 to 7), *Reoviridae*
Equine encephalosis virus, (EEV), *Reoviridae*
Equine infectious anemia virus, (EIAV), *Retroviridae*
Equine rhinitis A virus, (ERAV), *Picornaviridae*
Equine rhinitis B virus, (ERBV), *Picornaviridae*
Equine rhinopneumonitis virus, *Herpesviridae*

Equine rhinovirus 1, *Picornaviridae*
Equine rhinovirus 2, *Picornaviridae*
Equine rhinovirus 3, (ERV-3), *Picornaviridae*
Equine torovirus, (EqTV), *Coronaviridae*
Eret-147 virus, (E147V), *Bunyaviridae*
Eriborus terebrans ichnovirus, (EtIV), *Polydnaviridae*
Erinaceid herpesvirus 1, (ErHV-1), *Herpesviridae*
Eriogaster lanestris cypovirus 2, (ElCPV-2), *Reoviridae*
Eriogaster lanestris cypovirus 6, (E1CPV-6), *Reoviridae*
Erve virus, (ERVEV), *Bunyaviridae*
Erysimum latent virus, (ErLV), *Tymovirus*
Esocid herpesvirus 1, (EsHV-1), *Herpesviridae*
Essaouira virus, (ESSV), *Reoviridae*
Estero Real virus, (ERV), *Bunyaviridae*
Eubenangee virus, (EUBV), *Reoviridae*
Eubenangee virus, (EUBV), *Reoviridae*
Eucocytis meeki virus, (EmV), *Tetraviridae*
Euonymus fasciation virus, (EFV), *Rhabdoviridae*
Euonymus mosaic virus, (EuoMV), *Carlavirus*
Eupatorium yellow vein virus, (EpYVV), *Geminiviridae*
Euphorbia mosaic virus, (EuMV), *Geminiviridae*
Euphorbia ringspot virus, (EuRSV), *Potyviridae*
Euploea corea virus, (EcV), *Tetraviridae*
European bat lyssavirus 1, (EBLV-1), *Rhabdoviridae*
European bat lyssavirus 2, (EBLV-2), *Rhabdoviridae*
European brown hare syndrome virus, (EBHSV), *Caliciviridae*
European brown hare syndrome virus-BS89, (EBHSV-BS89), *Caliciviridae*
European brown hare syndrome virus-FRG, (EBHSV-FRG), *Caliciviridae*
European brown hare syndrome virus-GD, (EBHSV-GD), *Caliciviridae*
European brown hare syndrome virus-UK91, (EBHSV-UK91), *Caliciviridae*
European elk papillomavirus, (EEPV), *Papillomaviridae*
European ground squirrel cytomegalovirus, *Herpesviridae*
European hedgehog herpesvirus, *Herpesviridae*
European wheat striate mosaic virus, (EWSMV), *Tenuivirus*
Euxoa auxiliaris densovirus, (EaDNV), *Parvoviridae*
Euxoa scandens cypovirus 5, (EsCPV-5), *Reoviridae*
Everglades virus, (EVEV), *Togaviridae*
Eyach virus (France-577), (EYAV-Fr577), *Reoviridae*
Eyach virus (France-578), (EYAV-Fr578), *Reoviridae*
Eyach virus (Germany), (EYAV-Gr), *Reoviridae*
Eyach virus, (EYAV), *Reoviridae*

Faba bean necrotic yellows virus, (FBNYV), *Nanovirus*
Facey's Paddock virus, (FPV), *Bunyaviridae*
Falcon inclusion body diseases, *Herpesviridae*
Falconid herpesvirus 1, (FaHV-1), *Herpesviridae*
Farallon virus, (FARV), *Bunyaviridae*
Feldmannia irregularis virus a, (FiV-a), *Phycodnaviridae*
Feldmannia species virus a, (FsV-a), *Phycodnaviridae*
Feldmannia species virus, (FsV), *Phycodnaviridae*
Felid herpesvirus 1, (FeHV-1), *Herpesviridae*
Feline astrovirus 1, (FAstV-1), *Astroviridae*
Feline astrovirus, (FAstV), *Astroviridae*
Feline calicivirus CFI/68, (FCV-CFI/68), *Caliciviridae*
Feline calicivirus F9, (FCV-F9), *Caliciviridae*
Feline calicivirus, (FCV), *Caliciviridae*
Feline coronavirus, (FCoV), *Coronaviridae*
Feline foamy virus, (FFV), *Retroviridae*
Feline immunodeficiency virus (Oma), (FIV-O), *Retroviridae*
Feline immunodeficiency virus, (FIV), *Retroviridae*
Feline infectious peritonitis virus, (FIPV), *Coronaviridae*
Feline leukemia virus, (FeLV), *Retroviridae*
Feline panleukopenia virus, (FPLV), *Parvoviridae*
Feline parvovirus, (FPV), *Parvoviridae*
Feline rhinotracheitis virus, *Herpesviridae*
Fescue cryptic virus, (FCV), *Partitiviridae*
Festuca leaf streak virus, (FLSV), *Rhabdoviridae*
Festuca necrosis virus, (FNV), *Closteroviridae*
Fetal rhesus kidney virus, *Polyomaviridae*
Ficus carica virus, (FicCV), *Potyviridae*
Field mouse herpesvirus, *Herpesviridae*
Fig virus S, (FVS), *Carlavirus*
Figulus subleavis entomopoxvirus, (FSEV), *Poxviridae*
Figwort mosaic virus, (FMV), *Caulimoviridae*
Fiji disease virus, (FDV), *Reoviridae*
Fin V 707 virus, (FINV), *Bunyaviridae*
Finger millet mosaic virus, (FMMV), *Rhabdoviridae*
Finkel-Biskis-Jinkins murine sarcoma virus, (FBJMSV), *Retroviridae*
Flame chlorosis virus, (FlCV), Unassigned
Flanders virus, (FLAV), *Rhabdoviridae*
Flexal virus, (FLEV), *Arenaviridae*
Flock house virus, (FHV), *Nodaviridae*
Flounder lymphocystis disease virus, (FLDV), *Iridoviridae*
Flounder virus, *Iridoviridae*
Fomede virus, (FV), *Reoviridae*
Foot-and-mouth disease virus type A, (FMDV-A), *Picornaviridae*
Foot-and-mouth disease virus type Asia 1, (FMDV-Asia1), *Picornaviridae*

Foot-and-mouth disease virus type C, (FMDV-C), *Picornaviridae*
Foot-and-mouth disease virus type O, (FMDV-O), *Picornaviridae*
Foot-and-mouth disease virus type SAT 1, (FMDV-SAT1), *Picornaviridae*
Foot-and-mouth disease virus type SAT 2, (FMDV-SAT2), *Picornaviridae*
Foot-and-mouth disease virus type SAT 3, (FMDV-SAT3), *Picornaviridae*
Foot-and-mouth disease virus, (FMDV), *Picornaviridae*
Forecariah virus, (FORV), *Bunyaviridae*
Fort Morgan virus, (FMV), *Togaviridae*
Fort Sherman virus, (FSV), *Bunyaviridae*
Foula virus, (FOUV), *Reoviridae*
Fowl adenovirus 1 (CELO, 112, Phelps), (FAdV-1), *Adenoviridae*
Fowl adenovirus 10 (C-2B, M11, CFA20), (FAdV-10), *Adenoviridae*
Fowl adenovirus 11 (380), (FAdV-11), *Adenoviridae*
Fowl adenovirus 2 (GAL-1, 685, SR48), (FAdV-2), *Adenoviridae*
Fowl adenovirus 3 (SR49, 75), (FAdV-3), *Adenoviridae*
Fowl adenovirus 4 (KR-5, J-2), (FAdV-4), *Adenoviridae*
Fowl adenovirus 5 (340, TR22), (FAdV-5), *Adenoviridae*
Fowl adenovirus 6 (CR119, 168), (FAdV-6), *Adenoviridae*
Fowl adenovirus 7 (YR36, X-11), (FAdV-7), *Adenoviridae*
Fowl adenovirus 8a (TR59, T-8, CFA40), (FAdV-8a), *Adenoviridae*
Fowl adenovirus 8b (764, B3), (FAdV-8b), *Adenoviridae*
Fowl adenovirus 9 (A2, 90), (FAdV-9), *Adenoviridae*
Fowl adenovirus A, (FAdV-A), *Adenoviridae*
Fowl adenovirus B, (FAdV-B), *Adenoviridae*
Fowl adenovirus C, (FAdV-C), *Adenoviridae*
Fowl adenovirus D, (FAdV-D), *Adenoviridae*
Fowl adenovirus E, (FAdV-E), *Adenoviridae*
Fowl calicivirus, (FCV), *Caliciviridae*
Fowlpox virus, (FWPV), *Poxviridae*
Foxtail mosaic virus, (FoMV), *Potexvirus*
Fragaria chiloensis virus, (FClV), *Bromoviridae*
Frangipani mosaic virus, (FrMV), *Tobamovirus*
Fraser Point virus, (FPV), *Bunyaviridae*
Freesia leaf necrosis virus, (FLNV), *Varicosavirus*
Freesia mosaic virus, (FreMV), *Potyviridae*
Friend murine leukemia virus, (FrMLV), *Retroviridae*
Frijoles virus VP-161A, (FRIV), *Bunyaviridae*
Frijoles virus, (FRIV), *Bunyaviridae*
Frog adenovirus, (FrAdV-1), *Adenoviridae*

Frog herpesvirus 4, *Herpesviridae*
Frog virus 3, (FV-3), *Iridoviridae*
Fuchsia latent virus, (FLV), *Carlavirus*
Fujinami sarcoma virus, (FuSV), *Retroviridae*
Fukuoka virus, (FUKAV), *Rhabdoviridae*
Furcraea necrotic streak virus, (FNSV), *Tombusviridae*
Fusarium oxysporum Skippy virus, (FoxSkiV), *Metaviridae*

GA391 virus, *Arenaviridae*
Gabek Forest virus, (GFV), *Bunyaviridae*
Gadgets Gully virus, (GGYV), *Flaviviridae*
Gaeumannomyces graminis virus 019/6-A, (GgV-019/6-A), *Partitiviridae*
Gaeumannomyces graminis virus 45/101-C, (GGV-45/101C), Unassigned
Gaeumannomyces graminis virus 87-1-H, (GgV-87-1-H), *Totiviridae*
Gaeumannomyces graminis virus T1-A, (GgV-T1-A), *Partitiviridae*
Galinsoga mosaic virus, (GaMV), *Tombusviridae*
Galleria cell line virus, (GmCLV), Unassigned
Galleria mellonella densovirus, (GmDNV), *Parvoviridae*
Galleria mellonella MNPV, (GmMNPV), *Baculoviridae*
Gallid herpesvirus 1, (GaHV-1), *Herpesviridae*
Gallid herpesvirus 2, (GaHV-2), *Herpesviridae*
Gallid herpesvirus 3, (GaHV-3), *Herpesviridae*
Gamboa virus, (GAMV), *Bunyaviridae*
Gan Gan virus, (GGV), *Bunyaviridae*
Ganjam virus, *Bunyaviridae*
Garba virus, (GARV), *Rhabdoviridae*
Gardner-Arnstein feline sarcoma virus, (GAFeSV), *Retroviridae*
Garland chrysanthemum temperate virus, (GCTV), *Partitiviridae*
Garlic common latent virus, (GarCLV), *Carlavirus*
Garlic dwarf virus, (GDV), *Reoviridae*
Garlic latent virus, (GarLV), *Carlavirus*
Garlic mite-borne filamentous virus, (GarMbFV), *Allexivirus*
Garlic mite-borne latent virus, (GarMbLV), *Allexivirus*
Garlic mosaic virus, (GarMV), *Carlavirus*
Garlic virus 2, *Potyviridae*
Garlic virus A, (GarV-A), *Allexivirus*
Garlic virus B, (GarV-B), *Allexivirus*
Garlic virus C, (GarV-C), *Allexivirus*
Garlic virus D, (GarV-D), *Allexivirus*
Garlic virus X, (GarV-X), *Allexivirus*
Garlic virus, *Potyviridae*
Gazelle herpesvirus, *Herpesviridae*

GB virus A, (GBV-A), *Flaviviridae*
GB virus B, (GBV-B), *Flaviviridae*
GB virus C, (GBV-C), *Flaviviridae*
GBV-A-like agents, (GBV-A-like), *Flaviviridae*
Gentiana latent virus, (GenLV), *Carlavirus*
Geotrupes sylvaticus entomopoxvirus, (GSEV), *Poxviridae*
Gerbera symptomless virus, (GeSLV), *Rhabdoviridae*
Germiston virus, (GERV), *Bunyaviridae*
Getah virus, (GETV), *Togaviridae*
Giardia lamblia virus, (GLV), *Totiviridae*
Gibbon ape leukemia virus, (GALV), *Retroviridae*
Ginger chlorotic fleck virus, (GCFV), *Sobemovirus*
Gloriosa stripe mosaic virus, (GSMV), *Potyviridae*
Glycine mosaic virus, (GMV), *Comoviridae*
Glycine mottle virus, (GMoV), *Tombusviridae*
Glypta fumiferanae ichnovirus, (GfIV), *Polydnaviridae*
Glypta sp. ichnovirus, (GspIV), *Polydnaviridae*
Glyptapanteles flavicoxis bracovirus, (GflBV), *Polydnaviridae*
Glyptapanteles indiensis bracovirus, (GiBV), *Polydnaviridae*
Glyptapanteles liparidis bracovirus, (GlBV), *Polydnaviridae*
Goat adenovirus 1, 2, (GAdV-1, 2), *Adenoviridae*
Goat herpesvirus, *Herpesviridae*
Goatpox virus, (GTPV), *Poxviridae*
Goeldichironomus haloprasimus entomopoxvirus, (GHEV), *Poxviridae*
Golden shiner reovirus, (GSV), *Reoviridae*
Goldfish herpesvirus, *Herpesviridae*
Goldfish virus 1, (GFV-1), *Iridoviridae*
Gomoka virus, *Reoviridae*
Gomphrena virus, (GoV), *Rhabdoviridae*
Gonometa podocarpi virus, (GpV), Unassigned
Gonometa rufibrunnea cypovirus 3, (GrCPV-3), *Reoviridae*
Goose adenovirus 1 to 3, (GoAdV-1 to 3), *Adenoviridae*
Goose adenovirus, (GoAdV), *Adenoviridae*
Goose parvovirus, (GPV), *Parvoviridae*
Gordil virus, (GORV), *Bunyaviridae*
Gorilla herpesvirus, *Herpesviridae*
Gossas virus, (GOSV), *Rhabdoviridae*
Grand Arbaud virus, (GAV), *Bunyaviridae*
Grapevine Algerian latent virus, (GALV), *Tombusviridae*
Grapevine berry inner necrosis virus, (GINV), *Trichovirus*
Grapevine Bulgarian latent virus satellite RNA, Satellite
Grapevine Bulgarian latent virus, (GBLV), *Comoviridae*
Grapevine chrome mosaic virus, (GCMV), *Comoviridae*
Grapevine fanleaf virus satellite RNA, Satellite
Grapevine fanleaf virus, (GFLV), *Comoviridae*
Grapevine fleck virus, (GFkV), Unassigned
Grapevine leafroll-associated virus 1, (GLRaV-1), *Closteroviridae*
Grapevine leafroll-associated virus 2, (GLRaV-2), *Closteroviridae*
Grapevine leafroll-associated virus 3, (GLRaV-3), *Closteroviridae*
Grapevine leafroll-associated virus 4, (GLRaV-4), *Closteroviridae*
Grapevine leafroll-associated virus 5, (GLRaV-5), *Closteroviridae*
Grapevine leafroll-associated virus 6, (GLRaV-6), *Closteroviridae*
Grapevine leafroll-associated virus 7, (GLRaV-7), *Closteroviridae*
Grapevine Tunisian ringspot virus, (GTRSV), *Comoviridae*
Grapevine virus A, (GVA), *Vitivirus*
Grapevine virus B, (GVB), *Vitivirus*
Grapevine virus C, (GVC), *Vitivirus*
Grapevine virus D, (GVD), *Vitivirus*
Grapevine yellow speckle viroid 1, (GYSVd-1), *Pospiviroidae*
Grapevine yellow speckle viroid 2, (GYSVd-2), *Pospiviroidae*
Grass carp reovirus, (GCRV), *Reoviridae*
Grass carp rhabdovirus, *Rhabdoviridae*
Gray Lodge virus, (GLOV), *Rhabdoviridae*
Great Island virus, (GIV), *Reoviridae*
Great Island virus, (GIV), *Reoviridae*
Great Saltee Island virus, (GSIV), *Reoviridae*
Great Saltee virus, (GRSV), *Bunyaviridae*
Green lizard herpesvirus, *Herpesviridae*
Grey kangaroo poxvirus, (KXV), *Poxviridae*
Grey patch disease of turtles, *Herpesviridae*
Grimsey virus, (GSYV), *Reoviridae*
Ground squirrel hepatitis virus, (GSHV), *Hepadnaviridae*
Groundnut bud necrosis virus, (GBNV), *Bunyaviridae*
Groundnut chlorotic fan-spot virus, (GCFSV), *Bunyaviridae*
Groundnut crinkle virus, *Carlavirus*
Groundnut eyespot virus, (GEV), *Potyviridae*
Groundnut ringspot virus, (GRSV), *Bunyaviridae*
Groundnut rosette assistor virus, (GRAV), *Luteoviridae*
Groundnut rosette virus satellite RNA, Satellite
Groundnut rosette virus, (GRV), *Umbravirus*
Groundnut yellow spot virus, (GYSV), *Bunyaviridae*
Gruid herpesvirus 1, (GrHV-1), *Herpesviridae*

GU71U 344 virus, (GU344V), *Bunyaviridae*
GU71U 350 virus, (GU350V), *Bunyaviridae*
Guajara virus, (GJAV), *Bunyaviridae*
Guama virus, (GMAV), *Bunyaviridae*
Guanarito virus, (GTOV), *Arenaviridae*
Guar green sterile virus, *Potyviridae*
Guar symptomless virus, (GSLV), *Potyviridae*
Guaratuba virus, (GTBV), *Bunyaviridae*
Guaroa virus, (GROV), *Bunyaviridae*
Guinea grass mosaic virus, (GGMV), *Potyviridae*
Guinea pig adenovirus 1, (GPAdV-1), *Adenoviridae*
Guinea pig adenovirus, (GPAdV), *Adenoviridae*
Guinea pig Chlamydia phage, (GPCh), *Microviridae*
Guinea pig cytomegalovirus, *Herpesviridae*
Guinea pig herpesvirus 3, *Herpesviridae*
Guinea pig herpesvirus, *Herpesviridae*
Guinea pig type-C oncovirus, (GPCOV), *Retroviridae*
Guineafowl transmissible enteritis virus, (GTEV), *Picornaviridae*
Gumbo Limbo virus, (GLV), *Bunyaviridae*
Guppy virus 6, (GV6), *Iridoviridae*
Gurupi virus, (GURV), *Reoviridae*
Gynura latent virus, (GyLV), *Carlavirus*
Gypsy moth virus, (GMV), *Nodaviridae*

H-1 virus, (H-1PV), *Parvoviridae*
H-32580 virus, (H32580V), *Bunyaviridae*
Habenaria mosaic virus, (HaMV), *Potyviridae*
Haematopoietic necrosis herpesvirus of goldfish, *Herpesviridae*
Haemophilus phage HP1, (HP1), *Myoviridae*
Haemophilus phage S2, (S2), *Myoviridae*
Halobacterium phage Hs1, (Hs1), *Myoviridae*
Halobacterium phage φH, (φH), *Myoviridae*
Hamster herpesvirus, *Herpesviridae*
Hamster polyomavirus, (HaPyV), *Polyomaviridae*
Hantaan 76-118 virus, *Bunyaviridae*
Hantaan virus, (HTNV), *Bunyaviridae*
Harbour seal herpesvirus, *Herpesviridae*
Harbour seals picorna-like virus, (SPLV), *Picornaviridae*
Hard clam reovirus, (HCRV), *Reoviridae*
Hardy-Zuckerman feline sarcoma virus, (HZFeSV), *Retroviridae*
Hare fibroma virus, (FIBV), *Poxviridae*
Hart Park virus, (HPV), *Rhabdoviridae*
Hartebeest malignant catarrhal fever virus, *Herpesviridae*
Hart's tongue fern mottle virus, (HTFMoV), Unassigned
Harvey murine sarcoma virus, (HaMSV), *Retroviridae*
Hawaii virus, (HV), *Caliciviridae*
Hazara virus, (HAZV), *Bunyaviridae*

HB virus, (HBPV), *Parvoviridae*
HB55 virus, *Bunyaviridae*
HCV cluster 1, (HCV-1), *Flaviviridae*
HCV cluster 2, (HCV-J6), *Flaviviridae*
HCV cluster 3, (HCV-NZL1), *Flaviviridae*
HCV cluster 4, (HCV-ED43), *Flaviviridae*
HCV cluster 5, (HCV-EVH1480), *Flaviviridae*
HCV cluster 6, (HCV-EUHK2), *Flaviviridae*
Helenium virus S, (HVS), *Carlavirus*
Helenium virus Y, (HVY), *Potyviridae*
Helicoverpa armigera stunt virus, (HaSV) *Tetraviridae*
Helicoverpa zea SNPV, (HzSNPV), *Baculoviridae*
Heliothis armigera cypovirus ('B' strain), *Reoviridae*
Heliothis armigera cypovirus 11, (HaCPV-11), *Reoviridae*
Heliothis armigera cypovirus 14 ('A' strain), (HaCPV-14), *Reoviridae*
Heliothis armigera cypovirus 5, (HaCPV-5), *Reoviridae*
Heliothis armigera cypovirus 8, (HaCPV-8), *Reoviridae*
Heliothis armigera entomopoxvirus 'L', (HAVE), *Poxviridae*
Heliothis armigera iridescent virus, *Iridoviridae*
Heliothis virescens ascovirus 1a, (HvAV-1a), *Ascoviridae*
Heliothis zea cypovirus 11, (HzCPV-11), *Reoviridae*
Heliothis zea virus 1, (HzV-1), Unassigned
Heliothis/Helicoverpa zea iridescent virus, *Iridoviridae*
Helleborus mosaic virus, (HeMV), *Carlavirus*
Helminthosporium maydis virus, (HMV), Unassigned
Helminthosporium victoriae virus 145S, (HvV-145S), *Partitiviridae*
Helminthosporium victoriae virus 190S, (HvV-190S), *Totiviridae*
Henbane mosaic virus, (HMV), *Potyviridae*
Hepatitis A virus, (HAV), *Picornaviridae*
Hepatitis B virus, (HBV), *Hepadnaviridae*
Hepatitis C virus, (HCV), *Flaviviridae*
Hepatitis delta virus, (HDV), *Deltavirus*
Hepatitis E virus, (HEV), "HEV-like viruses"
Hepatitis G virus, (HGV-1), *Flaviviridae*
Hepatopancreatic parvo-like virus of shrimps, *Parvoviridae*
Heracleum latent virus, (HLV), *Vitivirus*
Heracleum virus 6, (HV-6), *Closteroviridae*
Heron hepatitis B virus, (HHBV), *Hepadnaviridae*
Herpes simplex virus 1, *Herpesviridae*
Herpes simplex virus 2, *Herpesviridae*
Herpesvirus aotus 1, *Herpesviridae*
Herpesvirus aotus 3, *Herpesviridae*
Herpesvirus ateles strain 73, *Herpesviridae*

Herpesvirus ateles, *Herpesviridae*
Herpesvirus cuniculi, *Herpesviridae*
Herpesvirus cyclopsis, *Herpesviridae*
Herpesvirus marmota, *Herpesviridae*
Herpesvirus pan, *Herpesviridae*
Herpesvirus papio 2, *Herpesviridae*
Herpesvirus papio, *Herpesviridae*
Herpesvirus pottos, *Herpesviridae*
Herpesvirus saimiri, *Herpesviridae*
Herpesvirus salmonis, *Herpesviridae*
Herpesvirus sanguinus, *Herpesviridae*
Herpesvirus scophthalmus, *Herpesviridae*
Herpesvirus simiae, *Herpesviridae*
Herpesvirus sylvilagus, *Herpesviridae*
Herpesvirus tamarinus, *Herpesviridae*
Heteronychus arator iridescent virus, *Iridoviridae*
Hibiscus chlorotic ringspot virus, (HCRSV), *Tombusviridae*
Hibiscus latent ringspot virus, (HLRSV), *Comoviridae*
Highlands J virus, (HJV), *Togaviridae*
Himetobi P virus, (HiPV), "CrPV-like viruses"
Hincksia hinckiae virus a, (HhV-a), *Phycodnaviridae*
Hippeastrum latent virus, *Carlavirus*
Hippeastrum mosaic virus, (HiMV), *Potyviridae*
Hippotragine herpesvirus 18, (HiHV-1), *Herpesviridae*
Hirame rhabdovirus, (HIRRV), *Rhabdoviridae*
Hog cholera virus, *Flaviviridae*
HoJo virus, *Bunyaviridae*
Holcus lanatus yellowing virus, (HLYV), *Rhabdoviridae*
Holcus streak virus, (HSV), *Potyviridae*
Hollyhock leaf curl virus, (HLCV), *Geminiviridae*
Honeysuckle latent virus, (HnLV), *Carlavirus*
Honeysuckle yellow vein mosaic virus, (HYVMV), *Geminiviridae*
Hop latent viroid, (HpLVd), *Pospiviroidae*
Hop latent virus, (HpLV), *Carlavirus*
Hop mosaic virus, (HpMV), *Carlavirus*
Hop stunt viroid, (HSVd), *Pospiviroidae*
Hop trefoil cryptic virus 1, (HTCV-1), *Partitiviridae*
Hop trefoil cryptic virus 2, (HTCV-2), *Partitiviridae*
Hop trefoil cryptic virus 3, (HTCV-3), *Partitiviridae*
Hordeum mosaic virus, (HoMV), *Potyviridae*
Hordeum vulgare BARE-1 virus, (HvuBar1V), *Pseudoviridae*
Horsegram yellow mosaic virus, (HgYMV), *Geminiviridae*
Horseradish curly top virus, (HrCTV), *Geminiviridae*
Horseradish latent virus, (HRLV), *Caulimoviridae*
Hosta virus X, (HVX), *Potexvirus*
HR80-39, *Bunyaviridae*
Hsiung kaplow herpesvirus, *Herpesviridae*
Hughes virus, (HUGV), *Bunyaviridae*

Human adenovirus 1, 2, 5, 6, (HAdV-1, 2, 5, 6), *Adenoviridae*
Human adenovirus 12, 18, 31, (HAdV-12, 18, 31), *Adenoviridae*
Human adenovirus 16, 21, 34, 35, 50, (HAdV-16, 21, 34, 35, 50), *Adenoviridae*
Human adenovirus 20, 22–30, 32, 33, (HAdV-20, 22–30, 32, 33), *Adenoviridae*
Human adenovirus 3, 7, 11, 14, (HAdV-3, 7, 11, 14), *Adenoviridae*
Human adenovirus 36-39, 42–49, 51, (HAdV-36–39, 42-49, 51), *Adenoviridae*
Human adenovirus 4, (HAdV-4), *Adenoviridae*
Human adenovirus 40, 41, (HAdV-40, 41), *Adenoviridae*
Human adenovirus 8–10, 13, 15, 17, 19, (HAdV-8–10, 13, 15, 17, 19), *Adenoviridae*
Human adenovirus A, (HAdV-A), *Adenoviridae*
Human adenovirus B, (HAdV-B), *Adenoviridae*
Human adenovirus C, (HAdV-C), *Adenoviridae*
Human adenovirus D, (HAdV-D), *Adenoviridae*
Human adenovirus E, (HAdV-E), *Adenoviridae*
Human adenovirus F, (HAdV-F), *Adenoviridae*
Human astrovirus 1, (HAstV-1), *Astroviridae*
Human astrovirus 2, (HAstV-2), *Astroviridae*
Human astrovirus 3, (HAstV-3), *Astroviridae*
Human astrovirus 4, (HAstV-4), *Astroviride*
Human astrovirus 5, (HAstV-5), *Astroviridae*
Human astrovirus 6, (HAstV-6), *Astroviridae*
Human astrovirus 7, (HAstV-7), *Astroviridae*
Human astrovirus 8, (HAstV-8), *Astroviridae*
Human astrovirus, (HAstV), *Astroviridae*
Human coronavirus 229E, (HCoV-229E), *Coronaviridae*
Human coronavirus OC43, (HCoV-OC43), *Coronaviridae*
Human coxsackievirus A1, (CV-A1), *Picornaviridae*
Human coxsackievirus A10, (CV-A10), *Picornaviridae*
Human coxsackievirus A11, (CV-A11), *Picornaviridae*
Human coxsackievirus A12, (CV-A12), *Picornaviridae*
Human coxsackievirus A13, (CV-A13), *Picornaviridae*
Human coxsackievirus A14, (CV-A14), *Picornaviridae*
Human coxsackievirus A15, (CV-A15), *Picornaviridae*
Human coxsackievirus A16, (CV-A16), *Picornaviridae*
Human coxsackievirus A17, (CV-A17), *Picornaviridae*
Human coxsackievirus A18, (CV-A18), *Picornaviridae*

Human coxsackievirus A19, (CV-A19), *Picornaviridae*
Human coxsackievirus A2, (CV-A2), *Picornaviridae*
Human coxsackievirus A20, (CV-A20), *Picornaviridae*
Human coxsackievirus A21, (CV-A21), *Picornaviridae*
Human coxsackievirus A22, (CV-A22), *Picornaviridae*
Human coxsackievirus A24, (CV-A24), *Picornaviridae*
Human coxsackievirus A3, (CV-A3), *Picornaviridae*
Human coxsackievirus A4, (CV-A4), *Picornaviridae*
Human coxsackievirus A5, (CV-A5), *Picornaviridae*
Human coxsackievirus A6, (CV-A6), *Picornaviridae*
Human coxsackievirus A7, (CV-A7), *Picornaviridae*
Human coxsackievirus A8, (CV-A8), *Picornaviridae*
Human coxsackievirus A9, (CV-A9), *Picornaviridae*
Human coxsackievirus B1, (CV-B1), *Picornaviridae*
Human coxsackievirus B2, (CV-B2), *Picornaviridae*
Human coxsackievirus B3, (CV-B3), *Picornaviridae*
Human coxsackievirus B4, (CV-B4), *Picornaviridae*
Human coxsackievirus B5, (CV-B5), *Picornaviridae*
Human coxsackievirus B6, (CV-B6), *Picornaviridae*
Human cytomegalovirus, *Herpesviridae*
Human echovirus 1, (E-1), *Picornaviridae*
Human echovirus 11, (E-11), *Picornaviridae*
Human echovirus 12, (E-12), *Picornaviridae*
Human echovirus 13, (E-13), *Picornaviridae*
Human echovirus 14, (E-14), *Picornaviridae*
Human echovirus 15, (E-15), *Picornaviridae*
Human echovirus 16, (E-16), *Picornaviridae*
Human echovirus 17, (E-17), *Picornaviridae*
Human echovirus 18, (E-18), *Picornaviridae*
Human echovirus 19, (E-19), *Picornaviridae*
Human echovirus 2, (E-2), *Picornaviridae*
Human echovirus 20, (E-20), *Picornaviridae*
Human echovirus 21, (E-21), *Picornaviridae*
Human echovirus 22, (E-22), *Picornaviridae*
Human echovirus 23, (E-23), *Picornaviridae*
Human echovirus 24, (E-24), *Picornaviridae*
Human echovirus 25, (E-25), *Picornaviridae*
Human echovirus 26, (E-26), *Picornaviridae*
Human echovirus 27, (E-27), *Picornaviridae*
Human echovirus 29, (E-29), *Picornaviridae*
Human echovirus 3, (E-3), *Picornaviridae*
Human echovirus 30, (E-30), *Picornaviridae*
Human echovirus 31, (E-31), *Picornaviridae*
Human echovirus 32, (E-32), *Picornaviridae*
Human echovirus 33, (E-33), *Picornaviridae*
Human echovirus 4, (E-4), *Picornaviridae*
Human echovirus 5, (E-5), *Picornaviridae*
Human echovirus 6, (E-6), *Picornaviridae*
Human echovirus 7, (E-7), *Picornaviridae*
Human echovirus 9, (E-9), *Picornaviridae*
Human enterovirus 68, (EV-68), *Picornaviridae*
Human enterovirus 69, (EV-69), *Picornaviridae*
Human enterovirus 70, (EV-70), *Picornaviridae*
Human enterovirus 71, (EV-71), *Picornaviridae*
Human enterovirus A, (HEV-A), *Picornaviridae*
Human enterovirus B, (HEV-B), *Picornaviridae*
Human enterovirus C, (HEV-C), *Picornaviridae*
Human enterovirus D, (HEV-D), *Picornaviridae*
Human foamy virus, HFV, *Retroviridae*
Human hepatitis A virus, (HHAV), *Picornaviridae*
Human herpesvirus 1, (HHV-1), *Herpesviridae*
Human herpesvirus 2, (HHV-2), *Herpesviridae*
Human herpesvirus 3, (HHV-3), *Herpesviridae*
Human herpesvirus 4, (HHV-4), *Herpesviridae*
Human herpesvirus 5, (HHV-5), *Herpesviridae*
Human herpesvirus 6, (HHV-6), *Herpesviridae*
Human herpesvirus 7, (HHV-7), *Herpesviridae*
Human herpesvirus 8, (HHV-8), *Herpesviridae*
Human immunodeficiency virus 1 90CR056, (HIV-1.90CR056), *Retroviridae*
Human immunodeficiency virus 1 93BR020, (HIV-1.93BR020), *Retroviridae*
Human immunodeficiency virus 1 ANT70, (HIV-1.ANT70), *Retroviridae*
Human immunodeficiency virus 1 ARV-2/SF-2, (HIV-1.ARV-2/SF-2), *Retroviridae*
Human immunodeficiency virus 1 BRU (LAI), (HIV-1.BRU(LAI)), *Retroviridae*
Human immunodeficiency virus 1 ELI, (HIV-1.ELI), *Retroviridae*
Human immunodeficiency virus 1 ETH2220, (HIV-1.ETH2220), *Retroviridae*
Human immunodeficiency virus 1 HXB2, (HIV-1.HXB2), *Retroviridae*
Human immunodeficiency virus 1 MN, (HIV-1.MN), *Retroviridae*
Human immunodeficiency virus 1 NDK, (HIV-1.NDK), *Retroviridae*
Human immunodeficiency virus 1 RF, (HIV-1.RF), *Retroviridae*
Human immunodeficiency virus 1 U455, (HIV-1.U455), *Retroviridae*
Human immunodeficiency virus 1, (HIV-1), *Retroviridae*
Human immunodeficiency virus 2 BEN, (HIV-2.BEN), *Retroviridae*
Human immunodeficiency virus 2 D205, (HIV-2.D205), *Retroviridae*
Human immunodeficiency virus 2 EHOA, (HIV-2.EHOA), *Retroviridae*
Human immunodeficiency virus 2 ISY, (HIV-2.ISY), *Retroviridae*
Human immunodeficiency virus 2 ROD, (HIV-2.ROD), *Retroviridae*

Human immunodeficiency virus 2 ST, (HIV-2.ST), *Retroviridae*
Human immunodeficiency virus 2 UC1, (HIV-2.UC1), *Retroviridae*
Human immunodeficiency virus 2, (HIV-2), Retroviridae
Human papillomavirus 1 to 82, (HPV-1 to 82), *Papillomaviridae*
Human papillomavirus, (HPV), Papillomaviridae
Human parainfluenza virus 1, (HPIV-1), Paramyxoviridae
Human parainfluenza virus 2, (HPIV-2), Paramyxoviridae
Human parainfluenza virus 3, (HPIV-3), Paramyxoviridae
Human parainfluenza virus 4, (HPIV-4), Paramyxoviridae
Human parainfluenza virus 4a, *Paramyxoviridae*
Human parainfluenza virus 4b, *Paramyxoviridae*
Human parechovirus 1, (HPeV-1), *Picornaviridae*
Human parechovirus 2, (HPeV-2), *Picornaviridae*
Human parechovirus, (HPeV), Picornaviridae
Human poliovirus 1, (PV-1), *Picornaviridae*
Human poliovirus 2, (PV-2), *Picornaviridae*
Human poliovirus 3, (PV-3), *Picornaviridae*
Human respiratory syncytial virus A2, *Paramyxoviridae*
Human respiratory syncytial virus B1, *Paramyxoviridae*
Human respiratory syncytial virus S2, *Paramyxoviridae*
Human respiratory syncytial virus, (HRSV), Paramyxoviridae
Human rhinovirus 1, (HRV-1), *Picornaviridae*
Human rhinovirus 10 to 13, (HRV-10 to 13), *Picornaviridae*
Human rhinovirus 11, (HRV-11), *Picornaviridae*
Human rhinovirus 14, (HRV-14), *Picornaviridae*
Human rhinovirus 15, (HRV-15), *Picornaviridae*
Human rhinovirus 16, (HRV-16), *Picornaviridae*
Human rhinovirus 17 to 20, (HRV-17 to 20), *Picornaviridae*
Human rhinovirus 2, (HRV-2), *Picornaviridae*
Human rhinovirus 21, (HRV-21), *Picornaviridae*
Human rhinovirus 22 to 28, (HRV-22 to 28), *Picornaviridae*
Human rhinovirus 29, (HRV-29), *Picornaviridae*
Human rhinovirus 3, (HRV-3), *Picornaviridae*
Human rhinovirus 30 to 38, (HRV-30 to 38), *Picornaviridae*
Human rhinovirus 36, (HRV-36), *Picornaviridae*
Human rhinovirus 39, (HRV-39), *Picornaviridae*
Human rhinovirus 4 to 6, (HRV-4 to 6), *Picornaviridae*
Human rhinovirus 40 to 48, (HRV-40 to 48), *Picornaviridae*
Human rhinovirus 49, (HRV-49), *Picornaviridae*
Human rhinovirus 50, (HRV-50), *Picornaviridae*
Human rhinovirus 51 to 57, (HRV-51 to 57), *Picornaviridae*
Human rhinovirus 58, (HRV-58), *Picornaviridae*
Human rhinovirus 59 to 61, (HRV-59 to 61), *Picornaviridae*
Human rhinovirus 62, (HRV-62), *Picornaviridae*
Human rhinovirus 63 to 64, (HRV-63 to 64), *Picornaviridae*
Human rhinovirus 65, (HRV-65), *Picornaviridae*
Human rhinovirus 66 to 71, (HRV-66 to 71), *Picornaviridae*
Human rhinovirus 7, (HRV-7), *Picornaviridae*
Human rhinovirus 72, (HRV-72), *Picornaviridae*
Human rhinovirus 73 to 84, (HRV-73 to 84), *Picornaviridae*
Human rhinovirus 8, (HRV-8), *Picornaviridae*
Human rhinovirus 85, (HRV-85), *Picornaviridae*
Human rhinovirus 86 to 88, (HRV-86 to 88), *Picornaviridae*
Human rhinovirus 89, (HRV-89), *Picornaviridae*
Human rhinovirus 9, (HRV-9), *Picornaviridae*
Human rhinovirus 90 to 100, (HRV-90 to 100), *Picornaviridae*
Human rhinovirus A, (HRV-A), Picornaviridae
Human rhinovirus B, (HRV-B), Picornaviridae
Human T-lymphotropic virus 1, (HTLV-1), *Retroviridae*
Human T-lymphotropic virus 2, (HTLV-2), *Retroviridae*
Human torovirus, (HuTV), Coronaviridae
Humpty Doo virus, (HDOOV), *Rhabdoviridae*
Humulus japonicus virus, (HJV), Bromoviridae
Huncho virus, (HUAV), *Reoviridae*
Hungarian datura innoxia virus, (HDIV), *Potyviridae*
HV114 virus, *Bunyaviridae*
Hyacinth mosaic virus, (HyaMV), Potyviridae
Hyalophora cecropia virus, (HcV), *Tetraviridae*
Hydra viridis Chlorella virus 1, (HVCV-1), Phycodnaviridae
Hydra viridis Chlorella virus 2, (HVCV-2), *Phycodnaviridae*
Hydra viridis Chlorella virus 3, (HVCV-3), *Phycodnaviridae*
Hydrangea latent virus, (HdLV), Carlavirus
Hydrangea mosaic virus, (HdMV), Bromoviridae
Hydrangea ringspot virus, (HdRSV), Potexvirus
Hyloicus pinastri cypovirus 2, (HpCPV-2), *Reoviridae*
Hyphomicrobium phage Hyφ30, (Hyφ30), *Podoviridae*
Hypochoeris mosaic virus, (HyMV), Furovirus

Hypocritae jacobeae virus, (HjV), *Tetraviridae*
Hypomicrogaster canadensis bracovirus, (HcBV), *Polydnaviridae*
Hypomicrogaster ectdytolophae bracovirus, (HecBV), *Polydnaviridae*
Hyposoter annulipes ichnovirus, (HaIV), *Polydnaviridae*
Hyposoter exiguae ichnovirus, (HeIV), *Polydnaviridae*
Hyposoter exiguae reovirus, (HeRV), *Reoviridae*
Hyposoter fugitivus ichnovirus, (HfIV), *Polydnaviridae*
Hyposoter lymantriae ichnovirus, (HlIV), *Polydnaviridae*
Hyposoter pilosulus ichnovirus, (HpIV), *Polydnaviridae*
Hyposoter rivalis ichnovirus, (HrIV), *Polydnaviridae*
Hypovirulence-associated virus, *Hypoviridae*

Iaco virus, (IACOV), *Bunyaviridae*
Ibaraki virus isolate 318, (IBAV), *Reoviridae*
Icoaraci virus, *Bunyaviridae*
Ictalurid herpesvirus 1, (IcHV-1), *Herpesviridae*
Ieri virus, (IERIV), *Reoviridae*
Ieri virus, (IERIV), *Reoviridae*
Ife virus, (IFEV), *Reoviridae*
Iguape virus, (IGUV), *Flaviviridae*
Ilesha virus, (ILEV), *Bunyaviridae*
Ilheus virus, (ILHV), *Flaviviridae*
Impatiens latent virus, (ILV), *Carlavirus*
Impatiens necrotic spot virus, (INSV), *Bunyaviridae*
Inachis io cypovirus 2, (IiCPV-2), *Reoviridae*
Indian cassava mosaic virus, (ICMV), *Geminiviridae*
Indian cobra herpesvirus, *Herpesviridae*
Indian peanut clump virus, (IPCV), *Pecluvirus*
Indian pepper mottle virus, (IPMoV), *Potyviridae*
Indian tomato bunchy top viroid, *Pospiviroidae*
Indian tomato leaf curl virus, (IToLCV), *Geminiviridae*
Indonesian soybean dwarf virus, (ISDV), *Luteoviridae*
Infectious bovine rhinotracheitis virus, *Herpesviridae*
Infectious bronchitis virus, (IBV), *Coronaviridae*
Infectious bursal disease virus 002-73, *Birnaviridae*
Infectious bursal disease virus 23/82, *Birnaviridae*
Infectious bursal disease virus 52/70, *Birnaviridae*
Infectious bursal disease virus Australian 002-73, *Birnaviridae*
Infectious bursal disease virus Cu-1, *Birnaviridae*
Infectious bursal disease virus Edgar, *Birnaviridae*
Infectious bursal disease virus Farragher, *Birnaviridae*
Infectious bursal disease virus GPF-1E, *Birnaviridae*
Infectious bursal disease virus KS, *Birnaviridae*
Infectious bursal disease virus OH, *Birnaviridae*
Infectious bursal disease virus OKYM attenuated, *Birnaviridae*
Infectious bursal disease virus OKYM, *Birnaviridae*
Infectious bursal disease virus P2, *Birnaviridae*
Infectious bursal disease virus PBG-98, *Birnaviridae*
Infectious bursal disease virus QC-2, *Birnaviridae*
Infectious bursal disease virus STC, *Birnaviridae*
Infectious bursal disease virus UK661, *Birnaviridae*
Infectious bursal disease virus, (IBDV), *Birnaviridae*
Infectious flacherie virus, (IFV), Unassigned
Infectious hematopoietic necrosis virus, (IHNV), *Rhabdoviridae*
Infectious laryngotracheitis virus, *Herpesviridae*
Infectious pancreatic necrosis virus DRT, *Birnaviridae*
Infectious pancreatic necrosis virus Jasper, *Birnaviridae*
Infectious pancreatic necrosis virus N1, *Birnaviridae*
Infectious pancreatic necrosis virus Sp, *Birnaviridae*
Infectious pancreatic necrosis virus, (IPNV), *Birnaviridae*
Influenza A virus, (FLUAV), *Orthomyxoviridae*
Influenza B virus, (FLUBV), *Orthomyxoviridae*
Influenza C virus, (FLUCV), *Orthomyxoviridae*
Ingwavuma virus, (INGV), *Bunyaviridae*
INH-95551 virus, *Arenaviridae*
Inini virus, (INIV), *Bunyaviridae*
Inkoo virus, (INKV), *Bunyaviridae*
Inner Farne virus, (INFV), *Reoviridae*
Insect iridescent virus 28, *Iridoviridae*
Invertebrate iridescent virus 1, (IIV-1), *Iridoviridae*
Invertebrate iridescent virus 10, *Iridoviridae*
Invertebrate iridescent virus 16, (IIV-16), *Iridoviridae*
Invertebrate iridescent virus 18, *Iridoviridae*
Invertebrate iridescent virus 2, (IIV-2), *Iridoviridae*
Invertebrate iridescent virus 21, (IIV-21), *Iridoviridae*
Invertebrate iridescent virus 22, (IIV-22), *Iridoviridae*
Invertebrate iridescent virus 23, (IIV-23), *Iridoviridae*
Invertebrate iridescent virus 24, (IIV-24), *Iridoviridae*
Invertebrate iridescent virus 29, (IIV-29), *Iridoviridae*
Invertebrate iridescent virus 3, (IIV-3), *Iridoviridae*
Invertebrate iridescent virus 30, (IIV-30), *Iridoviridae*
Invertebrate iridescent virus 31, (IIV-31), *Iridoviridae*
Invertebrate iridescent virus 32, *Iridoviridae*
Invertebrate iridescent virus 6, (IIV-6), *Iridoviridae*
Invertebrate iridescent virus 9, (IIV-9), *Iridoviridae*
Ippy virus, (IPPYV), *Arenaviridae*
Iranian wheat stripe virus, (IWSV), *Tenuivirus*
Iresine viroid 1, (IrVd-1), *Pospiviroidae*
Iris fulva mosaic virus, (IFMV), *Potyviridae*
Iris germanica leaf stripe virus, (IGLSV), *Rhabdoviridae*
Iris mild mosaic virus, (IMMV), *Potyviridae*
Iris severe mosaic virus, (ISMV), *Potyviridae*
Iris yellow spot virus, (IYSV), *Bunyaviridae*

Irituia virus, (IRIV), *Reoviridae*
Isachne mosaic virus*, (IsaMV), *Potyviridae*
Isfahan virus, (ISFV), *Rhabdoviridae*
Isla Vista virus, (ISLAV), *Bunyaviridae*
Isopod iridescent virus, *Iridoviridae*
Israel turkey meningoencephalomyelitis virus, (ITV), *Flaviviridae*
Issyk-Kul virus, (ISKV), *Bunyaviridae*
Itaituba virus, (ITAV), *Bunyaviridae*
Itaporanga virus, (ITPV), *Bunyaviridae*
Itaqui virus, (ITQV), *Bunyaviridae*
Itimirim virus, (ITIV), *Bunyaviridae*
Itupiranga virus, (ITUV), *Reoviridae*
Ivy vein clearing virus, (IVCV), *Rhabdoviridae*

Jaagsiekte sheep retrovirus, (JSRV), *Retroviridae*
Jacareacanga virus, (JACV), *Reoviridae*
Jamanxi virus, (JAMV), *Reoviridae*
Jamestown Canyon virus, (JCV), *Bunyaviridae*
Japanaut virus, (JAPV), *Reoviridae*
Japanese eel herpesvirus, *Herpesviridae*
Japanese encephalitis virus, (JEV), *Flaviviridae*
Japanese flounder nervous necrosis virus, (JFNNV), *Nodaviridae*
Japanese pear fruit dimple viroid, *Pospiviroidae*
Jari virus, (JARIV), *Reoviridae*
Jatropha mosaic virus, (JMV), *Geminiviridae*
JC polyomavirus, (JCPyV), *Polyomaviridae*
JD254 virus, (DGKV), *Bunyaviridae*
Joa virus, (JOAV), *Bunyaviridae*
Johnsongrass mosaic virus, (JGMV), *Potyviridae*
Johnston Atoll virus, (JAV), Unassigned
Joinjakaka virus, (JOIV), *Rhabdoviridae*
Jonquil mild mosaic virus, *Potyviridae*
Josiah virus, *Arenaviridae*
Juan Diaz virus, (JDV), *Bunyaviridae*
Jugra virus, (JUGV), *Flaviviridae*
Juncopox virus, (JNPV), *Poxviridae*
Junøn virus, (JUNV), *Arenaviridae*
Junonia coenia densovirus, (JcDNV), *Parvoviridae*
Jurona virus, (JURV), *Rhabdoviridae*
Jutiapa virus, (JUTV), *Flaviviridae*

K27 virus, *Bunyaviridae*
Kachemak Bay virus, (KBV), *Bunyaviridae*
Kadam virus, (KADV), *Flaviviridae*
Kadipiro virus (Java-7075), (KDV-Ja7075), *Reoviridae*
Kadipiro virus, (KDV), *Reoviridae*
Kaeng Khoi virus, (KKV), *Bunyaviridae*
Kaikalur virus, (KAIV), *Bunyaviridae*
Kairi virus, (KRIV), *Bunyaviridae*
Kaisodi virus, (KSOV), *Bunyaviridae*

Kala Iris virus, (KIRV), *Reoviridae*
Kalanchoe latent virus, (KLV), *Carlavirus*
Kalanchoë mosaic virus, (KMV), *Potyviridae*
Kalanchoe top-spotting virus, (KTSV), *Caulimoviridae*
Kamese virus, (KAMV), *Rhabdoviridae*
Kamiiso-8Cr-95 virus, *Bunyaviridae*
Kammavanpettai virus, (KMPV), *Reoviridae*
Kannamangalam virus, (KANV), *Rhabdoviridae*
Kao Shuan virus, (KSV), *Bunyaviridae*
Kaposi's sarcoma-associated herpesvirus, *Herpesviridae*
Karimabad virus, (KARV), *Bunyaviridae*
Karshi virus, (KSIV), *Flaviviridae*
Kasba virus (Chuzan virus), (KASV), *Reoviridae*
Kashmir bee virus, (KBV), Unassigned
Kasokero virus, (KASV), *Bunyaviridae*
Kawino virus, (KaV), Unassigned
Kazan virus, *Bunyaviridae*
Kedougou virus, (KEDV), *Flaviviridae*
Kelp fly virus, (KFV), Unassigned
Kemerovo virus, (KEMV), *Reoviridae*
Kenai virus, (KENV), *Reoviridae*
Kennedya virus Y, (KVY), *Potyviridae*
Kennedya yellow mosaic virus, (KYMV), *Tymovirus*
Kern Canyon virus, (KCV), *Rhabdoviridae*
Ketapang virus, (KETV), *Bunyaviridae*
Keterah virus, (KTRV), *Bunyaviridae*
Keuraliba virus, (KEUV), *Rhabdoviridae*
Keystone virus, (KEYV), *Bunyaviridae*
Khabarovsk virus, (KHAV), *Bunyaviridae*
Kharagysh virus, (KHAV), *Reoviridae*
Khasan virus, (KHAV), *Bunyaviridae*
KI-83-262 virus, *Bunyaviridae*
KI-85-1 virus, *Bunyaviridae*
KI-88-15 virus, *Bunyaviridae*
Kilham polyomavirus, (KPyV), *Polyomaviridae*
Kilham rat virus, (KRV), *Parvoviridae*
Kimberley virus, (KIMV), *Rhabdoviridae*
Kindia virus, (KINV), *Reoviridae*
Kinkajou herpesvirus, *Herpesviridae*
Kirsten murine sarcoma virus, (KiMSV), *Retroviridae*
Kismayo virus, (KISV), *Bunyaviridae*
Klamath virus, (KLAV), *Rhabdoviridae*
Kluyvera phage Kvp1, (Kvp1), *Podoviridae*
Kodzha virus AP92, *Bunyaviridae*
Kodzha virus C68031, *Bunyaviridae*
Kodzha virus, (CCHFV), *Bunyaviridae*
Kokobera virus, (KOKV), *Flaviviridae*
Kolongo virus, (KOLV), *Rhabdoviridae*
Konjac mosaic virus, (KoMV), *Potyviridae*
Koolpinyah virus, (KOOLV), *Rhabdoviridae*
Koongol virus, (KOOV), *Bunyaviridae*
Kotonkon virus, (KOTV), *Rhabdoviridae*
Koutango virus, (KOUV), *Flaviviridae*

Kowanyama virus, (KOWV), *Bunyaviridae*
Kunjin virus, (KUNV), *Flaviviridae*
Kurthia phage 6, (6), *Podoviridae*
Kurthia phage 7, (7), *Podoviridae*
Kwatta virus, (KWAV), *Rhabdoviridae*
Kyasanur Forest disease virus, (KFDV), *Flaviviridae*
Kyuri green mottle mosaic virus, (KGMMV), Tobamovirus
Kyzylagach virus, *Togaviridae*

L99 virus, *Bunyaviridae*
La Crosse virus, (LACV), *Bunyaviridae*
La Joya virus, (LJV), *Rhabdoviridae*
Lacanobia oleracea cypovirus 2, (LoCPV-2), *Reoviridae*
Lacertid herpesvirus, (LaHV-1), *Herpesviridae*
Lactate dehydrogenase-elevating virus, (LDV), *Arteriviridae*
Lactobacillus phage 222a, (222a), *Myoviridae*
Lactobacillus phage 223, (223), *Siphoviridae*
Lactobacillus phage fri, (fri), *Myoviridae*
Lactobacillus phage hv, (hv), *Myoviridae*
Lactobacillus phage hw, (hw), *Myoviridae*
Lactobacillus phage lb6, (lb6), *Siphoviridae*
Lactobacillus phage PL-1, (PL-1), *Siphoviridae*
Lactobacillus phage y5, (y5), *Siphoviridae*
Lactobacillus phage φFSW, (φFSW), *Siphoviridae*
Lactococcus phage 1358, (1358), *Siphoviridae*
Lactococcus phage 1483, (1483), *Siphoviridae*
Lactococcus phage 3ML, (3ML), *Siphoviridae*
Lactococcus phage 936, (936), *Siphoviridae*
Lactococcus phage 949, (949), *Siphoviridae*
Lactococcus phage bIL67, (bIL67), *Siphoviridae*
Lactococcus phage BK5-T, (BK5-T), *Siphoviridae*
Lactococcus phage c2, (c2), *Siphoviridae*
Lactococcus phage c6A, (PBc6A), *Siphoviridae*
Lactococcus phage KSY1, (KSY1), *Podoviridae*
Lactococcus phage ML3, (ML3), *Siphoviridae*
Lactococcus phage ml3, (ml3), *Siphoviridae*
Lactococcus phage P001, (P001), *Siphoviridae*
Lactococcus phage P107, (P107), *Siphoviridae*
Lactococcus phage P335, (P335), *Siphoviridae*
Lactococcus phage PO34, (PO34), *Podoviridae*
Lactococcus phage PO87, (PO87), *Siphoviridae*
Lactococcus phage φvML3, (φvML3), *Siphoviridae*
Laelia red leafspot virus, (LRLV), *Rhabdoviridae*
LaFrance isometric virus, (LFIV), Unassigned
Lagos bat virus, (LBV), *Rhabdoviridae*
Laguna Negra virus, (LANV), *Bunyaviridae*
Lake Clarendon virus, (LCV), *Reoviridae*
Lake victoria cormorant herpesvirus, *Herpesviridae*
Lamium mild mosaic virus, (LMMV), *Comoviridae*
Landjia virus, (LJAV), *Rhabdoviridae*
Landlocked salmon reovirus, (LSRV), *Reoviridae*

Langat virus, (LGTV), *Flaviviridae*
Langur virus, (LNGV), *Retroviridae*
Lanjan virus, (LJNV), *Bunyaviridae*
La-Piedad-Michoacan-Mexico virus, *Paramyxoviridae*
Lapine parvovirus, (LPV), *Parvoviridae*
Largemouth bass virus, (LMBV), *Iridoviridae*
Las Maloyas virus, (LMV), *Bunyaviridae*
Lasiocampa quercus cypovirus 6, (LqCPV-6), *Reoviridae*
Lassa virus, (LASV), *Arenaviridae*
Lates calcarifer encephalitis virus, (LcEV), *Nodaviridae*
Latino virus, (LATV), *Arenaviridae*
Lato river virus, (LRV), *Tombusviridae*
Latoia viridissima virus, (LvV), Unassigned
Launea arborescens stunt virus, (LArSV), *Rhabdoviridae*
Le Dantec virus, (LDV), *Rhabdoviridae*
Leanyer virus, (LEAV), *Bunyaviridae*
Lebombo virus 1, (LEBV-1), *Reoviridae*
Lebombo virus, (LEBV), *Reoviridae*
Lechiguanas virus, *Bunyaviridae*
Lednice virus, (LEDV), *Bunyaviridae*
Lee virus, *Bunyaviridae*
Leek white stripe virus, (LWSV), *Tombusviridae*
Leek yellow stripe virus, (LYSV), *Potyviridae*
Legume yellows virus, *Luteoviridae*
Leishmania RNA virus 1-1, (LRV1-1), *Totiviridae*
Leishmania RNA virus 1-10, (LRV1-10), *Totiviridae*
Leishmania RNA virus 1-11, (LRV1-11), *Totiviridae*
Leishmania RNA virus 1-12, (LRV1-12), *Totiviridae*
Leishmania RNA virus 1-2, (LRV1-2), *Totiviridae*
Leishmania RNA virus 1-3, (LRV1-3), *Totiviridae*
Leishmania RNA virus 1-4, (LRV1-4), *Totiviridae*
Leishmania RNA virus 1-5, (LRV1-5), *Totiviridae*
Leishmania RNA virus 1-6, (LRV1-6), *Totiviridae*
Leishmania RNA virus 1-7, (LRV1-7), *Totiviridae*
Leishmania RNA virus 1-8, (LRV1-8), *Totiviridae*
Leishmania RNA virus 1-9, (LRV1-9), *Totiviridae*
Leishmania RNA virus 2-1, (LRV2-1), *Totiviridae*
Lemon scented thyme leaf chlorosis virus, (LSTCV), *Rhabdoviridae*
Lentinus edodes virus, (LEV), Unassigned
Leonurus mosaic virus, (LeMV), *Geminiviridae*
Leporid herpesvirus 1, (LeHV-1), *Herpesviridae*
Leporid herpesvirus 2, (LeHV-2), *Herpesviridae*
Leporid herpesvirus 3, (LeHV-3), *Herpesviridae*
Lethocerus columbinae iridescent virus, *Iridoviridae*
Lettuce big-vein virus, (LBVV), *Varicosavirus*
Lettuce chlorosis virus, (LCV), *Closteroviridae*
Lettuce infectious yellows virus, (LIYV), *Closteroviridae*
Lettuce mosaic virus, (LMV), *Potyviridae*

Lettuce necrotic yellows virus, (LNYV), *Rhabdoviridae*
Lettuce speckles mottle virus, (LSMV), *Umbravirus*
Leuconostoc phage pro2, (pro2), *Siphoviridae*
Leucorrhinia dubia densovirus, (LdDNV), *Parvoviridae*
Lilac chlorotic leafspot virus, (LiCLV), *Capillovirus*
Lilac mottle virus, (LiMoV), *Carlavirus*
Lilac ring mottle virus, (LiRMoV), *Bromoviridae*
Lilac ringspot virus, (LiRSV), *Carlavirus*
Lilium henryi del1 virus, (LheDel1V), *Metaviridae*
Lily mild mottle virus, (LiMMoV), *Potyviridae*
Lily mottle virus, (LMoV), *Potyviridae*
Lily symptomless virus, (LSV), *Carlavirus*
Lily virus X, (LVX), *Potexvirus*
Limabean golden mosaic virus, (LGMV), *Geminiviridae*
Lipovnik virus, (LIPV), *Reoviridae*
Lisianthus necrosis virus, (LNV), *Tombusviridae*
Lissonota sp. ichnovirus, (LspIV), *Polydnaviridae*
Listeria phage 2389, (2389), *Siphoviridae*
Listeria phage 2671, (2671), *Siphoviridae*
Listeria phage 2685, (2685), *Siphoviridae*
Listeria phage 4211, (4211), *Myoviridae*
Listeria phage A511, (A511), *Myoviridae*
Listeria phage H387, (H387), *Siphoviridae*
Little cherry virus, (LChV), *Closteroviridae*
Liverpool vervet herpesvirus, *Herpesviridae*
Ljungan virus, (LV), *Picornaviridae*
Llano Seco virus, (LLSV), *Reoviridae*
Locusta migratoria entomopoxvirus 'O', (LMEV), *Poxviridae*
Lokern virus, (LOKV), *Bunyaviridae*
Lolium ryegrass virus, (LoRV), *Rhabdoviridae*
Lone Star virus, (LSV), *Bunyaviridae*
Lordsdale virus, (LDV), *Caliciviridae*
Lorisine herpesvirus 1, (LoHV-1), *Herpesviridae*
Lotus stem necrosis, (LoSNV), *Rhabdoviridae*
Louping ill virus British subtype, *Flaviviridae*
Louping ill virus Irish subtype, *Flaviviridae*
Louping ill virus Spanish subtype, *Flaviviridae*
Louping ill virus Turkish subtype, *Flaviviridae*
Louping ill virus, (LIV), *Flaviviridae*
LP virus, *Arenaviridae*
Lucerne Australian latent virus, (LALV), *Comoviridae*
Lucerne Australian symptomless virus, (LASV), *Comoviridae*
Lucerne enation virus, (LEV), *Rhabdoviridae*
Lucerne transient streak virus satellite RNA, Satellite
Lucerne transient streak virus, (LTSV), *Sobemovirus*
Lucké frog herpesvirus, *Herpesviridae*
Lucké triturus virus 1; CP4-4398B (276), *Iridoviridae*
LUIII virus, (LUIIIV), *Parvoviridae*
Lukuni virus, (LUKV), *Bunyaviridae*

Lumbo virus, (LUMV), *Bunyaviridae*
Lumpy skin disease virus, (LSDV), *Poxviridae*
Lundy virus, (LUNV), *Reoviridae*
Lupin leaf curl virus, (LLCV), *Geminiviridae*
Lupin yellow vein virus, (LYVV), *Rhabdoviridae*
Lychnis ringspot virus, (LRSV), *Hordeivirus*
Lychnis symptomless virus, (LycSLV), *Potexvirus*
Lymantria dispar cypovirus 1, (LdCPV-1), *Reoviridae*
Lymantria dispar cypovirus 11, (LdCPV-11), *Reoviridae*
Lymantria dispar MNPV, (LdMNPV), *Baculoviridae*
Lymantria dubia densovirus, (LdDNV), *Parvoviridae*
Lymantria ninayi virus (Greenwood), (LNV), *Nodaviridae*
Lymantria ninayi virus, (LnV), *Tetraviridae*
Lymantria ninayi virus, (LnV), Unassigned
Lymphocystis disease virus 1, (LCDV-1), *Iridoviridae*
Lymphocystis disease virus 2, (LCDV-2), *Iridoviridae*
Lymphocytic choriomeningitis virus, (LCMV), *Arenaviridae*

M'Poko virus, (MPOV), *Bunyaviridae*
M459 virus, (BWAV), *Bunyaviridae*
M67U5 virus, (MNTV), *Bunyaviridae*
Macaua virus, (MCAV), *Bunyaviridae*
Machupo virus, (MACV), *Arenaviridae*
Maciel virus, *Bunyaviridae*
Maclura mosaic virus, (MacMV), *Potyviridae*
Macropipus depurator P virus, (MdRV-P), *Reoviridae*
Macropodid herpesvirus 1, (MaHV-1), *Herpesviridae*
Macropodid herpesvirus 2, (MaHV-2), *Herpesviridae*
Macroptilium golden mosaic virus, (MGMV), *Geminiviridae*
Macrotyloma mosaic virus, (MaMV), *Geminiviridae*
Madrid virus, (MADV), *Bunyaviridae*
Maguari virus, (MAGV), *Bunyaviridae*
Mahogany Hammock virus, (MHV), *Bunyaviridae*
Maiden virus, (MDNV), *Reoviridae*
Main Drain virus, (MDV), *Bunyaviridae*
Maize chlorotic dwarf virus, (MCDV), *Sequiviridae*
Maize chlorotic mottle virus, (MCMV), *Tombusviridae*
Maize dwarf mosaic virus, (MDMV), *Potyviridae*
Maize mosaic virus, (MMV), *Rhabdoviridae*
Maize rayado fino virus, (MRFV), *Marafivirus*
Maize rough dwarf virus, (MRDV), *Reoviridae*
Maize stem borer virus, (MSBV), Unassigned
Maize sterile stunt virus, (MSSV), *Rhabdoviridae*
Maize streak virus, (MSV), *Geminiviridae*
Maize stripe virus, (MSpV), *Tenuivirus*
Maize white line mosaic satellite virus, Satellite
Maize white line mosaic virus, (MWLMV), Unassigned

Mal de Rio Cuarto virus, (MRCV), *Reoviridae*
Malacky/Ma32/94 virus, *Bunyaviridae*
Malacosoma disstria cypovirus 8, (MdCPV-8), *Reoviridae*
Malacosoma neustria cypovirus 2, (MnCPV-2), *Reoviridae*
Malacosoma neustria cypovirus 3, (MnCPV-3), *Reoviridae*
Malakal virus, (MALV), *Rhabdoviridae*
Malignant catarrhal fever virus, *Herpesviridae*
Malpais Spring virus, (MSPV), *Rhabdoviridae*
Malva silvestris virus, (MaSV), *Rhabdoviridae*
Malva vein clearing virus, (MVCV), *Potyviridae*
Malva veinal necrosis virus, (MVNV), *Potexvirus*
Malva yellows virus, *Luteoviridae*
Malvaceous chlorosis virus, (MCV), *Geminiviridae*
Mamestra brassicae cypovirus 11, (MbCPV-11), *Reoviridae*
Mamestra brassicae cypovirus 12, (MbCPV-12), *Reoviridae*
Mamestra brassicae cypovirus 2, (MbCPV-2), *Reoviridae*
Mamestra brassicae cypovirus 7, (MbCPV-7), *Reoviridae*
Mamestra brassicae MNPV, (MbMNPV), *Baculoviridae*
Mammalian orthoreovirus 1-Lang, (MRV-1), *Reoviridae*
Mammalian orthoreovirus 2-D5/Jones, (MRV-2), *Reoviridae*
Mammalian orthoreovirus 3-Dearing, (MRV-3), *Reoviridae*
Mammalian orthoreovirus, (MRV), *Reoviridae*
Manawa virus, (MWAV), *Bunyaviridae*
Manawatu virus, (MwV), *Nodaviridae*
Manitoba virus, (MNTBV), *Rhabdoviridae*
Manzanilla virus, (MANV), *Bunyaviridae*
Mapputta virus, (MAPV), *Bunyaviridae*
Maprik virus, (MPKV), *Bunyaviridae*
Mapuera virus, (MPRV), *Paramyxoviridae*
Maraba virus, (MARAV), *Rhabdoviridae*
Maracuja mosaic virus, (MarMV), *Tobamovirus*
Marble spleen disease virus, *Adenoviridae*
Marburg virus Marburg Ravn, *Filoviridae*
Marburg virus Musoke, *Filoviridae*
Marburg virus Ozolin, *Filoviridae*
Marburg virus Popp, *Filoviridae*
Marburg virus Ratayczak, *Filoviridae*
Marburg virus Voege, *Filoviridae*
Marburg virus, (MARV), *Filoviridae*
Marco virus, (MCOV), *Rhabdoviridae*
Marek's disease virus type 1, *Herpesviridae*
Marek's disease virus type 2, *Herpesviridae*
Marigold mottle virus, (MaMoV), *Potyviridae*
Marituba virus, (MTBV), *Bunyaviridae*

Marmomid herpesvirus 1, (MarHV-1), *Herpesviridae*
Marmoset cytomegalovirus, *Herpesviridae*
Marmoset herpesvirus, *Herpesviridae*
Marmosetpox virus, (MPV), *Poxviridae*
Marrakai virus, (MARV), *Reoviridae*
MARU 10962 virus, (GAMV), *Bunyaviridae*
Mason-Pfizer monkey virus, (MPMV), *Retroviridae*
Masou salmon reovirus MSV, (MSRV), *Reoviridae*
Matruh virus, (MTRV), *Bunyaviridae*
Matucare virus, (MATV), *Reoviridae*
Maus Elberfeld virus, *Picornaviridae*
Mayaro virus, (MAYV), *Togaviridae*
Mboke virus, (MBOV), *Bunyaviridae*
MC2 virus, *Arenaviridae*
Meaban virus, (MEAV), *Flaviviridae*
Measles virus, (MeV), *Paramyxoviridae*
Medical lake macaque herpesvirus, *Herpesviridae*
Megakepasma mosaic virus, (MegMV), *Closteroviridae*
Melandrium yellow fleck virus, (MYFV), *Bromoviridae*
Melanoplus sanguinipes entomopoxvirus 'O', (MSEV), *Poxviridae*
Melao virus, (MELV), *Bunyaviridae*
Meleagrid herpesvirus 1, (MeHV-1), *Herpesviridae*
Melilotus latent virus, (MeLV), *Rhabdoviridae*
Melilotus mosaic virus, (MeMV), *Potyviridae*
Melolontha melolontha entomopoxvirus, (MMEV), *Poxviridae*
Melon leaf curl virus, (MLCV), *Geminiviridae*
Melon necrotic spot virus, (MNSV), *Tombusviridae*
Melon rugose mosaic virus, (MRMV), *Tymovirus*
Melon variegation virus, (MVV), *Rhabdoviridae*
Melon vein-banding mosaic virus, (MVBMV), *Potyviridae*
Mengovirus, *Picornaviridae*
Mermet virus, (MERV), *Bunyaviridae*
Methanobacterium phage ΦF3, (ΦF3), *Siphoviridae*
Methanobacterium phage ΨM1, (ΨM1), *Siphoviridae*
Methanobrevibacter phage PG, (PG), *Siphoviridae*
Mexican papita viroid, (MPVd), *Pospiviroidae*
Mexico virus, (MXV), *Caliciviridae*
Mibuna temperate virus, (MTV), *Partitiviridae*
Mice minute virus, (MMV), *Parvoviridae*
Michigan alfalfa virus, *Luteoviridae*
Micrococcus phage N1, (N1), *Siphoviridae*
Micrococcus phage N5, (N5), *Siphoviridae*
Micromonas pusilla virus GM1, (MpV-GM1), *Phycodnaviridae*
Micromonas pusilla virus PB6, (MpV-PB6), *Phycodnaviridae*
Micromonas pusilla virus PB7, (MpV-PB7), *Phycodnaviridae*
Micromonas pusilla virus PB8, (MpV-PB8), *Phycodnaviridae*

Micromonas pusilla virus PL1, (MpV-PL1), *Phycodnaviridae*
Micromonas pusilla virus SG1, (MpV-SG1), *Phycodnaviridae*
Micromonas pusilla virus SP1, (MpV-SP1), *Phycodnaviridae*
Micromonas pusilla virus SP2, (MpV-SP2), *Phycodnaviridae*
Microplitis croceipes bracovirus, (McBV), *Polydnaviridae*
Microplitis demolitor bracovirus, (MdBV), *Polydnaviridae*
Microtus pennyslvanicus herpesvirus, *Herpesviridae*
Middelburg virus, (MIDV), *Togaviridae*
Milk vetch dwarf virus, (MDV), *Nanovirus*
Milker's nodule virus, *Poxviridae*
Mill Door virus, (MDRV), *Reoviridae*
Mimosa bacilliform virus, (MBV), *Caulimoviridae*
Minatitlan virus, (MNTV), *Bunyaviridae*
Mink calicivirus, (MCV), *Caliciviridae*
Mink enteritis virus, (MEV), *Parvoviridae*
Minnal virus, (MINV), *Reoviridae*
Mirabilis mosaic virus, (MiMV), *Caulimoviridae*
Mirim virus, (MIRV), *Bunyaviridae*
Miscanthus streak virus, (MiSV), *Geminiviridae*
Mitchell river virus, (MRV), *Reoviridae*
MM-2325 virus, (BAKV), *Bunyaviridae*
Mobala virus, (MOBV), *Arenaviridae*
Modoc virus, (MODV), *Flaviviridae*
Moju virus, (MOJUV), *Bunyaviridae*
Mojui Dos Campos virus, (MDCV), *Bunyaviridae*
Mokola virus, (MOKV), *Rhabdoviridae*
Molinia streak virus, (MoSV), *Tombusviridae*
Mollicutes phage Br1, (Br1), *Myoviridae*
Mollicutes phage C3, (C3), *Podoviridae*
Mollicutes phage L3, (L3), *Podoviridae*
Molluscum contagiosum virus, (MOCV), *Poxviridae*
Molluscum-like poxvirus, (MOV), *Poxviridae*
Moloney murine leukemia virus, (MoMLV), *Retroviridae*
Moloney murine sarcoma virus, (MoMSV), *Retroviridae*
Monkeypox virus, (MPXV), *Poxviridae*
Mono Lake virus, (MLV), *Reoviridae*
Monongahela virus, *Bunyaviridae*
Montana myotis leukoencephalitis virus, (MMLV), *Flaviviridae*
Monte Dourado virus, (MDOV), *Reoviridae*
Mopeia virus, (MOPV), *Arenaviridae*
Moravia/Ma5302V virus, *Bunyaviridae*
Moriche virus, (MORV), *Bunyaviridae*
Moroccan pepper virus, (MPV), *Tombusviridae*
Moroccan watermelon mosaic virus, (MWMV), *Potyviridae*
Mosqueiro virus, (MQOV), *Rhabdoviridae*
Mosquito iridescent virus, *Iridoviridae*
Mossuril virus, (MOSV), *Rhabdoviridae*
Mount Elgon bat virus, (MEBV), *Rhabdoviridae*
Mouse cytomegalovirus, *Herpesviridae*
Mouse herpesvirus strain 68, *Herpesviridae*
Mouse mammary tumor virus, (MMTV), *Retroviridae*
Mouse parvovirus 1, (MPV), *Parvoviridae*
Mouse thymic herpesvirus, *Herpesviridae*
Movar virus, *Herpesviridae*
MP 401 virus, (NDV), *Bunyaviridae*
MRM31 virus, (KOOV), *Bunyaviridae*
Mucambo virus, (MUCV), *Togaviridae*
Mudjinbarry virus, (MUDV), *Reoviridae*
Muir Springs virus, (MSV), *Rhabdoviridae*
Mulberry latent virus, (MLV), *Carlavirus*
Mulberry ringspot virus, (MRSV), *Comoviridae*
Mule deer poxvirus, (DPV), *Poxviridae*
Muleshoe virus, (MULV), *Bunyaviridae*
Mumps virus, (MuV), *Paramyxoviridae*
Mungbean mosaic virus, (MbMV), *Potyviridae*
Mungbean mottle virus, (MMoV), *Potyviridae*
Mungbean yellow mosaic virus, (MYMV), *Geminiviridae*
Munguba virus, (MUNV), *Bunyaviridae*
Murid herpesvirus 1, (MuHV-1), *Herpesviridae*
Murid herpesvirus 2, (MuHV-2), *Herpesviridae*
Murid herpesvirus 3, (MuHV-3), *Herpesviridae*
Murid herpesvirus 4, (MuHV-4), *Herpesviridae*
Murid herpesvirus 5, (MuHV-5), *Herpesviridae*
Murid herpesvirus 6, (MuHV-6), *Herpesviridae*
Murine adenovirus 1, (MAdV-1), *Adenoviridae*
Murine adenovirus 2, (MAdV-2), *Adenoviridae*
Murine adenovirus A, (MAdV-A), *Adenoviridae*
Murine adenovirus B, (MAdV-B), *Adenoviridae*
Murine hepatitis virus, (MHV), *Coronaviridae*
Murine leukemia virus, (MLV), *Retroviridae*
Murine parainfluenza virus 1, *Paramyxoviridae*
Murine pneumonia virus, (MPV), *Paramyxoviridae*
Murine pneumotropic virus, (MPtV), *Polyomaviridae*
Murine polyomavirus, (MPyV), *Polyomaviridae*
Murray Valley encephalitis virus, (MVEV), *Flaviviridae*
Murre virus, (MURV), *Bunyaviridae*
Murutucu virus, (MURV), *Bunyaviridae*
Musca domestica reovirus, (MdRV), *Reoviridae*
Muscovy duck parvovirus, (MDPV), *Parvoviridae*
Mushroom bacilliform virus, (MBV), *Barnaviridae*
Mushroom virus 4, *Partitiviridae*
Muskmelon vein necrosis virus, (MuVNV), *Carlavirus*
Mycobacterium phage I3, (I3), *Myoviridae*
Mycobacterium phage L5, (L5), *Siphoviridae*
Mycobacterium phage lacticola, (lacticola), *Siphoviridae*

Mycobacterium phage Leo, (Leo), *Siphoviridae*
Mycobacterium phage minetti, (minetti), *Siphoviridae*
Mycobacterium phage phlei, (GS4E), *Siphoviridae*
Mycobacterium phage R1-Myb, (R1-Myb), *Siphoviridae*
Mycobacterium phage ϕ17, (ϕ17), *Podoviridae*
Mycogone perniciosa virus, (MpV), *Totiviridae*
Mykines virus, (MYKV), *Reoviridae*
Mynahpox virus, (MYPV), *Poxviridae*
Myriotrichia clavaeformis virus a, (McV-a), *Phycodnaviridae*
Myrobalan latent ringspot virus (160), (MLRSV), *Comoviridae*
Myrobalan latent ringspot virus satellite RNA, Satellite
Myxoma virus, (MYXV), *Poxviridae*

Nairobi sheep disease virus, (NSDV), *Bunyaviridae*
Nandina mosaic virus, (NaMV), *Potexvirus*
Nandina stem pitting virus, (NSPV), *Capillovirus*
Naranjal virus, (NJLV), *Flaviviridae*
Narcissus degeneration virus, (NDV), *Potyviridae*
Narcissus late season yellows virus, (NLSYV), *Potyviridae*
Narcissus latent virus, (NLV), *Potyviridae*
Narcissus mosaic virus, (NMV), *Potexvirus*
Narcissus tip necrosis virus, (NTNV), *Tombusviridae*
Narcissus yellow stripe virus, (NYSV), *Potyviridae*
Nasoule virus, (NASV), *Rhabdoviridae*
Nasturtium mosaic virus, *Potyviridae*
Navarro virus, (NAVV), *Rhabdoviridae*
Ndelle virus, (NDEV), *Reoviridae*
Ndumu virus, (NDUV), *Togaviridae*
Neckar river virus, (NRV), *Tombusviridae*
Negro coffee mosaic virus, (NeCMV), *Potexvirus*
Nelson Bay orthoreovirus, (NBV), *Reoviridae*
Neodiprion sertifer NPV, (NeseNPV), *Baculoviridae*
Nepuyo virus, (NEPV), *Bunyaviridae*
Nerine latent virus, (NeLV), *Carlavirus*
Nerine virus X, (NVX), *Potexvirus*
Nerine virus Y, (NVY), *Potyviridae*
Nerine virus, (NV), *Potyviridae*
Nerine yellow stripe virus, (NeYSV), *Potyviridae*
Netivot virus, (NETV), *Reoviridae*
New Minto virus, (NMV), *Rhabdoviridae*
New York virus, (NYV), *Bunyaviridae*
New Zealand virus, (NZV), *Nodaviridae*
Newcastle disease virus, (NDV), *Paramyxoviridae*
Nezara viridula virus-1, (NVV-1), Unassigned
Ngaingan virus, (NGAV), *Rhabdoviridae*
Ngari virus, (NRIV), *Bunyaviridae*
Ngoupe virus, (NGOV), *Reoviridae*

Nicotiana glutinosa stunt viroid, (NGSVd), *Avsunviroidae*
Nicotiana tabacum Tnt1 virus, (NtaTnt1V), *Pseudoviridae*
Nicotiana tabacum Tto1 virus, (NtaTto1V), *Pseudoviridae*
Nicotiana velutina mosaic virus, (NVMV), Unassigned
Nilaparvata lugens reovirus, (NLRV), *Reoviridae*
Nile crocodile poxvirus, (CRV), *Poxviridae*
Nique virus, (NIQV), *Bunyaviridae*
Nkolbisson virus, (NKOV), *Rhabdoviridae*
NMH10 virus, *Bunyaviridae*
NMR-11 virus, *Bunyaviridae*
Noctua pronuba cypovirus 7, (NpCPV-7), *Reoviridae*
Nodamura virus, (NoV), *Nodaviridae*
Nola virus, (NOLAV), *Bunyaviridae*
North Clett virus, (NCLV), *Reoviridae*
North End virus, (NEDV), *Reoviridae*
Northern cereal mosaic virus, (NCMV), *Rhabdoviridae*
Northern pike herpesvirus, *Herpesviridae*
Northway virus, (NORV), *Bunyaviridae*
Norwalk virus, (NV), *Caliciviridae*
Norwalk virus, (NV), *Caliciviridae*
Nothoscordum mosaic virus, (NoMV), *Potyviridae*
Ntaya virus, (NTAV), *Flaviviridae*
Nudaurelia capensis β virus, (NβV) *Tetraviridae*
Nudaurelia capensis ε virusa, (NεV), *Tetraviridae*
Nudaurelia capensis ω virus, (NωV), *Tetraviridae*
Nudaurelia cytherea cypovirus 8, (NcCPV-8), *Reoviridae*
Nugget virus, (NUGV), *Reoviridae*
Nyabira virus, (NYAV), *Reoviridae*
Nyamanini virus, (NYMV), Unassigned
Nyando virus, (NDV), *Bunyaviridae*

O'nyong-nyong virus, (ONNV), *Togaviridae*
Oak-Vale virus, (OVRV), *Rhabdoviridae*
Oat blue dwarf virus, (OBDV), *Marafivirus*
Oat chlorotic stunt virus, (OCSV), *Tombusviridae*
Oat golden stripe virus, *Furovirus*
Oat mosaic virus, (OMV), *Potyviridae*
Oat necrotic mottle virus, (ONMV), *Potyviridae*
Oat sterile dwarf virus, (OSDV), *Reoviridae*
Oat striate mosaic virus, (OSMV), *Rhabdoviridae*
Obodhiang virus, (OBOV), *Rhabdoviridae*
Obuda pepper virus, (ObPV), *Tobamovirus*
Oceanside virus, (OCV), *Bunyaviridae*
Ockelbo virus, *Togaviridae*
Odontoglossum ringspot virus, (ORSV), *Tobamovirus*
Odrenisrou virus, (ODRV), *Bunyaviridae*

Oedaleus senigalensis entomopoxvirus 'O', (OSEV), *Poxviridae*
Oilseed rape mosaic virus, *Tobamovirus*
Oita virus, (OITAV), *Rhabdoviridae*
Okhotskiy virus, (OKHV), *Reoviridae*
Okola virus, (OKOV), *Bunyaviridae*
Okra leaf curl virus, (OLCV), *Geminiviridae*
Okra mosaic virus, (OkMV), *Tymovirus*
Olesicampe benefactor ichnovirus, (ObIV), *Polydnaviridae*
Olesicampe geniculatae ichnovirus, (OgIV), *Polydnaviridae*
Olifantsvlei virus, (OLIV), *Bunyaviridae*
Olive latent ringspot virus, (OLRSV), *Comoviridae*
Olive latent virus 1, (OLV-1), *Tombusviridae*
Olive latent virus 2, (OLV-2), *Bromoviridae*
Oliveros virus, (OLVV), *Arenaviridae*
Omo virus, (OMOV), *Bunyaviridae*
Omsk hemorrhagic fever virus, (OHFV), *Flaviviridae*
Oncorhynchus masou herpesvirus, *Herpesviridae*
Onion mite-borne latent virus, (OMbLV), *Allexivirus*
Onion yellow dwarf virus, (OYDV), *Potyviridae*
Ononis yellow mosaic virus, (OYMV), *Tymovirus*
Operophtera brumata cypovirus 2, (ObCPV-2), *Reoviridae*
Operophtera brumata cypovirus 3, (ObCPV-3), *Reoviridae*
Operophtera brumata entomopoxvirus 'L', (OBEV), *Poxviridae*
Opogonia iridescent virus, *Iridoviridae*
Oran virus, *Bunyaviridae*
Orangutan herpesvirus, *Herpesviridae*
Orchid fleck virus, (OFV), Unassigned
Orf virus, (ORFV), *Poxviridae*
Orgyia pseudosugata cypovirus 5, (OpCPV-5), *Reoviridae*
Orgyia pseudotsugata MNPV, (OpMNPV), *Baculoviridae*
Orgyia pseudotsugata SNPV, (OpSNPV), *Baculoviridae*
Oriboca virus, (ORIV), *Bunyaviridae*
Oriximina virus, (ORXV), *Bunyaviridae*
Ornithogalum mosaic virus, (OrMV), *Potyviridae*
Oropouche virus, (OROV), *Bunyaviridae*
Orungo virus 1 to 4, (ORUV-1 to 4), *Reoviridae*
Orungo virus, (ORUV), *Reoviridae*
Oryctes rhinoceros virus, (OrV), Unassigned
Ossa virus, (OSSAV), *Bunyaviridae*
Ostreid herpesvirus 1, (OsHV-1), *Herpesviridae*
Ouango virus, (OUAV), *Rhabdoviridae*
Oubi virus, (OUBIV), *Bunyaviridae*
Ourem virus, (OURV), *Reoviridae*
Ourmia melon virus, (OuMV), *Ourmiavirus*
Ovine adeno-associated virus, (OAAV), *Parvoviridae*
Ovine adenovirus 1, (OAdV-1), *Adenoviridae*
Ovine adenovirus 2-5, (OAdV-2 to 5), *Adenoviridae*
Ovine adenovirus 6, (OAdV-6), *Adenoviridae*
Ovine adenovirus A, (OAdV-A), *Adenoviridae*
Ovine adenovirus B, (OAdV-B), *Adenoviridae*
Ovine adenovirus C, (OAdV-C), *Adenoviridae*
Ovine adenovirus isolate 287, (OAdV-287), *Adenoviridae*
Ovine astrovirus 1, (OAstV-1), *Astroviridae*
Ovine astrovirus, (OAstV), *Astroviridae*
Ovine herpesvirus 1, (OvHV-1), *Herpesviridae*
Ovine herpesvirus 2, (OvHV-2), *Herpesviridae*
Ovine papillomavirus 1, (OPV-1), *Papillomaviridae*
Ovine papillomavirus 2, (OPV-2), *Papillomaviridae*
Ovine papillomavirus, (OPV), *Papillomaviridae*
Ovine pulmonary adenocarcinoma virus, *Retroviridae*
Owl hepatosplenitis herpesvirus, *Herpesviridae*

p2b-2 virus, *Arenaviridae*
p360 virus, *Bunyaviridae*
Pacific oyster herpesvirus, *Herpesviridae*
Pacific pond turtle herpesvirus, *Herpesviridae*
Pacora virus, (PCAV), *Bunyaviridae*
Pacui virus, (PACV), *Bunyaviridae*
Pahayokee virus, (PAHV), *Bunyaviridae*
Painted turtle herpesvirus, *Herpesviridae*
Pakistani cotton leaf curl virus, (PCLCuV), *Geminiviridae*
Palestina virus, (PLSV), *Bunyaviridae*
Palm mosaic virus, (PalMV), *Potyviridae*
Palyam virus, (PALV), *Reoviridae*
Palyam virus, (PALV), *Reoviridae*
Pampa virus, (PAMV), *Arenaviridae*
PAn 18400 virus, *Arenaviridae*
Pangola stunt virus, (PaSV), *Reoviridae*
Panicum mosaic satellite virus, Satellite
Panicum mosaic virus satellite RNA, Satellite
Panicum mosaic virus, (PMV), *Tombusviridae*
Panicum streak virus, (PanSV), *Geminiviridae*
Panolis flammea NPV, (PaflNPV), *Baculoviridae*
Papaya leaf curl virus, (PaLCV), *Geminiviridae*
Papaya leaf distortion mosaic virus, (PLDMV), *Potyviridae*
Papaya mosaic virus, (PapMV), *Potexvirus*
Papaya ringspot virus, (PRSV), *Potyviridae*
Papilio machaon cypovirus 2, (PmCPV-2), *Reoviridae*
Paprika mild mottle virus, (PaMMV), *Tobamovirus*
Paramecium bursaria Chlorella virus 1, (PBCV-1), *Phycodnaviridae*
Paramecium bursaria Chlorella virus A1, (PBCV-A1), *Phycodnaviridae*
Paramecium bursaria Chlorella virus AL1A, (PBCV-AL1A), *Phycodnaviridae*

Paramecium bursaria Chlorella virus AL2A, (PBCV-AL2A), *Phycodnaviridae*
Paramecium bursaria Chlorella virus AL2C, (PBCV-AL2C), *Phycodnaviridae*
Paramecium bursaria Chlorella virus B1, (PBCV-B1), *Phycodnaviridae*
Paramecium bursaria Chlorella virus BJ2C, (PBCV-BJ2C), *Phycodnaviridae*
Paramecium bursaria Chlorella virus CA1A, (PBCV-CA1A), *Phycodnaviridae*
Paramecium bursaria Chlorella virus CA1D, (PBCV-CA1D), *Phycodnaviridae*
Paramecium bursaria Chlorella virus CA2A, (PBCV-CA2A), *Phycodnaviridae*
Paramecium bursaria Chlorella virus CA4A, (PBCV-CA4A), *Phycodnaviridae*
Paramecium bursaria Chlorella virus CA4B, (PBCV-CA4B), *Phycodnaviridae*
Paramecium bursaria Chlorella virus CVBII, (PBCV-CVBII), *Phycodnaviridae*
Paramecium bursaria Chlorella virus CVK2, (PBCV-CVK2), *Phycodnaviridae*
Paramecium bursaria Chlorella virus CVU1, (PBCV-CVU1), *Phycodnaviridae*
Paramecium bursaria Chlorella virus G1, (PBCV-G1), *Phycodnaviridae*
Paramecium bursaria Chlorella virus IL2A, (PBCV-IL2A), *Phycodnaviridae*
Paramecium bursaria Chlorella virus IL2B, (PBCV-IL2B), *Phycodnaviridae*
Paramecium bursaria Chlorella virus IL3A, (PBCV-IL3A), *Phycodnaviridae*
Paramecium bursaria Chlorella virus IL3D, (PBCV-IL3D), *Phycodnaviridae*
Paramecium bursaria Chlorella virus IL5-2s1, (PBCV-IL5-2s1), *Phycodnaviridae*
Paramecium bursaria Chlorella virus M1, (PBCV-M1), *Phycodnaviridae*
Paramecium bursaria Chlorella virus MA1D, (PBCV-MA1D), *Phycodnaviridae*
Paramecium bursaria Chlorella virus MA1E, (PBCV-MA1E), *Phycodnaviridae*
Paramecium bursaria Chlorella virus NC1A, (PBCV-NC1A), *Phycodnaviridae*
Paramecium bursaria Chlorella virus NC1B, (PBCV-NC1B), *Phycodnaviridae*
Paramecium bursaria Chlorella virus NC1C, (PBCV-NC1C), *Phycodnaviridae*
Paramecium bursaria Chlorella virus NC1D, (PBCV-NC1D), *Phycodnaviridae*
Paramecium bursaria Chlorella virus NE8A, (PBCV-NE8A), *Phycodnaviridae*
Paramecium bursaria Chlorella virus NE8D, (PBCV-NE8D), *Phycodnaviridae*
Paramecium bursaria Chlorella virus NY2A, (PBCV-NY2A), *Phycodnaviridae*
Paramecium bursaria Chlorella virus NY2B, (PBCV-NY2B), *Phycodnaviridae*
Paramecium bursaria Chlorella virus NY2C, (PBCV-NY2C), *Phycodnaviridae*
Paramecium bursaria Chlorella virus NY2F, (PBCV-NY2F), *Phycodnaviridae*
Paramecium bursaria Chlorella virus NYb1, (PBCV-NYb1), *Phycodnaviridae*
Paramecium bursaria Chlorella virus NYs1, (PBCV-NYs1), *Phycodnaviridae*
Paramecium bursaria Chlorella virus R1, (PBCV-R1), *Phycodnaviridae*
Paramecium bursaria Chlorella virus SC1A, (PBCV-SC1A), *Phycodnaviridae*
Paramecium bursaria Chlorella virus SC1B, (PBCV-SC1B), *Phycodnaviridae*
Paramecium bursaria Chlorella virus SH6A, (PBCV-SH6A), *Phycodnaviridae*
Paramecium bursaria Chlorella virus XY6E, (PBCV-XY6E), *Phycodnaviridae*
Paramecium bursaria Chlorella virus XZ3A, (PBCV-XZ3A), *Phycodnaviridae*
Paramecium bursaria Chlorella virus XZ4A, (PBCV-XZ4A), *Phycodnaviridae*
Paramecium bursaria Chlorella virus XZ4C, (PBCV-XZ4C), *Phycodnaviridae*
Paramecium bursaria Chlorella virus XZ5C, (PBCV-XZ5C), *Phycodnaviridae*
Paramushir virus, *Bunyaviridae*
Paraná virus, (PARV), *Arenaviridae*
Parapoxvirus of red deer in New Zealand, (PVNZ), *Poxviridae*
Paravaccinia virus, *Poxviridae*
Pariacato virus, (PaV), *Nodaviridae*
Parietaria mottle virus, (PMoV), *Bromoviridae*
Parma wallaby herpesvirus, *Herpesviridae*
Paroo river virus, (PRV), *Reoviridae*
Parrot herpesvirus, *Herpesviridae*
Parry Creek virus, (PCRV), *Rhabdoviridae*
Parsley latent virus, (PaLV), Unassigned
Parsley virus 5, (PaV-5), *Potexvirus*
Parsley virus, (PaV), *Rhabdoviridae*
Parsnip mosaic virus, (ParMV), *Potyviridae*
Parsnip virus 3, (ParV-3), *Potexvirus*
Parsnip virus 5, (ParV-5), *Potexvirus*
Parsnip yellow fleck virus, (PYFV), *Sequiviridae*
Parvo-like virus of crabs, (PCV84), *Parvoviridae*
Paspalum striate mosaic virus, (PSMV), *Geminiviridae*
Passiflora latent virus, (PLV), *Carlavirus*
Passion fruit mottle virus, (PFMoV), *Potyviridae*
Passion fruit ringspot virus, (PFRSV), *Potyviridae*
Passion fruit woodiness virus, (PWV), *Potyviridae*

Passion fruit yellow mosaic virus, (PFYMV), *Tymovirus*
Pasteurella phage 22, (22), *Podoviridae*
Pasteurella phage 32, (32), *Siphoviridae*
Pasteurella phage AU, (AU), *Myoviridae*
Pasteurella phage AU, (AU), *Myoviridae*
Pasteurella phage C-2, (C-2), *Siphoviridae*
Pata virus, (PATAV), *Reoviridae*
Patas monkey herpesvirus deltaherpesvirus, *Herpesviridae*
Patchouli mild mosaic virus, (PatMMV), *Comoviridae*
Patchouli mottle virus, (PatMoV), *Potyviridae*
Patchouli virus X, (PatVX), *Potexvirus*
Pathum Thani virus, (PTHV), *Bunyaviridae*
Patois virus, (PATV), *Bunyaviridae*
Pea early-browning virus, (PEBV), *Tobravirus*
Pea enation mosaic virus satellite RNA, Satellite
Pea enation mosaic virus-1, (PEMV-1), *Luteoviridae*
Pea enation mosaic virus-2, (PEMV-2), *Umbravirus*
Pea green mottle virus, (PGMV), *Comoviridae*
Pea leafroll virus, *Luteoviridae*
Pea mild mosaic virus, (PMiMV), *Comoviridae*
Pea mosaic virus, *Potyviridae*
Pea necrosis virus, *Potyviridae*
Pea seed-borne mosaic virus, (PSbMV), *Potyviridae*
Pea streak virus, (PeSV), *Carlavirus*
Peach dapple viroid, *Pospiviroidae*
Peach latent mosaic viroid, (PLMVd), *Avsunviroidae*
Peach rosette mosaic virus, (PRMV), *Comoviridae*
Peacockpox virus, (PKPV), *Poxviridae*
Peanut bud necrosis virus, *Bunyaviridae*
Peanut chlorotic ring mottle virus, *Potyviridae*
Peanut chlorotic streak virus, (PCSV), *Caulimoviridae*
Peanut clump virus, (PCV), *Pecluvirus*
Peanut green mottle virus, (PeGMoV), *Potyviridae*
Peanut mild mottle virus, *Potyviridae*
Peanut mottle virus, (PeMoV), *Potyviridae*
Peanut stripe virus, *Potyviridae*
Peanut stunt virus satellite RNA, Satellite
Peanut stunt virus, (PSV), *Bromoviridae*
Peanut yellow mosaic virus, (PeYMV), *Tymovirus*
Peanut yellow spot virus, *Bunyaviridae*
Pear blister canker viroid, (PBCVd), *Pospiviroidae*
Pear rusty skin viroid, *Pospiviroidae*
Pear vein yellows virus, *Foveavirus*
Peaton virus, (PEAV), *Bunyaviridae*
Pecteilis mosaic virus, (PcMV), *Potyviridae*
Pectinophora gossypiella cypovirus 11, (PgCPV-11), *Reoviridae*
Pectinophora gossypiella virus, (PgV), Unassigned
Pelargonium flower break virus, (PFBV), *Tombusviridae*
Pelargonium leaf curl virus, (PLCV), *Tombusviridae*

Pelargonium vein clearing virus, (PVCV), *Rhabdoviridae*
Pelargonium zonate spot virus, (PZSV), Unassigned
Penaeus monodon NPV, (PemoNPV), *Baculoviridae*
Penguinpox virus, (PEPV), *Poxviridae*
Penicillium brevicompactum virus, (PbV), *Partitiviridae*
Penicillium chrysogenum virus, (PcV), *Partitiviridae*
Penicillium cyaneo-fulvum virus, (Pc-fV), *Partitiviridae*
Penicillium stoloniferum virus F, (PsV-F), *Partitiviridae*
Penicillium stoloniferum virus S, (PsV-S), *Partitiviridae*
Pepino latent virus, *Carlavirus*
Pepino mosaic virus, (PepMV), *Potexvirus*
Pepper huasteco virus, (PHV), *Geminiviridae*
Pepper leaf curl virus, (PepLCV), *Geminiviridae*
Pepper mild mosaic virus, (PMMV), *Potyviridae*
Pepper mild mottle virus, (PMMoV), *Tobamovirus*
Pepper mild tigré virus, (PepMTV), *Geminiviridae*
Pepper mottle virus, (PepMoV), *Potyviridae*
Pepper ringspot virus, (PepRSV), *Tobravirus*
Pepper severe mosaic virus, (PepSMV), *Potyviridae*
Pepper vein banding virus, (PVBV), *Potyviridae*
Pepper veinal mottle virus, (PVMV), *Potyviridae*
Perch hyperplasia virus, (PHV), *Retroviridae*
Percid herpesvirus 1, (PeHV-1), *Herpesviridae*
Perconia circinata virus, (PeCV), Unassigned
Perdicid herpesvirus 1, (PdHV-1), *Herpesviridae*
Pergamino virus, *Bunyaviridae*
Perilla mottle virus, (PerMoV, *Potyviridae*
Perinet virus, (PERV), *Rhabdoviridae*
Periplanata fuliginosa densovirus, (PfDNV), *Parvoviridae*
Peru tomato mosaic virus, (PTV), *Potyviridae*
Peste-des-petits-ruminants virus, (PPRV), *Paramyxoviridae*
Pestivirus of giraffe, *Flaviviridae*
Petevo virus, (PETV), *Reoviridae*
Petuluma, (FIV-P), *Retroviridae*
Petunia asteroid mosaic virus, (PetAMV), *Tombusviridae*
Petunia flower mottle virus, (PetFMV), *Potyviridae*
Petunia vein clearing virus, (PVCV), *Caulimoviridae*
Phalacrocoracid herpesvirus 1, (PhHV-1), *Herpesviridae*
Phalaenopsis chlorotic spot virus, (PhCSV), *Rhabdoviridae*
Phalera bucephala cypovirus 2, (PbCPV-2), *Reoviridae*
Phanerotoma flavitestacea bracovirus, (PfBV), *Polydnaviridae*
Pheasant adenovirus, (PhAdV-1), *Adenoviridae*

Phialophora radicicola virus 2-2-A, (PrV-2-2-A), *Partitiviridae*
Philosamia cynthia x ricini virus, (PxV), *Tetraviridae*
Phlogophera meticulosa cypovirus 3, (PmCPV-3), Reoviridae
Phlogophora meticulosa cypovirus 8, (PmCPV-8), *Reoviridae*
Phnom Penh bat virus, (PPBV), *Flaviviridae*
Phocid herpesvirus 1, (PhoHV-1), *Herpesviridae*
Phocine distemper virus, (PDV), *Paramyxoviridae*
Pholetesor ornigis bracovirus, (PoBV), *Polydnaviridae*
Physalis mottle virus, (PhyMV), *Tymovirus*
Physalis severe mottle virus, (PhySMV), *Bunyaviridae*
Physarum polycephalum Tp1 virus, (PpoTp1V), *Pseudoviridae*
Pichinde virus, (PICV), *Arenaviridae*
Picola virus, (PIAV), *Reoviridae*
Pieris brassicae granulovirus, (PbGV, ArGV-1), *Baculoviridae*
Pieris rapae cypovirus 12, (PrCPV-12), *Reoviridae*
Pieris rapae cypovirus 2, (PrCPV-2), *Reoviridae*
Pieris rapae cypovirus 3, (PrCPV-3), *Reoviridae*
Pieris rapae densovirus, (PrDNV), *Parvoviridae*
Pigeon adenovirus, (PiAdV), *Adenoviridae*
Pigeon circovirus, (PiCV), *Circoviridae*
Pigeon herpesvirus, *Herpesviridae*
Pigeon pea mosaic mottle viroid, (PPMMoVd), *Avsunviroidae*
Pigeon pea proliferation virus, (PPPV), *Rhabdoviridae*
Pigeonpox virus, (PGPV), *Poxviridae*
Pike fry rhabdovirus, (PFRV), *Rhabdoviridae*
Pineapple bacilliform virus, (PBV), *Caulimoviridae*
Pineapple chlorotic leaf streak virus, (PCLSV), *Rhabdoviridae*
Pineapple mealybug wilt-associated virus 1, (PMWaV-1), *Closteroviridae*
Pineapple mealybug wilt-associated virus 2, (PMWaV-2), *Closteroviridae*
Piper yellow mottle virus, (PYMoV), *Caulimoviridae*
Pirital virus, (PIRV), *Arenaviridae*
Piry virus, (PIRYV), *Rhabdoviridae*
Pisum virus, (PisV), *Rhabdoviridae*
Pittosporum vein yellowing virus, (PVYV), *Rhabdoviridae*
Pixuna virus, (PIXV), *Togaviridae*
Plantago asiatica mosaic virus, (PlAMV), *Potexvirus*
Plantago mottle virus, (PlMoV), *Tymovirus*
Plantago severe mottle virus, (PlSMoV), *Potexvirus*
Plantago virus 4, (PlV-4), *Caulimoviridae*
Plantain mottle virus, (PIMV), *Rhabdoviridae*
Plantain virus 6, (PlV-6), *Tombusviridae*
Plantain virus 7, (PlV-7), *Potyviridae*
Plantain virus 8, (PlV-8), *Carlavirus*

Plantain virus X, (PlVX), *Potexvirus*
Plautia stali intestine virus, (PSIV), "CrPV-like viruses"
Playas virus, (PLAV), *Bunyaviridae*
Pleioblastus mosaic virus, (PleMV), *Potyviridae*
Pleuronectid herpesvirus 1, (PlHV-1), *Herpesviridae*
Plodia interpunctella granulovirus, (PiGV), *Baculoviridae*
Plum dapple viroid, *Pospiviroidae*
Plum pox virus, (PPV), *Potyviridae*
Poa semilatent virus, (PSLV), *Hordeivirus*
Poinsettia cryptic virus, (PnCV), *Partitiviridae*
Poinsettia mosaic virus, (PnMV), *Tymovirus*
Pokeweed mosaic virus, (PkMV), *Potyviridae*
Poliovirus, (PV), *Picornaviridae*
Polistes hebraeus cypovirus 13, (PhCPV-13), *Reoviridae*
Pongine herpesvirus 1, (PoHV-1), *Herpesviridae*
Pongine herpesvirus 2, (PoHV-2), *Herpesviridae*
Pongine herpesvirus 3, (PoHV-3), *Herpesviridae*
Pongola virus, (PGAV), *Bunyaviridae*
Ponteves virus, (PTVV), *Bunyaviridae*
Poovoot virus, (POOV), *Reoviridae*
Poplar mosaic virus, (PopMV), *Carlavirus*
Populus virus, (PV), *Potyviridae*
Porcelio dilatatus reovirus, (PdRV), *Reoviridae*
Porcelio dilatatus iridescent virus, *Iridoviridae*
Porcine adenovirus 1-3, (PAdV-1 to 3), *Adenoviridae*
Porcine adenovirus 4, (PAdV-4), *Adenoviridae*
Porcine adenovirus 5, (PAdV-5), *Adenoviridae*
Porcine adenovirus A, (PAdV-B), *Adenoviridae*
Porcine adenovirus B, (PAdV-B), *Adenoviridae*
Porcine adenovirus C, (PAdV-C), *Adenoviridae*
Porcine astrovirus 1, (PAstV-1), *Astroviridae*
Porcine astrovirus, (PAstV), *Astroviridae*
Porcine circovirus, (PCV), *Circoviridae*
Porcine enteric calicivirus, (PECV), *Caliciviridae*
Porcine enterovirus 1, *Picornaviridae*
Porcine enterovirus 10, (PEV-10), *Picornaviridae*
Porcine enterovirus 11-13, (PEV-11 to 13), *Picornaviridae*
Porcine enterovirus 2-7, (PEV-2 to 7), *Picornaviridae*
Porcine enterovirus 8, (PEV-8), *Picornaviridae*
Porcine enterovirus 9, (PEV-9), *Picornaviridae*
Porcine enterovirus A, (PEV-A), *Picornaviridae*
Porcine enterovirus B, (PEV-B), *Picornaviridae*
Porcine epidemic diarrhea virus, (PEDV), *Coronaviridae*
Porcine hemagglutinating encephalomyelitis virus, (HEV), *Coronaviridae*
Porcine parvovirus, (PPV), *Parvoviridae*
Porcine respiratory and reproductive syndrome virus, *Arteriviridae*
Porcine respiratory coronavirus, (PRCoV), *Coronaviridae*

Porcine rotavirus Cowden, (PoRV-C/Cowden), *Reoviridae*
Porcine rotavirus DC-9, (PoRV-E/DC9), *Reoviridae*
Porcine rubulavirus, (PoRV), *Paramyxoviridae*
Porcine teschovirus 1, (PTV-1), *Picornaviridae*
Porcine teschovirus, (PTV), *Picornaviridae*
Porcine torovirus, (PoTV), *Coronaviridae*
Porcine type-C oncovirus, (PCOV), *Retroviridae*
Porton virus, (PORV), *Rhabdoviridae*
Potato aucuba mosaic virus, (PAMV), *Potexvirus*
Potato black ringspot virus, (PBRSV), *Comoviridae*
Potato leafroll virus, (PLRV), *Luteoviridae*
Potato mop-top virus, (PMTV), *Pomovirus*
Potato spindle tuber viroid, (PSTVd), *Pospiviroidae*
Potato virus A, (PVA), *Potyviridae*
Potato virus M, (PVM), *Carlavirus*
Potato virus S, (PVS), *Carlavirus*
Potato virus T, (PVT), *Trichovirus*
Potato virus U, (PVU), *Comoviridae*
Potato virus V, (PVV), *Potyviridae*
Potato virus X, (PVX), *Potexvirus*
Potato virus Y, (PVY), *Potyviridae*
Potato yellow dwarf virus, (PYDV), *Rhabdoviridae*
Potato yellow mosaic virus, (PYMV), *Geminiviridae*
Pothos latent virus, (PoLV) *Tombusviridae*
Potiskum virus, (POTV), *Flaviviridae*
Potosi virus, (POTV), *Bunyaviridae*
Powassan virus, (POWV), *Flaviviridae*
Precarious Point virus, (PPV), *Bunyaviridae*
Pretoria virus, (PREV), *Bunyaviridae*
Primate calicivirus, (VESV/Pan-1), *Caliciviridae*
Primate T-lymphotropic virus 1, (PTLV-1), *Retroviridae*
Primate T-lymphotropic virus 2, (PTLV-2), *Retroviridae*
Primate T-lymphotropic virus 3, (PTLV-3), *Retroviridae*
Primula mosaic virus, (PrMV), *Potyviridae*
Primula mottle virus, (PrMoV), *Potyviridae*
Prospect Hill virus, (PHV), *Bunyaviridae*
Protapanteles paleacritae bracovirus, (PpBV), *Polydnaviridae*
Prune dwarf virus, (PDV), *Bromoviridae*
Prunus necrotic ringspot virus, (PNRSV), *Bromoviridae*
Prunus virus S, (PruVS), *Carlavirus*
Pseudaletia includens densovirus, (PiDNV), *Parvoviridae*
Pseudaletia unipuncta cypovirus 11, (PuCPV-11), *Reoviridae*
Pseuderanthemum yellow vein virus, (PYVV), *Geminiviridae*
Pseudocowpox virus, (PCPV), *Poxviridae*
Pseudomonas phage 12S, (12S), *Myoviridae*
Pseudomonas phage 42, (42), *Myoviridae*

Pseudomonas phage 525, (525), *Podoviridae*
Pseudomonas phage 7s, (7s), *Leviviridae*
Pseudomonas phage D3, (D3), *Siphoviridae*
Pseudomonas phage F116, (F116), *Podoviridae*
Pseudomonas phage gh-1, (gh-1), *Podoviridae*
Pseudomonas phage Kf1, (Kf1), *Siphoviridae*
Pseudomonas phage M6, (M6), *Siphoviridae*
Pseudomonas phage PB-1, (PB-1), *Myoviridae*
Pseudomonas phage Pf1, (Pf1), *Inoviridae*
Pseudomonas phage Pf2, (Pf2), *Inoviridae*
Pseudomonas phage Pf3, (Pf3), *Inoviridae*
Pseudomonas phage PP7, (PP7), *Leviviridae*
Pseudomonas phage PP8, (PP8), *Myoviridae*
Pseudomonas phage PRR1, (PRR1), *Leviviridae*
Pseudomonas phage PS17, (PS17), *Myoviridae*
Pseudomonas phage PS4, (PS4), *Siphoviridae*
Pseudomonas phage PsP3, (PsP3), *Myoviridae*
Pseudomonas phage Pssy9220, (Psy9220), *Podoviridae*
Pseudomonas phage SD1, (SD1), *Siphoviridae*
Pseudomonas phage ϕ6, (ϕ6), *Cystoviridae*
Pseudomonas phage ϕCTX, (ϕCTX), *Myoviridae*
Pseudomonas phage ϕKZ, (ϕKZ), *Myoviridae*
Pseudomonas phage ϕPLS27, (ϕPLS27), *Podoviridae*
Pseudomonas phage ϕPLS743, (ϕPLS743), *Podoviridae*
Pseudomonas phage ϕW-14, (ϕW-14), *Myoviridae*
Pseudoplusia includens virus, (PiV), *Tetraviridae*
Pseudorabies virus, *Herpesviridae*
Psittacid herpesvirus 1, (PsHV-1), *Herpesviridae*
Psittacinepox virus, (PSPV), *Poxviridae*
Psophocarpus necrotic mosaic virus, *Carlavirus*
Pteroteinon laufella virus-1, (PlV-1), Unassigned
Puchong virus, (PUCV), *Rhabdoviridae*
Pueblo Viejo virus, (PVV), *Bunyaviridae*
Puffin Island virus, (PIV), *Bunyaviridae*
Puma lentivirus (PLV-14), (PLV), *Retroviridae*
Punta Salinas virus, (PSV), *Bunyaviridae*
Punta Toro virus D-4021A, (PTV), *Bunyaviridae*
Punta Toro virus, (PTV), *Bunyaviridae*
Purus virus, (PURV), *Reoviridae*
Puumala virus, (PUUV), *Bunyaviridae*
Python orthoreovirus, (PRV), *Reoviridae*

Qalyub virus, (QYBV), *Bunyaviridae*
Quail pea mosaic virus, (QPMV), *Comoviridae*
Quailpox virus, (QUPV), *Poxviridae*
Quaranfil virus, (QRFV), Unassigned
Queensland fruit fly virus, (QFFV), Unassigned
Quokka poxvirus, (QPV), *Poxviridae*

R22 virus, *Bunyaviridae*
Rabbit calicivirus, (RCV), *Caliciviridae*
Rabbit coronavirus, (RbCoV), *Coronaviridae*

Rabbit fibroma virus, (SFV), *Poxviridae*
Rabbit hemorrhagic disease virus, (RHDV), *Caliciviridae*
Rabbit hemorrhagic disease virus-AST89, (RHDV-AST89), *Caliciviridae*
Rabbit hemorrhagic disease virus-BS89, (RHDV-BS89), *Caliciviridae*
Rabbit hemorrhagic disease virus-FRG, (RHDV-FRG), *Caliciviridae*
Rabbit hemorrhagic disease virus-SD, (RHDV-SD), *Caliciviridae*
Rabbit hemorrhagic disease virus-V351, (RHDV-V351), *Caliciviridae*
Rabbit kidney vacuolating virus, (RKV), *Polyomaviridae*
Rabbitpox virus, (RPXV), *Poxviridae*
Rabies virus, (RABV), *Rhabdoviridae*
Raccoon parvovirus, (RPV), *Parvoviridae*
Raccoonpox virus, (RCNV), *Poxviridae*
Rachiplusia ou MNPV, (RoMNPV), *Baculoviridae*
Radi virus, (RADIV), *Rhabdoviridae*
Radish mosaic virus, (RaMV), *Comoviridae*
Radish vein clearing virus, (RaVCV), *Potyviridae*
Radish yellow edge virus, (RYEV), *Partitiviridae*
Rainbow trout virus, (RTV), *Iridoviridae*
Ranid herpesvirus 1, (RaHV-1), *Herpesviridae*
Ranid herpesvirus 2, (RaHV-2), *Herpesviridae*
Ranunculus mottle virus, (RanMoV), *Potyviridae*
Ranunculus repens symptomless virus, (RaRSV), *Rhabdoviridae*
Ranunculus white mottle virus, (RWMV), *Ophiovirus*
Raphanus virus, (RaV), *Rhabdoviridae*
Raspberry bushy dwarf virus, (RBDV), *Idaeovirus*
Raspberry ringspot virus, (RpRSV), *Comoviridae*
Raspberry vein chlorosis virus, (RVCV), *Rhabdoviridae*
Rat coronavirus, (RtCoV), *Coronaviridae*
Rat cytomegalovirus, *Herpesviridae*
Rat encephalomyelitis virus, (REV), *Picornaviridae*
Rat virus, *Parvoviridae*
Rattlesnake orthoreovirus, (RRV), *Reoviridae*
Raza virus, (RAZAV), *Bunyaviridae*
Razdan virus, (RAZV), *Bunyaviridae*
Red clover cryptic virus 2, (RCCV-2), *Partitiviridae*
Red clover mosaic virus, (RCIMV), *Rhabdoviridae*
Red clover mottle virus, (RCMV), *Comoviridae*
Red clover necrotic mosaic virus, (RCNMV), *Tombusviridae*
Red clover vein mosaic virus, (RCVMV), *Carlavirus*
Red deer herpesvirus, *Herpesviridae*
Red kangaroo poxvirus, (KPV), *Poxviridae*
Red pepper cryptic virus 1, (RPCV-1), *Partitiviridae*
Red pepper cryptic virus 2, (RPCV-2), *Partitiviridae*
Redfin perch virus, (RFPV), *Iridoviridae*

Redspotted grouper nervous necrosis virus, (RGNNV), *Nodaviridae*
Redwood Park virus, (RPV), *Iridoviridae*
Reed Ranch virus, (RRV), *Rhabdoviridae*
Regina ranavirus, (RRV), *Iridoviridae*
Reindeer herpesvirus, *Herpesviridae*
Rembrandt tulip breaking virus, (ReTBV), *Potyviridae*
Reptile calicivirus, (VESV/Cro-1), *Caliciviridae*
Resistencia virus, (RTAV), *Bunyaviridae*
Restan virus, (RESV), *Bunyaviridae*
Reston Ebola virus Philippines, *Filoviridae*
Reston Ebola virus Reston, *Filoviridae*
Reston Ebola virus Siena, *Filoviridae*
Reston Ebola virus Texas, *Filoviridae*
Reston Ebola virus, (REBOV), *Filoviridae*
Reticuloendotheliosis virus (strain T, A), (REV), *Retroviridae*
Rhesus EBV-like herpesvirus, *Herpesviridae*
Rhesus leukocyte associated herpesvirus strain 1, *Herpesviridae*
Rhesus monkey cytomegalovirus, *Herpesviridae*
Rhesus rhadinovirus, *Herpesviridae*
Rheumatoid arthritis virus, (RAV-1), *Parvoviridae*
Rhizidiomyces virus, (RZV), *Rhizidiovirus*
Rhizobium phage 16-2-12, (16-2-12), *Siphoviridae*
Rhizobium phage 16-6-2, (16-6-2), *Siphoviridae*
Rhizobium phage 2, (2), *Podoviridae*
Rhizobium phage 317, (317), *Siphoviridae*
Rhizobium phage 5, (5), *Siphoviridae*
Rhizobium phage 7-7-7, (7-7-7), *Siphoviridae*
Rhizobium phage CM$_1$, (CM$_1$), *Myoviridae*
Rhizobium phage CT4, (CT4), *Myoviridae*
Rhizobium phage m, (m), *Myoviridae*
Rhizobium phage NM1, (NM1), *Siphoviridae*
Rhizobium phage NT2, (NT2), *Siphoviridae*
Rhizobium phage S, (S), *Podoviridae*
Rhizobium phage WT1, (WT1), *Myoviridae*
Rhizobium phage ϕ2037/1, (ϕ2037/1), *Siphoviridae*
Rhizobium phage ϕ2042, (ϕ2042), *Podoviridae*
Rhizobium phage ϕgal-1/R, (ϕgal-1/R), *Myoviridae*
Rhizoctonia solani virus, (RsV), *Partitiviridae*
Rhododendron necrotic ringspot virus, (RoNRSV), *Potexvirus*
Rhopalosiphum padi virus, (RhPV), "CrPV-like viruses"
Rhubarb temperate virus, (RTV), *Partitiviridae*
Rhubarb virus 1, (RV-1), *Potexvirus*
Rhynchosia mosaic virus, (RhMV), *Geminiviridae*
RI-1 virus, *Bunyaviridae*
Ribgrass mosaic virus, (RMV), *Tobamovirus*
Rice black streaked dwarf virus, (RBSDV), *Reoviridae*
Rice dwarf virus, (RDV), *Reoviridae*
Rice gall dwarf virus, (RGDV), *Reoviridae*

rice giallume, *Luteoviridae*
Rice grassy stunt virus, (RGSV), *Tenuivirus*
Rice hoja blanca virus, (RHBV), *Tenuivirus*
Rice necrosis mosaic virus, (RNMV), *Potyviridae*
Rice ragged stunt virus, (RRSV), *Reoviridae*
Rice stripe necrosis virus, (RSNV), *Furovirus*
Rice stripe virus, (RSV), *Tenuivirus*
Rice transitory yellowing virus, (RTYV), *Rhabdoviridae*
Rice tungro bacilliform virus, (RTBV), *Caulimoviridae*
Rice tungro spherical virus, (RTSV), *Sequiviridae*
Rice wilted stunt virus, (RWSV), *Tenuivirus*
Rice yellow mottle virus satellite, Satellite
Rice yellow mottle virus, (RYMV), *Sobemovirus*
Rice yellow stunt virus, (RYSV), *Rhabdoviridae*
Rift Valley fever virus, (RVFV), *Bunyaviridae*
RIID 3229 virus, *Arenaviridae*
Rinderpest virus, (RPV), *Paramyxoviridae*
Rio Bravo virus, (RBV), *Flaviviridae*
Rio Grande cichlid virus, (RGRCV), *Rhabdoviridae*
Rio Grande virus, (RGV), *Bunyaviridae*
Rio Mamore virus, (RIOMV), *Bunyaviridae*
Rio Segundo virus, (RIOSV), *Bunyaviridae*
RM-97 virus, *Bunyaviridae*
RML 105355 virus, (RMLV), *Bunyaviridae*
Roan antelope herpesvirus, *Herpesviridae*
Robinia mosaic virus satellite RNA, Satellite
Robinia mosaic virus, *Bromoviridae*
Rochambeau virus, (RBUV), *Rhabdoviridae*
Rocio virus, (ROCV), *Flaviviridae*
Ross' goose hepatitis B virus, (RGHBV), *Hepadnaviridae*
Ross River virus, (RRV), *Togaviridae*
Rost Island virus, (RSTV), *Reoviridae*
Rotavirus A, (RV-A), *Reoviridae*
Rotavirus B, (RV-B), *Reoviridae*
Rotavirus C, (RV-C), *Reoviridae*
Rotavirus D, (RV-D), *Reoviridae*
Rotavirus E, (RV-E), *Reoviridae*
Rotavirus F, (RV-F), *Reoviridae*
Rotavirus G, (RV-G), *Reoviridae*
Rotifer birnavirus, (RBV), *Birnaviridae*
Rous sarcoma virus (Prague C), (RSV-Pr-C), *Retroviridae*
Rous sarcoma virus (Schmidt-Ruppin B), (RSV-SR-B), *Retroviridae*
Rous sarcoma virus (Schmidt-Ruppin D), (RSV-SR-D), *Retroviridae*
Rous sarcoma virus, (RSV), *Retroviridae*
Royal Farm virus, (RFV), *Flaviviridae*
RT parvovirus, (RTPV), *Parvoviridae*
Rubella virus, (RUBV), *Togaviridae*
Rubus Chinese seed-borne virus, (RCSV), *Comoviridae*

Rudbeckia mosaic virus, (RuMV), *Potyviridae*
Rupestris stem pitting-associated virus, (RSPaV), *Foveavirus*
Ryegrass cryptic virus, (RGCV), *Partitiviridae*
Ryegrass mosaic virus, (RGMV), *Potyviridae*

S 1954-847-32 virus, (TURV), *Bunyaviridae*
SA15 virus, *Herpesviridae*
SA6 virus, *Herpesviridae*
SAAAr 5133 virus, (OLIV), *Bunyaviridae*
SAAn 3518 virus, (TETEV), *Bunyaviridae*
SAAr 53 virus, (SIMV), *Bunyaviridae*
Sabiá virus, (SABV), *Arenaviridae*
Sabin virus, (SFNV), *Bunyaviridae*
Sabo virus, (SABOV), *Bunyaviridae*
Saboya virus, (SABV), *Flaviviridae*
Sacbrood virus, (SBV), Unassigned
Saccharomyces cerevisiae M virus, Satellite
Saccharomyces cerevisiae narnavirus 20S RNA, (ScNV-20S), *Narnaviridae*
Saccharomyces cerevisiae narnavirus 23S RNA, (ScNV-23S), *Narnaviridae*
Saccharomyces cerevisiae Ty1 virus, (SceTy1V), *Pseudoviridae*
Saccharomyces cerevisiae Ty2 virus, (SceTy2V), *Pseudoviridae*
Saccharomyces cerevisiae Ty3 virus, (SceTy3V), *Metaviridae*
Saccharomyces cerevisiae Ty4 virus, (SceTy4V), *Pseudoviridae*
Saccharomyces cerevisiae Ty5 virus, (SceTy5V), *Pseudoviridae*
Saccharomyces cerevisiae virus L-A (L1), (ScV-L-A), *Totiviridae*
Saccharomyces cerevisiae virus L-BC (La), (ScV-L-BC), *Totiviridae*
Sagiyama virus, *Togaviridae*
Saguaro cactus virus, (SgCV), *Tombusviridae*
Saimiriine herpesvirus 1, (SaHV-1), *Herpesviridae*
Saimiriine herpesvirus 2, (SaHV-2), *Herpesviridae*
Sainpaulia leaf necrosis virus, (SLNV), *Rhabdoviridae*
Saint-Floris virus, (SAFV), *Bunyaviridae*
Sakhalin virus, (SAKV), *Bunyaviridae*
Sal Vieja virus, (SVV), *Flaviviridae*
Salanga poxvirus, (SGV), *Poxviridae*
Salanga virus, (SGAV), *Bunyaviridae*
Salehebad I-81 virus, (SALV), *Bunyaviridae*
Salehebad virus, (SALV), *Bunyaviridae*
Salmon reovirus, (SSRV), *Reoviridae*
Salmonid herpesvirus 1, (SalHV-1), *Herpesviridae*
Salmonid herpesvirus 2, (SalHV-2), *Herpesviridae*
Sambucus vein clearing virus, (SVCV), *Rhabdoviridae*

Sammons's Opuntia virus, (SOV), *Tobamovirus*
San Angelo virus, (SAV), *Bunyaviridae*
San Juan virus, (SJV), *Bunyaviridae*
San Miguel sea lion virus, serotype 1, (VESV/SMSV-1), *Caliciviridae*
San Miguel sea lion virus, serotype 17, (VESV/SMSV-17), *Caliciviridae*
San Miguel sea lion virus, serotype 4, (VESV/SMSV-4), *Caliciviridae*
San Perlita virus, (SPV), *Flaviviridae*
Sand rat nuclear inclusion agents, *Herpesviridae*
Sandfly fever Naples virus, (SFNV), *Bunyaviridae*
Sandfly fever Sicilian virus, (SFSV), *Bunyaviridae*
Sandjimba virus, (SJAV), *Rhabdoviridae*
Sango virus, (SANV), *Bunyaviridae*
Santa Rosa virus, (SARV), *Bunyaviridae*
Santarem virus, (STMV), *Bunyaviridae*
Santee-Cooper ranavirus, (SCRV), *Iridoviridae*
Santosai temperate virus, (STV), *Partitiviridae*
Sapphire II virus, (SAPV), *Bunyaviridae*
Sapporo virus, (SV), *Caliciviridae*
Sapporo virus-Houston/86, (SV-Houston/86), *Caliciviridae*
Sapporo virus-Houston/90, (SV-Houston/90), *Caliciviridae*
Sapporo virus-London/29845, (SV-London/29845), *Caliciviridae*
Sapporo virus-Manchester, (SV-Manchester), *Caliciviridae*
Sapporo virus-Parkville, (SV-Parkville), *Caliciviridae*
Sapporo virus-Sapporo, (SV-Sapporo), *Caliciviridae*
Saraca virus, (SRAV), *Reoviridae*
Sarracenia purpurea virus, (SPV), *Rhabdoviridae*
Sathuperi virus, (SATV), *Bunyaviridae*
Satsuma dwarf virus, (SDV), *Comoviridae*
Saturnia pavonia virus, (SpV), *Tetraviridae*
Saumarez Reef virus, (SREV), *Flaviviridae*
Sawgrass virus, (SAWV), *Rhabdoviridae*
Schefflera ringspot virus, (SRV), *Caulimoviridae*
Schistocera gregaria entomopoxvirus 'O', (SGEV), *Poxviridae*
Schizosaccharomyces pombe Tf1 virus, (SpoTf1V), *Metaviridae*
Schizosaccharomyces pombe Tf2 virus, (SpoTf2V), *Metaviridae*
Sciurid herpesvirus 1, (ScHV-2), *Herpesviridae*
Sciurid herpesvirus 2, (ScHV-2), *Herpesviridae*
Scrophularia mottle virus, (ScrMV), *Tymovirus*
Sea-bass virus-1, (SBV), *Picornaviridae*
Seal distemper virus, *Paramyxoviridae*
Sealpox virus, *Poxviridae*
Seletar virus, (SELV), *Reoviridae*
Semliki Forest virus, (SFV), *Togaviridae*
Sena Madureira virus, (SMV), *Rhabdoviridae*
Sendai virus, (SeV), *Paramyxoviridae*
Seoul virus, (SEOV), *Bunyaviridae*
Sepik virus, (SEPV), *Flaviviridae*
Sericesthis iridescent virus, *Iridoviridae*
Serotype A of BCMV, *Potyviridae*
Serra do Navio virus, (SDNV), *Bunyaviridae*
Serrano golden mosaic virus, (SGMV), *Geminiviridae*
Sesame mosaic virus, *Potyviridae*
Setora nitens virus, (SnV), *Tetraviridae*
Setothosea asigna virus, (SaV), *Tetraviridae*
Shallot latent virus, (SLV), *Carlavirus*
Shallot mite-borne latent virus, (ShMbLV), *Allexivirus*
Shallot virus X, (ShV-X), *Allexivirus*
Shallot yellow stripe virus, (SYSV), *Potyviridae*
Shamonda virus, (SHAV), *Bunyaviridae*
Shark River virus, (SRV), *Bunyaviridae*
Sheep pulmonary adenomatosis associated herpesvirus, *Herpesviridae*
Sheep-associated malignant catarrhal fever virus, *Herpesviridae*
Sheeppox virus, (SPPV), *Poxviridae*
Shiant Islands virus, (SHIV), *Reoviridae*
Shokwe virus, (SHOV), *Bunyaviridae*
Shope fibroma virus, *Poxviridae*
Shuni virus, (SHUV), *Bunyaviridae*
Sialodacryoadenitis virus, (SDAV), *Coronaviridae*
Siamese cobra herpesvirus, *Herpesviridae*
Sibine fusca densovirus, (SfDNV), *Parvoviridae*
Sida golden mosaic virus, (SiGMV), *Geminiviridae*
Sida yellow vein virus, (SiYVV), *Geminiviridae*
Sigma virus, (SIGMAV), *Rhabdoviridae*
Sikhote-Alyn virus, (SAV), *Picornaviridae*
Silverwater virus, (SILV), *Bunyaviridae*
Simbu virus, (SIMV), *Bunyaviridae*
Simian adenovirus 1, 5, 7, 8, 12, 15, 17, 18, 20, 26?, 27?, (SAdV-1, 5, 7, 8, 12, 15, 17, 18, 20, 26?, 27?), *Adenoviridae*
Simian adenovirus 13, (SAdV-13), *Adenoviridae*
Simian adenovirus 16, 19, (SAdV-16, 19), *Adenoviridae*
Simian adenovirus 21, (SAdV-21), *Adenoviridae*
Simian adenovirus 22-25, (SAdV-22-25), *Adenoviridae*
Simian adenovirus 2-4, 6, (SAdV-2-4, 6), *Adenoviridae*
Simian adenovirus 9-11, 14, (SAdV-9-11, 14), *Adenoviridae*
Simian adenovirus, (SAdV), *Adenoviridae*
Simian enterovirus 1 to 18, (SEV-1 to 18), *Picornaviridae*
Simian enterovirus N125, (SEV-N125), *Picornaviridae*
Simian enterovirus N203, (SEV-N203), *Picornaviridae*
Simian foamy virus 1, (SFV-1), *Retroviridae*
Simian foamy virus 3, (SFV-3), *Retroviridae*

Simian hemorrhagic fever virus, (SHFV), *Arteriviridae*
Simian hepatitis A virus, (SHAV), *Picornaviridae*
Simian immunodeficiency virus African green monkey 155, (SIV-agm.155), *Retroviridae*
Simian immunodeficiency virus African green monkey 3, (SIV-agm.3), *Retroviridae*
Simian immunodeficiency virus African green monkey gr-1, (SIV-agm.gr), *Retroviridae*
Simian immunodeficiency virus African green monkey Sab-1, (SIV-agm.sab), *Retroviridae*
Simian immunodeficiency virus African green monkey Tan-1, (SIV-agm.tan), *Retroviridae*
Simian immunodeficiency virus African green monkey TYO, (SIV-agm.TYO), *Retroviridae*
Simian immunodeficiency virus African Green Monkey, (SIV-agm), *Retroviridae*
Simian immunodeficiency virus chimpanzee SIV, (SIV-cpz), *Retroviridae*
Simian immunodeficiency virus mandrill SIV, (SIV-mnd), *Retroviridae*
Simian immunodeficiency virus pig-tailed macaque, (SIV-mne), *Retroviridae*
Simian immunodeficiency virus red capped mangabey SIV, (SIV-rcm), *Retroviridae*
Simian immunodeficiency virus Rhesus (Maccaca mulatta), (SIV-mac), *Retroviridae*
Simian immunodeficiency virus sooty mangabey SIV-H4, (SIV-sm), *Retroviridae*
Simian immunodeficiency virus stump-tailed macaque (stm), (SIV-stm), *Retroviridae*
Simian immunodeficiency virus sykes monkey SIV, (SIV-syk), *Retroviridae*
Simian immunodeficiency virus, (SIV), *Retroviridae*
Simian retrovirus 1, (SRV-1), *Retroviridae*
Simian retrovirus 2, (SRV-2), *Retroviridae*
Simian rotavirus SA11, (SiRV-A/SA11), *Reoviridae*
Simian sarcoma virus, *Retroviridae*
Simian T-lymphotropic virus 1, (STLV-1), *Retroviridae*
Simian T-lymphotropic virus 2, (STLV-2), *Retroviridae*
Simian T-lymphotropic virus 3, (STLV-3), *Retroviridae*
Simian varicella virus, *Herpesviridae*
Simian virus 10, (SV-10), *Paramyxoviridae*
Simian virus 12, (SV-12), *Polyomaviridae*
Simian virus 40, (SV-40), *Polyomaviridae*
Simian virus 41, (SV-41), *Paramyxoviridae*
Simian virus 5, (SV-5), *Paramyxoviridae*
Simulium sp. iridescent virus, *Iridoviridae*
Simulium vittatum densovirus, (SvDNV), *Parvoviridae*
Sin Nombre virus, (SNV), *Bunyaviridae*

Sinaloa tomato leaf curl virus, (STLCV), *Geminiviridae*
Sindbis virus, (SINV), *Togaviridae*
Sint-Jem's onion latent virus, (SJOLV), *Carlavirus*
Sitke waterborne virus, (SWBV), *Tombusviridae*
Sitobion avenae virus, (SaV), Unassigned
Sixgun city virus, (SCV), *Reoviridae*
Skunk calicivirus, (VESV/SCV), *Caliciviridae*
Skunkpox virus, (SKPV), *Poxviridae*
Slow bee paralysis virus, (SBPV), Unassigned
Smelt reovirus, (SRV), *Reoviridae*
Smelt virus-1, (SmV-1), *Picornaviridae*
Smelt virus-2, (SmV-2), *Picornaviridae*
Smithiantha latent virus, (SmiLV), *Potexvirus*
Snake adenovirus, (SnAdV-1), *Adenoviridae*
Snakehead retrovirus, (SnRV), *Retroviridae*
Snakehead rhabdovirus, (SHRV), *Rhabdoviridae*
Snow Mountain virus, (SMV), *Caliciviridae*
Snowshoe hare virus, (SSHV), *Bunyaviridae*
Snyder-Theilen feline sarcoma virus, (STFeSV), *Retroviridae*
Soil-borne rye mosaic virus, (SBRMV), *Furovirus*
Soil-borne wheat mosaic virus, (SBWMV), *Furovirus*
Sokoluk virus, (SOKV), *Flaviviridae*
Solanum apical leaf curl virus, (SALCV), *Geminiviridae*
Solanum nodiflorum mottle virus satellite RNA, Satellite
Solanum nodiflorum mottle virus, (SNMoV), *Sobemovirus*
Solanum tomato leaf curl virus, (SToLCV), *Geminiviridae*
Solanum tuberosum Tst1 virus, (StuTst1V), *Pseudoviridae*
Solanum yellow leaf curl virus, (SYLCV), *Geminiviridae*
Solanum yellows virus, (SOLYV), *Luteoviridae*
Soldado virus, (SOLV), *Bunyaviridae*
Sonchus mottle virus, (SMoV), *Caulimoviridae*
Sonchus virus, (SonV), *Rhabdoviridae*
Sonchus yellow net virus, (SYNV), *Rhabdoviridae*
Sorghum chlorotic spot virus, (SrCSV), *Furovirus*
Sorghum mosaic virus, (SrMV), *Potyviridae*
Sorghum virus, (SrV), *Rhabdoviridae*
Sororoca virus, (SORV), *Bunyaviridae*
Sotkamo virus, *Bunyaviridae*
Soursop yellow blotch virus, (SYBV), *Rhabdoviridae*
South African cassava mosaic virus, (SACMV), *Geminiviridae*
South African passiflora virus, *Potyviridae*
South River virus, (SORV), *Bunyaviridae*
Southampton virus, (SHV), *Caliciviridae*
Southern bean mosaic virus, (SBMV), *Sobemovirus*
Southern cowpea mosaic virus, (SCPMV), *Sobemovirus*

Southern potato latent virus, (SoPLV), *Carlavirus*
Sowbane mosaic virus, (SoMV), *Sobemovirus*
Sowthistle yellow vein virus, (SYVV), *Rhabdoviridae*
Soybean chlorotic mottle virus, (SbCMV), *Caulimoviridae*
Soybean crinkle leaf virus, (SCLV), *Geminiviridae*
Soybean dwarf virus, (SbDV), *Luteoviridae*
Soybean mosaic virus, (SMV), *Potyviridae*
SPAr 2317 virus, (SPAV), *Bunyaviridae*
Sparrowpox virus, (SRPV), *Poxviridae*
Spartina mottle virus, (SpMV), *Potyviridae*
Spectacled caiman poxvirus, (SPV), *Poxviridae*
SPH114202 virus, *Arenaviridae*
Sphenicid herpesvirus 1, (SpHV-1), *Herpesviridae*
Spider monkey herpesvirus, *Herpesviridae*
Spinach latent virus, (SpLV), *Bromoviridae*
Spinach temperate virus, (SpTV), *Partitiviridae*
Spiroplasma phage 1-aa, (SpV1-aa), *Inoviridae*
Spiroplasma phage 1-C74, (SpV1-C74), *Inoviridae*
Spiroplasma phage 1-KC3, (SpV1/KC3), *Inoviridae*
Spiroplasma phage 1-R8A2B, (SpV1-R8A2B), *Inoviridae*
Spiroplasma phage 1-S102, (SpV1-S102), *Inoviridae*
Spiroplasma phage 1-T78, (SpV1-T78), *Inoviridae*
Spiroplasma phage 4, (Sp-4), *Microviridae*
Spiroplasma phage C1/TS2, (C1/TS2), *Inoviridae*
Spodoptera exempta cypovirus 11, (SexmCPV-11), *Reoviridae*
Spodoptera exempta cypovirus 12, (SexmCPV-12), *Reoviridae*
Spodoptera exempta cypovirus 3, (SexmCPV-3), *Reoviridae*
Spodoptera exempta cypovirus 5, (SexmCPV-5), *Reoviridae*
Spodoptera exempta cypovirus 8, (SexmCPV-8), *Reoviridae*
Spodoptera exempta MNPV, (SpexMNPV), *Baculoviridae*
Spodoptera exigua cypovirus 11, (SexgCPV-11), *Reoviridae*
Spodoptera exigua MNPV, (SeMNPV), *Baculoviridae*
Spodoptera frugiperda ascovirus 1a, (SfAV-1a), *Ascoviridae*
Spodoptera frugiperda MNPV, (SfMNPV), *Baculoviridae*
Spodoptera littoralis NPV, (SpliNPV), *Baculoviridae*
Spodoptera litura NPV, (SpltNPV), *Baculoviridae*
Spondweni virus, (SPOV), *Flaviviridae*
Spring beauty latent virus, (SBLV), *Bromoviridae*
Spring viremia of carp virus, (SVCV), *Rhabdoviridae*
Squash leaf curl virus - China, (SLCV-Ch), *Geminiviridae*
Squash leaf curl virus, (SLCV), *Geminiviridae*
Squash mosaic virus, (SqMV), *Comoviridae*
Squirrel fibroma virus, (SQFV), *Poxviridae*

Squirrel monkey retrovirus, (SMRV), *Retroviridae*
Squirrel parapoxvirus, (SPPV), *Poxviridae*
SR-11 virus, *Bunyaviridae*
Sri Lankan passion fruit mottle virus, (SLPMoV), *Potyviridae*
Sripur virus, (SRIV), *Rhabdoviridae*
St Abb's Head virus, (SAHV), *Reoviridae*
St. Abbs Head virus, (SAHV), *Bunyaviridae*
St. Louis encephalitis virus, (SLEV), *Flaviviridae*
Staphylococcus phage 107, (107), *Siphoviridae*
Staphylococcus phage 11, (11), *Siphoviridae*
Staphylococcus phage 1139, (1139), *Siphoviridae*
Staphylococcus phage 1154A, (1154A), *Siphoviridae*
Staphylococcus phage 187, (187), *Siphoviridae*
Staphylococcus phage 2848A, (2848A), *Siphoviridae*
Staphylococcus phage 392, (392), *Siphoviridae*
Staphylococcus phage 3A, (3A), *Siphoviridae*
Staphylococcus phage 44AHJD, (44AHJD), *Podoviridae*
Staphylococcus phage 77, (77), *Siphoviridae*
Staphylococcus phage B11-M15, (B11-M15), *Siphoviridae*
Staphylococcus phage P11, (P11), *Siphoviridae*
Staphylococcus phage ϕ11, (ϕ11), *Siphoviridae*
Starlingpox virus, (SLPV), *Poxviridae*
Statice virus Y, *Potyviridae*
Stickleback virus, (SBV), *Iridoviridae*
Stratford virus, (STRV), *Flaviviridae*
Strawberry crinkle virus, (SCV), *Rhabdoviridae*
Strawberry latent ringspot virus satellite RNA, Satellite
Strawberry latent ringspot virus, (SLRSV), *Comoviridae*
Strawberry mild yellow edge virus, (SMYEV), *Potexvirus*
Strawberry mild yellow edge associated virus, *Luteoviridae*
Strawberry pseudo mild yellow edge virus, (SPMYEV), *Carlavirus*
Strawberry vein banding virus, (SVBV), *Caulimoviridae*
Streptococcus phage 182, (182), *Podoviridae*
Streptococcus phage 24, (24), *Siphoviridae*
Streptococcus phage 2BV, (2BV), *Podoviridae*
Streptococcus phage A25, (A25), *Siphoviridae*
Streptococcus phage Cp-1, (Cp-1), *Podoviridae*
Streptococcus phage Cp-5, (Cp-5), *Podoviridae*
Streptococcus phage Cp-7, (Cp-7), *Podoviridae*
Streptococcus phage Cp-9, (Cp-9), *Podoviridae*
Streptococcus phage Cvir, (Cvir), *Podoviridae*
Streptococcus phage H39, (H39), *Podoviridae*
Streptococcus phage PE1, (PE1), *Siphoviridae*
Streptococcus phage VD13, (VD13), *Siphoviridae*
Streptococcus phage ω8, (ω8), *Siphoviridae*
Strigid herpesvirus 1, (StHV-1), *Herpesviridae*

Striped bass reovirus, (SBRV), *Reoviridae*
Striped jack nervous necrosis virus, (SJNNV), *Nodaviridae*
Stump-tailed macaque virus, *Polyomaviridae*
Subterranean clover mottle virus satellite RNA, Satellite
Subterranean clover mottle virus, (SCMoV), *Sobemovirus*
Subterranean clover red leaf virus, *Luteoviridae*
Subterranean clover stunt virus, (SCSV), *Nanovirus*
Sudan Ebola virus Boniface, *Filoviridae*
Sudan Ebola virus Maleo, *Filoviridae*
Sudan Ebola virus, (SEBOV), *Filoviridae*
Sugarcane bacilliform virus, (SCBV), *Caulimoviridae*
Sugarcane mild mosaic virus, (SMMV), *Closteroviridae*
Sugarcane mosaic virus, (SCMV), *Potyviridae*
Sugarcane streak virus, (SSV), *Geminiviridae*
Suid herpesvirus 1, (SuHV-1), *Herpesviridae*
Suid herpesvirus 2, (SuHV-2), *Herpesviridae*
Sulfolobus virus 1, (SSV-1), *Fuselloviridae*
Sulfolobus virus SIRV-1, (SIRV-1), *Rudiviridae*
Sulfolobus virus SIRV-2, (SIRV-2), *Rudiviridae*
Sulfolobus virus SNDV, (SNDV), "SNDV-like viruses"
Sunday Canyon virus, (SCAV), *Bunyaviridae*
Sunflower crinkle virus, (SuCV), *Umbravirus*
Sunflower mosaic virus, (SuMV), *Potyviridae*
Sunflower rugose mosaic virus, *Umbravirus*
Sunflower yellow blotch virus, (SuYBV), *Umbravirus*
Sunflower yellow ringspot virus, *Umbravirus*
Sunn-hemp mosaic virus, (SHMV), *Tobamovirus*
Sweet clover necrotic mosaic virus, (SCNMV), *Tombusviridae*
Sweet potato chlorotic leafspot virus, *Potyviridae*
Sweet potato chlorotic stunt virus, (SPCSV), *Closteroviridae*
Sweet potato feathery mottle virus, (SPFMV), *Potyviridae*
Sweet potato internal cork virus, *Potyviridae*
Sweet potato latent virus, (SPLV), *Potyviridae*
Sweet potato leaf speckling virus, (SPLSV), *Luteoviridae*
Sweet potato mild mottle virus, (SPMMV), *Potyviridae*
Sweet potato mild speckling virus, (SPMSV), *Potyviridae*
Sweet potato russet crack virus, *Potyviridae*
Sweet potato sunken vein virus, *Closteroviridae*
Sweet potato vein mosaic virus, (SPVMV), *Potyviridae*
Sweet potato virus A, *Potyviridae*
Sweet potato yellow dwarf virus, (SPYDV), *Potyviridae*
Sweetwater Branch virus, (SWBV), *Rhabdoviridae*
Swine calicivirus, (SwV-43), *Caliciviridae*
Swine cytomegalovirus, *Herpesviridae*
Swine vesicular disease virus, *Picornaviridae*
Swinepox virus, (SWPV), *Poxviridae*
Sword bean distortion mosaic virus, (SBDMV), *Potyviridae*
Synetaeris tenuifemur ichnovirus, (StIV), *Polydnaviridae*
Syr-Daria Valley fever virus, (SDFV), *Picornaviridae*

T.RVL.II 573 virus, *Arenaviridae*
Tacaiuma virus, (TCMV), *Bunyaviridae*
Tacaribe virus, (TCRV), *Arenaviridae*
Tadpole edema virus, *Iridoviridae*
Tadpole virus 2, *Iridoviridae*
Taggert virus, (TAGV), *Bunyaviridae*
Tahyna virus, (TAHV), *Bunyaviridae*
Tai virus, (TAIV), *Bunyaviridae*
Taiassui virus, (TAIAV), *Bunyaviridae*
Taino tomato mottle virus, (TToMoV), *Geminiviridae*
Tamana bat virus, (TABV), *Flaviviridae*
Tamarillo mosaic virus, (TamMV), *Potyviridae*
Tamdy virus, (TDYV), *Bunyaviridae*
Tamiami virus, (TAMV), *Arenaviridae*
Tamus red mosaic virus, (TRMV), *Potexvirus*
Tanapox virus, (TANV), *Poxviridae*
Tanga virus, (TANV), *Bunyaviridae*
Tanjong Rabok virus, (TRV), *Bunyaviridae*
Taro bacilliform virus, (TaBV), *Caulimoviridae*
Taro feathery mottle virus, (TFMoV), *Potyviridae*
Tataguine virus, (TATV), *Bunyaviridae*
Taterapox virus, (GBLV), *Poxviridae*
Taura syndrome virus, (TSV), *Picornaviridae*
TBRV-G serotype satellite RNA, Satellite
TBRV-S serotype satellite RNA, Satellite
Teasel mosaic virus, (TeaMV), *Potyviridae*
Tehran virus, (THEV), *Bunyaviridae*
Telfairia mosaic virus, (TeMV), *Potyviridae*
Telok Forest virus, (TFV), *Bunyaviridae*
Tembe virus, (TMEV), *Reoviridae*
Tembusu virus, (TMUV), *Flaviviridae*
Tench reovirus, (TNRV), *Reoviridae*
Tenebrio molitor iridescent virus, *Iridoviridae*
Tensaw virus, (TENV), *Bunyaviridae*
Tephrosia symptomless virus, (TeSV), *Tombusviridae*
Termeil virus, (TERV), *Bunyaviridae*
Tete virus, (TETEV), *Bunyaviridae*
Texas pepper virus, (TPV), *Geminiviridae*
Thailand virus, (THAIV), *Bunyaviridae*
Theiler's murine encephalomyelitis virus, (TMEV), *Picornaviridae*
Theilovirus, (ThV), *Picornaviridae*

Thermoproteus virus 1, (TTV1), *Lipothrixiviridae*
Thermoproteus virus 2, (TTV2), *Lipothrixiviridae*
Thermoproteus virus 3, (TTV3), *Lipothrixiviridae*
Thermoproteus virus TTV4, (TTV4), *Rudiviridae*
Thermus phage P37-14, (P37-14), *Tectiviridae*
Thiafora virus, (TFAV), *Bunyaviridae*
Thimiri virus, (THIV), *Bunyaviridae*
Thistle mottle virus, (ThMoV), *Caulimoviridae*
Thogoto virus, (THOV), *Orthomyxoviridae*
Thormodseyjarlettur virus, (THRV), *Reoviridae*
Thosea asigna virus, (TaV), *Tetraviridae*
Thottapalayam virus, (TPMV), *Bunyaviridae*
Tibrogargan virus, (TIBV), *Rhabdoviridae*
Tichoplusia ni cypovirus 5, (TnCPV-5), *Reoviridae*
Tick-borne encephalitis virus European subtype, *Flaviviridae*
Tick-borne encephalitis virus Far Eastern subtype, *Flaviviridae*
Tick-borne encephalitis virus Siberian subtype, *Flaviviridae*
Tick-borne encephalitis virus, (TBEV), *Flaviviridae*
Tiger puffer nervous necrosis virus, (TPNNV), *Nodaviridae*
Tiger salamander virus, *Iridoviridae*
Tillamook virus, (TILLV), *Bunyaviridae*
Tillamook virus, *Reoviridae*
Tilligerry virus, (TILV), *Reoviridae*
Timbo virus, (TIMV), *Rhabdoviridae*
Timboteua virus, (TBTV), *Bunyaviridae*
Tinaroo virus, (TINV), *Bunyaviridae*
Tindholmur virus, (TDMV), *Reoviridae*
Tipula iridescent virus, *Iridoviridae*
Tipula paludosa NPV, (TipaNPV), *Baculoviridae*
Tlacotalpan virus, (TLAV), *Bunyaviridae*
Tobacco bushy top virus, (TBTV), *Umbravirus*
Tobacco etch virus, (TEV), *Potyviridae*
Tobacco leaf curl virus, (TLCV), *Geminiviridae*
Tobacco leaf enation phytoreovirus, (TLEP), *Reoviridae*
Tobacco mild green mosaic virus, (TMGMV), *Tobamovirus*
Tobacco mosaic satellite virus, Satellite
Tobacco mosaic virus-U1, *Tobamovirus*
Tobacco mosaic virus-U2, *Tobamovirus*
Tobacco mosaic virus-vulgare, *Tobamovirus*
Tobacco mosaic virus, (TMV), *Tobamovirus*
Tobacco mottle virus, (TMoV), *Umbravirus*
Tobacco necrosis satellite virus, Satellite
Tobacco necrosis virus A, (TNV-A), *Tombusviridae*
Tobacco necrosis virus D, (TNV-D), *Tombusviridae*
Tobacco necrosis virus small satellite RNA, Satellite
Tobacco necrotic dwarf virus, (TNDV), *Luteoviridae*
Tobacco rattle virus, (TRV), *Tobravirus*
Tobacco ringspot virus satellite RNA, Satellite
Tobacco ringspot virus, (TRSV), *Comoviridae*
Tobacco streak virus, (TSV), *Bromoviridae*
Tobacco stunt virus, (TStV), *Varicosavirus*
Tobacco vein banding mosaic virus, (TVBMV), *Potyviridae*
Tobacco vein mottling virus, (TVMV), *Potyviridae*
Tobacco wilt virus, (TWV), *Potyviridae*
Tobacco yellow dwarf virus, (TYDV), *Geminiviridae*
Tobacco yellow vein virus, (TYVV), *Umbravirus*
Tobetsu-60Cr-93 virus, *Bunyaviridae*
Tomato apical stunt viroid, (TASVd), *Pospiviroidae*
Tomato aspermy virus, (TAV), *Bromoviridae*
Tomato black ring virus satellite RNA, Satellite
Tomato black ring virus, (TBRV), *Comoviridae*
Tomato bunchy top viroid, (ToBTVd), *Avsunviroidae*
Tomato bushy stunt virus satellite RNA, Satellite
Tomato bushy stunt virus, (TBSV), *Tombusviridae*
Tomato chlorosis virus, (ToCV), *Closteroviridae*
Tomato chlorotic spot virus, (TCSV), *Bunyaviridae*
Tomato golden mosaic virus, (TGMV), *Geminiviridae*
Tomato infectious chlorosis virus, (TICV), *Closteroviridae*
Tomato leaf crumple virus, (TLCrV), *Geminiviridae*
Tomato leaf curl virus-Australia, (ToLCV-Au), *Geminiviridae*
Tomato leaf curl virus-Bangalore I, (ToLCV-BanI), *Geminiviridae*
Tomato leaf curl virus-Bangalore II, (ToLCV-BanII), *Geminiviridae*
Tomato leaf curl virus-New Delhi, (ToLCV-NDe), *Geminiviridae*
Tomato leaf curl virus-Senegal, (ToLCV-Sn), *Geminiviridae*
Tomato leaf curl virus-Taiwan, (ToLCV-Tw), *Geminiviridae*
Tomato leaf curl virus-Tanzania, (ToLCV-Tz), *Geminiviridae*
Tomato leaf curl virus satellite DNA, Satellite
Tomato leafroll virus, (TLRV), *Geminiviridae*
Tomato mosaic virus, (ToMV), *Tobamovirus*
Tomato mottle virus, (ToMoV), *Geminiviridae*
Tomato pale chlorosis virus, *Carlavirus*
Tomato planta macho viroid, (TPMVd), *Pospiviroidae*
Tomato pseudo-curly top virus, (TPCTV), *Geminiviridae*
Tomato ringspot virus, (ToRSV), *Comoviridae*
Tomato severe leaf curl virus, (ToSLCV), *Geminiviridae*
Tomato spotted wilt virus, (TSWV), *Bunyaviridae*
Tomato top necrosis virus, (ToTNV), *Comoviridae*
Tomato vein yellowing virus, (TVYV), *Rhabdoviridae*

Tomato yellow dwarf virus, (ToYDV), *Geminiviridae*
Tomato yellow leaf curl virus-China, (TYLCV-Ch), *Geminiviridae*
Tomato yellow leaf curl virus-Israel, (TYLCV-Is), *Geminiviridae*
Tomato yellow leaf curl virus-Nigeria, (TYLCV-Ng), *Geminiviridae*
Tomato yellow leaf curl virus-Sardinia, (TYLCV-Sar), *Geminiviridae*
Tomato yellow leaf curl virus-Southern Saudi Arabia, (TYLCV-SSA), *Geminiviridae*
Tomato yellow leaf curl virus-Tanzania, (TYLCV-Tz), *Geminiviridae*
Tomato yellow leaf curl virus-Thailand, (TYLCV-Th), *Geminiviridae*
Tomato yellow leaf curl virus-Yemen, (TYLCV-Ye), *Geminiviridae*
Tomato yellow mosaic virus, (ToYMV), *Geminiviridae*
Tomato yellow mottle virus, (ToYMoV), *Geminiviridae*
Tomato yellow top virus, *Luteoviridae*
Tomato yellow vein streak virus, (ToYVSV), *Geminiviridae*
Tongan vanilla virus, (TVV), *Potyviridae*
Topografov virus, (TOPV), *Bunyaviridae*
Tortoise virus 5, (TV5), *Iridoviridae*
Toscana virus, (TOSV), *Bunyaviridae*
Tradescantia/Zebrina virus, (TZV), *Potyviridae*
Trager duck spleen necrosis virus, (TDSNV), *Retroviridae*
Tranosema rostrale bracovirus, (TrBV), *Polydnaviridae*
Tranosema rostrales ichnovirus, (TrIV), *Polydnaviridae*
Transmissible gastroenteritis virus, (TGEV), *Coronaviridae*
Tree shrew adenovirus 1, (TSAdV-1), *Adenoviridae*
Tree shrew adenovirus, (TSAdV), *Adenoviridae*
Tree shrew herpesvirus, *Herpesviridae*
Triatoma virus, (TrV), Unassigned
Tribec virus, (TRBV), *Reoviridae*
Tribolium castaneum Woot virus, (TcaWooV), *Metaviridae*
Trichomonas vaginalis T1 virus, Satellite
Trichomonas vaginalis virus, (TVV), *Totiviridae*
Trichoplusia ni ascovirus 1a, (TnAV-1a), *Ascoviridae*
Trichoplusia ni granulovirus, (TnGV), *Baculoviridae*
Trichoplusia ni MNPV, (TnMNPV), *Baculoviridae*
Trichoplusia ni SNPV, (TnSNPV), *Baculoviridae*
Trichoplusia ni TED virus, (TniTedV), *Metaviridae*
Trichoplusia ni virus, (TnV), *Tetraviridae*
Trichosanthes mottle virus, (TrMoV), *Potyviridae*

Tripneustis gratilla SURL virus, (TgrSurV), *Metaviridae*
Triticum aestivum chlorotic spot virus, (TACSV), *Rhabdoviridae*
Triticum aestivum WIS-2 virus, (TaeWis2V), *Pseudoviridae*
Trivittatus virus, (TVTV), *Bunyaviridae*
Trombetas virus, (TRMV), *Bunyaviridae*
Tropaeolum mosaic virus, (TrMV), *Potyviridae*
Tropaeolum virus 1, (TV-1), *Potyviridae*
Tropaeolum virus 2, (TV-2), *Potyviridae*
Trubanaman virus, (TRUV), *Bunyaviridae*
Tsuruse virus, (TSUV), *Bunyaviridae*
Tuberose mild mosaic virus, (TuMMV), *Potyviridae*
Tucunduba virus, (TUCV), *Bunyaviridae*
Tula virus, (TULV), *Bunyaviridae*
Tulare apple mosaic virus, (TAMV), *Bromoviridae*
Tulip band breaking virus, (TBBV), *Potyviridae*
Tulip breaking virus, (TBV), *Potyviridae*
Tulip chlorotic blotch virus, *Potyviridae*
Tulip mild mottle mosaic virus, (TMMMV), *Ophiovirus*
Tulip top breaking virus, *Potyviridae*
Tulip virus X, (TVX), *Potexvirus*
Tumor virus X, (TVX), *Parvoviridae*
Tunis virus, (TUNV), *Bunyaviridae*
Tupaia virus, (TUPV), *Rhabdoviridae*
Tupaiid herpesvirus 1, (TuHV-1), *Herpesviridae*
Turbot herpesvirus, *Herpesviridae*
Turbot reovirus, (TRV), *Reoviridae*
Turbot virus-1, (TuV-1), *Picornaviridae*
Turkey adenovirus 1, 2, (TAdV-1, 2), *Adenoviridae*
Turkey adenovirus, (TAdV), *Adenoviridae*
Turkey astrovirus 1, (TAstV-1), *Astroviridae*
Turkey astrovirus, (TAstV), *Astroviridae*
Turkey coronavirus, (TCoV), *Coronaviridae*
Turkey entero-like virus, (TELV), *Picornaviridae*
Turkey hemorrhagic enteritis virus (HEV), (TAdV-3), *Adenoviridae*
Turkey hepatitis virus, (THV), *Picornaviridae*
Turkey herpesvirus, *Herpesviridae*
Turkey pseudo enterovirus 1 to 2, (TPEV-1, 2), *Picornaviridae*
Turkey rhinotracheitis virus, (TRTV), *Paramyxoviridae*
Turkeypox virus, (TKPV), *Poxviridae*
Turlock virus, (TURV), *Bunyaviridae*
Turnaca rufisquamata virus, (TrV), Unassigned
Turnip crinkle virus satellite RNA, Satellite
Turnip crinkle virus, (TCV), *Tombusviridae*
Turnip mild yellows virus, *Luteoviridae*
Turnip mosaic virus, (TuMV), *Potyviridae*
Turnip rosette virus, (TRoV), *Sobemovirus*
Turnip vein-clearing virus, (TVCV), *Tobamovirus*
Turnip yellow mosaic virus, (TYMV), *Tymovirus*

Turuna virus, (TUAV), *Bunyaviridae*
Tyuleniy virus, (TYUV), *Flaviviridae*

Uasin Gishu disease virus, (UGDV), *Poxviridae*
Uganda S virus, (UGSV), *Flaviviridae*
Ulcerative disease rhabdovirus, (UDRV), *Rhabdoviridae*
Ullucus mild mottle virus, (UMMV), *Tobamovirus*
Ullucus mosaic virus, (UMV), *Potyviridae*
Ullucus virus C, (UVC), *Comoviridae*
Umatilla virus, (UMAV), *Reoviridae*
Umatilla virus, (UMAV), *Reoviridae*
Umbre virus, (UMBV), *Bunyaviridae*
Una virus, (UNAV), *Togaviridae*
Upolu virus, (UPOV), *Bunyaviridae*
UR2 sarcoma virus, (UR2SV), *Retroviridae*
Urmurtia/338Cg/92 virus, *Bunyaviridae*
Urochloa hoja blanca virus, (UHBV), *Tenuivirus*
Urucuri virus, (URUV), *Bunyaviridae*
Ustilago maydis killer M virus, Satellite
Ustilago maydis virus H1, (UmV-H1), *Totiviridae*
Usutu virus, (USUV), *Flaviviridae*
Utinga virus, (UTIV), *Bunyaviridae*
Utive virus, (UVV), *Bunyaviridae*
Uukuniemi virus S 23, (UUKV), *Bunyaviridae*
Uukuniemi virus, (UUKV), *Bunyaviridae*

Vaccinia virus, (VACV), *Poxviridae*
Vallota mosaic virus, (ValMV), *Potyviridae*
Vanilla mosaic virus, (VanMV), *Potyviridae*
Vanilla necrosis virus, *Potyviridae*
Varicella-zoster virus, *Herpesviridae*
Variola virus, (VARV), *Poxviridae*
VAV-488 virus, *Arenaviridae*
VAV-499 virus, *Arenaviridae*
Vearoy virus, (VAEV), *Reoviridae*
Vellore virus, (VELV), *Reoviridae*
Velvet tobacco mottle virus satellite RNA, Satellite
Velvet tobacco mottle virus, (VTMoV), *Sobemovirus*
Venezuelan equine encephalitis virus, (VEEV), *Togaviridae*
Vesicular exanthema of swine virus, (VESV), *Caliciviridae*
Vesicular exanthema of swine virus-A48, (VESV-A48), *Caliciviridae*
Vesicular stomatitis Alagoas virus, (VSAV), *Rhabdoviridae*
Vesicular stomatitis Indiana virus, (VSIV), *Rhabdoviridae*
Vesicular stomatitis New Jersey virus, (VSNJV), *Rhabdoviridae*
Vibrio phage 06N-22P, (06N-22P), *Myoviridae*
Vibrio phage 06N-58P, (06N-58P), *Corticoviridae*
Vibrio phage 06N-58P, *Tectiviridae*
Vibrio phage 493, (493), *Inoviridae*
Vibrio phage 4996, (4996), *Podoviridae*
Vibrio phage CTX, (CTX), *Inoviridae*
Vibrio phage fs1, (fs1), *Inoviridae*
Vibrio phage fs2, (fs2), *Inoviridae*
Vibrio phage I, (I), *Podoviridae*
Vibrio phage II, (II), *Myoviridae*
Vibrio phage III, (III), *Podoviridae*
Vibrio phage IV, (IV), *Siphoviridae*
Vibrio phage kappa, (kappa), *Myoviridae*
Vibrio phage KVP20, (KVP20), *Myoviridae*
Vibrio phage KVP40, (KVP40), *Myoviridae*
Vibrio phage nt-1, (nt-1), *Myoviridae*
Vibrio phage O6N-72P, (06N-72P), *Podoviridae*
Vibrio phage OXN-100P, (OXN-100P), *Podoviridae*
Vibrio phage OXN-52P, (OXN-52P), *Siphoviridae*
Vibrio phage P147, (P147), *Myoviridae*
Vibrio phage v6, (v6), *Inoviridae*
Vibrio phage VcA3, (VcA3), *Myoviridae*
Vibrio phage Vf12, (Vf12), *Inoviridae*
Vibrio phage Vf33, (Vf33), *Inoviridae*
Vibrio phage VP1, (VP1), *Myoviridae*
Vibrio phage VP11, (VP11), *Siphoviridae*
Vibrio phage VP3, (VP3), *Siphoviridae*
Vibrio phage VP5, (VP5), *Siphoviridae*
Vibrio phage VSK, (VSK), *Inoviridae*
Vibrio phage X29, (X29), *Myoviridae*
Vibrio phage α3α, (α3α), *Siphoviridae*
Vibrio phage φ149 (type IV), (φ149), *Siphoviridae*
Vibrio phage φVP253, (φVP253), *Myoviridae*
Vicia cryptic virus, (VCV), *Partitiviridae*
Vicia faba 447 cytolasmic male sterility-associated virus, (VfCMSaV), Unassigned
Vigna sinensis mosaic virus, (VSMV), *Rhabdoviridae*
Vilyuisk human encephalomyelitis virus, (VHEV), *Picornaviridae*
Vinces virus, (VINV), *Bunyaviridae*
Vindeln/L20Cg/83 virus, *Bunyaviridae*
Viola mottle virus, (VMoV), *Potexvirus*
Viper retrovirus, (VRV), *Retroviridae*
Viral hemorrhagic septicemia virus, (VHSV), *Rhabdoviridae*
Virgin River virus, (VRV), *Bunyaviridae*
Visna/maedi virus (strain 1514), (VISNA), *Retroviridae*
Voandzeia mosaic virus, *Carlavirus*
Voandzeia necrotic mosaic virus, (VNMV) *Tymovirus*
Vole poxvirus, (VPV), *Poxviridae*
Volepox virus, (VPXV), *Poxviridae*
Volvox carteri Osser virus, (VcaOssV), *Pseudoviridae*
Vranica virus, *Bunyaviridae*

W10777 virus, *Arenaviridae*
Wad Medani virus, (WMV), *Reoviridae*
Wad Medani virus, (WMV), *Reoviridae*
Wallal virus, (WALV), *Reoviridae*
Wallal virus, (WALV), *Reoviridae*
Walleye dermal sarcoma virus, (WDSV), *Retroviridae*
Walleye epidermal hyperplasia virus 1, (WEHV-1), *Retroviridae*
Walleye epidermal hyperplasia virus 2, (WEHV-2), *Retroviridae*
Walleye epidermal hyperplasia, *Herpesviridae*
Walrus calicivirus, (WCV), *Caliciviridae*
Wanowrie virus, (WANV), *Bunyaviridae*
Warrego virus, (WARV), *Reoviridae*
Warrego virus, (WARV), *Reoviridae*
Water buffalo herpesvirus, *Herpesviridae*
Watercress yellow spot virus, (WYSV), Unassigned
Watermelon bud necrosis virus, (WBNV), *Bunyaviridae*
Watermelon chlorotic stunt virus, (WmCSV), *Geminiviridae*
Watermelon curly mottle virus, (WmCMV), *Geminiviridae*
Watermelon mosaic virus 1, *Potyviridae*
Watermelon mosaic virus 2, *Potyviridae*
Watermelon mosaic virus, (WMV), *Potyviridae*
Watermelon silver mottle virus, (WSMoV), *Bunyaviridae*
WE virus, *Arenaviridae*
Weddel waterborne virus, (WWBV), *Tombusviridae*
Weldona virus, (WELV), *Bunyaviridae*
Welsh onion yellow stripe virus, *Potyviridae*
Wesselsbron virus, (WESSV), *Flaviviridae*
West Nile virus, (WNV), *Flaviviridae*
Western equine encephalitis virus, (WEEV), *Togaviridae*
Wexford virus, (WEXV), *Reoviridae*
Whataroa virus, (WHAV), *Togaviridae*
Wheat American striate mosaic virus, (WASMV), *Rhabdoviridae*
Wheat chlorotic streak virus, (WCSV), *Rhabdoviridae*
Wheat dwarf virus, (WDV), *Geminiviridae*
Wheat rosette stunt virus, (WRSV), *Rhabdoviridae*
Wheat spindle streak mosaic virus, (WSSMV), *Potyviridae*
Wheat streak mosaic virus, (WSMV), *Potyviridae*
Wheat yellow leaf virus, (WYLV), *Closteroviridae*
Wheat yellow mosaic virus, (WYMV), *Potyviridae*
White bryony mosaic virus, (WBMV), *Carlavirus*
White bryony virus, (WBV), *Potyviridae*
White clover cryptic virus 1, (WCCV-1), *Partitiviridae*
White clover cryptic virus 2, (WCCV-2), *Partitiviridae*
White clover cryptic virus 3, (WCCV-3), *Partitiviridae*
White clover mosaic virus, (WClMV), *Potexvirus*
White clover virus L, (WClVL), Unassigned
White lupin mosaic virus, *Potyviridae*
White sturgeon herpesvirus 1, *Herpesviridae*
White Sturgeon herpesvirus 2, *Herpesviridae*
Whitewater Arroyo virus, (WWAV), *Arenaviridae*
Wild cucumber mosaic virus, (WCMV), *Tymovirus*
Wild potato mosaic virus, (WPMV), *Potyviridae*
Winter wheat mosaic virus, (WWMV), *Tenuivirus*
Winter wheat Russian mosaic virus, (WWMV), *Rhabdoviridae*
Wiseana iridescent virus, *Iridoviridae*
Wissadula golden mosaic virus, (WGMV), *Geminiviridae*
Wisteria vein mosaic virus, (WVMV), *Potyviridae*
Witlesia iridescent virus, *Iridoviridae*
Witwatersrand virus, (WITV), *Bunyaviridae*
Wongal virus, (WONV), *Bunyaviridae*
Wongorr virus CS131, (WGRV- CS131), *Reoviridae*
Wongorr virus MRM13443, (WGRV- MRM13443), *Reoviridae*
Wongorr virus V1447, (WGRV- V1447), *Reoviridae*
Wongorr virus V195, (WGRV- V195), *Reoviridae*
Wongorr virus V199, (WGRV- V199), *Reoviridae*
Wongorr virus V595, (WGRV- V595), *Reoviridae*
Wongorr virus, (WGRV), *Reoviridae*
Woodchuck hepatitis virus, (WHV), *Hepadnaviridae*
Woodchuck herpesvirus, *Herpesviridae*
Woolly monkey sarcoma virus, (WMSV), *Retroviridae*
Wound tumor virus, (WTV), *Reoviridae*
Wyeomyia virus, (WYOV), *Bunyaviridae*

Xanthomonas phage Cf16, (Cf16), *Inoviridae*
Xanthomonas phage Cf1c, (Cf1c), *Inoviridae*
Xanthomonas phage Cf1t, (Cf1t), *Inoviridae*
Xanthomonas phage Cf1tv, (Cf1tv), *Inoviridae*
Xanthomonas phage Lf, (Lf), *Inoviridae*
Xanthomonas phage RR66, (RR66), *Podoviridae*
Xanthomonas phage Xf, (Xf), *Inoviridae*
Xanthomonas phage Xfo, (Xfo), *Inoviridae*
Xanthomonas phage Xfv, (Xfv), *Inoviridae*
Xanthomonas phage XP5, (XP5), *Myoviridae*
Xestia c-nigrum granulovirus, (XecnGV), *Baculoviridae*
Xiburema virus, (XIBV), *Rhabdoviridae*
Xingu virus, (XINV), *Bunyaviridae*
XJ virus, *Arenaviridae*

Y73 sarcoma virus, (Y73SV), *Retroviridae*
Yaba monkey tumor virus, (YMTV), *Poxviridae*
Yaba-1 virus, (Y1V), *Bunyaviridae*
Yaba-7 virus, (Y7V), *Bunyaviridae*
Yacaaba virus, (YACV), *Bunyaviridae*
Yam mosaic virus, (YMV), *Potyviridae*
Yaounde virus, (YAOV), *Flaviviridae*
Yaquina Head virus, (YHV), *Reoviridae*
Yata virus, (YATAV), *Rhabdoviridae*
Yellow fever virus, (YFV), *Flaviviridae*
Yellowtail ascites virus, (YTAV), *Birnaviridae*
Yogue virus, (YOGV), *Bunyaviridae*
Yoka poxvirus, (YKV), *Poxviridae*
Yokose virus, (YOKV), *Flaviviridae*
Youcai mosaic virus, (YoMV), *Tobamovirus*
Yucca bacilliform virus, (YBV), *Caulimoviridae*
Yug Bogdanovac virus, (YBV), *Rhabdoviridae*

Zaire Ebola virus Eckron, *Filoviridae*

Zaire Ebola virus Gabon, *Filoviridae*
Zaire Ebola virus Kikwit, *Filoviridae*
Zaire Ebola virus Mayinga, *Filoviridae*
Zaire Ebola virus Tandala, *Filoviridae*
Zaire Ebola virus Zaire, *Filoviridae*
Zaire Ebola virus, (ZEBOV), *Filoviridae*
Zaliv Terpeniya virus, (ZTV), *Bunyaviridae*
Zea mays Hopscotch virus, (ZmaHopV), *Pseudoviridae*
Zea mays virus, (ZMV), *Rhabdoviridae*
Zegla virus, (ZEGV), *Bunyaviridae*
Zika virus, (ZIKV), *Flaviviridae*
Zinnia leaf curl virus, (ZiLCV), *Geminiviridae*
Zirqa virus, (ZIRV), *Bunyaviridae*
Zoysia mosaic virus, (ZoMV), *Potyviridae*
Zucchini lethal chlorosis virus, (ZLCV), *Bunyaviridae*
Zucchini yellow fleck virus, (ZYFV), *Potyviridae*
Zucchini yellow mosaic virus, (ZYMV), *Potyviridae*
Zygocactus symptomless virus, (ZSLV), *Potexvirus*

INDEX

NOTE

Reference Locators

Reference locators are to page numbers and these are followed by a bold volume number. Page numbers followed by Table and Fig refer to tables and figures respectively.

Order

Entries are in word-by-word order (in which a group of letters followed by a space is filed before the same group of letters followed by further letters. Hyphens, are given an 'intermediate' value, and en-rules are placed after these. Characters within brackets are normally excluded from the alphabetization.

Entries

1. Bacteriophages are listed after the main index entry 'Bacteriophage', unless there are cross-references to other locations. ϕ is alphabetized as 'phi'. ψ is alphabetized as 'psi'.
2. Readers are advised to seek not only the genus, but also the group name e.g. *Baculovirus* and *Baculoviruses*.
3. US spelling is used.

Abbreviations

Abbreviations used in index subentries are as follows:

CMV	Cytomegalovirus
EBV	Epstein-Barr virus
FIV	Feline immunodeficiency virus
HBV	Hepatitis B virus
HCV	Hepatitis C virus
HIV	Human immunodeficiency virus
HPV	Human papillomavirus
HSV	Herpes simplex virus
IRES	Internal ribosome entry site
LCMV	Lymphocytic choriomeningitis virus
LDV	Lactate dehydrogenase-elevating virus
ORF	Open reading frame
RSV	Respiratory syncytial virus
SIV	Simian immunodeficiency virus
VSV	Vesicular stomatitis virus
VZV	Varicella zoster virus

INDEX

A

A20, expression activated by LMP-1 of EBV 1:499
2′-5′ A synthetase 3:1961
AaHIT toxin 2:848, 2:849
Abacavir 2:779
Abbreviations, virus names 3:1754
Abdominal pain, coxsackievirus infection 1:308
Abelson murine leukemia virus 2:995, 2:998
  apoptosis inhibition 1:74
  v-abl oncogene 3:1511
abl oncogene 3:1511–12
Abortion
  horses 1:508, 1:512, 1:513
  in Rift Valley fever 3:1993
  spontaneous, echoviruses causing 1:416
Abortive infections 3:1409–10, 3:1410, 3:1957
Abutilon, virus infections 2:1318, 2:1319(Fig)
Abutilon mosaic virus (AbMV) 1:600
Abutilon yellow virus (AYV), transmission 1:272
Ac elements 3:1503
Acalypha yellow mosaic virus (AYVV) 1:600
Acceptor sequences, parvovirus transcript splicing 2:1170
AccuSite 1:67
Acetylcholine
  receptors 1:250
  release blocked by botulinum toxins 2:1232
N-Acetylneuraminic acid 1:249
Acidianus ambivalens 1:88
Acidic hydrolases 1:250
Acinetobacter, ssRNA phage 3:1664
Acquired immunodeficiency syndrome feline see Feline immunodeficiency virus (FIV)
  see also AIDS
Acquired resistance by plants see Plant resistance to viruses, natural
Acquisition access time (AAT), sequiviruses 3:1624
Acridine orange stain 1:400
Acrolpiopsis assectella, (leek moth) 1:98
Actin microfilaments 1:253
  frog virus 3 (FV3)-infected cells 1:586
Actinic keratoses 2:1112
  HPVs causing 2:1110
Actinomycetes, phages infecting see Actinophage
Actinomycin D, birnavirus sensitivity 1:163
Actinophage
  detection in soil 2:1249
  half-life in soil 2:1252
  host interactions 2:1252
  types in soils 2:1250(Table)
Activating transcription factor (ATF) 1:24, 1:26, 1:27
  bovine leukemia virus (BLV) 1:192
Acute bee paralysis virus (ABPV) 2:1272
Acute hemorrhagic conjunctivitis see Conjunctivitis
Acute hemorrhagic cystitis, adenoviruses causing 1:5–6
Acute infections 1:484, 2:1175

Acute infectious dropsy see under Carp
Acute leukosis 2:945
Acute myeloid factor 1 (AML-1) 1:226
Acute paralysis virus (APV) 2:744(Table), 2:746–7
  infection and symptoms 2:746–7
Acute respiratory distress syndrome see Adult respiratory distress syndrome (ARDS)
Acyclovir
  CMV infections 3:1824, 3:1825
  EBV infection 1:493, 3:1826
  herpesvirus infections 1:62
  HSV infections 2:685, 3:1829
  oral, HSV infection treatment 2:685
  post-transplant HBV infection 3:1831
  resistance, varicella-zoster virus 3:1877
  VZV infections 3:1828, 3:1877
Acyclovir triphosphate, HSV infection treatment 2:685
Acyrthosiphon pisum (pea aphid), pea enation mosaic virus (PEMV) transmission 2:1194
Adansonian system 3:1732
Adaptation
  bromoviruses 1:203
  Vi phage 1:138
  see also Cell culture
Adapter proteins 3:1515–16
  cbl oncogene 3:1515–16
  crk 3:1516
Adefovir 2:779
Adefovir dipivoxil 1:60, 1:63
Adeno-associated viruses (AAV) 2:1152, 3:1885–6
AAV-2
  integration 2:1159
  nonstructural proteins 2:1158
  receptor 2:1153
  replication 2:1159
gene therapy role 2:1159
genome 2:1155, 3:1885
  inverted terminal repeats 3:1885
  structure 1:385(Fig)
infection, clinical features 2:1154
inverted terminal repeat 1:385
latent infection 3:1957
productive infection 3:1957
Rep protein 2:1158
serotypes 1:152
transcription 2:1157, 2:1157(Fig)
as vectors 3:1885–6
  advantages 3:1886
  applications 3:1885–6
  contamination 3:1885
  helper viruses 3:1885
Adenocarcinoma
  HPV causing 3:1845
  renal 1:51
Adenoid-degenerating (AD) agent 1:1
Adenopharyngo-conjunctival fever 1:5
Adenosine triphosphate, rotavirus transcription 3:1590
S-Adenosylmethionine (AdoMet; SAM) 1:336
  in host-controlled modification/restriction 2:758
Adenoviridae 1:1–7, 1:14–21, 1:444–5
  apoptosis inhibition/suppression 1:72
  apoptosis promotion 1:74
Aviadenovirus 1:1
  fish viruses 1:567–8

Adenoviridae (continued)
  Mastadenovirus 1:1
  see also Aviadenovirus; Mastadenovirus
Adenovirus 1 (Ad1) 1:4
  canine 1:5
Adenovirus 2 (Ad2) 1:4
  BHK21 cells infection 1:10
  canine, live attenuated virus 1:6
  as vector 3:1886
Adenovirus 3 (Ad3), epidemiology 1:4
Adenovirus 4 (Ad4) 1:4
  serological cross-reactivity 1:3
Adenovirus 5 (Ad5) 1:4
  human infection 1:19
  as vector 3:1886
Adenovirus 7 (Ad7)
  epidemic patterns 1:4
  epidemiology 1:4
  genomic types (Ad7c, Ad7b) 1:4
  pathogenicity 1:5
Adenovirus 8 (Ad8) 1:4
  epidemic keratoconjunctivitis 1:3
  pathogenicity 1:5
Adenovirus 9 (Ad9), subgroup D 1:22
Adenovirus 11 (Ad11) 1:4
  ocular disease 1:526
Adenovirus 12 (Ad12) 1:4
  history 1:1
  immunoescape 1:28
  oncogenicity 1:28
  see also Adenovirus, human
Adenovirus 14 (Ad14) 1:4
Adenovirus 18 (Ad18) 1:4
Adenovirus 19 (Ad19) 1:4
  pathogenicity 1:5
Adenovirus 21 (Ad21) 1:4
Adenovirus 31 (Ad31) 1:4
Adenovirus 34 (Ad34) 1:4
Adenovirus 35 (Ad35) 1:4
Adenovirus 37 (Ad37) 1:4
Adenovirus 40 (Ad40) 1:5
  enteric infections 1:445
  epidemiology 1:4
Adenovirus 41 (Ad41) 1:5
  enteric infections 1:445
  epidemiology 1:4
Adenovirus 1:1–7, 1:14–21
  abortive infection
    by Ad12 see Adenovirus, human (below)
    of hamster cells 1:9
  Altantic cod 1:567
  animal
    genome sequence 1:17
    host range and propagation 1:18
    hosts 1:14
    listing by species 1:15(Table)
    serological relationships 1:19
    tissue tropism 1:20
    as vaccine vectors 1:21
    see also Adenovirus infection; Mastadenoviruses
  antigens and antibodies 1:19
  apoptosis promotion 1:74
  avian 1:14
    see also Aviadenovirus
  bovine see Bovine adenoviruses (BAVs)
  canine see Canine adenoviruses
  capsids 1:3
  capsomers 1:16
    pentons 1:16
  chromosomal association with host 1:9
  complementation studies 1:10
  culture, cytopathic effects 1:397(Fig)
  death protein (ADP) 1:74

Adenovirus (continued)
  defective particles 3:1411
  DNA
    addition to maintenance medium 1:9
    fate in mammalian cells 1:7–9
    insertion in pseudo-tandem arrays 1:11
    integration and oncogenesis 1:11–12
    loss in host cells 1:9
    transfection by 1:9
  DNA polymerase (Ad pol) 1:10
  duck 1:20
  E1 region, foreign gene insertion 1:6
  E1A12S oncoprotein 1:23, 1:26(Fig), 1:72
    C-terminus function 1:30
    immortalization function 1:28
  E1A13S, p53 upregulation 1:72
  E1A gene 1:22–30, 1:23
    conserved regions (CR1-5) 1:23
    CR1 role 1:27, 1:29
    CR3 1:26
    CR5 1:26
    deletion in vectors 1:12, 3:1886
    expression 1:24–7
    N-terminal region 1:24, 1:25
    structure 1:23, 1:23(Fig)
    transformation 3:1821–2
  E1A protein 1:23, 2:860
    of Ad12 1:28
    antisense 1:28
    apoptosis by 1:28
    CD44 protein expression repressed 1:29
    cell cycle activation/proliferation 1:27
    cell cycle regulators affected 1:24(Table)
    cotransformation role 1:24, 1:28
    differentiation role 1:29
    effect on p53 action 1:27
    epithelialization 1:29
    gene regulatory protein affected 1:25(Table)
    immortalization 1:24, 1:24–7, 1:27–8, 1:29
    kinase activity 1:24
    mutant 1:24, 1:29
    oncogenicity 1:28–9
    p53 inhibition 1:72
    phosphorylation 1:24
    protein complexes/interactions 1:24, 1:24–7
    RB and CBP cooperativity 1:26
    structure and functional regions 1:23(Fig)
    transformation, modulation 1:29–30
  E1a-induced tumors 1:6
  E1B19K oncoprotein 1:22, 1:72
  E1B55K oncoprotein 1:22, 1:72
  E1B gene
    deletion in vectors 1:12, 3:1886
    transformation 3:1821–2
  E1B protein 1:22, 1:28
  E2 region 1:10
  E3 protein
    apoptosis inhibition 1:72
    apoptosis promotion 1:74
  E3 region 1:21
    foreign gene insertion 1:6
    immune response 1:6
  E4 protein, apoptosis promotion 1:74
  E4 region 1:22
    PDZ domain 1:22
  E4ORF1 gene 1:22
  E4ORF6 gene 1:22

Adenovirus (continued)
  E4ORF6 protein 1:22, 1:72
  early genes 1:1
    immune response
      modulation 1:6
  enteric 1:4, 1:5, 1:444
    structure 1:444(Fig)
  epidemiology 1:4
  epizootiology 1:19–20
  evolution 1:3, 1:19
  evolutionary variants 1:3
  fibers 1:3
  future perspectives 1:6–7
  gene transfer vectors 1:12–14
    DNA packaging limits 1:13
    first-generation 1:12–13
    high-capacity (gutless; helper-
      dependent) 1:13
    immune response to 1:12–13
    in vitro/in vivo
      experiments 1:13–14
    second-generation 1:13
    third-generation 1:13
    third-generation and
      advantages 1:14
  genetics 1:3, 1:19
  genome 1:14, 1:17–18, 1:444,
    3:1886
    inverted terminal repeats
      (ITRs) 1:10, 1:13, 1:17, 1:19
    ORFs 1:17, 1:18
    replication 1:18
    sequences 1:17, 1:19
  geographic/seasonal
    distribution 1:3
  guinea-pig 1:19
  hexons, epitopes 1:3
  history 1:1, 1:14–16
  host range 1:3, 1:18–19
  human
    classification 1:1
    genome sequence 1:17
  human (Ad12) 1:7–9
    abortive infection 1:7–9, 1:9
    abortive infection of BHK21
      cells 1:10
    abortive infection of hamster
      cells 1:9
    complementation studies 1:10
    DNA addition to medium 1:9
    DNA association in host 1:9
    DNA insertion in pseudo-
      tandem arrays 1:11
    DNA integration
      mechanism 1:11
    DNA integration and
      oncogenesis 1:11–12
    DNA loss from host cells 1:11–
      12, 1:12
    DNA persistence in host 1:12
    E1A and E1B proteins 1:10,
      1:11
    E2 region DNA 1:10
    early mRNAs 1:9
    lack of 34 kDa protein 1:9
    late fiber gene-derived
      mRNA 1:10
    late genes transcription 1:10
    major later promoter
      (MLP) 1:10
    methylation 1:11, 1:12
    productive infection 1:10
    superinfection 1:9
    terminal protein 1:9, 1:10
    transfection by 1:9
  identification, neutralization
    test 1:400
  immortalization of cells 1:22,
    1:24, 1:27–8, 1:29
  immune evasion
    mechanism 2:1204
  immune response 1:21

Adenovirus (continued)
  in immunodeficiency 1:445
  infections see Adenovirus
    infection
  malignant transformation 1:21–
    30, 3:1821–2
    E1A role 1:28–9
    suppression by E1A 1:29–30
  MHC repression 1:29
  molecular biology 1:7
  molecular weights 1:18
  monoclonal antibodies 1:3
  murine 1:17, 1:20
  nonenteric 1:445
  nuclear factors 1:10
  oncogenes 1:22
  oncogenicity 1:7, 1:21–30, 1:28–9
  oncoproteins 1:22
  ovine 1:14
    see also Ovine adenovirus
      isolate 287 (OAV287)
  pathogenicity 1:5
  penetration 1:252(Fig)
  phylogeny 1:14, 1:17(Fig), 1:19
  physical properties 1:18
  prevention and control 1:21
  productive infection of human
    cells 1:9
  propagation 1:3, 1:18–19
  properties 1:2(Table), 1:16–17
  proteins 1:16
    28K and 24K 1:17
    genes 1:17
    properties 1:18
    protein IX 1:16, 1:18
    protein V 1:16, 1:18
    see also specific proteins
      (above)
  recombinant viruses 1:3
  recombination 3:1886
  replication 1:18
    deficient and helper
      viruses 1:13
    discovery 2:722
    origin 1:13
  RNA polymerase III 1:18
  serological relationships and
    variability 1:3–4, 1:19
  serotypes and subgroups 1:1,
    1:21, 1:444, 3:1886
    tumorigenic
      potential 1:22(Table)
  simian, phylogeny 1:19
  sturgeon 1:567–8
  subgenera 1:444
  subgenus A 1:4, 1:5
    properties 1:2(Table)
  subgenus B:1 1:2(Table), 1:4
  subgenus B:2 1:2(Table), 1:4
  subgenus B 1:5
    properties 1:2(Table)
  subgenus C 1:4, 1:5
    properties 1:2(Table)
  subgenus D 1:4, 1:5
    properties 1:2(Table)
  subgenus E 1:4, 1:5
    properties 1:2(Table)
  subgenus F 1:4–5, 1:5
    properties 1:2(Table)
  taxonomy and classification 1:1–
    3
  tissue tropism 1:5, 1:19–20
  transcription, map 3:1886(Fig)
  transfection by Ad12 DNA 1:9
  transmission 1:5, 1:19–20
  ts mutants, intertypic
    crosses 3:1449
  tumor induction see Adenovirus,
    malignant transformation
  tumor/metastasis
    suppression 1:29–30

Adenovirus (continued)
  uncoating 1:252(Fig), 1:256,
    3:1472
  vaccine 1:6, 1:21, 3:1864
  as vaccine vectors 1:6
  as vectors 3:1886–7
    applications 3:1886–7
    cloning in bacterial
      plasmids 3:1886
    disadvantages 3:1887
    expression of transgenes 3:1886
    genes inserted 3:1886
    high titer preparations 3:1886
    homologous
      recombination 3:1886
    methods for gene
      insertion 3:1886
    toxicity to tumor cells 3:1887
    transgene expression
      duration 3:1887
  vertex capsomers 1:3, 1:6
  virus-associated (VA)
    RNAs 1:18, 1:19
Adenovirus infection 1:20–1
  animal 1:15(Table), 1:20, 1:445
  animal models 1:20
  avian 1:20
  clinical features 1:5–6, 1:20
  disseminated 1:20
  immune response 1:6
  ocular disease 1:4, 1:5, 1:526,
    1:528(Fig)
  target 1:527(Table)
  pathogenicity 1:20
  pathology/histopathology 1:6,
    1:20–1
  persistent, in kidney 2:1082
  pneumonia 3:1493
  post-transplant 3:1832–3
    clinical features 3:1832–3
    epidemiology and
      pathogenesis 3:1832
    incidence 3:1832
    treatment 3:1832–3
  prevention and control 1:6
  renal involvement 2:1082–3
β-Adrenergic receptors, reovirus
  type 3 receptor 1:250
Adsorption of viruses 3:1408
  see also Attachment of viruses;
    individual viruses
Adult respiratory distress
  syndrome (ARDS)
  HSV causing 2:681
  in Lassa fever 2:892
Adult T-cell leukemia (ATL) 2:792,
  2:794, 3:1821, 3:1845
  acute 2:792
  cell lines 2:788–9
  clinical features 2:792
  clinical forms 2:792
  history 2:788
  HTLV-1 association 3:1845
    genes involved 3:1845
  pathogenesis 3:1845
  without HTLV-1 2:792
  see also Human T-cell leukemia
    virus type 1 (HTLV-1)
Adult T-cell leukemia virus
  (ATLV) see Human T-cell
  leukemia virus type 1 (HTLV-
  1)
Aedes
  Ross River virus (RRV)
    transmission 3:1574
  Semliki Forest virus (SFV)
    transmission 3:1657
  Sindbis (SIN) virus
    transmission 3:1657
  subgenus Stegomyia, dengue
    virus transmission 1:377

Aedes (continued)
  Wesselsbron (WSL) virus
    transmission 1:431, 1:432,
    1:435
Aedes aegypti 1:380
  Chikungunya (CHIK) virus
    transmission 1:263
  control, problems 1:383
  dengue hemorrhagic fever/dengue
    shock syndrome (DHF/DSS)
    epidemics 1:376
  dengue virus transmission 1:375,
    1:377, 1:379, 1:380
  global distribution 1:376(Fig)
  habitats and lifecycle 1:380
  sources, reduction methods 1:383
  ultra low volume (ULV)
    insecticides 1:383
Aedes aegypti densovirus
  (AeDNV) 1:385, 1:385(Fig),
  1:386
Aedes albopictus
  emergence/re-emergence of
    diseases 1:422
  global spread 3:1996
  La Crosse virus
    transmission 1:209
Aedes albopictus densovirus
  (AaDNV) 1:386
Aedes triseriatus, La Crosse virus
  transmission 1:209
Aerophobia, rabies 3:1440
Aerosol transmission 2:1176,
  2:1183, 3:1488
  adenoviruses 1:5
  influenza viruses 2:827
  viruses 1:484
  zoonotic viruses 3:1987
Aferon see Interferon α (IFN-α)
Africa, zoonotic viruses 3:1993–4
African buffalo, lumpy skin disease
  (LSD) 3:1377
African cassava mosaic virus
  (ACMV) 1:600
African green monkey kidney cells
  (AGMK), rubella virus
  culture 3:1593
African green monkeys
  cytomegalovirus 1:357
  Marburg and Ebola virus
    infection 2:939
  simian immunodeficiency viruses
    (SIV) 3:1640
African horse sickness (AHS)
  clinical features 2:1057
  clinical forms 2:1057
  epidemiology 2:1055
  history 2:1043
  immune response 2:1059
  prevention and control 2:1059
African horse sickness virus
  (AHSV) 1:420(Table), 2:1043,
  2:1045(Table)
  baculovirus-expressed VP7
    protein 2:1061
  economic losses 2:1044
  epidemiology 2:1055
  host range and
    propagation 2:1049
  infectious subviral
    particles 2:1047(Fig)
  pathogenicity 2:1056
  species-specific 2:1056
  proteins, VP7 2:1059
  serologic relationships and
    variability 2:1052(Fig)
  serotypes 2:1052(Fig)
  structure and
    properties 2:1047(Fig)
  vaccines
    killed 2:1059
    polyvalent live 2:1060

African horse sickness virus
(AHSV) (*continued*)
virulence 2:1057
see also Orbiviruses
African swine fever
clinical features 1:36–7
history 1:30
immune response 1:37–8
genes regulating 1:37–8,
1:37(Table)
pathology/histopathology 1:37
prevention and control 1:38
African swine fever virus
(ASFV) 1:30–8
apoptosis inhibition 1:72
apoptosis promotion 1:74
BA71V strain, genome 1:32,
1:32(Fig), 1:36
DNA repair system 1:33
DNA replication 1:32–3
DNA-dependent RNA
polymerase 1:31, 1:34
evolution 1:36
genes 1:31, 1:33
A179L and *A224L* 1:38
early and late 1:34
functions and
homologies 1:33(Fig)
immune response
regulation 1:37–8,
1:37(Table)
genetic variability 1:35–6
genome 1:31, 1:31–2
hairpin loops 1:31, 1:32(Fig)
internal repetitions 1:31,
1:32(Fig)
organization 1:32(Fig)
terminal inverted repeats 1:31,
1:32(Fig)
geographic distribution 1:30
hemadsorption-inhibiting
antibodies 1:36
history 1:30
host range and propagation 1:35
infection *see* African swine fever
isolates and groups 1:36
LIS57 strain 1:36
Malawi Lil 20/1 strain 1:36
monoclonal antibodies 1:36
morphogenesis 1:35
mRNAs 1:31, 1:33–4
multigene families 1:35(Fig)
pathogenicity 1:36–7
PBCV-1 relationship 1:45
penetration 1:32
post-translational
processing 1:34–5
proteins 1:31
EP153R and adhesion 1:38
EP402R 1:37
immune evasion 1:37–8
induced in infected cells 1:34
p12 1:32
post-translational
processing 1:34–5
re-emergence of
disease 1:420(Table), 1:422
serologic relationships and
variability 1:36
structure and properties 1:31,
1:31(Fig)
taxonomy and
classification 1:30–1
tissue tropism 1:36
topoisomerase II 1:36
transcription 1:33–4
transmission 1:35, 1:36
Agar gel immunodiffusion,
morbilliviruses infection 3:1568
Age
coxsackievirus infection risk
factor 1:307

Age (*continued*)
effect on viral infection
outcome 2:1183
neural cell vulnerability
changes 2:1017
Aglaonema bacilliform virus
(AgBV) 1:1296
Agriculture, emerging viral diseases
associated 1:423
Agrobacterium
T-DNA transfer 3:1898
Ti plasmid vectors 1:606
geminivirus transmission 1:604
Agrobacterium tumefaciens 3:1893
T-DNA transfer 3:1894
transposable phage 2:987
Agroinoculation
geminivirus transmission 1:604
plant viruses and vectors 3:1893
viroid transmission by 3:1932
AIDS 2:822
B cell lymphomas
associated 3:1842
cancers 2:771
clinical features 2:1019
CMV infection 1:349, 1:350
CMV retinitis 1:528
dry eye 1:526
feline immunodeficiency virus
(FIV) as model 1:540
feline infection *see* Feline
immunodeficiency virus
(FIV)
HHV-6 isolation from
patient 2:697
history 2:763–4
HPV infections 2:1109
Kaposi's sarcoma 3:1842, 3:1848
long incubation period and
disease emergence 1:421
modeling of epidemic 1:487
neuro-ophthalmic lesions 1:529
non-Hodgkin's lymphoma
incidence 1:490
ocular complications 1:528–9
oligodendrocyte infection
in 2:1017
opportunistic infections 2:771,
2:823
pathogenesis 2:771–2
pericarditis 2:1077–8
SIV importance in
research 3:1646
vaccine, baculovirus-expressed
protein in 3:1889
varicella-zoster virus
infections 3:1876, 3:1877
see also HIV infection
Air pollution
economic significance of virus
diseases 2:1323
respiratory tract
infections 3:1488
Air travel
dengue transmission and
spread 1:379
MAY virus spread 1:265
Akabane virus, transmission 1:209
Akata cells, restricted latency of
EBV 1:500–1
AKR mice, murine leukemia
viruses (MuLVs)
leukemogenesis 2:999
AKT8 virus 2:995, 3:1516
akt oncogene 3:1516
Alagoas virus 1:257
Alanine aminotransferase (ALT)
changes in HBV infections 1:643
in hepatitis A 1:638
in Lassa fever 2:892
Alanine hydrogenase, in
cyanobacteria 1:331

Alastrim 3:1670
Alcelaphine herpesvirus 1 1:181
Alcelaphine
herpesviruses 1:181(Table)
infection 1:183
prevention and control 1:183
Aleutian mink disease 2:1153,
2:1160, 2:1165
clinical features 2:1154, 2:1165–6
immune responses 2:1166
pathology/histopathology 2:1166
prevention and control 2:1167
Aleutian mink disease virus
(AMDV) 2:1152, 2:1160
genome 2:1161
geographic/seasonal
distribution 2:1160
host range 2:1161
infection *see* Aleutian mink
disease
infectious plasmid clones 2:1161–
3
pathogenicity 2:1165
propagation 2:1161
shedding and transmission 2:1165
structure 2:1161
taxonomy and
classification 2:1160
vaccines 2:1155
variants 2:1164
see also Parvoviruses
Alfalfa cryptic virus 1
(ACV1) 1:314
Alfalfa mosaic virus (AlMV) 1:38–
43
buoyant density 1:40
cDNA of RNAs 1:42
coat protein 1:38, 1:40, 1:41, 1:42
monomer number 1:40
mutations 1:42
for RNA replication 1:41
coat protein-mediated
resistance 2:1309
composition 1:40–1
cytology of infected plants 1:42
economic significance 1:43
epidemiology and control 1:43
genetics and molecular
biology 1:42
genome 1:39
RNA3 1:41, 1:42
RNA4 1:39
RNAs 1:40, 1:41
sequence 1:39
structure 1:41
untranslated regions
(UTRs) 1:41, 1:42
geographical distribution 1:39–40
history 1:38
host range 1:39–40
particles 1:40
phylogeny 1:39
proteins
comparisons 2:810(Fig)
P1 and P2 1:41
P3 1:41, 1:42
RNAs encoding 1:41
in protoplasts 1:42, 1:43
RNA synthesis 1:41–2
replication 1:41–2, 1:42
resistance to 1:43
RNA synthesis 1:42
strains 1:39
structure 1:39, 1:40–1
taxonomy and
classification 1:38–9
in transgenic plants 3:1897
transmission 1:43
virus–host relationships 1:42–3
see also Ilarviruses

Alfamovirus 1:38
pathogen-derived engineered
resistance 2:1308(Table)
Algae
cytological changes after virus
infection 1:46
eucaryotic
ecology 1:49–50
virus-like particles
discovery 1:44
nuclear/chloroplast DNA
degradation by viruses 1:46
virus families/genera
infecting 3:1754(Fig)
Algal viruses 1:44–50, 1:44(Table)
assembly 1:46
carrier-state relationship 1:50
classification 1:45
composition 1:45
DNA site-specific (restriction)
endonuclease 1:48–9,
1:49(Table)
ecology 1:49–50
Ectocarpus (EsV) *see* Ectocarpus
(EsV) viruses
Feldmannia (FsV) *see* Feldmannia
(FsV) viruses
frog virus 3 (FV3) similarities/
differences 1:45
genes 1:48
genome 1:45, 1:46, 1:50
hairpin termini 1:45, 1:46
open reading frames 1:46, 1:48
terminal repeats 1:45, 1:46
history 1:44–5
lysogeny 1:50
methyltransferase enzymes 1:48–
9, 1:49(Table)
phylogenetic tree 1:45
proteins 1:45
replication 1:46–8
structure 1:45
taxonomy 1:45
transcription 1:48
see also Chlorella viruses;
Paramecium bursaria
Alimentary tract *see*
Gastrointestinal tract
Alkaline protease,
entomopoxviruses
(EPVs) 1:477
'All things in moderation'
hypothesis, interference by
dominant-negative
mutants 2:852
Alleles 2:753
Allograft recipients *see*
Transplantation
Allolevivirus 2:1227–8, 3:1663
Alpha nodaviruses *see*
Nodaviruses
Alpha-like plant viruses
replicase-associated
proteins 3:1839
tymovirus relationships 3:1853
Alphacryptovirus 1:312, 2:1147
characteristics and type
species 1:312–13
serologic relationships 1:314
species and possible
species 1:313(Table)
Alphaherpesvirinae 1:181, 1:509,
2:677, 2:707, 3:1421, 3:1872
baboon and chimpanzee
herpesviruses 2:707, 2:708
equine herpesviruses (EHV-1,
EHV-3 and EHV-4) 1:509
herpes simplex viruses 2:677
Simplexvirus 2:677
tissue tropism 2:711
Varicellovirus 3:1421

Alphaherpesvirinae (continued)
  see also *Simplexvirus*;
    Varicellovirus
Alphaherpesviruses 1:181(Table)
  clinical disease 1:182–3
  infection pathogenesis 1:182
  see also Bovine herpesviruses
Alpharetrovirus 1:112
Alphavirus 1:261, 3:1570, 3:1593,
    3:1657
  equine encephalitis viruses 1:502
  see also Equine encephalitis
    viruses; Semliki Forest virus
    (SFV); Sindbis (SIN) virus
Alphavirus encephalitis
  clinical features 1:506
  pathology/histopathology 1:506–
    7
  see also Eastern equine
    encephalitis (EEE);
    Venezuelan equine
    encephalitis (VEE); Western
    equine encephalitis (WEE)
Alphavirus 'supergroup' 1:317
Alphavirus-like superfamily 3:1596
Alphaviruses
  antigenic complexes
    (groups) 1:263
  antigenic determinants 1:263
  encephalitic, equine see Equine
    encephalitis viruses
  evolution 1:262, 1:504
  furovirus genome
    comparison 1:589(Table)
  genome, conserved regions 1:262
  ocular target 1:525(Table)
  proteins 1:262
  rubella virus relationship 3:1596–
    7
  as vectors 3:1891
  see also Chikungunya (CHIK)
    virus; Mayaro (MAY) virus;
    O'Nyong nyong (ONN)
    virus
Alstroemeria mosaic virus
    (ALMV) 1:38
ALVE proviral family 1:438–9,
    1:440
  ALVE21 1:439
Amantadine (Symmetrel) 1:63
  disadvantages of use 1:64
  respiratory virus
    infections 3:1495
Amapari virus 2:887, 2:888(Table)
Ambisense RNA 3:1476
  Bunyaviridae 1:215
  LCMV 2:916, 2:921
  tenuiviruses 3:1761
  Tospovirus 1:207
AMD3100 (bicyclam) 2:786
American plum line pattern virus
    (APLPV) 1:39
Americas, zoonotic viruses 3:1990–
    2
Aminopeptidase N, virus
    receptor 2:1181
Amphibian herpesviruses 1:51–3
  future prospects 1:53
  history 1:51
  taxonomy and classification 1:51
  see also Frog virus 4 (FV4); Lucké
    tumor herpesvirus (LTHV)
Amplicons 1:394–5
Amprenavir 1:60, 2:783, 2:785
Amsacta moorei entomopoxvirus
    (AmEPV) 1:475
  enzymes 1:477
  molecular biopesticides based
    on 1:480–1
  spheroidin genes 1:476, 1:480
  vaccinia virus gene
    homologue 1:477

Amsacta moorei entomopoxvirus
    (AmEPV) (continued)
  see also Entomopoxviruses
    (EPVs)
Amyloid plaques
  Creutzfeldt-Jakob disease
    (CJD) 3:1401
  Kuru 3:1401
  new variant CJD 3:1391(Fig)
  'florid plaques' 3:1391(Fig)
Amyloidosis, secondary, in
    ducks 1:655
Anabaena
  AB22 mutant 1:331
  cyanophage see Cyanophages
Andasibe virus
    (ANDV) 2:1045(Table)
Andean potato latent virus
    (APLV) 3:1850
Andean potato mottle virus
    (APMV) 1:285, 1:290
Andes virus (ANDV) 1:210, 1:621,
    3:1988
Anemia
  hemolytic, parvovirus B19
    infection 2:1154
  lymphoproliferative disease of
    turkeys 2:914
  see also Equine infectious anemia
    (EIA)
Animal cells 1:247, 1:248(Fig)
  see also Cell structure/function
Animal cytomegaloviruses see
  Cytomegalovirus (CMV),
    animal
Animal models, of virus infections
  see specific viruses
Animal papillomaviruses see
  Papillomaviruses, animal
Animal viruses
  biochemistry, history 2:722
  complementation 1:609
  cultivation, history 2:721–2
  enteroviruses see Enteroviruses
  gene product interactions 1:609–
    11
  genetic engineering
    applications 1:612
  genetic reassortment 1:609
  genetic recombination 1:608–9
    see also Genetic recombination
  genetics 1:606–13
  genomes 1:607
    mapping 1:611
    sequence analysis 1:612
    see also Genetic mapping
  history 1:606–7, 2:721–3
    see also History of virology
  molecular cloning (cDNA) 1:612
  molecular genetics 1:611–12
    recombinant DNA 1:611–12
  multiplicity reactivation 1:609
  mutagenesis 1:608
  mutations 1:607
    rates 1:607
    types 1:607–8
    see also Mutations
  phenotypic mixing 1:609
  polyploidy 1:610–11
  protein production 1:612
  replication 1:607
  structure, discovery 2:722
  tumor virology, history 2:722–3
Animals
  experimental, DI particles 1:373–
    4
  prion diseases see Prion diseases
  respiratory viruses 3:1494(Table)
  transport, in spread of
    zoonoses 3:1996
  see also Zoonoses

Anogenital infections see Human
  papillomavirus (HPV), genital;
  Warts
Anopheles funestus, O'Nyong
  nyong (ONN) virus
  transmission 1:263
Anthoxanthum latent bleaching
  virus (ALBV) 2:750
Anthraquinones 2:783
Anthriscus yellows virus
    (AYV) 3:1624, 3:1965
  genome 3:1966
  geographic distribution 3:1966
  as helper virus 3:1968
  host range 3:1625, 3:1966
  infections
    clinical features 3:1969
    pathology and
      histopathology 3:1969
    pathogenicity 3:1969
  taxonomy and
    classification 3:1965, 3:1970
  transmission 3:1968
Antibodies
  anti-idiotypic 1:109
  antigen interactions 2:814
  catalytic 2:1313
  in central nervous system 2:1014
  complement-fixing (CF)
    Tanapox and Yabapox
      viruses 3:1972
    yellow fever virus 3:1986
  cross-reacting 1:391
  detection see Diagnostic
    techniques
  effector functions 3:1862
  enhancing, visna-maedi
    viruses 3:1963
  enzyme-labeled 1:392
  expressed in plants 2:1313
    to nonstructural
      proteins 2:1313
    targeted to subcellular
      compartments 2:1313
  fetal response 1:390
  formation 2:1202
  history 2:812
  immune evasion
    mechanism 2:816
  neutralizing 2:814
    adenoviruses 1:6
    animal
      papillomaviruses 2:1128–9
    bluetongue virus (BTV) 2:1058
    bovine herpesviruses 1:183
    bovine leukemia virus
      (BLV) 1:197
    cardioviruses 1:237
    cowpox virus 1:304
    coxsackieviruses 1:310, 2:735
    detection 1:390
    EAV and LDV infection 1:96
    echoviruses 1:416
    equine encephalitis
      viruses 1:507
    equine herpesviruses 1:514
    hepatitis C virus 1:662–3
    herpesvirus sylvilagus 2:706
    hog cholera virus (HCV) 2:742
    human CMV infections 1:350
    infectious bursal disease virus
      (IBDV) 1:165–6
    measles 2:958
    rabies virus 3:1441
    respiratory viruses 3:1491
    rotaviruses 3:1581–2
    RSV 3:1487
    TMEV 3:1777
    Tupaia herpesviruses 3:1836
    vaccine-induced 3:1863
    vesicular stomatitis virus
      (VSV) 3:1918

Antibodies (continued)
  neutralizing (continued)
    viral epitopes 3:1862
    visna-maedi viruses 3:1963
    yellow fever virus 3:1986
  past *vs* current infection
    differentiation 1:390
  production, time for 1:390
  vaccine-induced
    production 3:1862, 3:1863
  viral, detection see Diagnostic
    techniques
  viral epitopes recognized
    by 3:1862
  yellow fever virus 3:1986
Antibody-dependent cellular
  cytotoxicity (ADCC),
  respiratory viruses 3:1491
Antibody-mediated enhancement
  (AME) 2:1179
Anticarsia gemmatalis NPV 2:847
Antigen(s)
  antibody interaction 2:814
  assays see under Diagnostic
    techniques
  binding sites, MHC class I
    molecules 2:839–40
  cellular immunity
    stimulation 2:821
  changes contributing to emerging
    viral diseases 1:421
  circulation 2:821
  requirement for antibody
    detection methods 1:390
  synthetic peptides, for antibody
    detection methods 1:390
  T cell-independent 2:814
  viral, detection see Diagnostic
    techniques
Antigen presentation 2:819–20,
    2:839, 2:1204
  endogenous (class I) 2:819
  exogenous (class II) 2:820,
    2:820(Fig)
  virus interference with 2:1204
Antigen presenting cells
    (APCs) 2:813
  autoimmunity pathogenesis 1:108
  cytokines produced 1:339
  properties 2:813(Table)
  T cell interaction 1:109(Fig)
Antigen processing 2:819–20, 2:840
  history 2:823
  influenza viruses 2:841
  pathway 2:820(Fig)
Antigenic determinants
    (epitopes) 2:838
  atomic structure 3:1945
  B cell 2:838
  cardioviruses 1:231
  crossreacting 1:110
  hidden 2:838
  influenza viruses see Influenza
    viruses
  native proteins 2:839
  T cell 2:838–9
  terminology 2:838
Antigenic drift 1:486, 2:816, 2:1203
  contributing to emerging viral
    diseases 1:421
  immune evasion
    mechanism 2:817
  influenza viruses 2:826, 2:829,
    3:1489
  mechanism 2:839
  polioviruses 2:1327
  West Nile virus 1:427
Antigenic shift 1:486, 2:816
  contributing to emerging viral
    diseases 1:421
  influenza A viruses 2:826

Antigenic sites, atomic
  structure 3:1945–6
Antigenic variation 2:816
  caliciviruses 1:219
  canine parvovirus (CPV) 2:1163–4
  Chikungunya (CHIK) virus 1:263
  echoviruses 1:413
  encephalitis viruses 1:427
  equine infectious anemia virus
    (EIAV) 1:518
    EIAV as model 1:515
  flaviviruses 1:434
  foot-and-mouth disease viruses
    (FMDVs) 1:574
  hepatitis A virus (HAV) 1:636
  immune evasion
    mechanism 2:816
  Newcastle disease virus 2:1024
  parvoviruses 2:1163–4, 2:1165
  RNA viruses 2:812, 2:816
  rotavirus group A 1:443
  vesicular stomatitis virus
    (VSV) 3:1916
Antigenome 1:214
  LCMV 2:922
Anti-idiotypic antibodies 1:109
Anti-idiotypic response,
  autoimmunity
  mechanism 1:109–10
Antioncogenes see Tumor
  suppressor genes
Antiretroviral agents 2:778–88
  approved drugs 2:786
  chemoprophylactic 2:787
  feline immunodeficiency virus
    (FIV) infection 1:540
  guidelines for use/evaluation in
    HIV infection 2:786–7
  integrase inhibitors 2:783
  new targets 2:785–6
  protease inhibitors see Protease
    inhibitors
  recommended regimen 2:787
  reverse transcriptase inhibitors
    see Reverse transcriptase
    inhibitors
  targets for drug
    development 2:778–9
  treatment commencement 2:786–7
  see also Antiviral agents
Antisense compounds, in HPV
  infections 1:67
Antisense RNA see RNA
Antisense-mediated resistance, in
  plants 2:1310–11
Antitermination, coliphage
  lambda 2:929
Antitoxin see Antibodies
Antiviral agents 1:54–68, 1:55–7(Table)
  atomic structure 3:1946
  Channel catfish virus (CCV)
    infection 1:557
  for coxsackieviruses 1:311
  delayed/accumulative
    toxicity 1:66
  design see Drug design
  dominant-negative mutants
    as 2:853–4
  equine herpesvirus
    infections 1:514
  exotic virus 1:67–8
  hepatitis viruses 1:65–6
  herpesviruses 1:61–3
  HIV infection see HIV infection
  HIV influence on
    development 1:54
  human cytomegalovirus
    (HCMV) 1:62–3
  human papillomaviruses 1:66–7

Antiviral agents (continued)
  influenza 2:829
  murine CMV infection 1:369
  myxoviruses 1:63–4
  new drugs and approaches 1:54
  ocular complications 1:529
  paramyxoviruses 1:64–5
  picornaviruses 1:66
  in progressive multifocal
    leukoencephalopathy
    (PML) 2:882
  quasispecies implications 3:1434
  see also Antiretroviral agents;
    specific agents
Antiviral mechanisms, of plants see
  Plant resistance to viruses,
  natural
α_1-Antrypsin gene, transfer by
  adenovirus vector 1:13, 1:13–14
AP-1 transcription factor
  (activating protein) 1:27
  HSV-1 reactivation 2:682
APAF1 1:71
Aphid(s)
  accessory salivary glands 3:1904
  alarm pheromone
    secretion 2:1303
  control 2:907, 2:1194
    potyviruses transmission
    prevention 3:1375
  endosymbiotic bacteria 3:1905
  hemocele and viruses
    acquisition 3:1904
  prediction of arrival and
    warning 2:907
  salivary glands 3:1904
  transmission by see Aphid
    transmission
  virus degradation, slowed by
    symbionin 3:1905
Aphid lethal paralysis virus
  (ALPV) 2:1273
Aphid transmission
  alfalfa mosaic virus (AMV) 1:43
  caulimovirus 2:1278
  closterovirus 1:268, 1:271
  cucumovirus 1:319
  dandelion yellow mosaic virus
    (DYMV) 3:1624
  fabaviruses 1:534
  heracleum virus (HLV) 3:1840
  luteoviruses 2:905, 2:905–6,
    3:1904
  pea enation mosaic virus
    (PEMV) 2:1191, 2:1193–4,
    3:1904
  plant rhabdoviruses 3:1538
  plant viruses 2:724, 3:1903
    barriers to 3:1904
  potyviruses 3:1374
  semipersistent transmission of
    viruses 1:271
  sequiviruses 3:1624
  umbraviruses 3:1858, 3:1859
  waikaviruses 3:1968
Aphid transmission factor (ATF),
  caulimoviruses 2:1278, 2:1282
Aphthovirus 1:568, 2:1326
  properties 1:568
Apical membrane 1:249
Apis cerana,
  sacbrood 2:744(Table), 2:746
Apis iridescent virus
  (AIV) 2:744(Table), 2:748–9
Apis mellifera 2:746, 2:748
APO-1 see FAS (APO-1)
Apoptin 1:74
Apoptosis 1:68–76, 2:1017
  activation/induction by
    viruses 1:70(Fig), 1:71, 1:74–6
    DNA viruses 1:74–5
    dsRNA 1:74

Apoptosis (continued)
  activation/induction by viruses
    (continued)
    HBV 1:74
    HIV 1:75, 3:1960
    immune-mediated,
      mechanism 1:69(Fig)
    late virus infections 1:72
    nervous system viruses 2:1017
    reoviruses 3:1461
    RNA viruses 1:75–6
    Sendai virus 3:1618
    see also other specific viruses
  defects 1:68
  definition 1:68
  function/role 1:68, 1:69–70
  increased 1:68
  inhibition/suppression 1:72–4
    Autographa californica nuclear
      polyhedrosis virus
      (AcMNPV) 1:73, 1:150
    DNA viruses 1:72–4
    E6 of HPV 2:1117
    EBV 3:1960
    gene products and
      targets 1:71(Table),
      1:72(Table)
    HBV 1:72–3
    HCV 3:1847
    RNA viruses 1:74
    see also other specific viruses
  inhibitor
    IAP 1:71, 1:73
    ITA 1:71
  p53-mediated, blocked by
    adenovirus E4ORF6 1:22
  pathway 1:70, 1:70–1, 1:70(Fig)
  response to viral
    infections 3:1960
  viruses and 1:72
    evasion by 1:72
Apoptosis-specific genes 1:68
Apoptotic bodies/cells 1:69
  viruses in 1:72
Apple chlorotic leaf spot virus
  (ACLSV) 3:1838(Table)
  capsid protein (CP) 3:1839
    variability 3:1841
  classification 3:1837, 3:1842
  coat protein 3:1839
  control measures 3:1841
  cytopathic effects 3:1840
  disease 3:1840–1
  genome 3:1839, 3:1839(Fig)
  geographic distribution 3:1838
  host range 3:1838
  host relations 3:1840
  molecular variability 3:1841
  ORF 1 (216 kDa) protein 3:1839,
    3:1840
  ORF 2 protein 3:1839
  particle structure/
    composition 3:1838
  phylogenetic relations 3:1840
  subgenomic messenger RNAs
    (sgRNA) 3:1840
  transmission 3:1840
Apple dimple fruit
  viroid 3:1930(Table)
Apple fruit crinkle
  viroid 3:1930(Table)
Apple mosaic virus (ApMV) 1:39
  virus–host relationships 1:42
Apple scar skin viroid
  (ASSVd) 3:1929, 3:1930(Table)
  epidemiology 3:1933
  symptomatology 3:1934(Fig)
Apple stem grooving virus
  (ASGV) 1:222
Aquabirnavirus 1:161
Aquabirnaviruses 1:558

Aquaculture 1:553
  baculovirus significance 3:1632
  infectious hematopoietic necrosis
    virus (IHNV) threat 3:1542
Ara A see Vidarabine
Arabidopsis
  as Cauliflower mosaic virus
    (CaMV) host 2:1280
  transgenic
    Apt8 expression 1:246
    turnip crinkle virus
      expression 1:246
    turnip crinkle virus
      interaction 1:246
Arabidopsis thaliana
  copia-like
    retrotransposons 2:1315
  ecotype Di-0 1:247
  retrotransposon sequences 2:1315
Arabis mosaic virus
  (ArMV) 2:1008(Table)
  satellite RNA 3:1611–12
Arboviruses 1:486
  Barmah Forest virus
    (BFV) 3:1570
  Bunyaviridae 1:204
  dengue viruses 1:376
  DNA containing, AFSV 1:35
  emergence and re-
    emergence 1:422
  encephalitis viruses see
    Encephalitis viruses
  encephalomyelitis 2:1018
  genetic resistance 2:753
  group A 1:261, 1:263, 1:424
    equine encephalitis
      viruses 1:502
  group B 1:424, 1:426, 1:430
    see also Encephalitis viruses;
      Flavivirus
  Japanese encephalitis (JE)
    virus 2:871
  limited epidemic potential 1:421
  maintenance 1:426
  origin of term 2:719
  plant-infecting 3:1906
  Ross River virus (RRV) 3:1570
  serological groups 1:424
  transmission 2:1184
Archaea 1:83
  thermophilic 1:76
Archaea phages and viruses 1:76–89
  of Crenarchaeota see
    Crenarchaeota
  of Euryarchaeota 1:77–83
  evolution 1:88–9
  future perspectives 1:88–9
  halophage see Halophage
  of methanogens 1:83, 1:84(Table)
  phylogeny 1:76–7
Arenaviridae 2:887–96, 2:888
  Arenavirus 2:887, 2:915
Arenavirus 2:887, 2:915
  see also Arenaviruses;
    Lymphocytic
    choriomeningitis virus
    (LCMV)
Arenavirus hemorrhagic fever (HF)
  viruses 3:1988–9
  diagnosis 3:1988–9
  prevention and control 3:1989
  see also Guanarito virus; Junin
    virus; Lassa virus;
    Lymphocytic
    choriomeningitis virus
    (LCMV); Machupo virus
Arenaviruses
  B cell epitope variability 2:889
  biological
    information 2:888(Table)
  classification 2:887

Arenaviruses (continued)
  epidemiology 2:890–1
  evolution 2:889–90
  future perspectives 2:896
  genome 2:887–8
    RNA segments 2:887–8
  GP1 and NP proteins 2:890
    antigenic sites 2:890
  GP2 proteins 2:890
  granules 2:888
  history 2:887
  infection
    clinical features 2:893–4
    immune response 2:895
    pathology/
      histopathology 2:894
    prevention and control 2:895
    renal involvement 2:1084
    therapy 1:68, 2:895–6
    see also Lassa fever
  monoclonal antibodies 2:890
  New World 2:887
  Old World 2:887, 2:890
    see also Lassa virus;
      Lymphocytic
      choriomeningitis virus
      (LCMV)
  pathogenesis 2:892–3
  properties 2:887–8
  ribosomal proteins 2:888
  serologic relationships and
    variability 2:890
  South American 2:887, 2:889
  tissue tropism 2:891–2
  transmission 2:890, 2:891, 2:891–2
  vaccines 2:895
  see also Guanarito virus; Junin
    virus; Lassa virus;
    Lymphocytic
    choriomeningitis virus
    (LCMV); Machupo virus;
    Sabia virus
Arg-Gly-Asp sequence see RGD
  motif
Argentine hemorrhagic fever
  (AHF) 2:891, 3:1989
  antibodies 2:891
  clinical features 2:893–4
  economic importance 2:891
  epidemiology 2:891
  immune response 2:895
  late neurological syndrome 2:896
  passive antibody therapy 2:896
  pathogenesis 2:892–3
  pathology/histopathology 2:894
  prevention and control 2:895
  therapy 2:896
  see also Junin virus
Arkansas bee virus
  (ABV) 2:744(Table), 2:749
Aroa virus group 1:433(Table)
Arracacha A virus 2:1008(Table)
Arracacha B virus 2:1009(Table)
Arrhenatherum blue dwarf virus
  (ABDV) 2:1263
Arteritis, murine CMV
  infection 1:367
Arteriviridae 1:89–97, 1:291, 3:1798
  apoptosis promotion 1:75
  in Nidovirales 1:90
  see also Arteriviruses
Arterivirus 1:90
Arteriviruses 1:89–97
  assembly 1:92
  buoyant density 1:90
  evolution 1:93–4
  genetics 1:93
  genome 1:90(Fig), 1:97
    coronaviruses similarity 1:90,
      1:93–4
    ORF5 1:96

Arteriviruses (continued)
  genome (continued)
    ORFs 1:91
    positive ssRNA 1:91
    properties 1:91
  geographic/seasonal
    distribution 1:92–3
  history 1:89–90
  host range and propagation 1:93
    new hosts 1:97
  immune response 1:96
  infection
    pathogenicity and clinical
      features 1:94–5
    pathology and
      histopathology 1:95–6
    prevention and control 1:96–7
  macrophage infection 1:92
  nucleocapsid (N) protein 1:90
  persistent infections 1:97
  physical properties 1:91
  properties 1:90
  proteins, properties 1:91
  replication 1:91–2
  RNA polymerase 1:91
  serologic relationships and
    variability 1:94
  subgenomic mRNAs 1:92
  taxonomy and classification 1:90
  tissue tropism 1:94
  transmission 1:94
  uptake and cytopathology 1:92
  see also Equine arteritis virus
    (EAV); Lactate
    dehydrogenase-elevating
    virus (LDV)
Arthralgia
  after rubella vaccine 3:1600
  Ross River virus (RRV) 3:1574
Arthritis
  after rubella vaccine 3:1600
  caprine arthritis encephalitis
    virus (CAEV) 1:227, 1:228
  see also Caprine arthritis
    encephalitis (CAE)
    syndrome
  rubella 3:1598
  see also Epidemic polyarthritis;
    Polyarthritis; Rheumatoid
    arthritis
Arthritis-myalgia syndrome,
  emergence in Fiji and
  Samoa 1:422
Arthritis-synovitis, in visna-maedi
  virus infections 3:1962
Arthropod-borne viruses 3:1987
  see also Arboviruses
Arthropods
  barrier to virus
    transmission 3:1906
  salivary gland 3:1906
  breeding, emergence and re-
    emergence of diseases 1:422
  feeding mechanics/
    behavior 3:1900–1,
    3:1903(Fig)
  migut infection and escape
    barriers 3:1906
  piercing–sucking
    mouthparts 3:1903(Fig)
  plant virus interactions 3:1906
  transmission cycles
    influence on viral
      infections 1:486
    mechanical and
      biological 1:486
  transmission of viruses
    Bunyaviridae 1:204, 1:208
    equine infectious anemia virus
      (EIAV) 1:519
    leporipoxviruses and
      suipoxvirus 3:1385

Arthropods (continued)
  transmission of viruses
    (continued)
    pathway 3:1903(Fig), 3:1906
    plant viruses,
      mechanisms 3:1899–900
    see also Arboviruses;
      Phytoarboviruses
    virus replication in 1:486
    virus vectors, discovery 2:723
Artichoke Aegian ringspot
  virus 2:1008(Table)
Artichoke Italian latent
  virus 2:1008(Table)
Artichoke mottled crinkle virus
  (AMCV) 3:1790, 3:1790(Table)
  antibodies 2:1313
Artichoke vein banding
  virus 2:1009(Table)
Artichoke yellow ringspot
  virus 2:1008(Table)
Artificial insemination, hog cholera
  virus (HCV)
  transmission 2:740
Ascospores, fungal partitiviruses
  transmission 2:1148
Ascoviridae 1:97
  insect killing by 2:844
  insect pest control by 2:844–5
Ascovirus 1:98
Ascoviruses 1:97
  cytopathology 1:101–2
  DNA polymerase gene 1:103
  ecology 1:100
  economic importance 1:97, 1:103
  evolution 1:103
  future perspectives 1:103
  genome 1:97
    linear dsDNA 1:98
    structure and composition 1:98
  geographical distribution 1:98
  history 1:98
  host range and propagation 1:100
  lipid membranes 1:98
  morphogenesis 1:102–3
  multilaminar layer 1:101, 1:102
  natural pest suppression 1:103
  pathology and
    pathogenesis 1:100–2
    stages 1:101(Fig)
  polypeptides 1:100
  prevalence rates in noctuid
    pests 1:100
  replication 1:102, 1:102–3
  structure and morphology 1:98,
    1:99(Fig)
  taxonomy and classification 1:98
  tissue tropism 1:102,
    1:102(Table)
  transmission 1:100
    in vesicles 1:99(Fig), 1:101, 1:102,
      1:103
Asfarviridae
  African swine fever virus
    (AFSV) 1:30–8
  Asfivirus 1:31
Asfivirus 1:31
Asia, zoonotic viruses 3:1994
Asparagus stunt virus 1:38
Asparagus virus 2 (AV-2) 1:38
Aspartate aminotransferase (AST)
  in hepatitis A 1:638
  in Lassa fever 2:892, 2:893
Assemblin 1:356
Assembly of viruses 1:252–3,
  3:1409, 3:1478
  at plasma membrane 3:1925
  atomic structure data 3:1945
  helical viruses 3:1478
  icosahedral viruses 3:1478, 3:1945
  membrane acquisition 3:1920,
    3:1924–5

Assembly of viruses (continued)
  see also Budding; individual
    viruses; Replication of
    viruses
Asthma, rhinovirus infections
  and 3:1549
Astrogliosis, reactive, Borna
  disease virus infection 1:172
Astroviridae 1:104, 1:445–6
Astroviruses 1:104–8, 1:445–6
  bovine (BAstV) 1:104
    pathology 1:107
  buoyant density 1:104
  culture 1:104
  enzyme immunoassay 1:446
  evolution 1:106
  experimental infections 1:446
  future prospects 1:108
  genetics 1:106
  genome 1:104–5
    human astrovirus 1:105(Fig)
    ORFs 1:104–5, 1:105,
      1:105(Fig)
  geographic/seasonal
    distribution 1:105
  history 1:104
  host range 1:106
  human see Human astrovirus
    (HAstV)
  immune response 1:107–8
  infection process 1:105
  infections
    diarrhea 1:442(Table), 1:446
    prevention and control 1:108
  ovine (OAstV), pathology 1:107
  pathogenicity 1:107
  pathology and
    histopathology 1:107
  phylogeny 1:106(Fig)
  physical properties 1:105
  propagation 1:106, 1:446
  properties 1:104
  proteins
    capsid 1:104
    synthesis 1:105
  replication 1:105
    site 1:105
  ribosomal frameshifting 1:104,
    1:106
  RNA (single-stranded plus
    strand) 1:104, 1:105
  subgenomic 1:105
  serologic relationships 1:106–7
  serotypes 1:106, 1:446
  structure, EM 1:446(Fig)
  taxonomy and
    classification 1:104
  tissue tropism 1:107
  transmission 1:107
Atadenovirus 1:14
  phylogeny 1:17(Fig)
Ateline herpesvirus see Herpesvirus
  ateles 2 (HVA-2)
Atherosclerosis
  human CMV and 1:349
  virus role 2:1076, 2:1077
Atkinsonella hypoxylon virus-1
  (AhV-1) 2:1147
  genome 2:1149
  serologic relationship 2:1150
Atkinsonella hypoxylon virus-2
  (AhV-2), genome 2:1149
Atlantic cod adenovirus 1:567
Atlantic salmon, infectious salmon
  anemia 1:564
Atomic structure 3:1943–6
  antigenic sites 3:1945–6
  antiviral drug design 3:1946
  assembly of viruses 3:1945
  evolution aspects 3:1945
  helical viruses 3:1944
  host receptors 3:1945

Atomic structure (continued)
  nucleic acid–protein
    interaction 3:1945
  spherical viruses 3:1944
  viral proteins 3:1944–5
ATP, rotavirus
  transcription 3:1590
Attachment proteins, viral 2:1181–
  2, 3:1960
Attachment of viruses 3:1408,
  3:1471–2
  membrane role 3:1921
  see also Receptors for viruses;
    Replication of viruses
attB site 2:1236
'Attractive genome' hypothesis,
  interference by dominant-
  negative mutants 2:853
Aujeszky's disease (AD) 3:1421
  see also Pseudorabies virus
    (PRV)
Aura virus 1:502, 1:503
Australia
  rabbit hemorrhagic disease virus
    as biocontrol agent 1:217,
    1:221
  zoonotic viruses 3:1994–5
Australia antigen 1:640
  see also Hepatitis B virus (HBV),
    surface antigen (HBsAg)
Australian bat
  lyssavirus 1:420(Table), 3:1987
Australian equine
  morbillivirus 1:420(Table)
Australian grapevine
  viroid 3:1930(Table)
Australian X disease 1:424
Autoantibodies, LDV infection
  causing 1:96
Autographa ascovirus 1:98
  tissue tropism 1:102,
    1:102(Table)
Autographa californica nuclear
  polyhedrosis virus
  (AcMNPV) 1:147
  apoptosis inhibition 1:73, 1:150
  DNA-binding protein 1:150
  genome 1:147–8
  insect-specific toxin genes 1:151
  life cycle and infection
    process 1:149–50
  polyhedrin gene 3:1888
  polyhedrin protein
    expression 3:1888
  recombinant, field trials 2:849
  see also Nuclear polyhedrosis
    viruses (NPVs)
Autoimmune diseases 2:817–18
  eye disease, hepatitis C virus
    (HCV) 1:524
  T-cell receptor association 2:756
Autoimmunity 1:108–12, 2:817–18
  hypotheses 1:108
  IDDM pathogenesis 2:1080,
    2:1081
  induced by nervous system
    viruses 2:1017
  models 1:110–12
    Oldstone 1:110–11
  murine CMV causing 1:368
  potential mechanisms 1:108–10
    anti-idiotypic response 1:109–
    10
    lymphoid cell infection 1:110
    molecular mimicry 1:110, 1:112
    neoantigens 1:109
Autoreactive cells, negative
  selection 1:110
Autoregulation, negative, animal
  CMV 1:361
Auzduk disease virus 2:1140
Avenavirus 3:1790

Aviadenovirus 1:1, 1:14
  atypical members 1:14
  phylogeny 1:17(Fig)
Aviadenoviruses
  genome 1:17
    E3 region 1:18
  host range and propagation 1:18
  infections
    clinical features 1:20
    pathology 1:20–1
  molecular weight 1:17
  proteins, properties 1:18
  replication 1:18
  serological relationships 1:19
  structure and properties 1:16
  terminal protein 1:16
  tissue tropism 1:20
  see also Adenovirus
Avian adenoviruses see
  Aviadenoviruses
Avian encephalomyelitis
  clinical features 1:467
  epidemiology 1:466
  geographic/seasonal
    distribution 1:464
  immune response 1:467
  pathology/histopathology 1:467
Avian encephalomyelitis virus
  (AEV) 1:461
  host range 1:464
  infections see Avian
    encephalomyelitis
  pathogenicity 1:466
  physical properties 1:463
  propagation 1:465
  proteins 1:462
  serotype 1:465
  transmission and tissue
    tropism 1:466
  vaccines 1:468
  see also Enteroviruses, animal
Avian erythroblastosis virus
  (AEV)
  oncogenes 3:1507
  v-erbB gene 3:1819
Avian erythroblastosis virus (AEV-
  ES4), erbB oncogene 3:1512
Avian erythroblastosis virus S13,
  oncogene 3:1514
Avian hepatitis B viruses see
  Hepatitis B viruses, avian
Avian infectious bronchitis virus
  (IBV) 1:294
  cell culture 1:294
  infections 1:296
  respiratory disease in
    chickens 1:296
  see also Coronaviruses
Avian influenza, fowlpox virus as
  vaccine vector 1:581–2
Avian influenza
  viruses 1:420(Table), 2:825
  infection, clinical features 2:828
  transmission 2:827
Avian leukemia virus (ALV)
  B cell lymphomas 3:1499–500
  E26 oncogene 1:74
Avian leukosis virus (ALV) 1:112
  budding 1:113
  c-myc activation 3:1818
  defective proviruses 1:116
  distribution and host range 1:113
  DNA integration 1:114
  endogenous proviruses 1:115
  env protein 1:114
  evolution 1:115
  gag gene 1:113
  Gag proteins 1:113
  Gag-Pro precursor 1:113
  genetics 1:115
  genome 1:113

Avian leukosis virus (ALV)
  (continued)
  genome (continued)
    long terminal repeats 1:113,
      1:114
    modification 1:113
    plus sense ssRNA 1:113
  helper virus 1:113, 1:115
  infection
    immune response 1:116
    pathogenesis 1:115–16
    prevention and control 1:116
  insertional activation of proto-
    oncogenes 1:116
  oncogenes 1:115, 1:116
  physical properties 1:114
  propagation 1:113
  properties 1:113
  proteins 1:113–14
  receptors 1:114
  replication 1:114–15
  reverse transcription 1:113,
    1:114, 1:115
  strategies for eradication 1:116
  superinfection resistance 1:116
  taxonomy and
    classification 1:112
  TM (transmembrane)
    protein 1:113, 1:114
  tolerance induction 1:116
  transformation 1:115
  transforming 1:113
  translation 1:114–15
  transmission and tissue
    tropism 1:115
Avian leukosis virus-type (ALV)
  elements 1:438
  alv6 1:440
Avian leukosis-sarcoma viruses
  (ALSV) 1:1496
Avian myeloblastosis virus (AMV)
  disease induced by 3:1510
  oncogene 3:1509
Avian myelocytomatosis virus
  (AMV) 3:1510
Avian nephritis virus (ANV) 1:461
  clinical features of infection 1:467
  epidemiology 1:466
  host range 1:464
  propagation 1:464–5
  serotype 1:465
  transmission and tissue
    tropism 1:466
Avian nephroblastoma
  NK24 3:1508
Avian paramyxoviruses 2:1139
  see also Newcastle disease virus
    (NDV)
Avian pneumovirus (APV) 3:1479
  gene order 3:1482
  RSV crossreactivity 3:1485
  see also Respiratory syncytial
    virus (RSV)
Avian pox see Fowlpox
Avian poxviruses 1:576
  see also Fowlpox virus
Avian reoviruses 1:1464
Avian reticuloendotheliosis virus
  strain T (REV-T) see
  Reticuloendotheliosis (RE)
  virus
Avian retrovirus E26,
  oncogene 3:1508
Avian retroviruses 3:1496
  see also Avian type C
    retroviruses;
    Reticuloendotheliosis (RE)
    viruses
Avian sarcoma virus 17 (ASV17),
  oncogene 3:1509
Avian sarcoma virus 31 (ASV31),
  oncogene 3:1511

Avian sarcoma viruses
  crk oncogene 3:1516
  yes oncogenes 3:1515
Avian sarcoma–leukemia viruses
  (ASLVs)
  lymphoproliferative disease virus
    (LPDV) relationship 2:912
  genome similarity 2:912
Avian type C retroviruses 1:112–17
  distribution and host range 1:113
  history 1:112
  propagation 1:113
  taxonomy and
    classification 1:112
  see also Avian leukosis virus
    (ALV)
Avibirnavirus 1:161
Avidin 1:392
Avihepadnavirus 1:650
  see also Duck hepatitis B virus
    (DHBV)
Avipoxvirus
  fowlpox virus 1:576
  members 1:576
Avirulent strains 2:1304
Avocado sunblotch viroid
  (ASBVd) 3:1556, 3:1929,
    3:1930(Table)
  cytopathic effects 3:1932
  evolution 3:1937
  geographic distribution 3:1932
  host range and
    transmission 3:1930, 3:1932
  replication 3:1935, 3:1936(Fig)
Avsunviroidae 3:1930,
  3:1930(Table)
Axon 2:1014
Axonal transport 2:1014
  virus spread 2:1180
Axoplasmic transport, virus
  spread 2:1180
Azidothymidine (AZT) see
  Zidovudine
Aziridines, in foot-and-mouth
  disease virus vaccines 1:575

B

B19 see Parvovirus B19
B cell lymphoma
  avian leukosis virus (ALV)
    causing 1:116
  EBV causing 1:490, 3:1844
  feline immunodeficiency virus
    (FIV) causing 1:538
  HIV associated 3:1842
  reticuloendotheliosis (RE)
    viruses inducing 3:1499–500
B cells 2:813
  activation 2:814–15, 2:814(Fig),
    2:839
  bovine leukemia virus
    (BLV) 1:196
  by T cells 2:814
  autoantibody production 1:109
  bovine leukemia virus (BLV)
    infection 1:196
  development 1:340
  EBV infection 2:900, 3:1826
  EBV tropism 1:491
  epitopes on arenaviruses 2:889
  functions 1:1202
  immortalization by EBV 1:495,
    1:497, 3:1843
    EBNA-2 role 1:498
    EBNA-3 role 1:498

B cells (continued)
　infectious bursal disease virus
　　(IBDV) replication 1:163,
　　1:166
　influenza virus antigenic
　　determinants 2:839–40
　LCMV infection 2:919
　memory 2:815
　　Ig expression 2:815
　MHC class II restriction 2:814
　mitogen response, defect in FIV
　　infection 1:539
　mouse mammary tumor virus
　　(MMTV) infection 2:968
　mumps virus tropism 2:994
　number latently infected by
　　EBV 1:500
　polyclonal activation 1:492
　　EBV infection 3:1844
　　by LDV 1:96
　proliferation 2:814
　　regulation by EBNA-2 1:498
　receptors 2:814, 2:820
　T cell interaction 2:820
B lymphoblastoid cell line 1:497
Babesia bovis virus (BBV),
　characteristics/
　properties 1:616(Table)
Baboon endogenous virus (BAEV)
　evolution 3:1496, 3:1497(Fig)
　receptor 3:1522
　reticuloendotheliosis (RE) viruses
　　relationship 3:1496
Baboons
　herpesvirus
　　antibodies 2:708(Table)
　herpesviruses *see* Herpesvirus
　　papio; Herpesviruses, baboon
　　and chimpanzee
Baby hamster kidney cell line
　(BHK), reporter genes 1:398
Bacilliform plant viruses
　features 2:1296
　see also Badnaviruses
Bacilliform virus (BV) 3:1633
Bacillus amyloliquefaciens H,
　bacteriophage φ29
　infection 1:119
Bacillus liqueniformis,
　bacteriophage φ29
　infection 1:119
Bacillus pumilus, bacteriophage
　φ29 infection 1:119
Bacillus subtilis 168 1:136
　phage 1:131
　phage φ29 *see* Bacteriophage φ29
　prophage PBSX 1:134
Bacillus subtilis
　linkage map 1:136
　protoplasts, transfection by
　　phage DNA 1:136
　RNase P reaction 3:1553
　SPO1 phage *see* SPO1 phage
　strains 1:131
Bacillus subtilis phage 1:119–30,
　1:130–7, 3:1681
　future perspectives 1:136
　genome 1:130
　icosahedral structure 1:130
　interaction in soil 2:1252
　prophage transformation 1:136
　pseudotemperate 1:130,
　　1:131(Table), 1:133
　PBS1 1:133
　temperate 1:130, 1:131(Table),
　　1:133–5
　　defective prophage 1:134–5
　　SPO2 1:134
　　see also Bacteriophage φ105;
　　Bacteriophage SBβ
　transduction
　　generalized 1:135

Bacillus subtilis phage (continued)
　transduction (continued)
　　specialized 1:135
　transfection 1:135–6
　　'direct' 1:136
　types 1:131(Table)
　as vectors for gene cloning 1:136
　　plasmid pCV1 1:136
　　strategies 1:136
　virulent 1:130, 1:131–3,
　　1:131(Table)
　　see also Bacteriophage φ29;
　　Bacteriophage SPO1
　see also Bacteriophage φ29
Bacillus subtilis W23
　phage PMB12 1:133
　prophage PBSX 1:134
Bacteria
　adhesion zones and phage
　　infection 3:1414
　DNA-bending factor IHF 2:1091
　effect of phage in industrial
　　fermentations 2:1244
　see also Bacteriophage in
　　industrial fermentations
　endosymbiotic, in aphids 3:1905
　growth, phage effect in industrial
　　processes 2:1244
　identification by use of phage *see*
　　Phage typing
　phage–host interactions in
　　soil 2:1251–2
　phage-resistant strain
　　development 2:1247–8
　propagation of viruses in *see*
　　Bacteriophage
　proteins produced by and effect
　　of phage 2:1246
　in soil 2:1248
　sporulation, phage
　　abundance 2:1251
　starter cultures 2:1246, 2:1254
　　failure 2:1245
　　judicial use 2:1246
　　Streptococcus thermophilus
　　　phage 2:1255(Fig)
　　*see also Streptococcus
　　　thermophilus*, phage
　toxinogenic 2:1228
　virus families/genera
　　infecting 3:1755(Fig)
Bacterial infections
　in caprine arthritis encephalitis
　　(CAE) syndrome 1:228
　interferon production 2:861
Bacterial restriction/methylation
　systems 1:49
Bacterial virus 2:1221
　see also Bacteriophage
Bacterial viruses *see* Bacteriophage
Bacteriocins
　PBSX prophage releasing 1:134
　phage SPβ releasing 1:134
Bacteriophage 3:1413
　adapted 1:138
　adsorption and infection 3:1414
　　cofactors 3:1414, 3:1417
　antirestriction
　　mechanisms 2:760–1
　assays, in industries 2:1245
　attachment mechanisms 3:1414
　*Bacillus subtilis see Bacillus
　　subtilis* phage
　bacterial identification *see* Phage
　　typing
　baseplates 3:1414
　burst size 3:1416–17
　chemicals controlling 2:1247
　as cloning vectors 2:1240–3
　　expression vectors 2:1242
　　hybrid systems 2:1243
　　insertion vectors 2:1241, 2:1243

Bacteriophage (continued)
　as cloning vectors (continued)
　　lambda vectors 2:1240–1
　　M13 2:1242
　　multicomponent 2:1243
　　for other bacteria 2:1243
　　phage P1 2:1242
　　plasmid/phage 2:1243
　　replacement vectors 2:1241,
　　　2:1241–2
　　requirements 2:1241
　　see also Insertion vectors
　complex, structures 3:1956
　concentration and
　　purification 3:1417
　conversion (lysogenic
　　conversion) 2:1228, 3:1415
　　definition 2:1228
　　see also Bacteriophage, toxins
　　　and phage conversion
　counts 2:1208
　culture conditions 3:1417
　of cyanobacteria *see*
　　Cyanophages
　densities 2:1208
　details 2:1223–8
　development prevention by
　　antisense mRNA 2:1248
　discovery 2:720, 2:725–6, 2:727–8
　display process, filamentous
　　phage 1:552
　DNA *see* DNA bacteriophage
　DNA modification/restriction *see*
　　Host-controlled modification
　　and restriction
　ecology 2:1208–9
　evolution 2:1209
　　gene clusters 2:1256
　exclusion, T4 *rII* mutants and
　　lambda *rex* genes 3:1715
　filamentous *see* Filamentous
　　phage
　frog virus 3 (FV3) shared
　　features 1:587(Table)
　genetics, history 2:721
　genome
　　fusion with cellular
　　　DNA 2:1236
　　integration at attachment
　　　sites 3:1415
　geographic distribution 2:1209
　growth 3:1414
　　measurement 3:1416–17
　head and tail, of
　　methanogens 1:83
　helper 2:1236–7
　history *see* History of virology
　homologies between genes and
　　host genes 2:1210
　homologous recombination *see*
　　Genetic recombination,
　　bacteriophage
　host–phage interactions, in
　　soil 2:1251–2, 2:1252–3
　immunity to
　　superinfection 3:1415
　as indicators of contamination by
　　bacteria 1:138
　killing efficiency 2:1244
　latent period 3:1416–17
　lysogenic *see* Bacteriophage,
　　temperate
　lysogenic conversion *see*
　　Bacteriophage, conversion
　lysogenic cycle 3:1415
　　maintenance 3:1415
　　see also Lysogeny; Prophage
　lytic, for phage typing 1:138,
　　1:139
　lytic cycle 3:1414–15
　　early gene
　　　transcription 3:1414–15

Bacteriophage (continued)
　lytic cycle (continued)
　　gene expression 3:1414
　　phage release 3:1415
　M/R systems *see* Host-controlled
　　modification and restriction
　maturation 3:1415
　media inhibiting 2:1247
　methyltransferases 2:761
　multiplication cycle 3:1413–14,
　　3:1414–16
　nonlytic multiplication 3:1415–16
　nucleic acid replication 3:1415
　packaging
　　genomes 2:1236–7
　　headful of DNA 2:1235–6
　plating and titration 3:1416–17
　population biology 2:1209
　propagation 3:1413–18
　　high-titre stocks 3:1417
　　liquid media 3:1417
　　solid media 3:1417
　prophage *see* Prophage
　protein coat, during infection
　　process 3:1414
　receptors 3:1414
　recombination 3:1446,
　　3:1448(Fig)
　　E. coli analogy 3:1449(Table)
　replication rate 2:1244
　repressors 3:1415
　resistance, *Streptococcus
　　thermophilus* 2:1260
　restriction 1:611
　RNA *see* RNA bacteriophage
　single-burst experiment 2:720
　single-stranded RNA *see* RNA
　　bacteriophage, single-
　　stranded
　in soil 2:1248–53
　　abundance and host
　　　abundance 2:1252
　　adsorption 2:1250, 2:1251
　　community dynamics 2:1253
　　detection 2:1249–50
　　direct counts 2:1249–50
　　ecology 2:1249
　　extraction method
　　　efficiency 2:1250
　　filamentous hosts 2:1252
　　filter sterilization 2:1250
　　host numbers and generation
　　　times 2:1252
　　host susceptibility 2:1251–2,
　　　2:1253
　　hosts 2:1249
　　numbers/counts 2:1249, 2:1250
　　single species dynamics 2:1252
　　species isolation by
　　　enrichment 2:1249
　　sporulation effect 2:1251,
　　　2:1252
　　stability 2:1250–1
　　virulent phage 2:1251
　speciation 2:1210
　species, definition 2:1222–3
　ssDNA, genetic recombination
　　see Genetic recombination,
　　bacteriophage
　storage 1:138
　of *Streptococcus thermophilus*
　　*see Streptococcus
　　thermophilus*, phage
　structure 3:1413
　T-even *see individual phage*
　tailed
　　assembly/maturation 3:1415
　　release 3:1415
　taxonomy and
　　classification 2:1209, 2:1221–
　　8
　　background 2:1221

Bacteriophage (continued)
  taxonomy and classification
      (continued)
    families 2:1223–4
    ICTV Universal
        System 2:1221–3
    new phage, description
        process 2:1223
    orders 2:1223
    outline 2:1222(Table)
  temperate 2:1209, 3:1413, 3:1415
    cultures 3:1417
    lambda as model 1:281
    for phage typing 1:138, 1:139
    plaque morphology 3:1416
    of *S. thermophilus* see
        Streptococcus thermophilus,
        phage
    see also Bacteriophage,
        lysogenic cycle; Lysogeny;
        Prophage
  therapy 2:726, 2:726–7
    in animals 2:729
    recent discovery 2:729–30
    trials 2:726–7
  toxins and phage
      conversion 2:1228–34
    botulinum 2:1232–3
    cholera 2:1233
    diphtheria 2:1228–9
    pyrogenic exotoxins of *S.
        aureus* 2:1230–2
    pyrogenic exotoxins of *S.
        pyogenes* 2:1230–2
    Shiga, of *E. coli* 2:1229–30
    types 2:1228
    see also Pyrogenic toxins;
        specific toxins
  transduction see Transduction
  transposable 2:981
    *Agrobacterium
        tumefaciens* 2:987
    evolution 2:986–7
    from *Pseudomonas* 2:986–7
    life cycle 2:981–3, 2:983(Fig)
    as model system 2:987
    use as genetic tools 2:987–8
    Vibrio cholera 2:987
    see also Coliphage D108;
        Coliphage Mu
  typing see Phage typing
  Vi 1:138
  virulent 3:1413
    in permanent equilibrium with
        hosts 2:1209
    plaque morphology 3:1416
    of *S. thermophilus* see
        Streptococcus thermophilus,
        phage
    in soil 2:1251
Bacteriophage 2C 3:1681
Bacteriophage 29-alpha 3:1716
Bacteriophage 186 2:1087
  *att*P sites 2:1092(Fig)
  genes, functions 2:1088(Table)
  genome organization 2:1089(Fig)
  lysogeny
    establishment 2:1091
    maintenance 2:1090
  lytic cycle, early
      transcription 2:1092–3
  lytic–lysogenic control
      features 2:1090(Fig)
  lytic–lysogenic
      promoters 2:1090(Fig)
  prophage induction 2:1091
  replication 2:1093
  site-specific recombination 2:1092
  SOS-inducible 2:1091
  tum gene 2:1091
  see also P2 bacteriophage

Bacteriophage 434, lysogens and
    sensitivity to coliphage
    lambda 2:928
Bacteriophage 933W 2:1230
Bacteriophage α3 1:274, 1:276
Bacteriophage β
  prophage map 2:1229
  toxinogenic conversion of *C.
      diphtheriae* 2:1229
Bacteriophage β22 1:131
Bacteriophage B103 1:119, 1:120
Bacteriophage BF23 3:1716
  genetic map 3:1717(Fig), 3:1718
  genome 3:1717
  receptor 3:1718
  see also T5-like phage
Bacteriophage BG3 3:1716
  see also T5-like phage
Bacteriophage CTXφ 1:547, 2:1233
  characteristics 2:1233
  ctx operon 2:1233
  see also Cholera toxin
Bacteriophage D20 3:1701
Bacteriophage D3112 2:987
  cip gene 2:984
  DNA transposition
      mechanism 2:985
  genetic map 2:981, 2:982(Fig)
  left end regulatory
      region 2:984(Fig)
  life cycle 2:981–3
  lytic cycle 2:981
  lytic/lysogenic decision 2:984
  repressor 2:984
  transposase gene 2:984
  see also Coliphage Mu
Bacteriophage f1 1:547
  genome organization 1:549(Fig)
  structure 1:548(Fig)
  see also Filamentous phage
Bacteriophage fd 1:547
  see also Filamentous phage
Bacteriophage FI 3:1663
Bacteriophage Fs1 1:547
Bacteriophage G4 1:274, 1:276
Bacteriophage GA 3:1663
Bacteriophage GA-1 1:119
Bacteriophage H19A 2:1230
Bacteriophage H19B 2:1230
Bacteriophage HF1 see Halophage
    HF1
Bacteriophage HF2 see Halophage
    HF2
Bacteriophage HP1 2:1087
  *att*P sites 2:1092(Fig)
  Cox repression 2:1092
  genome organization 2:1089(Fig)
  late gene transcription 2:1093
  lysogeny
    establishment 2:1091
    maintenance 2:1090
  lytic cycle, early
      transcription 2:1092–3
  lytic–lysogenic control
      features 2:1090(Fig)
  lytic–lysogenic
      promoters 2:1090(Fig)
  site-specific recombination 2:1092
  SOS-inducible 2:1091
  see also P2 bacteriophage
Bacteriophage Hs1 1:83
Bacteriophage If1 1:547
Bacteriophage If2 1:547
Bacteriophage in industrial
    fermentations 2:1244–8
  contamination source 2:1244
  continuous fermentations 2:1246
  control 2:1246–7
    by antiphage chemicals 2:1247
    by judicial starter use 2:1246–7
    by sanitation 2:1246
    by strain substitution 2:1245

Bacteriophage in industrial
    fermentations (continued)
  detection 2:1245, 2:1247
  factors predisposing 2:1244–5
    strains, spread and
        efficiency 2:1244
  impact during scale-up of
      starter 2:1244–5
  induction of prophage 2:1254
  industries affected 2:1245–6
  lysogenic phage 2:1254
  phage strain diversity 2:1245
  phage-resistant strains 2:1246–7
    development 2:1247–8
  production facilities 2:1245
  prophage curing of starter
      cultures 2:1247
  S. thermophilus phage 2:1254
    see also *Streptococcus
        thermophilus*, phage
  starter failures 2:1245
Bacteriophage K139 2:1087
Bacteriophage KU1 3:1663
Bacteriophage λ see Coliphage
    lambda
Bacteriophage M2Y 1:119
  DNA 1:120
Bacteriophage M13 1:547
  as cloning vector 2:1242
    cloning sites 2:1242
    plasmid with 2:1243
  genome 2:1242
  packaging, genome length 2:1238
  see also Filamentous phage
Bacteriophage MS2 3:1663
  attachment process and
      infection 3:1664
  coat protein 3:1663
  structure 3:1955, 3:1955(Fig)
  see also RNA bacteriophage,
      single-stranded
Bacteriophage Mu see Coliphage
    Mu
Bacteriophage Nf 1:119
  DNA 1:120
Bacteriophage NL95 3:1663
Bacteriophage P1 see P1
    Bacteriophage
Bacteriophage P2 see P2
    bacteriophage
Bacteriophage P3 1:455
Bacteriophage P4 see P4
    bacteriophage
Bacteriophage P7 see P7
    bacteriophage
Bacteriophage PB 3:1716
  see also T5-like phage
Bacteriophage PBS1 1:133, 1:135,
    1:136
Bacteriophage PBSX
  prophage 1:134–5
  transcription 1:135
Bacteriophage Pf1 1:547
Bacteriophage Pf3 1:547
Bacteriophage PG 1:84(Table)
Bacteriophage ΦH-like 2:1224
Bacteriophage φ3T 1:134
Bacteriophage φ6 2:1205–8
  classification 2:1205
  discovery 2:1205
  genetics 2:1206–7
  genome 2:1206–7
    map 2:1206(Fig)
  host range 2:1205
  hydrophobic membrane-
      associated proteins 2:1205
  in vitro assembly 2:1207(Fig),
      2:1208
  life cycle 2:1207–8, 2:1207(Fig)
  mutation rate 2:1206
  nucleocapsid 2:1205, 2:1207
  packaging 2:1207

Bacteriophage φ6 (continued)
  protein functions 2:1206(Table)
  protein P3 2:1207
  protein P5 2:1207
  protein P6 2:1207
  protein P8 2:1207
  replication 2:1207, 2:1207(Fig)
  spike protein 2:1205
  structure and properties 2:1205–
      6, 2:1205(Fig)
  transcription 2:1207
Bacteriophage φ15 1:119
  DNA 1:120
Bacteriophage φ29 1:119, 1:132–3
  adsorption 1:119, 1:120
  classification 1:119
  DNA
    in vitro amplification 1:125–6
    inverted terminal repeat 1:120
    p6 interaction 1:124
    structure/sequence 1:120
  DNA binding protein 1:121
  DNA encapsidation 1:129, 1:129–
      30
    chimeric proheads 1:130
  DNA polymerase 1:121, 1:122,
      1:126, 1:132
    amino acid sequence 1:123
    C-terminal domain 1:124
    consensus motifs 1:123–4
    eukaryotic homology 1:123
    functional domains 1:123–4
    inhibitors 1:123
    mutants 1:123, 1:124
    as proofreading enzyme 1:122
  EcoRI cleavage map 1:120
  gene expression regulation 1:126,
      1:136
  genes 1:121(Table), 1:132
    cloning in *E. coli* 1:122
  ORFs 1:120, 1:120–1
  genetic map 1:119
  genetics 1:119–20
  host range 1:119
  in vitro assembly system 1:129
  as lytic phage 1:119
  morphogenesis and assembly
      1:128–9, 1:132–3
  mutants
    gene 14 1:119
    spontaneous deletion 1:119
    sus 1:119
    ts 1:119, 1:124
  prohead RNA (pRNA), for DNA
      packaging 1:129–30
  proteins 1:120–1, 1:132
    p4 1:127–8
    p6 1:124–5, 1:128, 1:132
    p7 1:128
    p8 and p8.5 1:128, 1:129
    p9 (tail protein) 1:129
    p10 1:128
    p16 1:129, 1:133
    p17 1:121
    SSB (p5) 1:125
  related phage 1:119
  replication 1:121–6, 1:132
    of displaced strand 1:122
    DNA polymerase
        domains 1:123–4
    gene 5 product (p5; SSB) 1:125
    gene 6 product (protein
        p6) 1:124–5, 1:132
    initiation 1:125
    origins 1:122
    proteins involved 1:121–2
    replicative intermediates 1:121,
        1:122, 1:125
    sliding-back mechanism 1:126
    TP and DNA polymerase
        role 1:122
    TP domains 1:122–3

Bacteriophage φ29 (continued)
  replication (continued)
    TP–dAMP initiation complex 1:122, 1:124, 1:126, 1:132
    transcription relationship 1:128
  σ^A RNA polymerase 1:127
    carboxy-terminal domain (CTD) 1:127
  sporulating cell infection 1:119
  structure 1:120–1
  terminal protein (TP; p3) 1:120, 1:122, 1:132
    functional domains 1:122–3
    RGD motif 1:123
  TP–DNA complex 1:122, 1:125, 1:132
  in vitro packaging 1:129
  maturation pathway 1:129
  transcription 1:126–8, 1:132
    A2b and A2c promoters 1:127, 1:128, 1:132
    A3 promoter 1:127, 1:128, 1:132
    in vitro 1:127–8
    in vivo 1:127
    map 1:126–7
    model 1:127
    p4 role 1:127
    promoters 1:126, 1:127, 1:132
    regulation 1:127–8
    termination/terminators 1:126–7, 1:132
  transfection 1:136
Bacteriophage φ29-like viruses 2:1225
Bacteriophage φ105 1:133–4
  DNA and cohesive ends 1:133
  as gene cloning vector 1:136
  prophage insertion 1:134
  replication 1:134
  repressor gene cI 1:134
Bacteriophage φ105J119, as cloning vector 1:136
Bacteriophage φCTX 2:1087
Bacteriophage φF1 1:84(Table)
Bacteriophage φF3 1:84(Table)
Bacteriophage φH see Halophage φH
Bacteriophage φN see Halophage φN
Bacteriophage φR67 2:1087
  lytic–lysogenic promoters 2:1090(Fig)
Bacteriophage φR73 2:1104
  int gene 2:1104
  msDNA 2:1104
Bacteriophage φR86 2:1087
Bacteriophage φSfi21 2:1258
  DNA packaging 2:1261(Fig)
  gene cluster 2:1260
  genes 2:1261(Fig)
  genome 2:1258
    map 2:1259(Fig)
  lysogeny module 2:1258
  morphogenesis 2:1260, 2:1261(Fig)
  superinfection 2:1259
  transformation 2:1259
Bacteriophage φX174 1:274–81
  attachment and uncoating 1:275–6
  capsid and spikes 1:274–5
  cis-acting proteins 1:279–80
  as cloning vehicle 1:280
  DnaG primase 1:276
  ecology 1:274
  gene E 1:275, 1:280(Fig)
  gene expression 1:279–80
  gene K 1:275
  genetic map 1:275, 1:275(Fig)
  genome structure 1:275

Bacteriophage φX174 (continued)
  χ site 2:1213
  host range 1:274
  in vitro replication 1:280–1
  morphogenesis 1:279(Fig)
  mutations 1:275
  preprimosome and proteins 1:276
  promoters 1:279
  proteins 1:274–5
    B and D 1:278
    E protein 1:278, 1:280(Fig)
    F and G proteins 1:278
    gene A* protein 1:275, 1:276
    gene A protein 1:278, 1:279
    gene H protein 1:276
  recombination 1:280
    DNA replication with 2:1214
    RecA-independent 2:1214
  'reduction/incompatibility' sequence 1:276
  release 3:1415
  replication 1:275–9, 1:276(Fig)
    origin 1:278
    role in understanding 1:280
    stage I 1:276, 1:276–8, 1:276(Fig)
    stage II 1:276, 1:276(Fig), 1:278
    stage III 1:276, 1:276(Fig), 1:278
  replicative forms (RFI/RFII/RFIII) 1:276–8, 1:276(Fig)
  ribosomal frameshifting 1:278
  ssDNA binding protein (SSB) 1:276
  ssDNA (circular) 1:274
  structure 1:274–5, 1:274(Fig)
  superinfecting phage exclusion 1:276
  taxonomy and classification 1:274
  transcription and translation 1:275(Fig), 1:279–80
Bacteriophage pl1 1:134
  as cloning vector 1:136
Bacteriophage PMB12 1:133
Bacteriophage PRD1 2:1210–12
  assembly and release 2:1212
  classification 2:1210
  coat protein 2:1212
  discovery 2:1210
  DNA replication 2:1212
    protein-primed 2:1211–12, 2:1212
  future perspectives 2:1212
  genes 2:1211
  genetics 2:1211
  genome 2:1211, 2:1211(Fig)
    inverted terminal repeats 2:1211
  host range 2:1210
  life cycle 2:1211–12, 2:1212(Fig)
  proteins 2:1210–11
  receptor 2:1211
  structure and properties 2:1210–11, 2:1211(Fig)
Bacteriophage PRR1 3:1665
Bacteriophage ψM1 1:83, 1:84(Table)
  as general transducing element 1:83
  morphology 1:78(Fig)
Bacteriophage ψM1-like viruses 2:1225
Bacteriophage ψO1205 2:1258
  genome 2:1258
Bacteriophage PSM1 1:84(Table)
Bacteriophage PSP3 1:1087
  SOS-inducible 1:1091
Bacteriophage PZA 1:119
  DNA 1:120
Bacteriophage PZE 1:119

Bacteriophage Qβ 3:1663
  6S RNA accumulation 3:1667
  lysing protein 3:1666
  mutations 3:1432
  quasispecies concept and 3:1432
  recombination 3:1451
  replicase 3:1666
    binding sites 3:1667
    inaccuracy 3:1667
  replication 3:1666–7
    negative strand 3:1667
    positive strand 3:1667
  RNA variants 3:1667
  see also RNA bacteriophage, single-stranded
Bacteriophage S2 2:1087
Bacteriophage S13 1:274
Bacteriophage SBβ 1:133
Bacteriophage SF5 1:119
Bacteriophage Sfi11 2:1256
  genome and genes 2:1256–8, 2:1257(Fig)
  structure 2:1255(Fig)
Bacteriophage Sfi19 2:1256
  gene clusters 2:1256
  genome 2:1257(Fig)
  structure 2:1255(Fig)
Bacteriophage SP10 1:135
Bacteriophage SP15 1:135
Bacteriophage SP82 1:136, 3:1681
  transfection 1:135
Bacteriophage SP 3:1663
Bacteriophage SPβ 1:134
  DNA methyltransferases 1:134
  as gene cloning vector 1:136
  genes, order 1:134
  lysogens 1:134
  prophage insertion 1:134
Bacteriophage SPO1 1:131–2, 1:136
  DNA 1:131
  DNA polymerase 1:131
  DNA-binding protein (TF1) 1:132
  genes
    early, middle and late 1:131–2
    gene e3 1:132
  group I self-splicing intron 1:131
  host RNA/protein synthesis 1:132
  replication 1:131
  structure 1:131
  transcription 1:131
  transfection 1:135
Bacteriophage SPO2, prophage insertion 1:134
Bacteriophage St-1 1:274, 1:276
Bacteriophage T1 see T1-like phages
Bacteriophage T2 3:1706
Bacteriophage T3 see T3 phage
Bacteriophage T4 see T4-like phage
Bacteriophage T5 see T5-like phage
Bacteriophage T6 3:1706
Bacteriophage T7 see T7-like phage
Bacteriophage TP-13 1:133
Bacteriophage TW19 3:1663
Bacteriophage TW28 3:1663
Bacteriophage XP12 1:83
Bacteriophage Z 1:134
Baculoviridae 1:140–6
  biological control by 2:846–9
  characteristics 2:846–7
  genera 1:140, 2:846
  nuclear polyhedrosis viruses (NPVs) 1:146
  Nucleopolyhedrovirus 1:146
  occlusion bodies 2:846
Baculovirus
  phylogeny 1:140, 1:140(Fig)

Baculovirus (continued)
  see also Baculoviruses;
    Granuloviruses (GV);
    Nuclear polyhedrosis viruses (NPVs)
Baculovirus midgut gland necrosis virus (BMNV) 3:1632
  diagnosis structure and properties 3:1633
  host range 3:1632
  structure and properties 3:1633
Baculovirus p35, apoptosis inhibition 1:73
Baculovirus penaei (BP) 3:1625, 3:1630
  diagnosis and detection 3:1631
  distribution 3:1630
  epizootics 3:1630
  genome 3:1631
  infection cycle 3:1630
  pathogenesis 3:1630
  persistent infections 3:1630
  structure and properties 3:1630
Baculoviruses
  apoptosis inhibitors 2:865
  biological control by 2:846–9
    advantages/disadvantages 2:847–8
    commercial examples 2:847(Table)
    field trials of genetically modified viruses 2:849
    past and current uses 2:847
    production costs 2:848
  characteristics 2:846–7
  as expression vectors 3:1888–9
    applications 3:1888–9
    bluetongue virus VP7 protein 2:1061, 2:1065
    shuttle 3:1888
  genetic manipulation 2:848–9, 2:848(Table)
    AaHIT toxin 2:848, 2:849
    esterase insertion 2:848
    viral gene deletion 2:848–9
  host range 2:847, 2:848
  nonoccluded see Nonoccluded baculoviruses (NOB)
  occluded 3:1630
  resistance 2:848
  structure and components 1:147(Fig), 1:150–1
  uncoating 1:256
  UV sensitivity 2:848
  viruses included 1:146–7
  see also Granuloviruses (GV);
    Nuclear polyhedrosis viruses (NPVs)
Badnavirus 2:1293, 2:1296, 2:1314
  members 2:1296
Badnaviruses 2:1296–300
  absence of proteinaceous inclusion body 2:1298
  caulimoviruses differentiation 2:1276
  control 2:1299–300
  detection 2:1299–300
  economic importance 2:1298
  epidemiology 2:1299–300
  evolution 2:1296
  genome 2:1297
    ORFs 2:1297–8, 2:1297(Fig)
    terminal redundancy 2:1297
  geographic distribution 2:1298
  host range 2:1298
  host relationships 2:1298–9
  molecular biology 2:1297–8
  plant mitochondrial modification by 2:1298
  proteins 2:1296–7
  replication and multiplication 2:1297

Badnaviruses (continued)
  reverse transcription 2:1297
  serology 2:1298
  structure and composition 2:1296–7
  symptomatology 2:1298
  taxonomy and classification 2:1296
  transmission 2:1299
  viruses included 2:1296
Bamboo mosaic virus (BamV), satellite RNA 3:1612
Banana streak virus (BSV) 2:1296
  geographic distribution 2:1298
  integration into host chromosome 2:1298
  structure and composition 2:1296
BARE1 retrotransposon 2:1315
Barfin flounder nervous necrosis virus (BFNNV) 2:1026
Barley, seed production, screening for BSMV 2:750
Barley mild mosaic virus (BaMMV) 3:1374
Barley stripe mosaic virus (BSMV) 2:749
  CV42 strain 2:750, 2:752
  cytopathology 2:752
  economic significance 2:750
  genome 2:751
    organization 2:751(Table)
  host range 2:750
  hypersensitive response to 2:1187–8
  ND18 strain 2:752
  pathogenicity 2:752
  RNA-γ 2:1188
  transmission 2:750
  as vector 3:1897
  see also Hordeiviruses
Barley yellow dwarf virus (BYDV) 2:901
  economic significance 2:907
  geographic distribution 2:902
  pathogenicity 2:906
  PAV129 isolate 2:906
  prevention and control 2:907
  resistance gene Yd2 2:907
  serotypes 2:902
  transcription 2:904
  translation 2:904
  see also Luteoviruses
Barley yellow mosaic bymovirus (BaYMV), transmission 3:1909–10
Barley yellow striate mosaic virus (BYSMV) 3:1531
  replication and budding 3:1538
Barmah Forest virus (BFV) 3:1570–6
  assembly 3:1572
  epidemiology 3:1574
  genetics and evolution 3:1573–4
  genome 3:1571
  geographic/seasonal distribution 3:1572–3
  history 3:1570
  host range and propagation 3:1573
  infection
    clinical features 3:1574
    immune response 3:1575
    pathology/histopathology 3:1575
    prevention and control 3:1576
  pathogenicity 3:1575
  phylogenetic tree 3:1574
  proteins 3:1571–2
  replication 3:1572
  serologic relationships and variability 3:1574
  structure and properties 3:1570–1

Barmah Forest virus (BFV) (continued)
  taxonomy and classification 3:1570
Barnaviridae, Barnavirus 1:152
Barnavirus 1:152
Barnaviruses 1:152–4
  detection 1:154
  genome 1:153
    ORFs 1:153
    organization 1:153(Fig)
  geographic distribution 1:153–4
  history 1:152
  host range 1:153–4
  pathogenicity 1:154
  serology 1:154
  structure and composition 1:152–3, 1:153(Fig)
  taxonomy and classification 1:152
  transmission 1:154
β-barrel see beta-barrel
Basal cell carcinoma of skin, HPVs causing 2:1110, 3:1846
Basidiospores, fungal partitiviruses transmission 2:1148
Basolateral membrane 1:249
Bats
  control measures 3:1995
  rabies transmission 3:1987
  rabies-like viruses 3:1987
bax protein 1:71, 1:76
Bayou virus (BAYV) 1:621, 3:1988
bcl-2 1:22, 1:71
  adenovirus protein interaction 1:72
  apoptosis inhibition 1:71(Table), 1:72(Table)
  bovine leukemia virus (BLV) 1:196
  cleavage/downregulation, by HIV protein 1:75
  expression activated by LMP-1 of EBV 1:499
  homologue
    in African swine fever virus (ASFV) 1:72
    in EBV 1:73
  pro-death members 1:71
  promoter 1:74
  upregulation, EBV 1:73
bcl-2 homology (BH) domains 1:71
Bdellomicrovirus 2:1227
Bean common mosaic virus (BCMV)
  host range 2:1303
  resistance to 2:1301
    mechanisms 2:1304
Bean dwarf mosaic virus (BDMV) 1:600
Bean golden mosaic virus (BGMV) 1:597
Bean golden mosaic virus-Puerto Rico (BGMV-PR) 1:600
Bean leafroll virus (BLRV) 2:1194, 3:1856(Table)
Bean mild mosaic virus (BMMV) 1:244
Bean pod mottle virus (BPMV) 1:285, 1:290
  economic importance 1:291
  genome structure 1:287
    RNAs 1:286, 1:286–7
  nucleic acid–protein interaction 3:1945
  structure 1:286–7
Bean rugose mosaic virus (BRMV) 1:285, 1:290
Bean yellow dwarf virus (BeYDV), genome structure 1:597

Bean yellow vein banding virus (BYVBV) 2:1194, 3:1856, 3:1856(Table), 3:1858
Beans, snap, economic significance of virus diseases 2:1323
Bee virus X (BVX) 2:744(Table), 2:748
Bee virus Y (BVY) 2:744(Table), 2:748
Bee viruses see Honey bee viruses
Bees, picorna-like viruses 2:1271–2
Beet
  cryptoviruses 1:312
  yellowing disease 1:272
Beet cryptic virus 1 (BCV1) 1:314
  virus–host relationships 1:313
Beet cryptic virus 2 (BCV2) 1:314
Beet cryptic virus 3 (BCV3) 1:314
Beet cryptic virus (BCV) 1:312
  fungal partitiviruses relationship 2:1147
Beet curly top virus (BCTV) 1:597
  genome organization/expression 1:597, 1:598
Beet leaf curl virus 3:1538
Beet mild yellowing virus (BMYV)
  economic significance 2:907
  evolution 2:905
  host range 2:903
  prevention and control 2:907
  see also Poleroviruses
Beet necrotic yellow vein virus (BNYVV) 1:154, 1:588, 3:1608
  coat protein 3:1909–10
  dispersal 1:156
  ecology and control 3:1363
  genetics and replication 1:593
  genome 3:1362
    organization 1:156(Fig)
    structure/expression 1:590(Fig), 1:592
  infection features 1:594
  ORFs 1:155
  replicase 1:593
  RNA1 and RNA2 1:593
  RNA3 and RNA4 1:593
  transmission 1:595
  RNA5 1:593
  RNA polyadenylation (3'-) 1:155
  satellite-like ssRNAs 3:1613
  serological relationships and variability 1:158
  survival in soil 1:159
  transmission 1:159, 1:595, 3:1362
    fungi 3:1909–10
    types A, B and P 1:158
  as vectors 3:1897
  see also Benyviruses
Beet pseudo-yellows virus (BPYD), transmission 1:272
Beet soil-borne mosaic virus (BSBMV) 1:155, 1:588
  infection 1:158
  serological relationships and variability 1:158
  see also Benyviruses
Beet soil-borne virus (BSBV) 1:588, 3:1361
  ecology and control 3:1363
  genetics and replication 1:593
  genome 3:1361, 3:1361(Fig)
    structure/expression 1:590(Fig)
  host range and distribution 3:1362
  RNA1, RNA2 and RNA3 1:591–2
  see also Pomoviruses
Beet virus Q (BVQ) 3:1361
  genome 3:1361
  host range and distribution 3:1362
  see also Pomoviruses

Beet western yellows virus (BWYV) 2:901, 3:1856(Table), 3:1857
  economic significance 2:907
  evolution 2:905
  geographic distribution 2:902
  host range 2:903
  RNA 3:1614
  satellite RNAs 2:904
  ST9 RNA 2:904
  see also Poleroviruses
Beet yellows stunt virus (BYSV) 1:269
  genome 1:267, 1:269(Fig)
Beet yellows virus (BYV) 1:267
  cell-to-cell movement 1:269, 1:270
  classification 3:1837
  diseases and economic significance 1:272
  epidemiology and control 1:273
  genome 1:269–70, 1:269(Fig)
    ORFs 1:269–70
  host range and distribution 1:271
  HSP70 homologue 1:269, 1:270
  inclusions 1:271
  proteins 1:269–70
  RNA 1:267
  RNA polymerase (POL) 1:269, 1:270
  transmission 1:271
    reduction 2:1303
  vector ranges 1:272
  see also Closteroviruses
Beetles
  bromovirus transmission 1:203
  carmovirus transmission 1:243
  chrysomelid 1:1853
  comovirus transmission 1:290
  inoculation of plant viruses 3:1900–1
  pill 3:1853
Begamovirus 1:597
Begamoviruses
  bipartite genome 1:600
  gene functions 1:599(Table)
  coat protein replacement vectors 1:604
  evolution 1:605
  genes, functions 1:600–1
  genome organization/expression 1:600–1
    DNA A ORFs 1:600–1
    DNA B ORFs 1:601
  monopartite genome 1:598(Fig), 1:600
    gene functions 1:599(Table)
  pathogen-derived engineered resistance 2:1308(Table)
  proteins 1:600–1
  transmission 1:603
Belladonna mottle virus 3:1850
  genome 3:1851
  Iowa strain 3:1850
Benevirus 1:588
  genetics and replication 1:593
  genome structure/expression 1:589(Table), 1:592
  see also Beet necrotic yellow vein virus (BNYVV); Furoviruses
Benyvirus 1:155
Benyviruses 1:154–60
  cell-to-cell movement 1:157
  characteristics 1:155
  coat protein 1:156, 1:157
  control 1:159–60
  detection and diagnosis 1:158–9
  economic importance 1:155–6
  epidemiology 1:159
  experimental infection 1:157
  genetics 1:157–8

Benyviruses (continued)
  genome organization 1:156(Fig)
  genome structure 1:156–7
    ORF N (necrosis) 1:157
    ORFs 1:156
  geographic distribution 1:155
  host range 1:158
  infections, symptoms and
      diseases 1:157, 1:158
  members 1:155
  molecular biology 1:156–7
  particles 1:156
  proteins
    sequence motifs 1:157
    synthesis 1:157
  resistant cultivars 1:160
  RNA 1:156
    3′-polyadenylated tail 1:158
    3′-polyadenylation 1:156
    functions 1:157
    replication 1:157
    RNA1 1:156, 1:157
    RNA2 1:156–7, 1:157, 1:159
    RNA3 1:157, 1:158
    RNA4 1:157, 1:158, 1:159
    RNA5 1:157, 1:158
    sequences 1:158
  serological relationships and
      variability 1:158
  structure 1:156
  taxonomy and
      classification 1:154–5
  transmission 1:159
    by fungus 1:159
  triple gene block (TGB) 1:157
  see also Beet necrotic yellow vein
      virus (BNYVV)
Benzimidazole derivatives, in CMV
    infection 1:63
Berkeley bee paralysis virus
    (BBPV) 2:1272
Berkeley bee virus 2:744(Table),
    2:749
Bermuda grass etched line
    virus 3:1852
Berne virus 3:1798
  coronavirus homology 1:295
  infections 1:447
  see also Equine torovirus (ETV)
Beta nodaviruses see Nodaviruses
β-barrel
  bromovirus coat proteins 1:199
  capsid proteins of spherical
      viruses 3:1944
  enterovirus structure 2:738
  evolutionary aspects 3:1945
  nodavirus structure 2:1027,
      2:1028
  poliovirus protein
      structure 2:1330–1,
      2:1333(Fig)
  tymoviruses 3:1851
β-barrel subunits 3:1947(Fig),
    3:1955
  T=3 symmetry 3:1953
Betacin, phage SPβ releasing 1:134
Betacryptovirus 1:312, 2:1147
  characteristics and type
      species 1:313
  serologic relationships 1:314
  species and possible
      species 1:313(Table)
β-cylinder, polioviruses 2:1331
Betaherpesvirinae 1:344, 1:357,
    1:363, 2:698, 2:707
  baboon and chimpanzee
      herpesviruses 2:707
  characteristics 1:344, 1:345
  cytomegaloviruses 1:344
  genera 1:357
  Roseolovirus 2:698
  transmission 2:711

Betaherpesviruses 1:345
  beta-1 subgroup 1:357, 1:358
  beta-2 subgroup 1:357, 1:358
  characteristics 1:358
  homologous genes 1:363
  M25 protein 1:363
  prototype species 1:357
  species 1:358(Table)
  see also Cytomegalovirus
      (CMV)
Betaretrovirus 3:1496, 3:1518
  see also Reticuloendotheliosis
      (RE) viruses; Retroviruses,
      type D
β-sheets, orbivirus proteins 2:1068
β-strands, bromovirus coat
    proteins 1:199
Betatetravirus (β-type
    viruses) 3:1765, 3:1767(Table)
  see also Tetraviruses
BHK21 cells, adenovirus infections
  abortive with Ad12 1:7, 1:10
  Ad2 infection 1:10
  Ad2/5 and Ad12 1:10
  Ad12 DNA addition 1:9
  complementation studies 1:10
BHK21-C131 hamster cells,
    adenovirus Ad12 infection 1:10
BI-RG-587 (Viramune,
    nevirapine) 1:59
Bicyclam 2:786
Bidens mottle virus (BMoV) 3:1539
Bidensovirus 1:386
Bile salts, viral entry
    inhibition 2:1177
Bilirubin, in hepatitis A 1:638
Biocontrol see Biological control
Biohazard classification see
    Biosafety
Biological control 2:842–9
  of aphids 2:907
  by ascoviruses 1:103
  by cypoviruses 1:332
  by densoviruses 1:387
  DNA viruses 2:844–9
    Ascoviridae 2:844–5
    Baculoviridae see
        Baculoviruses
    Densovirinae 2:844
    Entomopoxvirinae 2:845
    Iridoviridae 2:845
    non-occluded viruses 2:845–6
  effect of toxins on nontarget
      organisms 2:849
  by entomopoxviruses
      (EPVs) 1:480–1
  by granuloviruses 1:145–6
  history 2:726
  by hypoviruses 2:804, 2:806–7
  insect picorna-like viruses
      for 2:1274
  by iridoviruses 2:868
  by nonoccluded baculoviruses
      (NOB) 2:1031
  by nuclear polyhedrosis viruses
      (NPVs) 1:151–2
  by Oryctes virus (Or-1V) 2:1033–
      4, 2:1034
  polydnaviruses role 2:1351
  rabbit hemorrhagic disease
      as 1:217
  RNA viruses 2:843–4
    Nodaviridae 2:843
    picorna-like viruses 2:843–4
    Reoviridae 2:844
    Tetraviridae 2:843
  by satellite RNAs of
      cucumoviruses 1:319
  tetraviruses for 3:1771
  see also Biopesticides;
      Insecticides
Biological warfare 1:423

Biopesticides
  entomopoxviruses in 1:480–1
  see also Biological control
Biosafety
  classification, Ebola and Marburg
      viruses 2:940, 2:944
  concerns over cypoviruses 1:338
  Level 4 category,
      hantaviruses 1:628
  recommendations, LCMV 2:917,
      2:919
Biphasic milk fever 1:435
Bipolar disorders, Borna disease
    virus association 1:169
BIR (Baculovirus IAP repeat)
    domains 1:73
Birds
  migrations, emergence/re-
      emergence of diseases 1:422
  Newcastle disease virus
      transmission 3:1996
  poxviruses see Avian poxviruses
  see also entries beginning avian
Birnaviridae 1:160–7
  fish viruses 1:563–4
  genera 1:161
  see also Birnaviruses
Birnavirus-like agents 1:161
Birnaviruses 1:160–7
  antigenic structure 1:165–6
  cell tropism 1:162–3
  clinical signs and pathology 1:162
  failure to block host
      synthesis 1:163
  genome 1:160, 1:161
    noncoding regions 1:164–5
    ORF1 1:164, 1:165
    ORF2 1:164
    organization 1:161(Fig), 1:164–
        5, 1:164(Fig)
    segment B 1:164–5, 1:165
    genome-linked protein 1:160,
        1:163(Fig), 1:165
  history and definition 1:160–1
  host range and
      epidemiology 1:161–2
  immune response 1:166
  in vitro replication 1:163–4
  RNA (24S and 14S) 1:163
  laboratory diagnosis 1:166
  pathogenic properties 1:162
  polyproteins 1:160
  prevention and control 1:166
  properties 1:161
  proteins 1:161
    synthesis 1:163–4
    VP1 1:165
    VP1–GMP complex 1:165
    VP2 1:164
    VP4 1:163–4
  RNA polymerase 1:165
  stability 1:162
  taxonomy and
      classification 1:161
  see also Infectious bursal disease
      of chickens (IBDV);
      Infectious pancreatic necrosis
      virus of fish (IPNV)
BIS45BS 1:62
Bis-1 retrotransposon 2:1315
Bismuth subsalicylate 2:1040
BK virus 2:876–83
  antibodies 2:878, 2:882
  classification 2:876
  detection, ELISAs 2:880
  epidemiology 2:880
  evolution 2:878–80
  genetics 2:878–80
  genome 2:876, 2:877(Fig)
    'archetype' 2:879, 2:879(Fig)
    sequence
      hypervariability 2:878–9

BK virus (continued)
  geographic/seasonal
      distribution 2:877–8
  history 2:876
  host range and propagation 2:878
  infection 2:876
    post-transplant 3:1831
    prevention and control 2:882–3
    renal involvement 2:1083
  nomenclature 2:876
  pathogenicity 2:881
  properties 2:876
  proteins
    BELP (BK early leader
        protein) 2:877
    large T and small t
        antigens 2:877
    properties 2:877
  reactivation 3:1831
  serologic relationships and
      variability 2:880
  serotypes 2:880
  tissue tropism 2:880–1
  transmission 2:880
  typing schemes 2:879–80
Black beetle virus (BBV) 2:1026
  coat protein 2:1027
  three-dimensional
      structure 2:1027–8
Black Creek Canal virus
    (BCCV) 1:621, 3:1988
Black Queen cell virus
    (BQCV) 2:744(Table), 2:747,
    2:1272
Black raspberry latent virus 1:38
Blackgram mottle virus
    (BMoV) 1:244
Blaschenausschlag (coital
    exanthema) 1:180, 1:182
Bleeding
  Argentine hemorrhagic fever
      (AHF) 2:894
  Bolivian hemorrhagic fever
      (BHF) 2:894
  Lassa fever 2:892, 2:893
  Venezuelan hemorrhagic
      fever 2:894
  see also Hemorrhage;
      Hemorrhagic fever
Blindness, Borna disease virus
    causing 1:172
Blood
  agglutination by
      coxsackieviruses 1:306
  hepatitis A virus
      transmission 1:637
  virus exit from 2:1179
  virus spread by 2:1178–9
Blood donors, HTLV-2
    infection 2:796
Blood products, CMV infection
    from 3:1823
Blood transfusions
  emerging viral diseases
      associated 1:423
  hepatitis C virus (HCV)
      transmission 1:661–2, 1:663
  human CMV transmission 1:348
Blood–brain barrier 2:1013–14,
    2:1015
  disruption 2:1014
  increased permeability 2:1015
Blood–cerebrospinal fluid
    barrier 2:1013
Blue fox parvovirus 2:1164(Fig)
Blue-green algae 1:324
  classification 1:324
  see also Cyanobacteria
Blueberry leaf mottle virus
    (BLMV) 2:1008(Table)
'Blueberry muffin'
    syndrome 3:1598

Blueberry red ringspot virus
    (BRRV) 2:1276
Blueberry scorch virus (BBSV),
    genome 1:239
Blueberry shock virus (BShV) 1:39
Blueberry shoe string virus
    (BSSV) 3:1674
  symptomatology 3:1677
  see also Sobemoviruses
Bluetongue 2:1017
  clinical features 2:1057
  distribution 2:1048
  economic losses 2:1054
  epidemiology 2:1054–5
  history 2:1044
  immune response 2:1058–9
    VP5 role 2:1064
  mortality 2:1056
  outbreaks 2:1054–5
  pathology/histopathology 2:1058
  prevention and control 2:1059–60
Bluetongue virus
    (BTV) 1:420(Table), 2:1043,
    2:1045(Table)
  antigen, VP2 2:1064
  assembly and release 2:1073
  attachment and entry 2:1056,
    2:1072
    VP2 role 2:1064
  baculovirus-expressed VP7
    protein 2:1061, 2:1065
  core particle 2:1066(Fig)
    crystallographic
      structure 2:1068–72,
      2:1072(Fig)
  infectivity 2:1059
  core-associated enzymes
    activation 2:1072
  evolution 2:1051, 2:1053(Fig),
    2:1063
  future perspectives 2:1061, 2:1073
  genome 2:1046, 2:1050, 2:1062–3
    coding assignments 2:1063,
      2:1063(Table)
    conserved sequences 2:1063
    serotype 10 virus 2:1062
    structure 2:1063
  geographic/seasonal
    distribution 2:1048,
    2:1049(Fig)
  germline transmission 2:1044
  host range and vector
    range 2:1049
  infection process 2:1072
  modification and infectivity
    increase 2:1055–6
  neutralization epitopes 2:1058
  pathogenicity 2:1056–7
  phylogenetic
    associations 2:1053(Fig)
  propagation 2:1050, 2:1072
  proteins 2:1053, 2:1063–7
    capsid 2:1052
    major core proteins 2:1064–5
    minor core proteins 2:1065–6
    non-structural 2:1066–7
    NS1 2:1066–7, 2:1073
    NS2 2:1067
    NS3 2:1067, 2:1073
    outer capsid 2:1064
    topography 2:1067(Fig)
    VP see below
  receptor 2:1072
  release 2:1055
  replication 2:1058, 2:1072–3
    sites 2:1055, 2:1058
  resistance to 2:1056
  RNA polymerase 2:1072
  serotype 10 virus 2:1054, 2:1062
  serotypes 2:1068
    evolutionary
      relationships 2:1063

Bluetongue virus (BTV)
    (continued)
  structure and properties 2:1044–
    6, 2:1062(Table), 2:1065,
    3:1956
    three-dimensional 2:1062(Fig)
  topotypes 2:1051
  transcription 2:1072
  transmission 2:1048, 2:1049,
    2:1055
    barriers 2:1055
    vertical 2:1057
  'tubule' formation 2:1058,
    2:1066, 2:1073
  vaccines
    attenuated 2:1059–60
    serotype 10 (BTV10) 2:1060
  viral inclusion bodies
    (VIBs) 2:1058, 2:1073
  virulence strain BTV3 2:1057
  virus-like particles (VLPs) 2:1073
  VP1 protein 2:1065, 2:1073
  VP2 protein 2:1052, 2:1053,
    2:1064, 2:1073
    function 2:1064
    structure 2:1064
  VP3 protein 2:1064–5,
    2:1070(Fig)
    crystallographic
      structure 2:1070–2,
      2:1070(Fig)
    subcore shell 2:1070,
      2:1071(Fig)
  VP4 protein 2:1065, 2:1073
    function 2:1072
  VP5 protein 2:1052, 2:1064,
    2:1073
  VP6 protein 2:1066, 2:1073
  VP7 protein 2:1061, 2:1065
    adherence to VP3 2:1070
    crystal structure 2:1068,
      2:1068(Fig)
    function 2:1065
    structure 3:1949(Fig)
    synthesis 2:1065
    trimer 2:1068, 2:1068–70,
      2:1068(Fig)
  X-ray crystallographic
    structure 2:1068–72,
    2:1069(Fig)
  see also Orbiviruses
B-lymphocytes see B cells
Bolivian hemorrhagic fever
    (BHF) 2:891, 3:1989
  clinical features 2:893–4
  epidemiology 2:891
  immune response 2:895
  pathogenesis 2:892–3
  pathology/histopathology 2:894
  prevention and control 2:895,
    3:1995
  therapy 2:896
  transmission 2:891
  see also Machupo virus
Bollinger bodies 1:579
Bombyx mori
  cytoplasmic polyhedrosis virus
    (CPV) 1:332, 1:333(Fig),
    1:334(Fig), 1:335
  viruses 2:1274
Bombyx mori densovirus
    (BmDNV) 1:386
  disease due to 1:387
  distribution 1:387
  genome structure 1:385,
    1:385(Fig)
  host range 1:386
Bombyx mori
  nucleopolyhedrovirus
    (BmNPV) 1:143, 1:147
  genome 1:147–8
  polyhedrin gene 1:141

Bone marrow depression, equine
    infectious anemia (EIA) 1:520
Bone marrow transplantation
    (BMT)
  adenovirus infection after 1:6,
    3:1832
  BK virus and JC virus
    infections 2:1083, 3:1831
  CMV infection after 1:349
  CMV infections after 3:1824,
    3:1825
  EBV infections after 3:1826
    prevention 3:1827
  EBV-associated B cell lymphomas
    after 1:490
  echovirus infection after 1:416
  HBV reactivation 3:1830
  passive immunization 3:1833
  RSV pneumonia after 1:65
  vaccination after 3:1833
  VZV infection after 3:1828
  see also Transplantation
Boolarra virus (BoV) 2:1026
Border disease virus (BDV) 1:173–
    80, 2:738
  antigenic relationships 1:174
  epidemiology 1:178
  genetics 1:177
  genome, organization 1:175(Fig)
  geographic/seasonal
    distribution 1:176
  history 1:174
  hog cholera virus similarity 2:740
  host range and
    propagation 1:176–7
  infection
    immune response 1:179–80
    pathology and
      histopathology 1:179
    prevention and control 1:180
    reproductive problems 1:179
  noncytopathic 1:177
  pathogenicity 1:178
  physical properties 1:175
  properties 1:174
  proteins 1:174
    properties 1:175
  replication 1:175–6
  serologic relationships and
    variability 1:177–8
  tissue tropism 1:178
  transmission 1:178
  see also Bovine viral diarrhea
    virus (BVDV); Pestiviruses
Bordet, J. 2:727
Borel bodies see under Fowlpox
    virus
Borna disease see Borna disease
    virus, infection
Borna disease virus 1:167–73
  antibodies 1:171, 1:172, 1:173
  antigens 1:173
  carrier animals 1:172
  cDNA clones 1:168
  classification 1:168
  envelope 1:168
  epidemiology 1:170
  experimental infection and
    model 1:169–70, 1:170–1,
    1:172
  future perspectives 1:173
  genome structure 1:168
    ORFs 1:168
    overlapping ORFs 1:168, 1:169
  geographic distribution 1:169
  history 1:167–8
  host range and
    propagation 1:169–70
  human infections 1:169, 1:173
  in situ hybridization 1:169
  infection 1:167, 1:171–2
    clinical features 1:171–2

Borna disease virus (continued)
  infection (continued)
    immune response 1:171
    intracerebral 1:170
    pathogenicity 1:171
    pathology/
      histopathology 1:172
    route 1:170
  noncytolytic virus 1:171
  persistent infection 1:170, 1:171
  physical properties 1:168
  prevention and control 1:172–3
  properties 1:168
  proteins
    intracellular localization 1:168
    properties 1:168
    sequences 1:168
  replication 1:169
  RNA splicing 1:169
  serological relationships and
    variability 1:170
  synonyms 1:167
  target cells 1:169
  tissue tropism 1:170–1
  transcription 1:167, 1:169
  transmission 1:170–1, 1:173
  variants 1:171
Bornaviridae 1:167–73
Bornavirus 1:168
Bornholm disease 1:308
  history 2:734
  see also Coxsackieviruses
Botulinum toxins 2:1232–3
  C1 and D 2:1232
  mechanism of action 2:1232,
    2:1232–3
  phage conversion to
    produce 2:1232
  serotypes and 2:1232
  synthesis and structure 2:1232
  types 2:1232
Botulism 2:1232
  forms 2:1232
  symptoms and treatment 2:1232
'Boules hyaline' 1:145
Bovidae 1:180, 1:181, 1:183
  members 1:181(Table)
Bovine adenoviruses (BAVs) 1:14
  genetics and evolution 1:19
  serotype 2 (BAV-2) 1:19
  serotype 6 (BAV-6),
    replication 1:18
  serotype 9 (BAV-9) 1:19
  serotype 10 (BAV-10) 1:17, 1:19,
    1:20
  serotypes 1:14
  structure and properties 1:16
  vaccines 1:21
Bovine astrovirus (BAstV) see
    under Astroviruses
Bovine coronavirus (BCV) 1:294
  infections 1:295
Bovine encephalitis herpesvirus see
    Bovine herpesvirus 5 (BHV5)
Bovine enteroviruses (BEVs) 1:461
  epidemiology 1:465–6
  evolution 1:465
  genome 1:462
    ORFs and untranslated
      regions 1:462
  host range 1:464
  propagation 1:464
  proteins 1:462
    structure 1:463
  receptors 1:463
  serotypes 1:463
  transmission and tissue
    tropism 1:466
  see also Enteroviruses, animal
Bovine foamy virus (BFV)
  infection 3:1691
  see also Spumaviruses

INDEX

Bovine herpesvirus 1 (BHV1) 1:180,
1:181(Table)
  infection 1:182
  prevention and control 1:183
Bovine herpesvirus 2 (BHV2) 1:181,
1:181(Table)
  infection 1:182–3
  prevention and control 1:183
Bovine herpesvirus 3 (BHV3) 1:181
Bovine herpesvirus 4 (BHV4) 1:181,
1:181(Table), 1:357
  infection pathogenesis 1:182
Bovine herpesvirus 5 (BHV5) 1:181,
1:181(Table), 1:182
Bovine herpesviruses 1:180–4
  antigenic relationships 1:182
  Bovidae members 1:181(Table)
  classification 1:181
  epidemiology 1:182
  future perspectives 1:183
  genome
    dsDNA 1:181
    short region 1:182
  geographical distribution 1:182
  glycoproteins 1:181
  history 1:180–1
  infection
    clinical features 1:182–3
    immune response 1:183
    pathogenesis 1:182
    prevention and control 1:183
    latency 1:182
    replication 1:182
  structure 1:181–2
  tegument 1:181
  vaccines 1:183
Bovine immunodeficiency virus
(BIV) 1:184–90
  assembly 1:185
  cell lines infected 1:188
  cross-reactions 1:188
  as cytopathic virus 1:187
  discovery 1:184
  envelope 1:185
  evolution 1:188, 1:189(Fig)
  future perspectives 1:190
  Gag precursor 1:185, 1:187
  Gag–Pol precursor 1:185, 1:187
  genes 1:185–6, 1:186
    accessory 1:185
  genome 1:185–6
    ORFs 1:185, 1:186
    organization 1:186, 1:186(Fig)
  geographic distribution 1:187
  history 1:184
  HIV-1 relationship 1:186,
1:186(Fig), 1:188
  host range and
    propagation 1:187–8
  immune response 1:189–90
  isolation 1:184
  long terminal repeats
    (LTRs) 1:185
  morphogenesis 1:185, 1:185(Fig)
  mRNA classes 1:186
  pathogenicity 1:189, 1:190
  prevention and control 1:190
  protease 1:185
  proteins
    capsid (CA) 1:187, 1:188,
1:190(Fig)
    envelope (Env) 1:187
    nucleocapsid (NC) 1:187
    surface (SU) 1:185, 1:187
    Tat protein 1:186
    transmembrane (TM) 1:185,
1:187
  serologic relationship and
    variability 1:188, 1:190(Fig)
  shedding and budding 1:185
  structure and properties 1:185

Bovine immunodeficiency virus
(BIV) (continued)
  taxonomy and
    classification 1:184–5
  tissue tropism 1:187, 1:188–9
  tmx gene 1:186
  transcription 1:186–7
    Northern blot
      analysis 1:187(Fig)
  translation 1:186–7
  transmission 1:188–9
    iatrogenic 1:188
  vaccination 1:190
Bovine lentivirus 1:184
Bovine leukemia virus (BLV) 1:184,
1:191–8
  antibodies 1:196, 1:197
    cross-reactive 1:195
  apoptosis inhibition 1:74
  assembly and RNA
    encapsidation 1:194
  cell tropism 1:195
  envelope 1:192
  epidemiology 1:194
  evolution 1:194
  future perspectives 1:197–8
  genes 1:191, 1:193(Fig)
    orf III and *orf IV* 1:192
    tax and *rex* 1:192, 1:194
  genetic and serologic
    variability 1:195
  genome structure 1:191–2,
1:193(Fig)
    dsDNA proviral 1:191
    sequence 1:191
    ssRNA plus strand 1:191–2
  geographic distribution 1:194
  history 1:191
  host range and
    propagation 1:194–5
  HTLV comparison 1:194
  infections
    clinical/pathological
      features 1:196–7
    immune response 1:197
    pathogenesis 1:195–7
    persistent 1:196
    prevention and control 1:197
    process/initiation 1:192
    tumors 1:194, 1:196, 1:197
  integrase 1:192
  molecular clones 1:195
  proteins 1:192, 1:193(Fig)
    aspartyl protease
      (p14PR) 1:192
    capsid (p24CA) 1:192
    Gag polyproteins 1:194
    matrix (p15MA) 1:192
    nucleocapsid (p12NC) 1:192
    R3 and G4 1:192
    Rex 1:192, 1:193, 1:194
    surface (gp60SU) 1:192
    Tax 1:191, 1:192, 1:193, 1:196
    transmembrane
      (pg30TM) 1:192
  proviral DNA integration 1:192
  replication 1:192–4, 1:196
    sites 1:196
  reverse transcriptase 1:192
  structure and properties 1:191–2
  taxonomy and
    classification 1:191
  transcription 1:192–3, 1:196
    trans-activation by Tax 1:192,
1:194
    transcription factors 1:192–3
  translation 1:193–4
  transmission 1:195
  tumorigenesis 1:191, 1:196–7
  vaccine 1:197
  viremia 1:196

Bovine leukemia/
  lymphosarcoma 1:184
  see also Bovine leukemia virus
    (BLV), infections
Bovine leukosis 1:191
Bovine malignant catarrhal
  fever 1:181, 1:182, 1:183
  prevention and control 1:183
  sheep-associated 1:181
  virus 1:420(Table)
Bovine papillomavirus 1 (BPV-1)
  E1 protein 2:1124
  E2 protein 2:1123–4
  E2TA protein 2:1124
  E4 protein 2:1124
  E5 protein 2:1124
  E6 and E7 proteins 2:1124
  future perspectives 2:1130
  genetics 2:1123–4
  genome 2:1123(Fig)
  host range 2:1122
  importance 2:1130
  infection 2:1122, 2:1125
    pathology/
      histopathology 2:1127–8
    treatment 2:1129
  proteins 2:1123–4
  transgenic mice 2:1123
  see also Bovine papillomaviruses
    (BPV); Papillomaviruses,
    animal
Bovine papillomavirus 2 (BPV-2),
  host range 2:1122
Bovine papillomavirus 3 (BPV-3),
  infection 2:1125
Bovine papillomavirus 4 (BPV-4)
  geographic distribution 2:1122
  infection 2:1125, 2:1127
  pathogenicity 2:1127
  tissue tropism 2:1125
Bovine papillomavirus 5 (BPV-5),
  infection 2:1125
Bovine papillomavirus 6 (BPV-6),
  infection 2:1125
Bovine papillomaviruses (BPV)
  E7 protein 2:1128
  genetics, ORFs 2:1123
  genomic rearrangements 2:1124
  host range 2:1122
  infection
    clinical features 2:1127
    pathology/
      histopathology 2:1127–8
  life cycle 2:1128
  serologic relationship and
    variability 2:1124–5
  tissue tropism 2:1125–6
  transmission 2:1125–6
  types 2:1121
  vaccination 2:1129
  see also *individual viruses*;
    Papillomaviruses, animal
Bovine papular stomatitis
  virus 2:1140
  history 2:1140
  host range 2:1144
  see also Parapoxviruses
Bovine parainfluenza virus 3 (BPIV-
  3) 2:1134
  epidemiology 2:1139
  evolution 2:1139
Bovine parvovirus (BPV) 2:1152
  genome 2:1169
    ORFs 2:1170
  geographic distribution 2:1171
  history 2:1168
  host range and
    propagation 2:1172
  infection, clinical features 2:1154,
2:1174
  structure 2:1168

Bovine parvovirus (BPV)
(continued)
  tissue tropism and
    pathogenicity 2:1173
  transcription strategy 2:1170–1
  vaccine 2:1174
  see also Parvoviruses
Bovine respiratory syncytial virus
  (BRSV) 3:1479
  RSV crossreactivity 3:1484–5
Bovine rhinoviruses 3:1545
Bovine spongiform encephalopathy
  (BSE) 3:1388, 3:1396
  as common source
    epidemic 1:421
  epidemic (UK) 3:1396
  incubation time 3:1396
  monitoring cattle for
    prions 3:1397
  prions 1:420(Table)
  origin 3:1396–7
  relationship with new variant
    CJD 3:1397
  see also Prion diseases; Prions
Bovine syncytial virus (BSV) 1:184
Bovine torovirus (BTV)
  antibodies 3:1802, 3:1803
  antigen 3:1803
  defective interfering (DI) 3:1801
  epidemiology 3:1802
  hemagglutinin esterase 3:1799
  history/discovery 3:1798
  infection
    clinical features 3:1802
    diagnosis 3:1803
    immune response 3:1803
    pathology/
      histopathology 3:1802–3
  intracellular, dimensions 3:1801
  peplomers and spikes 3:1799
  propagation difficulty 3:1798,
3:1801
  proteins 3:1799
  serologic relationships and
    variability 3:1802
  serotypes 3:1802
  structure and properties 3:1799
  transmission and tissue
    tropism 3:1802
  see also Toroviruses
Bovine viral diarrhea virus
  (BVDV) 1:173–80, 2:738
  antigenic relationships 1:174
  antigenic variation 1:177
  apoptosis promotion 1:76
  assembly 1:176
  classical swine fever virus (CSFV)
    comparison 1:177
  cytopathic 1:178
  DI particles 1:176, 1:177, 1:374
  envelope and glycoproteins 1:174,
1:175, 1:4
  epidemiology 1:178
  evolution 1:177
  future perspectives 1:180
  genetics 1:177
  genome 1:174–5
    ORFs 1:174, 1:176
    RNA (positive strand) 1:174
    sequence analysis 1:176
  geographic/seasonal
    distribution 1:176
  history 1:174
  hog cholera virus
    differentiation 2:742
  similarities 2:740
  host range and
    propagation 1:176–7
  infection
    clinical features 1:178, 1:179
    immune response 1:179–80

Bovine viral diarrhea virus (BVDV) (continued)
infection (continued)
pathology and histopathology 1:179
prevention and control 1:180
reproductive problems 1:179
monoclonal antibodies 1:177
noncytopathic 1:177
pathogenicity 1:178
persistently infected animals 1:179
physical properties 1:175
plaque assay for 1:174
properties 1:174
proteins 1:174
E2 1:175, 1:176, 1:178
E^{RNS} and E1 1:175, 1:176
nonstructural 1:175, 1:176, 1:177
N^{PRO} (autoprotease) 1:175, 1:176
NS3 1:176, 1:177, 1:180
NS23 1:177
properties 1:175
replication 1:175–6, 1:178
serologic relationships and variability 1:177–8
taxonomy and classification 1:174
tissue tropism 1:178
transcription and translation 1:176
transmission 1:178
vaccines 1:180
see also Pestiviruses
Bovine viral diarrhea–mucosal disease (BVD–MD) 1:174
Bowen's disease 2:1112
HPVs causing 2:1110, 2:1111(Table)
papules 2:1111(Table), 2:1112
pathology 2:1112
Braconidae 2:1349
Bracoviruses 2:1349
genome 2:1350
structure 2:1349, 2:1349(Fig)
see also Polydnaviruses
Brain
CMV in 1:350
JC virus tropism 2:881
virus invasion 2:1015
see also Central nervous system
'Brain fever' 1:424
Branched DNA (bDNA)
amplification method 1:392, 1:394, 1:394(Fig)
Breast feeding
cessation in HTLV-1 prevention 2:794
HHV-6 not transmitted by 2:701
HTLV-1 transmission 2:791
rotavirus infection prevention 3:1582
Breda virus
discovery 3:1798
infections 1:447
see also Bovine torovirus (BTV)
Brevidensovirus 1:385–6, 1:386
'Bridge' hypothesis, plant virus transmission 3:1901
Broad bean mottle virus (BBMV) 1:198
defective-interfering (DI) RNAs 3:1453–4
pathology 1:203
proteins, comparisons 2:810(Fig)
see also Bromoviruses
Broad bean necrosis virus (BBNV) 1:588, 3:1361
ecology and control 3:1363

Broad bean necrosis virus (BBNV) (continued)
host range and distribution 3:1362
see also Pomoviruses
Broad bean stain virus (BBSV) 1:285, 1:290
Broad bean true mosaic virus (BBTMV) 1:285, 1:290
Broad bean wilt disease 1:531
Broad bean wilt virus (BBWV) 1:290, 1:531
BBWV-1 1:531, 1:533
BBWV-2 1:531, 1:533–4
cytopathology 1:532, 1:533(Fig)
genome 1:532
host range 1:531, 1:533
serotypes 1:533
structure 1:532(Fig)
taxonomy and classification 1:531
transmission 1:534
see also Fabaviruses
Broccoli necrotic yellows virus (BNYV) 1:1531
Brome mosaic virus (BMV) 1:198, 1:322, 3:1974, 3:1974(Table)
movement protein-mediated resistance 2:1310
mutations 1:202
pathology 1:203
proteins, comparisons 2:810(Fig)
recombination 3:1450, 3:1451(Fig)
see also Bromoviruses
Bromoviridae 1:38–43, 1:39, 1:198–204
characteristics 2:809
Closteroviridae affinity 1:271
cucumoviruses 1:315–20
evolution 1:317, 2:811
Idaeovirus 2:809
proteins, comparisons 2:810(Fig)
see also Alfalfa mosaic virus (AlMV); Ilarviruses
Bromovirus 1:39
Bromoviruses 1:198–204
capsid structure 1:199
cDNA 1:200
classification 1:198–9
coat protein 1:199, 1:200
amino acids 1:199
gene 1:203
linkage C-termini 1:199
cucumoviruses relationship 1:198–9
evolution 1:202
gene exchanges between 1:201
gene expression 1:200
genes, 3a 1:203
genetics and recombination 1:202
genome structure 1:200, 1:200(Fig)
host range 1:203
host-specific adaptation 1:203
infection spread 1:203
mRNAs 1:200, 1:201
packaging 1:199
pathogen-derived engineered resistance 2:1308(Table)
pathology 1:203–4
proteins 1a and 2a 1:200, 1:201
protoplast experiments 1:201
RNA 1:199
amplification 1:201–2
RNA1 1:200, 1:203
RNA2 1:200
RNA3 1:200, 1:203
RNA4 1:200, 1:201, 1:202
tRNA-like 1:201
RNA replication 1:200–1
cis-acting sequences 1:201–2

Bromoviruses (continued)
RNA replication (continued)
host gene dependence 1:202
template switching 1:202
structure and properties 1:199
transcription and translation 1:200
internal initiation 1:202
transmission 1:202–3
see also Broad bean mottle virus (BBMV)
Bronchiolitis 3:1493, 3:1493(Table)
RSV 3:1491
Bronchitis 3:1492
Bronchus-associated lymphoid tissue (BALT) 2:1176
Bryopsis, dsRNA in chloroplasts 1:312
BS69 protein 1:26
Buchnera 3:1905
Budding (of viruses) 3:1478, 3:1920
avian leukosis virus (ALV) 1:113
bovine immunodeficiency virus (BIV) 1:185
Bunyaviridae 1:216
cytorhabdoviruses 3:1538
Ebola and Marburg viruses 2:942
Equine torovirus (ETV) 3:1800–1
fowlpox virus 1:577
granuloviruses (GV) 1:142(Fig), 1:143–4
hantaviruses 1:216
herpes simplex viruses (HSV) 2:678
influenza viruses 1:253(Fig), 2:835
measles virus 2:957
mumps virus 2:991
plant rhabdoviruses 3:1537
process 3:1924, 3:1925(Fig)
rubella virus 3:1596
Sendai virus 3:1618, 3:1620
type D retroviruses 3:1522
see also other specific viruses
Buffalopox virus 1:304, 1:3:1869, 3:1870
Buffers
plant virus extraction 3:1420
propagation of plant viruses 3:1419
Bugs, picorna-like viruses 2:1273–4
Bulbus olfactorius, edema 1:172
Bunyamwera virus 1:209
Bunyaviridae 1:204–12
genera 1:204, 1:206(Table), 1:212
hantaviruses 1:621
viruses included 1:622(Table)
see also Hantaviruses
serogroups 1:205, 1:206(Table)
Tospovirus 3:1804
see also Bunyavirus; Bunyaviruses; Hantaviruses; Nairovirus; Phlebovirus; Tospoviruses
Bunyavirus 1:204, 1:209
California serogroup 1:208, 1:209, 3:1991
epidemiology 1:208
proteins 1:207
reassortant viruses 1:209
serogroups 1:206(Table), 1:209
Simbu serogroup 1:209
transmission 1:209
viruses included 1:206(Table)
see also La Crosse virus
Bunyaviruses
apoptosis promotion 1:75
budding 1:216
cell culture 1:207
characteristics 1:204
defective interfering virus 1:208
ecology and epidemiology 1:208–9

Bunyaviruses (continued)
envelope 1:205
epizootics and epidemics 1:209
G2 1:207
genetics 1:207–8
genome
coding strategies 1:213–14, 1:213(Fig)
ORFs 1:214
replication 1:215, 1:215(Fig)
terminal complementarity 1:207
terminal nucleotide sequences 1:213(Table)
glycoproteins 1:207, 1:212, 1:213, 1:216
G1 1:207, 1:212, 1:214
G2 1:214
immune response 1:208
infections 1:205, 1:209
therapy 1:68
invertebrate infections 1:208, 1:216
mRNA, 3' ends 1:215
nucleocapsids 1:207, 1:212
persistent infections 1:204, 1:216
physical properties 1:207
proteins 1:212, 1:214, 1:216
L 1:213
N protein 1:207, 1:214
N protein synthesis block 1:216
NSs 1:207, 1:214
replication 1:205, 1:212–16
assembly and release 1:216
attachment/entry and uncoating 1:214
of genome 1:215, 1:215(Fig)
transcription 1:214–15
reverse genetics 1:216
RNA
ambisense 1:215
defective L RNA 1:216
L RNA 1:207, 1:212, 1:213, 1:213(Fig)
M RNA 1:207, 1:212, 1:213–14, 1:213(Fig)
reassortment of segments 1:207–8, 1:208
S RNA 1:207, 1:212, 1:213(Fig), 1:214, 1:215, 1:216
terminal complementarity 1:212
structure and properties 1:205–7, 1:212–13
susceptibility 1:208
target organs 1:208
taxonomy and classification 1:205
transcription 1:215(Fig)
primary 1:214
secondary 1:214
translation 1:214, 1:215
transmission 1:208, 1:208–9
by arthropods 1:204, 1:208
ts mutants 1:207–8
vertebrate infections 1:208, 1:216
Burdock mottle virus (BdMV) 1:155
infection 1:158
serological relationships and variability 1:158
see also Benyviruses
Burdock stunt viroid 3:1930(Table)

Burkitt's lymphoma (BL) 1:487, 1:488(Table), 3:1822
  B cell polyclonal expansion 3:1844
  chromosomal translocations 1:490, 3:1844
  clinical features 1:492, 3:1843
  EBV and 3:1843–4
  EBV gene expression 1:497
  EBV latent protein expression 1:492
  endemic form 1:489
  epidemiology 1:489–90, 3:1843
  malaria association 1:489, 1:494
  pathology/histopathology 1:493
  risk factor 3:1843
  treatment 1:494
  see also Epstein–Barr virus (EBV)
Burkitt's lymphoma (BL) cell line 1:497
Burmah Forest virus 3:1995
Bursa of Fabricius (BF) 1:161
  infectious bursal disease virus (IBDV) 1:162
  tropism 1:162, 1:166
Bursectomy, tolerant reticuloendotheliosis (RE) virus infection 3:1497
Burst size, bacteriophage 3:1416–17
Buschke–Loewenstein tumors 2:1107, 2:1110
Butterflies, picorna-like viruses 1:1274
Button-ulcers, hog cholera 2:741
Bymoviruses
  genome 3:1371
    map 3:1371(Fig)
  pathogenicity 3:1374
  structure and properties 3:1369
  transmission 3:1369, 3:1374
    fungi 3:1910
bZIP transcription factor 1:27

C

c2-like viruses 2:1225
C3H mice, MMTV infection 2:969
C3Hf mice, MMTV infection 2:967, 2:969
C57BL mice, resistance to mouse mammary tumor virus (MMTV) 2:969
c-abl gene 3:1511
c-Abl protein 3:1511
c-Akt protein 3:1516
  structure 3:1516
c-Cbl protein 3:1515–16
c-Ets 3:1508
c-fms oncogene 3:1513
c-Fms protein 3:1513
c-Fos 3:1509
c-jun
  adenovirus E1A action 1:27
  oncogenic activation 3:1509
c-Kit protein 3:1514
c-myc
  activation
    by avian leukosis virus 3:1818
    by reticuloendotheliosis (RE) viruses 3:1500
  chromosome translocations in Burkitt's lymphoma 3:1844
c-Raf protein 3:1517
c-rel 3:1500
  functional domains 3:1501(Fig)
c-Ros protein 3:1514
c-Sea protein 3:1514–15

c-sis gene, platelet-derived growth factor gene 3:1819
c-Src protein 3:1514, 3:1819
CAAT box 1:192
  lymphoproliferative disease virus (LPDV) 2:912
Cacao industry, economic significance of cacao swollen shoot virus 2:1318, 2:1321
Cacao swollen shoot virus (CSSV) 2:1296
  control and costs of 2:1324
  economic significance 2:1318, 2:1321
  geographic distribution 2:1298
  structure and composition 2:1296
  see also Badnaviruses
Cacao yellow mosaic virus 3:1850
Cache Valley virus 1:205(Fig), 1:209
Caco-2 cells, astrovirus propagation 1:106
Cadang-cadang, economic significance 2:1321–3
Caenorhabditis elegans, ced-3 1:71
Calchaqui virus 1:257
Calcium
  rotavirus maturation dependence on 3:1591
  T5 phage DNA transfer and 3:1718
Calcium channel, KP4 killer toxin effect 3:1814
Caliciviridae 1:218, 1:445
  genera 2:1035
  hepatitis E virus (HEV) declassification 1:669
  Lagovirus 2:1035
  Norwalk virus 2:1035
  Norwalk-like viruses 2:1035, 2:1035–41
  Sapporo-like viruses 2:1035
  Vesiculovirus 2:1035
Caliciviruses 1:217–21, 1:445, 2:1035
  antigen variation 1:219
  antigenic relationships 2:1036(Table)
  astroviruses similarity 1:106
  capsids and capsomers 1:218
  classical 1:445
  classification and genera 1:218, 2:1036(Table)
  epidemiology 1:219, 2:1038–9
  feline see Feline calicivirus
  future perspectives 1:220–1
  genome 1:218
    ORFs 1:218
    organization 2:1036–8
  geographic distribution 1:218–19
  history 1:217–18
  host range and propagation 1:219
  human (HuCV)
    immune response 1:448
  immune response to 1:448, 2:1039–40
  immunity to 1:448
  infections
    clinical features 1:220
    immunity 1:220
    pathogenesis 1:219
    prevention and control 1:220
  pathogenicity 2:1039
  picornaviruses relationship 2:1037(Fig), 2:1038
  proteins 1:218
  replication 1:221
  serologic relationships and variability 1:219
  serologic/phylogenetic relationships 2:1038

Caliciviruses (continued)
  structure and properties 1:218, 1:445(Fig), 2:1036
  transmission 1:219, 2:1039
  see also Norwalk-like viruses; Rabbit hemorrhagic disease virus; Sapporo-like viruses; Vesicular exanthema virus
California encephalitis, as 'delayed emerging disease' 1:422
California encephalitis virus 3:1991
California group encephalitis viruses 3:1991
Californian mule deer 1:20
Californian volepox virus 1:304
Callitrichid arenavirus, in tamarins 1:420(Table)
Calnexin 2:819
Calomys rodents
  arenavirus infections 2:888, 2:889
  Junin virus transmission 2:891
  Machupo virus transmission 2:891
Calopo yellow mosaic virus (CYMV) 3:1675, 3:1679(Table)
  host range 3:1677
  symptomatology 3:1677
  see also Sobemoviruses
Calopogonium yellow mosaic virus 3:1850
Calreticulin 2:819, 3:1594
Camel contagious ecthyma virus 2:1141
Camelpox, evolution 3:1670
cAMP responsive element (CRE) see Cyclic AMP responsive element (CRE)
Canarypox 1:576
Canarypox virus
  infection 1:579
  vaccine 1:581
  vector 3:1888
Cancer
  virus-associated, latency periods 3:1849(Table)
  viruses causing see Tumor viruses, human
  see also Carcinogenesis; Oncogenesis; Transformation; Tumors
Cancer cells, properties 3:1818
Cancer-inducing mutations, signaling pathway as direct target 3:1818
Canine adenoviruses 1:20
  serotypes (CAV-1 and CAV-2) 1:20
Canine coronavirus (CCV) 1:294
Canine distemper 3:1562
  clinical features 3:1567
  geographic distribution 3:1560
  pathology 3:1567
Canine distemper virus (CDV) 2:953
  biotypes 3:1566
  in black-footed ferret 1:420(Table)
  epizootiology 3:1565–6
  evolution 3:1564
  history 3:1560
  host range 3:1562
  isolation 3:1562
  properties and genome 3:1562
  vaccines 3:1569
  see also Morbilliviruses
Canine fetal thymus (Cf2Th), BIV infection 1:188
Canine minute virus see Minute virus of canines (MVC)
Canine oral papillomavirus (COPV) 2:1122

Canine parainfluenza virus 5 (CPIV-5) 2:1139
Canine parvovirus (CPV) 2:1152, 2:1160
  antigenic variants 2:1163–4, 2:1165
  emergence/re-emergence 1:420(Table)
  epidemiology 2:1164–5
  evolution 2:1153
  genetics 2:1161
  genome 2:1161, 2:1163(Fig)
  geographic/seasonal distribution 2:1160
  host range 2:1160
  infections
    clinical features 2:1154, 2:1165
    immune responses 2:1166
    pathology/histopathology 2:1166
    prevention and control 2:1167
  infectious plasmid clones 2:1161–3
  monoclonal antibodies 2:1163
  pathogenicity 2:1165
  phylogeny 2:1164(Fig)
  propagation 2:1161
  properties 2:1155
  in red wolf 1:420(Table)
  structure 2:1155, 2:1161, 2:1162(Fig)
    canyon 2:1161
  taxonomy and classification 2:1160
  transmission 2:1164–5
  vaccines 2:1167
  see also Parvoviruses
Canine parvovirus type 2, evolution from feline parvovirus 1:420
Canna yellow mottle virus (CaYMV) 2:1296
Cannibalism
  cessation 3:1401
  iridovirus transmission 2:866
  Kuru transmission 3:1392, 3:1399, 3:1400, 3:1401
Canyon hypothesis 1:231
Canyon structure 3:1945
  animal enteroviruses 1:463
  polioviruses 2:1331
Cap snatching 3:1762
CAP-binding complex, foot-and-mouth disease virus translation 1:571
Capillary leakage
  Argentine hemorrhagic fever (AHF) 2:892
  Bolivian hemorrhagic fever (BHF) 2:892
  Lassa fever 2:892
Capillovirus 1:222
Capilloviruses 1:222
  detection and control 1:222
  geographic distribution 1:222
  host range and symptoms 1:222
  structure and properties 1:222
  taxonomy and classification 1:222
  transmission 1:222
Caprine arthritis encephalitis (CAE) syndrome 1:223
  bacterial/parasitic infections in 1:228
  clinical features 1:227
  future perspectives 1:228
  histopathology 1:227–8
  immune response 1:228
  pathogenesis 1:227
Caprine arthritis encephalitis virus (CAEV) 1:223–9, 3:1962
  apoptosis promotion 1:76
  assembly 1:226

Caprine arthritis encephalitis virus
    (CAEV) (continued)
  capsid proteins 1:223
  classification 1:223
  dUTPase (pseudoprotease)
      gene 1:225
  env gene 1:223
    hypervariable domain 1:227
  Env precursor 1:226
  epidemiology 1:227
  gag and *pol* genes 1:223, 1:225–6
  gene expression
      regulation 1:225(Fig)
  genetic variation 1:226
  genetics and evolution 1:226–7
  genome 1:223
    organization 1:224(Fig)
    positive-strand ssRNA 1:223
  history 1:223
  host range and
      epizootiology 1:226, 3:1962–3
  in vivo expression 1:226
  infection *see* Caprine arthritis
      encephalitis (CAE)
      syndrome
  as model for macrophage-tropic
      lentivirus infections 1:228
  pathogenicity 1:227
  propagation 1:226
  replication 1:225–6, 1:227
  rev gene 1:224–5
  structure and properties 1:223–5
  tat gene 1:224
  taxonomy and
      classification 3:1963
  transcription and
      translation 1:225–6
  transmission 1:226
  vaccination 1:228
  vaccines 1:228
  vif gene 1:224
Caprine herpesvirus 1 1:181(Table)
  disease 1:183
Caprine respiratory syncytial virus
    (CRSV) 3:1479
Capripoxvirus 3:1376
Capripoxviruses 3:1376–81
  antibodies 3:1380
  cell lines and isolates 3:1377
  enveloped 3:1380
  epidemiology 3:1378
  evolution 3:1377
  future perspectives 3:1381
  genetics 3:1377
  genome, comparisons 3:1377
  geographic/seasonal
      distribution 3:1376
  history 3:1376
  host range and
      propagation 3:1376–7
  infection
    clinical features 3:1379–80,
        3:1380(Fig)
    immune response 3:1380
    incubation period 3:1379
    pathology/
        histopathology 3:1380,
        3:1380(Fig)
    prevention and control 3:1380–
        1
  pathogenicity 3:1379
  serologic relationships and
      variability 3:1377–8
  taxonomy and
      classification 3:1376
  tissue tropism 3:1378–9
  transmission 3:1376, 3:1378–9
  use of term 3:1376
  vaccines 3:1377, 3:1381
  viruses in scabs 3:1379

Capripoxviruses (continued)
  see also Goatpox; Lumpy skin
      disease of cattle (LSD);
      Sheeppox
Capsids 3:1946
  all-pentamer 3:1951
  antiparallel β sandwich 3:1948
  assembly 3:1947–8
  cell attachment proteins 2:1181
  folds used 3:1948, 3:1955,
      3:1955(Fig)
  icosahedral *see* Icosahedral
      symmetry
  maturation 3:1409
  proteins
    atomic structure 3:1944
    evolutionary aspects 3:1945
    in RNA viruses,
        functions 3:1946(Table)
  T=4 quasi-symmetry 3:1766
Capsules, phage adsorption 3:1414
2′-Carbodeoxyguanosine, duck
    hepatitis B virus (DHBV)
    infection 1:656
Carbohydrate, in glycocalyx 1:249
Carbon dioxide sensitivity 1:259,
    1:260
  Drosophila 3:1635, 3:1639
Carbon fixation, cyanobacteria
    role 1:325–30, 1:330, 1:332
Carcinogenesis
  oncogenes role 3:1507
  SV40 model 3:1647
  see also Oncogenesis;
      Tumorigenesis
Carcinogens, acute transforming
    retroviruses as 3:1818
Cardamine chlorotic fleck virus
    (CCFV) 1:244
  genome 1:245
Cardiac disease
  chronic 2:1076
  clinical features 2:1077–8
  epidemiology 2:1076
  etiology (viral) 2:1074,
      2:1075(Table)
  intrauterine/perinatal 2:1074–5
  laboratory diagnosis 2:1078
  pathogenesis 2:1076–7
  see also Dilated cardiomyopathy;
      Myopericarditis
Cardiac transplantation
  CMV infection after 2:1078
  virus infection after 2:1076
Cardiomyopathy
  dilated (DCM) *see* Dilated
      cardiomyopathy
  infants, HIV-1 causing 2:1075
Cardiovirus 1:229, 2:1326, 3:1773
  see also Theiler's murine
      encephalomyelitis viruses
      (TMEV)
Cardioviruses 1:229–38
  3D^{pol} polymerase 1:233, 1:234
  antigenic determinants 1:231
  assembly 1:235
  capsid 1:230
    three-dimensional
        structure 1:230–1
  cytopathology 1:237
  evolution 1:235–6
  genetics and serotype
      stability 1:235–6
  genome 1:231–2
    poly(A) tail 1:232
    poly(C) segment 1:232, 1:237
    positive ssRNA 1:230, 1:231
    sequences 1:231–2,
        1:236(Table), 1:237
    untranslated regions 1:231–2,
        1:232

Cardioviruses (continued)
  genome-linked protein
      (VPg) 1:231, 1:234
  geographic distribution 1:235
  history 1:229
  host range 1:235
  host RNA/protein synthesis
      inhibition 1:234–5
  human infections 1:236
  immune response 1:237
  infection initiation 1:234
  infectious unencapsidated
      virus 1:232
  internal ribosomal entry site
      (IRES) 1:232
  pathogenicity in laboratory
      mice 1:236–7
  physicochemical
      properties 1:230(Table)
  polyproteins 1:230, 1:230–1,
      1:236(Table)
  organization 1:233–4
  prevention and control 1:237
  propagation 1:235
  properties 1:230
  protease 3C^{pro} 1:233
  proteins 1:233–4, 1:234
    1AB peptide (VP0)
        maturation 1:233
    3B *see* Cardioviruses, genome-
        linked protein (VPg)
    expression and
        processing 1:232–3
    secondary processing 1:233
    'suicide' activity 1:233
  replication 1:236
    regulation 1:234(Fig)
  replicative intermediates
      (RIs) 1:234
  ribosome modification 1:235
  RNA sequences,
      comparisons 1:230
  synthesis of components 1:234
  taxonomy and
      classification 1:229–30
  tissue tropism 1:236
  translation 1:232, 1:234
  transmission 1:236
  vaccines 1:237
  see also Encephalomyocarditis
      (EMC) virus; Mengo virus
Carlavirus 1:238
  members and possible
      members 1:241(Table)
Carlavirus potato virus M
    (PVM) 1:238
Carlaviruses 1:238–42
  cytopathology 1:240–1
  economic significance and
      ecology 1:242
  epidemiology and control 1:241–
      2
  evolution 1:242
  genome 1:239, 1:239(Fig)
    expression 1:240
    noncoding regions 1:239
    ORFs 1:239, 1:240
    positive ssRNA 1:239
  geographic distribution 1:241
  history 1:238
  host range 1:242
  multiplication 1:239–40
  pathogen-derived engineered
      resistance 2:1308(Table)
  physicochemical
      properties 1:238–9
  RNA replicase 1:239, 1:240
  serology 1:241
  structure and composition 1:238
  subgenomic RNAs 1:238, 1:240
  symptomatology 1:242

Carlaviruses (continued)
  taxonomy and
      classification 1:238
  translation 1:240
  transmission 1:240
Carmovirus 1:243
  members 1:244(Table)
Carmoviruses 1:243–7
  assembly 1:245
  coat proteins (CP) 1:245, 1:247
    satellite RNA C
        interactions 1:247
  defective-interfering (DI)
      RNAs 3:1453
  RNA recombination 1:246
  distribution 1:243–5
  double-stranded RNAs 1:246
  economic significance 1:243–5
  evolutionary relationships 1:243
  gene expression 1:246
  genome
    ORFs 1:243, 1:245, 1:246
    organization 1:244(Fig)
    sequences 1:243
    ssRNA (positive) 1:243
    structure 1:245
  host range 1:243–5
  machlomoviruses
      similarity 2:937, 2:938
  mutagenesis studies 1:246
  propagation 1:243
  R and P domains 1:245
  replicase 1:247
  replication 1:246
  RNA–CP complex (rp-
      complex) 1:245
  RNA-dependent RNA
      polymerase (RDRP) 1:243,
      1:246
  structure 1:245
  taxonomy and
      classification 1:243
  tombusviruses similarity 1:243
  transmission 1:243–5
  virus–host interactions 1:246–7
  see also Turnip crinkle virus
      (TCV)
Carnation cryptic virus
    (CCV) 1:312
Carnation etched ring virus
    (CERV) 2:1276, 2:1289
Carnation Italian ringspot virus
    (CIRV) 3:1790, 3:1790(Table)
Carnation latent virus (CLV) 1:238
  genome 1:239
Carnation mottle virus
    (CarMV) 1:243
  genome 1:245
  propagation 1:243
Carnation necrotic fleck virus
    (CNFV), coat proteins 1:267
Carnation ring spot virus
    (CRSV) 1:403
  aggregation properties of
      strains 1:404–5
  capsid proteins, species
      homology 1:404(Table)
  epidemiology 1:407
  features of infection 1:406
  genome properties 1:405
  geographic/seasonal
      distribution 1:403
  host range and propagation 1:406
  movement protein 1:407(Table)
  pathogenicity 1:408
  pathology and
      histopathology 1:408
  prevention and control 1:408
  replicase, species
      homology 1:406(Table)
  strains and serologic
      relationship 1:407

Carnation ring spot virus (CRSV) (continued)
  transmission and tissue tropism 1:407
  see also Dianthoviruses
Carnation small viroid-like RNA (CarSV RNA) 3:1556, 3:1930
Carnations, CRSV infection 1:408
Carp
  acute infectious dropsy 1:562, 3:1543
  spring viremia of carp virus infection 1:562, 1:562–3
  see also Spring viremia of carp virus (SVCV)
Carp pox herpesvirus 1:553
Carrier cultures 3:1409
Carrot fly 3:1859
Carrot motley dwarf disease 3:1855, 3:1858
Carrot mottle mimic virus (CMoMV) 3:1855, 3:1856(Table)
  genome 3:1856, 3:1857(Fig)
  propagation 3:1858
  replication 3:1857
Carrot mottle virus (CMoV) 3:1855, 3:1856(Table)
  epidemiology 3:1858
  pathology 3:1858
  propagation 3:1858
  properties 3:1855–6
Carrot red leaf luteovirus (CaRLV) 3:1855, 3:1856(Table), 3:1858
Carrot red leaf virus (CRLV)
  geographic distribution 2:902
  satellite RNAs 2:904
  see also Poleroviruses
Cas NS-1 murine retrovirus 3:1516
Case-control studies 1:482–3
  retrospective 1:482
Case-fatality rates 1:482
Casein kinase II 1:258
Caspase 8 1:71
Caspase, apoptosis inhibition 1:71(Table)
Casphalia extranea, biological control by densoviruses 1:387
Cassava American latent virus 2:1008(Table)
Cassava green mottle virus 2:1008(Table)
Cassava vein mosaic virus (CsVMV) 2:1285–9
  aspartic proteinase (PR) 2:1286
  coat protein 2:1286
  economic significance 2:1285–6
  genome 2:1281, 2:1286
    comparison with CaMV 2:1288(Fig)
    gag and pol genes 2:1286
    ORFs 2:1286
    genomic map 2:1287(Fig)
  geographic distribution 2:1285–6
  history 2:1285
  host range 2:1285–6
  inclusion bodies 2:1286(Fig)
  movement protein (MP) 2:1286, 2:1288
  promoter function/ organization 2:1288, 2:1288(Fig)
  propagation 2:1285–6
  replication 2:1286–8
  reverse transcriptase 2:1287
  structure and properties 2:1286, 2:1286(Fig)
  symptom of infection 2:1286
  taxonomy and classification 2:1285
Cassia yellow blotch virus 1:198

Castleman's disease 3:1848
Cathepsin, granulovirus 1:143
Cations, phage adsorption 3:1414
Cats
  calicivirus infection see Feline calicivirus
  cowpox virus infection 1:301, 1:302, 1:302–3, 1:303, 1:303(Fig), 1:304, 3:1992
  feline immunodeficiency virus see Feline immunodeficiency virus (FIV)
  immunity to feline calicivirus 1:220
  leukemia viruses see Feline leukemia viruses (FeLVs)
  rabies transmission 3:1987
  see also entries beginning Feline
Cattle
  cowpox virus infection 1:301, 1:302
  foot-and-mouth disease virus infection 1:572, 1:574
  lumpy skin disease see Lumpy skin disease of cattle (LSD)
  monitoring for BSE and prions 3:1397
  parapoxviruses 2:1144
  persistent lymphocytosis 1:184
  prion protein (PrP) gene polymorphisms 3:1396
  pseudorabies virus (PRV) infection 3:1425
  vesicular stomatitis 3:1910, 3:1918
  see also entries beginning Bovine
Cattle plague see Rinderpest
Cauda equina neuritis, adenoviruses causing 1:6
Caudovirales 2:1223, 3:1731, 3:1750
  families included 3:1750
  new families 2:1223
Cauliflower, transgenic 2:1280, 2:1281
Cauliflower mosaic virus (CaMV) 2:1275, 2:1314–15
  amorphous inclusion bodies 2:1279–80, 2:1279(Fig)
  control 2:1280
  economic significance 2:1280
  gene VI protein 2:1277, 2:1279, 2:1280
  genes 2:1277
    involved in resistance 2:1186(Table)
  genome 2:1275, 2:1277, 2:1278(Fig), 2:1281–2
    comparison with cassava vein mosaic virus (CsVMV) 2:1288(Fig)
    ORFs 2:1314–15, 3:1894
    supercoiled DNA 2:1279
    genomic map 2:1282(Fig), 2:1287(Fig)
  Hepadnaviridae relationship 1:641
  history 2:724
  host range 2:1276–7
  hypersensitive defense response in hosts 2:1277
  impact on plant biotechnology 2:1275
  P18 and aphid transmission 2:1278
  pathogenicity 2:1277, 2:1278(Fig)
  pathology 2:1279–80
  polyadenylation signal 2:1284
  promoter 2:1307
    35S 2:1284
    35S, in plant genetic engineering 2:1275, 2:1280–1

Cauliflower mosaic virus (CaMV) (continued)
  promoter (continued)
    in RNA virus vectors 3:1895
  propagation 2:1276–7
  recombination 3:1449, 3:1894
  replication 2:1275, 2:1279, 2:1295
  resistance and cross-protection 2:1280
  RNA processing 2:1284
  serologic relationships 2:1278, 2:1289
  symptoms of infections 2:1279
    chlorosis 2:1188
  tissue tropism 2:1279
  transgenic 2:1188
  translation 2:1284
  transmission 3:1901–3
    'bridge' hypothesis 3:1901
    as vector 2:1275, 3:1894
    criteria/requirements 3:1894
  see also Caulimoviruses
Caulimoviridae 2:1285, 2:1289
  Badnavirus 2:1293
  Caulimovirus 2:1275
  characteristics 2:1275–6
  legume caulimoviruses features 2:1290
Caulimovirus 2:1275, 2:1285, 2:1314
  characteristics 2:1275–6
  members 2:1276(Table), 2:1282(Table)
Caulimoviruses 2:1275–81
  35S RNA and promoter 2:1284
  amorphous inclusion bodies 2:1279–80, 2:1281
  aphid transmission factor (ATF) 2:1278, 2:1282
  badnaviruses differentiation 2:1276
  capsid proteins 2:1282–3
  disease control 2:1280
  economic significance 2:1280
  epidemiology 2:1280
  evolution 2:1277–8
  future perspectives 2:1280–1
  general features 2:1275–81
  genetic recombination 2:1277
  genetics 2:1277
  genome 2:1277, 2:1281–2, 2:1286
    gag and pol genes 2:1277–8
    ORFs 2:1281–2, 2:1283(Fig)
    sequence 2:1281–2
    supercoiled DNA 2:1279, 2:1281
  genomic map 2:1282(Fig)
  geographic distribution 2:1276
  history 2:1275
  host range 2:1276–7
  inclusion body protein 2:1283
  legume see Legume caulimoviruses
  minichromosome 2:1281
  molecular biology 2:1281–5
  pathogenicity 2:1279
  pathology 2:1279–80
  plasmodesmata enlargement due to 2:1280
  Pol polyprotein 2:1283, 2:1285
  promoter (35S) 2:1275, 2:1280
  propagation 2:1276–7
  protease 2:1283, 2:1285
  proteins 2:1282–3
    movement protein 2:1282
    p37 and p44 2:1282–3
    processing 2:1284–5
    small nucleic acid binding protein 2:1282
  replication 2:1283–4
  reverse transcriptase 2:1283

Caulimoviruses (continued)
  ribosome shunt mechanism 2:1284
  RNA processing 2:1284
  serologic relationships and variability 2:1278
  stability 2:1283
  structure and properties 2:1281
  symptoms of infections 2:1279
  taxonomy and classification 2:1275–6
  terminal redundancy 2:1281, 2:1284
  tissue tropism 2:1278–9
  trans-activation 2:1283, 2:1284
  transcription 2:1284
  translation 2:1284
  transmission 2:1278–9, 3:1901–3
  viruses included 2:1276(Table), 2:1282(Table)
  see also Cassava vein mosaic virus (CsVMV); Cauliflower mosaic virus (CaMV)
Caulobacter, ssRNA phage 3:1664
cbl oncogene 3:1515–16
CBP (CREB binding protein) 1:25
CC chemokines see Chemokine families
CCR5 receptor, HIV coreceptor 1:537, 2:768
CD4, HIV receptor 1:250, 2:774–5, 2:779, 3:1921, 3:1926
CD4 T cells 1:339, 3:1862
  activation by Nef of HIV 2:768–9
  in adult T-cell leukemia (ATL) 2:792
  apoptosis, HIV causing 1:75–6
  in autoimmunity model 1:111
  CD8 T cell ratio, FIV infection 1:538
  functions 2:1202
  in HIV infection 2:772
  HTLV-1 infection 2:791
  IL-2 synthesis 1:341
  loss
    in FIV infection 1:537, 1:538
    in HIV infection 2:822
  measles 2:958–9
  MHC-II restriction 1:340, 2:813
  protective function 3:1863
  reovirus infection 3:1462
  respiratory virus control 3:1491
  in RSV infection 3:1484
  in SIV infection 3:1645
  SIV receptor 3:1642, 3:1643
  support of CD8 T cell response 2:1202
  Theiler's murine encephalomyelitis viruses (TMEV) infection 3:1778
    demyelination 3:1779
  see also T cells, helper
CD8 T cells 1:339, 2:813, 2:818–19, 2:840, 3:1862
  action in virus infections 1:70
  antiviral cytokines 2:1201
  Borna disease virus infection 1:171
  bovine leukemia virus (BLV) infection 1:195, 1:196
  CD4 cells function 2:1202
  crossreactivity 2:823
  cytotoxic see Cytotoxic T lymphocytes
  Fas ligand upregulation 2:1201
  functions 2:1201–2
  in HIV infection 2:772
  IDDM development in autoimmunity model 1:110–11
  measles 2:958–9
  murine CMV infection 1:367

CD8 T cells (continued)
  properties 2:813(Table)
  reovirus infection 3:1462
  in simian immunodeficiency virus infection 3:1645
  stimulation and MHC-1 restriction 1:339
  virus killing mechanism 2:1201
  see also Cytotoxic T lymphocytes (CTL)
CD9, in feline immunodeficiency virus (FIV) infection 1:537
CD21 (CR2)
  EBV receptor 1:491
  monoclonal antibodies, in EBV infection 3:1827
CD24, monoclonal antibodies, in EBV infection 3:1827
CD44 protein, adenovirus E1A repression 1:29
CD46, measles virus (MV) receptor 2:955
CD55 see Decay accelerating factor (DAF)
CD95 see FAS (APO-1)
CD155
  gene 2:1334
  receptor of polioviruses 2:1333–5, 2:1348
  transgenic mice and poliovirus susceptibility 2:1335
  see also Poliovirus
cdks, adenovirus E1A protein complex 1:24
cDNA clones
  equine encephalitis viruses 1:507
  RNA viruses, infectivity 3:1895–6
  see also individual viruses
ced-3 1:71
ced-4 1:71
ced-9 1:71
Cell
  animal 1:247, 1:248(Fig)
  cytoskeleton, virus transport to nucleus 3:1473
  differentiation, adenovirus E1A induction 1:29
  division, parvovirus replication requirement 2:1173
  homeostasis 1:250
  polarity and shape 1:253
  polarization 1:249
  rounding 3:1959
  signaling see Signal transduction
  susceptibility to viruses and virus isolation 1:397
  terminal differentiation, inhibition by adenovirus E1A 1:29
Cell adhesion molecules see ICAM-1
Cell culture 1:395
  adaptation to, by CMV strains 1:346
  centrifugation culture in shell vials 1:397–8, 1:398(Fig)
  CMV strains 1:346
    human CMV 1:346
  conditions 3:1411
  coronaviruses 1:294
  definition 3:1410
  hepatitis A virus (HAV) 1:631, 1:635–6
  history 2:735
  Kuru 3:1400
  lymphocyte see Lymphocytes, culture
  monolayers, virus isolation 1:396
  primary 3:1410–11
  reasons for failure 3:1411
  three-dimensional systems 3:1411–12

Cell culture (continued)
  tube culture 1:396–7
  types 3:1410–11
  virus propagation 3:1410–12
  viruses not cultured 1:388
  see also individual viruses
Cell cycle, adenovirus E1A protein action 1:27
Cell fusing agent (CFA) 1:427
Cell fusion
  from within (FFWI) 3:1619
  from without (FFWO) 3:1619
  sendai virus 3:1619
  type D retroviruses inducing 3:1522
Cell lines
  adult T-cell leukemia (ATL) 2:788–9
  continuous 1:396, 3:1411
  ELVIS 1:398
  fish 1:554
  genetically modified 1:398, 1:402
  hepatitis delta virus (HDV) 1:667
Cell lysis
  of bacteria, by phage see Bacteriophage
  by cytotoxic T cells see Cytotoxic T lymphocytes (CTL)
  by nervous system viruses 2:1017
Cell membrane see Plasma membrane
Cell receptors see Receptors
Cell structure/function, in virus infections (animal cells) 1:247–57
  cytoskeleton 1:253–4
  cytosol 1:253–4
  membrane network 1:251–3
  nuclear–cytoplasmic exchanges 1:255–6
  nucleus 1:254–5
  schematic representation 1:248(Fig)
  surface 1:249–51
    extracellular coats 1:249
    organization and polarity 1:249
    plasma membrane 1:249–51
  see also Plasma membrane
Cell-free de novo synthesis of viruses, polioviruses 1:1347
Cell-mediated immune response 2:818–24, 3:1862–3
  antigen presentation 2:819–20
  antigen processing 2:819–20, 2:820(Fig)
  crossreactivity of CD8+ T cells 2:823
  effector mechanism 2:818
  history 2:823
  general features 2:818–19
  history 2:823
  immune evasion see Immune evasion
  immunopathology 2:821–2
  levels of response 2:819–20
  stimulation 2:820–1
  vaccine-induced 3:1863
  in viral infections
    African swine fever virus 1:37
    bluetongue virus (BTV) 2:1059
    Borna disease virus 1:171
    capripoxvirus 3:1380
    coronaviruses 1:297
    cowpox virus 1:304
    dengue virus 1:383
    Ebola and Marburg viruses 2:944
    enteric viruses 1:449
    Epstein–Barr virus (EBV) 1:493
    equine encephalitis viruses 1:507
    fowlpox virus 1:581

Cell-mediated immune response (continued)
  in viral infections (continued)
    hantavirus 1:629
    hepatitis A virus 1:638–9
    hepatitis B virus 1:643, 1:644
    hepatitis C virus 1:663
    herpes simplex virus 2:684
    HIV 2:822–3
    human CMV 1:350
    human herpesvirus 6 (HHV-6) 2:702
    human papillomavirus 2:1113
    lymphocytic choriomeningitis virus (LCMV) 2:918–19, 2:919–20
    Marek's disease 2:950
    measles 2:958–9
    mousepox 2:977–8
    mumps 2:994
    parapoxvirus 2:1145
    reoviruses 3:1462
    reticuloendotheliosis (RE) viruses 3:1498
    Theiler's murine encephalomyelitis viruses (TMEV) 3:1778
    varicella-zoster virus 3:1876
    vesicular stomatitis virus (VSV) 3:1918
    yellow fever 3:1986
  see also T cells
Cell-mediated lysis see Cell lysis
Cell-to-cell movement
  cucumoviruses 1:322
  cypoviruses 1:336
  dianthoviruses 1:406–7
  furoviruses 1:591
  geminiviruses 1:604
  machlomoviruses 2:937
  plant viruses 2:1185, 2:1186
  for resistance to plant viruses 2:1301, 2:1303
  tobacco necrosis virus (TNV) 2:1005
  tospoviruses 1:1805
Cell-to-cell spread
  animal parainfluenza viruses 2:1139
  viruses in CNS 2:1016–17
Cellular suicide see Apoptosis
CELO virus 1:18
  GAM-1 gene product 1:72
  polypeptide 1:18
Central European encephalitis 1:429
Central European encephalitis virus (CEEV) 1:426
  epidemiology 1:428
  features 1:425(Table)
  genetic stability 1:427
  geographic/seasonal distribution 1:426
  vaccine 1:429
Central European tick-borne encephalitis (CETBE) virus 3:1992
Central nervous system
  anatomy and virus infections 2:1013–14
  antibodies 2:1014
  as immune privileged site 2:1203
  involvement in measles 2:956
  neural transport mechanisms 2:1180
  Reovirus type 3 cellular receptor 3:1928
  TMEV persistence 3:1777
  viral infections
    animal enteroviruses 1:467
    Borna disease virus spread 1:170

Central nervous system (continued)
  viral infections (continued)
    enterovirus 70 (EV70) 1:472
    equine herpesvirus 1 (EHV-1) 1:513
    feline immunodeficiency virus (FIV) 1:539
    herpes simplex viruses 2:680
    Japanese encephalitis (JE) virus 2:874
    poliovirus 2:1327, 2:1328, 2:1330, 2:1348
    reoviruses 3:1461
    Theiler's murine encephalomyelitis virus (TMEV) 3:1776
    virus infection and viremia association 2:1179
    virus invasion 2:1179–80
    pathways 2:1014–15, 2:1016(Fig)
  see also Brain; Nervous system viruses
Centrifugation
  equilibrium 3:1412
  virus purification 3:1412
Centrifugation culture in shell vials 1:397–8
Centrocytes 2:814
Cercopithecine herpesvirus 2 2:708
Cereal tillering disease virus (CTDV) 2:1263
Cereal yellow dwarf virus (CYDV)
  economic significance 2:907
  evolution 2:905
  geographic distribution 2:902
  pathogenicity 2:906
  RPV helper virus 2:904
  satellite RNAs 2:904
  structure and composition 2:903
  see also Poleroviruses
Cereal yellow dwarf virus-RPV 2:902
Cerebellar ataxia
  Kuru 3:1400
  in prion diseases 3:1390
Cerebellum, in Kuru 3:1401
Cerebral capillaries 1:1013
  virus invasion 2:1015, 2:1016
Cerebral infections, murine CMV 1:367
Cerebrospinal fluid
  in alphavirus encephalitis 1:506
  in Japanese encephalitis (JE) 2:874
Cervical cancer 1:67
  HPVs causing 2:1105, 2:1110–11, 2:1114, 2:1119, 3:1845
  HSV-2 role 2:684
  mortality 2:1119
  prevalence and geographic distribution 2:1106
  risk factors 2:1111
  types and HPV types associated 3:1845
  vaccines and therapy 2:1114
Cervical intraepithelial neoplasia (CIN)
  clinical features 2:1112
  HPVs causing 2:1111, 2:1111(Table), 2:1114
  immunologic/genetic factors 2:1111–12
Cervicovaginal smears, Bethesda System nomenclature 2:1112
Cervid herpesviruses 1:181(Table)
Cetacean morbillivirus 3:1560
Chamois contagious ecthyma virus 2:1141

Chandipura (CHP) virus 1:257–60
  antibodies 1:259
  classification 1:257
  crossreactivity with vesicular
    stomatitis virus 1:257
  genetics 1:260
  genome organization 1:257–9,
    1:259(Table)
  genome sequence 1:258
  geographic distribution 1:259
  history 1:257
  host range 1:259
  human infections 1:259
  mRNAs 1:257, 1:259(Table)
  proteins 1:257–8, 1:259(Table)
    G protein 1:258
    N protein 1:258
    P protein 1:258
    phosphorylation of P 1:258
    vesicular stomatitis virus
      similarity 1:258
  structure 1:258(Fig)
  transcription 1:257
  transmission 1:259
  ts mutants 1:260
Changuinola virus species
  (CGLV) 2:1045(Table)
Channel catfish virus (CCV) 1:553
  evolution 1:555
  genome 1:555
    organization 1:556(Fig)
    sequence 1:555
  geographic/seasonal
    distribution 1:554
  history 1:553
  host range and
    propagation 1:554–5
  infection
    clinical features 1:557
    immune response 1:557
    pathology 1:557
    prevention and control 1:557
    treatment 1:557
  isolates and comparisons 1:555
  latency 1:556–7
  pathogenesis 1:555–7
  proteins 1:555
  structure 1:554(Fig)
  transmission 1:555
  vaccines 1:557
Chaperones, in prion
  propagation 3:1407
Chaperonins
  discovery 3:1708
  symbionin 3:1905
  T4-like phages head
    assembly 1:1709
  see also GroEL; GroES
Chase, M. 2:728
Chayote mosaic virus 3:1850
Cheese, phage in cultures 2:1254,
  2:1256, 2:1256(Table)
Cheetahs, cowpox virus
  infection 1:303
Chemical toxicants, emergence and
  re-emergence of diseases 1:422
Chemokine families 1:343–4
  CC (β-chemokines) 1:343
    receptors 1:343
  CXC (α-chemokines) 1:343
    receptors 1:343
    receptors as drug targets 2:786
  see also CCR5 receptor; CXCR4
Chemokines 1:339–44
  definition 1:339
  functions 1:339
  immune evasion
    mechanism 2:1204
  receptors 1:339, 1:343–4
    HHV-6 and HHV-7
      proteins 2:700–1

Chemokines (continued)
  receptors (continued)
    HIV see CCR5 receptor;
      CXCR4
  see also CCR5 receptor; CXCR4
Chenopodiaceae, benyvirus
  infections 1:158
Chenopodium, pea enation mosaic
  virus (PEMV)
  symptoms 2:1194
Chenuda virus species
  (CNUV) 2:1045(Table), 2:1047
Cherry leaf roll virus
  (CLRV) 2:1008(Table)
Cherry mottle leaf virus
  (CMLV) 3:1838(Table)
  classification 3:1838, 3:1842
  coat protein 3:1838
  disease 3:1841
  geographic distribution 3:1838
  host range 3:1838
  host relations 3:1840
  transmission 3:1840
Cherry rasp leaf
  virus 2:1009(Table)
Cherry rugose mosaic virus 1:38
Cherry small circular RNA 3:1556
Chest pain, retrosternal, Lassa
  fever 2:893
Chestnut blight fungus 2:804
  control 2:804
Chick embryo cells (CEC)
  infectious bursal disease virus
    culture 1:162
    replication 1:163
Chicken(s)
  adenoviruses see
    Aviadenoviruses
  avian type C retrovirus
    infections 1:113
  erythroblastosis 3:1508
  infectious bursal disease see
    Infectious bursal disease of
    chickens; Infectious bursal
    disease virus (IBDV)
  late-feathering 1:439
  loci for avian leukosis virus
    (ALV) receptors 1:114
  'Marble spleen disease' 1:20
  Marek's disease 2:948
    see also Marek's disease
  myeloid leukemia 3:1510
  Newcastle disease 2:1023
  respiratory disease, infectious
    bronchitis virus (IBV)
    causing 1:296
  see also Poultry
Chicken anemia virus (CAV),
  apoptosis promotion 1:74
Chicken fibroblast cells, resistance
  to poliovirus 3:1960
Chicken herpesvirus see Marek's
  disease virus (MDV)
Chicken influenza virus, DI
  particles 1:374
Chicken syncytial virus
  (CSV) 3:1496
  env gene 3:1499
  immunosuppressive peptide
    (ISP) 3:1499
  nonneoplastic disease 3:1499
Chickenpox (varicella) 1:61
  clinical features 3:1875,
    3:1875(Fig)
  complications 3:1875–6
  epidemiology 3:1874
  geographic and seasonal
    distribution 3:1873
  history 3:1872
  immune response 3:1876
  pathology and histology 3:1876

Chickenpox (varicella) (continued)
  prevention and control 3:1876–7,
    3:1877
  transmission 3:1874
  see also Varicella-zoster virus
    (VZV)
Chickenpox (varicella)-like
  illnesses, in non-human
  primates 3:1873
Chicks, Marek's disease virus
  isolation 2:947–8
Chicory yellow mottle virus
  (CYMV) 2:1008(Table)
  satellite RNA 3:1611
Chikungunya (CHIK) fever 1:261
  clinical features 1:264
  epidemics 1:263
  immune response 1:264–5
  pathology/histology 1:264
  prevention and control 1:265
  treatment 1:264
Chikungunya (CHIK) virus 1:261–
  5, 1:375, 3:1989, 3:1992
  antibodies 1:262
  antigenic variation 1:263
  cell culture 1:262
  classification 1:261
  epidemiology 1:263
  evolution 1:262
  experimental vaccine 1:265
  genetics 1:262
  genome structure 1:262
  geographic/seasonal
    distribution 1:261
  history 1:261
  host range and propagation 1:262
  human infections 1:261–2
    see also Chikungunya (CHIK)
      fever
  O'Nyong nyong virus and 3:1994
  pathogenicity 1:264
  serodiagnosis 1:263
  serologic relationships and
    variability 1:263
  subgenomic mRNA 1:262
  tissue tropism 1:263–4
  transcription and
    translation 1:262
  transmission 1:263–4
  viremia 1:263
Childhood diseases, re-
  emergence 1:423
Children
  gastroenteritis,
    astroviruses 1:104, 1:107
  human CMV infections 1:348
    transmission 1:346
  Lassa fever 2:893
  torovirus infections 3:1801
Chilo iridescent virus (CIV) 2:862
  cypovirus infection with 1:337
  economic importance 2:868
  genes 2:865
  host macromolecular
    shutdown 2:867
  replication 2:867
  types 2:866
  see also Iridoviruses
Chimpanzee herpesvirus see
  Herpesvirus pan;
  Herpesviruses, baboon and
  chimpanzee
Chimpanzees
  coxsackievirus infections 2:735
  hepatitis C virus serology 1:661
  herpesvirus
    antibodies 2:708(Table)
  herpesviruses see Herpesviruses,
    baboon and chimpanzee
  poliovirus infections 2:732
  see also Primates

China, Japanese encephalitis (JE)
  virus 2:873
Chinese baculovirus (CBV) 3:1633
Chinese hamster ovary (CHO)
  cells, cowpox virus
  growth 1:299
Chlamydia, isolation 1:397
Chlamydiamicrovirus 2:1227
Chlorella viruses 1:44
  ecology 1:50
  functions of endonucleases 1:49
  glycosylation of proteins 1:50
  NC64A viruses 1:47
  Paramecium bursaria Chlorella
    virus 1 see PBCV-1
  Pbi viruses 1:48
  vaccinia virus similarities 1:45
  see also Algal viruses
Chlorine 1:311
Chloriridovirus 2:862, 2:868
  insect pest control by 2:845
Chloris striate mosaic virus
  (CSMV)
  capsids 1:597
  genome structure 1:597
Chlorophyll, decrease 2:1188
Chloroplasts
  furoviruses effect 1:594
  hordeivirus infection effect 2:752
  potato virus Y (PVY) coat
    protein effect 2:1189
Chlorosis, of plants 2:1188–90
  geminiviruses causing 1:605
Chobar Gorge virus species
  (CGV) 2:1045(Table)
Cholera toxin 2:1233
  CTX genetic element 2:1233
  genes (ctxA and ctxB) 2:1233
  phage conversion to
    produce 2:1233
  see also Bacteriophage CTXφ
  production 2:1233
  structure 2:1233
Cholestasis, in hepatitis E 1:674
Chordopoxvirinae 1:298, 1:475,
  2:960, 2:1140, 3:1376, 3:1383,
  3:1865
  Capripoxvirus 3:1376
  characteristics 2:1141
  genera 1:475
  Orthopoxvirus 3:1668
  see also Capripoxviruses;
    Orthopoxvirus
Chorioallantoic membrane (CAM)
  cowpox virus propagation 1:300,
    1:303
  fowlpox virus propagation 1:576,
    1:580
  inoculation method 1:399
Chorioretinitis, HSV-1
  causing 2:681
Choristoneura biennis
  entomopoxvirus
  (CbEPV) 1:477
  see also Entomopoxviruses
    (EPVs)
Choristoneura fumiferana
  entomopoxvirus (CfEPV) 1:476
  see also Entomopoxviruses
    (EPVs)
Choroid plexus
  blood–CSF barrier 2:1013
  virus invasion 2:1015
Chromatin 1:255
Chromosomal translocation
  Burkitt's lymphoma 1:490, 3:1844
  v-abl oncogene and 3:1512
Chromosomes 1:255
Chronic fatigue syndrome (post-
  viral fatigue syndrome) 1:308
  HHV-6 infection
    associated 2:702

Chronic fatigue syndrome (post-viral fatigue syndrome) (continued)
  Ross River virus (RRV) and 3:1574
Chronic infections 2:897, 2:1175, 2:1200
  see also Persistent infections
Chronic leukemia virus, genome 2:789(Fig)
Chronic paralysis virus (CPV) 2:744(Table), 2:745–6
  pathology and epizootiology 2:745–6
  syndromes caused by 2:745
  transmission 2:745–6
Chronic paralysis virus associate (CPVA) 2:744(Table), 2:745–6
Chronic wasting disease (CWD) of mule deer and elk 1:420(Table), 3:1388
Chroococcales 1:325, 1:325(Table)
Chrysanthemum aspermy virus 1:316
Chrysanthemum chlorotic mottle viroid 3:1930(Table)
Chrysanthemum stunt viroid (CSVd) 3:1930(Table)
Chrysanthemum virus B (CVB), genome 1:239
Chrysochromulina brevifilum, viruses 1:48
Chrysovirus 1:313, 2:1147
  dsRNA components 2:1149
  members 2:1148(Table)
CHV1-EP713 2:804
  cDNA clone 2:804, 2:806
  G-protein accumulation 2:806
  genome 2:805
  ORFs 2:805
  see also Hypoviruses
CHV2-NB58 2:805
CHV-1-EP747 2:805
Chysochromulina (CbV) viruses 1:44
Chytridiomycetes, plant virus transmission 3:1907
cI repressor see Coliphage lambda; P22 bacteriophage; Repressor
Cidofovir
  CMV infections 1:63
  HPV infections 1:67
  HSV infection therapy 2:685
  human CMV infections 1:351
  monkeypox virus therapy 1:68
Circoviridae
  apoptosis promotion 1:74
  geminiviruses similarities 1:606
Circulative-propagative viruses 3:1758
Cirrhosis, Laennec's 3:1830
Cisternae 1:251
Citrus bent leaf viroid 3:1930(Table)
Citrus cachexia viroid 3:1930(Table)
Citrus exocortis viroid (CEVd) 3:1930(Table), 3:1933(Fig)
  geographic distribution 3:1932
  pathogenicity 3:1935
Citrus leaf rugose virus (CiLRV) 1:38
  genome 1:39
  structure 1:41
  host range and distribution 1:40
  proteins, comparisons 2:810(Fig)
  replication 1:42
  virus–host relationships 1:42
Citrus mosaic badnavirus (CMBV) 2:1296

Citrus tatter leaf virus (CTLV) 1:222
Citrus tristeza virus (CTV)
  diseases and economic significance 1:272
  epidemiology and control 1:273
  gene blocks 1:270
  genome 1:269, 1:269(Fig), 1:270
  resistance 1:273
  RNA 1:267
  transmission 1:271
  vector ranges 1:272
Citrus variegation virus (CVV) 1:38
  replication 1:42
  virus–host relationships 1:42
Citrus viroid III (CVd-III) 3:1930(Table)
Citrus viroid IV (CVd-IV) 3:1930(Table)
Clara cells, Sendai virus infection 3:1618, 3:1620
Classes
  polythetic 3:1939, 3:1939(Fig), 3:1940–1
  species as 3:1938–9
Classical swine fever virus (CSFV) 1:173
  antigenic relationships 1:174
  comparison with bovine viral diarrhea virus (BVDV) 1:177
  genome, sequence analysis 1:176
  serologic relationships and variability 1:177–8
  taxonomy and classification 1:174
  see also Bovine viral diarrhea virus (BVDV); Hog cholera virus (HCV); Pestiviruses
Classification of viruses see Taxonomy of viruses
Clathrin 1:250
Clathrin-coated pits 3:1472
Climate change, global 3:1996
Clinically inapparent infections 1:484
Clitoria yellow vein virus 3:1850
Clonal selection, negative 1:110
Clonal Selection Theory 2:812
Cloning of genes, T5-like phage 3:1721
Cloning vectors
  Bacillus subtilis phage 1:136
  bacteriophage φX174 1:280
  coliphage lambda see Coliphage lambda
  densoviruses 1:387
  filamentous phage 1:552
  herpesviruses saimiri and ateles 2:718
  nuclear polyhedrosis viruses (NPVs) 1:152
  phage see Bacteriophage requirements 2:1241
  SPO1 phage 3:1685
Cloning of viruses
  animal viruses 1:612
  see also *individual viruses*
Closteroviridae 1:238, 1:266–73, 3:1837
  Bromoviridae affinity 1:271
  carloviruses 1:238–42
  characteristics 1:266
  genera 1:266
  genome size 1:271
  taxonomy and classification 1:266–7
  see also *Closterovirus; Crinivirus*
Closterovirus 1:266, 1:267
  transmission 1:267, 1:268
  Trichovirus versus 3:1837

Closterovirus (continued)
  viruses included 1:268
  see also Closteroviruses
Closteroviruses 1:266–73
  cDNA clones 1:273
  coat proteins 1:267
    duplicate 1:267, 1:270–1, 1:271
    coronavirus similarities 1:270
  defective-interfering (DI) RNAs 3:1454
  diseases and economic significance 1:272–3
  epidemiology and control 1:273
  future perspectives 1:273
  gene expression 1:269–71, 1:270
  genome
    comparisons 1:270
    organization 1:269–71, 1:269(Fig)
    sequences 1:269
    structure 1:267–9
  heat shock protein (HSP70) homologue 1:266, 1:269, 1:270
  history 1:266
  host range and distribution 1:271
  inclusions 1:271
  physical properties 1:267
  properties 1:266
  proteins 1:269–70
  RNA content 1:267
  structure and particle composition 1:267
  taxonomy and classification 1:266, 1:266–7, 1:268
  transmission 1:266, 1:267, 1:268, 1:271–2
  virus–host relation (cytopathic effects) 1:271
  see also Beet yellows virus (BYV); *Crinivirus*
Clostridium botulinum 2:1232
  toxins see Botulinum toxins
Cloudy wing virus (CWV) 2:744(Table), 2:748
Clover yellow mosaic virus (CYMV), genome 3:1366
Clump disease 2:1196
Clustering disease 2:748
CMV see Cytomegalovirus (CMV); Human cytomegalovirus (HCMV)
CNS see Central nervous system
Coat proteins 2:1309
  linkage by C-terminal extensions 1:199
  plant resistance mediated by 2:1309
Cocal virus 1:257
Cockle agent 1:446
Cocksfoot mild mosaic virus (CMMV) 3:1675
Cocksfoot mottle virus (CfMV) 3:1674
  host range 3:1677
  see also Sobemoviruses
Cocoa necrosis virus 2:1008(Table)
Coconut cadang-cadang viroid (CCCVd) 3:1929, 3:1930(Table), 3:1932, 3:1933
Coconut tinangaja 3:1930(Table)
Codons
  start (initiation) 1:612
    ATG 1:120
  stop (termination) 1:612
Cofactors, phage adsorption 3:1414
Coffee ringspot virus 3:1538
Coggins assay 1:521
Cohen, S. 2:728
Cohort studies 1:482–3

Coital exanthema 1:180, 1:182, 1:512, 1:513
  see also Equine herpesvirus 3 (EHV-3)
Cold sores (herpes labialis) 1:61, 2:680
Colds, common see Common cold
Coleoptera, entomopoxviruses (EPVs) 1:476, 1:478–9
Coleus blumei viroid 1 (CbVd 1) 3:1929, 3:1930(Table)
Coleus blumei viroid 2 (CbVd 2) 3:1929, 3:1930(Table)
Coleus blumei viroid 3 (CbVd 3) 3:1929, 3:1930(Table)
Coleus blumei viroids (CbVd) 3:1932
ColIb, T5-like phage abortive infection 3:1720–1
Colicinogenic plasmids, ColIb 3:1720
Coliphage, as cloning vectors 2:1240
Coliphage B278 2:987
Coliphage D108 2:981–8
  attachment and DNA entry 2:981
  discovery 2:981
  DNA maturation/encapsidation 2:985
  DNA modification 2:985–6
  DNA transposition 2:981–2, 2:982, 2:983–4
  mechanisms 2:985
  early gene expression regulation 2:983–4
  genetic map 2:981, 2:982(Fig)
  left end regulatory region 2:984(Fig)
  genome 2:981
  invertible G-loop 2:986
  late gene expression 2:985
  life cycle 2:981–3, 2:983(Fig)
  lysogeny 2:982
  lytic cycle 2:981, 2:982, 2:983
  lytic/lysogenic decision 2:983–4
  mom and *mod* genes 2:985–6
  promoter P_c 2:983
  repressor 2:982
  see also Coliphage Mu
Coliphage lambda 1:281–5, 2:1209, 2:1240
  abortive transcription 2:929
  antitermination 2:929
  att site 1:283, 1:284, 2:926, 2:928, 2:932, 2:932(Fig)
    recombination with *attB* 2:932–3, 2:932(Fig)
    sequence 2:932
  attachment sites 2:1236
  *att*P sites 2:1092(Fig)
  capsid proteins 1:281
  cI repressor, see also Coliphage lambda, repressor (cI)
  cI (repressor) gene 2:927
  cII and cIII genes 1:283, 2:927, 2:928
  cII protein 2:929, 2:930
  as cloning vector 1:284–5, 2:1241
    M13 and plasmid 2:1243
    multicomponent 2:1243
    replacement 2:1241–2
  cos sequence 2:1241
  Cro protein 1:282, 1:283, 2:927–8, 2:930
    binding to oR 2:931, 2:931(Fig)
    structure 2:931
  DNA 2:925
    base composition 1:282
    cohesive ends 1:281, 1:282
  DNA integration 2:926, 2:932–3
  DNA replication 2:925
    modes 2:1214

INDEX I xxiii

Coliphage lambda (*continued*)
  DNA replication (*continued*)
    rolling-circle 2:1214
    gam mutant 2:1214, 2:1216
    recombination essential 2:1214
  gene expression, regulation 2:930
  gene map 1:282, 2:926, 2:929(Fig)
    function–site specificity 2:926
    order of genes 2:925
  gene N and gpN 1:282
  gene Q 1:282
  genes
    late 2:926
    lysogeny establishment 2:926
    lysogeny maintenance 2:926
    see also specific genes (above/below)
  genome 2:1241
    sequence 1:282
    sequences in enterobacteria 1:281
    structure 1:282
  λdv 1:284
  gpcII protein 1:283
  gpO and gpP proteins 1:284
  gpP and dnaB interactions 2:1210
  gpS and pgR 1:282
  χ site 2:1215, 2:1216
  head assembly 1:282
  heteroimmune 2:928
  history 1:281
  host mutations affecting repression 2:928
  host range 1:281
  hybridization of genome with host's 2:1237, 2:1238
  in vitro replication 1:284
  int and *xis* genes 1:284, 2:928
  Int and Xis proteins 2:928, 2:930, 2:932
  integrase 1:283
  lysis 2:1094
  lysogeny 1:283–4, 2:925, 2:933
    advantages 2:926
    establishment 2:926, 2:929–30, 2:1091
    frequency 2:926
    maintenance 2:926, 2:930–1
    mass depression 1:283
    mutations affecting establishment 2:928
  lysogeny *vs* lytic cycle 1:283
  lytic cycle 1:282, 2:1092
    regulation 2:930(Fig)
  as model temperate phage 1:281
  mutations/mutants 2:926, 2:926–9
    affecting repression 2:926–8
    clear plaques (λc mutants) 2:926
    complementation patterns 2:927
    cY 2:927
    gam mutant *see above*
    λcI 2:927
    λcII 2:927
    λcIII 2:927
    λpRM 2:927
    int 2:928
    integration and excision 2:928
    virulence 2:931
  N gene product 2:929
  nut sites 1:282
  operators 2:927
  oR 2:930–1, 2:931(Fig)
  Orf protein 2:1215
  packaging 1:282, 1:284–5, 2:1214, 2:1236, 2:1241
    genome length 2:1237
  phage P22 relationship 3:1604
  plaque 2:925–6
  plasmid formation 1:284

Coliphage lambda (*continued*)
  proheads with phage φ29 connector 1:130
  promoters
    pI 2:929
    pL and pR 2:929, 2:930
  prophage 2:925, 2:1236
    excision 1:283, 2:931, 2:932–3
    excision, model 1:1237
    induction 2:926, 2:931
    maintenance 2:930–1
    mutations affecting integration 2:928
    testing for presence 1:139
    transposon insertion 2:1237–8
  Q protein action 2:929
  receptor 3:1414
  recombination 1:283, 1:284, 2:1214–16
    double-strand breaks for 2:1215
    localization 2:1216
    pathways 2:1214–16
    RecBCD pathway 2:1215, 2:1215–16
    RecE and RecF pathway 2:1215
    Red pathway 2:1214, 2:1214–15, 2:1215, 2:1220
    use as model for 2:1215
  red genes 2:1214
  red mutant 2:1215
  repressor (cI) 1:283, 2:926, 2:927, 2:930, 2:931
    binding to oR 2:931, 2:931(Fig)
    dimers 2:930
    host mutations affecting 2:928
    mutations 2:927
    prophage maintenance 2:930–1
    structure 2:931
  restriction/modification 1:284
  site-specific recombination 2:1091–2
  structure 1:281–2
  tail 1:282
  taxonomy and classification 1:281
  temperate phage 2:925
  transcription
    early 1:282, 2:930(Fig)
    promoters 1:282
    regulation 2:930(Fig)
  transducing phage 2:1236–7
    gal or *bio* genes 2:1237, 2:1238
    mechanisms 2:1236–7
    transduction 2:1236–7
    see also Transduction
  vector construction 1:285
  xis gene 2:930
Coliphage lambda-like viruses 2:1224
Coliphage Mu 2:981–8
  attachment and DNA entry 2:981
  B gene 2:983, 2:984
  C gene 2:985
  com gene 2:986
  discovery 2:981
  DNA, G-segment 1:460
  DNA maturation/encapsidation 2:985
  DNA modification 2:985–6
  DNA transposition 2:981–2, 2:982, 2:983–4
    A and B proteins required 2:984
    mechanism 2:984–5, 2:985
  early gene expression regulation 2:983–4
  Fis protein 2:986
  genetic map 2:981, 2:982(Fig)
    left end regulatory region 2:984(Fig)
  genome 2:981

Coliphage Mu (*continued*)
  gin gene 2:986
  Gin protein 2:986
  IAS (internal activating sequence) 2:984
  invertible G-loop 2:986
  late gene expression 2:985
  life cycle 2:981–3, 2:983(Fig)
  lysogeny 2:982
  lytic cycle 2:981, 2:982, 2:983
  lytic/lysogenic decision 2:983–4
  mini-Mu 2:987
  mom and *mod* genes 2:985–6
  Mu-1 2:981
  ner gene 2:982, 2:983
  Ner protein 2:985
  pac gene and pacase 2:985
  promoter P_c 2:983
  repressor 2:982, 2:983
  transposase (A protein) 2:982, 2:983, 2:984
  transposase-binding sites 2:984
Coliphage Mu-like phage *see* Mu-like phage
Coliphage N4 1:450–4
  adsorption and infection process 1:450, 1:454
  DNA polymerase 1:453
  effect on host cell 1:453
  5′-3′ exonuclease 1:453
  future perspectives 1:454
  gene expression 1:450–2
  genetic and physical map 1:452–3
  genome 1:450
    3′ extensions 1:450, 1:453, 1:454
    hairpin structures 1:451
  growth cycle and morphogenesis 1:450
  host range 1:454
  mutants 1:452–3
  proteins
    p4 and p7 1:451
    p17 1:451
  receptor 1:454
  recombination 1:452
  replication 1:453
    in vitro 1:453
    in vivo 1:453
    initiation 1:453
    RNA primer 1:453
  restriction endonuclease resistance 1:454
  RNA polymerase 1:450
    early transcripts 1:450, 1:451
    gene 1:452
    host σ70 for late transcripts 1:451, 1:452
  RNA polymerase II 1:451, 1:454
  ssDNA binding protein (SSB) 1:450, 1:452, 1:454
    mutants 1:452
    RNA polymerase interaction 1:452
    specificity 1:452
  structure 1:450
  taxonomy and classification 1:450
  transcription
    blocks in mutants 1:452
    early 1:450, 1:450–1
    in vitro 1:451
    initiation 1:450
    late 1:450, 1:451–2
    middle 1:450, 1:451
    promoters 1:451
    templates 1:451
  ts mutants 1:452
Colony stimulating factor 1 (CSF-1), receptor, EBV lytic cycle gene 1:496

Colorado tick fever (CTF) 3:1991
  case numbers 2:1060
  clinical features 2:1057–8
  history 2:1044
  pathology/histopathology 2:1058
  prevention and control 2:1060
Colorado tick fever virus (CTFV) 2:1043, 2:1046(Table), 3:1991–2
  geographic/seasonal distribution 2:1048, 2:1049(Fig)
  humans as 'dead-end' hosts 2:1044
  ocular target 1:525(Table)
  serotypes 2:1047
  spread in bloodstream 2:1178
  structure and properties 2:1047
  transmission 2:1054
  see also Coltiviruses
Colostrum
  bovine leukemia virus (BLV) transmission 1:195
  caprine arthritis encephalitis virus (CAEV) transmission 1:226
  feline immunodeficiency virus (FIV) transmission 1:537
Coltivirus 2:1044, 3:1991
Coltiviruses 2:1043–61
  classification 2:1044–8, 2:1048(Fig)
  epidemiology 2:1054–5
  evolution 2:1051–2
  future perspectives 2:1060–1
  genetic reassortment 2:1050
  genome segments 2:1048(Fig)
  geographic/seasonal distribution 2:1048
  group A 2:1046(Table), 2:1047
  group B 2:1046(Table), 2:1048
  history 2:1043–4
  infection
    clinical features 2:1057–8
    pathology/histopathology 2:1058
    prevention and control 2:1059–60
  molecular biology 2:1062–74
  nucleotypes 2:1046, 2:1048
  pathogenicity 2:1056–7
  replication 2:1056
  structure and properties 2:1047–8
  tissue tropism 2:1055–6
  transmission 2:1048, 2:1055–6
  viruses included 2:1046(Table)
  see also Colorado tick fever virus (CTFV)
Columbia-SK 1:229
Columnea latent viroid (CLVd) 3:1929, 3:1930(Table), 3:1936
Commelina yellow mottle virus (ComYMV) 2:1296
  genome 2:1288(Fig)
  structure and composition 2:1296
Committee on Enteroviruses 2:736
Common cold (coryza) 3:1492
  coronaviruses causing 1:295
  coxsackievirus infection 1:309
  history 3:1545
  prophylaxis 1:66
  rhinoviruses causing 3:1545
  see also Rhinoviruses
  symptoms 3:1549
  transmission of viruses 3:1488
Comoviridae 1:285–91
  Comovirus 1:285
  Fabavirus 1:531
  fabaviruses 1:531–4
  Nepovirus 2:1007
Comovirus 1:285, 2:1007

Comoviruses 1:285–91
  biological properties 1:285
  capsid, structure 3:1954(Fig)
  coat proteins 1:285, 1:286,
    1:287(Fig)
    subunits 1:286
  components (top/middle/
    bottom) 1:285, 1:286(Fig)
  cytopathology 1:291
  economic importance 1:291
  epidemiology 1:290
  fabaviruses relationship 1:290
  genome expression 1:287–8,
    1:288(Fig)
  genome structure 1:287
    RNAs 1:285–6, 1:287,
      1:288(Fig)
    VPg linked to 5' termini 1:287
  geographic distribution 1:290
  host range 1:290
  nepoviruses differences 2:1010
  P=3 shells 3:1953
  pathogen-derived engineered
    resistance 2:1308(Table)
  physical properties 1:285–6
  polyamines in 1:286
  proteins 1:287–8
    32K 1:287, 1:288–9
    48K 1:288, 1:289
    58K 1:288, 1:289
    87K 1:289
    105K and 95K 1:288
    110K 1:287
    170K 1:287
    encoded by RNA1 1:288–9
    encoded by RNA2 1:289
    functions 1:288–9
  relationships with other virus
    groups 1:290
  replication 1:289–90
  serology 1:285
  structure 1:286–7, 1:286(Fig)
  symptomatology 1:291
  taxonomy and
    classification 1:285
  translation 1:287–8
  transmission 1:290
  see also Bean pod mottle virus
    (BPMV); Cowpea mosaic
    virus (CPMV)
Compartmentalization, of virus
  replication 3:1434
Complement 1:390
  activation 2:812
  decreased in Argentine
    hemorrhagic fever
    (AHF) 2:893
  fixation, antiviral antibody
    detection 1:390
Complementation 1:609
  animal viruses 1:609
  dominant-negative mutants 2:853
  ts mutants, Chandipura (CHP)
    virus 1:260
Complementation groups 1:611
Computer modeling, epidemiology
  of viral diseases 1:487
Concatemers
  bacteriophage P22 3:1603
  frog virus 3 (FV3) 1:584, 1:585
  T4-like phages 3:1707
Concentration of virus
  preparations 3:1412
Condyloma acuminata see Genital
  warts
Congenital infections 1:484
  fetal antibody response
    lacking 1:390
Congenital rubella syndrome
  (CRS) 3:1593, 3:1597
  clinical features 3:1598
  IgM response 3:1599

Congenital rubella syndrome (CRS)
  (continued)
  incidence 3:1600
  insulin-dependent diabetes
    mellitus 2:1080
  neuropathology 3:1599
  ocular abnormalities 1:524
  pathology 3:1598–9
  progressive consequences 3:1598
  see also Rubella
Conidiospores, fungal
  partitiviruses
  transmission 2:1148
Conjunctiva
  follicular hypertrophy 1:472
  immune response in 1:524
  squamous cell carcinoma 1:523
  virus entry 2:1178
Conjunctivitis
  acute hemorrhagic (AHC) 1:469,
    1:526
    clinical features 1:472
    enterovirus 70 (EV70) 1:526
    epidemics 1:472
    epidemiology 1:471
    outbreaks 1:469–70, 1:471
    pandemic 1:470
    treatment 1:473
  clinical features 1:523
  coxsackievirus infection 1:309
  follicular 1:526
  Lassa fever 2:893
  RNA viruses causing 1:524
  swimming pool 2:1178
  viral causes 1:523
Consensus sequence,
  definition 3:1433(Table)
Contagious ecthyma virus see Orf
  virus
Contagious pustular dermatitis
  virus see Orf virus
Contagium vivum fluidum 2:719
Control of viral disease,
  quasispecies implication 3:1436
Convulsions
  Chikungunya (CHIK) fever 1:264
  see also Febrile seizures
copia retroelement 2:1295
copia-like
  retrotransposons 2:1315–16
  genome 2:1316, 2:1316(Fig)
Copper, effect on
  cyanobacteria 1:331
Copy-choice template mechanism,
  recombination 3:1451
Corethrella brakeleyi 2:868
Corky bark disease,
  grapevines 3:1841
Corky rugose wood,
  grapevines 3:1841
Corn lethal necrosis (CLN) 2:935
  pathogenesis and
    symptoms 2:937–8
  pathology/histopathology 2:938
  prevention and control 2:938
  see also Maize chlorotic mottle
    virus (MCMV)
Corn rootworms 2:937
Corn stunt agent, Ohio (VSA-
  OH) 3:1965
  see also Maize chlorotic dwarf
    virus
Cornea
  anesthesia 1:526
  as immune-privileged site 1:524
  squamous cell carcinoma 1:523,
    1:523(Fig)
  stromal infection 1:523
  ulceration 1:526
  viral infections 1:523

Coronaviridae 1:291–8, 1:446–7,
  3:1801
  apoptosis promotion 1:75
  in Nidovirales 1:90
  Torovirus 3:1798, 3:1798–803
  see also Coronaviruses;
    Toroviruses
Coronavirus, E1 protein 3:1921
Coronavirus JHM, microtubules
  interaction 1:254, 1:256(Fig)
Coronavirus-like particles 1:446,
  1:447(Fig)
Coronaviruses 1:291–8
  assembly 1:249
  attachment and entry 1:294
  cDNA 1:297
  cell lines 1:294
  classification 1:291
  closteroviruses similarities 1:271
  cytopathic effects 1:295
  defective interfering RNAs 1:294
  economic importance 1:297
  enteric infections 1:442(Table),
    1:446–7
  enterotropic 1:296
  epidemiology 1:295–6
  evolution 3:1801
  future perspectives 1:297
  genetic recombination 1:294,
    1:295
  genetics 1:294
  genome
    arteriviruses similarity 1:90,
      1:93–4
    deletions 1:294
    intergenic sequences (IS) 1:293
    map 1:293(Fig)
    ORFs 1:292–3
    structure 1:292–3
  geographic distribution 1:296
  glycoproteins 1:294
    M and E 1:292
    S glycoprotein 1:292, 1:294,
      1:295
  host range 1:294
  human 1:294
  infections 1:294, 1:297, 3:1492
    clinical features 1:296
    diagnostic tests 1:297
    epidemics 1:294
    epidemiology 1:295–6
    immune response 1:297
    immunocompromised 1:295
    neonatal 1:295
    outbreaks 1:295–6
    pathology 1:296–7
    prevention and control 1:297
    RT-PCR 1:296
  macrophage infection 1:297
  murine 1:292
    see also Mouse hepatitis virus
      (MHV)
  mutation frequency 1:293–4
  ocular target 1:525(Table)
  persistence 1:296, 1:297
  proteins 1:291–2
  receptors 1:294
  recombination 3:1451
  reinfection 1:296
  replication 1:293–4
    sites 1:294, 1:296
  respiratory, human 1:296
  serogroups 1:295
  serologic/evolutionary
    relationships 1:295
  shedding 1:296
  structure 1:291–2
    model 1:292(Fig)
  tissue tropism 1:296
  toroviruses relationship 3:1801
  transcription 1:293–4
  translation 1:293–4

Coronaviruses (continued)
  vaccines 1:297
Corriparta virus species
  (CORV) 2:1045(Table)
Corticosteroids, in herpes
  zoster 3:1877
Corticoviridae 2:1226
  characteristics 2:1226
  phage included 2:1226
Corynebacterium diphtheriae
  infection, lesions 2:1228
  toxinogenic conversion 2:1229
  toxins see Diphtheria toxin
Corynephage, tox^+ 2:1229
cos site 2:1236
Cosmids 2:1243
Costelytra zealandica iridescent
  virus (CzIV), genome 2:868
Cosuppression of genes see Gene
  silencing
Cotton leaf curl virus- Pakistan
  (CLCuV-Pk) 1:600
Cottontail rabbit herpesvirus
  (CTHV) 2:703
Cottontail rabbit papillomavirus
  (CRPV)
  genetics 2:1124
  geographic distribution 2:1122
  history/discovery 2:1121
  infection
    clinical features 2:1127
    endemic 2:1122
    pathology/
      histopathology 2:1127
    treatment 2:1129
  pathogenicity 2:1127
  proteins 2:1124
  tissue tropism 2:1126
  transgenic rabbits 2:1123
  transmission 2:1126
  see also Papillomaviruses,
    animal
Cottontail rabbits
  herpesvirus sylvilagus 2:704
  isolation from 2:703
  lymphoma-like disease 2:703,
    2:705
Councilman bodies 1:382
COUP-TF 1:29
Cowpea chlorotic mottle virus
  (CCMV) 1:198
  capsid structure 1:199
  coat protein gene 1:203
  infection spread 1:203
  pathology 1:203
  protein subunit
    structure 3:1949(Fig)
  recombination 1:202
  structure 1:199(Fig), 3:1948
  see also Bromoviruses
Cowpea mild mottle virus
  (CPMMV) 1:240
  genome 1:239
Cowpea mosaic virus
  (CPMV) 1:285, 1:290, 3:1966,
  3:1967(Table)
  economic importance 1:291
  gene expression 1:287–8
  genome structure 1:287
    RNA 1:287
  protease, inhibitor 2:1305
  proteins 1:287–8
  resistance mechanisms
    against 2:1305
  structure and coat proteins 1:286
  translation 1:287–8
  see also Comoviruses
Cowpea mottle virus (CPMoV),
  genome 1:245
Cowpea severe mosaic virus
  (CPSMV) 1:285, 1:290
  genome structure 1:287

Cowpox 2:1140
  see also Cowpox virus, infections
Cowpox virus 1:298–304, 3:1865, 3:1870, 3:1992–3
  A-type inclusions (ATI) 1:298, 1:299, 1:299(Fig), 1:300, 1:303
  animal reservoirs 1:301(Fig)
  antigenic crossreactivity 1:301
  apoptosis inhibition 1:74
  B-type inclusions 1:300
  Brighton strain 1:299, 1:301
  C (capsule) form 1:299
  cell culture 1:299, 1:300
  CmrA gene, loss 1:300
  crmA 1:74
  'd' antigen 1:300, 1:301
  digestion with *Hind* III 1:298, 1:299
  envelope 1:299
  evolution 1:300–1
  extracellular enveloped (EEV) 1:299, 1:304
  future perspectives 1:304
  genetics 1:300
  genome structure 1:299
  geographic/seasonal distribution 1:300
  hemagglutinin gene 1:299
  history 1:298
  host range 1:298, 1:300, 1:301–2, 1:301(Fig)
  immune response evasion 1:300
  infections
    cats 1:301, 1:302, 1:302–3, 1:303, 1:303(Fig), 1:304
    cattle 1:301, 1:302
    clinical features 1:302–3, 1:303(Fig)
    epidemiology 1:301–2, 1:302(Fig)
    human 1:301, 1:302, 1:303(Fig), 1:304
    immune response 1:303–4
    pathogenicity 1:302
    pathology/histopathology 1:303, 1:303(Fig)
    prevention and control 1:304
  intracellular naked virus (INV) 1:299
  M (mulberry) form 1:299
  Moscow Zoo strain 1:300, 1:301
  mutations 1:299
  orthopoxviruses differentiation 1:298
  physical properties 1:300
  propagation 1:300
  proteins, properties 1:299–300
  replication 1:300
  serologic relationship and variability 1:301
  structure and properties 1:298–9, 1:299(Fig)
  taxonomy and classification 1:298
  transmission and tissue tropism 1:302
  vaccination 1:304
  vaccinia virus relationship
    differences 1:299, 1:300
    similarities 1:300
  virulence factors 1:300, 1:302
  white pock mutants 1:299, 1:300, 1:302, 1:303
Cowpox virus cytokine response modifier (crmA) 1:74
Cowpox-like viruses 1:298
Coxsackievirus A4, discovery 2:733
Coxsackievirus A16, evolution 1:465

Coxsackievirus A21, receptors and co-receptors 2:1181
Coxsackievirus A23 1:305, 2:736, 2:737
Coxsackievirus A24 1:305, 1:307, 1:309
  acute hemorrhagic conjunctivitis (AHC) 1:526
  variant (CA24v) 1:469
Coxsackievirus A 1:305
  history/discovery 2:734
  infections
    enteric 1:447
    pathology/histopathology 1:309, 1:310(Fig)
  receptors 1:305
  serotypes 1:307
Coxsackievirus and adenovirus receptor (CAR) 1:305
Coxsackievirus B3 1:308, 1:309
  genetic susceptibility 2:756–7
  infectious myocarditis 2:756
  resistance genes 2:755(Table)
Coxsackievirus B5 1:305
  swine vesicular disease virus (SVDV) similarity 1:464, 1:465
Coxsackievirus B 1:305
  cardiac disease due to 2:1075
    neonatal 2:1074
    pathogenesis 2:1076–7
  echoviruses relationship 1:413
  history/discovery 2:734
  infections
    clinical features 1:308
    diabetes mellitus and 1:308, 2:1080
    of heart 1:308
    pancreatitis 2:1079
    pathology/histopathology 1:310(Fig)
  receptors 1:305
  serotypes 1:307
  tissue tropism 2:1077
Coxsackieviruses 1:305–11
  antibodies 2:735
  classification 1:306(Table)
  coreless particles 1:306
  defective particles 1:307
  dense virion 1:306
  detection, suckling mice 1:399
  epidemiology 1:307
  epitopes 1:310
  evolution 1:307
  experimental infections 1:309
  future perspectives 1:311
  genetics 1:306–7
  genome organization 1:306(Fig)
  genome sequence 1:306
  geographic/seasonal distribution 1:305
  heat inactivation 1:311
  history 1:305, 2:734–5
    discovery 2:734
    tissue culture 2:735–6
  host range 1:305–6
  host susceptibility 1:307
  infections
    antiviral agents 1:311
    clinical features 1:307–9
    immune response 1:309–10
    neonates 1:309
    pathology/histopathology 1:309, 1:310(Fig)
    persistent 1:307, 1:308, 1:311
    in pregnancy 1:309
    prevention and control 1:310–11
  internal ribosome entry site 1:306
  nomenclature 2:737

Coxsackieviruses (*continued*)
  pathogenicity 1:307
  propagation 1:305–6
  proteins 1:306–7
  provirion 1:306
  receptors 1:305–6, 1:306(Table)
  serologic relationship and variability 1:307
  spread in environment 1:307
  in suckling mice 1:305
  taxonomy and classification 1:305
  transmission and tissue tropism 1:307
  vaccines 1:311
CPP32 cysteine protease 1:71, 1:75
CR2 (CD21) *see* CD21 (CR2)
CRE binding protein (CREB) 2:800
  binding protein (CBP) *see* CREB binding protein (CBP)
  bovine leukemia virus (BLV) 1:192
  HTLV-1 Tax protein binding 2:790
Cre-*Lox* system, bacteriophage P1 2:1242
CREB binding protein (CBP) 1:25, 2:800
  HTLV-1 Tax protein binding 2:790
  in HTLV-2 2:800
Crenarchaeota 1:76
  viruses 1:85–8, 1:88
    of *Sulfolobus* 1:86–8
    of *Thermoproteus tenax* 1:85–6
    see also SSV1 virus
Creutzfeldt–Jakob disease (CJD) 2:1018, 3:1388, 3:1402
  aetiology and prion concept 3:1402
  amyloid plaques 3:1401
  background 1:1402
  familial 3:1392
  iatrogenic 3:1390, 3:1392
  infectious 3:1392
  pathology/histopathology 3:1401
  sporadic 3:1390–2
    Kuru origin 3:1399
    neuropathology 3:1391(Fig)
    transmission, to apes 3:1388
Creutzfeldt–Jakob disease (CJD), new variant (nvCJD) 1:421, 3:1392, 3:1397, 3:1401
  age of onset 3:1390
  bovine prions causing 3:1397
  case number prediction problems 3:1397
  emerging viral disease 1:419(Table)
  etiology 3:1392
  neuropathology 3:1391(Fig), 3:1397
  prion transmission 1:485(Table)
  PrP amyloid plaques 3:1390
  PrP^{Sc} conformation 3:1397
  relationship with BSE 3:1397
Crick, F. 2:729
Cricket paralysis virus (CrPV) 2:844, 2:1268–71
  biological control by 2:1274
  cell cultures 1:1274
  cross-reactivity with *Drosophila* C virus (DCV) 2:1269
  genome 2:1271
  host protein synthesis shutoff 2:1271
  host range 2:1269
  isolate CrPV$_{ARK}$ 2:1271
  isolates and groups 2:1269–71
  isolation and outbreaks 2:1268
  replication 2:1269
  structure 2:1269(Fig)

Crimean–Congo hemorrhagic fever 1:209
Crimean–Congo hemorrhagic fever (CCHF) virus 1:211, 1:419(Table), 3:1990
  transmission 1:211
Crimson clover latent virus 2:1008(Table)
Crinivirus 1:266, 1:267
  transmission 1:272
  viruses included 1:268(Table)
Crixivan (indinavir) 1:60
crk oncogene 1:116, 3:1516
Crop
  failures, virus diseases 2:1321
  production
    impact of plant viruses 2:1318
    see also Plant virus disease
  total losses due to viral infections 2:1321
Cross-protection 2:851, 3:1694
  plant resistance mechanism 2:1306
  see also Interference, viral
Cross-reactivation of viruses 1:609
Croup 1:65, 3:1492, 3:1493(Table)
  parainfluenza viruses (PIVs) causing 2:1133
Cruciferae, cauliflower mosaic virus (CaMV) infection 2:1276–7
Cryphonectria hypovirus (CHV) 2:805
  see also CHV1-EP713
Cryphonectria parasitica 2:804
  G-protein 2:806
  transgenic hypovirulent strains 2:806
Crypt cell, hyperplasia 1:448
Cryptic viruses *see* Cryptoviruses
Cryptophlebia leucotreta 1:141
Cryptotopes 2:838
Cryptoviridae 1:312
  classification 2:1147
  fungal virus affinities 1:313
Cryptovirus 1:312
Cryptoviruses 1:312–15
  economic importance 1:315
  evolution 1:315
  future perspectives 1:314–15
  genome (RNA1 and RNA2) 1:312, 1:313, 1:314
    sequences 1:314
  graft non-transmissibility 1:313
  history 1:312
  host range 1:312
  as minimal self-sufficient virus 1:314
  molecular biology 1:314
  RNA-dependent RNA polymerases (RDRPs) 1:314
  sectoring 1:313
  serologic relationships and variability 1:314
  structure and properties 1:312
  taxonomy and nomenclature 1:312
  transmission 1:313–14
  transport function absent 1:313
  virus–host relationships 1:313–14
CtBP 1:26
  E1A protein interaction 1:24, 1:28
CTX genetic element 2:1233
Cucumber green mottle mosaic virus (CGMMV), structure 3:1781
Cucumber leaf spot virus (CLSV) 1:244, 3:1790, 3:1790(Table)
  genome 3:1791(Fig)
  host range 3:1792

Cucumber leaf spot virus (CLSV) (*continued*)
   proteins 3:1791(Table)
Cucumber mosaic virus (CMV) 1:315
   as adaptable virus 1:318
   classification 1:316
   coat protein 1:319
   control strategies 3:1615
   evolution 1:317
   genome, nucleotide sequences 1:317, 1:318(Fig)
   geographic/seasonal distribution 1:316
   graft transmission 1:319
   host range and propagation 1:316
   IB strains 1:318
   nucleic acid-mediated resistance 2:1311
   P1/HC-Pro region and synergism 3:1696, 3:1697(Fig)
   pathogenicity and symptoms 1:319
   proteins, comparisons 2:810(Fig)
   replication 1:322–3
   resistance to 1:319
   RNA-dependent RNA polymerase 1:323
   RNAs
      defective 1:321
      sequences 1:317(Table)
      satellite RNAs 1:317, 1:323, 3:1612
         'chlorosis domain' 2:1190
         chlorosis induction 2:1190
         necrotic response 2:1190
         replication 3:1614
         secondary structure 1:321(Fig)
   serologic relationships and variability 1:318
   strains 1:318
   subgroups 1:316, 1:317(Table)
   transmission 1:319
   see also Cucumoviruses
Cucumber necrosis tombusvirus (CNV) *see* Cucumber necrosis virus (CNV)
Cucumber necrosis virus (CNV) 3:1790, 3:1790(Table)
   coat protein 3:1796
   transmission 3:1909
   transmission specificity 3:1793
   multivesicular bodies 3:1793(Fig)
   promoter sequences 3:1795(Fig)
   serologic relationships 3:1792
   transmission 3:1792–3
      by fungi 3:1909
      in vitro 3:1909
   see also Tombusviruses
Cucumber pale fruit viroid 3:1930(Table)
Cucumber plants, economic significance of virus diseases 2:1323
Cucumber soil-borne virus (CSBV) 1:244
Cucumovirus 1:39, 1:316, 1:317
   species included 1:316
Cucumoviruses 1:315–20, 1:320–4
   bromoviruses relationship 1:198–9
   cDNA clones 1:316, 1:317, 1:324
   cell-to-cell movement 1:322
   epidemiology 1:318–19
   evolution 1:317–18, 1:318(Fig)
   future perspectives 1:320
   genetic mapping of symptom determinants 1:323–4
   genetics 1:316–17
   genome 1:321(Fig)
      nucleotide sequences 1:317, 1:318(Fig)

Cucumoviruses (*continued*)
   genome (*continued*)
      ORFs 1:321, 1:323
      properties 1:320–1
   geographic/seasonal distribution 1:316
   history 1:315–16
   host range and propagation 1:316
   inclusion body formation 1:319
   pathogen-derived engineered resistance 2:1308(Table)
   pathogenicity and cytopathology 1:319
   physical properties 1:320, 1:322
   prevention and control 1:319–20
   proteins 1:321(Table), 1:322
      1a and 2a proteins 1:317, 1:322, 1:323
      2b protein 1:317, 1:322
      3a protein 1:317, 1:323
      coat protein 1:319, 1:322
   reassortment 1:317, 1:323
   replication 1:322–3, 1:323
   resistant plants 1:319
   RNAs 1:316, 1:317(Table), 1:320, 1:321(Table)
      3′ termini 1:322–3
      5′ termini 1:323
      defective 1:321
      RNA1 and RNA2 1:316, 1:320–1
      RNA3 1:317, 1:321
      RNA3 exchange 1:317
      RNA4 1:317, 1:321, 1:323
      RNA4a 1:323
      RNA5 1:321
   satellite RNAs 1:316, 1:317, 1:320, 1:321–2
      attenuation for biocontrol 1:319
      D4 satellite 1:321–2
      longevity 1:318
      as model for RNA virus evolution 1:318, 1:322
      origin 1:318
      replication 1:323
      secondary structure 1:321(Fig)
      symptoms associated 1:319
   serologic relationships and variability 1:318
   structure and properties 1:320
   taxonomy and classification 1:316
   transcription and translation 1:323
   transmission and tissue tropism 1:319
   see also Cucumber mosaic virus (CMV); Peanut stunt virus (PSV); Tomato aspermy virus (TAV)
Cucurbit aphid-borne yellows virus (CABYV)
   evolution 2:905
   transcription 2:904
   see also Poleroviruses
Cucurbit chlorotic spot virus (CCSV), transmission 1:272
Cucurbit yellow stunting disorder virus (CYSDV), transmission 1:272
Culex species
   St Louis encephalitis virus transmission 1:428
   Sindbis (SIN) virus transmission 3:1657
Culex tritaeniorhynchus
   Japanese encephalitis (JE) virus transmission 2:871, 2:872, 2:873
   overwintering 2:875
   reduction 2:873

Culicoides
   bluetongue virus (BTV) transmission 2:1048, 2:1049, 2:1055
      barriers 2:1055
      orbivirus vector 2:1054
   Oropouche virus transmission 1:209, 3:1992
   spread 3:1996
Cultivar resistance 2:1304–5
Culture of viruses *see* Cell culture; Tissue culture
Curtovirus 1:597
Curtoviruses
   genes, functions 1:598–600, 1:599(Table)
   genome organization/expression 1:598, 1:598–600
   transmission 1:603
'Cutter incident' 2:1182
Cvm-1 gene 2:757
CXC chemokines *see* Chemokine families
CXCR4, HIV coreceptor 1:537, 2:768, 2:775
Cyanobacteria 1:324, 1:331
   carbon fixation role 1:325–30, 1:330, 1:332
   characteristics 1:324
   classification 1:324
   copper effect 1:331
   DNA viruses *see* Cyanophages
   enzymes, cyanophages effect 1:331
   filamentous 1:327(Table)
   freshwater 1:325
   importance 1:325
   marine 1:325–31
   taxa 1:325(Table)
   unicellular 1:325, 1:326(Table)
   see also Synechococcus
Cyanophages 1:324–32
   A-1 1:327(Table), 1:331
   A-2 1:327(Table)
   A-4(L) 1:327(Table)
      Anabaena resistance 1:331
   AC-1 1:327(Table)
   AN-11 to AN-22 1:327(Table)
   Anabaena 1:331
      infection prevention by lipopolysaccharide 1:331
   AS-1 1:325, 1:326(Table), 1:331
   AS-1M 1:326(Table)
   AS-2 1:326(Table)
   carbon cycling role 1:330, 1:332
   DNA repair 1:330
   ecology 1:325–31
   filamentous cyanobacteria 1:327(Table)
   freshwater 1:325
   inactivation by sunlight 1:330
   LPP-1, LPP-2 and LPP-3A 1:327(Table)
   LPP-3 1:331
   lysogeny in phosphate-depletion 1:330
   marine
      cyanobacterial interactions 1:330, 1:332
      distribution pattern 1:330
      metabolism 1:331
      morphology 1:325
      ms-1 1:331
      N-1 1:327(Table), 1:331
      osmotic stress effect 1:331
      ts mutants 1:331
   NP-1T 1:327(Table)
   physiology–genetics 1:331
   replication 1:331
   role as control agent 1:325
   S-1, S-2L, S-3L, S-4L and S-5L 1:326(Table)

Cyanophages (*continued*)
   S-PM2 1:330
   SM-1 and SM-2 1:326(Table)
   Synechococcus 1:325–30
      concentrations 1:328, 1:329, 1:329(Fig)
      contact rates 1:329–30
      phosphate status effect 1:330–1
      resistance 1:328–9
   types and classification 1:325
   unicellular cyanobacteria 1:326(Table)
Cycas necrotic stunt virus 2:1008(Table)
Cyclic AMP responsive element (CRE) 1:26, 2:800
   binding protein *see* CRE binding protein (CREB)
   bovine leukemia virus (BLV) 1:192
   HTLV-1 2:790
Cycling of viruses 3:1418
Cyclins, adenovirus E1A protein complex 1:24
Cydia pomonella 1:141
   granuloviruses (GV) 1:145
Cymbidium ringspot virus (CyRSV) 3:1790, 3:1790(Table)
   coat protein 3:1796
   nucleic acid-mediated resistance in plants 2:1311
   proteins 3:1795–6
   see also Tombusviruses
Cynomolgus monkeys
   Ebola-Reston virus isolation 2:939
   monkeypox 3:1672
Cynosurus mottle virus (CyMV) 3:1675
CYP3A4, protease inhibitor metabolism 2:785
Cypovirus 1:332, 2:844
Cypoviruses 1:332–9
   applications 1:338
   as biocontrol agent 1:332
   biosafety concerns 1:338
   Bombyx mori 1:333(Fig), 1:334(Fig), 1:335
   cell-to-cell movement 1:336
   Dendrolimus spectabilis 1:338
   epidemiology 1:334
   Euxoa scandens 1:334(Fig), 1:335
   evolution 1:334
   gene
      mutations 1:333, 1:334
      polyhedrin 1:333
   genetic reassortment 1:334
   genome properties 1:333
      dsRNA segments 1:333, 1:334, 1:335
   'dwarf gene' 1:333
   geographic/seasonal distribution 1:332
   Heliothis armigera 1:336
   history 1:332
   host range and propagation 1:334
   inclusion bodies 1:332, 1:334(Fig)
   insect resistance 1:337
   internalization 1:337
   latency 1:334
   lethality 1:337
   mixed infections 1:336–7
   morphogenesis and cytopathology 1:334–5
   mRNA synthesis 1:336
   nomenclature 1:332
   occlusion bodies 2:844
   pathogenicity 1:337–8
   persistence 1:335–6, 1:338
   physical properties 1:333–4
   polyhedrin formation 1:333
   prevention and control 1:338

Cypoviruses (continued)
  protein and antigen
    synthesis 1:336
  release 1:335
  replication 1:336–7
    abortive 1:337
    factors affecting 1:336
  serologic relationships 1:334
  strain interactions 1:337
  structure and properties 1:332–3,
    1:333(Fig)
  synergism, insecticides 1:338
  taxonomy and
    classification 1:332
  tissue culture 1:336
  transcriptase 1:333, 1:336
  transcription 1:336
  transmission 1:334, 1:335–6
  virulence 1:338
  virus–host interactions 1:337–8
  see also Polyhedra
Cysteine proteases
  aspartate-specific 1:71
  inhibitor 1:75
  poliovirus 2A^{pro} and
    3CD^{pro} 2:1340
  see also CPP32 cysteine protease
Cystitis, hemorrhagic 2:876
  adenoviruses causing 1:5–6
Cystoviridae 2:1227
  characteristics 2:1227
  Cystovirus 2:1205
  phage included 2:1227
Cystovirus 2:1205
  see also Bacteriophage φ6
Cytokines 1:339–44
  anti-inflammatory 1:342
  antiviral 2:1201
  chemotactic see Chemokines
  definition 1:339
  families 1:340–3
  feline immunodeficiency virus
    (FIV) infection 1:539–40
  functions 1:339
  immune evasion
    mechanism 2:1204
  induction in HIV infection 2:772
  murine CMV inducing 1:367–8
  networks 1:339–40, 1:340(Fig)
  in parapoxvirus infections 2:1145
  phagocytic cells producing 1:339
  receptors 1:339
    mpl oncogene 3:1515
    oncogenes 3:1515
  release in HPV infections 2:1113
  viruses encoding
    homologues 1:339
  see also Interferons; specific
    interleukins, interferons,
    tumor necrosis factors
Cytomegalia 1:363
Cytomegalic inclusion
  disease 1:344, 1:349, 1:356
Cytomegalovirus 1:345, 1:357
Cytomegalovirus (CMV) 1:344–51
  animal see Cytomegalovirus
    (CMV), animal (below)
  apoptosis induction 1:73
  cytopathic effect 1:397(Fig)
  cytotoxic T lymphocytes
    generation 3:1825
  detection, centrifugation culture
    method 1:397
  epidemiology 1:347–8
  evolution 1:347
  genetics 1:346–7
  geographic/seasonal
    distribution 1:345–6, 2:709
  history 1:344–5
  host range and
    propagation 1:346, 2:709
    adaptation to cell culture 1:346

Cytomegalovirus (CMV)
    (continued)
  host species barrier
    crossing 1:362
  human see Human
    cytomegalovirus (HCMV)
  IE1 and IE2 1:73
  infection see Human
    cytomegalovirus (HCMV)
    infection
  lymphoproliferative
    herpesviruses
    relationship 2:707
  murine see Murine
    cytomegalovirus (MCMV)
  'owl's eye' inclusions 1:346, 1:349
  reactivation 2:1081
  simian see Cytomegalovirus
    (CMV), animal
  strains and sequence
    homologies 1:345
  taxonomy and
    classification 1:345, 2:708
  tissue tropism 1:348
  transmission 1:345, 1:347, 1:348
  UL89 terminase 1:63
  UL97 gene 1:54
  unstable in environment 1:347
Cytomegalovirus (CMV),
    animal 1:344–5, 1:357–63
  African green monkeys
    (AgCMV) 1:357, 1:359, 1:360
  cell culture 1:359, 1:360(Fig)
  classification 1:357–8
  DNA binding proteins 1:359
  DNA replication proteins 1:358
  epidemiology 1:359
  evolution 1:357–8
  gene expression control 1:360–1
  genome sequence 1:359
  genome structure 1:358–9
  guinea pigs (GpCMV) 1:357
  history 1:357
  IE1 proteins 1:361
  IE2 proteins 1:361
  IE2 region 1:359
  immediate early genes 1:362(Fig)
  major immediate early (MIE)
    region 1:359, 1:360–1
  MIE promoter/enhancer 1:361
  as model of virus
    reactivation 1:361
  monkey (SCMV) 1:357, 1:359,
    1:360
  murine see Murine
    cytomegalovirus (MCMV)
  physical properties 1:359
  rat (RCMV) see Rat
    cytomegalovirus (RCMV)
  replication 1:359–60
    origins 1:361
  simian 2:707, 2:709
    clinical features 2:712
    immune response 2:712–13
    structure 1:358
    transcription 1:360–1
Cytopathic effects
    (CPE) 1:397(Fig), 1:399
  animal enteroviruses 1:464
  animal viruses 3:1409
  arenaviruses 2:889
  Chandipura and Piry
    viruses 1:259
  closteroviruses 1:271
  definition 3:1409
  Drosophila C virus
    (DCV) 2:1269
  echoviruses 1:411, 1:413
  enterovirus 68 (EV68) 1:469
  enterovirus 70 (EV70) 1:472
  hepatitis A virus (HAV) 1:635
  history 2:722

Cytopathic effects (CPE)
    (continued)
  inclusions see Inclusions
  LCMV 2:889
  lymphocystis virus 1:566
  measles virus (MV) 2:955
  molluscum contagiosum virus
    (MCV) 2:962–3
  mumps virus (MuV) 2:991
  nepoviruses 2:1012
  nodaviruses 2:1030
  nonoccluded baculoviruses
    (NOB) 2:1032
  orbiviruses 2:1056
  pea enation mosaic virus
    (PEMV) 2:1195
  plaques 3:1412
  polioviruses 2:1344–5
  polyomaviruses 2:1354, 2:1360
  pomoviruses 3:1362
  reoviruses 3:1456, 3:1470–1
  reticuloendotheliosis (RE)
    viruses 3:1499
  RSV 3:1485
  rubella virus 3:1593
  trichoviruses 3:1840
  in tube culture 1:396–7
  type D retroviruses 3:1522
  vaccinia virus 3:1868
  varicella-zoster virus 3:1884
  vesicular stomatitis virus
    (VSV) 3:1914
  viroid infections 3:1932
  see also Cytopathology; other
    specific viruses
Cytopathic inclusions see
    Inclusions
Cytopathic virus, bovine
    immunodeficiency virus
    (BIV) 1:187
Cytopathology
  arteriviruses 1:92
  cardiovirus-infected cells 1:237
  carlaviruses 1:240–1
  cell rounding 3:1959
  host membrane damage 3:1959
  iridoviruses 2:867
  Japanese encephalitis (JE)
    virus 2:872
  leporipoxviruses 3:1384–5
  luteoviruses 2:906–7
  plant rhabdoviruses 3:1536–8
  poleroviruses 2:906–7
  potyviruses 3:1370(Fig)
  sendai virus 3:1618–19
  sobemoviruses 3:1679
  spumaviruses 3:1685, 3:1690
  tombusviruses 3:1793
  tospoviruses 3:1807
  see also Cytopathic effects (CPE)
Cytoplasm, modification in
    cucumovirus-infected
    cells 1:319
Cytoplasmic polyhedrosis viruses
    (CPVs) 1:332, 2:844
  see also Cypoviruses
Cytorhabdovirus 3:1531
  see also Plant rhabdoviruses
Cytorhabdoviruses
  budding 3:1538
  polymerases 3:1536
  replication cycle 3:1537(Fig)
  see also Plant rhabdoviruses
Cytoskeleton 1:253–4
  host
    changes induced by frog virus 3
      (FV3) 1:586
    effects of virus infection 3:1960
  virus transport to nucleus 3:1473
Cytosol 1:253–4

Cytotoxic T lymphocytes
    (CTL) 3:1862
  adoptive therapy, EBV
    infection 1:493, 1:494
  antigenic drift as immune evasion
    mechanism 2:817
  apoptosis activation
    mechanism 1:69(Fig)
  bluetongue virus (BTV) 2:1059
  CMV infections (human) 1:350
  CMV-specific 1:1825
  coxsackievirus infection 1:309
  EBV infection 1:493
  effector molecules 2:818
  elimination of viral-infected
    cells 1:69
  feline immunodeficiency virus
    (FIV) infection 1:539
  functions/actions 2:818–19, 2:819
  herpesvirus sylvilagus
    infection 2:706
  HIV infection 2:772
  HPV infections 2:1113
  HSV infections 2:684
  IFN-γ action 1:339
  immune response to respiratory
    viruses 3:1491
  influenza virus 2:829
  LCMV infection 2:919, 2:920
  MHC class I restriction 2:813,
    2:818, 2:819
  MHC glycoproteins
    involved 2:820
  neutralizing 1:310
  primary response 2:822(Fig)
  protective function 3:1863
  pseudorabies virus (PRV) 3:1427
  receptor 2:819
  reoviruses 3:1462
  reticuloendotheliosis (RE) virus
    infection 3:1498
  RSV infection 3:1484
  resistance 3:1486
  secondary response by 2:816
  Sendai virus infection 3:1621
  transfer
    experiments 3:1863(Table)
  vaccine-induced
    production 3:1863
  viral epitopes 3:1863
  in viral infections 2:819–20
    circulation 2:821
  virus evasion 2:1204
  virus killing mechanism 2:1201
  visna-maedi viruses 3:1963
  see also CD8 T cells; T cells

D

d4T (Stavudine, Zerit) see
    Stavudine (d4T)
Dacryoadenitis, mumps virus 1:524
DAFV (Desulfurolobus ambivalens
    filamentous virus) 1:78(Fig),
    1:88
Dahlia mosaic virus
    (DaMV) 2:1276
  transmission 2:1279
Dairy fermentations
  phage in 2:1246
  phage-resistant strain
    development 2:1247
  Streptococcus thermophilus
    phage 2:1255(Fig)
  see also Streptococcus
    thermophilus, phage
  Streptococcus thermophilus
    role 2:1253

Dam methylase 3:1715
Dandelion yellow mosaic virus (DYMV) 3:1622
  host range and propagation 3:1624
  prevention and control 3:1625
  properties 3:1622
  serology 3:1623
  symptoms of infections 3:1624
  transmission 3:1624
  see also Sequiviruses
Dane particles see under Hepatitis B virus (HBV)
Danish plum line pattern virus 1:39
Dapple apple viroid 3:1930(Table)
Dasheen mosaic virus, economic significance 2:1323
Database, viruses (ICTVdB) 3:1731
Datura yellow vein virus (DYVV) 3:1531
Daycare, emerging viral diseases associated 1:423
DBA/2 mice, coxsackievirus B3 infection 2:756
ddC (Zalcitabine) 1:58–9, 2:779
  resistance 1:59
  toxicity 1:59
ddCTP 1:58
ddI (didanosine) 1:59, 2:779
  half-life 1:59
  toxicity 1:59
  US guidelines 1:59
DEAD box protein family 1:201
Death domains 1:71
Death effector domains (DED) 1:70(Fig)
  protein see DED proteins
Death proteases 1:71
Death receptors 1:71
  apoptosis inhibition 1:71(Table), 1:72(Table)
Decay accelerating factor (DAF; CD55)
  coxsackievirus receptor 1:305, 2:1183–4
  echovirus receptor 1:411
  enterovirus 70 (EV70) receptor 1:471
DED proteins, apoptosis inhibition 1:71(Table)
Defective interfering (DI) viruses/RNAs 1:371–5, 1:608, 2:1311, 3:1453–4, 3:1607
  animal parainfluenza viruses 2:1137
  assays 1:373
    deficulties 1:374
  biological effects 1:373
  in carmoviruses 1:246
  carmoviruses 1:246
  co-infection of cells with 1:372
  comparison with St particles 1:371
  coronaviruses 1:294
  cyclic variations 1:372–3, 1:373(Fig)
  defective viruses vs 1:372
  definition 1:371
  equine herpesviruses 1:511–12
  equine torovirus (ETV) 3:1801
  in experimental animals 1:373–4
  future perspectives 1:374
  genome
    defectiveness 1:371–2
    generation 1:371, 1:372(Fig)
  history 1:371
  Hz-1V 2:1033, 2:1034
  influenza viruses 2:830, 2:835
  interference by 1:372, 2:851
  LCMV 2:916, 2:923, 2:924
  M protein 1:373

Defective interfering (DI) viruses/RNAs (continued)
  as mutational drivers for evolution 1:373
  in natural infections 1:374
  origin 1:371
  phytoreoviruses 2:1264
  plant resistance mechanism 2:1311
  plant rhabdoviruses 3:1536
  potexviruses 3:1366
  properties 1:608
  recombination see Recombination of viruses
  replication 1:371, 1:372–3
  RNA viruses 1:608
  Semliki Forest virus (SFV) 3:1662
  sindbis (SIN) virus 3:1662
  single deletion-type 3:1453
  structure 1:371
  tobraviruses 3:1786–7, 3:1787(Fig)
  tombusviruses see Tombusviruses
  tospoviruses 3:1805
  types 3:1453–4
Defective particles
  adenoviruses 3:1411
  multiplication 3.1411
  parvoviruses 3:1411
Defective RNAs 3:1607
Deforestation, emergence and re-emergence of diseases 1:422
Deformed wing virus (DWV) 2:744(Table), 2:747
Delavirdine (Rescriptor, U90152) 1:60
Delayed-type hypersensitivity 2:821
  in conjunctiva 1:524
  HSV infections 2:684
  respiratory viruses 3:1491
  TMEV-induced demyelination 3:1778(Fig), 3:1779
Delbruck, M. 2:728
Delta antigen 1:664, 3:1614
  see also Hepatitis delta virus (HDV)
Delta herpesvirus 3:1873
Delta regulator, P4 bacteriophage 2:1095, 2:1101
Deltaretrovirus 1:191, 2:795
  proviral DNA integration 1:191
Deltavirus 1:664
Dementia
  HIV infection 1:76
  in prion diseases 3:1390
  in slow virus infections 2:1018–19
Demyelination
  immune-mediated by TMEV 3:1773, 3:1778–9
  Marek's disease 2:949
  mechanism 3:1778, 3:1778(Fig)
  in virus infections 2:1017
DEN virus see Dengue viruses
Dendritic cells 2:813
  follicular see Follicular dendritic cells (FDCs)
  Orf virus infection 2:1145
Dendrolimus spectabilis
  control by cytoplasmic polyhedroviruses (CPVs) 2:844
  cytoplasmic polyhedrosis virus 2:338
Dengue fever 1:375
  classical 1:380, 1:381
  epidemics 1:379
  etiology 1:375
  history 1:375
  prevalence 1:376

Dengue fever (continued)
  see also Dengue viruses, infection
Dengue hemorrhagic fever/dengue shock syndrome (DHF/DSS) 1:376
  classical disease 1:380
  clinical features 1:381–2
  critical stage 1:381–2
  Cuban epidemic 1:378, 1:381
  emergence and spread 1:379–80, 1:383
  epidemics 1:376, 1:380
  grades and severity 1:382
  pathogenesis 1:380
  pathology and histopathology 1:382
  treatment 1:382
  WHO diagnostic criteria 1:382, 1:382(Table)
Dengue viruses 1:375–84, 1:433(Table)
  antibodies and crossreactions 1:382–3
  antigenic and biologic variation 1:379
  antigenic determinants 1:379
  antigenic differences 1:377
  antigens 1:376
  apoptosis promotion 1:75
  classification 1:375–7
  DEN1 1:375, 1:381
  DEN2 1:375, 1:376, 1:381
    Cuban epidemic 1:378, 1:381
    genetic differences 1:378–9
    genotypes 1:378
    Jamaica genotype 1:378
    Puerto Rico genotype 1:378
  DEN3 1:375, 1:377
    antigenic variation 1:379
  DEN4 1:375, 1:377
    antigenic variation 1:379
  emerging 1:419(Table)
  epidemics 1:381
  epidemiology 1:376(Fig), 1:379–80
  evolution 1:378–9
  experimental infections 1:377
  future perspectives 1:383–4
  genetic drift 1:378
  genetics 1:377–8
  genotypes 1:378
  geographic/seasonal distribution 1:376(Fig), 1:377
  as global public health problem 1:376
  history 1:375–6
  host range 1:377
  hyperendemicity 1:376, 1:378, 1:379, 1:381, 1:381(Fig)
  iceberg concept 1:379(Fig), 1:380, 1:381
  immune enhancement 2:817
  infection
    clinical features 1:381–2
    immune response 1:382–3
    incubation period 1:381
    pathogenesis 1:380–1
    pathology and histopathology 1:382
    secondary 1:380, 1:382
    see also Dengue fever; Dengue hemorrhagic fever/dengue shock syndrome (DHF/DSS)
  maintenance cycles 1:378(Fig), 1:379
    forest cycle 1:378, 1:379
    rural cycle 1:379
    urban cycle 1:378, 1:379
  oligonucleotide fingerprinting 1:377
  pathogenicity 1:380–1

Dengue viruses (continued)
  prevention and control 1:383
  propagation 1:377
    cell lines and baby mice 1:377
  proteins 1:376
  replication, sites 1:380
  RNA genome 1:376
  serologic relationships and variability 1:379
  serotypes 1:376, 1:379
  structure and properties 1:376–7
  surveillance systems 1:383
  target cell type 1:75
  tissue tropism 1:380
  transmission 1:375, 1:377, 1:378(Fig), 1:379, 1:380, 1:485(Table)
    epidemic 1:377
  vaccine development 1:383
  viremia 1:377, 1:380
  virulence 1:380
  yellow fever virus cross-protection 1:1983, 3:1986
Densonucleosis viruses (DNVs) 1:384–8
  see also Densoviruses
Densovirinae 1:384, 2:844, 2:1152, 2:1168
  biological control by 2:844
  characteristics 2:844
  classification 1:384–6
  genera 1:384–6, 2:1168
  genome structures 1:384–6
    diversity 1:386
  insect pest control by 2:844
  taxonomy 1:386
  see also Densoviruses
Densovirus 1:386
  genome structure 1:386
Densoviruses 1:384
  autonomously replicating 1:385
  biological control by 1:387
  capsomers 1:384
  characteristics 1:384
  classification 1:384–6
  composition and structure 1:384–6
  density classes 1:384
  disease caused by 1:387
  ecology 1:387
  economic significance 1:387
  gene expression 1:384–6
  as gene vectors 1:387–8
  genome structure 1:384–6, 1:385(Fig)
    terminal hairpins 1:384
  histopathology 1:387
  host range 1:386
  propagation 1:386–7
  protein synthesis 1:386
  proteins 1:384
  tissue specificity 1:387
  types 1:386
  UV radiation sensitivity 1:387
2-Deoxy-2′-fluoroguanosine 1:64
Deoxyuridine triphosphatase, HSV 2:693
Dependovirus 2:1152, 2:1168
  genetics 2:1152–3
  members 2:1152
Derzsy andersoni, Powassan (POW) virus
  transmission 1:435
Dermacentor marginatus 1:426, 1:428
Dermacentor pictus 1:426, 1:428
Dermatitis
  infectious, HTLV association 2:802
  smallpox vaccine-induced 3:1871
Derzsy's disease 2:1168
Descriptors, viruses 3:1750, 3:1751

Desmodium yellow mosaic virus 3:1850
Desmodium yellow mottle virus 3:1850
Desulfurolobus ambivalens filamentous virus (DAFV) 1:78(Fig), 1:88
Detection of early antigen fluorescent foci (DEAFF) 2:1085
Detection of viral antigens *see* Diagnostic techniques
Detergents, nonionic 3:1420
DFF (DNA fragmentation factor) 1:71
d'Herelle, F. 2:720, 2:725–7, 2:1221
DI particles *see* Defective interfering (DI) viruses/RNAs
Diabetes mellitus, insulin-dependent (type 1)
  as autoimmune disease 2:1080, 2:1081
  HLA associations 2:1080
  molecular mimicry mechanism 1:110–11
  Oldstone model of autoimmunity 1:110–11
  viral pathogenesis 2:1079–81
    after acute infections 2:1080
    coxsackievirus B 1:308, 2:1080
    evidence 2:1079–80
    hypotheses 2:1080–1
    mumps virus 2:992, 2:1080
    seroepidemiology 2:1080
    viruses associated 2:1079
Diadromus ascovirus 1:98
  DNA as episome in wasp 1:100
  evolution 1:103
  genome 1:98
  host range and propagation 1:100
  tissue tropism 1:102, 1:102(Table)
  transmission and ecology 1:100
Diadromus pulchellus 1:98
Diagnosis, virus species 3:1941–3, 3:1942(Table)
Diagnostic probes
  animal viruses 1:612
  see also DNA probes
Diagnostic techniques 1:388–95, 1:395–403
  antibodies (viral) 1:389–91, 1:390(Table)
    complement fixation 1:390
    enzyme immunoassays and ELISA 1:391
    hemagglutination inhibition 1:390
    immunoblot 1:391
    immunofluorescence 1:391
    method advantages 1:389
    method limitations 1:389–90
    neutralization 1:390
    particle agglutination 1:391
    pitfalls 1:391
    radioimmunoassays 1:391
  antigens (viral) 1:388–9, 1:390(Table)
    centrifugation culture method 1:397
    concentration limitation 1:388
    enzyme immunoassays 1:389
    immunoenzyme staining 1:389
    immunofluorescence 1:389
    method advantages 1:388–9
    method limitations 1:388
    particle agglutination 1:389
    radioimmunoassay 1:389
  direct observation
    electron microscopy *see* Electron microscopy
    light microscopy 1:400

Diagnostic techniques (*continued*)
  flow chart 1:396(Fig)
  future perspectives 1:402
  identification of virus 1:399–400
    immunofluorescence 1:399
    immunoperoxidase 1:399–400
    neutralization 1:400
  in vitro virus isolation 1:388
  isolation of plant viruses 3:1418–21
    preserving infectivity during 1:1420
  nucleic acids (viral) 1:391–5, 1:392(Table)
    amplification *see* Nucleic acids, amplification
    hybridization technique 1:391–2
    potential problems 1:394–5
  primary virus isolation/identification 1:396–9
    cell culture *see* Cell culture
    conventional techniques 1:396–7
    embryonated eggs 1:399
    genetically modified cell lines 1:398, 1:402
    infant mice 1:399
    shell vial centrifugation culture 1:397–8, 1:398(Fig)
  rapid assays 1:402
  see also individual techniques; Purification of viruses
Dianthovirus 1:243, 1:403
Dianthoviruses 1:403–9
  capsid protein 1:403–4, 1:408
    domains 1:404
    gene encoding 1:406
    species homology 1:404(Table)
  cell-to-cell movement 1:406–7, 1:407
  epidemiology 1:407
  evolution 1:408–9
  future perspectives 1:409
  genetics 1:406–7
  genome structure 1:403, 1:405
    RNA-1 and RNA-2 1:405, 1:406
  geographic/seasonal distribution 1:403
  history 1:403
  host range and propagation 1:406
  movement proteins 1:406–7, 1:408
    species homology 1:407(Table)
  p88 protein 1:405
  pathogenicity 1:408
  pathology and histopathology 1:408
  physical properties 1:405
  prevention and control 1:408
  proteins 1:405, 1:406
  pseudorecombination 1:407
  replicase 1:405, 1:406, 1:408
    species homology 1:406(Table)
  replication 1:405–6, 1:406
  serologic relationships and variability 1:407
  structure and properties 1:403–5
  T=3 symmetry 1:403
  taxonomy and classification 1:403
  transmission and tissue tropism 1:406, 1:407–8
  see also Carnation ring spot virus (CRSV); Red clover necrotic mosaic virus (RCNMV)
Dianthus 1:403
Diapedesis 2:1179
Diarrhea 3:1576
  adenoviruses causing 1:5, 1:442(Table), 1:445

Diarrhea (*continued*)
  astroviruses causing 1:107, 1:442(Table), 1:446
  bovine viral diarrhea virus causing 1:178
  caliciviruses causing 1:442(Table), 1:445
  coronaviruses causing 1:296, 1:442(Table)
  enteric viruses causing 1:448
  epidemic, coronaviruses causing 1:446
  etiology 1:442(Table), 1:447
    developing/developed countries 1:443(Fig)
  in hepatitis A 1:638
  infantile, adenoviruses causing 1:4, 1:5
  Lassa fever 2:893
  mechanisms 2:1177
  neonatal
    astroviruses causing 1:446
    rotaviruses causing 1:443
  Norwalk virus causing 2:1035, 2:1039
  parvoviruses causing 1:442(Table)
  pathogenesis, rotaviruses 3:1581
  picobirnaviruses causing 1:442(Table)
  rotaviruses causing 1:442(Table), 1:443
  torovirus-associated in calves 3:1802
  toroviruses causing 1:442(Table), 1:447, 3:1801
  watery 1:448
  see also Gastroenteritis
Dicaffeoylquinic acids 2:783
Dicentrarchus labrax encephalitis virus (DLEV) 2:1026
Didanosine *see* ddI (didanosine)
Dieffenbachia, economic significance of virus infections 2:1323, 2:1324
Digitaria streak virus (DSV), genome structure 1:597
Dilated cardiomyopathy
  clinical features 2:1078
  coxsackievirus infection 1:308
  laboratory diagnosis 2:1078
  pathogenesis 2:1077
  virus infections causing 2:1076, 2:1077
Diodia vein chlorosis virus (DVCV), transmission 1:272
Dioscorea bacilliform virus (DBV) 2:1296
2,4-Dioxobutanoic acid derivatives 1:64
Dip (Delta antigen-interacting protein) 1:667
Diphtheria
  features and treatment 2:1228–9
  respiratory 2:1228
Diphtheria toxin 2:1228–9
  gene 2:729
  production 2:1229
  regulation 2:1229
  repressor (DtxR) 2:1229
  structure 2:1229
Diptera
  biological control by *Iridoviridae* 2:845
  entomopoxviruses (EPVs) 1:479
  picorna-like viruses 1:1272–3
'Direct competition' hypothesis 2:852–3
Disinfectants, coxsackievirus infection control 1:311

Disseminated intravascular coagulation, dengue viruses causing 1:381
Distemper viruses 3:1559–69
  epizootiology 3:1565–6
  evolution 3:1564
  future perspectives 3:1569
  genome 3:1562
  geographic distribution 3:1560
  history 3:1560
  host range and propagation 3:1561–2
  infection
    clinical features 3:1567
    immune response 3:1567
    pathology/histopathology 3:1567
  pathogenicity 3:1566
  replication 3:1562–3
  serologic relationships and variability 3:1564
  structure and properties 3:1562
  taxonomy and classification 3:1560
  transmission and tissue tropism 3:1566
  vaccination 3:1569
  see also Canine distemper virus; Morbilliviruses; Phocid distemper virus
DN19 virus 2:737
DNA
  amplification 1:392
    ligase chain reaction (LCR) 1:393
    polymerase chain reaction (PCR) 1:392–3
    strand displacement amplification (SDA) 1:393
    see also Nucleic acid; Polymerase chain reaction (PCR)
  branched (bDNA), amplification method 1:392, 1:394, 1:394(Fig)
  in cell nucleus 1:255
  circular permutation
    frog virus 3 (FV3) 1:583
    lymphocystis disease virus (LCDV) 2:909
  concatemers *see* Concatemers
  covalently closed circular
    avian hepatitis B viruses 1:650, 1:652(Fig), 1:656
    hepatitis B virus *see* Hepatitis B virus (HBV)
    JC and BK viruses 2:876
  crossovers 3:1446
  double-stranded
    algal virus genomes 1:45
    animal papillomaviruses 2:1123
    bacteriophage PRD1 2:1210
    caulimoviruses 2:1275
    coliphage N4 1:450
    Epstein–Barr virus (EBV) 1:494
    hepatitis B virus (HBV) 1:645
    herpesvirus of turkeys 2:947
    Iridoviridae 2:864
    leporipoxviruses and suipoxvirus 3:1383
    Marek's disease virus 2:947
    nuclear polyhedrosis viruses (NPVs) 1:147
    P2 bacteriophage 2:1087
    P4 bacteriophage 2:1094
    parapoxvirus 2:1143
    rice tungro bacilliform virus (RTBV) 2:1294
    SPO1 phage 3:1681
    Tanapox and Yabapox viruses 3:1971
    Tupaia herpesviruses 3:1834

DNA (continued)
  double-stranded (continued)
    vaccinia virus 3:1866
  double-stranded circular
    badnaviruses 2:1296
    human papillomaviruses
      (HPVs) 2:1105, 2:1115
    polyomaviruses 2:1352, 2:1356
    SV40 3:1648
    see also DNA, covalently
      closed circular
  double-stranded linear
    African swine fever virus
      (AFSV) 1:31
    cowpox virus 1:299
    entomopoxviruses
      (EPVs) 1:477
    equine herpesviruses 1:509
    fowlpox virus 1:576
    frog virus 3 (FV3) 1:583
    herpesvirus sylvilagus 2:704
    HHV-6 and HHV-7 2:698
    HSV 2:686
    human CMV 1:352
    lymphocystis disease virus
      (LCDV) 2:908
    molluscum contagiosum virus
      (MCV) 2:961
    pseudorabies virus
      (PRV) 3:1421
  double-stranded segmented,
    polydnaviruses 2:1349
  HMC-containing,
    restriction 2:761
  integration into host
    chromosome 2:897, 3:1446
    bacteriophage P1 1:460
    bacteriophage P4 2:1098–9
    bacteriophage P22 3:1605
    badnaviruses 2:1298
    bovine leukemia virus
      (BLV) 1:192
    coliphage lambda 1:283–4,
      2:926
    coliphages Mu and
      D108 2:981–2
    DNA tumor viruses 1:609
    feline immunodeficiency virus
      (FIV) 1:538
    Hepadnaviridae 1:642
    hepatitis B virus
      mechanism 1:649
    HIV 2:765
    HPV 2:1119
    HPV18 3:1846
    murine leukemia viruses
      proviral DNA 2:996
    oncogenesis 3:1843
    parvoviruses 2:1159
    Retroviridae 1:641–2
    transduced donor DNA 2:1238
    Ty3 and Ty1 elements 3:1506
  methylation see DNA
    methylation (below)
  modification
    phage isolation 1:138
    see also DNA methylation
  modification/restriction
    bacteriophage P1 1:455, 1:459–60
    see also Host-controlled
      modification and restriction
  modular exchange in
    streptococcal phage 2:1260
  recombinant see Recombinant
    DNA technology
  recombination 1:1446
    homologous 3:1446, 3:1449
    nonhomologous (site-
      specific) 3:1446
    see also Recombination of
      viruses

DNA (continued)
  repair
    African swine fever virus
      (AFSV) 1:33
    cyanophages 1:330
    replication see DNA replication
      (below)
  restriction
    function 2:760
    see also Host-controlled
      modification and restriction
  restriction endonuclease
    digestion, history 2:720,
      2:729
  satellite 3:1609(Table), 3:1611
    tomato leaf curl virus-Australia
      (ToLCV-Au) 1:601
  sequencing, history 2:720
  single-stranded
    densoviruses 1:384
    parvoviruses 2:1152, 2:1155,
      2:1156, 2:1161, 2:1167
  single-stranded circular
    filamentous phage 1:550
    geminiviruses 1:597
  supercoiled, SV40 3:1648
  transposition 2:981
DNA adenine methyltransferase
  (dam) methylation sites,
  bacteriophage P1 1:457
DNA bacteriophage
  dsDNA
    lambda 1:281
    see also Coliphage lambda; T1-
      like phage
  evolution 2:1209
  φX174 1:274
  ssDNA circular 1:274
DNA binding proteins
  coliphage N4 1:450
  SV40 T-ag 3:1649, 3:1651
DNA fragmentation factor
  (DFF) 1:71
DNA gyrase, Escherichia coli 1:451
DNA methylation 2:758, 3:1478
  DNA restriction
    dependence 2:761
  eukaryotic viruses 2:763
  frog virus 3 (FV3) 1:583
  functions in prokaryotic
    cells 2:762
  M.dam and M.dcm 2:762
  prokaryotic cells 2:762
  promoters 2:762
DNA methyltransferase
  algal viruses 1:49, 1:49(Table)
  bacteriophage SPβ 1:134
  T1-like phage 3:1702
DNA polymerase 3:1477
  coliphage N4 1:453
  Hepadnaviridae 1:641
  hepatitis B virus (HBV) 1:645,
    1:647
  herpes simplex viruses
    (HSV) 2:693
  varicella-zoster virus 3:1879
DNA polymerase II 3:1472
DNA probes 1:139, 1:391
DNA replication
  bacteriophage φX174 role in
    elucidating 1:280
  bidirectional 2:1214
  human CMV 1:355
  T7-like phage 3:1727
  error rate 1:607
  hairpin transfer
    mechanism 1:1156
  'leading strand' 1:280
  methylation 2:758
  models in parvoviruses 2:1156
  not associated with latent
    infections 2:899

DNA replication (continued)
  Okazaki fragments 2:729
  protein priming mechanism 2:722
  rolling circle model 3:1477
    bacteriophage 186 2:1093
    bacteriophage φX174 1:278
    bacteriophage P22 3:1605
    coliphage lambda 1:282
    equine herpesviruses 1:511
    filamentous phage 1:551
    human CMV 1:355
    human papillomaviruses
      (HPVs) 2:1117
    murine cytomegalovirus
      (MCMV) 1:364
    P2 bacteriophage 2:1093
    T5-like phage 3:1720
  rolling-circle model 2:1214
  sliding-back mechanism 1:126
  theta mode, human
    papillomaviruses
      (HPVs) 2:1117
DNA site-specific (restriction)
  endonuclease, algal
    viruses 1:48–9, 1:49(Table)
DNA tumor viruses
  JC and BK viruses 2:876
  proviral DNA integration 1:609
  transformation by 3:1821–2
  see also Transformation
DNA vaccine
  dengue viruses 1:383
  Ebola virus 2:944
  influenza viruses 2:842
DNA viruses 3:1477–8, 3:1735–9(Table)
  antisense-mediated resistance in
    plants 2:1311
  apoptosis inhibition/
    suppression 1:72–4
  apoptosis promotion 1:74–5
  Baculoviridae 1:140
  double-stranded 3:1735–7(Table), 3:1745
    algae, fungi and
      protozoa 3:1754
    Bacillus subtilis phage 1:130
    bacterial 3:1755
    bacteriophage φ29 1:132
    insect 1:97
    see also Ascoviruses
    invertebrates 3:1752
    plants 3:1753
    vertebrates 3:1751
  eye infections 1:526–8
    see also Eye infections; specific
      viruses
  fish see Fish viruses
  gene expression regulation 3:1477
  insect pest control by 2:844–9
    see also Biological control
  interferon induction 2:856
  latency 2:897
    see also Epstein–Barr virus
      (EBV); Herpes simplex virus
  light microscopy 1:400
  non-occluded 2:845–6
  recombination see
    Recombination of viruses
  replication 1:255, 3:1409, 3:1477–8
  reverse transcribing 3:1738–9(Table), 3:1746(Table)
  RNA virus recombination 3:1500
  shrimp viruses 3:1630–5
  single-stranded 3:1737–8(Table), 3:1746
    bacterial 3:1755
    invertebrates 3:1752
    plants 3:1753
    replication 3:1477
    vertebrates 3:1751

DNA viruses (continued)
  small, replication 3:1477
  in thin-sectioned cells 1:400(Fig)
  transcription 3:1472, 3:1477
  transformation by 3:1960
  as vectors 3:1892
DNA-dependent DNA
  polymerase 3:1472
DNA-dependent RNA polymerase,
  African swine fever virus
    (AFSV) 1:31, 1:34
Dobrava virus 1:210
Dobrava-Belgrade virus
  (DOBV) 1:621, 3:1988
Dogs
  pseudorabies virus (PRV)
    infection 3:1425
  rabies transmission 3:1987
Dogwood mosaic
  virus 2:1008(Table)
Dolphin morbillivirus
  (DMV) 1:420(Table), 2:953,
    3:1560
Dominant-negative mutants 2:851–4
  as antiviral agents 2:853–4
  interference with virulent
    viruses 2:853–4
  in gene therapy 2:853
  genotypic dominants 2:852
  interference by 2:851
  'all things in moderation'
    hypothesis 2:852
  'attractive genome'
    hypothesis 2:853
  complementation 2:853
  'direct competition'
    hypothesis 2:852–3
  mechanisms 2:852–3
  reassortment inhibition 2:853
  'road block' hypothesis 2:852
  'rotten apple' hypothesis 2:852
  'intracellular
    immunization' 2:853
  live virus vaccines 2:854
  origin/source 2:851
  phenotypes 2:851
  phenotypic dominance 2:852
Donkeys, equine arteritis virus
  (EAV) 1:93
Dorsal root ganglia
  HSV infection 2:680
  HSV replication 2:682
DP1 transcription factors 1:25
Droplets, virus transmission 1:484
Drosophila
  carbon dioxide sensitivity 3:1635,
    3:1639
  retroviruses see Drosophila
    melanogaster gypsy virus
  sigma virus 3:1635
  see also Sigma rhabdoviruses
Drosophila A virus (DAV) 2:1273
Drosophila C virus (DCV) 2:844,
  2:1268, 2:1268–9
  cross-reactivity with cricket
    paralysis virus (CrPV) 2:1269
  cytopathic effects 2:1269
  genome 2:1269(Fig), 2:1271
  sequence analysis 2:1271
  host protein synthesis
    reduced 2:1271
  host range 2:1269
  isolates 2:1269
Drosophila iota virus (DiV) 2:1273
Drosophila line 1 virus
  (DLV) 2:1026
Drosophila melanogaster
  carbon dioxide sensitivity 1:259,
    1:260
  cell cultures 3:1528

Drosophila melanogaster
(*continued*)
defective Gypsy
proviruses 3:1530
flamenco gene 3:1526, 3:1528,
3:1529
ref(2)P protein 3:1638
ref alleles 3:1637
ref(2)P 3:1638
resistance to sigma viruses 3:1637
Drosophila melanogaster gypsy
virus 3:1526–30
characteristics of particles 3:1528
control by host genome 3:1526–7
defective 3:1530
distribution 3:1529
env gene products 3:1528
gag gene 3:1527
genome
cis sequences 3:1527
ORF3 3:1527, 3:1528, 3:1529
provirus sequence 3:1527,
3:1527(Fig)
as germline parasite 3:1527,
3:1529
history 3:1526
insertional mutations 3:1529
integration and excision 3:1529
long-terminal repeat 3:1527,
3:1528
post-translational
processing 3:1528
provirus 3:1527, 3:1527(Fig)
regulation by *flamenco*
gene 3:1529
replication strategy 3:1527
reverse transcription 3:1528–9
structure and
properties 3:1529(Fig)
taxonomy and
classification 3:1526
tissue specificity 3:1529
transcription 3:1527–8,
3:1527(Fig)
leader region 3:1528
regulation 3:1528
translation 3:1528
transmission 3:1529
Drosophila P virus (DPV) 2:1273
Drosophila X virus (DXV) 1:161
Drug abusers
hepatitis A virus infection 1:637
HTLV-2 infection 2:797
Drug design 3:1495
atomic structure data 3:1946
HIV protease inhibitors 3:1946
rhinovirus antiviral drugs 3:1551,
3:1551(Fig), 3:1946
Drugs, antiviral *see* Antiviral
agents
dsRNA-specific adenosine
deaminase (dsRAD) 2:859
Duchenne muscular dystrophy,
gene transfer model 1:13
Duck(s)
Newcastle disease 2:1024
secondary amyloidosis 1:655
see also Poultry
Duck adenovirus 1:20
Duck hepatitis B virus
(DHBV) 1:640, 1:650
antibodies 1:655
c antigen 1:652
e antigen 1:652
future perspectives 1:656
genetics 1:653
genome, map 1:651(Fig)
geographic/seasonal
distribution 1:641, 1:652–3
host range and
propagation 1:641, 1:653
immune response 1:654

Duck hepatitis B virus (DHBV)
(*continued*)
infection
clinical features 1:654–5
hepatocellular carcinoma
and 1:650, 1:654
immune response 1:655
incidence 1:652
pathology/histobiology 1:655
prevention and control 1:655–6
as model of human hepatitis B
virus 1:655, 1:656
pathogenicity 1:654–5
polymerase 1:651
proteins 1:651–2
L and S proteins 1:651
M protein 1:651
receptors 1:653
replication 1:650, 1:652(Fig),
1:656
in Ross goose 1:650
serologic relationship and
variability 1:653–4
surface antigen particles 1:651
tissue tropism 1:654
transmission 1:652–3, 1:654
congenital 1:654
vaccines 1:656
see also Hepadnaviridae
Duck hepatitis virus (DHV) 1:461,
1:467
clinical features of infection 1:467
epidemiology 1:466
geographic/seasonal
distribution 1:464
serotype 1:465
transmission and tissue
tropism 1:107, 1:466
vaccines 1:468
see also Enteroviruses, animal
Duck infectious anemia virus
(DIAV) 3:1496
Duck parvovirus (DPV),
history 2:1168
Dulcamara mottle virus 3:1850,
3:1851
Duncan syndrome 3:1844
Dura mater grafts, CJD
after 3:1392
Dust, fowlpox virus
transmission 1:579
Duvenhage virus 3:1439, 3:1442,
3:1443
host range 3:1443
infection
clinical features 3:1445
immune response 3:1445
prevention and control 3:1445
see also Rabies-like viruses
Dwarfing, phytoreoviruses
causing 2:1266
Dynamin family 2:858
Dysentery, bacteriophage
discovery 2:725

E

E1A *see under* Adenoviruses
E2F transcription factor 1:25, 1:26
E1A inhibition of
breakdown 1:27
overexpression 1:25
E26 avian retrovirus
disease induced by 3:1508
oncogene 3:1508
Ear
CMV infection (human) 1:350
murine CMV infection 1:366

Eastern equine encephalitis (EEE)
animal infection
clinical features 1:506
pathology/
histopathology 1:506
epidemiology 1:504
epizootic and enzootic
vectors 1:504
evolution 1:504
geographic/seasonal
distribution 1:503
history 1:502
host range 1:503
human infections 1:504
clinical features 1:506
fatality rate 1:505
overwintering 1:504
pathogenicity 1:505–6
replication, in CNS 1:505
subtypes 1:502
transmission 1:504, 1:505
vaccine 1:507
see also Equine encephalitis
viruses
Eastern equine encephalitis (EEE)
virus 3:1990–1
diagnosis 3:1991
in whooping crane 1:420(Table)
EAV *see* Equine arteritis virus
(EAV)
EBERs 2:1200
Ebola virus 1:67, 2:939–45, 3:1993
biosafety level 2:940, 2:944
DNA vaccination 2:944
effect on host immune
system 2:944
emerging/re-emerging viral
disease 1:419(Table)
evolution 2:942–3
genome 2:940–1
geographic distribution 2:942
history 2:939
host range and propagation 2:942
inclusion bodies and
budding 2:942
infection
clinical features 2:943, 3:1993
diagnosis 2:944–5
epidemiology 2:943
hyperimmune polyclonal
equine antibody 1:68
immune response 2:944
outbreaks 1:68
passive immunization 2:944
pathogenesis 2:943–4
pathology/
histopathology 2:943–4
prevention and control 2:944
therapy 1:68
mRNA 2:941
pathogenicity 2:943
physical properties 2:940
proteins 2:941
GP protein 2:941, 2:944
L protein 2:941
nucleoprotein 2:941
sGP 2:941, 2:944
VP40 2:941
replication 2:941–2
Reston outbreak 1:89
serologic relationship 2:943
stability 2:940
structure and properties 2:940
subtypes 2:939
sequence differences 2:942
taxonomy and
classification 2:939–40
tissue tropism 2:943
transcription 2:941–2
transmission 1:485(Table), 2:943,
3:1993

Ebola-Reston virus 2:942
discovery 2:939
infection
immune response 2:944
pathology 2:944
outbreak 2:942
Ebola-Sudan virus 2:942
Ebola-Zaire virus 2:940, 2:942
EBV *see* Epstein–Barr virus (EBV)
Ecdysteroid UDP-glucosyl
transferase (EGT) 2:848
Echinochola hoja blanca virus
(EHBV) 3:1756
Echinochola ragged stunt virus
(ERSV) 2:1263
Echovirus type 4, infection 1:416
Echovirus type 6 1:415
enterovirus 69 (EV69)
crossreaction 1:469
Echovirus type 7 1:416
Echovirus type 9 1:414, 2:736
Barty strain 1:415
motor paralysis due to 1:415
RGD motif in capsid
protein 1:415
Echovirus type 11, infection
features 1:415, 1:416
Echovirus type 22 1:411, 1:413
Echovirus type 23 1:411, 1:413
Echovirus type 30 1:413
Echovirus type 34 2:737
Echoviruses 1:411–17
antigenic variation 1:413
attenuated variants 1:414–15
capsid proteins 1:413
sequences 1:412(Fig)
cytopathic effects 1:411, 1:413
distribution 1:414
epidemic strains 1:414
evolution 1:413
experimental infections 1:415
future perspectives 1:417
genetics 1:412–13
genome 1:412
sequence comparisons 1:412–13
untranslated regions
(UTR) 1:412, 1:414
geographic/seasonal
distribution 1:411
history 1:411, 2:736
host range and
propagation 1:411–12
cell lines 1:411
identification 1:414
infections
after bone marrow
transplant 1:416
clinical features 1:415–16,
1:415(Table)
epidemiology 1:413–14
gastrointestinal 1:447
immune response 1:416
neonatal 1:414, 1:415–16, 1:416
outbreaks and
prevalence 1:413–14
pathology and
histopathology 1:416
persistent 1:415, 1:416
prevention and control 1:416–17
surveillance 1:417
pathogenicity 1:414–15
proteins 1:412
receptors 1:411, 1:412(Fig), 1:417
replication site 1:414
resistance 1:417
serologic relationships and
variability 1:413
shedding 1:414
taxonomy and
classification 1:411
tissue culture 1:411

Echoviruses (continued)
  tissue tropism 1:414
  transmission 1:414
  types 1:411
  vaccines 1:417
  variability and rapid evolution 1:413
  viremia 1:414
  virus-encoded protein (VPg) 1:412
Ecological factors
  emergence and re-emergence of diseases 1:422
  zoonotic disease spread and 3:1995–6
Ecological niche
  definition 3:1941
  occupancy 3:1941
Ecology, *Streptococcus thermophilus* phage 2:1254
Economic aspects, plant virus disease *see* Plant virus disease
Economic significance
  bacteriophage in industrial fermentations 2:1244
  cacao swollen shoot virus 2:1318, 2:1321
  Cadang-cadang 2:1321–3
  coronaviruses 1:297
  crop losses in USA 2:1320(Fig)
  Dasheen mosaic virus 2:1323
  entomopoxviruses (EPVs) 1:480–1
  Fiji disease virus 2:1321
  fish rhabdoviruses 3:1542, 3:1543
  fowlpox virus 1:579
  idaeovirus 2:811
  insects 2:842–3
  Iridoviridae 2:868
  pea enation mosaic virus (PEMV) 2:1194
  pecluviruses 2:1197
  plant viruses 2:1300
  potato virus M 2:1321
  potato virus X 2:1321
  potyviruses 3:1369
  rhinoviruses 3:1549
  rubella virus 3:1600
  shrimp viruses 3:1632
  tenuiviruses 3:1758
  tobacco mosaic virus (TMV) 2:1321
  tobacco ringspot virus 2:1323
  tobraviruses 3:1787
  tospoviruses 3:1807
  virus examples and yield losses 2:1322(Table)
  white clover 2:1323
  see also other individual viruses
Economic use, tetraviruses 3:1771–2
*Eco*P15 2:761
*Eco*RII enzyme, requirement for DNA restriction 2:761
Ectocarpus (EsV) viruses 1:44, 1:48, 1:50
  genome 1:46
Ectromelia (mousepox) virus 2:973–80
  classification 2:973
  clinical inapparent infections 2:974
  enzootic mousepox 2:974
  epidemiology 2:973–4
  experimental 2:974
  future perspectives 2:978
  geographic/seasonal distribution 2:973
  history 2:973
  host range and propagation 2:973
  infection *see* Mousepox
  as model system 2:974

Ectromelia (mousepox) virus (continued)
  pathogenesis 2:974
  prevention and control 2:978
  resistance genes 2:755(Table)
  susceptibility of mice strains 2:974
  transmission 2:973
Eczema *see* Dermatitis
Eczema herpeticum 2:680
Edema
  Lassa fever 2:892, 2:893
  pulmonary *see* Pulmonary edema
Edge Hill virus 1:376
Education, STDs, HPV infection prevention 2:1113
Eels virus *see* European eels virus (EV)
Efavirenz 1:60
Egg drop syndrome (EDS) virus 1:14, 1:18
Eggplant latent viroid 3:1930(Table)
Eggplant mosaic virus 3:1850
Eggplant mottled crinkle virus (EMCV) 3:1790(Table)
Eggplant mottled dwarf virus (EMDV) 3:1531
Egypt bee virus (EBV) 2:744(Table), 2:747, 2:1272
eIF-4 *see* Initiation factors
Eimeria stiedae virus (ESV) 1:613
  characteristics/properties 1:616(Table)
El Niño-southern oscillation, zoonotic diseases and 3:1996
Elderly
  astrovirus infections 1:107
  pneumonia 3:1493
Electrocardiography (ECG), Lassa fever 2:893
Electroencephalography (EEG), measles 2:958
Electron density map (EDM) 3:1943
  see also Atomic structure
Electron microscopy 1:402
  negative staining 1:402
  particle counting 3:1413
  thin sectioning 1:400(Fig), 1:402
  virus structure, history 2:720
Elephants, hemorrhagic disease 1:357
Elicitors
  definition 2:1186
  hypersensitive responses (HR) 2:1186
ELISA
  antiviral antibody detection 1:391
  Barmah Forest virus (BFV) 3:1575
  benyviruses detection 1:158
  birnavirus detection 1:166
  Borna disease virus detection 1:172
  bovine immunodeficiency virus (BIV) 1:190
  carlavirus detection 1:242
  Chikungunya (CHIK) fever 1:265
  Ebola and Marburg viruses 2:945
  equine infectious anemia (EIA) 1:521
  fowlpox virus 1:581
  hepatitis E detection 1:675
  HPV virus-like particles 2:1113
  iridoviruses 2:866
  JC and BK viruses 2:880
  morbilliviruses infection 3:1568
  Norwalk-like viruses 2:1040

ELISA (continued)
  pseudorabies virus (PRV) detection 3:1428
  Ross River virus (RRV) 3:1575
  viral antigen detection 1:389
Elm mottle virus (EMoV) 1:38
  genome 1:39
  host range and distribution 1:40
  virus–host relationships 1:42
ELVIS (enzyme-linked inducible system) 1:398
Embedding, for electron microscopy 1:402
Embryonal carcinoma (EC) cells, adenovirus E1A induction of differentiation 1:29
Embryonated eggs
  herpesvirus of turkeys (HVT) culture 2:948
  Marek's disease virus culture 2:948
  virus isolation/identification 1:399
  virus propagation 3:1410
Embryonic fibroblasts, *Tupaia* herpesviruses 3:1834(Fig), 3:1835
Embryonic lung fibroblasts, coxsackievirus infection 1:305
Embryonic rabbit epithelial (EREp) cell line, bovine immunodeficiency virus (BIV) infection 1:188
Embryonic tissue, virus isolation 1:396
Emergent properties 3:1938
Emerging viral diseases 1:418–23
  animals 1:420(Table)
  characterization and assessment 1:418, 1:418–19
  'delayed' 1:422
  ecological change and 3:1995–6
  endangered/threatened species 1:420(Table)
  epidemiological considerations 1:421–2
    common source epidemics 1:421
    propagated epidemics 1:421
  factors contributing 1:418
    behavioral and societal 1:422–3
    ecological and zoonotic 1:421, 1:422
    host determinants 1:418, 1:422–3
    host range 1:420–1
    long incubation periods 1:421
    natural determinants 1:418, 1:421, 1:422
    persistent infections 1:421
    viral determinants 1:418, 1:419–20
  frequency and reasons for acceleration 1:418
  human infections 1:419(Table)
  inevitability but unpredictability 1:418–19
  international organization for prevention 1:423
  new recognition of existing diseases 1:422
  prevention and control 1:423
  professional response network 1:418
  risk assessment 1:418
  social change and 3:1997
  tospoviruses 3:1806
  zoonoses 3:1995–7
Emperor moths
  viruses of 3:1764
  see also Tetraviruses

Enamovirus 2:901, 2:902(Table), 2:1191, 3:1855
  see also Pea enation mosaic virus (PEMV)
Enation
  features 2:1194
  see also Pea enation mosaic virus (PEMV)
Encephalitis 2:1018
  acute during measles (AME) 2:957
  adenoviruses causing 1:6
  arthropod-borne 1:424
  bovine herpesviruses causing 1:181, 1:182
  BHV1 1:182
  Central European 1:429
  coxsackievirus A (CA) infection 1:309
  echoviruses causing 1:415
  equine *see* Equine encephalitis
  herpes simplex virus 2:679–80, 2:681, 2:1018, 3:1829
  Japanese *see* Japanese encephalitis (JE) virus
  La Crosse virus causing 1:209
  mumps virus causing 2:992
  Murray Valley 1:429
  neonatal, echoviral 1:416
  old dog 3:1567
  polioviruses causing 2:1328
  Russian spring summer *see* Russian spring summer encephalitis
  St Louis *see* St Louis encephalitis
  SIV 3:1645
  subacute measles 2:956
  summer 1:424
  tick-borne *see* Tick-borne encephalitis (TBE) virus complex
  in visna-maedi virus infections 3:1962
  see also Encephalomyelitis
Encephalitis viruses 1:424–30
  in Americas 3:1990–1
  antibodies 1:429
  antigen 1:429
  envelope glycoprotein E 1:428, 1:429
  epidemiology 1:428
  evolution 1:427, 1:430
  features 1:425(Table)
  genetic variation 1:427
  genetics 1:427
  genome 1:426
  geographic/seasonal distribution 1:426
  hemorrhagic disease due to 1:424–30
  history 1:424–6, 1:430
  host range and propagation 1:426–7
  infections
    clinical features 1:428–9
    history of outbreaks 1:424–6
    immune response 1:429
    mortality 1:428
    pathology/histopathology 1:429
    prevention and control 1:429
  mosquito-borne 1:433
    see also Wesselsbron (WSL) virus
  pathogenicity 1:428
  properties 1:426
  serologic relationships and variability 1:427–8, 1:430
  taxonomy and classification 1:424, 1:426, 1:430
  tick-borne 1:430–7, 1:433

Encephalitis viruses (continued)
 transmission and tissue
  tropism 1:428
 see also Flaviviruses
Encephalomyelitis 2:1018
 caprine arthritis encephalitis
  virus 1:223, 1:227
 pigs 1:297
 TMEV see Theiler's murine
  encephalomyelitis viruses
  (TMEV)
 see also Encephalitis
Encephalomyocarditis (EMC)
 virus 1:229, 3:1773
 antibodies 1:235
 EMC(D) variant 1:236–7
 genetics and evolution 1:235–6
 genome, sequence 1:236(Table)
 host range and distribution 1:235
 infection, pancreas 2:1079
 internal ribosome entry site
  (IRES) 2:1337
 L proteins 1:233
 polyprotein processing 1:233
 see also Cardioviruses
Encephalomyocarditis (EMC)-like
  viruses 1:230
 receptor 1:231
Encephalopathy
 dengue virus infection 1:380,
  1:381
 spongiform see Spongiform
  encephalopathy
Endemic diseases 1:482
Endemic transmission 1:486
Endocytosis 1:250
 coated pit-mediated 3:1408
 receptor-mediated see Receptor-
  mediated endocytosis
Endogenous proviruses 1:437–41
 ALVE 1:438–9, 1:440
 association with host 1:437
 characteristics 1:438(Table)
 colonization 1:439
 complete 1:437
 distribution 1:437
 evolution 1:437, 1:439–40
 expression and effect on immune
  response 1:440
 intragenomic spread 1:439–40
 nomenclature 1:438
 pathogenicity 1:440
 polymorphisms 1:439
 prevention and control 1:441
 profiling of humans 1:441
 rapid diagnostic tests 1:441
 receptor blocking by 1:440
 standardization of
  nomenclature 1:438
 taxonomy and
  classification 1:437–9
 vertical transmission 1:439
 viral interference 1:439
Endogenous viral elements
  (EAV) 1:438
Endogenous viruses 1:437–41
 see also Endogenous proviruses;
  Retroviruses
Endoplasmic reticulum (ER) 1:251
 functions 1:251–3
 membrane synthesis and virus
  budding 3:1924(Fig), 3:1925
 protein modification 1:251
 protein synthesis 1:251
 rough 1:251
 smooth 1:251
 TAP 2:841
Endosomes 1:250, 3:1472, 3:1922
 acidification 3:1589
 virus sequestration 1:251
Endothelial cells
 virus exit from blood and 2:1179

Endothelial cells (continued)
 virus infection 2:1016
Engineered resistance see Plant
  resistance to viruses
Enhancers 2:1182
 polyomavirus DNA
  replication 2:1359
Enhancin 1:143
enhancin gene 1:141
Enrichment, isolation of phage in
  soil 2:1249
Enteric cytopathogenic human
  orphan (ECHO) viruses see
  Echoviruses
Enteric viruses 1:441–9,
  1:442(Table)
 adenoviruses 1:442(Table),
  1:444–5
 antibodies 1:448
 astroviruses 1:442(Table), 1:445–
  6
 caliciviruses 1:442(Table), 1:445
 coronaviruses 1:442(Table),
  1:446–7
 crossinfection control 1:449
 enterocytes as target cells 2:1176
 enteroviruses 1:447
 entry route 2:1176
 history 1:442
 infection mechanisms 2:1177
 infections
  clinical features 1:448
  immune response 1:448–9
  pathology/
   histopathology 1:448
  prevention and control 1:449
  treatment 1:448
 miscellaneous viruses 1:447
 parvoviruses 1:446
 'Picobirnaviruses' 1:447
 reoviruses 1:447
 rotaviruses see Rotaviruses
 toroviruses 1:447
 see also individual viruses
Enteritis
 hemorrhagic, adenoviruses
  causing 1:445
 see also Diarrhea;
  Gastroenteritis
Entero-hepatic-renal syndrome, in
  trout 1:561
Enterobacteria phage N4 see
  Coliphage N4
Enterobacteria phage P1 see P1
  bacteriophage
Enterocytes, target of enteric
  viruses 2:1176
'Enteroviral' syndrome 2:736
Enterovirus 1:305, 1:411, 1:461,
  1:468, 2:1326, 2:1330
 characteristics 1:412
 classification 1:306(Table)
 see also Coxsackieviruses;
  Echoviruses; Enteroviruses;
  Picornaviruses; Poliovirus
Enterovirus 68 (EV68) 1:468, 2:737
 California strain 1:469
 discovery and features 1:469
 EV70 relationship 1:470
 genome 1:469
 Rhyne strain 1:469
 transmission and cytopathic
  effects 1:469
Enterovirus 69 (EV69) 1:468, 1:469
 transmission and infection 1:469
Enterovirus 70 (EV70) 1:309, 1:468,
  1:469–73, 2:737
 conjunctivitis see Conjunctivitis,
  acute hemorrhagic (AHC)
 cytopathic effects 1:472
 EV68 relationship 1:470
 genetics and evolution 1:471

Enterovirus 70 (EV70) (continued)
 genome properties 1:470
  noncoding regions 1:470
 geographic/seasonal
  distribution 1:470
 growth temperature 1:471
 history 1:469–70
 host range and propagation 1:471
 infections
  clinical features 1:472
  conjunctival 2:1178
  epidemiology 1:471
  immune response 1:472
  pathology/histology 1:472
  prevention and control 1:473
 J670/71 strain 1:470
 pathogenicity 1:471–2
 properties 1:470
 proteins 1:470–1
 receptor 1:471
 replication 1:471
 serologic properties 1:471
 tissue tropism 1:471
 transmission 1:471–2
 VPg protein 1:470
Enterovirus 71 (EV71) 1:469,
  1:473–4
 BrCr/1970 strain 1:473
 genome 1:473
 geographic/seasonal
  distribution 1:473
 history and classification 1:473
 host range and propagation 1:473
 infections
  clinical features 1:473
  epidemiology 1:473, 1:473–4
  immune response 1:474
  meningitis 2:737
  pathology/histology 1:474
  see also Hand–foot–mouth
   disease (HFMD)
 pathogenicity 1:474
 properties 1:473
 serologic relationships and
  variability 1:473
 transmission and tissue
  tropism 1:473–4
Enterovirus 72 (EV72) 1:468
 hepatitis A virus as 2:737
 see also Hepatitis A virus (HAV)
Enteroviruses 1:468–74
 cardiac disease due to 2:1075–6
  dilated cardiomyopathy 2:1076,
   2:1077
 classification
  history 2:734
  modifications 2:737
  problems 2:736–7
 future perspectives 2:737–8
 history 2:730–8, 2:736
 infections 3:1492
  clinical features 1:307
  enteric 1:447
  heart muscle 2:1074
  IgM 2:1078
  laboratory diagnosis 2:1078
  pancreatic 2:1079
 new types 2:736–7
 nomenclature 2:737
 ocular target 1:525(Table)
 properties 1:462
 proteins, processing 1:233
 RNA phage as index organisms
  for 3:1665
 taxonomy and
  classification 1:468–9
 transmission 2:1076
 see also Coxsackieviruses;
  Echoviruses; Poliovirus
Enteroviruses, animal 1:461–8
 assembly and release 1:464
 canyon structures 1:463

Enteroviruses, animal (continued)
 classification 1:461–2
 cytopathic effects 1:464
 epidemiology 1:465–6
 evolution 1:465
 future perspectives 1:468
 genetics 1:465
 genome 1:462
 geographic/seasonal
  distribution 1:464
 history 1:461
 host range and
  propagation 1:464–5
 infections
  clinical features 1:466–7
  immune response 1:467
  pathology/
   histopathology 1:467
  prevention and control 1:467–8
 pathogenicity 1:466
 physical properties 1:463
 post-translational
  processing 1:463–4
 proteins 1:462, 1:462–3
 replication 1:463
 RNA-dependent RNA
  polymerase 1:463
 serologic relationships 1:465
 translation 1:463
 transmission and tissue
  tropism 1:466
 vaccines 1:467–8
 VPg 1:462
 see also Avian encephalomyelitis
  virus (AEV); Bovine
  enteroviruses (BEVs); Porcine
  enteroviruses (PEVs)
Entomobirnavirus 1:161
Entomopoxvirinae 1:475, 3:1865
 genera 1:475
 insect pest control by 2:845
 see also Entomopoxviruses
  (EPVs)
Entomopoxvirus A 1:475
Entomopoxvirus B 1:475
Entomopoxvirus C 1:475
Entomopoxviruses (EPVs) 1:474–
  81
 alkaline protease 1:477
 cell culture 1:479–80
 economic importance 1:480–1
 filament-associated late protein
  (FALPE) 1:477
 fusolin (spindle body
  protein) 1:476–7
 gene expression regulation 1:480
 in gene therapy 1:481
 genome 1:474, 1:477
  gene order 1:477
  homologies between
   EPVs 1:477
  organization 1:478(Fig)
 geographic distribution 1:475
 history 1:475
 host range 1:475
 infections
  characteristics 1:477–9
  pathology 1:477–9
 lateral bodies 1:475
 occlusion bodies 1:475, 1:476
 polypeptides and proteins 1:476–
  7
 recombinant 1:481
 replication 1:479–80
 size 1:475–6
 spheroidin 1:475, 1:476
  gene 1:476, 1:480
 structure and properties 1:475–6,
  1:476(Fig)
 taxonomy and
  classification 1:475
 thymidine kinase 1:480

Entomopoxviruses (EPVs) (*continued*)
  topoisomerase 1:477
  transcription 1:480
  vertebrate poxvirus similarity 1:474–5
  viropexis 1:479
  viroplasm 1:479
  virulence enhancing factor 1:477
Entry of viruses 1:483, 2:1176–8, 3:1922
  CNS pathways 2:1014
  conjunctiva 2:1178
  gastrointestinal tract 2:1176–7
  genitourinary system 2:1177–8
  neural route 2:1014
  respiratory tract 2:1176, 3:1488, 3:1490(Fig)
  routes 1:483
  skin 2:1176
  specific viruses 1:485(Table)
  see also Pathogenesis of viral infections; Penetration of viruses
env gene
  caprine arthritis encephalitis virus (CAEV) 1:223, 1:227
  equine infectious anemia virus (EIAV) 1:516
  HTLV-2 *see* Human T-cell leukemia virus type 2 (HTLV-2)
  human foamy virus (HFV) 3:1689
  insect endogenous retroviruses 3:1530(Table)
  lymphoproliferative disease virus (LPDV) 2:913
  lymphoproliferative disease virus (LPDV) of turkeys 2:913
  murine leukemia viruses (MuLVs) 2:995
  reticuloendotheliosis (RE) viruses 3:1497, 3:1499
  simian foamy virus (SFV) 3:1689
  simian immunodeficiency virus *see* Simian immunodeficiency viruses (SIV)
  visna-maedi viruses 3:1963
Env protein
  expression in retroviral vectors 3:1890
  Eyk fusion protein 3:1512
  Sea protein fusion 3:1514
Envelope
  cell attachment proteins 2:1181
  glycoprotein synthesis 1:252
  interaction with receptors 2:1181, 2:1182
Envelope–cell membrane fusion 2:1181, 2:1182
Enveloped viruses
  uncoating 3:1472
  see also individual viruses
Envelopment, of viruses 3:1478
Environment
  coxsackievirus infection spread risk factor 1:307
  influence on quasispecies 3:1434
Enviroxime 1:66
Enzyme immunoassays (EIA)
  antiviral antibody detection 1:391
  respiratory viruses 3:1494
  viral antigen detection 1:389
Enzyme-linked immunosorbent assay *see* ELISA
Enzyme-linked virus inducible system (ELVIS) 1:398
  advantages 1:398
Eotaxin 1:343
Ependymal cells 2:1014
  virus infection 2:1017

Epidemic(s)
  common source 1:421
  definition 1:482
  potential and role of transmission 1:421
  propagated 1:421
  virgin-soil 1:486
Epidemic curves 1:487
Epidemic gastroenteritis 1:442
Epidemic hemorrhagic fever *see* Hemorrhagic fever with renal syndrome (HFRS)
Epidemic keratoconjunctivitis (EKC) 1:526, 1:528(Fig)
  clinical features 1:5
  geographic/seasonal distribution 1:3
  history 1:1
  prevention and treatment 1:6
  see also Adenovirus; Adenovirus 8 (Ad8)
'Epidemic myalgia' 1:308
Epidemic polyarthritis 3:1570, 3:1572, 3:1575
  see also Ross River virus (RRV)
Epidemic transmission 1:486
Epidemiology 1:482
  history 1:482
  role and uses 1:482
Epidemiology of viral diseases 1:482–7
  assessment of disease occurrence/outcome 1:482
  case-control studies 1:482–3
  cohort studies 1:482–3
  implications for disease prevention 1:487
  mathematical modeling 1:486–7
  molecular epidemiology studies 1:483
  perpetuation of viruses in nature 1:484–6
    influence of arthropod transmission cycle 1:486
    influence of clinical status of host 1:484–5
    influence of host immunity 1:486
    influence on population size 1:486
    influence of virulence of virus 1:485–6
    influence of zoonotic transmission cycle 1:486
  prospective studies 1:483
  sentinel studies 1:483
  seroepidemiologic studies 1:483
  vaccine trials 1:483
  virus transmission 1:483–4
  see also Transmission of viruses
Epidermal cells, animal papillomavirus pathology 2:1128
Epidermal growth factor receptor (EGFR) 3:1819
  v-ErbB as mutant form 3:1819
  v-*erbB* oncogene as truncated version 3:1512
  vaccinia virus binding 3:1926
Epidermodysplasia verruciformis (EV) 2:1107, 3:1846
  clinical features 2:1112
  epidemiology 2:1109
  HPV causing 2:1109, 2:1111(Table)
  HPV5 2:1105
  types 2:1110, 2:1111(Table)
Epithelial cells
  bovine, bovine immunodeficiency virus (BIV) infection 1:188
  HPVs infection 2:1115, 2:1116

Epithelial–mesenchymal transitions, adenovirus E1A12S role 1:30
Epithelioma papulosum cyprini (EPS) 3:1627
Epitope library, construction using filamentous phage 1:552
Epitopes *see* Antigenic determinants
Epizootic hemorrhagic disease
  clinical features 2:1057
  history 2:1043
Epizootic hemorrhagic disease virus (EHDV) 2:1043, 2:1045(Table), 2:1047
  epidemiology 2:1055
  evolution and topotypes 2:1051
  genome 2:1050
  host range and propagation 2:1049
  pathogenicity 2:1056
  proteins, VP5 2:1064
  serotypes 2:1055
  vaccine development 2:1060
  see also Orbiviruses
Epsilon, RNA packaging signal, hepatitis B virus 1:648, 1:648(Fig)
Epsilonvirus 1:511
Epstein–Barr virus (EBV) 1:487–94
  adoptive CTL therapy 1:493, 1:494
  antibodies 1:493
    in primates 2:711
  antigens 1:493, 2:710, 2:712
  early (EA) and antibodies 1:490
  apoptosis inhibition 3:1960
  autoantibody production 1:109
  B cell proliferation 3:1826
  B lymphocytes immortalization 3:1843
  baboon/chimpanzee herpesvirus comparison 2:709, 2:709–10, 2:710
  BARTs 1:497, 1:500
    functions in restricted latency 1:497(Table), 1:500
  BHRF1 expression 1:73
  BZLF1 1:73
  capsid antigen (VCA), antibodies 1:490
  carrier state 1:492, 1:493
  cell lines 3:1843
  cell transformation by 1:492
  classification 2:708
  detection, lymphocyte cultures 1:398
  discovery 3:1843
  diseases associated 1:489–94
    B cell lymphomas 1:490
    diffuse B cell lymphomas 3:1844
    epidemiology 1:489–91
    gastric adenocarcinoma 1:490
    Hodgkin's disease 1:490–1
    T cell lymphomas 1:490
    tumors 1:488, 1:488(Table), 1:493
    see also Burkitt's lymphoma (BL); Epstein–Barr virus (EBV) infection; Infectious mononucleosis; Nasopharyngeal carcinoma (NPC)
  early genes 1:496
  EBERs, EBER-1 and EBER-2 RNAs 1:497, 1:497(Table)
  EBNA 1:489, 1:495, 2:900, 3:1843
    genes encoding 1:497
    promoter (Qp) 1:500
    promoters (Cp and Wp) 1:500
  'EBNA type' of isolates 1:489

Epstein–Barr virus (EBV) (*continued*)
  EBNA-1 1:495, 1:497(Table), 2:1200, 3:1826, 3:1845
  EBNA-2 1:497, 1:498, 3:1845
    B cell proliferation regulation 1:498
    expression with EBNA-LP 1:499
    functions 1:497(Table), 1:498
    gene encoding 1:489
    Notch mimicked by 1:498
    role in cell transformation 1:492
    targeting to promoters by Jκ 1:498
    targeting to promoters by Spi-1 and Spi-B 1:498
  EBNA-3 1:497, 1:497(Table), 1:498–9
    genes 1:498
    Jκ interaction 1:498
  EBNA-3A 1:497(Table), 1:498
  EBNA-3B 1:497(Table), 1:499
  EBNA-3C 1:497(Table), 1:498–9
  EBNA-5 1:73
  EBNA-LP (leader protein) 1:497, 1:497(Table), 1:499
  EBV-1 1:489, 1:494
    EBV-2 relationship 1:489
  EBV-2 1:489, 1:494
    EBV-1 relationship 1:489
  envelope 1:494
  evolution 1:489, 3:1874
  future perspectives 1:494, 2:713
  genetics 1:489
  genome 1:488, 1:494–5
    episome formation 1:495
    in Hodgkin's disease 3:1844
    microheterogeneity over repeat regions 1:489
    organization 1:495(Fig)
    terminal repeats 1:495
    variations in isolates 1:489
  geographic/seasonal distribution 1:488
  glycoproteins 1:494
  gp42 1:496
  het DNA 1:374
  history 1:487–8
  host range and propagation 1:488–9, 2:709
  immediate early genes 1:496
  infection *see* Epstein–Barr virus (EBV) infection
  late genes 1:496
  latency 1:495, 1:496–501
    EBNA-2 expression 1:498
    EBNA-3 expression 1:498–9
    EBNA-LP expression 1:499
    gene expression 1:492, 1:497
    genes downregulation 1:492
    genome organization 1:495(Fig)
    growth program (type III) 1:497–9, 1:501
    in vitro models 1:496
    initiation 1:496
    LMP-1 expression 1:499
    long-term 1:500, 1:501
    models 1:497
    periodic reactivation of growth program 1:500
    regulation and function 1:500–1
    restricted program *see* Epstein–Barr virus (EBV), restricted latency
    type II *see* Epstein–Barr virus (EBV), restricted latency
  latency-associated genes 1:494, 1:497, 1:500
    expression 1:497, 1:497–9

Epstein–Barr virus (EBV) (continued)
  latency-associated genes (continued)
    functions 1:497(Table)
    repression 1:500
    see also Epstein–Barr virus (EBV), EBNA-1, EBNA-2, EBNA-3, EBNA-LP, LMP-1
  latent infections 2:900, 2:1200
  latent membrane proteins (LMP) 3:1843
    see also Epstein–Barr virus (EBV), LMP-1
  LMP1 gene 1:489
  LMP-1 1:73, 1:497, 1:497(Table), 1:499
    activation by EBNA-3C 1:498
    downregulation in restricted latency 1:500
    expression and functions 1:497(Table), 1:499
    interaction with TNFR 1:499
    role in cell transformation 1:492
    transformation effector sites (TES) 1:499
  LMP-2A, functions in restricted latency 1:497(Table), 1:500
  LMP-2B 1:497(Table), 1:500
  lymphoproliferative herpesviruses relationship 2:707
  lymphoproliferative syndrome 3:1844
  lytic cycle
    activation 1:496
    apoptosis 1:73
    BARF1 gene 1:496
    BHRF1 gene 1:496
    BZLF2 gene 1:496
    gene functions 1:496
    vIL-10 1:496
    Zta and Rta proteins 1:496
  maintenance 1:495, 1:496
  membrane antigen (MA) 1:491
    in vaccine 1:493
  molecular biology 1:494–501
  multidrug resistance, mechanism 1:73
  nuclear antigen see EBNA (above)
  P3HR-1 virus 1:489
  pathogenicity 1:492, 3:1826
  persistence, sites 1:491
  persistent infection 2:1200
  properties 1:494
  proteins 2:900
  reactivation 1:491(Fig), 2:900
  receptors 1:491, 1:494
  recombinants 1:494
  recombination 3:1449
  replication 1:491, 1:495, 1:495–6
    origins 1:495, 1:496
  restricted latency 1:497, 1:499–501
    in Akata cells 1:500–1
    methylation 1:500
    regulation and function 1:500–1
  Rta protein 1:496
  seroconversion during infancy 3:1843
  serologic relationship and variability 1:489, 2:710
  shedding 1:491
  spread in bloodstream 2:1178
  taxonomy and classification 1:488
  tegument 1:494
  terminal consensus sequence 3:1835

Epstein–Barr virus (EBV) (continued)
  tissue tropism 1:491, 2:711
  transformation by 3:1822
  transmission 1:491
    oropharyngeal 1:491
  tumor pathogenesis 2:900, 3:1843–4
  tumor production 2:707
  vaccine development 1:493, 1:494
  variants 3:1449
  as vector 3:1889
  ZEBRA protein 2:900
  Zta protein 1:496
Epstein–Barr virus (EBV) infection 2:1200
  acute 1:492
  chronic 2:1200
  chronic active 1:492
  clinical features 1:492, 2:712
  eye 1:526–8, 1:527(Table)
  immune response 1:493, 2:712–13
  model 1:491(Fig)
  pancreas 2:1078–9
  pathology/histopathology 1:492–3, 2:712
  pharyngitis 3:1492
  post-transplant 3:1825
    clinical course 3:1826
    clinical features 3:1826
    diagnosis 3:1826
    incidence 3:1826
    pathogenesis 3:1826
    treatment 3:1826–8
  prevention and control 1:493–4
  primary 1:488, 1:489, 1:491(Fig), 3:1843
  see also Epstein–Barr virus (EBV), diseases associated
Equilibrium sedimentation, bacteriophage purification 3:1417
Equine abortion virus see Equine herpesvirus 1 (EHV-1)
Equine animals see Horses
Equine arteritis virus (EAV) 1:89
  antibodies 1:96
  evolution 1:93
  genome 1:90(Fig), 1:91, 1:93
  geographic/seasonal distribution 1:92
  host range and propagation 1:93
  immune response 1:96
  infection
    pathogenicity and clinical features 1:95
    pathology and histopathology 1:96
  macrophage infection 1:92
  proteins 1:92(Fig)
  taxonomy and classification 1:90
  tissue tropism 1:94
  transmission 1:94
  vaccine 1:94, 1:96
  virulence mutants 1:93
  virulent and avirulent strains 1:94
Equine coital exanthema virus (ECE) 1:508
  see also Equine herpesvirus 3 (EHV-3)
Equine encephalitis
  clinical features 1:506
  epidemiology 1:504
  immune response 1:507
  pathology/histopathology 1:506–7
  prevention and control 1:507
  vaccines 1:507
Equine encephalitis viruses 1:501–7
  attachment and entry 1:503
  cDNA clones 1:507
  epidemiology 1:504–5

Equine encephalitis viruses (continued)
  evolution 1:504
  experimental infection 1:504, 1:506
  future perspectives 1:507
  genetics 1:504
  genome 1:502
  geographic/seasonal distribution 1:503
  glycoproteins 1:502
  history 1:501–2
  host range and propagation 1:503–4
    epidemic periods 1:503
  infections see Equine encephalitis
  pathogenicity 1:505–6
  physical properties 1:503
  properties 1:502
  proteins 1:502–3
    capsid 1:502
  replication 1:503
  subtypes 1:502
  taxonomy and classification 1:502
  tissue tropism 1:505
  translation and transcription 1:503
  transmission 1:503, 1:505
  see also Eastern equine encephalitis (EEE); Venezuelan equine encephalitis (VEE); Western equine encephalitis (WEE)
Equine encephalosis virus (EEV) 2:1045(Table), 2:1047
Equine herpesvirus 1 (EHV-1) 1:508
  abortion storm 1:509
  abortions 1:508, 1:512, 1:513
  defective interfering particles 1:511–12
  genome 1:512
  envelope 1:511
  genetics 1:509
  genome 1:509(Table), 1:510
  geographic/seasonal distribution 1:509
  history 1:508
  infection
    clinical features 1:513
    epidemiology 1:512
    immune response 1:514
    pathology/histopathology 1:513
    prevention and control 1:514
  Kentucky A strain 1:510
  replication 1:510–11
  latency 1:511–12, 1:514
  pathogenicity 1:512–13
  persistent infections 1:512
  strain Ab4 1:510
  taxonomy and classification 1:508–9
  transmission and tissue tropism 1:512
Equine herpesvirus 2 (EHV-2) 1:357
  as factor in EHV-1 and EHV-4 infections 1:508
  genetics 1:509
  genome 1:509(Table), 1:510
  geographic/seasonal distribution 1:509
  history 1:508
  infection 1:508
    clinical features 1:513
    epidemiology 1:512
    immune response 1:514
    pathology/histopathology 1:514

Equine herpesvirus 2 (EHV-2) (continued)
  pathogenicity 1:513
  taxonomy and classification 1:508–9
Equine herpesvirus 3 (EHV-3)
  genetics 1:509
  genome 1:509(Table)
  geographic/seasonal distribution 1:509
  history 1:508
  infection
    clinical features 1:513
    epidemiology 1:512
    immune response 1:514
    pathology/histopathology 1:514
  pathogenicity 1:513
  taxonomy and classification 1:508–9
Equine herpesvirus 4 (EHV-4) 1:508
  genetics 1:509
  genome 1:509(Table), 1:510
  geographic/seasonal distribution 1:509
  history 1:508
  infection
    clinical features 1:513
    epidemiology 1:512
    immune response 1:514
    pathology/histopathology 1:513
    prevention and control 1:514
  pathogenicity 1:512–13
  taxonomy and classification 1:508–9
  transmission and tissue tropism 1:512
Equine herpesvirus 5 (EHV-5) 1:357
  genetics 1:509
  genome 1:509(Table)
  geographic/seasonal distribution 1:509
  history 1:508
  infection
    clinical features 1:513
    epidemiology 1:512
    immune response 1:514
    pathology/histopathology 1:514
  pathogenicity 1:513
  taxonomy and classification 1:508–9
Equine herpesviruses 1:508–15
  assembly and release 1:511
  capsids 1:511
  defective interfering particles 1:511–12
  envelope 1:511
  epidemiology 1:512
  evolution 1:512
  future perspectives 1:514
  genetics 1:509–10
  genome structure 1:509, 1:509(Table), 1:510
    inverted repeat (IR) sequences 1:510
    ORFs 1:510
    unique long (UL) region 1:510
  geographic/seasonal distribution 1:509
  history 1:508
  host range and propagation 1:509
  infection
    clinical features 1:513
    immune response 1:514
    pathology/histopathology 1:513–14
    prevention and control 1:514
    therapy 1:514

Equine herpesviruses (continued)
  latency associated transcripts
      (LATs) 1:512
  oncogenic transformation 1:511
  pathogenicity 1:512–13
  persistent infection 1:511–12
  proteins 1:510–11
  replication 1:510–11
  serologic relationship and
      variability 1:512
  serotypes 1:512
  taxonomy and
      classification 1:508–9
  tegument 1:511
  tissue culture 1:509
  transactivation domain 1:510
  transcription 1:510–11
  transmission and tissue
      tropism 1:512
  vaccines 1:514
Equine infectious anemia (EIA)
  acute 1:520
  chronic 1:519(Fig), 1:520
  clinical features 1:519–20,
      1:519(Fig)
    classical signs 1:520
  diagnostic assays 1:521
  epidemiology 1:519
  history 1:515
  immune response 1:520–1, 1:522
  pathology/histopathology 1:520
  prevention and control 1:521
  transmission and tissue
      tropism 1:519
Equine infectious anemia virus
    (EIAV) 1:515–22
  antibodies 1:520, 1:520–1
  antigenic variability 1:518
  antigenic variants 1:518
  assembly and release 1:517
  attachment and entry 1:517
  bovine immunodeficiency virus
      (BIV) cross-reaction 1:188
  capsid 1:517
  carriers 1:520
  classification 1:515
  cytopathicity 1:517
  envelope 1:516
  evolution 1:518
  field strains 1:518
  future perspectives 1:521–2
  genes 1:516
    env 1:516
    gag and pol 1:516
    tat and rev 1:516
  genetics 1:518
  genome organization 1:516(Fig)
  genome properties 1:516
  geographic/seasonal
      distribution 1:517–18
  history 1:515
  host range and propagation 1:518
  infection see Equine infectious
      anemia (EIA)
  integrase 1:517
  model of antigenic
      variation 1:515
  pathogenicity 1:519
  proteins 1:516–17
    Env 1:516, 1:517
    gag-encoded 1:517
    pol-encoded 1:517
    structural 1:516–17
    SU (gp90) 1:516, 1:517
    synthesis 1:517
    transmembrane (TM;
        gp45) 1:516, 1:517
  proviral DNA 1:517
  transcription 1:517
  receptor 1:517
  replication 1:517, 1:518
    in acute disease 1:520

Equine infectious anemia virus
    (EIAV) (continued)
  replication (continued)
    error rate 1:518
    site 1:518
    reverse transcriptase 1:517, 1:518
  serologic relationship and
      variability 1:518–19
  structure and properties 1:515–
      16, 1:516(Fig)
    oblong core 1:515
  tricistronic messenger RNA 1:517
  vaccine development 1:515, 1:521
Equine morbillivirus,
    infection 3:1494
Equine rhinopneumonitis virus see
    Equine Herpesvirus 4 (EHV-4)
Equine rhinoviruses 3:1545
Equine torovirus (ETV)
  assembly and budding 3:1800–1
  defective interfering (DI) 3:1801
  genome 3:1799, 3:1801–2
    ORFs 3:1800, 3:1801
  history/discovery 3:1798
  host range and
      propagation 3:1801
  infection, clinical features 3:1802
  mRNAs 3:1800
  physical properties 3:1800
  post-translational
      processing 3:1800
  proteins 3:1799
    M (membrane) protein 3:1799
    nucleocapsid and N
        protein 3:1799
    S (spike) protein 3:1799
  relationship to human
      toroviruses 3:1801
  replication 3:1800
  serologic relationships and
      variability 3:1802
  structure and properties 3:1798–9
  transcription 3:1800
  translation 3:1800
  see also Toroviruses
erb genes 3:1508
ErbA 3:1507–8
erbB oncogene 3:1512
Errantivirus 3:1526
  see also Drosophila melanogaster
      gypsy virus
Error threshold relationship 3:1431
Erysimum latent virus 3:1850,
    3:1851
Erythema infectiosum 2:1153,
    2:1154
Erythema multiforme
  HSV-1 causing 2:681
  parapoxviruses causing 2:1145
Erythroblastosis, chicken 3:1508
Erythrocytes
  agglutination
    cardioviruses 2:231
    enterovirus 70 (EV70) 1:471
  viral erythrocytic necrosis in
      fish 1:567
Erythrocytic necrosis virus see
    Viral erythrocytic necrosis
    virus (VENV)
Erythrovirus 2:1152
  members 2:1152
Erythroviruses 2:1154
Escherichia coli
  analogy with phage
      recombination
      proteins 3:1449(Table)
  attB site 2:926, 2:932, 2:1236
  β-galactosidase, enzyme-linked
      inducible system
      (ELVIS) 1:398
  bacteriophage φ29 genes
    cloned 1:122

Escherichia coli (continued)
  coliphage lambda infection 1:281
  conjugative plasmids 1:547
  DNA gyrase 1:451
  dnaF, lig and gyrB 1:453
  enterhemorrhagic (EHEC)
    hemorrhagic colitis 2:1230
    prototype converting
        phage 2:1230
  GroEL, luteovirus and PEMV
      binding 3:1905
  hfl gene mutations 2:928
  him/hip 2:928
    mutants 2:928
  Hsd system 2:761, 2:762(Table)
  insulin production 2:1247–8
  integrative host factor
      (IHF) 2:928
  McrA and McrBC systems 2:761
  methylation-dependent
      restriction 2:761
  Mrr system 2:761
  mutations
    affecting coliphage lambda
        lysogeny 2:928
    lambda integration/excision
        blocked 2:928–9
  nfrA, nfrB genes 1:454
  nfrC gene 1:454
  P4 bacteriophage infection see P4
      bacteriophage
  reporter genes 1:398
  restriction of nonglucosylated
      HMC-containing DNA 2:761
  Rgl system 2:761, 2:762(Table)
  RNA phage see RNA
      bacteriophage, single-
      stranded
  RNase P reaction 3:1553
  rnc (RNase III) 2:928
  Shiga toxins see Shiga-like
      toxins
  ssDNA binding protein (Eco
      SSB) 1:451
Escherichia coli B
  coliphage 1:1722
  coliphage N4 resistant 1:454
  T1-like phages 3:1701
  T7 phage infection 3:1722
Escherichia coli K-12 1:281
  coliphage N4 1:450
    see also Coliphage N4
  lambda isolation 1:281
  lambda phage 2:1209
Ets family of transcription
    factors 1:498
ets oncogene 3:1508
Eubenangee virus
    (EUBV) 2:1045(Table), 2:1047
Eucaryotic transposable
    elements 3:1503
Eukaryotic viruses, nonclassical
    restriction/modification 2:762–
    3
Europe
  rubella vaccination
      program 3:1600
  zoonotic viruses 3:1992–3
European bat lyssavirus
    (EBL) 3:1442, 3:1443, 3:1988
  geographic distribution 3:1443
  host range 3:1443
European brown hare
    syndrome 1:217, 1:218
European eels virus (EV) 1:161
  genome and proteins 1:161
European honeybee, viruses 2:1272
European seal morbillivirus 3:1560
  geographic distribution 3:1560
Euryarchaeota 1:76
  phage 1:88
  viruses 1:77–83

Euryarchaeota (continued)
  viruses (continued)
    see also Halophage
Euxoa scandens, cytoplasmic
    polyhedrosis virus 1:334(Fig),
    1:335
Evolution of viruses
  Archaea phage and viruses 1:88–
      9
  atomic structure data 3:1945
  bacteriophage 2:1209
  cassette 3:1374
  DI particles as mutational
      drivers 1:373
  head and tail viruses 1:88–9
  RNA viruses 3:1435
  significance of nonviral
      retroelements 2:1317
  transduction as element 2:1239–
      40
  see also individual viruses
Evolutionary species 3:1940
Evolutionary variants,
    definition 1:3
Exanthem subitum 2:701, 2:702
Exanthems
  Chikungunya (CHIK) fever 1:264
  echoviruses causing 1:415
Excisionase
  coliphage lambda 1:283
  in SSV1 virus 1:86
Exocytosis, viruses 1:253
Exogenous viruses 1:438
Exons 1:255
Experimental autoimmune
    encephalomyelitis (EAE) 1:111
Expression vectors 2:1242
  see also Cloning vectors
Extracellular matrix 1:249
Extrahepatic biliary atresia
    (EHBA), reovirus
    infection 3:1461
Eyach virus (EYAV) 2:1046(Table),
    2:1047–8, 3:1991
  history 2:1044
Eye
  anatomy 1:522, 1:522(Fig)
  dry, in AIDS 1:526
Eye infections 1:522–30
  acute 1:523
  adenovirus 1:4, 1:5, 1:526,
      1:528(Fig)
  in AIDS/HIV infection 1:528–9,
      1:529
  coxsackievirus 1:309
  DNA viruses 1:526–8,
      1:527(Table)
  targets 1:527(Table)
  enterovirus 70 (EV70) 1:471
  see also Conjunctivitis
  Epstein–Barr virus 1:526–8
  herpes simplex viruses
      (HSV) 1:523, 2:678
  HSV-1 2:681
  herpes viruses 1:526
  human cytomegalovirus
      (HCMV) 1:528
  human papillomaviruses 1:523–4,
      1:523(Fig), 1:528
  immunology 1:524
  infection route 1:522–3
  molluscum contagiosum
      virus 1:528
  murine CMV 1:367
  pathogenic mechanisms 1:523–4
  RNA viruses 1:524–6
    targets 1:525(Table)
  smallpox virus 1:528
  varicella zoster virus 1:526
eyk oncogene 3:1512
Eyk protein 3:1512

F

F9 teratocarcinoma, adenovirus
  E1A induction of
  differentiation 1:29
F-dda (2′-á-á-fluoro-2′3′-
  dideoxyadenosine) 2:779
Fabavirus 1:531, 2:1007
  species 1:531
Fabaviruses 1:531–4
  assisted transmission 1:534
  bioassay hosts 1:533
  comoviruses relationship 1:290
  cytopathology 1:532, 1:533(Fig)
  genome structure 1:532
  history 1:531
  host range 1:532–3
    experimental 1:533
  nepoviruses differences 2:1010
  serology 1:533–4
  structure and composition 1:531–2
  symptomatology 1:532–3
  taxonomy and
    classification 1:531
  transmission 1:534
  virus-like particles (VLPs) 1:532
  viruses included 1:531
  X bodies 1:532
Famciclovir (Famvir)
  in hepatitis B 1:66
  herpesvirus infections 1:62
  in varicella-zoster virus
    infection 3:1877
Families, virus *see* Taxonomy of
  viruses
FAP1 (FAS-associated phosphatase-1) 1:71
FAS (APO-1; CD95) 1:70, 1:70–1
  activation 1:71
  apoptosis activation
    mechanism 1:69(Fig)
  apoptosis of CD4+ T cells 1:75
FAS associated death domain
  protein 1:71
FAS ligand (FASL) 1:70
  upregulation 2:1201
Fas/FasL pathway 2:1201
Fatal familial insomnia
  (FFI) 3:1388
  prion protein
    conformation 3:1393
  PrP^{Sc}
    neuronal targeting 3:1395–6
    protease-resistant
      fragment 3:1393
Fatal sporadic insomnia
  (FSI) 3:1388, 3:1393
FBJ murine sarcoma virus (FBJ-MSV) 2:995, 3:1508–9
FBR murine sarcoma virus (FBR-MSV) 3:1508–9
Fc receptors, HSV glycoprotein
  function 2:694
Febrile seizures, HHV-6 infection
  associated 2:701
Fecal–oral transmission 1:484
  caliciviruses 2:1039
  coxsackieviruses 1:307
  echoviruses 1:414
  hepatitis A virus (HAV) 1:637
  human astrovirus (HAstV) 1:107
  polioviruses 1:1327
  reoviruses 3:1459
  rotaviruses 3:1580
  Theiler's murine
    encephalomyelitis viruses
    (TMEV) 3:1776
Feces
  noncultivable viruses 1:442

Feces (*continued*)
  nonenteric adenoviruses in 1:445
  viruses excreted in 1:441, 1:442
Feldmannia (FsV) viruses 1:45,
  1:48, 1:50
  genome 1:46
Feline autoimmune deficiency
  syndrome (FAIDS) 1:544
Feline calicivirus (FCV) 1:217,
  1:218
  antigenic variation 1:219, 1:220
  genome 1:218
    comparison with
      picornaviruses 2:1037(Fig)
  geographic distribution 1:219
  infection
    clinical features 1:220
    pathogenesis 1:219
    prevention and control 1:220
  transmission 1:219
Feline endogenous virus
  (RD114) 3:1496
Feline enteric coronavirus
  (FECV) 1:294, 1:295
  infection 1:297
Feline foamy virus (FeFV)
  genome 3:1687, 3:1687(Fig)
  isolates 3:1690
  pathogenicity 3:1692
  see also Spumaviruses
Feline immunodeficiency virus
  (FIV) 1:420(Table), 1:535–41
  antibodies 1:537, 1:539
    cross-reactivity 1:537
  AZT-resistant mutants 1:540
  diagnostic kit for 1:537
  DNA integration 1:538
  dual infection with feline
    leukemia viruses
    (FeLVs) 1:543
  enzymes 1:536
  FIV-Ple 1:535, 1:536
  future perspectives 1:540–1
  genetics and evolution 1:536–7
  genome organization 1:536(Fig)
  genome structure 1:536
    ORFs 1:536
  geographic distribution 1:535
  history 1:535
  host range and propagation 1:536
  infection
    B cell lymphomas due to 1:538
    clinical features 1:538
    epidemiology 1:537
    experimental 1:538
    immune response 1:539, 1:539–40
    pathology/
      histopathology 1:538–9
    prevention and control 1:540
    treatment 1:540
    as model for AIDS 1:540
  proteins 1:536, 1:536(Fig)
    MA protein 1:536
  receptors 1:537
  related viruses 1:536
  structure and properties 1:535–6
  subtypes (clades) 1:535, 1:536
  taxonomy and
    classification 1:535
  tissue tropism 1:537, 1:538
  transmission 1:536, 1:537
  vaccines 1:540
    trials 1:540
Feline infectious peritonitis
  (FIP) 1:296, 1:297
Feline infectious peritonitis virus
  (FIPV) 1:294, 1:295
  in cheetah 1:420(Table)
Feline leukemia viruses
  (FeLVs) 1:541–6

Feline leukemia viruses (FeLVs)
  (*continued*)
  antitumor antibodies
    (FOCMA) 1:545
  assembly 1:542
  DI particles 1:374
  dual infection with FIV 1:543
  envelope 1:542
    antibodies 1:545
    gene variation 1:544
  epidemiology 1:543
  evolution 1:544–5
  FeLV-A 1:543, 1:543(Table), 1:544
    transmission 1:545
  FeLV-B 1:543, 1:543(Table), 1:544
    transmission 1:545
  FeLV-C 1:543, 1:544
  future perspectives 1:546
  gag and *pol* genes 1:542
  genome organization 1:542(Fig)
  genome structure 1:541–2
  geographic distribution 1:543
  history 1:541
  host range and
    propagation 1:543–4
  infection
    categories 1:543
    clinical features 1:544
    immune response 1:545
    pathology 1:544
    prevention and control 1:546
    thymic tumors due to 1:545
  long terminal repeats 1:542, 1:545
  lymphosarcomas 1:544
  in multicat households 1:543, 1:546
  oncogenesis 1:544, 1:544–5
    insertional mutagenesis 1:545, 1:545(Table)
    transduction mechanism 1:544–5, 1:545(Table)
  pathogenicity 1:544
  properties 1:543(Table)
  proteins 1:542
  replication 1:542–3
  resistance (age-related) 1:545
  shedding 1:543, 1:546
  structure 1:541–2
  subgroups 1:543, 1:543(Table)
    oncogenesis relationship 1:544
  superinfection prevention 1:543
  taxonomy and
    classification 1:541
  transmission 1:541, 1:545–6
  vaccines and vaccine
    strategies 1:546, 1:546(Table)
  viremia 1:543
Feline panleukopenia virus
  (FPV) 1:1152, 1:1159
  canine parvovirus 2 evolution
    and 1:420
  epidemiology 2:1164–5
  evolution 2:1153
  genetics 2:1161
  genome 2:1161, 2:1163(Fig)
  geographic/seasonal
    distribution 2:1160
  host range 2:1160
  infections
    clinical features 2:1154, 2:1165
    immune responses 2:1166
    pathology/
      histopathology 2:1166
    prevention and control 2:1167
  infectious plasmid clones 2:1161–3
  pathogenicity 2:1165
  phylogeny 2:1164(Fig)
  propagation 2:1161

Feline panleukopenia virus (FPV)
  (*continued*)
  structure and properties 2:1155, 2:1162(Fig)
  taxonomy and
    classification 2:1160
  transmission 2:1164–5
  vaccines 2:1167
  see also Parvoviruses
Feline parvovirus (FPV) *see* Feline
  panleukopenia virus (FPV)
Feline sarcoma viruses
  (FeSVs) 1:541–6
  history 1:541
  see also Feline leukemia viruses
    (FeLVs)
Feline spongiform encephalopathy
  (FSE) 3:1388
Fermentations, industrial 2:1244, 2:1245–6
  continuous 2:1246
  phage impact *see* Bacteriophage
    in industrial fermentations
  prophage curing of starter
    cultures 2:1247
Fermon virus 1:469, 2:737
  see also Enterovirus 68 (EV68)
fes/fps oncogene 3:1512–13
Festuca leaf streak virus
  (FLSV) 3:1531
  transmission and infection 3:1539
Fetal bovine serum, contamination,
  with bovine viral diarrhea virus
  (BVDV) 1:176
Fetus
  border disease virus (BDV)
    infection 1:179
  bovine viral diarrhea virus
    (BVDV) infection 1:179
  damage by rubella virus
    infection 3:1597, 3:1598
  see also Congenital rubella
    syndrome (CRS)
Feulgen reaction 1:400
Fever blisters (herpes labialis) *see*
  Herpes labialis
fgr oncogene 3:1513
fhuA, receptor for T5-like
  phage 3:1718
Fialuridine (FIAU), in hepatitis
  B 1:66
Fibroblasts
  avian leukosis virus 1:113
  human CMV culture 1:359, 1:360(Fig)
  human CMV growth 1:346
  human diploid (HDF) 1:397
  immortalization, v-Myc
    protein 3:1510
  lifespan, Tax protein from BLV
    affecting 1:196
  transformation by Fos 3:1509
Fibromas, leporipoxviruses and
  suipoxvirus causing 3:1386, 3:1387
Fibromatosis, squirrels 3:1383
Fibropapillomas 2:1128
  cattle 2:1122
Fibrosarcomas
  gibbon ape leukemia virus
    (GaLV) causing 1:618
  Src causing 3:1514
  v-Fms causing 3:1513
Fifth disease 2:1153, 2:1154
Figwort mosaic virus
  (FMV) 2:1276
  cell-to-cell transport 2:1291
Figwort virus (FWV) 2:1289
Fiji disease virus (FDV) 2:1263
  economic significance 2:1321
Fijivirus 2:1262
  characteristics 2:1263

Fijuvirus (continued)
  conserved sequences 2:1263
  genome, sequence 2:1263–4
  members 2:1263
Filamentous phage 1:547–52, 3:1414
  assembly 1:551–2, 3:1415
    elongation 1:551
    initiation 1:551
    termination 1:551–2
  capsid proteins 1:548
    interaction with bacterial proteins 1:550
  classification 1:547
  as cloning vectors 1:552
  coat protein 3:1416
  conjugative plasmids 1:547
  CTX genetic element from 2:1233
  DNA replication 1:551
  epitope library construction using 1:552
  gene expression 1:548–50
  genome 1:547, 1:548–50
    hairpin loop 1:548, 1:552
    intergenic region 1:550, 1:552
  genome organization 1:549(Fig)
  infection and life cycle 1:550–2
    binding to F conjugative pilus 1:550
    dsDNA formation 1:550–1
    infection initiation 1:550
  nonlytic multiplication 3:1415–16
  in phage display 1:552
  phage included 1:547
  plaque morphology 3:1416
  polyphage 1:552
  promoters 1:549
  proteins 1:548–9
    gene I 1:549
    gene II 1:548–9, 1:551
    gene III 1:547, 1:548
    gene VI 1:547
    gene VII 1:547
    gene IX 1:547
    gene XI 1:549
    for membrane-associated assembly 1:549
    in phage packaging 1:551
    synthesis 1:550, 1:551
  release 3:1415
  replicative forms 1:550, 1:551
  ssDNA binding protein 3:1416
  structural classes 1:547
  structure 1:547, 1:547–8, 1:548(Fig)
  transcription 1:549–50
  translation 1:550
  uses 1:552
Filamentous virus (FV) 2:744(Table), 2:748
Filamentous viruses *see* Helical viruses
Filoviridae, Filovirus 2:939
Filovirus 2:939
Filoviruses
  biohazard classification 2:940, 2:944
  epidemiology 2:943
  evolution 2:942–3
  genetics 2:941
  genome 2:940–1
    complexity 2:942
  geographic distribution 2:942
  host range and propagation 2:942
  mRNA 2:941
  physical properties 2:940
  proteins 2:941
  replication 2:941–2
  serologic relationship 2:943
  structure and properties 2:940

Filoviruses *(continued)*
  taxonomy and classification 2:939–40
  tissue tropism 2:943
  transcription 2:941–2
  transmission 2:943
  see also Ebola virus; Marburg virus
Finkel–Biskis–Jinkins (FBJ-MSV) murine osteogenic sarcoma virus *see* FBJ murine sarcoma virus (FBJ-MSV)
Finkel–Biskis–Reilly (FBR-MSV) murine osteogenic sarcoma virus 3:1508–9
FIS (factor for inversion stimulation) 1:460
Fish
  aquaculture 1:558
  beta nodaviruses 2:1026
  cell hypertrophy 1:566
  cell lines 1:554
  eggs, certification as pathogen-free 1:558
  infectious pancreatic necrosis 1:161
    clinical signs and pathology 1:162
    see also Infectious pancreatic necrosis virus of fish (IPNV)
  lymphocystis *see* Lymphocystis disease (LD)
Fish herpesviruses 1:553–7
  evolution 1:555
  genetics 1:555
  geographic/seasonal distribution 1:554
  history 1:553–4
  host range and propagation 1:554–5
  infection
    clinical features 1:557
    immune response 1:557
    pathology 1:557
    prevention and control 1:557
  pathogenesis 1:555–7
  taxonomy and classification 1:553–4
  types and new viruses 1:553
  see also Channel catfish virus (CCV)
Fish rhabdoviruses 3:1541–4
  economic significance 3:1543
  see also Infectious hematopoietic necrosis virus (IHNV); Spring viremia of carp virus (SVCV); Viral hemorrhagic septicemia virus (VHSV)
Fish virology, history 1:558
Fish viruses 1:558
  classification 1:560(Table)
  control strategies 1:558
  DNA viruses 1:559(Table), 1:566–8
    Adenoviridae 1:567–8
    Iridoviridae 1:566–7
  genomes 1:558
  infection outbreaks 1:558
  RNA viruses 1:558, 1:558–65, 1:559(Table)
    Birnaviridae 1:563
    Orthomyxoviridae 1:564–5
    Reoviridae 1:564
    Retroviridae 1:565
    Rhabdoviridae 1:558
  skin lesions associated 1:565
  transmission models 1:558
  types 1:560(Table)
  vaccines 1:558
  see also individual viruses; Infectious pancreatic necrosis virus of fish (IPNV)

Fitness of virus 3:1435–6
  concept 3:1435
  definition 3:1433(Table)
Fixation, for electron microscopy 1:402
flamenco gene, *Drosophila melanogaster* 3:1526, 3:1528, 3:1529
Flaviviridae 1:426, 3:1980
  border disease virus 1:173–80
  bovine viral diarrhea virus 1:173–80
  encephalitis viruses 1:424–30
  Flavivirus 1:376, 2:871
  Hepacivirus 1:657
  hog cholera virus 2:738–43
  Japanese encephalitis (JE) virus 2:871
  Pestivirus 1:657, 2:738
  Pestivirus reclassification 1:174
  Tombusviridae relationship 1:243
  see also Flaviviruses
Flavivirus 1:174, 1:376, 1:424, 1:426, 1:430, 2:871, 3:1980
  see also Dengue viruses; Encephalitis viruses; Yellow fever virus
Flaviviruses 1:376–7, 1:430
  antigenic relationships 1:376
  antigenic variability 1:434
  apoptosis
    inhibition 1:74
    promotion 1:75
  characteristics 1:376
  classification of groups 1:433
  conservation 1:427
  detection, suckling mice 1:399
  encephalitis 2:1018
  see also Encephalitis viruses
  evolution 1:430
  genetic variability 1:432–4
  mosquito-borne 1:433
    epidemiology 1:428
    evolution 1:427
    see also Encephalitis viruses; Japanese encephalitis virus (JEV); St Louis encephalitis virus (SLEV); West Nile virus (WNV)
  ocular target 1:525(Table)
  tick-borne 1:376, 1:433
    epidemiology 1:428
    serologic relationships 1:428
    stability 1:427
    see also Central European encephalitis virus (CEEV); Dengue viruses; Encephalitis viruses; Omsk hemorrhagic fever virus (OHFV)
Flexal virus 2:887, 2:888(Table)
FLICE (FADD-like ICE) 1:71, 1:73
Flies, picorna-like viruses 2:1272–3
Flock house virus (FHV) 2:1026, 3:1974
  cDNA clones 2:1029–30
  coat protein 2:1027
  host range 2:1027
  packaging 2:1030
  persistent infections 2:1031
  protein subunit structure 3:1949(Fig)
Flumadine *see* Rimantadine (Flumadine)
Fluorescein isothiocyanate (FITC) 1:389
Fluorescence *see* Immunofluorescence
5-Fluorouracil, in HPV infections 1:67
fms oncogene 3:1513
Foamy viruses *see* Spumaviruses

Follicular dendritic cells (FDCs) 2:814, 2:821
  HIV attachment 2:814–15
Fomites 1:484
Fomiversen 1:63
Food industry
  centralization, emerging viral diseases associated 1:423
  phage in industrial fermentations 2:1246
Food poisoning, *Staphylococcus aureus* toxins causing 2:1230
Food processing, emerging viral diseases associated 1:423
Food-borne infections, hepatitis A 1:423
Foot-and-mouth disease viruses (FMDVs) 1:420(Table), 1:568–75
  antibodies 1:574
  antigenic variation 1:574
  assembly and release 1:571–2
  attachment to cell receptors 1:572
  encapsidation 1:570
  endemic/nonendemic infection areas 1:574
  epidemiology 1:574
  field isolates 1:574
  gene triplication 1:569
  genetics and evolution 1:572–4
  genome 1:568, 1:569–70
    leader protein 1:570
    ORF 1:570
    organization 1:569(Fig)
    P1 and P2 regions 1:570
    P3 region 1:570
  geographic distribution 1:572, 1:573(Fig)
  history 1:568, 2:719
  host range and propagation 1:572
  infections
    clinical features 1:574
    immune response 1:574–5
    mass vaccination 1:572, 1:575
    prevention and control 1:575
    vaccination frequency 1:575
    vaccines 1:575
  infectious RNA (nature of) 1:571
  mutation rate 1:572
  pathogenicity 1:574
  persistent infections 1:572
  post-translational processing 1:571
  properties 1:568–9
  protective immunity against 1:569
  proteins 1:569, 1:570
  structural 1:568, 1:571
  VP1 (G–H loop) 1:569, 1:572
  VP1 truncation 1:569
  RNA replication 1:570–1
  SAT3 1:573(Fig)
  serologic relationships and variability 1:574
  serotypes 1:572, 1:574
  taxonomy and classification 1:568
  tissue tropism 1:574
  translation 1:571
  transmission 1:574
  virulence 1:574
  virus infection-associated (VIA) antigen 1:575
  VPg 1:569, 1:570, 1:572
Fort Morgan virus 1:502, 1:503
Fortovase 1:60
fos oncogene 3:1508, 3:1820
Fos protein 3:1508–9
  DNA binding activity 3:1509
  structure 3:1508–9
  transformation of fibroblasts 3:1509

Fos-related antigens (FRA) 3:1509
Foscarnet (Foscavir)
  CMV infections 1:63
  herpesvirus infections 1:62
  HHV-6 infection 2:703
  human CMV infections 1:351
Fowl see Chicken(s); Duck(s); Poultry
Fowl paralysis 2:945, 2:948
Fowl pest see Newcastle disease
Fowl plague 2:824
Fowlpox 1:576
  clinical features 1:579
  cutaneous form 1:579, 1:580(Fig)
  diagnosis 1:579–80
  diphtheritic form 1:579, 1:580(Fig)
  immune response 1:581
  outbreaks 1:581
  pathology/histopathology 1:579
  prevention and control 1:581
  synonyms 1:576
Fowlpox virus 1:576–82
  budding 1:577
  chemical composition 1:576
  DNA replication 1:577
  economic importance 1:579
  elementary bodies (Borel bodies) 1:577, 1:578, 1:579
  enzymes 1:577
  epidemiology 1:578
  evolution 1:578
  future perspectives 1:581–2
  genetics 1:576–7
  genome 1:576, 1:577
    characterization methods 1:577
  geographic/seasonal distribution 1:576
  history 1:576
  host range and propagation 1:576
  inclusion bodies 1:577, 1:579, 1:580(Fig)
  infection see Fowlpox
  Marek's disease virus infection with 1:578
  pathogenicity 1:579, 1:580
  persistent infections 1:578
  promoters 1:581
  re-emerging strains 1:578
  replication 1:577–8
  reticuloendotheliosis virus sequences 1:578
  serologic relationships and variability 1:578
  structure and properties 1:577(Fig)
  taxonomy and classification 1:576
  thymidine kinase 1:577
  transmission and tissue tropism 1:578–9
  vaccine 1:581
  as vector for vaccines 1:581–2
    avian influenza and Newcastle disease 1:581–2
Foxes, rabies vaccination 3:1988, 3:1995
Foxtail mosaic virus (FoMV), genome 3:1366
Fragaria chilensis virus (FCV) 1:39
Frameshifting see Ribosomal frameshifting
Friend murine leukemia virus 2:995
Fringed viruses 1:446, 1:447
Frog virus 3 (FV3) 1:582–7
  algal virus similarities/differences 1:45
  assembly and release 1:585–6
    assembly sites 1:585–6
    microvillus-like projections 1:586

Frog virus 3 (FV3) (continued)
  bacteriophage shared features 1:587(Table)
  budding and microfilaments role 1:586
  cytoskeletal changes induced by 1:586
  DNA
    circular permutation 1:583
    concatemer 1:584
    functions of concatemers 1:585
    methylation 1:583
    nucleus and cytoplasm stages 1:584
    replication 1:584
  envelope 1:582
  evolution 1:587
  Feulgen-positive inclusion bodies 1:583(Fig)
  future perspectives 1:587
  genetics 1:586
  genome 1:45, 1:583
  history 1:582
  mRNA 1:45, 1:585
    methylation 1:585
  packaging, 'headful' 1:585
  pathogenicity 1:586–7
  properties and structure 1:582–3
  protein properties 1:583
  temperature sensitivity 1:584
  protein synthesis 1:585
  recombination frequencies 1:586
  replication 1:45, 1:583–4, 1:587, 2:867
    general characteristics 1:583–4
    proposed cycle 1:584(Fig)
  structure, EM 1:583
  taxonomy and classification 1:582
  transcription 1:585
    immediate-early/delayed-early/late 1:585
  uncoating 1:585
Frog virus 4 (FV4) 1:51, 1:52–3
  discovery 1:52
  DNA 1:52–3
  histology of infected cells 1:52(Fig)
  intranuclear inclusions in cells 1:53(Fig)
  properties 1:52–3
  replication 1:53
  transmission 1:53
  see also Amphibian herpesviruses
Fujinami-PRCII Sarcoma 3:1512
Fulminant hepatitis see Hepatitis, fulminant
Fungal partitiviruses see Partitiviruses
Fungal viruses 1:313
  see also Hypoviruses; Mycoviruses; Partitiviruses, fungal
Fungi
  heterokaryon incompatibility see Heterokaryon incompatibility
  hypovirus-mediated changes 2:806
  plant virus transmission mechanisms 3:1908–10
    in vitro 3:1909
    in vivo 3:1909–10
    as plant virus vectors 3:1907–8
  prions see Prions
  retrotransposons see Retrotransposons of fungi
  spores see Spores
  susceptibility in plants after virus infection 2:1323

Fungi (continued)
  virus families/genera infecting 3:1754(Fig)
  virus transmission
    carmoviruses 1:243, 1:244
    cucumber necrosis tombusvirus (CNV) 3:1909
    furoviruses 1:594–5
    partitiviruses 2:1148
    pomoviruses 3:1361, 3:1362
    properties of vectors 3:1907–8
    tobacco necrosis virus (TNV) 2:1003, 3:1909
Fungus-transmitted rod-shaped plant viruses see Furoviruses
Furcraea necrotic streak virus (FNSV) 1:403, 1:409
  pathology and histopathology 1:408
  strains and serologic relationship 1:407
  see also Dianthoviruses
Furin, animal parainfluenza viruses 2:1135
Furovirus 1:154, 1:587
  genetics and replication 1:592–3
  genome structure/expression 1:589(Table), 1:591
  see also Furoviruses; Oat golden stripe virus (OGSV)
Furoviruses 1:587–96
  capsid protein 1:590
  cell-to-cell movement 1:591
  coat protein 1:589, 3:1909–10
  economic significance 1:595–6
  epidemiology and control 1:595–6
  genetics and replication 1:592–3
    Benevirus 1:593
    Furovirus 1:592
    Pecluvirus 1:593
    Pomovirus 1:593
  genome structure/expression 1:588, 1:589(Table), 1:590–2
    Benevirus 1:592
    Furovirus 1:591
    genetic map 1:590(Fig)
    Pecluvirus 1:591
    Pomovirus 1:591–2
  tobamoviruses and alphaviruses comparison 1:589(Table)
  geographic distribution 1:588(Table), 1:596
  host interactions 1:593–4
  host range 1:588(Table)
  infections, effects on host 1:593–4
  particles 1:588, 1:589(Table)
  relationship to tobamo-/alphavirus families 1:588, 1:590
  replication 1:590
  serology 1:589–90
  species 1:588
  structure and composition 1:588–9
  taxonomy and classification 1:587–8
  transmission 1:594–5
    fungi 3:1909–10
    vectors 1:594–5
  viruses included 1:588
Fuselloviridae 1:86, 2:1226
  characteristics 2:1226
  phage included 2:1226
Fusin 2:786

Fusion of host/viral membranes 3:1921
  mechanism 3:1924(Fig)
  see also Influenza virus
Fusion proteins 3:1922
  measles virus (MV) 2:953, 2:954
  synthesis by ribosomal frameshifting 3:1975–7
  see also Hemagglutinin (HA); Influenza virus
Fusogenic activity, envelope and cell membrane 2:1182
Fusogenic proteins 1:249
Fusogens, viral 1:251
Fuzzy sets, species as 3:1939–40

G

G:C content
  animal CMV 1:358
  coliphage lambda 1:282
  cypoviruses 1:333
  human CMV genome 1:352
G-protein, Cryphonectria parasitica 2:806
G-protein coupled receptors (GCP), HHV-6 and HHV-7 proteins 2:700
Gadget's Gully virus 1:435
Gaeumannomyces graminis virus (GgV)
  genome 2:1149
  transcription 2:1150
gag gene
  caprine arthritis encephalitis virus (CAEV) 1:223, 1:225–6
  caulimoviruses 2:1277–8
  equine infectious anemia virus (EIAV) 1:516
  HIV see HIV
  HTLV-2 see Human T-cell leukemia virus type 2 (HTLV-2)
  lymphoproliferative disease virus (LPDV) of turkeys 2:912
  see also other specific viruses
Gag protein
  HIV see HIV
  Ty elements 3:1505
gag-pol gene, type D retroviruses 3:1519–20
Gait spasticity, Theiler's murine encephalomyelitis viruses (TMEV) 3:1777
Galinsoga mosaic virus (GaMV) 1:245
Galleria mellonella densovirus (GmDNV) 1:384, 1:386
  histopathology 1:387
  host range 1:386
  immunity 1:387
  tissue culture 1:386
Gamma activated sequences (GAS) 2:857
Gammaherpesvirinae 1:181, 1:488, 1:509, 2:707, 2:715
  classification 2:703
  equine herpesviruses (EHV-2 and EHV-5) 1:509
  gamma-1 subgroup 2:704
    see also Epstein–Barr virus (EBV)
  gamma-2 subgroup 2:704
    see also Herpesvirus sylvilagus
  host range and propagation 2:709
  Lymphocryptovirus 1:488, 2:707, 2:708

Gammaherpesvirinae (*continued*)
  Lymphocryptovirus and
    Rhadinovirus
    comparison 2:704(Table)
Gammaherpesviruses 1:181(Table)
  infection pathogenesis 1:182
  see also Bovine herpesviruses
Gammaretrovirus, murine
  leukemia viruses
  (MuLVs) 2:995
Ganciclovir (GCV)
  CMV infections 1:62–3, 1:351
    prophylaxis 2:1076, 2:1082
  CMV resistance 1:54
  HHV-6 infection 2:703
  HHV-6 susceptibility 2:700
GAPs (GTPases activating
  protein) 3:1517
Garbage
  hog cholera virus (HCV)
    transmission 2:740
  vesicular exanthema virus
    spread 1:217
Gardner–Rasheed feline sarcoma
  virus (GR-FSV),
  oncogene 3:1513
Garlic common latent virus
  (GaCLV), genome 1:239
Gastric adenocarcinoma, EBV
  association 1:490
Gastroenteritis
  acute nonbacterial
    discovery of Norwalk
      virus 2:1035
    epidemiology 2:1038
    outbreaks 2:1038
  astroviruses causing 1:104, 1:107,
    1:446
  coxsackievirus infection 1:308
  epidemic 1:442
  Norwalk virus causing 2:1039
    clinical features 2:1039
    diagnosis 2:1040
    treatment 2:1040
    see also Norwalk virus
  'Picobirnaviruses' causing 1:447
  rotaviruses causing 3:1576,
    3:1577
    clinical features 3:1580,
      3:1581(Table)
    epidemiology 3:1579–80
    pathology 3:1580–1
  see also Diarrhea; Rotaviruses
Gastrointestinal hemorrhage,
  dengue viruses causing 1:381
Gastrointestinal tract
  colonization by viruses 1:441
  coxsackievirus infection 1:308
  entry route for viruses 1:441
  immune system 2:1177
  local infections and
    symptoms 2:1177
  proteolytic enzymes 2:1177
  shedding of viruses 2:1177
  virus entry 2:1176–7
    inhibition 2:1177
GBV-A 1:660
GBV-A-like viruses 1:660
GBV-B 1:660
  hepatitis C virus
    relationship 1:660
GBV-C 1:660
GDD motif 3:1785
  tombusviruses 3:1795
Geese
  duck hepatitis B virus
    infection 1:653
  Newcastle disease 2:1024
GEFs (guanine nucleotide exchange
  factor) 3:1517
GEM 132 1:63

Geminiviridae 1:597–606
  characteristics 1:597
  diagnostic criteria 3:1942,
    3:1942(Table)
  establishment 1:597
  genera 1:597
Geminivirus 1:597
Geminiviruses 1:597–606, 3:1894
  cell-to-cell movement 1:604
  Circoviridae similarities 1:606
  coat proteins 3:1895
    replacement vectors 1:604,
      3:1895
    role in transmission 3:1905
    vector specificity 1:603
  components A and B 3:1895
  of dicotyledonous plants 3:1894
  DNA replication 1:601–3
    minus-strand 1:602
    plus-strand 1:602
    stages 1:602
  evolution 1:605–6
  gene amplification vectors based
    on 1:604–5
  genes, functions 1:597–601,
    1:599(Table)
  genome organization/
    expression 1:597–601
    Begamovirus 1:599(Table),
      1:600–1
    bound oligodeoxyribo-
      nucleotides 1:598
    conserved stem–loop
      structure 1:602
    Curtovirus 1:598–600
    large intergenic region
      (LIR) 1:597, 1:602
    Mastrevirus 1:597–8
  geographic distribution 1:603–4
  history 1:597
  host range 1:603–4
  infections, symptoms 1:605
  of monocotyledonous
    plants 3:1895
  Nanovirus similarities 1:606
  nucleic acid-mediated resistance
    to 2:1311
  pathogenesis 1:605
  proteins
    begamoviruses 1:600–1
    ORF C1 and ORF C2
      products 1:598
    ORF V1 and ORF V2
      products 1:597–8
  recombination 3:1449
  Rep proteins 1:598, 1:602, 1:604
    binding sites 1:603
  replication 3:1895
    in vectors 3:1905
  replication enhancer 1:599
  ssDNA, infectious nature 1:602
  structure 1:597
  taxonomy and
    classification 1:597
  transcription, *Mastrevirus* 1:597
  transmission 1:603–4
  as vectors 3:1894–5,
    3:1895(Table)
    observations/
      requirements 3:1895
GemStar^{TM} 2:847
Gene(s)
  acquisition
    evolution 2:1239
    see also Transduction
  amplification *see* DNA,
    amplification; Polymerase
    chain reaction (PCR)
  chimeric 2:1307
  duplication, coat protein in
    closteroviruses 1:270
  nomenclature 2:1211

Gene(s) (*continued*)
  overlapping, discovery 1:275
  proteins encoded by same
    sequence 3:1473
  resistance *see under* Host genetic
    resistance
  triple gene block *see* Triple gene
    block
  viral disease relationships 2:753
Gene amplification vectors, based
  on geminivirus replicons 1:604–
  5
Gene cloning *see* Cloning
Gene expression
  cis- and *trans*-acting
    sequences 3:1473
  regulation in viruses 3:1472–3
    DNA viruses 3:1477
  vectors *see* Cloning vectors
Gene gun, vaccine delivery 3:1495
Gene probes
  shrimp viruses 3:1635
  see also DNA probes
Gene reassortment *see* Genetic
  reassortment
Gene regulation 3:1472–3
Gene silencing 2:1310, 3:1368,
  3:1375
  potexviruses 3:1368
Gene therapy 1:12
  adeno-associated viruses (AAV)
    use 3:1885
  adenovirus vectors *see*
    Adenovirus
  disorders 1:12
  dominant-negative mutants 2:853
  entomopoxviruses (EPVs) 1:481
  murine dystrophin 1:13
  parvoviruses 2:1159
Gene transfer
  α_1-antrypsin gene 1:13, 1:13–14
  murine dystrophin 1:13
  virus-mediated 2:1240
Gene vectors *see* Cloning vectors
Gene-for-gene relationship 2:1304,
  2:1304(Table)
Genera, virus 2:1222, 2:1223
  definition 2:1223
  see also Taxonomy of viruses
Genetic diversity 2:753, 3:1446
  HIV-1 2:770
Genetic drift
  dengue viruses 1:378
  St Louis encephalitis virus 1:427
Genetic engineering 1:612
  animal viruses,
    applications 1:612
  crops, furovirus control 1:595
  luteovirus resistant crops 2:907
  see also Cloning vectors
Genetic factors, effect on viral
  infection outcome 2:1183
Genetic mapping
  animal virus genomes 1:611
  complementation groups 1:611
  recombination maps 1:611
    three-factor crosses 1:611
    two-factor crosses 1:611
  restriction maps 1:611
Genetic plasticity 3:1431, 3:1433,
  3:1961
Genetic reassortment 1:606, 1:609,
  3:1478
  animal viruses 1:609
  Bunyaviridae RNA 1:207–8,
    1:208
  coltiviruses 2:1050
  cucumoviruses 1:317, 1:323
  cypoviruses 1:334
  emerging viral diseases
    associated 1:419
  genetic mapping by 1:611

Genetic reassortment (*continued*)
  immune evasion
    mechanism 2:816
  influenza viruses 2:825, 2:826
  inhibition, dominant-negative
    mutants 2:853
  LCMV 2:916, 2:923–4
  orbiviruses 2:1046, 2:1050,
    2:1054, 2:1058
  recombination by 3:1450
  reoviruses 3:1458, 3:1470
  rotaviruses 3:1578
Genetic recombination,
  bacteriophage 2:1213–21
  bacteriophage ϕX174 1:280
  bacteriophage P22 3:1606
  coliphage λ *see* Coliphage
    lambda
  coliphage N4 1:452
  DNA replication
    dependence 2:1220
  DNA signals 2:1220
  double-stranded breaks 2:1220
  homologous 2:1213
  P2 bacteriophage *see* P2
    bacteriophage
  P4 bacteriophage 2:1098
  parallels between phage 2:1219–
    20
  phage T4 *see* T4 bacteriophage
  phage T7 *see* T7-like
    bacteriophage
  SPO1 phage 3:1684
  ssDNA annealing 2:1220
  ssDNA phage 2:1213–14
    hotspot at replication
      origin 2:1213
    models 2:1213
    RecA-dependent 2:1213
    RecA-independent 2:1213–14
    see also Bacteriophage ϕX174
  T4-like phages 3:1711(Fig),
    3:1713–14
Genetic recombination, viruses *see*
  Recombination of viruses
Genetic variation 1:486
  caprine arthritis encephalitis
    virus (CAEV) 1:226
  quasispecies 3:1431
Genetically engineered resistance,
  of plants *see* Plant resistance to
  viruses
Genetically modified viruses, field
  trials of baculoviruses 2:849
Genetics
  animal viruses *see* Animal
    viruses
  phage, history 2:721
Genital cancer 3:1845–6
Genital infections, HSV-2
  causing 2:679, 2:681, 2:681(Fig)
Genital warts (condyloma
  acuminata) 1:67, 2:1110,
  2:1111(Table), 2:1112
  interferon use 2:860
  therapy 2:1114
  treatment 1:67
Genitourinary system, virus
  entry 2:1177–8
Genome
  animal viruses 1:607
    partial sequencing 1:483
  replication *see* DNA replication;
    RNA replication
  segmented, reassortment 1:609
  sequence analysis 1:612
    animal viruses 1:612
  variation and emerging
    diseases 1:419–20
  virus 3:1938
    classification 3:1941
    variability 3:1941

'Genome activation' 1:39
Genome type, definition 1:3
Genome-linker protein (Vpg) see specific viruses
Genomic clusters 1:3
Genomic libraries, screening 2:1242
Germ-line, virus transmission 1:484
German measles see Rubella
Germline proviruses, *Drosophila melanogaster* gypsy virus 3:1527, 3:1529
Gerstmann–Straussler disease 2:1018
Gerstmann–Sträussler–Scheinker (GSS) disease 3:1388
  neuropathology 3:1391(Fig)
  PrP amyloid plaques 3:1390
  PrP gene mutations 3:1392
  sporadic 3:1390
Getah virus 3:1570
Giant cells
  HSV infections 2:683
  measles 2:957, 2:958
  syncytium see Syncytium
Giardia lamblia virus see Giardiavirus (GLV)
Giardiavirus 1:613, 3:1808, 3:1974
  viruses included 3:1809(Table)
  see also Giardiavirus (GLV)
Giardiavirus (GLV) 1:613–16, 3:1808
  characteristics/properties 1:616, 1:616(Table)
  evolution 1:616
  genome (dsRNA) 1:614, 1:615(Fig), 3:1809–10
    ORFs 1:614
    organization and molecular biology 1:614–15
    overlap fragment 1:615
    sequence 1:614
    ssRNA with 1:616
  geographic distribution 1:613–14
  history 1:613
  host range 1:613–14
  human isolates 1:614
  infected cell pathology 1:615(Fig)
  infection process 1:615–16
  number per infected cell 1:615
  physical/biochemical characteristics 1:614
  replication 1:615–16
  RNA-dependent RNA polymerase (RDRP) 1:614
  structure 1:614, 1:614(Fig)
  taxonomy and classification 1:613
  as vector 1:615
    foreign genes inserted 1:615
  see also Totiviruses
Gibbon ape leukemia virus (GaLV) 1:617–19, 3:1496
  evolution 3:1496, 3:1497(Fig)
  from UCD-144 cell line 1:617
  GaLV-Br 1:617
  GaLV-H 1:617
  GaLV-SEATO 1:617, 1:619
  GaLV-SF (San Francisco strain) 1:617
  gene delivery vector system 1:619
  infections
    clinical features 1:617
    specificity 1:618
  murine leukemia viruses relationship 1:617
  pathogenicity 1:618–19
  receptor 1:617
  serologic relationships and variability 1:617–18
  simian sarcoma virus (SSV) relationship 1:617, 1:618
  sis gene 1:618

Gibbon ape leukemia virus (GaLV) (continued)
  taxonomy and classification 1:617
  transmission 1:617
Ginger fleck virus (GCFV) 3:1675
Gingivostomatitis, HSV-1 causing 2:679, 2:680
Glandular fever see Infectious mononucleosis
Global warming, emergence and re-emergence of diseases 1:422
Glomerulonephritis 1:249
  in hepatitis B 2:1082
Glomerulonephropathy, in hepatitis B 2:1082
Glutamate synthetase, in cyanobacteria 1:331
Glycine mosaic virus (GMV) 1:285, 1:290
Glycine mottle virus (GMoV) 1:244, 1:245
Glycocalyx 1:249
Glycophorin A 1:231
Glycoproteins 1:249
  in plasma membrane 1:249
  sorting and transfer in cells 1:249
  synthesis 1:251
Glycosaminoglycans, as virus receptor 2:1181
Glycosylation 1:252
  African swine fever virus (AFSV) proteins 1:34
  Asn-linked, PrP^{Sc} prion protein 3:1395
  Chlorella viruses 1:50
  human CMV 1:356
Glycosyltransferases 1:251, 1:252
Goat(s)
  caprine arthritis encephalitis virus infection 1:223
  pox disease see Goatpox
  see also entries beginning caprine
Goatpox 3:1376
  clinical features 3:1379
  epidemiology 3:1378
  transmission 3:1378
  see also Capripoxviruses
Golden shiner reovirus (GSV) 1:564
  clinical features of infection 1:564
  genome and proteins 1:564
  geographic/seasonal distribution 1:564
  history 1:564
  host range and propagation 1:564
  taxonomy and classification 1:564
  transmission and tissue tropism 1:564
Golgi apparatus 1:251
  Bunyaviridae glycoprotein accumulation 1:216
  cis and *trans* faces 1:251–2
  functions 1:252
  hantavirus assembly 1:625
  membrane synthesis and budding of viruses 3:1924(Fig), 3:1925
Gonad-specific virus (GSV) 2:1032
Gonadotropin, iatrogenic CJD after 3:1390, 3:1392
Gonometa podocarpi, biological control 2:1274
Gonometa virus (GV) 2:844, 2:1274
Goose parvovirus (GPV)
  geographic distribution 2:1171–2
  history 2:1168
  host range and propagation 2:1172
  infection, clinical features 2:1174
  see also Parvoviruses

Gossas virus 3:1541
Graaf Reinet disease 3:1962
Graft-versus-host disease 3:1823, 3:1824
Grafting, propagation of plant viruses 3:1419
Graham 293 cells 1:445
Granulin 1:141
  gene 1:141
  granulovirus 1:141, 1:144
Granulocyte-macrophage colony-stimulating factor (GM-CSF) 1:342
Granulosis 1:140
Granulosis viruses see Granuloviruses (GV)
Granulovirus 2:846
  see also Baculoviruses
Granuloviruses (GV) 1:140–6, 1:147
  budding 1:142(Fig), 1:143–4
  cathepsin 1:143
  Cydia pomonella 1:141, 1:145
  ecology 1:145
  EGT protein 1:143
  enhancin protein 1:143
  'fast' and 'slow' 1:145
  gene expression 1:143
  genes 1:141–3
    enhancin 1:141
    granulin 1:141
    iap 1:141–3
    number 1:141
  genome
    homologous repeats (*hrs*) 1:143
    organization and expression 1:141–3
    transposable element insertion 1:141
  granulin 1:141, 1:144
  host range 1:145, 1:147
  infection mechanism 1:143
  as insecticides 1:145–6
  nuclear 'clearing' 1:143
  occlusion bodies (capsules/granules) 1:141, 1:142(Fig), 1:144–5
  ODVP-6E protein 1:143
  parasitoid interaction 1:145
  pathology 1:145
  phylogeny 1:140
  replication 1:143–5, 1:144(Fig)
    in fat body 1:145
  species 1:140
  structure 1:140–1, 1:142(Fig)
  supercoiled dsDNA 1:140
  taxonomy and classification 1:140
  tissue tropism and GV types 1:145
  see also Baculoviruses
Granzyme B 1:300
Granzymes (serine proteases) 2:818, 2:1201
Grapevine Algerian latent virus (GALV) 3:1790(Table)
Grapevine berry inner necrosis virus (GBINV) 3:1838(Table)
  classification 3:1838
  coat protein 3:1839
  cytopathic effects 3:1840
  disease 3:1841
  genome 3:1839, 3:1839(Fig)
  geographic distribution 3:1838
  host range 3:1838
  host relations 3:1840
  phylogenetic relations 3:1840
  transmission 3:1840
Grapevine chrome mosaic virus (GCMV) 2:1008(Table)
Grapevine fanleaf 2:1012

Grapevine fanleaf virus (GFLV) 2:1008(Table)
  host range 2:1011
  satellite RNA 3:1611–12
Grapevine leafroll associated virus 2 (GLRaV-2) 1:269
  disease and economic significance 1:272–3
  structure 1:267(Fig)
Grapevine leafroll associated virus 3 (GLRaV-3) 1:269
  disease and economic significance 1:272–3
  transmission 1:272
Grapevine leafroll associated viruses (GLRaVs) 1:267
Grapevine viroid 1B (now grapevine yellow speckle 2 viroid) 3:1930(Table)
Grapevine virus A (GVA) 3:1838(Table)
  classification 3:1837, 3:1842
  coat protein 3:1839
  control measures 3:1841–2
  cytopathic effects 3:1840
  disease 3:1841
  genome 3:1839, 3:1839–40, 3:1839(Fig)
  geographic distribution 3:1838
  host range 3:1838
  host relations 3:1840
  phylogenetic relations 3:1840
  serological relationships 3:1841
  transmission 3:1840
Grapevine virus B (GVB) 3:1838(Table)
  classification 3:1837, 3:1842
  coat protein 3:1839
  control measures 3:1841–2
  cytopathic effects 3:1840
  disease 3:1841
  genome 3:1839, 3:1839–40, 3:1839(Fig)
  geographic distribution 3:1838
  host range 3:1838
  host relations 3:1840
  phylogenetic relations 3:1840
  serological relationships 3:1841
  transmission 3:1840
Grapevine virus C (GVC) 3:1838(Table)
  classification 3:1837, 3:1842
  disease 3:1841
  geographic distribution 3:1838
  host relations 3:1840
Grapevine virus D (GVD) 3:1838(Table)
  classification 3:1838, 3:1842
  coat protein 3:1839
  control measures 3:1841
  cytopathic effects 3:1840
  disease 3:1841
  genome 3:1839, 3:1839(Fig), 3:1840
  geographic distribution 3:1838
  host range 3:1838
  host relations 3:1840
  phylogenetic relations 3:1840
  serological relationships 3:1841
  transmission 3:1840
Grapevine yellow speckle 1 viroid (GVYSVd 1) 3:1930(Table)
Grapevine yellow speckle 2 viroid (GVYSVd 2) 3:1930(Table)
Grapevines
  mosaic disease 3:1841
  new viruses 1:273
  rugose wood complex of diseases 3:1841
  virus-free plants 3:1841
Grass carp, golden shiner reovirus (GSV) infection 1:564

Great Island virus
(GIV) 2:1045(Table), 2:1047,
2:1050
immune response to 2:1058
neurovirulence 2:1057
see also Orbiviruses
Greenhouse effect, zoonotic disease
spread and 3:1996
Grimsby virus
detection 2:1040
serologic relationships 2:1038
GroE 1:282
GroEL 3:1708, 3:1709
GroES 3:1709
Groundnut rosette disease 2:907
'Ground glass cells' 1:643
Ground squirrel hepatitis virus
(GSHV) 1:640, 1:645
carcinogenic mechanism 1:643
genome 1:645–6
geographic/seasonal
distribution 1:641
host range and propagation 1:641
transcription 1:649
see also Hepadnaviridae
Groundnut chlorotic spot
virus 3:1804
Groundnut rosette assistor virus
(GRAV) 2:903, 3:1855,
3:1856(Table), 3:1857, 3:1858
Groundnut rosette disease 3:1855,
3:1857, 3:1858
control 3:1859
epidemiology 3:1858
Groundnut rosette virus
(GRV) 3:1608, 3:1613, 3:1855,
3:1856(Table), 3:1858
disease see Groundnut rosette
disease
genome 3:1856, 3:1857(Fig)
propagation 3:1858
properties 3:1855–6
replication 3:1857
satellite RNA 3:1857
satellite-like ssRNAs 3:1613
Groundnuts, clump disease 2:1196
Grouse
louping ill 1:432
tick-borne encephalitis (TBE)
virus complex
transmission 1:435
Growth, plant, reduction in virus
diseases 2:1321–3
Growth factors, oncogenes 3:1511
Growth hormone, human,
iatrogenic CJD 3:1390, 3:1392
Growth retardation, intrauterine,
in HSV infections 2:683
GTP-binding proteins
dynamin family 2:858
Ras proteins as 3:1820
GTPase activity, Ras
proteins 3:1517, 3:1820
Guanarito virus 1:419(Table),
2:887–96, 2:888(Table), 3:1988
antibodies 2:895
classification 2:887
genetics 2:889
geographic/seasonal
distribution 2:888
history 2:887
host range 2:889
propagation 2:889
see also Venezuelan hemorrhagic
fever
Guanyltransferase,
rotaviruses 3:1583, 3:1587
Guarneri bodies 2:980, 3:1868
Guillain–Barré syndrome 2:1019
Duvenhage virus
association 3:1445
echoviruses causing 1:415

Guinea pigs cytomegalovirus
(GpCMV) 1:357
Guinea-pig adenovirus 1:19
Gumboro disease 1:160
GUS gene 3:1897
Gypcheck 2:847
gypsy-like retrotransposons 2:1316
genome 2:1316, 2:1316(Fig)

H

H-1 virus 2:1167
infection 2:1174
H-2D gene, MCMV
resistance 2:754
H-2^k haplotype 2:754
HAART see Highly active
antiretroviral therapy
(HAART)
HADEN (hemadsorbing enteric)
virus 2:1168
Haemagogus janthinomys, Mayaro
(MAY) virus
transmission 1:263
Hagovirus 1:218
Hairpin loops
African swine fever virus (AFSV)
genome 1:31, 1:32(Fig)
densovirus genome 1:384
filamentous phage 1:548, 1:552
parvoviruses 2:1156, 2:1169
Hairpin ribozyme 3:1557–8,
3:1557(Fig)
history 3:1552
Hairpin transfer mechanism, DNA
replication in
parvoviruses 2:1156
Hairy cell leukemia
HJTLV-2 3:1845
interferon use 2:860
Mo T cell virus 2:795
Hairy leukoplakia 1:491
'Hairy root' phenotype, furovirus
infection 1:594
Hairy-shaker syndrome 1:179
Halobacterium saccharovorum
1:82
Halobacterium salinarum
1:81(Table)
genetic instability 1:82
genetic variability 1:77
halophage HF1 and HF2 1:82
phage φN 1:82
phage Hs1 1:83
Haloferax 1:82
Haloferax volcanii 1:82
Halophage 1:77–83
DNA genome 1:77
hosts and
characteristics 1:80(Table)
other 1:82–3
protein profiles 1:77
see also Halophage φH
Halophage φCh1 1:80(Table), 1:83
Halophage φH 1:77, 1:77–83
antisense transcript T$_{ant}$ 1:82
gene expression 1:77–82
genome 1:81(Fig)
insertion element ISH1.8 1:77
L region 1:77
organization 1:77
terminal redundancy 1:77
hosts and
characteristics 1:80(Table)
immunity to superinfection 1:81–2
lysogenic state 1:77–82
lytic cycle 1:77–81

Halophage φH (continued)
morphology 1:77, 1:78(Fig)
post-transcriptional
modification 1:82
prophage 1:77
rep gene product 1:81, 1:82
repressor 1:82
transcript T1 1:82
transcript T4 1:81
transcription 1:77–82
variant φH1 1:77, 1:82
variant φH2 1:77
variant φH5 1:77
variants 1:77, 1:81(Table)
Halophage φN 1:82–3
hosts and
characteristics 1:80(Table)
Halophage HF1 1:82
genome organization 1:82
hosts and
characteristics 1:80(Table)
replication strategy 1:82
Halophage HF2 1:82
genome organization 1:82
hosts and
characteristics 1:80(Table)
replication strategy 1:82
Halophage Hh1 1:80(Table)
Halophage Hh3 1:80(Table)
Halophage Ja1 1:77, 1:80(Table)
Halophage S45 1:80(Table)
Hammerhead ribozyme 3:1556–7,
3:1556(Fig)
crystal structure 3:1557,
3:1557(Fig)
hammerhead reaction in
trans 3:1556(Fig), 3:1557
history 3:1552
size 3:1557
stem III and I 3:1557
viroids/satellite RNAs
with 3:1556
Hamming distance 3:1431
Hand–foot–mouth disease
(HFMD) 1:308
clinical features 1:473
enterovirus 71 (EV71)
causing 1:473
outbreaks 1:473
Hantaan virus (HTNV) 1:210,
1:621, 3:1988
geographic/seasonal
distribution 1:626
infection 2:1083(Table), 2:1084
structure, EM 1:623(Fig)
see also Hantaviruses
Hantavirus 1:204, 1:210, 1:621,
3:1988
Arvicolinae subfamily-associated
viruses 1:622(Table)
groups and viruses 1:210
human-to-human
transmission 1:210
insectivore-associated
virus 1:621, 1:622(Table)
Murinae subfamily-associated
viruses 1:622(Table)
proteins 1:207
serogroups and
viruses 1:206(Table)
Sigmodontinae subfamily-
associated
viruses 1:622(Table)
transmission and
epidemiology 1:208, 1:210
viruses included 1:621–2,
1:622(Table)
Hantavirus hemorrhagic
fevers 3:1988
Hantavirus pulmonary syndrome
(HPS) 1:68, 1:210, 1:621, 3:1988
activities associated 1:627

Hantavirus pulmonary syndrome
(HPS) (continued)
clinical features 1:628
ecological change and 3:1996
epidemiology 1:627
geographic/seasonal
distribution 1:626
immune response 1:629
mortality rate 1:627
outbreaks 1:621
pathology/histopathology 1:629
see also Hantaviruses
Hantaviruses 1:68, 1:209, 1:621–30,
2:1083(Table), 3:1988
antigenic diversity 1:627
assembly and transport 1:625–6
Biosafety Level 4 category 1:628
budding 1:216
cytopathology 1:626
as emerging viruses 1:418,
1:419(Table)
epidemiology 1:627
evolution 1:626–7
natural reservoirs
association 1:627(Fig)
future perspectives 1:630
genetics 1:626
genome 1:623
coding strategy 1:623(Fig)
panhandle structures 1:623,
1:624(Fig)
geographic/seasonal
distribution 1:626
history 1:621
host range and propagation 1:626
infections 1:209
clinical features 1:628
immune response 1:629
pathology/
histopathology 1:628–9
prevention and control 1:630
renal involvement 2:1083–4
respiratory distress
syndrome 1:421
therapy 1:68
see also Hantavirus pulmonary
syndrome (HPS);
Hemorrhagic fever with renal
syndrome (HFRS)
pathogenicity 1:628
physical properties 1:622–3
post-translational
processing 1:625
proteins
glycoproteins (G1 and
G2) 1:623–4, 1:625, 1:625–6
properties 1:623–4
replication 1:624–5, 1:624–6
RNA-dependent RNA
polymerase 1:622
serologic relationships and
variability 1:627
structure and properties 1:622
EM 1:623(Fig)
taxonomy and
classification 1:621
tissue tropism 1:627–8
transcription 1:624–5, 1:624(Fig)
translation 1:625
transmission 1:204, 1:621, 1:627–
8, 2:1083
vaccine development 1:629, 1:630
genetically engineered
vaccine 1:630
Hardy–Zuckerman 4 feline
sarcoma virus (HZ4-
FSV) 3:1513
Hare fibroma virus (HFV),
history 3:1383
Hare sarcoma 3:1383
Harvey murine sarcoma virus (Ha-
MuSV) 2:995, 3:1517, 3:1820

Hawaii virus 2:1038
  detection 2:1040
  pathogenicity 2:1039
'Head disease' 3:1544
Health care workers, hepatitis C
  risk 1:662
Heart
  coxsackievirus infection 1:308
  murine CMV infection 1:367
  viruses affecting 2:1074–8,
    2:1075(Table)
Heart disease see Cardiac disease
Heat shock proteins
  DnaJ–DnaK–GrpE 1:284
  Hsp70, homologue in
    closteroviruses 1:266, 1:269,
    1:270
  Hsp104, [PSI] prion loss 3:1405
  T cell activation 1:109
Helenium virus S (HVS) 1:238
  genome 1:239, 1:240
Helical viruses 3:1943
  atomic structure 3:1944
  structure 3:1946–7
Helicase 1:322
  iridoviruses 2:865
Helicoverpa armigera stunt virus
  (HaSV) 3:1772
  assembly in protoplasts 3:1772
  genome 3:1768
  host range 3:1770
  mutants 3:1769
  replication 3:1769
  transmission and
    symptoms 3:1770
  tropism 3:1771
  see also Tetraviruses
Helicoverpa ascovirus 1:98
Helicoverpa zea 1:98, 1:102
  biological control 2:847
  nonoccluded
    baculoviruses 2:1032
  viruses see Hz-1V; Hz-2V
Helicoverpa zea virus 1 (Hz-
  1V) 2:845–6
Helicoverpa zea virus 2 (Hz-
  2V) 2:845–6
Heliothine caterpillars, HaSV in
  biological control of 3:1772
Heliothis armigera
  biological control 2:847(Fig)
  cytoplasmic polyhedrosis virus
    (CPV) 1:336
Heliothis armigera entomopoxvirus
  (HaEPV) 1:475, 1:476, 2:845
  see also Entomopoxviruses
    (EPVs)
Heliothis armigera stunt virus
  (HaSV) 2:843
Heliothis ascovirus 1:102(Table)
Helix–loop–helix family
  Fos protein 3:1508
  v-Myc protein 3:1510
Helix-turn-helix DNA binding
  (HTH) motif 2:1090
Helminthosporium victoriae 190S
  virus (Hv190SV) 3:1808, 3:1812
  190S-1 and 190S-2 3:1808
  coat protein 3:1810
  genome 3:1809–10
    organization 3:1809(Fig)
  life cycle 3:1810–11, 3:1810(Fig)
  RNA replication 3:1810
  RNA-dependent RNA
    polymerase 3:1811
  structure and properties 3:1808
  see also Totiviruses
Helper bacteriophage 2:1236–7
  see also P2 bacteriophage; P4
    bacteriophage
Helper component (HC) protein, in
  waikavirus transmission 3:1968

Helper dependence, pea enation
  mosaic virus (PEMV) 2:1194
Helper viruses 3:1607, 3:1948
  for acute transforming
    viruses 1:995
  for adeno-associated viruses
    (AAV) as vectors 3:1885
  avian leukosis virus (ALV) 1:113
  caulimovirus
    transmission 3:1901–3
  defective-interfering
    carmoviruses 1:246
  hepatitis B virus as 1:664
  heracleum latent virus
    (HLV) 3:1840
  potyviruses transmission 3:1901
    see also Potyviruses
  satellites dependence on 3:1614
    see also Satellite RNAs
  symptoms, effect of satellite
    RNAs 3:1612
  tobacco necrosis virus (TNV)
    as 2:1003
  umbraviruses 3:1855,
    3:1856(Table), 3:1858
  waikaviruses 3:1968
  see also Parsnip yellow fleck virus
    (PYFV)
Hemadsorption, virus isolation/
  identification 1:397
Hemadsorption virus type 2
  (HV2) 3:1616
  see also Sendai virus
Hemagglutinating
  encephalomyelitis virus see
    Porcine hemagglutinating
    encephalomyelitis virus (HEV)
Hemagglutinating virus of Japan
  (HVJ) 3:1616
  see also Sendai virus
Hemagglutination
  adenovirus identification 1:19
  assay 3:1413
Hemagglutination inhibition
  (HAI)
  antirubella virus
    antibodies 3:1599
  antiviral antibody detection 1:390
  cowpox virus 1:303
Hemagglutinin (HA)
  atomic structure 3:1944
  fusion mediated by 3:1922
  fusion-competent form 3:1922
  gene, cowpox virus 1:299
  HA1 3:1922
  HA2 3:1922
    fusion peptide 3:1922
    transmembrane domain 3:1923
  influenza virus see Influenza
    viruses
  measles virus (MV) 2:953
  rotaviruses 3:1589
  synthesis 3:1924
  three-stranded coiled-coil
    stem 3:1922
  see also Influenza virus
Hemagglutinin esterase, bovine
  torovirus (BTV) 3:1799
Hemagglutinin–neuraminidase
  (HN)
  mumps virus (MuV) see Mumps
    virus
  Newcastle disease virus 2:1022
  parainfluenza viruses
    (PIVs) 2:1131
Hematogenous spread see
  Pathogenesis of viral infections;
  Spread of viruses
Hematoxylin and eosin
  (H&E) 1:400
Hemipterans, picorna-like
  viruses 2:1273–4

Hemolysis, equine infectious
  anemia (EIA) 1:520
Hemorrhages
  African swine fever 1:37
  Chikungunya (CHIK) fever 1:264
  see also Bleeding; Hemorrhagic
    fever
Hemorrhagic disease
  dengue see Dengue hemorrhagic
    fever/dengue shock syndrome
    (DHF/DSS)
  elephants 1:357
Hemorrhagic enteritis
  adenoviruses causing 1:6, 1:20
  turkey 1:20
Hemorrhagic fever 2:1084
  Crimean-Congo 3:1990
  Ebola virus 2:939, 2:943, 3:1993
  ecology 2:890
  hantavirus 3:1988
  Marburg virus 2:939, 2:943,
    3:1993
  Omsk 3:1992
  renal involvement 2:1084
Hemorrhagic fever with renal
  syndrome (HFRS; Korean
  hemorrhagic fever) 1:210,
  1:621, 2:1083–4, 2:1084
  activities associated 1:627
  clinical features 1:628
  epidemiology 1:627
  geographic/seasonal
    distribution 1:626
  immune response 1:629
  incubation period and
    phases 1:628
  laboratory-acquired 1:627
  pathology/histopathology 1:628–
    9
  rural and urban forms 1:627
  vaccine development 1:630
  see also Hantaviruses
Henderson–Paterson bodies 2:963
Hepacivirus 1:657
  see also Hepatitis C virus (HCV)
Hepadnaviridae 1:640–5
  antigens 1:642
    c and e antigens 1:642
    surface antigen 1:642
  apoptosis promotion 1:74
  Avihepadnavirus 1:650
    see also Duck hepatitis B virus
      (DHBV)
  cauliflower mosaic virus
    relationship 1:641
  DNA integration 1:642
  envelope 1:640, 1:641
  evolution 1:641–2
  genetics 1:641
  genome 1:650
    size 1:650
  geographic/seasonal
    distribution 1:641
  host range 1:640, 1:641
  infections see Hepatitis B
  mammalian and avian virus
    comparisons 1:641
  Orthohepadnavirus 1:650
  pathogenicity 1:643
  persistent infections 1:640
  propagation 1:641
  Retroviridae relationship 1:641
  reverse transcription 1:641
  serologic relationships and
    variability 1:642
  transmission and tissue
    tropism 1:640, 1:642–3
  viruses included 1:640
  see also Hepatitis B virus (HBV)

Hepadnaviruses 1:640–5
  apoptosis inhibition 1:72–3
  avian see Hepatitis B viruses,
    avian
  mammalian 1:645
    genome 1:645–6
    see also Hepatitis B virus
      (HBV)
  receptors 3:1411
  replication 1:656
  transfection studies 3:1411
  see also Hepadnaviridae;
    Hepatitis B virus (HBV)
Heparnavirus 2:737
Hepatic necrosis, dengue virus
  infection 1:380, 1:382
Hepatitis
  acute infectious see Hepatitis A
  adenoviruses causing 1:6
  autoimmune chronic, hepatitis A
    virus causing 1:638
  chronic, hepatitis B 1:642, 1:643,
    1:644
  chronic active
    hepatitis B 1:643, 3:1830
    non-A, non-B 3:1830
  CMV 3:1824
  delta 1:668
    acute 1:668
    chronic 1:668
    see also Hepatitis delta virus
      (HDV)
  duck virus see Duck hepatitis
    virus (DHV)
  fulminant
    echovirus type 11 and 1:416
    hepatitis B 1:643
    hepatitis delta 1:668
    hepatitis E 1:674
  HSV 3:1829
  mouse hepatitis virus
    causing 1:296–7
  murine CMV 1:367
  non-A non-B 1:65, 1:657
    enterically transmitted see
      Hepatitis E virus (HEV)
    see also Hepatitis C virus
      (HCV)
  serum see Hepatitis B
  transfusion-associated see
    Hepatitis C virus (HCV)
  turkey virus see Turkey hepatitis
    virus (THV)
  in yellow fever 3:1985
Hepatitis A
  age-related infections 1:637
  chronic 1:637, 1:638
  clinical features 1:634(Table),
    1:638
  daycare centers 1:423
  drug abusers 1:637
  immune response 1:638–9
  incubation period 1:638
  outbreaks and epidemics 1:637
  passive
    immunoprophylaxis 1:639
  pathology/histopathology 1:638
  prevention and control 1:639
  severity and factors
    affecting 1:637
  sporadic 1:637
  vaccines see under Hepatitis A
    virus (HAV)
Hepatitis A virus (HAV) 1:631–9
  antibodies 1:637, 1:638, 1:639
  antigenic site 1:631
  antigenic variability 1:636
  assembly and release 1:635
  attachment and entry 1:634
  cDNA clone (infectious) 1:631
  cell culture 1:631, 1:635–6
  cytopathic effects 1:635

Hepatitis A virus (HAV)
(continued)
DI particles 1:374
as enterovirus 72 2:737
epidemiology 1:637
evolution 1:636
food-borne 1:423
genetics 1:636
genome 1:631–2
3′NTR 1:632
5′NTR 1:632, 1:633(Table)
cloning 1:631
ORF 1:632
P2 region mutations 1:636
'pY1' 1:632
genome
organization 1:632(Table)
genotypes 1:636
geographic/seasonal
distribution 1:635
history 1:631
host range and
propagation 1:635–6
infection see Hepatitis A
internal ribosome entry site
(IRES) 1:632, 1:635
eIF-4G requirement 1:635
isolation in cell culture 1:635–6
maize chlorotic dwarf virus strain
TN (MCDV-TN)
vs 3:1967(Table)
mutations 1:636
pathogenicity 1:637–8
physical properties 1:634
polypeptides 1:631
1A 1:631
1B, 1C and 1D 1:631
cleavage 1:632
proteins 1:632–4
2A 1:633
2B and 2C 1:633
3A, 3B and 3C 1:633–4
functions 1:632–4
pX protein 1:631
receptor 1:634
replication 1:634–5
RNA synthesis 1:634–5
RNA encapsidation 1:634
serologic relationship 1:636
simian 'biotypes' 1:635
simian isolates 1:636
structure and properties 1:631
taxonomy and
classification 1:468, 1:631
tissue tropism 1:637
translation 1:635
GAPDH role 1:635
PTB role 1:635
transmission 1:485(Table), 1:637
vaccines 1:639
candidates 1:636, 1:639
viremia 1:637
VPg 1:631
Hepatitis B
acute 1:643
chronic 1:642, 1:643
hepatocellular carcinoma
and 3:1847
immune response 1:644
chronic active hepatitis 3:1830
clinical features 1:643
glomerulonephritis and nephrosis
with 2:1082
hepatitis delta virus infection
with 1:668
hepatocellular carcinoma
and 1:642, 1:643, 1:649,
3:1847
mechanism 3:1847
immune response 1:644
pathogenic mechanisms 1:643

Hepatitis B (continued)
pathology and
histopathology 1:644
post-transplant infections 3:1829
clinical features 3:1830–1
epidemiology and
pathogenesis 3:1830
incidence 3:1829
prevention 3:1831
treatment 3:1831
prevention and control 1:644
therapy
approved agents 1:57, 1:65–6
experimental agents 1:57, 1:66
interferon use 2:860
vaccines see under Hepatitis B
virus (HBV)
Hepatitis B immune globulin (H-
BIG) 1:65
Hepatitis B virus (HBV) 1:65,
1:640–5
antigens 1:642
apoptosis inhibition 1:72–3
apoptosis promotion 1:74
assembly and release 1:647–8
C-mRNA 1:649
carcinogenic mechanism 1:643,
1:649
carriers 1:65, 1:642, 1:643
chronic hepatitis see Hepatitis B
chronic liver cell necrosis
by 1:643
core antigen (HBcAg) 1:642,
1:645, 1:646, 1:664
antibodies 1:644
structure 1:646
Dane particle 1:640, 1:645, 1:648
assembly 1:648
delta virus with 1:664
see also Hepatitis delta virus
(HDV)
DNA integration
mechanism 1:649
DNA polymerase 1:645, 1:647
duck hepatitis B virus (DHBV) as
model 1:655, 1:656
e antigen (HBeAg) 1:642, 1:644,
1:646
structure 1:646
translation 1:649
envelope 1:645, 1:646, 1:647
epidemiology 1:642
future perspectives 1:644
genome 1:645–6
complete strand
(negative) 1:645, 1:647–8
covalently closed circular
(CCC) 1:647, 1:648
incomplete positive
strand 1:645
interrupted precore
antigen 1:374
map 1:646(Fig)
ORFs 1:646
relaxed circular (RC) 1:647
geographic/seasonal
distribution 1:641
hepatocellular carcinoma and see
under Hepatitis B
history 1:640
host range and propagation 1:641
immune complex disease 1:643
immunization 3:1831
infection see Hepatitis B
liver injury mechanism 1:643
molecular biology 1:645–50
nucleocapsid 1:645
pathogenicity 1:643
persistent infection 1:643
physical properties 1:646
precore polypeptide see Hepatitis
B virus (HBV), e antigen

Hepatitis B virus (HBV)
(continued)
pregenome 1:647
pregenomic (pg) RNA 1:647,
1:649
preS$_2$/S protein 3:1847
properties 1:645
proteins
L (pre-S1) and M (pre-
S2) 1:645, 1:646, 1:646–7
properties 1:646–7
S protein (HBsAg) see surface
antigen (HBsAg) (below)
pX 1:74, 1:647, 3:1847
as oncogene 1:72
p53 interaction 1:72
translation 1:649
reactivation 3:1830
receptors 1:647
replication 1:647–8
model 1:648(Fig)
negative-strand DNA 1:647–8
pancreas 2:1078
rev response element (RRE)
similarity 1:648
reverse transcriptase 1:647
RNA packaging 1:647
epsilon signal 1:648, 1:648(Fig)
screening for 1:644
subviral structures 1:645
surface antigen (HBsAg) 1:640,
1:642, 1:645, 1:646, 3:1829
antibodies 1:644
carriers 1:642
detection by enzyme
immunoassay 1:389
subtypes 1:642
taxonomy and
classification 1:640–1
tissue tropism 1:642–3, 1:647
transactivators 3:1847
transcription 1:647, 1:648–9
covalently closed circular
template 1:648–9
transformation by 3:1822
translation 1:646–7, 1:649
transmission 1:642
prevention 1:644
vaccination 3:1847
vaccines 1:65, 1:644, 2:723,
2:1204
history 3:1861
as universal childhood vaccine
in US 1:644
virion numbers in blood 1:645
X protein see Hepatitis B virus
(HBV), pX
X-mRNA 1:649
Hepatitis B viruses, avian 1:650–6
classification 1:650
DNA replication 1:650–1,
1:652(Fig)
epidemiology 1:654
evolution 1:653
future perspectives 1:656
genetics 1:653
genome 1:650–1
complete strand
(negative) 1:650
covalently closed
circular 1:650, 1:652(Fig),
1:656
incomplete strand
(positive) 1:650
ORFs 1:650
X ORF absence 1:650
geographic/seasonal
distribution 1:652–3
history 1:650
host range and propagation 1:653
infections
clinical features 1:654–5

Hepatitis B viruses, avian
(continued)
infections (continued)
immune response 1:655
pathology/histobiology 1:655
prevention and control 1:655–6
low mutation rate 1:653
pathogenicity 1:654–5
pregenome 1:650
proteins 1:651–2
replication 1:656
reverse transcription 1:650
serologic relationship and
variability 1:653–4
transmission and tissue
tropism 1:654
see also Duck hepatitis B virus
(DHBV)
Hepatitis C
chronic 1:662
clinical features 1:662
community-acquired 1:662
hepatocellular carcinoma
association 1:662, 3:1847
mechanism 3:1847
immune response 1:662–3
incidence 1:65
pathology/histopathology 1:662
post-transplant infections 3:1829
clinical features 3:1831
epidemiology and
pathogenesis 3:1830
incidence 3:1830
prevention 3:1831
treatment 3:1831
prevention and control 1:663
therapy
approved agents 1:57, 1:65–6
experimental agents 1:57, 1:66
Hepatitis C immune globulin (H-
CIG) 1:65
Hepatitis C virus (HCV) 1:65,
1:657–63
animal model 1:661, 1:663
antibodies
assays 3:1830
detection 1:391
antigenic differences 1:661
apoptosis inhibition 1:74, 3:1847
apoptosis promotion 1:75
assembly 1:659
autoimmune eye disease 1:524
carriers 1:65
cytoplasmic tubular
structures 1:659
detection methods 1:663
economic burden 1:662
emerging/re-emerging
virus 1:419(Table)
epidemiology 1:661–2
evolution 1:660–1
rate 1:660
future perspectives 1:663
genetics 1:660
genome 1:657
internal ribosomal entry
site 1:657
mutations 1:660
ORFs 1:657
genotypes 1:660, 1:661
geographic/seasonal
distribution 1:659, 1:661(Fig)
history 1:657
host range and
propagation 1:659–60
hypervariable regions 1:660,
1:662
immunization 3:1831
infection see Hepatitis C
pathogenicity 1:662
physical properties 1:659
polyprotein 1:657, 1:658(Fig)

Hepatitis C virus (HCV)
  (continued)
  post-transplant infection 3:1829
    see also Hepatitis C
  proteins 1:657–9
    envelope 1:658
    nonstructural 1:657, 1:659
    post-translational
      cleavage 1:659
    properties 1:657–9
    structural 1:657
  quasispecies 1:660
  ras oncogene and 3:1847
  reactivation 3:1830
  replication 1:659, 1:660
  screening for 1:663
  serine protease 1:66
  serologic relationships and
    variability 1:661
  structure and properties 1:657,
    1:658(Fig)
  subtypes 1:660
  taxonomy and
    classification 1:657
  tissue tropism 1:662
  transmission 1:661–2, 1:662
    by grafts 3:1830
  vaccine development 1:65, 1:663
  virus-like particles 1:658(Fig)
Hepatitis C-like viruses 1:174
Hepatitis delta virus (HDV) 1:664–
  9, 3:1608, 3:1613–14
  antibodies 1:668
  assembly 1:667
  cell lines 1:667
  delta antigen see Hepatitis delta
    virus (HDV), HDAg
  envelope 1:666
  epidemiology 1:667
  evolution 1:667
  future perspectives 1:668–9
  genetics 1:667
  genome 1:664, 1:665
    sequence 1:665
  genotypes 1:667
    distribution 1:664, 1:667
  geographic distribution 1:664
  HBV as helper virus 1:664
  HDAg 1:665, 1:665–6, 1:667,
    3:1614
    functional domains 1:666
    RNA encoding 1:666
    RNA-binding motif 1:666
    small and large species 1:665
  history 1:664
  host range and
    propagation 1:664–5
  infection
    clinical features 1:668
    in HBV carrier 1:668
    HBV with 1:668
    immune response 1:668
    pathology/
      histopathology 1:668
    prevention and control 1:668
  isolation/discovery 1:664
  mutation rates 1:667
  pathogenicity 1:667–8
    cytocidal 1:667
    immune-mediated 1:667–8
  properties 1:665
  protein 1:665, 1:665–6
    see also Hepatitis delta virus
      (HDV), HDAg
  pseudoknot ribozyme 3:1552,
    3:1558
  replication 1:666–7
    inhibition 1:668
  RNA 1:665(Fig)
    editing 1:666–7
    genomic-/antigenomic-
      sense 1:665, 1:666

Hepatitis delta virus (HDV)
  (continued)
  RNA (continued)
    replication 1:665–6, 1:666(Fig)
    ribozyme activity 1:665, 1:667
    viroids and 3:1931(Fig)
  as satellite-related agents 3:1613–
    14
  serologic relationships and
    variability 1:667
  taxonomy and
    classification 1:664
  transmission 1:667
Hepatitis E 1:672
  acute 1:673–4
  clinical course 1:674
  clinical features 1:673–4
  epidemics 1:669, 1:672(Fig), 1:673
  fulminant 1:674
  future perspectives 1:676
  history of outbreaks 1:669
  immune response 1:674–5
  immunodiagnosis 1:674–5
  imported cases 1:672, 1:673,
    1:676
  pathology/histopathology 1:674
  prevention and control 1:675–6
  serologic markers 1:674–5
  sporadic outbreaks 1:673
  vaccination, experimental 1:675–
    6
  vaccine development 1:675–6
    capsid protein 1:676
Hepatitis E virus (HEV) 1:218,
  1:669–76
  African strains 1:671
  animal reservoir 1:672
  Asian strains 1:671
  biophysical properties 1:670–1
  cDNA cloning 1:671
  discovery 1:669
  emerging/re-emerging
    virus 1:419(Table)
  epidemiology 1:673
  epitopes 1:674
  evolution 1:671–2, 1:672(Fig)
  excretion 1:673
  genetics 1:671–2
  genome organization 1:670(Fig)
  genome structure 1:671
    domains X and Y 1:671
    ORFs 1:671, 1:675(Fig)
  geographic heterogeneity 1:671–2
  HEVAg staining method 1:673
  history 1:669
  host range and
    propagation 1:672–3
  infection see Hepatitis E
  Mexico isolates 1:671
  nucleic acid diagnosis 1:675
  phylogeny 1:672(Fig)
  physiochemical properties 1:670–
    1
  proteins 1:671
  replication, sites 1:673
  strains 1:671
  structure and
    properties 1:670(Fig)
  subgenomic RNA
    transcripts 1:671
  taxonomy and
    classification 1:669
  tissue tropism 1:673
  transmission 1:673
    animal model 1:672
  viremia 1:673
Hepatitis E-like viruses 1:669
Hepatitis G virus (GBV-C) 1:660
Hepatitis viruses 1:65–6
  post-transplant infections 3:1829
  see also individual viruses
    (above)

Hepatocellular carcinoma 3:1847
  duck hepatitis B virus (DHBV)
    and 1:650, 1:654
  hepatitis B virus (HBV)
    and 1:642, 1:643, 1:649
  hepatitis C virus (HCV)
    and 1:662, 3:1847
Hepatocyte growth factor (HGF)
  receptors 3:1515
c-Sea protein 3:1514–15
Hepatocytes
  degeneration, in hepatitis E 1:674
  hepatitis C virus detection 1:659,
    1:660
Hepatoma see Hepatocellular
  carcinoma
Hepatopancreatic parvo-like virus
  (HPV) 3:1634–5
  structure and properties 3:1635
Hepatovirus 1:631, 2:1326
  hepatitis A virus (HAV) 1:631
HER agent 2:1174
Heracleum latent virus
  (HLV) 3:1838(Table)
  classification 3:1838, 3:1842
  coat protein 3:1839
  disease 3:1841
  geographic distribution 3:1838
  host range 3:1838
  host relations 3:1840
  serological relationships 3:1841
  transmission 3:1840
Heracleum virus 6 (HV6) 3:1840
Herd immunity 1:486
Heron hepatitis B virus 1:650
  epidemiology 1:654
  serologic relationship and
    variability 1:654
  transmission and tissue
    tropism 1:653, 1:654
Herpangina 1:308
  echoviruses causing 1:415
Herpes dermatitis 2:680
Herpes genitalis 1:61
Herpes labialis (cold sores) 1:61,
  2:680
'Herpes pac homology'
  sequence 1:355
Herpes saimiri see Herpesvirus
  saimiri
Herpes simplex virus (HSV) 2:677–
  86
  α0 null mutants 2:693
  alkaline exonuclease gene 2:694
  anti-PKR mechanisms 2:860
  assembly and release 2:678,
    2:695–6
  attachment and entry 2:694–5
  budding 2:678, 2:678(Fig)
  capsid 2:677, 2:677(Fig), 2:686
    formation 2:693–4, 2:695
    hexons and pentons 2:686
    proteins 2:693
  cell lines 2:678
  characteristics 2:678
  core 2:677
  cytopathology 2:696
  detection, ELVIS method 1:398
  DNA 2:677
    episomal 2:682, 2:696
    packaging 2:694, 2:695–6
    U_L 2:677
    U_S 2:677
  DNA binding protein 2:693
  DNA polymerase 2:693
  DNA replication 2:695, 2:697
    effect on HSV gene
      expression 2:697
    role in productive cycle 2:695
    effect on nuclear membrane 2:696
  envelope 2:677, 2:677(Fig), 2:686

Herpes simplex virus (HSV)
  (continued)
  future perspectives/trends 2:685–
    6, 2:697
  genes 2:677
    α22 2:694
    classes 2:678
    early 2:678
    functions of each 2:691(Table)
    ICP34.5 2:688
    immediate early 2:678, 2:690
    late 2:678
    RR1 2:678, 2:682, 2:684
  genetic map 2:687(Fig)
  genetics 2:679
  genome 2:686–90
    'a' sequences 2:687
    arrangement 2:686–8
    circularization 2:686
    long repeat 2:688
    ORFs 2:687, 2:688–9
    sequence 2:686
    sequence inversions 2:688
    short repeats 2:688
    unique long region (U_L) 2:688
    unique short region (U_S) 2:688
  glycoproteins 2:678, 2:686, 2:693,
    2:694
    for HSV internalization 2:694
    VSV homologues 3:1879
  helicase/primase, inhibitor 1:62
  history 2:677
  host range 2:678
  host shut-off protein 2:695
  immune evasion
    mechanism 2:1204
  immunity 2:684
  infection see Herpes simplex
    virus (HSV) infection
  latency 2:682–3
  latency-associated transcripts
    (LAT) 2:688, 2:689, 2:697,
    2:899, 2:1200
    primary 2:697
    promoter 2:689, 2:690(Fig),
    2:696
  latent infections 2:696–7, 2:899–
    900
    establishment 2:696, 2:899
    maintenance 2:696, 2:899–900
    mechanism 2:899
    lytic cycle 2:899
    maturation 2:693–4
    modification of nuclear
      compartmentalization 2:695
    molecular biology 2:686–97
    mRNAs 2:688
      α0 2:697
    neoplastic transformation 2:684
    neurotropism 2:697
    pathogenicity 2:680, 2:899
    persistence, sites 2:686
    physical properties 2:694
    post-translational
      processing 2:695
    promoters 2:688–9
      LATs 2:689, 2:690(Fig), 2:696
    productive cycle 2:689(Fig)
      TATA box homologies 2:688
    properties and structure 2:686
    proteins 2:678, 2:686, 2:690–4
      α0 protein 2:693
      α4 protein 2:690–3, 2:695
      α27 protein 2:693
      α47 protein 2:694
      αTIF 2:690, 2:693, 2:695
      β proteins 2:693
      βγ 2:693
      capsid formation and
        maturation 2:693–4
      for DNA replication 2:693

Herpes simplex virus (HSV) (continued)
proteins (continued)
functional classification 2:690–4
functions of specific proteins 2:691(Table)
ICP0 and ICP4 2:899
ICP27 2:689
ICP34.5 2:694, 2:695
ICP47 2:678
immediate early 2:690–3, 2:694
nomenclature and properties 2:690
in pathogenesis/cytopathology 2:694
regulatory 2:690–3, 2:697
scaffolding 2:694, 2:695
sizes 2:690
structural 2:693
tegument 2:686
VSV homologues 3:1878, 3:1879, 3:1880(Table)
reactivation 2:682, 2:696, 3:1828
stimuli 2:682
triggers 2:696
receptors and co-receptors 2:1181
recurrent lesions 2:682
replication 2:678, 2:694–6
origins 2:689–90
sites 2:682, 2:697
replication-defective 2:696
ribonucleoside reductase inhibitor (348U87) 1:62
serologic relationships 2:678–9
shedding 2:685
spread through nerves 2:1179
nonstructural proteins effect 2:1180
taxonomy and classification 2:677–8
tegument 2:677, 2:686, 2:693
in HSV assembly 2:696
thymidine kinase 2:693
inhibitor 1:62
tissue tropism 2:680, 2:697
transcription
cis-acting sequences 2:688
enhancement 2:688
map 2:687(Fig), 2:688
regulation 2:695
TATGARAT sequence role 2:688, 2:690
transcriptional activator (α4 protein) 2:690–3
transcripts 2:688–9
latent-phase 2:697
splicing 2:689
see also latency-associated transcripts (above)
translation 2:695
transmission 1:485(Table), 2:680
vaccines 2:685
gd-2 gene 2:685
novel vectors 2:685
as vector 3:1889
helper-dependent 3:1889
for vaccines 2:697
see also Herpes simplex virus 1 (HSV-1); Herpes simplex virus 2 (HSV-2)
Herpes simplex virus 1 (HSV-1)
apoptosis inhibition 1:73
apoptosis promotion 1:74–5
dominant-negative mutants 2:853
encephalitis 679–80
evolution 3:1873–4
genome
LAT 2:682
ORFs 2:678, 2:682
sequence 2:678
ICP4 1:73

Herpes simplex virus 1 (HSV-1) (continued)
immune response 2:684
infection route 2:680
infections
acute rhinitis 2:681
clinical features 2:680–1
epidemiology 2:679
eye 1:526, 2:681
genital 2:680
oral 2:679, 2:680
pathology 2:683–4
sites 2:679
skin 2:678, 2:680–1
late γ34.5 gene 1:73
ocular target 1:527(Table)
proteins
HHV-6 and HHV-7 protein similarity 2:699
VSV homologues 3:1879
reactivation 2:680
mechanism 2:682
RRI PK 2:684
shedding 2:680
terminal consensus sequence 3:1835
transmission 2:680
US3 gene 1:73
Herpes simplex virus 2 (HSV-2)
acyclovir resistance 2:681, 2:681(Fig), 2:685
DNA, oncogene 2:684
evolution 3:1873–4
factors influencing acquisition 2:679
genome 2:678
HIV-1 and HTLV-1 infection with 2:679
immune response 2:684
infections
CNS 2:681
epidemiology 2:679
female 2:681
fetal 2:679
genital 2:679, 2:681, 2:681(Fig)
male 2:681
meningitis 2:681
mucosal 2:678
ocular 1:526
pathology 2:678(Fig), 2:683–4
latency 2:682(Fig)
neoplastic transformation 2:684
ocular target 1:527(Table)
oncogenicity, concerns over long-term therapy 2:685
reactivation 2:682(Fig)
replication sites 2:680
RR1 PK 2:682, 2:682(Fig), 2:684
RAS signaling pathway activation 2:682, 2:683(Fig)
shedding 2:679, 2:680
terminal consensus sequence 3:1835
transmission 2:680
vertical 2:679, 2:680
Herpes simplex virus (HSV) infection 1:61
acyclovir-resistance 3:1829
in chimpanzees 2:707, 2:708
clinical features 2:680–2, 3:1828
CNS 2:680
encephalitis 2:679–80, 2:681, 2:1018
epidemiology 2:679–80
eye infections 1:523, 1:527, 2:678
immune response 2:684
neonatal 2:683
prevention and therapy 2:685
pathology 2:683–4
pharyngitis 2:1492
post-transplant 3:1828–9
clinical features 3:1828–9

Herpes simplex virus (HSV) infection (continued)
post-transplant (continued)
epidemiology 3:1828
incidence 3:1828
pathogenesis 3:1828
treatment 3:1829
in pregnancy 2:683
prevention and therapy 2:685
therapy
approved agents 1:55–6(Table), 1:62
experimental agents 1:55–6(Table), 1:62
visceral dissemination 3:1829
see also Herpes simplex virus 1 (HSV-1); Herpes simplex virus 2 (HSV-2)
Herpes viruses see Herpesviruses
Herpes zoster ophthalmicus 1:526, 1:529
Herpes zoster (shingles) 1:61
clinical features 3:1876
complications 3:1876
disseminated 3:1875(Fig), 3:1876
epidemiology 3:1874, 3:1874(Fig)
eye involvement 1:526
geographic and seasonal distribution 3:1873
history 3:1872
immune response 3:1876
pathogenesis 3:1875
pathology and histology 3:1876
post-transplant 3:1828
prevention and control 3:1876–7, 3:1877
transmission 3:1874
see also Varicella-zoster virus (VZV)
Herpesviridae 3:1872
Alphaherpesvirinae see Alphaherpesvirinae
amphibian herpesviruses 1:51, 1:51–3
apoptosis inhibition 1:73
apoptosis promotion 1:74–5
baboon and chimpanzee herpesviruses 2:707–14
see also Herpesviruses, baboon and chimpanzee
Betaherpesvirinae see Betaherpesvirinae
bovine herpesviruses 1:180–4
characteristics 2:707
classification 2:707, 2:708
equine herpesviruses 1:508–15
Gammaherpesvirinae see Gammaherpesvirinae
herpesvirus ateles 2:714
herpesvirus saimiri 2:714
Ictalurovirus 1:553
Marek's disease virus 2:945–52
Rhadinovirus 2:718
tree shrew 3:1834–7
see also Herpesviruses
Herpesvirus 6 see Human herpesvirus 6 (HHV-6)
Herpesvirus 7 see Human herpesvirus 7 (HHV-7)
Herpesvirus ateles 1 (HVA-1) 2:714
nomenclature 2:714–15
serological relationship 2:715
unclassified 2:715
Herpesvirus ateles 2 (HVA-2) 2:714–18
antibodies 2:717
future perspectives 2:718
as gene vector 2:718
genome 2:717
growth/propagation in laboratory 2:717–18
history 2:714–15

Herpesvirus ateles 2 (HVA-2) (continued)
host range 2:714
immune response to 2:717
nomenclature 2:714–15
serological relationship 2:715
structure and properties 2:715–16
taxonomy and classification 2:715, 2:717
transformation-associated genes 2:718
transmission 2:716–17
Herpesvirus cercopithecus 2 (SA8) 2:707, 2:708
classification 2:708
epidemiology 2:711
genetics 2:710
geographic/seasonal distribution 2:709
host range and propagation 2:709
infection
clinical features 2:712
immune response 2:713
pathology/histopathology 2:712
pathogenicity 2:711
serologic relationship and variability 2:710
transmission 2:711
Herpesvirus pan 2:707, 2:708
characteristics 2:708
epidemiology 2:711
future perspectives 2:713
genetics 2:709–10
geographic/seasonal distribution 2:709
host range and propagation 2:709
infection
clinical features 2:712
pathology/histopathology 2:712
prevention and control 2:713
serologic relationship and variability 2:710
tissue tropism 2:711
transmission 2:711
Herpesvirus papio 2:707, 2:708
cell transformation by 2:709
characteristics 2:708
epidemiology 2:710
future perspectives 2:713
genetics 2:709–10
geographic/seasonal distribution 2:709
host range and propagation 2:709
infection 2:713
clinical features 2:712
pathology/histopathology 2:712
prevention and control 2:713
lymphocyte infection 2:711
pathogenicity 2:711
serologic relationship and variability 2:710
simian T-cell leukemia virus (STLV-1) relationship 2:710
tissue tropism 2:711
transmission 2:711
Herpesvirus papio 2 (HVP-2) 2:707, 2:708
classification 2:708
epidemiology 2:711
genetics 2:710
host range and propagation 2:709
infection
clinical features 2:712
immune response 2:713
pathology/histopathology 2:712
pathogenicity 2:711
serologic relationship and variability 2:710

Herpesvirus papio 2 (HVP-2) (continued)
  transmission 2:711
Herpesvirus platyrrhinae (HVP) 2:715
Herpesvirus saimiri 1 (HVS-1) 2:714
  nomenclature 2:714–15
  serological relationship 2:715
Herpesvirus saimiri 2 (HVS-2) 2:714–18
  antibodies 2:717
  future perspectives 2:718
  as gene vector 2:718
  genome 2:715–16
    H-DNA 2:715–16
    M genome 2:715–16
  growth/propagation in laboratory 2:717–18
  history 2:714–15
  host range 2:714, 2:715
  immune response to 2:717
  intrastrain variation 2:717
  isolates, SMKI-83 2:717–18
  latency 2:715
  nomenclature 2:714–15, 2:717
  permanent cell lines 2:718
  persistence 2:716
  serological relationship 2:715
  structure and properties 2:715–16
  taxonomy and classification 2:715
  transformation by 2:716
  transformation-associated genes 2:718
  transmission 2:716–17
Herpesvirus saimiri
  apoptosis inhibition 1:73
  ORF16 1:73
Herpesvirus salmonis 1:553
  see also Salmonid herpesvirus 1 (SalHV-1)
Herpesvirus sylvilagus 2:703–6
  classification 2:703–4
  future perspectives 2:706
  genome 2:705
    latent episomal form 2:705
    organization 2:704(Fig)
    structure 2:704
  geographic distribution 2:704
  history 2:703
  host range 2:705
  infection
    clinical features 2:705
    immune response 2:706
    lymphoproliferative disease 2:705
    pathogenicity 2:705
    prevalence 2:704
    treatment 2:706
  macrophage-like cell immortalization 2:705–6
  propagation 2:705
  proteins 2:704
  replication 2:705, 2:706
  transforming ability 2:706
  transmission 2:705
Herpesvirus tamarinus (HVT) 2:714
Herpesvirus of turkeys (HVT) 2:945–6
  cell culture 2:948
  classification 2:946
  distribution 2:948
  epizootiology 2:948
  genome 2:946–7
  isolation and propagation 2:947–8
  physical properties 2:947
  productive/nonproductive infections 2:947
  proteins 2:947

Herpesvirus of turkeys (HVT) (continued)
  replication 2:947
  semiproductive infections 2:947
  transmission and risk factors 2:948
  see also Marek's disease virus (MDV)
Herpesvirus-associated ubiquitin specific protease (HAUSP) 2:693
Herpesviruses
  amphibian see Amphibian herpesviruses
  in Bovidae 1:181(Table)
  class E isomerizing genome 1:352
  crossing species barrier 2:707
  diversity 2:707
  fish see Fish herpesviruses
  gamma-2 2:715
  genome groups 1:363
  group F genome 1:363
  infections
    eye 1:523, 1:526, 1:527(Table)
    interferon use 2:861
    latent infections 2:897–900
    lymphoproliferative 2:707
      EBV relationship 2:707
      see also Gammaherpesvirinae
  MHC-like molecules, autoimmunity mechanism 1:112
  pathogenicity 1:618(Table)
  pongine 2:708
  post-transplant infections 3:1823–9
    see also Epstein–Barr virus (EBV); Herpes simplex virus (HSV); Human cytomegalovirus (HCMV); Varicella Zoster virus (VZV)
  T lymphocyte tropic 2:715
  therapy 1:61–3
    approved agents 1:62
    experimental agents 1:62
  tree shrews see Tupaia herpesvirus 1 (THV-1); Tupaia herpesvirus 2 (THV-2)
  as vectors 3:1889
    helper-dependent/helper-independent 3:1889
  see also Herpesviridae
Herpesviruses, baboon and chimpanzee 2:707–14, 3:1873
  antibodies 2:708(Table)
  baboon viruses 2:707–8
  cell cultures 2:707
  classification 2:707, 2:708
  crossing species barrier 2:707
  EBV comparison 2:709, 2:709–10, 2:710
  epidemiology 2:710–11
  evolution 2:710
  future perspectives 2:713–14
  genetics 2:709–10
  geographic/seasonal distribution 2:709
  history 2:707
  host range and propagation 2:709
  infection
    clinical features 2:712
    immune response 2:712–13
    pathology/histopathology 2:712
    prevention and control 2:713
    pathogenicity 2:711
  pongine 2:708
  serologic relationship and variability 2:710

Herpesviruses, baboon and chimpanzee (continued)
  taxonomy and classification 2:708–9
  transmission and tissue tropism 2:711
  xenotransplantation concerns 2:714
Herpetic whitlow 2:681
[Het-S] 3:1406
  features 3:1406
  genetic properties indicating 3:1406
  as prion form of het-s protein 3:1406
  reverse curability 3:1406
het-s protein
  features 3:1406
  see also [Het-s]; Heterokaryon incompatibility
Heterokaryon 3:1406
  formation 3:1406
Heterokaryon incompatibility 3:1406, 3:1406(Fig)
  definition 3:1406
  genetic control 3:1406
  het genes 3:1406
  het-s strains and prion form 3:1406
Heteropolyploid viruses 1:611
Hexamers 3:1949
Hexons 1:16, 3:1945
  peripentonal 1:16
Hibiscus chlorotic ringspot virus (HCRSV) 1:244
Hibiscus latent ringspot virus 2:1008(Table)
High Point virus 2:733
Highlands J virus 1:502, 1:503
  epidemiology 1:505
  evolution 1:504
  pathogenicity 1:506
Highly active antiretroviral therapy (HAART) 1:58, 2:773, 2:787
  drugs included 1:58
  interleukin-2 with 1:61
  US DHHS guidelines 1:58, 1:59
  viral replication reduced 1:58
Himetobi P virus (HiPV) 2:1273
Hirame rhabdovirus (HIRRV) 3:1544
Histiocytes, in Yabapox virus infections 3:1973
Histones 1:255
  polyomavirus DNA 2:1356
  SV40 DNA association 3:1648
History of virology 2:718–25
  animal viruses 2:721–3
    biochemistry 2:722
    cultivation 2:721–2
    purification 2:722
    structure 2:722
    see also Coxsackieviruses; Echoviruses; Poliovirus
  bacterial viruses 2:720–1, 2:721, 2:725–30
    discovery 2:720, 2:725–6, 2:727–8
    lysogeny 2:721
    molecular biology/genetics 2:721
    Phage Group 2:720–1, 2:728
    phage therapy 2:725, 2:726–7, 2:729–30
    phage therapy in animals 2:729
    process of infection of bacteria 2:721
  chemical composition 2:720
  early investigations 2:719
  future perspectives 2:724–5
  immunology 2:723

History of virology (continued)
  invertebrate viruses 2:723
  origin of term 'virus' 2:719
  physical studies 2:720
  plant viruses 2:723–4
    transmission 2:724
    types 2:724
    taxonomy and nomenclature 2:724
  tissue culture 2:721–2
  tumor virology 2:722–3
  use of animals for virus research 2:721
  vaccines and disease control 2:723
  virus structure 2:720
'Hit and run' oncogenesis mechanism 3:1842
HIV (HIV-1) 1:54–8, 2:763–73, 2:774–8
  AIDS pathogenesis 2:771–2
  ancillary genes 2:777–8
  animal models 1:535, 1:540
  antibodies, detection methods 1:391
  apoptosis induced by/promotion 1:75–6, 3:1960
  assembly and release 2:764–5, 2:777
  attached to follicular dendritic cells (FDCs) 2:814–15
  attachment and entry 2:774–6
  bovine immunodeficiency virus (BIV) relationship 1:186, 1:186(Fig), 1:188
  budding 2:777
  cardiac disease due to 2:1075–6
  cardiomyopathy in infancy 2:1075
  CD4 receptor see HIV (HIV-1), receptor
  clades 2:770
  co-receptors 2:768, 2:774–5, 2:779, 2:1181
    action 2:775–6
    as drug targets 2:786
    in vesicular stomatitis virus clones 3:1919
  cross-reactions 1:188
  cytotoxic T cells (CTLs) specific for 3:1863
  detection, lymphocyte cultures 1:398–9
  DI particles 1:374
  differentiation with HIV-2 2:771
  DNA synthesis 2:765
  dominant-negative mutants 2:853
  drug resistance 2:787
    AZT 1:58
    ddC 1:59
    protease inhibitors 2:785, 2:785(Fig)
    reverse transcriptase inhibitors 2:781–3, 2:782(Fig)
  as emerging and new virus 1:418, 1:419(Table), 1:421
  env glycoprotein 2:766, 2:768, 2:814–15
  env recombinant, vaccinia virus-based 3:1888
  envelope, as drug target 2:779, 2:786
  evolution 3:1643
  fusion of membrane with cell membrane 2:768, 2:775
  gag gene 2:778
    conservation 2:769
    as drug target 2:778
  Gag polyprotein 2:767, 2:777
    cleavage 2:777
    function 2:764
  Gag protein 2:766, 2:767–8

HIV (HIV-1) (continued)
  gag-pol polyproteins 1:60, 2:777
  gene expression 2:776–7
    regulation 2:765–7
  genes 2:774
  genetic diversity 2:770
  genetic variability 2:769
  genetics 2:769–70
  genome 2:765, 2:766(Fig), 2:774, 2:775(Fig), 2:778–9
    cis-acting elements 2:765, 2:774
    differential splicing 2:774
    drug targets 2:778–9
    HIV-1 and HIV-2 comparison 2:766(Fig)
    long terminal repeats 2:765, 2:776, 2:1182
    long terminal repeats promoter 2:766
    polypurine tract 2:765
    splice donor (SD) and acceptor (SA) 2:776
  geographic distribution 2:770
  gp41 2:768
    potential drug target 2:786
    T-20 2:786
  gp120 2:768
    MHC interaction 3:1926
  history 2:763–4
  host range 2:771
  infection route 2:1177
  influence on antiviral development 1:54
  integrase 2:765, 2:776
    functions 2:783
    inhibitors 2:783
  integration 2:765, 2:987
    process 2:776
  interaction with immune system 2:772
  isolates 2:770
  latency and chronic infections 2:1200
  maturation 2:774
  molecular biology 2:774–8
  morphogenesis 2:764–5
  mRNA 2:776–7
  mRNA processing 2:777
    regulation 2:766–7
  nef gene 2:778, 2:779
    deletions 1:374
  Nef protein 2:768–9, 2:777, 2:778
    CD4 T cell activation 2:768–9
    costimulation of T cells 2:769
    as drug target 2:786
    functions 2:768–9, 2:778
    nuclear export signals (NES) 2:765
  nucleocapsid protein (NCP7), as drug target 2:785–6
  origin 2:770
  p24, structure 3:1955(Fig)
  pathogenicity 2:779
  physical properties 2:765, 2:774
  pol gene 2:779
    conservation 2:769
  Pol protein 2:766, 2:767–8
  polypurine tract 2:776
  Pr55^{gag} 2:777
  preintegration complex 2:775
    transport to nucleus 2:775
  promoters 2:766
  protease 1:60, 2:779, 2:783
    atomic structure 3:1944
    inhibitors see Protease inhibitors
    structure 2:783
  proviral DNA 2:765, 2:776
  receptor 1:250, 2:768, 2:774–5, 2:779, 2:1181, 3:1921, 3:1926
    cDNA 2:1181

HIV (HIV-1) (continued)
  receptor (continued)
    co-receptors see HIV (HIV-1), co-receptors
    therapeutic strategies 1:61
    in vesicular stomatitis virus (VSV) clones 3:1919
  receptor-binding antagonist 1:61
  replication 1:54, 1:57, 2:774
    Nef role 2:778
  rev gene, function 2:779
  Rev protein 2:766–7, 2:776, 3:1477
    as drug target 2:786
  rev response element (RRE) 2:776
    HBV factor similarity 1:648
    structure 2:766
  reverse transcriptase (RT) 2:776, 2:779
    as drug target 2:779
    error rates 2:776
    inhibitors see Reverse transcriptase inhibitors
    lysine tRNA as primer 2:765, 2:774
    mutations and drug resistance 2:781–2, 2:782–3, 2:782(Fig)
    p66 and p51 subunits 2:779
    structure 2:779
  reverse transcription 2:765–6, 2:776
    efficiency/errors 2:765
  spread in bloodstream 2:1178
  structural proteins 2:767–9, 2:767(Table)
    HIV-1 and HIV-2 comparison 2:767(Table)
    precursors 2:767
    see also specific proteins (above/below)
  structure and properties 2:764, 2:764(Fig), 2:774
  SU glycoprotein 2:774
  T cell epitopes 3:1863
  TAR (trans-acting response element) 2:776
  tat gene
    defective 1:374
    function 2:779
  Tat protein 2:776, 3:1477
    actions 1:76
    cofactors 2:766
    as drug target 2:786
    expression 2:776
    trans-activation of JC virus late promoter 2:881
    transactivation by 2:776
    transcription regulation 2:766
  taxonomy and classification 2:764
  trans-esterification reaction 2:776
  transcription 2:765–6, 2:776
    activators 2:765
    crosstransactivation of HIV-1/HIV-2 2:766
    see also HIV (HIV-1), reverse transcription
  transcriptional regulation 2:766
    negative elements (NREs) 2:765
  transmission 1:485(Table), 2:771
    perinatal 2:787
    prevention 2:773
    sexual 2:771
    vertical 2:771
  vif gene 2:777
  Vif protein 2:769, 2:777
    defective 2:777
  vpr gene 1:76, 2:777
  Vpr protein 2:769, 2:777, 2:777–8
    functions 2:769, 2:777
  vpu gene 2:778

HIV (HIV-1) (continued)
  Vpu protein 2:769, 2:778
    functions 2:769, 2:778
  vpx gene 2:777–8
  Vpx protein 2:769, 2:778
    functions 2:778
HIV infection
  acute, transcripts produced 2:766, 2:767
  astrovirus infections, diarrhea 1:107
  cardiac disease due to, dilated cardiomyopathy 2:1076
  cell-mediated immune response 2:822–3
  chemoprophylaxis 2:787
  copy number of viral DNA 2:765
  cures 2:787
  dementia mechanism 1:76
  enteropathy 1:447
  epidemic 2:770
  epidemiology, sex differences 2:1183
  HSV-2 infection associated 2:679
  human CMV infection in 1:349
  immune response 2:772
  immunization, gp160 and T cell memory 2:822
  immunosuppression by 2:816
  latency 2:772
  natural history 2:771
  nephropathy 2:1082
  neural cell damage 2:1017
  neurological features 2:772, 2:1019, 2:1019(Fig)
  number of infected persons 2:770
  ocular disease 1:526
  ocular target 1:525(Table)
  opportunistic ocular infections 1:529
  pandemic 2:770
  prevention and control 2:773, 2:778–88
  primary infection 2:771–2
  progressive multifocal leukoencephalopathy (PML) 2:882
  renal involvement 2:1082
  resistance to 2:773
  retinopathy 1:528–9
  serologic relationships 2:770–1
  therapy 2:772–3
    antiviral agents 2:772–3
    approved agents 1:55, 1:58–60
    changing in suspected failure 2:787
    combination 1:54, 2:773, 2:783
    experimental agents 1:55, 1:60–1
    goal 1:58
    initiation 2:786–7
    monotherapy 2:772
    new drug targets 1:54–7
    recommended regimen 2:787
    see also Antiretroviral agents
  thyroid involvement 2:1085
  vaccines 1:61
    development 2:773
    effectiveness limitations 2:822
  see also AIDS
HIV protease inhibitors see Protease inhibitors
HIV-1 see HIV (HIV-1)
HIV-2
  differentiation with HIV-1 2:771
  as emerging and new virus 1:419(Table), 1:421
  evolution 3:1643
  genetics 2:770
  genome 2:765, 2:766(Fig)
  geographic distribution 2:770
  history 2:764, 2:770

HIV-2 (continued)
  host range 2:771
  structure and properties 2:764, 2:764(Fig)
Hivid see ddC (Zalcitabine)
HLA, insulin-dependent diabetes mellitus 2:1080
HMC 2:761
  DNA containing, restriction 2:761
Hodgkin's disease 1:488(Table)
  clinical features 1:492
  EBV infection association 1:490–1, 3:1844
  pathology/histopathology 1:493
  treatment 1:494
Hodgkin's-like disease, Tupaia herpesvirus-associated 3:1834, 3:1836, 3:1837
Hog cholera
  chronic 2:741
  clinical features 2:741
  congenital 2:740, 2:741
  congenital persistent 2:742
  epidemics 2:739
  epidemiology 2:740
  eradication programs 2:742
  history 2.738
  immune response 2:742
  late-onset 2:741
  pathology/histopathology 2:741
  postnatal infection 2:740
  prevention and control 2:742
  rapid diagnosis 2:742
  vaccination 2:742, 2:743
    large-scale programs 2:742
Hog cholera virus (HCV) 2:738–43
  antibodies 2:742
  bovine virus diarrhea virus (BVDV)
    differentiation 2:742
    similarity 2:740
  economic significance 2:742–3
  epidemiology 2:740
  eradication program 2:739
  fringe-like projections 2:738
  future perspectives 2:742–3
  genetics and evolution 2:740
  genome properties 2:739
  geographic/seasonal distribution 2:739
  high-virulent strains 2:740
  history 2:738
  host range and propagation 2:739–40, 2:741
  infection see Hog cholera
  infection route 2:740
  intermediate-virulent strains 2:741
  low-virulent strains 2:740, 2:741
  pathogenicity 2:741
  physical properties 2:739
  proteins 2:739
    E1 and E2 2:739
    E^{rns} 2:739
    N^{pro} (protease) 2:739
    p7 2:739
  serologic relationships and variability 2:740
  structure and properties 2:738–9
  taxonomy and classification 2:738
  tissue tropism 2:740–1
  transmission 2:740, 2:740–1
    oronasal 2:740
  vaccines and strains for 2:742
  virulence 2:741
  see also Classical swine fever virus (CSFV)
Holin 2:1259
  bacteriophage P1 1:457
  bacteriophage P22 3:1605

Holin (continued)
  phage release 3:1415
Holliday structure 1:283
Homosexual men
  hepatitis A virus
    transmission 1:637
  HPV infections 2:1109
  HSV-2 infection 2:679, 2:681
Honey bee
  ilarvirus transmission 1:43
  paralysis 2:743, 2:745
  sacbrood see Sacbrood
Honey bee viruses 2:743–9
  acute paralysis virus
    (APV) 2:744(Table), 2:746–7
  Apis iridescent virus
    (AIV) 2:744(Table), 2:748–9
  Arkansas bee virus
    (ABV) 2:744(Table), 2:749
  bee virus X (BVX) 2:744(Table), 2:748
  bee virus Y (BVY) 2:744(Table), 2:748
  Berkeley bee virus 2:744(Table), 2:749
  Black Queen cell virus
    (BQCV) 2:744(Table), 2:747
  characteristics 2:743
  chronic paralysis
    virus 2:744(Table), 2:745–6
  chronic paralysis virus (CPV)
  chronic paralysis virus associate
    (CPVA) 2:744(Table), 2:745–6
  cloudy wing virus
    (CWV) 2:744(Table), 2:748
  deformed wing virus
    (DWV) 2:744(Table), 2:747
  Egypt bee virus
    (EBV) 2:744(Table), 2:747
  filamentous virus
    (FV) 2:744(Table), 2:748
  future perspectives 2:749
  history 2:743
  Kashmir bee virus
    (KBV) 2:744(Table), 2:747
  physicochemical
    properties 2:743–5
  properties 2:744(Table)
  sacbrood 2:744(Table), 2:746
  slow paralysis virus
    (SPV) 2:744(Table), 2:747
  see also individual viruses
Hop latent viroid 3:1930(Table)
Hop stunt viroid
    (HSVd) 3:1930(Table)
  epidemiology 3:1933
  geographic distribution 3:1932
  host range and
    transmission 3:1932
Hop trefoil cryptic virus 1
    (HTCV1) 1:314
Hop trefoil cryptic virus 2
    (HTCV2) 1:314
Hop trefoil cryptic virus 3
    (HTCV3) 1:314
Hop virus C 1:38
Hordeivirus 2:749
  benyviruses comparison 1:155
Hordeiviruses 2:749–53
  coat proteins 2:749
  cytopathology 2:752
  economic significance 2:750
  future perspectives 2:752
  genome organization 2:750, 2:751(Table)
  genome structure 2:750–1
    α RNA 2:750
    β RNA 2:750, 2:750–1
    distinguishing features 2:750–1
    γ RNA 2:750
  host range 2:750

Hordeiviruses (continued)
  molecular biology 2:751–2
  pathogenicity 2:752
  physical properties 2:750
  proteins 2:750–1
    αa 2:752
    βa (coat protein) 2:751
    βb 2:751, 2:751–2
    βc and βd 2:752
    γa and γb 2:750, 2:751
  replication 2:752
  taxonomy and
    classification 2:749–50
  triple gene block 2:750
  see also Barley stripe mosaic
    virus (BSMV)
Hormone-response element (HRE)
  see under Mouse mammary
    tumor virus (MMTV)
Hormones, effect on viral infection
    outcome 2:1183
Horse-flies, equine infectious
    anemia virus (EIAV)
    transmission 1:519, 1:521
Horseradish curly top virus
    (HrCTV), genome
    organization/expression 1:598
Horseradish latent virus
    (HRLV) 2:1276
Horses
  abortions 1:508, 1:512, 1:513
  Borna disease virus
    infection 1:169, 1:170, 1:172
  equine arteritis virus (EAV) 1:93
  influenza virus infection, clinical
    features 2:828
  orthopoxvirus infections 1:304
  Venezuelan equine encephalitis
    see Venezuelan equine
    encephalitis (VEE)
  vesicular stomatitis 3:1918
  see also entries beginning Equine;
    Equine arteritis virus (EAV)
Host
  cytoskeletal changes see
    Cytoskeleton
  defense
    interferons 3:1961
    respiratory tract
      mechanisms 3:1490(Fig)
    see also Immune response
  DNA degradation
    T1-like phage infection 3:1702, 3:1704(Fig)
    T4-like phages infection 3:1706
    T5-like phage 3:1719
  DNA synthesis, effects of virus
    infection 3:1958
  effects of virus infection 3:1958–60
  factors affecting tropism of
    viruses 2:1182–3
  gene transcription, bovine
    leukemia virus (BLV)
    affecting 1:196
  'helper' functions for plant
    viruses 2:1303
  hypovirus-mediated phenotype
    alteration 2:806
  inclusion bodies see Inclusion
    bodies
  macromolecular shutdown
    effects of virus infection 3:1958
    frog virus 3 (FV3) 1:584, 1:585
    HSV 2:695
    iridoviruses 2:867
    by phage 3:1414
    Semliki Forest virus
      (SFV) 3:1661–2
    Sindbis (SIN) virus 3:1661–2
    SPO1 phage 3:1684
    T1-like phage 3:1701

Host (continued)
  membranes
    effects of virus
      infection 3:1959–60
    phases of damage by
      viruses 3:1959
    see also Plasma membrane
  metabolism changes, human
    CMV infection 1:356
  mitochondrial modification by
    badnaviruses 2:1298
  morphology and viability, virus
    infection effect 3:1958
  mRNA degradation, T4-like
    phages infection 3:1706
  nuclear compartmentalization,
    HSV-induced
    modification 2:695
  protein synthesis
    shutdown 3:1473
    bacteriophage SPO1 1:132
    cardioviruses 1:234–5
    cricket paralysis virus
      (CrPV) 2:1271
    echoviruses 1:411
    effects of virus
      infection 3:1958–9
    foot-and-mouth disease
      virus 1:571
    polioviruses 2:1344
  range, changes contributing to
    emerging viral
    diseases 1:420–1
  resistance to virus
    infections 3:1960–1
    see also Host genetic resistance
  RNA synthesis shutdown 3:1473
    bacteriophage SPO1 1:132
    cardioviruses 1:234–5
    effects of virus infection 3:1958
  T5-like phage effect 3:1719
  transformation see
    Transformation
  virus interactions 3:1957–61
  viruses as probes for
    studies 3:1961
Host Factor, bacteriophage Qβ
  replication 3:1667
Host genetic resistance 2:753–7
  characteristics 2:754
  future perspectives 2:757
  genetic loci 2:753
    mapping 2:754
  history 2:753–4
  Hv-2 locus 2:754–6
  polymorphous 2:754, 2:755(Table)
  resistance genes
    constitutive expression 2:754, 2:754–6
    expression through host
      antiviral effectors 2:756–7
    expression by unknown
      mechanisms 2:757
    H-2D 2:754
    inducible expression 2:754, 2:756
Host-controlled modification and
  restriction 2:758–63, 2:758(Fig)
    antirestriction by phage 2:760–1
    phage inhibitory
      proteins 2:760–1
    barrier to transduction 2:1238–9
    biological functions 2:760, 2:1239
    in prokaryotic cells 2:762
    classes in prokaryotes (M/
      R) 2:758–60, 2:759(Table)
    type I enzymes 2:758–60, 2:759(Table)
    type II (IIS) 2:759(Table), 2:760

Host-controlled modification and
  restriction (continued)
    classes in prokaryotes (M/R)
      (continued)
      type II restriction
        endonucleases
        (IIE) 2:759(Table), 2:760
      type II restriction
        enzymes 2:760
      type III enzymes 2:759(Table), 2:760
    cofactor requirements 2:758
    coliphage lambda 1:284
    DNA methylation
      eukaryotic viruses 2:763
      prokaryotic cells 2:762
    history 2:758
    Hsd system 2:761, 2:762(Table)
    McrBC system 2:759(Table), 2:760, 2:761
    methylation 2:758
    methylation-dependent DNA
      restriction 2:761
    nonclassical restriction/
      modification 2:762–3
    restriction 2:758
      of nonglucosylated HMC-
        containing DNA 2:761
    Rgl system 2:761, 2:762(Table)
    T1-like phages 3:1704–5
Host–virus interactions
  concept, polydnaviruses
    significance 2:1351
  pseudotemperate phage 1:133
Hs1 phage 1:80(Table)
Hsd system 2:758, 2:761, 2:762(Table)
Hsp104, [PSI] prion loss 3:1404
HTLV-1 see Human T-cell
  leukemia virus type 1 (HTLV-1)
Human adenoviruses see
  Adenovirus
Human astrovirus (HAstV) 1:104
  antibodies 1:107
  epidemiology 1:107
  genome, organization 1:105(Fig)
  immune response 1:107–8
  incubation period 1:107
  infection
    clinical features 1:107
    histopathology 1:107
    mortality 1:107
    pathology 1:107
    prevention and control 1:108
  monoclonal antibodies 1:106
  pathogenicity 1:107
  phylogeny 1:106(Fig)
  serologic relationships 1:106–7
  serotypes 1:106
    serotype 1 1:107
    serotypes 2-5 1:107
    serotypes 6 and 7 1:106, 1:107
  structure 1:104(Fig)
  tissue tropism 1:107
  transmission 1:107
  vaccine potential 1:108
  see also Astroviruses
Human B lymphotropic virus
  (HBLV) 2:697
Human caliciviruses (HuCV) see
  Caliciviruses
Human carcinoma cell line (Hep-
  2) 1:397(Fig)
Human cytomegalovirus
  (HCMV) 1:351–7
  AD169 1:345
  genome 1:346, 1:352
  antibodies 1:350
    to tegument proteins 1:350
  assembly 1:356
  binding and penetrating 1:356

Human cytomegalovirus (HCMV)
(continued)
  capsid and capsid proteins 1:353,
    1:354(Table)
  capsomeres and 'triplexes' 1:352
  cytopathology 1:356
  dense bodies 1:356
  DNA polymerase 1:353
  DNA replication 1:355
  DNA-binding
    phosphoproteins 1:353
  drug-resistant mutants 1:351
    ganciclovir 1:54
  early proteins 1:352, 1:353
  early RNAs (βRNAs) 1:355
  envelope 1:352, 1:353–5
    proteins 1:353–5, 1:354(Table)
  enzymes 1:352
  epidemiology 1:347–8
  evolution 1:347
  genes 1:345, 1:346
    functions 1:347
    homology to host genes 1:347,
      1:352
    murine CMV homology 1:364
  genetics 1:346–7
  genome 1:346–7
    animal CMV
      comparisons 1:359
    ORFs 1:352
    properties 1:352
    sequence 1:352
  geographic/seasonal
    distribution 1:345–6
  glycoprotein B (gpB) 1:345
  glycoprotein complex gcII 1:354,
    1:356
  glycoprotein complex gcIII 1:355
  glycoproteins 1:353–5
    gpB 1:353, 1:356
    gpH 1:354, 1:356
  homology with other
    herpesviruses 1:345
  host range and propagation 1:346
    permissive cells 1:346
    semipermissive cells 1:346
  immediate early (IE)
    genes 1:362(Fig)
  immediate early (IE)
    proteins 1:352, 1:352–3
    IE2 1:352–3
    major (MIEP; IE1) 1:352
  immediate early (IE) RNA
    (αRNAs) 1:355
  immune evasion 1:353, 2:1204
  impact 1:344
  kinase 1:351
  late proteins 1:352
  late RNAs (γRNAs) 1:355
  latency 1:348
    in mononuclear
      leukocytes 1:348
  maturation and encapsidation of
    DNA 1:346
  monoclonal antibodies 1:351
  mRNAs 1:355
  murine CMV as model 1:366–7
  noninfectious enveloped
    (NIEPs) 1:356
  nucleocapsid 1:351
  ocular target 1:527(Table)
  pathogenicity 1:348
  phospholipids 1:352
  physical properties 1:355
  post-translational
    modification 1:356
  progeny viruses released 1:356
  promoters 1:352, 1:355
  propagation 1:359, 1:360(Fig)
  properties 1:351–2
  proteins 1:352–5, 1:354(Table)

Human cytomegalovirus (HCMV)
(continued)
  proteins (continued)
    high molecular weight
      (HMWP) 1:353
    integral membrane protein
      (IMP) 1:355
    MIE 1:364
    nonvirion 1:352–3
    nuclear DNA-binding
      (DB52) 1:353
    nuclear DNA-binding
      (DB140) 1:353
    upper/lower matrix 1:353,
      1:355
    virion 1:353–5
  reactivation 1:344, 1:348, 3:1823–5
  replication 1:346, 1:347, 1:355
    origin (ori-Lyt) 1:352
  seven-membrane spanning
    receptors (GCR)
    encoded 1:359
  shedding 1:347, 1:348
  strains 1:345
  tegument 1:352
    proteins 1:353, 1:354(Table)
  tissue tropism 1:348
  Toledo strain 1:351
  Towne strain 1:345, 1:346, 1:351
  transcription 1:355
  translation 1:355–6
  transmission 1:347, 1:348
    to children 1:346
  vaccines 1:351
  virus–host interactions 1:348
Human cytomegalovirus (HCMV)
  infection 1:62, 1:344, 3:1823
  after cardiac
    transplantation 2:1076
  laboratory diagnosis 2:1078
  children 1:348
  clinical features 1:348–9
  congenital and neonatal 1:62,
    1:347, 1:348, 1:349
  detection/diagnosis 2:1084–5,
    3:1823
  diarrhea due to 1:447
  eye 1:528
  fetus 1:344
  hepatitis 3:1824
  immune response 1:350, 3:1823
  immunity 1:350
  immunocompromised
    hosts 1:348, 1:349, 1:350
  incidence 3:1823–4
  intravenous
    immunoglobulin 1:351,
    3:1824, 3:1825
  kidney 2:1081–2
  opportunistic 1:349
  pancreas 2:1079
  pathology/histopathology 1:348,
    1:349–50
  pneumonia 3:1493
  pneumonitis 3:1824
  post-transplant 1:347, 1:349,
    3:1823–5
    bone marrow transplant 1:349
    cardiac see above
    clinical features 3:1824
    diagnosis 3:1824
    from blood products 3:1823
    from bone marrow
      transplants 3:1824
    from organ grafts 3:1823–4
    immunomodulation 3:1825
    pathogenesis 3:1824
    pathology 3:1827(Fig)
    prophylaxis 3:1825,
      3:1825(Table)
    renal transplant 2:1082

Human cytomegalovirus (HCMV)
  infection (continued)
  post-transplant (continued)
    treatment 3:1824–5
  prevention and control 1:349,
    1:350–1
    prophylaxis 2:1076, 2:1082
  reinfection 1:350
  retinitis 1:62, 1:63, 1:528, 1:529,
    1:529(Fig)
  serological diagnosis/tests 1:349,
    2:1085, 3:1824
  therapy 1:350–1
    approved agents 1:62–3
    experimental agents 1:63
  toddlers 1:347
  transfusion recipients 1:348
Human diploid fibroblast
  (HDF) 1:397(Fig)
Human disturbance, zoonotic
  diseases and 3:1995–6
Human embryonic kidney (HEK)
  cells, astrovirus culture 1:104
Human endogenous retrovirus
  (HERV) 1:438
Human enteric cornaviruses see
  Coronaviruses
Human foamy virus (HFV) 3:1686
  env glycoprotein 3:1689
  genome 3:1687, 3:1687(Fig)
  pathogenicity 3:1692
  propagation 3:1691
  prototype, isolation 3:1692
  serologic
    relationships 3:1688(Table)
Human herpesvirus 4 (HHV-4) see
  Epstein–Barr virus (EBV)
Human herpesvirus 5 (HHV-
  5) 1:345
  see also Cytomegalovirus
    (CMV)
Human herpesvirus 6 (HHV-
  6) 1:345, 1:358, 2:697–703
  detection, lymphocyte
    cultures 1:398
  DNA replication 2:699–700
    origin binding protein
      (OBP) 2:699
  emerging/re-emerging
    virus 1:419(Table)
  future perspectives 2:703
  genome 1:359, 2:698–9
    comparison to animal
      CMVs 1:359
    direct terminal repeats 2:698
    organization 2:699(Fig)
  HHV-6A 2:698
  HHV-6B 2:698
    infection 2:701–2, 2:702
    latent infections 2:702
    in saliva 2:701
  history 2:697–8
  host range and propagation 2:698
  HSV-1 protein similarity 2:699
  infection
    clinical features 2:701–2
    epidemiology 2:701
    immune response 2:702
    latent/persistent 2:702
    post-transplant 3:1829
    prevention and control 2:703
  major ssDNA-binding protein
    (MDBP) 2:699
  ocular target 1:527(Table)
  organ transplant pathogen 2:702
  pathogenesis 2:701
  persistent infection 2:702
  phosphotransferase 2:699
  properties and structure 2:698
  proteins 2:699–701
    capsid, tegument and
      assembly 2:700

Human herpesvirus 6 (HHV-6)
(continued)
  proteins (continued)
    chemokine receptors 2:700–1
    for DNA replication 2:699–700
    glycoprotein U18 2:700
    glycoprotein U20 2:700
    glycoprotein U85 2:700
    glycoproteins 2:700
  reactivation 2:701
  rep gene homologue 2:698
  REP protein 1:359, 2:698
  spread in bloodstream 2:1178
  susceptibility to ganciclovir 2:700
  taxonomy and
    classification 2:698
  tegument layer 2:698
  transmission and tissue
    tropism 2:701
Human herpesvirus 7 (HHV-
  7) 1:345, 1:358, 2:697–703
  detection, lymphocyte
    cultures 1:398
  DNA replication 2:699–700
  emerging/re-emerging
    virus 1:419(Table)
  future perspectives 2:703
  genome 2:698–9
    comparison to animal
      CMVs 1:359
    direct terminal repeats 2:698
    organization 2:699(Fig)
  history 2:697–8
  host range and propagation 2:698
  HSV-1 protein similarity 2:699
  infection
    clinical features 2:702
    epidemiology 2:701
    immune response 2:702
    latent/persistent 2:702
    post-transplant 3:1829
    prevention and control 2:703
  phosphotransferase 2:699
  properties and structure 2:698
  proteins 2:699–701
    capsid, tegument and
      assembly 2:700
    chemokine receptors 2:700–1
    for DNA replication 2:699–700
    glycoprotein U85 2:700
    glycoproteins 2:700
  in saliva 2:701
  in salivary glands 2:702
  spread in bloodstream 2:1178
  taxonomy and
    classification 2:698
  tegument layer 2:698
  transmission and tissue
    tropism 2:701
Human herpesvirus 8 (HHV-8;
  KSHV) 2:706
  cell lines 3:1848
  genes 3:1848
  genome structure and
    function 3:1848
  herpesvirus sylvilagus
    relationship 2:706
  Kaposi's sarcoma
    associated 3:1848
  ocular target 1:527(Table)
  post-transplant infection 3:1829
Human immunodeficiency virus see
  HIV
Human papillomavirus 1 (HPV1),
  structure 2:1105(Fig)
Human papillomavirus 5
  (HPV5) 1:1105
  infections 2:1109
  skin cancer 2:1105, 2:1110, 3:1846
  variants 2:1107
Human papillomavirus 6 (HPV6),
  variants 2:1107

INDEX

Human papillomavirus 7 (HPV7), warts due to 2:1109
Human papillomavirus 8 (HPV8), skin cancer 3:1846
Human papillomavirus 16 (HPV16)
  cervical cancer 2:1111
  epidermoid carcinoma 3:1845
  evolution 2:1108
  genetic map 2:1106(Fig)
  genome organization 2:1115(Fig)
  keratinocyte immortalization 3:1845–6
  replication 2:1110(Fig)
  tumors associated 2:1111, 2:1112
  vaccine development 2:1114
  variants 2:1108
Human papillomavirus 18 (HPV18) 2:1111
  adenocarcinoma 3:1845
  genome integration 3:1846
Human papillomavirus 33 (HPV33) 2:1112
Human papillomavirus (HPV) 1:66–7, 2:1105–14
  antibodies 2:1113
  apoptosis inhibition 1:73
  assembly and release 2:1116
  attachment and entry 2:1115
  capsid 2:1118–19
  carcinogenesis 2:1119–20
    anogenital 2:1112
    E6 and E7 role 2:1111, 2:1119–20
    E6 and E7 synergy 2:1118(Fig), 2:1120
  cutaneous types 2:1108
    pathogenicity 2:1110, 2:1111(Table)
    transmission 2:1109
  detection methods 2:1108, 2:1110
  DNA
    detection by PCR 2:1108, 2:1114
    frequency in skin cancers 2:1110, 2:1114
    integration into host 2:1119
  DNA replication 2:1109
    modes 2:1117
    switching 2:1117
  E1 and E2 disruption during integration 3:1846
  E1 protein 2:1117
  E1OE4 gene 2:1116
  E2 gene product (E2 transactivator; E2TA) 1:75, 2:1116, 2:1117
  E6 associated protein (E6-AP) 2:1120
  E6 gene 3:1846
    epidermodysplasia verruciformis 3:1846
    p53 and Rb interaction 3:1846
    suppression and cancer inhibition 3:1846
  E6 protein 1:73, 2:1117, 2:1120
    antibodies 2:1113
    binding/inactivation of p53 2:1120
    carcinogenic mechanism 2:1120
    cytotoxic T lymphocyte response 2:1113
    oncogenic action in culture 2:1120
    'progression' stage of carcinogenesis 2:1120
    structure 2:1120
    synergy with E7 2:1118(Fig), 2:1120
    transgenic mice 2:1120
    vaccine development 2:1114

Human papillomavirus (HPV) (continued)
  E6-AP (E6 associated protein) 1:73
  E7 gene 3:1846
    p53 and Rb interaction 3:1846
    suppression and cancer inhibition 3:1846
  E7 protein 2:1117, 2:1119–20
    antibodies 2:1113
    binding to p21 and p27 2:1119
    conserved regions and domains 2:1119
    cytotoxic T lymphocyte response 2:1113
    increased in cervical cancer 2:1119
    pRb degradation by 2:1119
    promotion phase of carcinogenesis 2:1119
    synergy with E6 2:1118(Fig), 2:1120
    as transforming protein 2:1119–20
    transgenic mice 2:1120
    vaccine development 2:1114
  emerging viruses 1:419(Table)
  epidemiology 2:1108–9
  evolution 2:1107–8, 2:1107(Fig), 2:1125(Fig)
  future perspectives 2:1114
  gene expression 2:1116–17
  genetic map 2:1106(Fig)
  genetics 2:1106–7
  genital see Human papillomavirus (HPV) infection
  genome 1:67, 2:1105
    amplification 2:1117
    conserved regions 2:1106
    E1OE4 gene 2:1115
    early region 2:1105, 2:1115
    as episome 2:1110
    late region 2:1105, 2:1115
    long control region (LCR) 2:1105, 2:1115
    ORFs 2:1106, 2:1115
    transcription factors binding 2:1117
  genome organization 2:1115, 2:1115(Fig)
  genotypes 2:1106
    number 2:1105
    relationship 2:1106
  geographic/seasonal distribution 2:1106
  high-risk types 2:1110
  history 2:1105
  host range and propagation 2:1106
  immune evasion 2:1116
  infection process 2:1115–16
  keratinocyte immortalization 2:1106
  L1 and L2 proteins 2:1108, 2:1118–19
  life cycle 2:1115–16, 2:1116(Fig)
    early/nonproductive stage 2:1115
    in keratinocytes 2:1109–10, 2:1109(Fig)
    replicative 2:1117
  low-risk types 2:1110
  molecular biology 2:1115–20
  monoclonal antibodies 2:1108
  novel types identification 2:1106
  ocular target 1:527(Table)
  oncogenic 2:1106
    detection tests 2:1114
    nucleotide sequences 2:1106
    transmission 2:1109

Human papillomavirus (HPV) (continued)
  pathogenicity 2:1110–12, 2:1111(Table)
  phylogenetic tree 2:1107(Fig)
  promoters 2:1116
  promyelocytic leukemia oncogenic domains (PODs) 2:1119
  receptors 2:1106, 2:1109
  replication 2:1106, 2:1110(Fig), 2:1112–13, 2:1117
  serologic relationships and variability 2:1108
  serotypes 2:1108
  stability 2:1107
  structure and properties 2:1105(Fig), 2:1118–19
  supergroup A 2:1107
  supergroup B 2:1108
  supergroup E 2:1108
  taxonomy and classification 2:1105–6
  terminal differentiation of infected cells 2:1116
  tissue tropism 2:1109–10, 2:1115, 2:1116
  transcription 2:1116–17
    regulation 2:1116–17
    transactivators 2:1116
  transformation by 3:1822
  transmission 2:1109–10
  type-common epitopes 2:1108
  types
    diseases associated (summary) 2:1111(Table)
    growth patterns 2:1112
  vaccine development 2:1113–14
  variants 2:1106
  virus-like particles (VLPs) 2:1108, 2:1118
    ELISA 2:1113
Human papillomavirus (HPV) infection 2:1115
  anal 2:1109, 2:1112
  anogenital see Human papillomavirus (HPV), genital
  cancer associated 2:1105, 2:1111(Table), 2:1115
  clinical features 2:1112
  control, immune factors 2:1109
  cutaneous 2:1110
    clinical features 2:1112
    therapy 2:1114
    see also Warts
  epidermodysplasia verruciformis (EV) 3:1846
  eye 1:523–4, 1:523(Fig), 1:528
  genital 2:1107, 2:1108
    clinical features 2:1112
    pathogenicity 2:1110–11, 2:1111(Table)
    pathology/histopathology 2:1112
    prevalence 2:1108–9
    transmission 2:1109
    see also Cervical cancer; Cervical intraepithelial neoplasia
  genital cancer 3:1845–6
  immune response 2:1113
  invasive carcinomas 2:1110
  oral 2:1109, 2:1111(Table)
    carcinoma 3:1846
    clinical features 2:1112
  papilloma, formation mechanism 2:1115, 2:1116(Fig)
  pathology/histopathology 2:1112–13

Human papillomavirus (HPV) infection (continued)
  prevention and control 2:1113–14
  skin cancer 3:1846–7
  therapy 1:66–7
    approved agents 1:67
    experimental agents 1:67
    interferon use 2:860
Human parainfluenza viruses see Parainfluenza viruses (PIVs)
Human parvovirus B19 see Parvovirus B19
Human polyomavirus infections, renal involvement 2:1083
Human respiratory coronaviruses (HCV) 1:294
Human respiratory syncytial virus (RSV) see Respiratory syncytial virus (RSV)
Human rhinoviruses (HRVs)
  serotypes 3:1545
  type 2 (HRV2), IRES 2:1334, 2:1337
  see also Rhinoviruses
Human spumaretrovirus (HSRV) 3:1686
Human spumavirus (HSpV) 3:1686
Human T-cell leukemia virus (HTLV)
  bovine leukemia virus (BLV) comparison 1:194
  bovine leukemia virus (BLV) as model 1:197
  emerging/re-emerging virus 1:419(Table)
  taxonomy and classification 1:191
Human T-cell leukemia virus type 1 (HTLV-1) 2:788–94, 2:1019
  adult T-cell leukemia 3:1845
  antibodies 2:790, 2:792
  apoptosis inhibition 1:74
  cAMP-responsive element 2:790
  cell culture 2:795
  cell cycle inhibitor inactivation 2:793
  cytokines induced 2:792
  detection, lymphocyte cultures 1:398
  epidemiology 2:790–1
    age and family factors 2:791
    geographic clustering 2:790–1
  future perspectives 2:794
  gene expression 2:789–90
    regulation 2:789–90, 2:790(Fig)
    Rex protein action 2:790
    trans-activation and Tax 2:790
  genes, rex 2:800–1
  genome 2:789, 2:789(Fig), 2:795
    long terminal repeat (LTR) 2:789, 2:790
    ORFs 2:789
    proviral 2:789
    pX sequence 2:789
  genomic stability 2:791
  history 2:788–9, 2:794–5
  host range 2:791–2
  HTLV-2 discrimination 2:803
  HTLV-2 relationship 2:789
  HTLV-2 serologic crossreactivity 2:796, 2:798
  in vitro infection 2:791
  in vivo expression 2:794
  infection 2:791–2, 2:791–4
    clinical features 2:1019–20
    diseases associated 2:792–3
    HAM 2:792–3
    HSV-2 infection associated 2:679
    prevention and control 2:793–4

Human T-cell leukemia virus type 1 (HTLV-1) (continued)
  infection (continued)
    see also Adult T-cell leukemia (ATL); Human T-cell leukemia virus type 1 (HTLV-1)-associated myelopathy (HAM) tropical spastic paraparesis (TSP) 2:792–3
    integration into host chromosome 2:792, 2:793
    lack of variation between isolates 2:797, 2:797–8
    leukemogenesis 2:793, 2:794
      Tax role 2:793
    molecular biology 2:789–90, 2:793
    origin 2:791
    P21^x protein 2:789
    pathogenicity 2:792–3
    pX region 2:793
    receptor 2:797
    rex gene and Rex protein 2:789, 2:790
      binding to cis-acting element 2:790
      transformation 3:1845
    simian T-cell leukemia virus similarity 2:713, 2:789
    spread in bloodstream 2:1178
    subtypes 2:789
    T cell stimulation 2:803
    Tax gene 1:74
    Tax protein 2:789, 2:790, 2:793
      actions 2:793, 2:793(Fig)
      functions 3:1821
      ICAM-1 trans-activation by 2:800
      leukemogenesis role 2:793
      trans-activation 2:790, 2:793, 2:794
      transformation 3:1845
    taxonomy and classification 2:789
    tissue tropism 2:791
    transcription 2:789–90, 2:790(Fig), 2:793
      splicings 2:789, 2:790(Fig)
      trans-activation 2:790, 2:793, 2:794
      trans-repression 2:793, 2:794
    transformation 2:791, 3:1821
    transmission 2:791–2
      breast milk 2:791
      prevention 2:793–4
      sexual 2:791–2
      VSV pseudotypes 2:797
    see also Adult T-cell leukemia (ATL)
Human T-cell leukemia virus type 1 (HTLV-1)-associated myelopathy (HAM) 2:792–3, 2:795
Human T-cell leukemia virus type 2 (HTLV-2) 2:794–804
  in blood donors 2:796
  carriers 2:803
  cell lines 2:797
    Mo T cell line 2:795
  cell-to-cell contact for infection 2:797
  cocultivation 2:799, 2:802
  detection 2:803
  epidemiology 2:795, 2:796, 2:796–7, 2:801–2
    drug users 2:797
  future perspectives 2:803
  genes
    env 2:796, 2:798(Fig), 2:799
    gag 2:796, 2:799
    pol 2:796, 2:798, 2:799

Human T-cell leukemia virus type 2 (HTLV-2) (continued)
  genes (continued)
    protease 2:799
    regulatory 2:798–9
    rev 2:801
    rex 2:795, 2:798, 2:799–801, 2:800–1
    tax 2:795, 2:798, 2:799–801
  genome 2:789, 2:795–6, 2:796–7
    long terminal repeat 2:797
    ORFs 2:799
    X region 2:796, 2:798
  hairy cell leukemia 3:1845
  history 2:794–5, 2:798
  host range 2:797
  HTLV-1 discrimination 2:803
  HTLV-1 relationship 2:789
  HTLV-1 serologic crossreactivity 2:796, 2:798
  HTLV-2 Mo (HTLV-2a) 2:795
  infection 2:795
    clinical features 2:798–9
    control 2:803
    disorders associated 2:802
    endemic 2:802
    malignancy 2:798, 2:802
    progressive spastic myelopathy 2:802
    risks 2:803
  as model for transformation 2:795, 2:803
  molecular genetics 2:797–8
  mRNA 2:798
  as 'new World' virus 2:796
  polymerase 2:799
  proteins 2:795–7, 2:796(Fig), 2:799
    p12 2:801
    Rex see below
    Tax see below
  receptor 2:797
  replication 2:798
  Rex protein 2:800, 2:801
    nuclear protein binding 2:801
  Rex-responsive element (RxRE) 2:801
  serological assays 2:803
  structure and properties 2:795–6
  subtypes
    epidemiology 2:801
    HTLV-2a and HLTV-2b 2:795–6, 2:797
    HTLV-2c 2:801
    isolate sources 2:801
  T cell stimulation 2:803
  T cell transformation 2:797, 2:802–3
    mechanism 2:802–3
    Tax role 2:800
  Tax expression vectors 2:800
  Tax protein 2:799–800
    ICAM-1 trans-activation by 2:800
    trans-activation by 2:800, 2:800(Fig)
  taxonomy and classification 2:795–6
  trans-regulatory genes 2:799–801
  transcription
    promoters 2:800
    Tax protein action 2:800
    trans-activation by Tax 2:800, 2:800(Fig)
Human T-cell leukemia virus type III (HTLV-IIIB) 2:770
Humoral immunity
  African swine fever virus 1:37
  bovine immunodeficiency virus (BIV) 1:190
  capripoxvirus infections 3:1380
  dengue virus infection 1:382–3

Humoral immunity (continued)
  echovirus infection 1:416
  Epstein–Barr virus (EBV) 1:493
  equine encephalitis viruses 1:507
  equine infectious anemia virus (EIAV) 1:520–1
  fowlpox virus 1:581
  hantavirus infections 1:629
  hepatitis A 1:638
  HSV infections 2:684
  HVP infections 2:1113
  influenza 2:828
  Japanese encephalitis (JE) virus 2:874
  LCMV 2:919
  Marek's disease 2:950
  mousepox 2:977
  mumps 2:993–4
  Newcastle disease virus 2:1025
  orbiviruses 2:1058–9
  polioviruses 2:1328
  reticuloendotheliosis (RE) viruses 3:1497–8
  vaccine-induced 3:1862
  varicella-zoster virus 3:1876
  vesicular stomatitis virus (VSV) 3:1918
  yellow fever 3:1986
Humpty Doo virus 3:1637
Humulus japonicus virus (HJV) 1:39
Hv-2 locus, MHV4 susceptibility and 2:754, 2:754–6
HVEM, co-receptor for HSV 2:1181
Hyalomma ticks, Crimean–Congo hemorrhagic fever (CCHF) virus 3:1990
Hybridization
  in situ assays 3:1412–13
  nucleic acid 1:391–2
    benyviruses detection 1:158
    solid-phase 1:392
    solution-phase 1:392
    sandwich assay 1:394
Hydra viridis 1:48
Hydrangea mosaic virus (HdMV) 1:38
Hydrophobia, rabies 3:1440
Hydroxycoumarin complexes 2:783
Hydroxymethylcytosine (HMC), T4 phage 3:1706, 3:1715
Hydroxymethyluracil, in SPO1 phage 3:1681
Hydroxyurea, HIV infection therapy 1:61
Hygiene, coxsackievirus infection prevention 1:310
Hymenoptera, picorna-like viruses 2:1271–2
Hyperendemicity, dengue viruses 1:376, 1:378, 1:379, 1:381, 1:381(Fig)
Hypergammaglobulinaemia, Aleutian mink disease 2:1166
Hypermutation, caprine arthritis encephalitis virus (CAEV) 1:226
Hyperplasia, virus-induced, animal papillomaviruses 2:1128
Hyperplastic alveolar nodules (HANs) 2:969
Hypersensitive response (HR) 2:1186–8
  plant resistance to viruses 2:1311
    mechanism 2:1304–5, 2:1306
  plant viruses 2:1186–8
    coat protein of TMV 2:1186–7, 2:1187(Fig)
    elicitors 2:1186–8
    PVX coat protein 2:1187
    replicase of TMV 2:1187

Hypersensitivity, delayed see Delayed-type hypersensitivity
Hypervariable regions, hepatitis C virus (HCV) genome 1:660, 1:662
Hypochoeris mosaic virus (HMV) 1:588
Hypotension, hemorrhagic fever with renal syndrome (HFRS) 1:628
Hypoviridae, Hypovirus 2:805
Hypovirulence 2:804
Hypovirus 2:805
Hypoviruses 2:804–7
  biological control 2:804, 2:806–7
  CPG-1 (G-protein α subunit) in cultures 2:806
  future perspectives 2:807
  gene expression strategy 2:805–6, 2:805(Fig)
  genome
    organization 2:805–6, 2:805(Fig)
    replicative dsRNA form 2:805
    short dsRNAs 2:806
  history 2:804
  host phenotype alteration 2:806
  persistent infection 2:804
  proteins
    p29 2:806
    roles 2:806
  prototypic virus (CHV1-EP713) 2:804
  taxonomy 2:804–5
  transmission 2:805, 2:806–7
  see also CHV1-EP713
Hypovolemic shock
  Argentine hemorrhagic fever (AHF) 2:892
  Bolivian hemorrhagic fever (BHF) 2:892
  Lassa fever 2:893
Hz-1V 2:1032
  cytopathic effects 2:1032
  defective interfering particles 2:1033, 2:1034
  genes and promoters 2:1033
  genome 2:1032
  persistent infection 2:1032, 2:1033, 2:1034
  persistently associated transcript (PAT1) 2:1034
  proteins 2:1032, 2:1033
  replication and stages 2:1032–3
  transcription 2:1033
Hz-2V 2:1032
  agonadal condition due to 2:1034
  genome 2:1032
  host–virus association 2:1034
  replication 2:1034
  transmission 2:1034

I

IAP (inhibitor of apoptosis) 1:71, 1:73
Ibaraki virus, vaccine 2:1060
ICAM-1
  rhinovirus receptor 1:66, 3:1545, 3:1547
    blocking 3:1551
  soluble, rhinovirus infection prophylaxis 1:66
  trans-activation by HTLV-1 and HTLV-2 2:800
ICE (interleukin-1β converting enzyme) 1:71
  apoptosis inhibition 1:71(Table)

Ichneumonidae 2:1349
Ichnoviruses 2:1349
  ascoviruses similarity 1:103
  genome 2:1350
  structure 2:1349, 2:1349(Fig)
  see also Polydnaviruses
Icosahedral symmetry 3:1947(Fig)
  all-pentamers 3:1951
  capsid assembly 3:1947–8
  capsid structure 3:1947–8
  Caspar and Klug
    hypothesis 3:1948–51
  high resolution
    crystallography 3:1948–53
  P=3 3:1953
  protein subunit
    structures 3:1949(Fig)
  quasi-equivalence 3:1948–51,
    3:1951(Fig)
  T=3 3:1951, 3:1952(Fig), 3:1953–5, 3:1953(Fig)
    picornavirus vs comovirus
      capsid 3:1954(Fig)
  T=7 3:1951
Icosahedral viruses 3:1943, 3:1947–55
  assembly 3:1945
  atomic structure 3:1944
  capsid proteins, atomic
    structure 3:1944
Ictalurovirus 1:553
ICTV see International Committee
  on Taxonomy of Viruses
  (ICTV)
ICTVdB 3:1731
Idaeovirus 2:809–11
  economic significance 2:811
  evolution 2:811
  genes 2:810–11
  genome 2:809–10
    organization 2:810(Fig)
    properties 2:810–11
    RNA1 2:809–10, 2:810
    RNA2 2:809–10, 2:810–11
    RNA3 2:811
  geographic distribution 2:809
  history 2:809
  host range and propagation 2:809
  pathogenicity 2:811
  prevention and control 2:811
  proteins, comparisons 2:810(Fig)
  resistant cultivars 2:811
  serologic relationship and
    variability 2:811
  structure and properties 2:809
  taxonomy and
    classification 2:809
  transmission and tissue
    tropism 2:811
Idaeovirus 2:809
Idiotypic–anti-idiotypic antibody
  network 2:815
Idoxuridine, HSV infection
  treatment 2:685
Ieri virus (IERIV) 2:1045(Table)
Ife virus (IFEV) 2:1045(Table)
Igbo Ora virus 3:1994
IkB
  interferon induction 2:858
  proteolysis by interferons 2:856
IkB-α, activation by
  reticuloendotheliosis (RE) virus
  strain T 3:1500–1
IKe phage 1:547
Ilarvirus 1:38
  taxonomy 1:38–9
Ilarviruses 1:38–43
  capsids 1:40
  economic significance 1:43
  epidemiology and control 1:43
  genome 1:39
    structure 1:41

Ilarviruses (continued)
  geographical distribution 1:39–40
  host range 1:39–40
  replication 1:42
  RNAs 1:40, 1:41
  structure 1:40–1
  transmission 1:43
  virus–host relationships 1:42–3
  see also Alfalfa mosaic virus
    (AlMV)
IMC-Hz-1 cells 2:1032
Imiquimod (Aldara) 1:67
Immune blotting see Immunoblot
Immune complexes
  deposition 1:249
  formation 2:817
  hepatitis B virus (HBV)
    infection 1:643
  lactate dehydrogenase-elevating
    virus (LDV) 1:95, 1:96
  in lymphocytic
    choriomeningitis 2:915
Immune diseases, viral infections
  associated/
  causing 2:817(Table)
Immune enhancement 2:817
  dengue viruses 1:380
  see also Immunomodulators
Immune evasion 2:816–18, 2:1175,
  2:1202–4, 2:1203(Table)
  African swine fever virus (AFSV)
    proteins 1:37–8
  anti-cytokine and chemokine
    proteins 2:1204
  antibody 2:816
    by antigenic variation 2:816
    by immunosuppression 2:816
  antigen suppression 2:1204
  cell-mediated response 2:816–17
    antigenic drift 2:817
    infection of effector cells 2:817
    latency 2:816
    MHC class I regulation 2:816
    sanctuary sites 2:816
    tolerance 2:817
  cowpox virus 1:300
  human cytomegalovirus
    (HCMV) 1:353
  human papillomaviruses
    (HPVs) 2:1116
  immune privileged sites 2:1203
  interference with antigen
    presentation/
    processing 2:1204
  mechanisms 2:897
  persistent viremia
    mechanisms 2:1015
  summary of
    mechanisms 2:1203(Table)
  T cell receptor
    antagonism 2:1204
  Theiler's murine
    encephalomyelitis viruses
    (TMEV) 3:1778
  viral genome mutations
    causing 2:1203–4
Immune exhaustion, hog cholera
  virus (HCV) causing 2:741,
  2:742
Immune interferon see Interferon-γ
  (IFN-γ)
Immune modulators see
  Immunomodulators
Immune privileged site,
  cornea 1:524
Immune privileged sites 2:1203
Immune response/system 2:812–18,
  2:1200–2, 2:1202(Table)
  adaptive (specific) 2:813–15
    antigen-presenting cells 2:813
    B cell activation 2:814–15
    evolution 2:812–13

Immune response/system
  (continued)
  adaptive (specific) (continued)
    T cell activation 2:813–14
  to adenovirus gene transfer
    vectors 1:12–13
  adverse reactions to viral
    infections 2:817
    immune complexes 2:817
    immune enhancement 2:817
    immunopathology 2:817
  antibody-mediated 3:1862
  apoptosis function 1:69–70
  autoimmunity 2:817–18
  caprine arthritis encephalitis
    (CAE) syndrome 1:228
  cytokines role 1:339–40,
    1:340(Fig)
  effector T cells and 3:1862–3
  endogenous provirus expression
    effect 1:440
  evasion see Immune evasion
  eye 1:524
  gastrointestinal tract 2:1177
  history 2:812
  indirect neural cell
    damage 2:1017
  influence on perpetuation of
    viruses 1:486
  innate see Immune response/
    system, nonadaptive
  interference by Ebola and
    Marburg viruses 2:944
  levels of protection and
    overlapping features 2:821
  memory see Immunological
    memory
  modulators see
    Immunomodulators
  molecular mimicry 2:817–18
  mucosal, stimulation by
    interferon 2:861
  nature 2:812–16
  nonadaptive (innate) 1:69, 2:812–13
    cytokines 1:339, 1:340(Fig)
    evolution 2:812–13
  normal, for antibody production/
    detection 1:390
  plant viruses 2:1185
  respiratory tract 2:1176
  secondary 3:1863
  self-reactive see Autoimmunity
  sequence, influenza virus
    infection 2:815(Table)
  sequence of response in acute
    viral infection 2:815–16
    primary 2:815–16
    secondary 2:816
  specific see Immune response/
    system, adaptive
  to superantigens 2:1231–2
  vaccines and 3:1861–5
  viruses as tool for
    elucidating 2:812
  see also individual virus
    infections
Immune surveillance, suppression
  after transplants 3:1823
Immunity, temperate
  phage 2:1099–100
Immunization
  passive, post-transplant 3:1833
  pre/post transplant 3:1833
  routes, immune responses
    and 3:1864
  secondary response 3:1863
  see also Vaccines
Immunization challenge test,
  rabies-like viruses 3:1444

Immunoassays
  PrP^{Sc} prion protein 3:1394,
    3:1394(Fig), 3:1397
  viral antigen detection 1:389
  see also ELISA; Enzyme
    immunoassays (EIA)
Immunoblot
  antiviral antibody detection 1:391
  Borna disease virus
    detection 1:172
Immunocompromised hosts
  adenovirus infections 1:6, 1:20
  coronavirus infections 1:295
  herpes zoster 3:1874, 3:1876
  HPV infections 2:1109
  HSV infections 2:681–2
  human CMV infection 1:348,
    1:349, 1:350
  parvovirus B19 infection 2:1154
  VZV infections 3:1877
Immunodeficiency
  adenovirus infections 1:445
  echovirus infection 1:416
  lymphomas, EBV
    association 1:490
  T cell deficiency, respiratory
    virus infections 3:1491
Immunoelectron microscopy
  (IEM) 1:402
  Norwalk virus 2:1035, 2:1040
Immunoenzyme staining, viral
  antigen detection 1:389
Immunofluorescence 1:389
  antiviral antibody detection 1:391
  direct 1:389, 1:399
  indirect see Indirect
    immunofluorescence
  monoclonal antibodies in 1:399
  polyclonal antiserum 1:399
  viral antigen detection 1:389
  virus identification method 1:399
Immunoglobulin A (IgA)
  coxsackievirus infection 1:309
  in respiratory tract 2:1176
  RSV infection 3:1486
  secretory 2:816
  Sendai virus infection 3:1621
Immunoglobulin E (IgE), HHV-6
  glycoprotein U20 sequence
  similarity 2:700
Immunoglobulin G (IgG)
  Chikungunya (CHIK)
    fever 1:264–5
  dengue virus infection 1:382,
    1:383
  echovirus infection 1:416
  enterovirus 70 (EV70) 1:472
  hantavirus infections 1:629
  in hepatitis A 1:638
  respiratory tract 2:1176
  rubella 3:1599
  yellow fever virus 3:1986
Immunoglobulin M (IgM)
  assays
    false-negative 1:391
    false-positive 1:391
  bovine leukemia virus (BLV)
    infection 1:197
  Chikungunya (CHIK) fever 1:264
  coxsackievirus infection 1:309
  dengue virus infection 1:382,
    1:383
  detection, by enzyme
    immunoassays 1:391
  echovirus infection 1:416
  enterovirus 70 (EV70) 1:472
  hantavirus infections 1:629
  in hepatitis A 1:638
  Japanese encephalitis (JE)
    virus 2:874
  rubella 3:1599
  yellow fever virus 3:1986

Immunoglobulin M (IgM)-capture technique 1:391
Immunoglobulin-like domains, tetravirus capsid 3:1766
Immunological memory 2:815
  B cells 2:815
    respiratory tract infections 3:1491
  T cells 2:815, 2:822
Immunological techniques
  viral antigen detection 1:388
  see also Diagnostic techniques; Immunoassays
Immunological tolerance 2:817, 2:915
Immunology
  history 2:723
  LCMV as model system 2:915
  ocular 1:524
Immunomodulation, by murine CMV 1:368, 1:369
Immunomodulators
  HIV infection 1:61
  virus-encoded 1:72
    parapoxviruses 2:1145–6
  see also Immune enhancement
Immunopathology 2:817, 2:821
  Borna disease virus infection 1:171
  T cell-mediated 2:821–2
Immunoperoxidase test 1:399–400
Immunostimulatory complexes (ISCOMs) 3:1495
Immunosuppression
  immune evasion mechanism 2:816
  in transplantation 3:1823
  by viruses
    baboon and chimpanzee herpesviruses 2:712
    feline leukemia viruses (FeLVs) 1:544
    HIV 2:771
    lactate dehydrogenase-elevating virus 1:95
    LCMV 2:917
    measles virus 2:959
    murine CMV 1:368
    reticuloendotheliosis (RE) viruses 3:1499
    simian immunodeficiency viruses 3:1644
    type D retroviruses 3:1518
Immunosuppressive therapy, emerging viral diseases associated 1:423
Immunotherapy, HPV infections 2:1114
Impatiens necrotic spot virus (INSV) 3:1803
  see also Tospoviruses
Incidence rates 1:482
Inclusion bodies 3:1960
  ascoviruses 1:102
  caulimoviruses see Caulimoviruses
  Iridoviridae 2:866–7
  mousepox 2:976
  nepovirus infections 2:1012
  orbiviruses 2:1046, 2:1058
  potexvirus infections 3:1367–8
  Tanapox and Yabapox virus infections 3:1973
  vaccinia virus 3:1868
  varicella-zoster virus 3:1875(Fig), 3:1876, 3:1884
  viral erythrocytic necrosis 1:566, 1:567
  waikaviruses 3:1969
Inclusion body myositis, mumps virus (MuV) and 2:994
Inclusion body protein 2:1286

Inclusions
  dianthovirus infections 1:408
  electron microscopy 1:400(Fig)
  'owl's eye' 1:346, 1:349
  tombusviruses 3:1793
Incompatibility, of heterologous viruses 2:850–1
Incubation periods, long, emerging viral diseases associated 1:421
Indian peanut clump virus (IPCV) 2:1196
  alternative hosts 2:1199
  coat protein 2:1199
  control recommendations 2:1199
  genome 2:1197, 2:1198(Fig), 2:1199
  host range 2:1197
  life cycle 2:1198(Fig)
  resistance 2:1199
  transmission 2:1197
  see also Pecluviruses
Indinavir (Crixivan) 1:60
  structure 2:784(Fig)
Indirect immunofluorescence 1:389
  antiviral antibody detection 1:391
  dengue viruses 1:379
  virus identification 1:399
  see also Immunofluorescence
Industrial fermentations, phage in see Bacteriophage in industrial fermentations
Infants
  HHV-6 infection 2:701
  ribavirin therapy 1:65
  rotavirus infections 3:1580
  RSV infection 3:1486
Infectious bovine rhinotracheitis (IBR) 1:180, 1:182
Infectious bulbar paralysis see Aujeszky's disease (AD)
Infectious bursal disease of chickens
  causes of death 1:166
  clinical signs and pathology 1:162
  prevention and control 1:166
Infectious bursal disease virus (IBDV) 1:160, 1:162(Fig)
  antigenic structure 1:165–6
  cell tropism 1:162–3, 1:166
  culture 1:162
  dsRNA–protein complexes 1:163(Fig)
  genome 1:161, 1:161(Fig)
    noncoding regions 1:164–5
    organization 1:164–5, 1:164(Fig)
  host range and epidemiology 1:162
  immune response 1:166
  in vitro replication 1:163
  laboratory diagnosis 1:166
  neutralizing antibodies to 1:165–6
  pathogenic properties 1:162
  proteins 1:161
  replication 1:163
  serotypes 1:162, 1:165–6
  stability 1:162
  VP5-defective mutant 1:164
  see also Birnaviruses
Infectious canine hepatitis (Rubarth's disease) 1:20
Infectious ectromelia 2:973
Infectious falchering virus (IFV) 1:1267
Infectious hematopoietic necrosis virus (IHNV) 1:558, 3:1542
  genome and proteins 1:560, 3:1542
  geographic/seasonal distribution 1:560
  history 1:560

Infectious hematopoietic necrosis virus (IHNV) (continued)
  host range and propagation 1:560
  infection
    clinical features 1:561, 3:1542
    immune response 1:561
    pathology 3:1542
  taxonomy and classification 1:560
  transmission and tissue tropism 1:560–1, 3:1542
    by eggs 1:560
Infectious hepatitis see Hepatitis A
Infectious hypodermal and hematopoietic necrosis virus (IHHNV) 3:1626, 3:1634
  diagnosis 3:1634
  infections 3:1634
  structure and properties 3:1634
Infectious icterus (jaundice) 1:640
Infectious mononucleosis (glandular fever) 1:488, 3:1492
  EBV latent protein expression 1:492
  epidemiology 1:489
  fatal 1:492
  see also Epstein–Barr virus (EBV)
Infectious pancreatic necrosis virus of fish (IPNV) 1:160, 1:563
  antigenic structure 1:165
  genome 1:161, 1:161(Fig), 1:563
    organization 1:165
  geographic/seasonal distribution 1:563
  history 1:563
  host range and epidemiology 1:161–2, 1:563
  in vitro replication 1:163
    undiluted passage 1:164
  infection 1:563
    clinical signs and pathology 1:162, 1:563
    history 1:160
    immune response 1:564
    prophylaxis 1:166
  laboratory diagnosis 1:166
  pathogenic properties 1:162
  polypeptides 1:563
  propagation 1:563
  proteins 1:161
  stability 1:162
  taxonomy and classification 1:563
  transmission and tissue tropism 1:563
    in eggs 1:563
  vaccine 1:564
  see also Birnaviruses
Infectious proteins see Prions
Infectious pustular vulvovaginitis (IPV) 1:180
Infectious salmon anemia 1:564
  clinical features 1:565
Infectious salmon anemia virus (ISAV) 1:564
  geographic/seasonal distribution 1:564
  history 1:564
  host range and propagation 1:564–5
  taxonomy and classification 1:564
  transmission and tissue tropism 1:565
Infectious subviral particles (SIVPs), reoviruses 2:1177
Infectivity assays 1:1412
Inflammatory infiltrates, Borna disease virus infection 1:172
Inflammatory response 2:821

Influenza 1:63
  antigenic drift 3:1489
  bronchiolitis 3:1493
  clinical features 2:828
  epidemics 2:824, 2:828
  geographic/seasonal distribution 2:825
  history 2:824
  immune response 2:828–9
    class II-associated 2:841
    Ig response to HA 2:828
  pandemics 1:421, 2:824, 2:826
    emergence of viruses 2:827(Fig)
    H5N1 pandemic 2:826
    planning for 2:829
  pathology/histopathology 2:828
  pharyngitis 3:1492
  prevention and control 2:829
  as re-emerging disease 1:421
  therapy 1:63–4
    antiviral agents 2:829
    approved agents 1:63–4
    experimental agents 1:64
  vaccination 2:828
  vaccines 2:829
  as winter disease 2:825
Influenza A
  epidemic 3:1489(Fig)
  immune response 2:829
  M2 protein, inhibition 1:63
  pathology/histopathology 2:828
  prophylaxis 1:64
Influenza A virus
  1968 strain (H3N2) 2:836
  antigenic shift 2:826
  dominant-negative mutants 2:853
  emergence of pandemics 2:827(Fig)
  evolution 2:826, 2:826(Fig)
  H2N2 2:827(Fig)
  H3N8 2:827(Fig)
  hemagglutinin (HA)
    of H3N2 strain 2:836
    structure 2:836
  Hong Kong (H3N2) strain 2:836, 2:837(Fig)
  host range 2:825
  mutation rate 2:825
  productive infection 3:1957
  replication 3:1476
  reservoir 2:825(Fig)
  resistance genes 2:755(Table)
  RNA segments 2:830
  serologic relationships 2:826
  structure and properties 2:830, 2:830(Fig)
  subtypes 2:825, 2:836
    antigenic shift 2:826
    cyclic appearance 2:826
    maintenance 2:827
  transcription 3:1476
  VSV interference 2:850
Influenza B
  clinical features 2:828
  cytopathic effect 1:397(Fig)
Influenza B virus
  BM2 protein 2:833
  host range 2:825
  M1 protein synthesis 2:834
  NA and NB protein synthesis 2:834
  serologic relationships 2:826
  structure and properties 2:830
Influenza C virus
  hemagglutinin esterase (HEF) 2:830, 2:832
  host range 2:825
  receptors 2:832
  structure and properties 2:830
Influenza viruses 2:824–9, 3:1488
  anti-antiviral mechanisms 2:860
  antigen processing 2:840, 2:841

Influenza viruses (continued)
   antigen structure 2:836–42
   antigenic determinants
      (epitopes) 2:838–9
      B cell epitopes 2:838, 2:839–40
      criteria for 2:842
      in infections 2:840–1
      T cell see below
   antigenic drift 2:826, 2:829
      mechanism 2:839
   apoptosis promotion 1:75
   assembly and release 1:249, 2:835
   attachment and entry 3:1923
      HA role 2:830, 2:836
   avian 1:420(Table), 2:825, 3:1494
      transmission 2:827
   budding 1:253(Fig), 2:835
   cDNA-derived RNA 2:835,
      2:836(Fig)
   cRNA 2:833
   defective interfering (DI)
      particles 2:830, 2:835
   DNA vaccination 2:842
   emergence of new strains 3:1996
   emerging/re-emerging
      virus 1:419(Table)
   epidemiology 2:826–7
   escape mutants 2:839
   evolution 2:826
   experimental hosts 2:825
   eye infection 1:524
   fusion mechanism 3:1922–3,
      3:1924(Fig)
      see also Hemagglutinin (HA)
   fusion pore
      enlargement 3:1923
      formation 3:1923
   fusion protein 3:1922–3
      activation 3:1923, 3:1923(Fig)
      hemifusion 3:1923
      penetration 3:1923
      relocation 3:1923
   future perspectives 2:829
   genetic manipulation 2:835–6,
      2:836(Fig)
   genetic reassortment 2:825, 2:826
   genetics 2:825–6
   genome 2:830
      panhandle structures 2:830,
         2:833
      RNA segments 2:830
   geographic/seasonal
      distribution 2:825
   H1N1 strain 2:815
   hemagglutinin (HA) 2:824, 2:830,
      3:1921
      antibody response 2:828
      antigenic drift 2:826
      antigenic sites 2:828
      in attachment 2:830
      attachment role 2:836
      epitopes 2:814, 2:839
      epitopes location 2:839
      escape mutants 2:839
      functions 2:830–1
      fusion activity 2:831
      HA1 and HA2 2:830, 2:835
      N-terminal of HA2 2:831
      in pathogenicity 2:828
      post-translational
         modification 2:834–5
      structure 2:830–1, 2:836–7,
         2:837(Fig)
      three-dimensional
         structure 2:831(Fig), 2:836–7
   history 2:824
   host range and propagation 2:825
      cell lines 2:825
      embryonated eggs 2:825
      immune response, in
         mice 2:815(Table)
   in vitro reconstitution 2:835–6

Influenza viruses (continued)
   infection see Influenza
   interpandemic variants 2:828
   isolation/identification
      embryonated eggs 1:399
      hemadsorption 1:397
   matrix protein, atomic
      structure 3:1944
   molecular biology 2:830–6
   mRNA 2:833
      synthesis 2:833
   mutation rate 2:825
   neuraminidase (NA) 2:824, 2:830
      antigenic drift 2:826
      apoptosis promotion 1:75
      complementarity-determining
         regions (CDR) 2:839
      as drug target 1:64
      epitopes 2:839
      functions 2:831–2, 2:837–8
      head structure 2:831
      inhibitors 2:825
      mutants lacking 2:837–8
      NC41 epitope 2:838(Fig), 2:839
      orientation 2:838
      in pathogenicity 2:828
      post-translational
         modification 2:835
      release 2:832
      RNA segment encoding 2:832
      structure and synthesis 2:831–
         2, 2:837–8, 2:837(Fig)
      three-dimensional
         structure 2:831(Fig), 2:838
   ocular target 1:525(Table)
   p58 activation 2:860
   pathogenicity 2:828
   peptide transport 2:841
   physical properties 2:833
   plasmid-derived RNA
      system 2:835
   polymerase, as drug target 1:64
   post-translational
      processing 2:834–5
   promoters 2:833
   proteins 2:830–3
      BM2 2:833
      CM2 2:830
      M1 2:832, 2:834, 2:835
      M2 2:824, 2:830, 2:832, 2:834
      NA 2:834
      NB 2:830, 2:832, 2:834
      NEP (nuclear export
         protein) 2:833, 2:834
      NEP role 2:835
      NP 2:829, 2:832–3
      NS1 2:833, 2:834
      NS2 2:833
      polymerase proteins BP1, BP2
         and PA 2:832
      post-translational
         modifications 2:835
      synthesis 2:834
   replication 1:255, 2:833–5
      replicative cycle 2:834(Fig)
   resistance, Mx1 gene role 2:756
   ribonucleoprotein (RNP)
      core 2:830
   in vitro reconstitution 2:835–6
   RNA polymerase 2:833
   RNA replication 2:833
   seasonal distribution 3:1488
   serologic relationships and
      variability 2:826
   structure and properties 2:830,
      2:830(Fig)
   spikes 2:824
   T cell epitopes 2:839–40, 3:1863
      binding class I molecules 2:841
      criteria for 2:842
      general characteristics 2:840–1

Influenza viruses (continued)
   T cell epitopes (continued)
      nonoverlapping
         sequences 2:842
      recognition 2:841
      sequential 2:839
      specific characteristics 2:841–2
   taxonomy and
      classification 2:824–5
   tissue tropism 2:827
   transcription 2:833–4
   translation 2:834
   transmission 1:485(Table), 2:827
   vaccination, DNA encoding viral
      proteins 2:842
   vaccine, history 3:1861
   vRNA 2:833
      mRNA synthesis 2:833
      packaging 2:835
   see also Influenza A virus;
      Influenza B virus; Influenza C
      virus
Influenzavirus A 2:824, 2:825
Influenzavirus B 2:824, 2:825
Influenzavirus C 2:825
Ingestion–egestion model, plant
   virus transmission 3:1901
Ingestion–salivation model, plant
   virus transmission 3:1901
Initiation factors
   eIF4GI, rotavirus NSP3 protein
      interaction 3:1587
   eIF-2α, inactivation in interferon
      action 2:858
   eIF-4 2:1344
   eIF-4G 2:1344
   virus-mediated
      inactivation 3:1959
Innate immune response see
   Immune response/system
'Innocent bystander' response,
   TMEV-induced
   demyelination 3:1779
Inoculation access time (IAT),
   sequiviruses 3:1624
Inoculation, plant viruses
   insect feeding mechanics/
      behavior 3:1900
   propagation 3:1419
   see also Mechanical
      transmission
Inoviridae 2:1226–7
   characteristics 2:1226–7
   filamentous phage 1:547–52
   Inovirus 1:547, 2:1227
   phage included 2:1227
   Plectrovirus 2:1227
Inovirus 1:547, 2:1227
Insect pest control by viruses see
   Biological control
Insect picorna-like
   viruses 2:1268(Table)
   biological control by 2:843–4,
      2:1274
   CrPV/DV complex 2:1268–71
   di-cistronic 2:1268
   of dipterans 2:1272–3
   genome
      properties 2:1267–8
      RNA 2:1267
   of hemipterans 2:1273–4
   of hymenopterans 2:1271–2
   of lepidopterans 2:1274
   RNA-dependent RNA
      polymerase 2:1268
Insect picornaviruses 2:1267–75
   misuse of term 2:1267
   see also Insect picorna-like
      viruses
Insect transmission, of plant
   viruses 3:1899–910
   circulative 3:1900, 3:1904–7

Insect transmission, of plant viruses
   (continued)
   circulative (continued)
      feeding mechanics/
         behavior 3:1900
      nonpropagative 3:1904–5
      propagative 3:1906–7
   feeding mechanics/
      behavior 3:1900–1
      prolonged feeding 3:1900
   general mechanisms 3:1899–900
   noncirculative 3:1900, 3:1901–4
      'bridge' hypothesis 3:1901
      feeding mechanics/
         behavior 3:1900
      helper viruses 3:1901–3
      ingestion–egestion
         model 3:1901
      ingestion–salivation
         model 3:1901
      mechanics theories 3:1901–4
      nonpersistent 3:1900
      potyviruses and
         caulimoviruses 3:1901–3
      semipersistent 3:1901, 3:1903–4
      transmission efficiency 3:1901
   nontransmissible viruses 3:1901
   terminology 3:1900
   virus–vector associations 3:1900
Insect viruses 1:97, 2:843(Table)
   classification 2:843(Table)
   DNA viruses 2:844–9
   flaviviruses evolutionary
      link 1:427
   history 2:723
   non-occluded 2:845–6
   RNA viruses 2:843–4
   see also Ascoviruses;
      Baculoviruses; Iridoviruses;
      Nodaviruses; Tetraviruses
Insecticides 3:1995
   aphid control, potyviruses
      transmission
      prevention 3:1375
   caulimovirus spread
      control 2:1280
   cypovirus synergism 1:338
   development 1:338
   from Bacillus subtilis 1:136
   granuloviruses as 1:145–6
   luteovirus prevention and
      control 2:907
   nuclear polyhedrosis viruses
      (NPVs) comparison 1:151
   rice tungro bacilliform virus
      transmission control 2:1293
   ultra low volume (ULV) 1:383
   viral 2:843
   see also Biological control
Insects
   control
      biocontrol see Biological
         control
      phytoreovirus transmission
         prevention 2:1265
   cypoviruses, pathogenicity and
      interactions 1:337–8
   economic significance 2:842–3
   hibernation resistance 1:338
   metabolism, cypovirus
      effects 1:337
   nucleic acid synthesis, cypovirus
      effects 1:337
   resistance to cypoviruses 1:337
   small RNA
      viruses 2:1268(Table), 2:1271
   in vesicular stomatitis virus
      (VSV) cycle 3:1915
   vesicular stomatitis virus (VSV)
      tropism 3:1917

Insects (continued)
  virus transmission
    bovine leukemia virus
      (BLV) 1:195
    bromoviruses 1:203
    fowlpox virus 1:579
    geminivirusvirus 1:603
Inserted sequences (IS)
  elements 2:1237
  bacteriophage P1 1:455
Insertion vectors 2:1241, 2:1243
  applications 2:1241
  screening 2:1241
Insertional mutagens
  murine leukemia viruses
    (MuLVs) as 2:997–8
  transposable phage as 2:987
Insulin
  impaired secretion, after
    echovirus infection 1:416
  processing 3:1978, 3:1978(Fig)
  production by E. coli 2:1247–8
Intasome 1:283
Integrase
  coliphage lambda 1:283
  see also individual viruses
Integrated pest management 3:1995
Integration of DNA into host
  genome see DNA
Integration host factor (IHF) 1:283
Integrative suppression 1:460
Integrins
  α6β4 2:1128
  $α_vβ_3$, coxsackievirus
    receptor 1:306
  foot-and-mouth disease virus
    receptor 1:572
  HPV attachment 2:1115
Intercellular adhesion molecule 1
  see ICAM-1
Interference, viral 2:850–4, 2:854
  endogenous proviruses 1:439
  heterologous 2:850
  history 2:850
  homologous 2:850
  types 2:850–1
    DI particles 1:372, 2:851
    dominant-negative
      mutants 2:851
    incompatibility of heterologous
      viruses 2:850–1
    interferons 2:850
    multimeric complexes 2:850–1
    superinfection exclusion 2:851
  see also Dominant-negative
    mutants; Interferons
Interferon 2:850, 2:854–62
  administration at low
    doses 2:861
  anti-antiviral mechanisms 2:860
  antiviral state and 2:857–9
    2-5 oligoadenylate synthetase/
      2-5(A)RNase L system 2:858
    Mx proteins 2:858–9
    PKR 2:858
    proteins associated 2:859
    receptor binding 2:857
    signal transduction 2:857–8
    systems activated/actions 2:858
  in bacterial infections 2:861
  clinical uses 2:855, 2:860–1
    as antiviral agent 2:855
    cautions 2:861
    hepatitis B and C therapy 1:65–6
    results 2:861
  cloning and expression 2:855
  in CMV infections 3:1824, 3:1825
  discovery 2:854–5
  EBV infection 3:1826
  future perspectives 2:861–2
  genes 2:855–6

Interferon (continued)
  in genital warts 2:1114
  history 2:854–5
  as host defense system 3:1961
  in HSV-1 infections 2:684
  immune see Interferon-γ (IFN-γ)
  inducers 1:67
    polyribonucleotides 2:861
  inducible genes 2:859
  induction 2:850, 2:856–7
    acquisition during
      development 2:857
    DNA viruses 2:856
    RNA viruses 2:856
    by Sendai virus 3:1621
    by SV40 3:1656
  levels in Argentine hemorrhagic
    fever (AHF) 2:893
  mechanisms of action 2:859–60
    virus replication blocked 2:859
  molecule structures 2:855–6
  mRNA 2:856–7
  murine CMV inducing 1:367–8
  nonadaptive immune
    response 2:812
  production
    enhanced by 'priming'
      cells 2:857
    vesicular stomatitis virus
      infection 3:1918
    viral hemorrhagic septicemia
      virus infection 3:1543
    rhinovirus prevention 3:1550
  signal transduction
    pathways 2:857–8
  thymosin $α_1$ with 1:66
  type I
    IFNs α, β, ω, τ, δ 2:855–6
    proteins induced by 2:859
    receptors (IFNAR) 2:857
    signal transduction
      pathway 2:857
    type II synergy 2:861
  type II (IFN-γ) 2:856
    proteins induced by 2:859
    receptor (IFNGR) 2:857
    signal transduction
      pathway 2:857–8
  vaccinia virus proteins
    targeting 3:1871
  viral replication inhibition 2:754
  in VZV infections 3:1877
Interferon α (IFN-α) 2:855
  biologically active
    molecules 2:855
  genes 2:855
  hepatitis B and C therapy 1:65
  HHV-6 inducing 2:702
  in HPV infections 1:67
  induced in virus infections 1:339
  LCMV infection 2:919
  murine 2:855
  recombinant 2:860–1
  respiratory virus
    infections 3:1495
  ribavirin with 1:66
  structure and synthesis 2:855
  in VZV infections 3:1828
Interferon β (IFN-β)
  expression 2:856
  regulators 2:856
  genes 2:855
  induced in virus infections 1:339
  recombinant 2:860–1
  structure and synthesis 2:855
Interferon σ (IFN-σ), structure and
  synthesis 2:856
Interferon γ (IFN-γ) 1:341, 2:813
  activation of caprine arthritis
    encephalitis virus
    (CAEV) 1:226
  cells producing 1:341

Interferon γ (IFN-γ) (continued)
  as dimer 1:341
  functions 1:341, 2:1202
  in hepatitis A 1:639
  leporipoxvirus homologs 3:1387
  production 1:340
  proteins induced by 2:859
  receptors 1:341, 2:857
  reovirus sensitivity 3:1463
  structure and synthesis 2:856
  Th1 and Th2 response 1:341
Interferon γ-responsive element
  (GAS) 1:226
Interferon τ, structure and
  synthesis 2:856
Interferon ω (IFN-ω), structure and
  synthesis 2:855–6
Interferon regulatory factor
  (IRF) 2:857, 2:859
  bovine leukemia virus
    (BLV) 1:193
  types and actions 2:859
Interferon stimulated gene factors
  (ISGF) 2:857
  regulatory factors see Interferon
    regulatory factor (IRF)
Interferon stimulated genes 2:857
Interferon stimulated response
  elements (ISRE) 2:857
Interferon-induced 2-5A
  system 2:1312
  2-5A synthetase 2:1312
  2-5A-dependent RNAase
    L 2:1312
Interferon-induced protein ISG-
  15 2:859
Interferon-inducible protein (IP-
  10) 1:343
Intergenic 'gene-junction'
  sequences, plant
  rhabdoviruses 3:1534,
  3:1534(Fig)
Intergenic sequences (IS) 3:1534
  coronavirus 1:293
  sigma rhabdoviruses 3:1636
Interleukin-1 (IL-1) 1:339
  IL-1α 1:341
  IL-1β 1:341
  nonadaptive immune
    response 2:812
  receptors 1:341
  vaccinia virus proteins
    targeting 3:1871
Interleukin-1 (IL-1) family 1:341
Interleukin-1 (IL-1) receptor
  antagonist (IL-1Ra) 1:341
Interleukin-1β, HHV-6
  inducing 2:702
Interleukin-1β-converting enzyme
  (ICE) 1:341
Interleukin-2 (IL-2) 1:340, 1:341–2
  bovine leukemia virus (BLV)
    infection 1:196
  cells synthesing 1:341
  defects 1:342
  functions 1:341–2
  HAART with 1:61
  IL-2Rα and IL-2Rβ 1:341
  receptor 1:341
  signal transduction 1:341
Interleukin-3 (IL-3) 1:342
Interleukin-4 (IL-4) 1:342
  functions 1:342
  type 2 response 2:813
Interleukin-4 (IL-4) family 1:342
Interleukin-5 (IL-5) 1:342
  cells producing 1:342
  receptor 1:342
Interleukin-6 (IL-6) 1:339, 1:342
  functions and synthesis 1:342

Interleukin-7 (IL-7) 1:342
  functions and synthesis 1:342
  receptor 1:342
Interleukin-8 (IL-8) 1:343
Interleukin-10 (IL-10) 1:342
  functions and synthesis 1:342
  homolog in Orf virus 2:1146
  homolog in EBV lytic cycle 1:496
Interleukin-12 (IL-12) 1:339, 1:342–3, 2:813
  functions and synthesis 1:339, 1:342
  heterodimer 1:342
  murine CMV inducing 1:367
  receptors 1:342
Interleukin-13 (IL-13) 1:342
Interleukin-15 (IL-15) 1:343
Interleukin-18 (IL-18) 1:339, 1:343
Intermediate filaments 1:253
  changes, induced by frog virus 3
    (FV3) 1:586
  frog virus 3 (FV3) assembly 1:586
  functions 1:253
Intermediate subviral particles
  (ISVPs), reoviruses 3:1459, 3:1463
Internal replication sequence,
  parvovirus genome 2:1157
Internal ribosome entry site (IRES)
  animal enteroviruses 1:463
  cardioviruses 1:232
  coxsackieviruses 1:306
  encephalomyocarditis virus
    (EMCV) 2:1337
  enterovirus 70 (EV70) 1:470
  foot-and-mouth disease viruses
    (FMDVs) 1:571
  hepatitis A virus (HAV) 1:632, 1:635
  hepatitis C virus (HCV) 1:657
  pestiviruses 1:174
  polioviruses see Poliovirus
  Theiler's murine
    encephalomyelitis viruses
    (TMEV) 3:1774
International Committee on
  Nomenclature of Viruses
  (ICNV) 3:1730
  establishment 2:724
International Committee on
  Taxonomy of Viruses
  (ICTV) 3:1730, 3:1731, 3:1937–8
  definitions of virus species 3:1940
  guidelines for virus
    identification 3:1754–5
  Luteoviridae 2:901
  Report 1999 3:1745(Table)
  reports 3:1731
  structure and functions 3:1731
  study groups and
    subcommittees 3:1731
  virus database project 3:1731
  virus descriptors 3:1733(Table)
  virus families and genera 3:1732, 3:1734
  virus orders 3:1732
  virus species concept 3:1732–4
  virus species definition 3:1732–4, 3:1734
  see also Taxonomy of viruses
International Committee for
  Taxonomy of Viruses (ICTV)
  Universal System 2:1221–3
  description of new phage 2:1223
  families 2:1223
  genus definition 2:1223
  nomenclature rules 3:1753–4
  orders 2:1223
  species definition 2:1222–3
International Enterovirus Study
  Group 2:736

Intervening sequences
    (IVS) 3:1553–5
Intestine, virus replication 1:441,
    1:448
'Intracellular immunization' 2:853
Intracytoplasmic A-type particles
    (ICAPs), type D
    retroviruses 3:1518, 3:1520,
    3:1522
Intranuclear inclusions, adenovirus
    infections 1:21
Intraocular infections 1:523
    see also Eye infections
Intrauterine infections, cardiac
    disease due to 2:1074–5
Intravenous immunoglobulin,
    cytomegalovirus (CMV)
    infection 3:1824, 3:1825
Intron see Interferon α
Introns 1:255
    Group I 3:1552
    Group II 3:1552
    as ribozymes see Ribozymes
    self-splicing 3:1552
        group I 1:131
        SPO1 phage 3:1681
Invertebrates
    virus families/genera
        infecting 3:1752(Fig)
    see also Insect viruses
Inverted repeat (IR) sequences,
    equine herpesviruses 1:510
Inverted terminal repeats (ITRs)
    see Terminal inverted repeats
    (TIRs)
Invirase see Saquinavir (invirase)
Ion pumps 1:250
Ipomoviruses 3:1369
    structure and properties 3:1369
    transmission 3:1374
Ippy virus 2:888
Iresine viroid 3:1930(Table)
Iridescence 2:868
Iridescent viruses 2:862
    Apis (AIV) 2:744(Table), 2:748–9
    see also Iridoviruses
Iridocorneal adhesions 1:523
Iridolenticular adhesions 1:523
Iridoviridae 2:862–9
    apoptosis inhibition 1:73
    characteristic features 1:582
    fish viruses 1:566–7
    genera 1:582, 2:862
    insect pest control by 2:845
    lymphocystis disease virus 2:908–11
    Ranavirus 1:582
        see also Frog virus 3 (FV3)
    taxonomy and
        classification 2:863(Table)
    viruses included 2:863(Table)
    see also Iridoviruses
Iridovirus 2:862, 2:868
    classification 2:864
    evolution 2:864(Fig), 2:868
    insect pest control by 2:845
    types 2:864(Table)
Iridoviruses 2:862–9
    assembly 3:1478
    characteristics 2:862, 2:908
    composition 2:865
    covert and patent
        infections 2:869
    cytopathology 2:867
    DNA replication 3:1478
    ecology 2:868–9
    economic importance 2:868
    enzymes 2:865
    evolution 2:864(Fig), 2:868
    genes 2:865

Iridoviruses (continued)
    genome 2:864–5
        terminal redundancy 2:864,
        2:868
    helicase 2:865
    icosahedral capsid 2:865
    inclusion bodies 2:866–7
    lipid membrane 2:865
    MCP genes 2:865
    pathology 2:867
    replication 2:867, 3:1478
        model 2:867
        site 2:867
    serology 2:866
    structure and properties 2:864–5
    taxonomy and
        classification 2:862–4
    temperature-dependent
        pathogenicity 2:867
    transmission 2:865
    types 2:863–4, 2:866
    virus–host interactions 2:865–6
    viruses included 2:863(Table)
    see also Chilo iridescent virus
        (CIV); *Tipula* iridescent virus
        (TIV)
Iris atrophy, sectoral 1:526
Iris yellow spot virus (IYSV) 3:1804
ISCOM vaccines, rinderpest and
    distemper viruses 3:1567,
    3:1569
Isfahan virus 1:257–60
    antibodies 1:259
    classification 1:257
    history 1:257
    host range 1:259
ISIS 2922 1:63
ISIS 13312 1:63
Isle of Wight disease 2:745
Isolation of viruses see Diagnostic
    techniques
Isosporalen 1:395
Isoxazole compounds 1:66
ITA (inhibitor of T cell
    apoptosis) 1:71
Iteravirus 1:385, 1:386
Iterons 1:603
Itupiranga virus
    (ITUV) 2:1045(Table)
Ixodes persulcatus 1:424
Ixodes ricinus
    louping ill virus
        transmission 1:434
    Russian spring summer
        encephalitis virus (RSSEV)
        transmission 1:424
    tick-borne encephalitis (TBE)
        virus complex
        transmission 1:435

J

Jaagsiekte sheep retrovirus
    (JSRV) 3:1524
Jamestown Canyon (JC)
    virus 3:1991
Japan
    benyvirus distribution 1:155
    rubella vaccination
        program 3:1600
Japanaut virus
    (JAUT) 2:1045(Table)
Japanese encephalitis (JE)
    virus 2:871–6, 3:1994
    cell culture 2:872
    cytopathology 2:872
    emergence in new areas 1:422

Japanese encephalitis (JE) virus
        (continued)
    emerging/re-emerging
        virus 1:419(Table)
    epidemics 2:873
    epidemiology 2:873
    future perspectives 2:875
    genetics 2:872
    genome 2:871
    glycoprotein NS1 2:872
    history/discovery 1:424, 2:871
    host range and propagation 2:872
    infection
        clinical features 2:874
        epidemiology 3:1994
        experimental 2:872
        fatality rate 2:874
        history 2:871
        immune response 2:874
        pathology 2:873–4, 2:874
        prevention and control 2:874–
        5, 3:1994
    neuroinvasiveness 2:873
    overwintering 2:875
    pathogenicity 2:873
    physical properties 2:872
    prevention and control 2:873
    proteins 2:871
        E protein 2:872
        E protein epitopes 2:871
        NS3 and NS5 2:872
        structural 2:871
    RNA replication 2:872
        intermediate RNA 2:872
        site 2:872
    serologic relationship and
        variability 2:873
    serotype 2:872
    structure and properties 2:871
    taxonomy and
        classification 2:871
    tissue tropism 2:873
    transmission 2:871, 2:873
        prevention 2:873
    vaccination 2:873
        swine 2:874–5
    vaccine 2:874–5
        bivalent 2:874
        formalin-inactivated 2:874
        immunity 2:874
        live-attenuated 2:875
        recombinant 2:875
    viremia 2:873
Japanese encephalitis (JE) virus
    group 1:433(Table)
Japanese flounder nervous necrosis
    virus (JFNNV) 2:1026
Jasminum, economic significance of
    virus infections 1:1323
Jaundice, infectious 1:640
Jaw tumors, in endemic Burkitt's
    lymphoma (BL) 1:492, 1:493
JC virus 2:876–83
    antibodies 2:878, 2:882
    classification 2:876
    cloning 2:878–9
    detection, ELISAs 2:880
    epidemiology 2:880
    evolution 2:878–80
    genetics 2:880
    genome 2:876, 2:877(Fig)
        'archetype' 2:879, 2:879(Fig),
        2:880
        promoter–enhancer
        sequences 2:879, 2:880, 2:881
        sequence
        hypervariability 2:878–9
    geographic/seasonal
        distribution 2:877–8
    history 2:876
    host range and propagation 2:878
    infection

JC virus (continued)
    infection (continued)
        post-transplant 3:1831
        renal involvement 2:1083
        see also Progressive multifocal
            leukoencephalopathy (PML)
    isolates 2:877
    nomenclature 2:876
    pathogenicity 2:881
    properties 2:876
    proteins 2:880
        functional domains of T
            antigen 2:878(Fig)
        JELP (JC early leader
            protein) 2:877
        large T and small t
            antigens 2:877, 2:880, 2:1182
        properties 2:877
    reactivation 3:1831
    serologic relationships and
        variability 2:880
    serotypes 2:880
        Mad1 2:876, 2:880
        Mad11 2:880
    tissue tropism 2:880–1
    trans-activation of late promoter
        by HIV *tat* 2:881
    transmission 2:880–1
    typing schemes 2:879–80
Jellyroll β barrel
    dianthovirus capsid
        protein 1:404, 1:408
    evolution 2:938
Jenner, Edward 1:298, 3:1861
    vaccination technique 3:1870
    virus used by 3:1865, 3:1870
Jκ transcription factor, in EBV
    latency 1:498
JKT-6423 virus 2:1046(Table)
JKT-7075 virus 2:1046(Table)
Joest–Degen inclusion bodies 1:172
jun oncogene 1:116, 3:1509, 3:1820
Junin virus 2:887–96, 2:888(Table),
    2:1084, 3:1988
    antibodies 2:895
    classification 2:887
    emerging/re-emerging
        virus 1:419(Table)
    genetics 2:889
    geographic/seasonal
        distribution 2:888
    history 2:887
    host range 2:889
    propagation 2:889
    transmission 2:891
    vaccine 2:895
    see also Argentine hemorrhagic
        fever (AHF)
Junonia coenia densovirus
    (JcDNV) 1:386
    genome structure 1:385(Fig),
    1:386
    host range 1:386
    tissue culture 1:386
    as vector 1:387
Juquitiba virus 1:210
Jurona virus 1:257

K

Kalanchoë top-spotting virus
    (KTSV) 2:1296
Kammavanpettai virus
    (KMPV) 2:1045(Table)
Kaposi's sarcoma 3:1848
    in AIDS 3:1848
    classic form 3:1848
    disseminated form 3:1848

INDEX

Kaposi's sarcoma (continued)
 eyelids and conjunctiva 1:529
 HHV-8 associated 3:1848
 HIV associated 3:1842
 pathogenesis 3:1848
Kaposi's sarcoma-associated
 herpesvirus (HSHV) see
 Human herpesvirus 8 (HHV-8)
Kashmir bee virus
 (KBV) 2:744(Table), 2:747,
 2:1272
 geographic distribution 2:1272
 pathology and
 epizootiology 2:747
 persistence 2:747
Kawino virus (KV) 2:1272, 2:1273
Kennedya yellow mosaic
 virus 3:1850, 3:1852
Kennel cough syndrome 1:20
Keratinocytes
 HPV infection 2:1109–10
 HPV life cycle 2:1109–10,
  2:1109(Fig)
 HPV-infected, cytokine
  release 2:1113
 immortalization by HPVs 2:1106
 HPV16 3:1845–6
 molluscum contagiosum virus
  (MCV)
  culture 2:963
  infection 2:964
 virus maturation 2:1176
Keratitis
 Epstein–Barr virus causing 1:526
 HSV-1 causing 1:526
 necrotizing herpes stromal 1:523
 punctate epithelial 1:523
 recurrent lytic epithelial 1:523
Keratoconjunctivitis see Epidemic
 keratoconjunctivitis (EKC)
Keratopathy, measles 1:524
KEX1 protease, yeast 3:1978,
 3:1978(Fig)
KEX2 protease, yeast 3:1978,
 3:1978(Fig)
Kidney
 adenocarcinoma, amphibian
  herpesviruses causing 1:51
 failure see Renal failure
 transplantation see Renal
  transplantation
 viruses affecting 2:1081–5,
  2:1081(Table)
Killer toxin
 helper totiviruses
  requirement 3:1808
 Saccharomyces cerevisiae 3:1611
 satellite dsRNA encoding 3:1808,
  3:1812
 yeast RNA viruses see Yeast
  RNA viruses, killer toxins
 yeast and smut fungus 3:1808,
  3:1812
 see also Ustilago maydis viruses
Killing phenomenon,
 totiviruses 3:1813
Kinesin 1:254
Kirsten murine sarcoma virus (Ki-
 MuSV) 2:995, 3:1517
kit oncogene 3:1513
KITC box, potyvirus helper
 factors 3:1901
Klamath virus 3:1541
Kober stem grooving,
 grapevines 3:1841
Kokobera virus group 1:433(Table)
Koplik's spots 2:957
Korea, Japanese encephalitis (JE)
 virus 2:873

Korean hemorrhagic fever see
 Hemorrhagic fever with renal
 syndrome (HFRS)
Kozak rule 3:1469
KP4 killer toxins see Ustilago
 maydis viruses
KP6 killer toxins see Ustilago
 maydis viruses
KTER motif 1:157
Kunjin virus 3:1995
Kupffer cells
 LDV infection 1:94
 necrosis, dengue virus
  infection 1:382
 virus uptake/entry 2:1179
Kuru 2:1018, 3:1388, 3:1392,
 3:1398–402, 3:1402
 classification 3:1398
 clinical features 3:1400–1
 geographic/seasonal
  distribution 3:1398–9
 history 3:1398
 host range and
  propagation 3:1399
 immune response 3:1401
 incidence 3:1400
  reduction 3:1401
 incubation 3:1400
 origin 3:1399
 pathology/histopathology 3:1401
 prevention and control 3:1401
Kuru agent
 cell cultures 3:1400
 epidemiology 3:1400
 evolution 3:1399
 experimental
  transmission 3:1399, 3:1400
 genetics 3:1399
 pathogenicity 3:1400
 serologic relationships and
  variability 3:1400
 strains 3:1399
  adaptation 3:1399
 tissue tropism 3:1400
 transmission 3:1399, 3:1400
 see also Prion protein (PrP)
Kyasanur Forest disease 1:429,
 1:430, 1:434, 3:1994
 pathology/histopathology 1:436
Kyasanur Forest disease virus
 (KFDV) 3:1994
 features 1:425(Table)
 geographic/seasonal
  distribution 1:426
 history/discovery 1:426
 tissue tropism 1:435
 transmission 1:435

L

L5-like viruses 2:1225
L-A virus 3:1974, 3:1974(Table),
 3:1975(Fig)
 expression/ribosomal
  frameshifting 3:1975–7,
  3:1976(Fig)
 future perspectives 3:1979
 Gag protein 3:1975, 3:1975(Fig),
  3:1977
  acetylation 3:1977
  expression 3:1975, 3:1976(Fig)
 Gag-Pol protein 3:1975
  synthesis 3:1975–7, 3:1976(Fig)
 host functions 3:1977–8,
  3:1977(Table)
 M satellite viruses see M satellite
  viruses

L-A virus (continued)
 replication cycle 3:1975,
  3:1976(Fig)
 satellites 3:1974
L-BC virus 3:1974, 3:1974(Table)
 host functions 3:1977,
  3:1977(Table)
La Bouhite disease 3:1962
La Crosse virus 3:1760, 3:1991
 apoptosis promotion 1:75
 'delayed emergence' 1:422
 infection 1:208
  encephalitis 1:68, 1:209
  pathogenesis 1:209
 morphology 1:212(Fig)
 transmission 1:209
La France isometric virus
 (LIV) 1:154
La Joya virus 1:257
Lactate dehydrogenase, elevation in
 LDV infection 1:94, 1:95
Lactate dehydrogenase-elevating
 virus (LDV) 1:89
 antibodies 1:95, 1:96
 evolution 1:93
 genome 1:90(Fig), 1:91, 1:93
  ORF5 1:96
 geographic/seasonal
  distribution 1:92
 host range and propagation 1:93
 immune complexes 1:94, 1:95,
  1:96
 immune response 1:95, 1:96
 infection
  pathogenicity and clinical
   features 1:94–5
  pathology and
   histopathology 1:95–6
 LDV-C 1:93, 1:94, 1:95
 macrophage infection 1:93, 1:94
 morphology 1:91(Fig)
 persistent infection 1:94
 receptor 1:92
 replication 1:95
  in vitro 1:93
 T-independent antigen 1:96
 taxonomy and classification 1:90
 transmission 1:94
 virulence mutants 1:93
Lactic acid bacteria 2:1253
Lactobacillus casei, phage-
 resistant 2:1247
Lactose malabsorption, enteric
 virus infections 1:448
lacZ gene
 insertion vectors 2:1241
 M13 vectors 2:1242
Laennec's cirrhosis 3:1830
Lagos bat virus 3:1439, 3:1443,
 3:1445
 discovery 3:1442
 epidemiology 3:1444
 host range 3:1443
 infections 3:1442
 propagation 3:1443
Lagovirus 2:1035
 genome 2:1038
Laguna Negra virus 1:210, 1:621,
 3:1988
Lake Clarendon virus
 (LCV) 2:1045(Table)
Lambda bacteriophage see
 Coliphage lambda
Lambdoid phages 1:281
 SSV1 virus similarity 1:88
Laminated inclusion components
 (LIC), potexvirus
 infections 3:1368
Laminin receptor, Sindbis (SIN)
 virus 3:1658

Lamium mild mosaic virus
 (LMMV) 1:531
 genome 1:532
 host range 1:533
 serology 1:534
 transmission 1:534
 see also Fabaviruses
Lamivudine (3TC, Epivir) 1:59,
 2:779
 feline immunodeficiency virus
  (FIV) infection 1:540
 hepatitis B 1:66
 post-transplant HBV
  infection 3:1831
Langerhans cells, in HSV
 infections 2:684
Laryngeal papillomatosis, HPVs
 causing 2:1111(Table), 2:1112
Laryngotracheobronchitis see
 Croup
Lassa fever
 antibodies 2:890, 2:895
 clinical features 2:892, 2:893
 complications 2:893
 drug prophylaxis 2:895
 epidemiology 2:890
 immune response 2:895
 incubation 2:892, 2:893
 mortality rate 2:890
 pathogenesis 2:892
 pathology/histopathology 2:892,
  2:894
 prevention and control 2:895,
  3:1989
 therapy 2:895, 2:895–6
 viremia 2:892, 2:896
Lassa virus 2:887–96, 2:888(Table),
 2:1084, 3:1988
 B cell epitope variability 2:889
 emerging/re-emerging
  virus 1:419(Table)
 genetics 2:889
 geographic/seasonal
  distribution 2:888–9
 history 2:887
 host range 2:889
 LCMV relationship 2:916
 propagation 2:889
 reservoir 2:889
 transmission 1:485(Table), 2:890,
  2:891–2, 3:1988
 vaccines 2:895
Lassa virus complex,
 evolution 2:889
Latency 2:897–901
 immune evasion
  mechanism 2:816
 mechanisms 2:897
 see also Latent infections
Latency-associated transcripts
 (LATs) 2:1200
 equine herpesviruses 1:512
 HSV see Herpes simplex virus
  (HSV)
 pseudorabies virus
  (PRV) 3:1423–4
Latent infections 2:897–901,
 2:1175, 2:1200, 3:1410, 3:1957
 cell types involved 2:897,
  2:898(Table)
 consequences 2:897
 definition 2:897
 DNA replication not
  associated 2:899
 establishment 2:899
 features 2:897
 future perspectives 2:900–1
 herpesvirus model 2:897–900
 maintenance 2:899–900
 neoplastic alteration 2:897
 neuronal functions 2:899

Latent infections (continued)
  re-activation 2:897, 2:899–900, 2:1200
  viruses establishing 2:897, 2:898(Table)
  see also individual viruses; Latency; Persistent infections
Latent period, bacteriophage 3:1416–17
Lates calcarifer (barramundi) encephalitis virus (LcEV) 2:1026
Latex agglutination, viral antigen detection 1:389
Latex particles, virus particle assay 3:1413
Latino virus 2:887, 2:888(Table)
Lato river virus (LRV) 3:1790(Table)
Latoia viridissima virus (LvV) 2:1274
Leaf
  abnormal morphology in virus infections 2:1318–19
  abrasion, sobemovirus transmission 3:1677
  early fall due to virus infections 2:1323
  epinasty, in viroid infections 3:1932, 3:1933(Fig)
  propagation of plant viruses 3:1419
Leafhoppers
  badnavirus transmission 2:1299
  geminivirus transmission 1:603, 3:1905
  phytoreoviruses transmission 2:1266
  plant rhabdoviruses relationship 3:1538
  plant symptoms caused by 3:1969
  rice tungro bacilliform virus transmission 2:1293
  waikavirus transmission 3:1968
Leaky scanning, tombusviruses 3:1795
Lebombo virus (LEBV) 2:1045(Table)
Lechiguanas virus 3:1988
Lederberg, J. 2:729
Leek white stripe virus (LWSV) 2:1003
  genome 2:1004
  infection 2:1003
  see also Necroviruses
Leek yellow stripe potyvirus 1:242
Legume caulimoviruses 2:1289–92
  caulimoviruses differential features 2:1290
  control 2:1292
  gene products 2:1291
  genome 2:1290, 2:1290(Fig)
    ORF1 2:1290
  geographic distribution 2:1289
  history 2:1289
  host range 2:1289, 2:1290(Table)
  intergenic region 2:1290
  molecular biology 2:1290–2
  serologic relationships 2:1289
  strains 2:1289
  structure and proteins 2:1289
  symptoms 2:1289
  taxonomy and classification 2:1289
  transactivation 2:1291–2
  transcription 2:1290–1
  transmission 2:1289–90
  tRNA primer binding site (PBS) 2:1290

Legume caulimoviruses (continued)
  see also Peanut chlorotic streak virus (PClSV); Soybean chlorotic mottle virus (SoyCMV)
Leishmania braziliensis, totiviruses 3:1808
Leishmania braziliensis virus (LBV) 1:613
Leishmania RNA virus (TRV), characteristics/properties 1:616(Table)
Leishmaniavirus 3:1808, 3:1974
  life cycle and replication 3:1811, 3:1811(Fig)
  viruses included 3:1809(Table)
Lelystad virus 1:420(Table)
Lenti-retroviruses 3:1963
Lentivirus 1:535, 2:774, 2:789, 2:795, 3:1640
  caprine arthritis encephalitis virus (CAEV) 1:223
  equine infectious anemia virus (EIAV) 1:515
  HTLV-1 2:789
  human immunodeficiency viruses 2:774
    nucleotide divergences 1:226
  simian immunodeficiency viruses (SIV) 3:1640
  see also individual viruses
Lentiviruses 1:184, 1:223, 2:764, 3:1963
  animal, serologic relationships 2:771
  animal models 1:535
  apoptosis promotion 1:75
  bovine 1:184
    see also Bovine immunodeficiency virus (BIV)
  characteristics 3:1640
  evolution and relationships 1:188, 1:518
  genes 3:1641(Table)
  mutation rates 3:1643
  persistent infections 1:223
  phylogenetic tree 1:535
  primate
    genome 3:1644(Fig)
    groups 3:1641(Fig)
    see also Simian immunodeficiency viruses (SIV)
  in sheep and goats see Visna-maedi viruses
Lepidopterans
  entomopoxviruses (EPVs) 1:476, 1:478
  picorna-like viruses 2:1274
  tetravirus infections 3:1770
Leporipoxvirus 3:1383
  characteristics 3:1383
  members 3:1382(Table)
Leporipoxviruses 3:1381–8
  cytopathology 3:1384–5
  DNA replication 3:1384
  evolution 3:1385
  future perspectives 3:1387–8
  genetic variability 3:1385
  genome 3:1383–4
    terminal inverted repeat (TIR) 3:1383
  geographic/seasonal distribution 3:1384
  history 3:1381–3
  host range and propagation 3:1384–5
  immune evasion 3:1384
  infection
    clinical features 3:1386
    immune response 3:1387

Leporipoxviruses (continued)
  infection (continued)
    pathology/histopathology 3:1386–7
    prevention and control 3:1387
  members 3:1382(Table)
  pathogenic mechanisms 3:1384
  pathogenicity 3:1385–6
  proteins 3:1383–4
  replication
    sites 3:1385
    in virosomes 3:1384
  structure and properties 3:1383
  taxonomy and classification 3:1383
  transcription and translation 3:1384
  transmission and tissue tropism 3:1385
  tumors 3:1386
  viroceptors 3:1384
  virokines 3:1384
  virulence 3:1384, 3:1385
  see also Myxoma virus (MYX)
Leptin, murine, cDNA transfer 1:14
Lettuce infectious yellows virus (LIYV) 1:267
  disease and economic significance 1:272
  genome 1:269, 1:269(Fig)
  RNA 1:267
    RNA1 and RNA2 1:270
  transmission 1:272
Lettuce necrotic yellows virus (LNYV) 3:1531
  genome 3:1534
  outbreaks 3:1540
  proteins 3:1534–6
    nucleocapsid (N) 3:1535
  replication and budding 3:1538
  see also Plant rhabdoviruses
Lettuce speckles mottle virus (LSMV) 3:1856, 3:1856(Table), 3:1858
Leucine zipper, v-Myc protein 3:1510
Leukemia 1:197
  adult T-cell see Adult T-cell leukemia
  chronic myelogenous, v-Abl role 3:1512
  gibbon ape leukemia virus (GaLV) causing 1:617, 1:618
  hairy cell see Hairy cell leukemia
Leukemia viruses, transmission, 1:485(Table)
Leukemogenesis
  HTLV-1 see Human T-cell leukemia virus type 1 (HTLV-1)
  murine leukemia viruses (MuLVs) see Murine leukemia viruses (MuLVs)
Leukopenia
  LCMV 2:918
  measles 2:956, 2:959
  morbillivirus infections 3:1567
Leukoplakia, hairy 1:491
Leviviridae 2:1227–8, 3:1663
  characteristics 2:1227–8
  phage included 2:1227–8
  Tombusviridae relationship 1:243
  see also RNA bacteriophage, single-stranded
Levivirus 2:1227, 3:1663
LexA protein 1:283
Lidakol 1:62
Ligase chain reaction (LCR) 1:392, 1:393

Light microscopy, virus identification 1:400
Lilac chlorotic leafspot virus (LCLV) 1:222
Lilac ring mottle virus (LRMV) 1:39
Lily, Enchantment, growth failure 2:1321
Lily symptomless virus (LSV), genome 1:239
Lily virus X (LVX), genome 3:1366
LINEs (long interspersed nuclear elements) 1:437, 1:438(Table), 2:1316–17, 2:1316(Fig)
Linnean system 3:1731–2
Lipids
  functions 3:1920
  viral membranes 3:1920, 3:1924
Lipopolysaccharide
  bacteriophage ϕX174 receptor 1:275
  prevention of cyanophage infection of Anabaena 1:331
Lipothrixviridae 1:85, 2:1226
  characteristics 2:1226
  phage included 2:1226
Lipothrixvirus 1:86
Little cherry virus (LChV)
  coat proteins 1:267
  genome 1:269, 1:269(Fig)
  RNA 1:267
Liver
  cancer see Hepatocellular carcinoma
  coxsackievirus infection 1:308
  damage, Lassa fever 2:892, 2:894
  necrosis see Hepatic necrosis
  transplantation, HBV infection 3:1830
  yellow fever pathology 3:1985
Livestock transportation, emergence/re-emergence of diseases 1:422
LLCMK2 cells, astrovirus culture 1:104
LN33 stem grooving, grapevines 3:1841
Lobucavir 1:63
Local acquired resistance (LAR), in plants 2:1306
'Local suicide' hypothesis, plant resistance 2:1305
Locus diarrhoea 2:726
Locusts, biological control by Entomopoxvirinae 2:845
Lodenosine 1:60
Lolium enation viruses (LEV) 2:1263
Long interspersed nuclear elements see LINEs
Long terminal repeat (LTR) 3:1503
  avian leukosis virus (ALV) 1:113, 1:114
  bovine immunodeficiency virus (BIV) 1:185
  bovine leukemia virus (BLV) 1:191
  Drosophila melanogaster gypsy virus 3:1527, 3:1528
  feline leukemia viruses (FeLVs) 1:542, 1:545
  fungal retrotransposons 3:1503–4, 3:1504(Fig)
  HIV see HIV
  HTLV-1 2:789, 2:790
  HTLV-2 2:797
  lymphoproliferative disease virus (LPDV) 2:912
  mouse mammary tumor virus (MMTV) 2:966, 2:967, 2:969
  murine leukemia viruses (MuLVs) 2:996

Long terminal repeat (LTR) (*continued*)
  prototype 1:438
  retrotransposons 2:1315
  retroviruses 3:1476
  simian immunodeficiency viruses (SIV) 3:1642
  spumaviruses 3:1689
  type D retroviruses 3:1521
Lordsdale virus 2:1037
Louping ill (LI) 1:432
  epidemics 1:434
  prevention and control 1:436
Louping ill (LI) virus 1:431, 1:433(Table)
  escape mutants 1:434
  host range and propagation 1:432
  transmission 1:434
  vaccine 1:434, 1:436
Low density lipoprotein, rhinovirus receptor 3:1545
Lox-cre site-specific recombination system, bacteriophage P1 1:455, 1:456, 1:458, 1:460
Lucerne Australian latent virus 2:1008(Table)
Lucerne Australian symptomless virus 2:1009(Table)
Lucerne transient streak virus (LTSV) 3:1556, 3:1674
  genome 3:1678
  host range 3:1677
  properties 3:1675–6
  see also Sobemoviruses
Luciferase 3:1897
  firefly 1:398
Lucké tumor herpesvirus (LTHV) 1:51, 1:51–2
  culture failure 1:51, 1:53
  DNA 1:51
  gene expression 1:51–2
  geographic distribution 1:51
  histology of tumors 1:51(Fig)
  oncogenicity 1:52
  properties 1:51
  replication 1:51–2
    temperature relationship 1:52
  transmission 1:52
  see also Amphibian herpesviruses
Lucké tumors 1:51(Fig), 1:52
Lumpy skin disease of cattle (LSD)
  in African buffalo 3:1377
  clinical features 3:1379
  epidemiology 3:1378
  geographic distribution 3:1376
  history 3:1376
  transmission 3:1377, 3:1378
  vaccines 3:1380
  see also Capripoxviruses
Lung
  murine CMV infection 1:366
  see also Respiratory tract
Luria, S. 2:728
Luteoviridae 2:901–8
  economic significance 2:907–8
  Enamovirus 2:901
  epidemiology 2:905
  genera 2:901
  genome organization 2:903(Fig)
  Luteovirus 2:901
    pea enation mosaic virus 1 (PEMV 1) 3:1855, 3:1857
  Polerovirus 2:901
  serological relationships 2:905
  structure and properties 2:903
  taxonomy 2:901–2, 2:902(Table)
  tissue tropism 2:906
  transmission 2:905–6
  umbravirus helper viruses 3:1855, 3:1858
  vectors 2:901

Luteoviridae (*continued*)
  see also Luteoviruses; Poleroviruses
Luteovirus 1:243, 2:901–8, 2:902(Table)
Luteoviruses 1:272, 2:902
  astroviruses similarity 1:106
  binding to *E. coli* GroEL 3:1905
  coat protein 3:1904
    readthrough 3:1904, 3:1905
  cross-enhancing RNA interactions 2:904
  cytopathology 2:906–7
  economic significance 2:907–8
  epidemiology 2:905
  evolution 2:905
  genome organization 2:903, 2:903(Fig)
  geographic distribution 2:902–3
  host range 2:903
  pathogen-derived engineered resistance 2:1308(Table)
  pathogenicity 2:906–7
  prevention and control 2:907
  protein functions 2:903–4
  replication 2:903–4
  RNA1 of pea enation mosaic virus (PEMV) similarity 2:1192–3
  RNA-dependent RNA polymerase (RDRP) genes 2:903, 2:905
  satellite RNAs 2:904, 3:1554(Table)
  serological relationships 2:905
  structure and composition 2:903
  subgenomic (sg) RNAs 2:904
  taxonomy 2:902, 2:902(Table)
  tissue tropism 2:906
  transcription 2:904
  translation 2:904
    initiation 2:904
  transmission 2:905, 2:905–6, 3:1904–5
  vector specificity 2:906
  virus-like particles (VLPs) 3:1904–5
  viruses included 2:901–2
Luxury functions of cells 2:1017
Lychnis ringspot virus (LRSV) 2:749
  host range 2:750
Lymantria dispar, biological control 2:847
Lymantria dispar MNPV (LpMNPV) 1:147
  genome 1:147–8
Lymantria ninayi virus (LNV$_G$) 2:1026, 2:1274
Lymph nodes 2:820, 2:821(Fig)
  cell:cell interactions 2:814(Fig)
Lymphadenopathy, Hodgkin's disease 1:492
Lymphatic vessels 2:814
  virus growth 2:1015
Lymphoblastoid cell lines, EBV culture 1:488
Lymphocryptovirus 1:488, 2:707, 2:708
  Rhadinovirus comparison 2:704(Table)
Lymphocystis cells 2:909(Fig), 2:910
Lymphocystis disease (LD) 1:566, 2:908
  clinical features 1:566, 2:910
  fish 2:908, 2:910
  geographic/seasonal distribution 2:910
  pathology/histopathology 2:910–11

Lymphocystis disease virus (LCDV) 1:566, 2:908–11
  cytopathic effects 1:566
  enzymes 2:910
  evolution 2:910
  future perspectives 2:911
  genome 2:908–9
    circular permutation 2:909
    methylation 2:909
    organization 2:909(Fig)
    replication 2:909
  geographic/seasonal distribution 1:566, 2:910
  history 1:566, 2:908
  host range and propagation 1:566, 2:910
  infection *see* Lymphocystis disease (LD)
  properties 2:908
  proteins 2:909
  structure 2:909(Fig)
  taxonomy and classification 1:566, 2:908
  transmission and tissue tropism 1:566, 2:910
  types 1 and 2 2:908
Lymphocystivirus 1:566, 2:908, 2:910
Lymphocytes
  cultures 1:398–9
    viruses detected using 1:398
  immortalization with herpesvirus sylvilagus 2:706
  measles virus (MV) infection 2:955
  necrosis, LDV infection 1:95
  viruses persistent in 2:707
Lymphocytic choriomeningitis virus (LCMV) 2:888, 2:915–20, 2:920–5
  anti-genomes 2:922
  antibodies 2:915, 2:919
    functions 3:1862
  Armstrong strain 2:915, 2:916
  autoimmunity model 1:110–11
  Biosafety Level recommendation 2:917, 2:919
  cDNAs 2:924–5
  cytopathic effect 2:889
  defective interfering mechanism 2:916
  defective-interfering RNAs 2:923, 2:924
  enzyme activities 2:921
    polymerase 2:923
  epidemiology 2:917
  evolution 2:889, 2:916–17
  experimental infections (mice) 2:915, 2:916, 2:920
    variant LCMVs 2:924
  future perspectives 2:919–20
  general features 2:915–20
  genes, expression in novel environments 2:924–5
  genetic reassortment 2:916
  genetics 2:916
  genome 2:916, 2:921
    ambisense 2:916, 2:921
    L and S RNAs 2:921, 2:923
    replication 2:922
    Z protein sequence 2:921, 2:923
  geographic/seasonal distribution 2:916
  glycoproteins 2:916
  history 2:887, 2:915
  host range 2:889, 2:916
  human infections 2:917, 3:1988
    acute, progression 2:923
    clinical features 2:918
    immune response 2:817, 2:918–19, 2:919–20, 2:1202
    immunopathology 2:817

Lymphocytic choriomeningitis virus (LCMV) (*continued*)
  human infections (*continued*)
    pancreas 2:1079
    pathology/histopathology 2:918
    prevention and control 2:919
  immune response history and 2:823
  immune response (in mice) 2:918(Fig)
  immunosuppression by 2:917
  in situ hybridization 2:924
  loss of 'luxury' functions in cells 2:917, 2:919
  as model system 2:915
  molecular biology 2:920–5
  mutation frequency 2:916
  pathogenicity 2:917–18, 2:918(Fig)
  persistent carrier state 2:823
  persistent infections 2:916, 2:917, 2:924
    in situ hybridization and 2:924
    regulation 2:923
    in tissue culture 2:923
  polymerase activity 2:923
  propagation 2:889, 2:916, 2:924
  proteins 2:921–2
    glycoprotein precursor (GPC) 2:921–2
    GP-1 and GP-2 2:921–2
    L-encoded 2:922
    nucleoprotein 2:921
    ribonucleoprotein (RNP) 2:921
    Z (zinc-binding) 2:916, 2:921, 2:922
  purification 2:920–1
  reassortant viruses 2:923–4
  receptors 2:916
  replication 2:922
  serologic relationship and variability 2:917
  strains 2:923–4
  structure and properties 2:920–1
    spikes 2:920
  taxonomy and classification 2:915–16
  tissue tropism 2:917
  transcription 2:922–3
  transgenic mice 2:925
  transmission 2:917
  Traub strain 2:915
  variants 2:916, 2:917, 2:924
    clone 13 2:916, 2:924
    Clone 13-like 2:924
    'docile' or viscerotropic 2:917
  WE strain 2:915, 2:917
  zinc-binding proteins *see* proteins, Z (*above*)
Lymphocytosis, persistent, bovine leukemia virus (BLV) infection 1:184, 1:189, 1:196
Lymphoepithelioma 1:493
Lymphoid cells
  reovirus type 3 cellular receptor 3:1927–8
  virus infection, autoimmune development 1:110
Lymphoid tissues, SIV infection 3:1645
Lymphoidal parvo-like virus (LOV) 3:1635
Lymphokines 2:819
Lymphomas
  B cell *see* B cell lymphoma
  baboon and chimpanzee herpesviruses causing 2:712
  body cavity-based (BCBL) 3:1848
  bovine leukemia virus (BLV) causing 1:197

Lymphomas (continued)
  Burkitt's see Burkitt's lymphoma (BL)
  EBV-associated 1:490
    clinical features 1:492
  Hodgkin's disease see Hodgkin's disease
  immunoblastic, EBV association 1:488(Table)
  in immunodeficient patients, EBV association 1:490
  Marek's disease 2:946(Fig), 2:949–50, 2:949(Fig)
  model, Marek's disease as 2:946
  mouse mammary tumor virus (MMTV) causing 2:970
  non-Hodgkin's, in AIDS 1:490
  reticuloendotheliosis (RE) viruses causing 3:1499–500
    REV-T 3:1500
  T cell, EBV-associated 1:488(Table), 1:490
  Tupaia herpesvirus-associated 3:1834, 3:1836, 3:1836–7
Lymphopenia 2:821
  measles 2:959
Lymphoproliferative disease (LPD)
  in baboons 2:711
  clinical features 2:913–14
  diagnosis and laboratory tests 2:914
  etiology 2:911
  history 2:911
  pathology/histopathology 2:913–14, 2:913(Fig)
Lymphoproliferative disease virus (LPDV) of turkeys 2:911–15
  antigen detection 2:914
  evolution 2:912(Fig)
  future perspectives 2:914
  genome 2:912–13, 2:914
    avian sarcoma–leukemia virus similarity 2:912
    env gene 2:913
    gag ORF 2:912
    long terminal repeats (LTR) 2:912
    ORFs 2:912–13, 2:913(Fig)
    pol ORF 2:913
    pro ORF 2:912–13
    proviral 2:912
  history 2:911
  host range and propagation 2:913
  infection see Lymphoproliferative disease (LPD)
  isolation 2:914
  leukemogenic action 2:914
  organotropism 2:914
  pathogenicity 2:913–14
  proteins 2:912–13
    Gag 2:912
  replication 2:911
  RT assay 2:914
  structure and properties 2:911–12
  taxonomy and classification 2:912
Lymphoproliferative syndrome 3:1844
  EBV-induced 3:1825, 3:1826
Lymphosarcomas
  bovine leukemia virus (BLV) causing 1:197
  feline leukemia viruses (FeLVs) causing 1:544
Lymphotactin 1:343
Lymphotoxin
  LT-α 1:340
  LT-β 1:340
  production 1:340

Lysine tRNA, as primer for HIV reverse transcriptase 2:765, 2:774
Lysogenic conversion 3:1415
  definition 2:1228
Lysogenic cycle, phage see Bacteriophage
Lysogenic state, definition 2:925
Lysogeny 2:925–33, 2:1251, 3:1415
  algal viruses 1:50
  coliphage lambda see Coliphage lambda
  detection 2:925
  general features 2:925–6
  P2 bacteriophage see P2 bacteriophage
  P4 bacteriophage see P4 bacteriophage
  phage, history 2:721
Lysosomes 1:250
Lysosomotropic amines 3:1922
Lysozyme, bacteriophage P22 3:1605
Lyssavirus 3:1442, 3:1987
  characteristics 3:1443
  rabies-like viruses 3:1439
  viruses included 3:1439
  see also Rabies-like viruses
Lyssaviruses
  epidemiology 3:1444
  evolution 3:1444
  history 3:1442
  serologic relationships 3:1444
  serotypes 3:1443
  transmission 3:1444
Lytic cycle, phage see Bacteriophage
Lytic infections, pseudolysogeny as variation 1:133
Lytic viruses, infectivity assays 3:1412

M

M_1 satellite virus 3:1974, 3:1974(Table)
  killer toxin (K_1)
    action 3:1978
    processing 3:1978
    replication 3:1975
M_2 satellite virus 3:1974, 3:1974(Table)
M_3 satellite virus 3:1974, 3:1974(Table)
M satellite viruses 3:1974, 3:1974(Table)
  host functions 3:1977, 3:1977(Table)
  replication 3:1975, 3:1976(Fig)
  see also M_1 satellite virus; M_{28} satellite virus
M_{28} satellite virus 3:1974, 3:1974(Table)
  killer toxin (K_{28}) 3:1978
M (microfold) cells
  enteric viruses in 1:448
  reovirus infection 3:1459
  rotavirus internalization 3:1582
'M' tropic viruses 2:775
M/R enzymes 2:758–60
  see also Host-controlled modification and restriction
Macaques, simian hemorrhagic fever virus infection 1:95
MACH (MORT1 associated CED-3/ICE homolog) 1:71

Machlomovirus 1:243, 2:935
  see also Machlomoviruses; Maize chlorotic mottle virus (MCMV)
Machlomoviruses 2:935–9
  carmoviruses similarity 2:937, 2:938
  cell-to-cell movement 2:937, 2:938
  epidemiology 2:937
  future perspectives 2:938
  genome 2:935–6
    ORFs 2:935–6, 2:937
  geographic/seasonal distribution 2:936
  history 2:935
  host range and propagation 2:936–7
  as monotypic genus 2:935, 2:938
  serologic relationship and variability 2:937
  structure and properties 2:935
  see also Maize chlorotic mottle virus (MCMV)
Machupo virus 2:887–96, 2:888(Table), 2:1084, 3:1988
  antibodies 2:895
  classification 2:887
  emerging/re-emerging virus 1:419(Table)
  genetics 2:889
  geographic/seasonal distribution 2:888
  history 2:887
  host range 2:889
  prevention and control 3:1995
  propagation 2:889
  see also Bolivian hemorrhagic fever (BHF)
Macluraviruses 3:1369
  structure and properties 3:1369
Macrolide antibiotics 2:786
Macrophage
  arterivirus infection 1:92, 1:94
  caprine arthritis encephalitis virus (CAEV) 1:226
  coronavirus infection 1:297
  echovirus infection 1:416
  equine infectious anemia virus (EIAV) infection 1:519
  in HSV-2 infections 2:684
  IL-10 action 1:342
  LDV receptor and infection 1:92, 1:94
  TNF synthesis 1:340–1
  tropic lentivirus infections, model 1:228
  virus uptake/entry 2:1179
  visna-maedi virus infection 3:1963–4
Macrophage inflammatory protein (MIP)-1 1:343
Macrophage-like cells, immortalization with herpesvirus sylvilagus 2:705–6
'Mad-itch' disease 3:1421
Maden–Darby bovine kidney cells, Mengo virus infection 1:235
Maedi 3:1961–2
  clinical/pathological criteria 3:1962
  pathology 3:1962
  see also Visna-maedi viruses
maf oncogene 3:1509
Maf response element (MARE) 3:1509
Magnesium ions (Mg^{2+}), *Tupaia* herpesvirus protein kinase and 3:1835
Mahoney leukemia virus, receptor 3:1471
Maize, agroinoculation 3:1894

Maize chlorotic dwarf virus (MCDV) 3:1965
  epidemiology 3:1968
  genome 3:1966
  geographic distribution 3:1965
  host range 3:1966
  infections 3:1965, 3:1968–9, 3:1969
    clinical features 3:1969
    pathology and histopathology 3:1969
    prevention and control 3:1969
  M1 strain 3:1967, 3:1970
  Ohio (OH) strain 3:1967, 3:1967(Table), 3:1970
  pathogenicity 3:1968–9
  seasonal distribution 3:1966
  serologic relationships and variability 3:1967
  TN strain 3:1967, 3:1967(Table), 3:1970
  transmission 3:1968
  type (T) strain 3:1967, 3:1967(Table)
  white stripe (WS) strain 3:1967
Maize chlorotic mottle virus (MCMV)
  capsid protein 2:938
  cDNA clone 2:938
  co-infection with potyviruses 2:937–8
  epidemiology 2:937
  evolution 2:938
  future perspectives 2:938
  genetics 2:937
  genome 2:935–6, 2:936(Fig)
    ORFs 2:935–6, 2:937
  geographic/seasonal distribution 2:936
  history 2:935
  host range and propagation 2:936–7
  infection see Corn lethal necrosis (CLN)
  Kansas serotypes 2:937
  pathogenicity 2:937–8
  physical properties 2:936
  prevention and control 2:938
  replicase 2:936, 2:938
  replication 2:936
  resistant varieties of maize 2:938
  serotypes 2:937
  structure and properties 2:935
  taxonomy and classification 2:935
  tissue tropism 2:937
  transmission 2:936, 2:937
  see also Machlomoviruses
Maize dwarf mosaic potyvirus (MDMV) 2:937
Maize mosaic virus (MMV) 3:1531
  resistance 3:1540
  see also Plant rhabdoviruses
Maize rayado fino virus 3:1852
Maize rough dwarf virus (MRDV) 2:1263
  genome 2:1264
  see also Phytoreoviruses
Maize streak virus (MSV) 1:597
  genome organization/expression 1:597
  genome structure 1:597
  transcripts (V-sense) 1:598
Maize stripe virus (MSpV) 3:1756
  genomic RNAs 3:1759
  glycoproteins 3:1907
  morphology 3:1763(Fig)
  serologic relationships 3:1763
  transmission 3:1907
  see also Tenuiviruses

Major histocompatibility complex (MHC)
  in CD8+ T cell response 2:820
  class I antigens 2:813, 2:819, 2:839–40
    antigen binding site 2:839–40
    CD8 T cell response 1:339
    cytotoxic T cell interaction 1:69
    decreased by murine CMV 1:368
    expression regulation in immune evasion 2:816
    human CMV proteins interfering 1:353
    influenza virus peptides 2:841
    m144 modulator 1:368
    peptide binding and 'dominant anchors' 2:840
    peptide loading 2:841
    T cell receptor interactions 2:840
    T cell recognition 2:841
    upregulation in inflammation 1:110
  class I restriction 2:813, 2:819
    history 2:823
  class II antigens 2:813, 2:820, 2:839
    α- and β-chains 2:820
    autoimmunity pathogenesis 1:108
    CD4 T cells response 1:340
    invariant chain 2:820
    peptide binding site 2:840
    structure 2:840
    upregulation in inflammation 1:110
  class II restriction 2:813, 2:814, 2:819, 2:820, 2:841
  discovery 2:723
  genetic resistance to Marek's disease 2:950–1
  gp120 interaction 3:1926
  immune response to respiratory viruses 3:1491
  repression by adenovirus E1A 1:29
  resistance genes association 2:757
  restriction 2:818, 2:839–40, 2:840, 2:1201–2
  superantigen action 2:1231
  T cell restriction 2:1201–2
  TCR–peptide interaction 1:108, 1:109(Fig)
  viral vaccines and 3:1863
MAK genes
  mutants, yeast 3:1977
  yeast 3:1812, 3:1977
MAK3 gene, yeast 3:1977, 3:1977(Table)
Malaria, Burkitt's lymphoma (BL) association 1:489, 1:494
'Malarial catarrhal fever' 2:1044
Malignancy, see also Cancer; Carcinogenesis; Tumors
Malignant catarrhal fever see Bovine malignant catarrhal fever
Malignant rabbit fibroma virus (MRV)
  history 3:1383
  replication, sites 3:1385
  see also Myxoma virus
Mammary tumors, MMTV causing see Mouse mammary tumor virus (MMTV)
Mammillitis 1:181, 1:182
Manawatu virus (MwV) 2:1026
Manchester virus 2:1037
  genome organization 2:1037(Fig), 2:1038

Manchester virus (continued)
  genome organization (continued)
    comparison with picornaviruses 2:1037(Fig)
    see also Sapporo-like viruses
MAP-4, N protein of coronavirus JHM interaction 1:254, 1:256(Fig)
Maraba virus 1:257
Marafiviruses
  phylogenetic relationships 3:1852, 3:1852–3, 3:1852(Fig)
  replicase protein (RP) 3:1853
'Marble spleen disease' of chickens 1:20
Marburg virus 2:939–45, 3:1993
  biosafety level 2:940, 2:944
  budding 2:940(Fig), 2:942
  carbohydrate structures 2:941
  effect on host immune system 2:944
  emerging/re-emerging virus 1:419(Table)
  epidemiology 2:943
  evolution 2:942–3
  genome 2:940–1
  geographic distribution 2:942
  Golgi-specific precursor (preGP) 2:941
  history 2:939
  host range and propagation 2:942
  inclusion bodies 2:942
  infection
    clinical features 2:943, 3:1993
    diagnosis 2:944–5
    immune response 2:944
    pathogenesis 2:943–4
    pathology/histopathology 2:943–4
    prevention and control 2:944
  pathogenicity 2:943
  physical properties 2:940
  proteins 2:941
    GP protein 2:941, 2:944
    L protein 2:941
    nucleoprotein 2:941
    VP40 2:941
  receptor (asialoglycoprotein) 2:941
  replication 2:941–2
  serologic relationship 2:943
  stability 2:940
  strains 2:939
    sequence comparisons 2:942
  structure and properties 2:940, 2:940(Fig)
  taxonomy and classification 2:939–40
  tissue tropism 2:943
  transcription 2:941–2
  transmission 1:485(Table), 2:943, 3:1993
Marburg/Ebola-like filovirus 3:1993
Marek's disease 2:945
  acute form 2:945, 2:948
  acute mortality syndrome 2:948
  classical form 2:948
  clinical features 2:945(Fig), 2:948
  forms and nomenclature 2:945
  genetic resistance 2:950–1
  history 2:945
  immune response 2:950
  lymphoma 2:946(Fig), 2:949–50, 2:949(Fig)
  as lymphoma model 2:946
  pathogenesis 2:950
  pathology 2:946(Fig), 2:948–50, 2:949(Fig)
  prevention and control 2:951
  transient paralysis 2:948

Marek's disease (continued)
  vaccinations 2:945
  vaccine see Marek's disease virus (MDV)
Marek's disease tumor-associated surface antigen (MATSA) 2:949
Marek's disease virus (MDV) 2:945–52
  antibodies to 2:950
  apoptosis promotion 1:75
  atherosclerosis due to 2:1077
  cell culture 2:948
  cell line derived from 2:950(Fig)
  classification 2:946
  contamination, RE viruses 3:1498
  distribution 2:948
  epizootiology 2:948
  fowlpox virus infection with 1:578
  future perspectives 2:951–2
  genome 2:946–7, 2:947(Fig)
    direct terminal repeats 2:698
  history 2:945–6
  infection see Marek's disease
  isolates 2:946
  isolation and propagation 2:947–8
  oncogenicity 2:947
  PCR studies 2:948
  physical properties 2:947
  productive/nonproductive infections 2:947
  proteins 2:947
  recombination with RE virus 3:1500
  replication 2:947
  semiproductive infections 2:947
  serotypes 2:946
  structure and properties 2:946–7
  transmission and risk factors 2:948
  vaccines 2:951, 2:1025
    failure 2:951
    serotype 1 (attenuated) 2:951
    serotype 2 2:951
    serotype 3 2:951
Marine green algae, dsRNA in chloroplasts 1:312
Marker rescue 1:609, 1:612
Marmoset herpesvirus (MHV) 2:714
Marmosets, cotton-top, herpesvirus ateles 2:715
Mason Pfizer monkey virus (M-PMV) 2:912, 3:1518
  crossreactivity and evolution 3:1523–4
  gag gene 3:1521(Fig)
  genome 3:1519, 3:1523
  intracytoplasmic A-type particles (ICAPs) 3:1518, 3:1520
  protease gene 3:1520–1
  structure and properties 3:1520(Fig)
  see also Retroviruses, type D
Mastadenovirus 1:1
  adenoviruses 1:3
  atypical members 1:14
  epitopes on hexons 1:3
  phylogeny 1:17(Fig)
Mastadenoviruses
  genome 1:17
    E3 region 1:17
    organization 1:17
    polypeptide IX 1:16
  proteins, properties 1:18
Master sequence 3:1431
  definition 3:1433(Table)
Mastitis
  cattle, vesicular stomatitis virus (VSV) causing 3:1918

Mastitis (continued)
  mumps virus causing 2:992
Mastoadenovirus 1:14
Mastomys
  Lassa fever transmission 2:890
  Lassa virus reservoir 2:889
Mastrevirus 1:597
Mastreviruses
  evolution 1:605
  gene functions 1:597–8, 1:599(Table)
  genome organization/expression 1:597, 1:597–8
  transmission 1:603
Mathematical modeling 1:486–7
Matucare virus (MATV) 2:1045(Table)
Maus-Elberfeld (ME) virus see Mouse encephalomyelitis viruses
MAY virus see Mayaro (MAY) virus
Mayaro (MAY) virus 1:261–5, 3:1992
  antibodies 1:262
  classification 1:261
  epidemiology and transmission 1:263
  evolution 1:262
  genetics 1:262
  geographic/seasonal distribution 1:261
  history 1:261
  host range and propagation 1:262
  infection 1:261–2
    clinical features 1:264
    emergence 1:422
    outbreaks 1:261
    pathology/histology 1:264
    prevention and control 1:265
  transcription and translation 1:262
mdx mice, gene transfer 1:13
Mealybugs
  badnavirus transmission 2:1299
  closterovirus transmission 1:268(Table), 1:272
  control 2:1299
  trichovirus transmission 3:1840
Measles 2:952
  acute encephalitis 2:957
  atypical 2:956
  case number estimates (WHO) 2:956
  clinical features 1:524, 2:956–7, 2:957
  complications 2:956, 2:956–7, 2:957(Table)
  diarrhea in 1:447
  diseases associated 2:957(Table)
  epidemics 2:954
  epidemiology 2:955–6
  eradication 3:1861
  eye infections 1:524
  immune response 2:958–9
  incubation period 2:956
  mortality 2:952, 2:959
  natural immunity 2:956
  pathology/histopathology 2:957–8
  pneumonia 2:956, 2:957
  prevention and control 2:959
  SSPE see Subacute sclerosing panencephalitis (SSPE)
  subacute encephalitis 2:956
  vaccine see under Measles virus (MV)
Measles, mumps and rubella (MMR) vaccine 2:994
  meningitis after 2:994

Measles virus (MV) 2:952–60, 3:1560
  antibodies to 2:958
  apoptosis promotion 1:75
  assembly and release 2:953–4
  budding 2:957
  cytopathic effects 2:955
  DI particles 1:374
  diseases associated 2:957(Table)
  emerging/re-emerging virus 1:419(Table)
  envelope 2:953, 2:954
  epidemiology 2:955–6
  eradication progress 2:959
  evolution 2:955
  fusion protein 2:953, 2:954
  future perspectives 2:959–60
  genetics 2:955
  genome 2:953
    organization 2:954(Fig)
  geographic/seasonal distribution 2:954
  history 2:952–3
  host range and propagation 2:954–5
  intracerebral infection 2:954
  isolates 2:955
  isolation 2:955
  molecular biology 2:953–4
  monotypic 2:955
  ocular target 1:525(Table)
  pathogenicity 2:956
  persistence 2:952
    gene expression 2:958(Fig)
    influence on population size 1:486
  physical properties 2:954
  polymerase 2:953
  prevention and control 2:959
  proteins 2:953, 2:958(Fig)
  receptor 2:955
  replication 2:953–4, 2:954(Fig), 2:956
  serologic relationships and variability 2:955
  structure and properties 2:953
  taxonomy and classification 2:953
  tissue tropism 2:954–5, 2:956
  transcription 2:954(Fig)
  transmission 2:955–6, 2:956
    efficiency 2:954
    interruption by vaccination 2:959–60
  vaccination program 2:959
  vaccine 2:952, 2:959, 3:1864
    Edmonston strain 2:959
    Edmonston Zagreb strain 2:959
    strains 2:955, 2:959
  viremia 2:956
  see also Morbilliviruses
Meat and bone meal (MBM), BSE epidemic 3:1396
Mechanical transmission 3:1899
  bromoviruses 1:202
  caulimoviruses 2:1278–9
  geminiviruses 1:604
  maize chlorotic mottle virus (MCMV) 2:937
  molluscum contagiosum virus (MCV) 2:963
  nepoviruses 2:1012
  pea enation mosaic virus (PEMV) 2:1194
  pecluviruses 2:1197
  plant viruses and vectors 3:1893
  propagation of plant viruses 3:1418
  sequiviruses 3:1624
  tombusviruses 3:1792
  viral entry into skin 2:1176

Mechanical transmission (continued)
  see also Inoculation, plant viruses
Medical Lake macaque virus 3:1873
Melandrium yellow fleck virus 1:198
Melanoma cell line, metastasis suppression by adenovirus E1A 1:29
Melolontha melolontha entomopoxvirus (MmEPV) 1:476
Melon necrotic spot virus (MNSV) 1:244
  genome 1:245
Melon rugose mosaic virus 3:1850
Membranes, host see Host; Plasma membrane
Membranes, viral 3:1920–5
  acquisition during assembly 3:1920, 3:1924–5
  attachment to host cells 3:1921
  bilayer 3:1920, 3:1920–1
  enveloped viruses 3:1920
  host/viral membrane fusion 3:1921–3
  impermeability to proteases 3:1920
  Iridoviruses 2:865
  membrane proteins 3:1920, 3:1921
    targeted to cellular locations 3:1924, 3:1924(Fig)
  peripheral proteins attached 3:1921
  reconstituted 3:1921
  synthesis 3:1923–4
    lipids 3:1924
  transmembrane (membrane-spanning; anchoring) 3:1921
Membranous vesicles, closterovirus infections 1:271
Mengo virus 1:229
  capsid structure 1:231(Fig)
  cDNA 1:237
  genetics and evolution 1:235–6
  genome 1:232(Fig)
    sequence 1:236(Table)
  immune response 1:237
  infection in Maden–Darby bovine kidney cells 1:235
  L proteins 1:233
  receptor 1:231
  structure 1:230–1, 1:231(Fig)
  TMEV structure differences 3:1773
    similarities 3:1773
  see also Cardioviruses
Meningitis
  acute aseptic 2:915, 2:918, 2:1018
  aseptic
    coxsackievirus infection 1:308
    echoviruses causing 1:415
    enterovirus 71 (EV71) causing 1:473, 2:737
    St Louis encephalitis virus causing 1:428
    West Nile virus causing 1:428
    HSV-2 causing 2:681
    LCMV causing 2:917, 2:918
    viral 2:1018
Meningoencephalitis, Borna disease virus infection 1:172
Meningoencephalomyelitis, LCMV causing 2:918
Metapneumovirus 2:1131
Metaviridae, Errantivirus 3:1526
Methanobacterium thermoautotrophicum 1:83
Methanobacterium wolfei 1:83

Methanococcus voltae, virus-like particle (VLP) 1:83
Methanococcus voltae strain A3, virus-like particle 1:83, 1:84(Table)
Methanogens, viruses 1:83, 1:84(Table)
Methyladenine, Chlorella NC64A viruses 1:48
Methylases 2:762
Methylation
  adenovirus (Ad12) DNA 1:11, 1:12
  DNA see DNA methylation
  of EBV promoters in restricted latency 1:500
  frog virus 3 (FV3) DNA 1:583
  lymphocystis disease virus (LCDV) genome 2:909
  mRNA, frog virus 3 (FV3) 1:585
  PBCV-1 (Paramecium bursaria Chlorella virus 1) genome 1:46
5-Methylcytosine 2:763
  Chlorella NC64A viruses 1:48
Methyltransferases
  algal viruses 1:48–9
  DNA see DNA methyltransferase
  phage 2:761
Mexican papita viroid 3:1930(Table)
Mexico virus
  detection 2:1040
  serologic relationships 2:1038
Mice
  demyelinating disease 2:756
  echovirus infections 1:415
  laboratory, Ectromelia (mousepox) virus infection 2:973
  LCMV propagation 2:915, 2:916, 2:920
  LDV infection see Lactate dehydrogenase-elevating virus (LDV)
  poliovirus model 2:731
  poliovirus resistance 2:1335
  SCID see SCID mice
  suckling
    coxsackievirus discovery 2:734
    dengue virus propagation 1:377
    echovirus infection 1:411
    virus isolation/identification 1:399
  transgenic see Transgenic mice
  see also entries beginning Mouse, Murine; Rodents
Microfilaments
  actin 1:253
  changes induced by frog virus 3 (FV3) 1:586
  frog virus 3 (FV3) budding 1:586
β_2-Microglobulin 2:819
  human CMV binding 1:356
Micromonas pusilla (MpV) viruses 1:44, 1:48, 1:50
Microtubules 1:253–4
  changes, induced by frog virus 3 (FV3) 1:586
  damage by viruses 3:1959
  functions 1:253–4
  N protein of coronavirus JHM interaction 1:254, 1:256(Fig)
  reovirus inclusions 1:1471
  use by viruses 1:254
Microvilli 1:249
Microvillus-like projections, frog virus 3 (FV3) 1:586
Microviridae 2:1227
  bacteriophage φX174 1:274–81
  characteristics 2:1227

Microviridae (continued)
  phage included 2:1227
Microvirus 1:274, 2:1227
Midges see Culicoides
Military personnel, adenovirus infections 1:4
Milk
  fermentation, effect of phage 2:1244, 2:1246
  RSSEV and CEEV transmission 1:428
  tick-borne encephalitis (TBE) virus complex transmission 1:435
  visna-maedi viruses transmission 3:1962, 3:1962–3
  see also Breast feeding
Milker's nodule virus see Pseudocowpox virus
Mini-Mu phage 2:987
Minichromosome, caulimoviruses 2:1281
Mink
  Aleutian disease see Aleutian mink disease
  mink enteritis virus infection see Mink enteritis virus (MEV)
Mink enteritis virus (MEV) 2:1152, 2:1159–60
  antigenic variants 2:1163, 2:1165
  epidemiology 2:1164–5
  evolution 2:1153
  geographic/seasonal distribution 2:1160
  host range 2:1160
  infections 2:1153
    clinical features 2:1154, 2:1165
    immune responses 2:1166
    pathology/histopathology 2:1166
    prevention and control 2:1167
  infectious plasmid clones 2:1161–3
  pathogenicity 2:1165
  phylogeny 2:1164(Fig)
  propagation 2:1161
  taxonomy and classification 2:1160
  transmission 2:1164–5
  vaccines 2:1154, 2:1167
  see also Parvoviruses
Minute virus of canines (MVC) 2:1160
  genome 2:1163
  geographic/seasonal distribution 2:1160
  host range 2:1160
  see also Parvoviruses
Minute virus of mice (MVM)
  genome structure 1:385, 1:385(Fig)
  geographic distribution 2:1171
  history 2:1167–8
  host range 2:1172
  MVMi, tissue tropism 2:1173
  nonstructural proteins 2:1158
    Sp1 interaction 2:1158
  pathogenicity 2:1173
  receptor 2:1153
  replication 2:1157, 2:1159
  structure and properties 2:1155, 2:1168, 2:1168–9
  transcription 2:1157, 2:1157(Fig), 2:1169–70, 2:1170(Fig)
  see also Parvoviruses
Mirabilis mosaic virus (MMV) 2:1276
Miscanthus streak virus (MiSV), genome structure 1:597
Mississippi corn stunt 3:1965

Mitochondria 1:251
    functions, L-A virus and 3:1977–8, 3:1977(Table)
    modification by badnaviruses 2:1298
MM viruses 1:229
Mo T cell line 2:795
Mo T cell virus 2:795
    see also Human T-cell leukemia virus type 2 (HTLV-2)
Mobala virus 2:888(Table)
Modeling, epidemiology of viral diseases 1:486–7
Models, autoimmunity 1:110–12
Modification
    host-controlled see Host-controlled modification and restriction
    of proteins see Post-translational processing
Modoc virus group 1:433(Table)
Moesin, measles virus (MV) receptor 2:955
Mokola virus 3:1439, 3:1443
    concerns over 3:1445
    discovery 3:1442
    epidemiology 3:1444
    genetics 3:1438
    genome 3:1443
    host range 3:1443
    infection 3:1442
        clinical features 3:1445
        immune response 3:1445
        pathology 3:1445
        prevention and control 3:1445
    isolation 3:1442
    propagation 3:1443
    transmission 3:1444
Molecular biology, history 2:721
Molecular cloning see Cloning
Molecular epidemiology 1:483
    definition 1:483
Molecular mimicry 2:817–18
    autoimmunity mechanism 1:110, 1:112
    eye infections 1:524
    microtubules and N protein of coronavirus JHM 1:254, 1:256(Fig)
Molluscipoxvirus 2:960
    apoptosis inhibition 1:74
Molluscum bodies 2:963
Molluscum contagiosum 2:960
    clinical features 2:963
    complications 2:963
    immune response 2:964–5
    incubation period 2:963
    ocular infection 1:528
    pathology/histopathology 2:963–4, 2:964(Fig)
    prevention and control 2:965
    tumors 2:964
Molluscum contagiosum virus (MCV) 2:960–5
    culture and keratinocyte requirement 2:963
    cytopathic effects 2:962–3
    epidemiology 2:963
    evolution 2:963
    genetics 2:963
    genome 2:961
        colinearity 2:961
        ORFs 2:961, 2:962
        terminal invert repeats 2:961
    geographic/seasonal distribution 2:962
    history 2:960
    host range and propagation 2:962–3
    as host-dependent conditional lethal mutant 2:963

Molluscum contagiosum virus (MCV) (continued)
    infection see Molluscum contagiosum
    isolates 2:963
    keratinocyte infection 2:964
    ocular target 1:527(Table)
    pathogenicity 2:963
    proteins 2:961–2
        vaccinia virus homology 2:961
    replication 2:962
    serologic relationship and variability 2:963
    structure and properties 2:960
    subtypes 2:960, 2:961, 2:961(Fig)
        distribution 2:962
    taxonomy and classification 2:960
    tissue tropism 2:963
    transcriptional control 2:962
    transmission 2:963
    vaccinia virus similarity 2:962
    see also Molluscipoxvirus
Moloney murine sarcoma virus (M-MSV) 2:995
Monkey(s)
    CMV see Cytomegalovirus (CMV), animal
    Ebola and Marburg viruses 2:939, 2:943
    Kyasanur Forest disease 1:434
    poliovirus susceptibility 2:1334
    see also entries beginning Simian; Primates
Monkeypox
    clinical features 3:1673
    human infections 3:1673
    immune response 3:1673–4
    natural infections 3:1672–3
    pathology/histopathology 3:1673
    prevention and control 3:1674
    therapy 1:68
Monkeypox virus 1:304, 3:1672–4, 3:1993–4
    epidemiology 3:1673
    evolution 3:1673
    experimental infections 3:1672
    future perspectives 3:1674
    genetics 3:1673
    genome 3:1672
    geographic/seasonal distribution 3:1672
    history 3:1672
    host range and propagation 3:1672–3
    infection see Monkeypox
    properties and replication 3:1672
    taxonomy and classification 3:1672
    transmission 3:1673, 3:1993
        human-to-human 3:1673
    vaccination 3:1674
    'white pock' mutants 3:1673
Monoclonal antibodies
    adenoviruses 1:3
    African swine fever virus (AFSV) 1:36
    arenaviruses 2:890
    CD21 and CD24, in EBV infection 3:1827
    expressed in plants 2:1313
    human papillomaviruses (HPVs) 2:1108
    in immunofluorescence methods 1:399
    parvoviruses 2:1163
    reovirus type 3 cellular receptor 3:1927, 3:1927(Fig)
    reoviruses 3:1462
    rinderpest virus 3:1563
    RSV 3:1487

Monoclonal antibodies (continued)
    RSV (continued)
        F glycoprotein 1:65
Monocyte chemoattractant protein (MCP-1) 1:343
Monocyte chemoattractant protein (MCP-4) 1:343
Monocyte chemotactic proteins (MCP) 1:339
Monocytes
    caprine arthritis encephalitis virus (CAEV) 1:226
    measles virus (MV) infection 2:955
    see also Macrophage
Mononegavirales 3:1479, 3:1731, 3:1750
    families included 2:1021, 3:1750
    families and subfamilies 3:1480(Table)
    filoviruses 2:939
    vesicular stomatitis virus (VSV) classification 3:1911
Mononuclear cells, accumulation, Borna disease virus infection 1:172
Montana lung disease 3:1962
Mopeia virus 2:888(Table)
Morbillivirus 2:953, 2:1021, 2:1130, 2:1134, 2:1135(Fig), 3:1560
    members 2:1021
Morbilliviruses
    evolution 3:1563–4, 3:1564(Fig)
    genome 3:1563(Fig)
    prevention and control 3:1567
    propagation 3:1562
    structure and properties 3:1563(Fig)
    transmission 3:1566
    viruses included 2:953, 2:953(Table)
    see also Canine distemper virus; Distemper viruses; Measles virus (MV); Rinderpest virus
Moroccan pepper virus (MPV) 3:1790(Table)
MORT1-MACH pathway 1:71
MORT1/FADD 1:71
Mosaic disease, grapevines 3:1841
Mosquito transmission
    Bunyavirus 1:209
    Chandipura and Piry viruses 1:259
    Chikungunya (CHIK) virus 1:263, 3:1989
    dengue virus 1:375, 1:377, 1:379, 1:380
    encephalitis viruses see Encephalitis viruses
    equine encephalitis viruses 1:503, 1:505
    Japanese encephalitis (JE) virus 2:872, 3:1994
    La Crosse (LAC) virus 3:1991
    Mayaro (MAY) virus 1:263
    Murray Valley encephalitis (MVE) virus 3:1994
    O'Nyong nyong (ONN) virus 1:263, 3:1994
    Rift Valley fever virus 1:210, 3:1993
    Ross River virus (RRV) 3:1574, 3:1995
    St Louis encephalitis virus 1:428
    Sindbis virus 3:1989
    Tanapox and Yabapox viruses 3:1971, 3:1972
    Venezuelan equine encephalitis virus 3:1990
    yellow fever virus 2:719, 3:1980, 3:1984, 3:1984–5, 3:1989

Mosquitoes
    carbon dioxide sensitivity 1:259
    control 1:265, 1:507, 3:1986
    geographic spread 3:1996
    habitat changes 3:1996
    susceptibility to encephalitis viruses 1:427
Moths, picorna-like viruses 2:1274
Motor neurons, ventral, LDV infection 1:94
Mottles 3:1853
Mouse cytomegalovirus see Murine cytomegalovirus (MCMV)
Mouse encephalomyelitis viruses 1:229, 3:1773
    resistance genes 2:755(Table)
    see also Theiler's viruses
Mouse hepatitis virus (MHV) 1:292, 1:294
    apoptosis promotion 1:75
    attachment and infection process 1:295
    genome map 1:293(Fig)
    HE glycoprotein 1:295
    immune response 1:297
    infection 1:295
        clinical features 1:296–7
    receptors 1:294
    see also Coronaviruses
Mouse hepatitis virus type 4 (MHV4)
    resistance genes 2:755(Table)
    susceptibility, Hv-2 locus role 2:754, 2:754–6
Mouse mammary tumor virus (MMTV) 2:965–72
    attachment and entry 2:966–7
    B-particles 2:966
    C particles 2:967
    endogenous (germline) 2:968, 2:969
    envelope 2:967
    future perspectives 2:972
    genetic experiment difficulties 2:969
    genetics 2:968–9
    genome 2:966, 2:966(Fig), 2:967
        long terminal repeat 2:966
    glycoproteins, gp52 2:966
    history 2:965–6
    immune response to 2:972
    int gene 2:970
        transcription 2:970
    integrase (IN protein) 2:967
    integration 2:967
        common sites in tumors 2:970(Table)
    intracytoplasmic A particles 2:967
    life cycle 2:968(Fig)
    mammary tumors 2:969
        factors influencing 2:968–9
        incidence 2:968–9
        pathogenesis 2:969–70
    milk-borne virus (exogenous) 2:966, 2:968
    life cycle 2:968(Fig)
    resistance to 2:969
    as model 2:966(Fig)
    mRNA 2:967
    pathogenicity 2:969–70
    primer-binding site (PBS) 2:966
    promoters 2:966(Fig), 2:967, 2:970
    protease 2:966, 2:967
    provirus 2:967, 2:970
    receptor (MTVR) 2:966
    replication 2:966–7
    resistance to 2:969
    reverse transcriptase 2:967
    ribosomal frameshifting 2:967
    sag gene 2:966

Mouse mammary tumor virus
(MMTV) (continued)
  sag mRNA 2:967
  Sag protein 2:966, 2:968, 2:969, 2:972
    C-terminus
      polymorphism 2:972
    T cell receptor
      interaction 2:972, 2:972(Fig)
    structure and properties 2:966
  T-cell lymphomas 2:970
  taxonomy and
    classification 2:966
  tissue tropism 2:968
  transcription 2:967, 2:970
    termination 2:967
  transcription regulation 2:970–2
    enhancer elements 2:971
    factors involved 2:971
    hormone-response element
      (HRE) 2:971
    location of
      sequences 2:971(Fig)
    negative elements 2:971–2
    transcription factors 2:971
  transmission 2:968
  tumors types 2:970
Mouse neurofilament protein
  (NFP) 1:368
Mousepox (ectromelia)
  active and passive
    immunity 2:977
  clinical features 2:974, 2:975(Fig)
  distribution 2:973
  enzootic 2:974
  immune response 2:977–8
  intracytoplasmic inclusion
    bodies 2:976
  laboratory diagnosis 2:978
  pathology/
    histopathology 2:975(Fig),
    2:976–7, 2:977(Fig)
    hepatic lesions 2:976
    lesions after intranasal
      inoculation 2:977
    lesions after intraperitoneal
      inoculation 2:976
    skin lesions 2:976
    spleen lesions 2:976
  prevention and control 2:978
  screening tests 2:978
  spread in bloodstream 2:1178
  see also Ectromelia (mousepox)
    virus
Mousepox virus 2:973–80
  see also Ectromelia (mousepox)
    virus
Mouth see Oral cavity
Movement proteins (MPs) 2:1185,
  2:1301, 3:1839
  dominant-negative
    mutations 2:1310
  plant resistance
    mechanism 2:1309–10
  in RNA virus vectors 3:1896
Mozzarella industry 2:1254
mpl oncogene 3:1515
mRNA 1:255
  3' polyadenylation 1:255
  5' caps 1:255
  methylation, frog virus 3
    (FV3) 1:585
  transcapping 1:255
  transgenic 2:1310
  viral 3:1473
    effect on host protein
      synthesis 3:1959
  see also Host; individual viruses
Mu-1 phage see Coliphage Mu
Mu-like phage 2:981–8, 2:1224
  genomes 2:981
  life cycle 2:981–3

Mu-like phage (continued)
  see also Bacteriophage D3112;
    Coliphage D108; Coliphage
    Mu
Mucociliary clearance 2:1176
Mucosal disease 1:174
  bovine viral diarrhea virus
    causing 1:178
  clinical features 1:179
  pathology and
    histopathology 1:179
Mucosal disease (MD) virus 1:173
  see also Bovine viral diarrhea
    virus (BVDV)
Mucosal immune system
  stimulation by interferon 2:861
  vaccine-induced immunity 3:1864
Mucosal infections
  coxsackieviruses 1:308
  HSV-2 2:678
Mulberry latent virus (MLV) 1:240
Mulberry pyralid, Bombyx mori
  densovirus (BmDNV) 1:387
Mulberry ringspot
  virus 2:1008(Table)
Muller's ratchet effect 3:1436
Multifocal
  leukoencephalopathy 3:1831
Multiple sclerosis
  HHV-6 infection
    associated 2:702
  IFN-γ treatment, Th1 cell
    enhancement 1:110
  model 1:111
  TMEV as model 3:1773, 3:1776
Multiplication cycle of
  viruses 3:1408–9
  blocking 3:1410
  respiratory viruses 3:1490
  see also Pathogenesis of viral
    infections; Propagation of
    viruses
Multiplicity of infection
  (moi) 3:1411
Multiplicity reactivation 1:609
Multivesicular bodies (MVB),
  tombusviruses 3:1793,
  3:1793(Fig)
Mumps
  clinical features 2:988, 2:992,
    2:993(Table)
  complications 2:993(Table)
  dacryoadenitis 1:524
  epidemics 2:992
  epidemiology 2:992
  history 2:988
  immune response 2:993–4
  incubation period 2:992
  insulin-dependent diabetes
    mellitus after 2:1080
  pancreatitis after 2:1079
  pathogenesis 2:993
  pathology/histopathology 2:992–
    3, 2:993(Table)
  prevention and control 2:994
  prognosis 2:993(Table)
  transmission and attack
    rates 2:992
  vaccines 2:994
    attenuated 2:994
Mumps virus (MuV) 2:988–94
  attachment and entry 2:989–90
  budding 2:991
  cDNA clone 2:994
  cytopathic effects 2:991
  Enders strain 2:989, 2:994
  epidemiology 2:992
  evolution 2:991
  future perspectives 2:994
  genetics 2:992
  genome 2:988, 2:989
    gene order 2:989(Fig)

Mumps virus (MuV) (continued)
  genome (continued)
    intergenic sequences 2:990
    replication 2:990
  genotypes 2:992
  geographic/seasonal
    distribution 2:991
  hemagglutinin-neuraminidase
    (HN) 2:989, 2:990, 2:991,
    2:991(Table)
  history 2:988
  host range and
    propagation 2:991–2
  inclusion body myositis
    and 2:994
  as monotypic virus 2:992
  mRNA 2:990
    polyadenylated 2:990
  mutants 2:992
  ocular target 1:525(Table)
  pathogenicity 2:993
  perinatal exposures 2:994
  persistent infection 2:992
  physical properties 2:989
  prevention and control 2:994
  proteins 2:989
    functions 2:990, 2:991(Table)
    fusion protein 2:989, 2:991,
      2:991(Table)
    N protein 2:990, 2:991(Table)
    nonstructural 2:989, 2:990,
      2:991(Table)
    properties 2:991(Table)
    SH protein 2:989, 2:990,
      2:991(Table)
    structural 2:989
  replication 2:989–91
  RNP complex 2:988
  serologic relationships and
    variability 2:992
  structure and properties 2:988–9
  spikes 2:988
  syncytium formation 2:991
  taxonomy and
    classification 2:988
  tissue tropism 2:992, 2:994
  transcription 2:989(Fig), 2:990
    cotranscriptional editing 2:990
  translation 2:990
  transmission 2:992
  see also Paramyxoviruses
Murid herpesvirus 1 1:363
  see also Murine cytomegalovirus
    (MCMV)
Murine acquired immunodeficiency
  syndrome (MAIDS) 1:367,
  2:1000
Murine adenovirus (MAV) 1:20
  type 1 (MAV-1) 1:17
Murine cytomegalovirus
  (MCMV) 1:357, 1:363–9
  antibodies 1:368
  assembly site and release 1:365
  cell cultures 1:365
  classification 1:363
  Cmv1 locus 1:364
  cross-resistance 1:369
  cytokines induced 1:367–8
  cytopathology 1:365
  drug-resistant 1:369
  early transcripts 1:364
  evolution 1:365
  Fc receptor homologue 1:368
  G-protein coupled receptor
    homologue 1:364
  genes, human CMV
    homology 1:364
  genetics 1:363–4
  genome organization 1:363
  genome structure 1:359
  glycoproteins 1:365
  history 1:363

Murine cytomegalovirus (MCMV)
  (continued)
  host range and propagation 1:365
  IE1 and IE2 regions 1:364
  immediate early genes 1:364
  immune modulation 1:368
    genes 1:368
  immune modulators 1:369
  immunotherapy 1:368–9
  inclusion bodies 1:365
  infection
    embryonic 1:366
    features 1:366–7
    immune response 1:367–8
    pathology/
      histopathology 1:366
    prevention and control 1:368–9
    response to 1:367–8
    treatment 1:369
  late transcripts 1:364
  latent infections 1:366
  MIE protein 1:364
  MIE region 1:364
  as model of human CMV
    infection 1:366–7
  pathogenicity 1:365–6
  persistent infection 1:366
  properties 1:363
  proteins 1:364–5
    genome replication and
      repair 1:364–5
    regulatory functions 1:364
    structural 1:365
  replication 1:363, 1:364, 1:366
    DNA replication 1:364
    origin (ori-Lyt) 1:364
  replication and
    propagation 1:360
  resistance 1:367
  resistance genes 2:755(Table)
    Cmv1 locus 1:367
    Cvm-1 gene action 2:757
    H-2D gene 2:754
  Smith strain 1:365
  genome 1:363
  tissue tropism 1:366
  transcription 1:364
  translation 1:364
  transmission 1:365
  uptake 1:365
  vaccines 1:368
  see also Cytomegalovirus
    (CMV)
Murine dystrophin, cDNA
  transfer 1:13
Murine leptin, cDNA transfer 1:14
Murine leukemia viruses
  (MuLVs) 2:995, 2:997
  amphotropic receptor 2:997
  attachment and entry 2:995–6
  defective genome and
    MAIDS 2:1000
  DI particles 1:374
  distribution 2:996–7
  ecotropic 2:997
  endogenous 2:997
  env gene 2:995
  enzymes 2:995, 2:996
  Friend–Moloney–Rauscher
    (FMR) group 2:996
  Fv-1 restriction (N/B
    tropism) 2:997
  gag gene 2:995
  Gag protein 2:995, 2:996
    mutants 2:996
  Gag-Pol fusion protein 2:996
  gene order 2:995
  genome 2:995, 2:996(Fig)
    long terminal repeats 2:996
  gibbon ape leukemia virus
    (GaLV) relationship 1:617
  Gross virus group 2:996

Murine leukemia viruses (MuLVs) (continued)
history 2:995, 2:1352
host range 2:997
control 2:997
immunodeficiency 2:1000
infection
neonatal 2:997
'potentially leukemic cells' 2:999
as insertional mutagens 2:997–8
integration of viral DNA 2:996
leukemogenesis 2:997–9
control by LTR enhancer specificity 2:998–9
insertion sites 2:998(Table)
long latency 2:999
LTR activation of proto-oncogenes 2:997–8, 2:998(Fig), 2:998(Table)
MCF recombinant viruses 2:997, 2:999
preleukemic changes 2:999
proximal leukemogens 2:999
neuropathic 2:999
oncogenes 2:995
packaging and maturation 2:996
pol gene 2:995
Pol protein 2:996
polymorphism 2:997
polytropic 2:997
receptor 2:997
amphotropic 2:997
replication 2:995–6
retroviral vectors based on 2:1000–1, 2:1000(Fig)
reverse transcriptase 2:996
reverse transcription 2:996
sites of infection 2:997
structure and properties 2:995–6
taxonomy and classification 2:995, 2:996
tissue tropism 2:997
transcription 2:996
type-specific antigens 2:996
xenotropic 2:997
Murine mammary tumor virus-related (MuMTV)
proviruses 1:438
Murine myeloproliferative virus (MPLV), oncogenes 3:1515
Murine osteogenic sarcoma viruses, oncogenes 3:1508
Murine polioviruses *see* Theiler's viruses
Murine polyomavirus *see* Polyomaviruses, murine
Muromegalovirus 1:357, 1:363
Murray Valley encephalitis (MVE) 1:429, 3:1994
Murray Valley encephalitis virus (MVEV) 3:1994–5
features 1:425(Table)
genetics 1:427
geographic/seasonal distribution 1:426
history/discovery 1:424
host range 1:427
Muscles, striated, coxsackievirus infection 1:308
Muscovy duck parvovirus (MDPV)
history 2:1168
infection, clinical features 2:1174
Mushroom bacilliform virus (MBV) 1:152
see also Barnaviruses
Mushrooms, mushroom bacilliform virus (MBV) infection 1:153
Muskrats, Omsk hemorrhagic fever 1:428, 1:434, 3:1992

Mutagenesis 1:608
animal viruses 1:608
insertional
adenovirus (Ad12) DNA 1:11
feline leukemia viruses (FeLVs) causing 1:545, 1:545(Table)
mouse mammary tumor virus (MMTV)-induced 2:969–70
localized random, transduction application 2:1239
site-directed 1:608
Mutagens, viruses as 3:1842
Mutant spectrum 3:1431
definition 3:1433(Table)
Mutations
animal viruses 1:607
cold-adapted 1:608
conditional lethal 1:608
defective-interfering (DI) 1:608
fixation rate, definition 3:1433(Table)
frequency 1:419
coronaviruses 1:293–4
definition 3:1433(Table)
immune evasion due to 2:1203–4
phenotypic expression 1:608
point 1:607
polioviruses 2:1327
rate
animal viruses 1:607
bacteriophage φ6 2:1206
definition 3:1433(Table)
foot-and-mouth disease viruses (FMDVs) 1:572
hepatitis delta virus (HDV) 1:667
polioviruses 2:1327, 2:1335, 2:1346
RNA viruses 2:1335, 3:1449, 3:1489
simian immunodeficiency viruses (SIV) 3:1643
spontaneous 1:608
Streptococcus thermophilus phage 2:1260
suppressor, [PSI] discovery 3:1404
temperature sensitive 1:608
types 1:607–8
viable 1:607
see also Quasispecies
Mutator phage *see* Coliphage Mu
Mx1 gene, resistance to influenza viruses 2:756
Mx1 protein 2:756
Mx proteins, interferon-inducible 2:858–9
Mx system 2:858–9
Myalgia, coxsackievirus infection 1:308
Myalgic encephalomyelitis (ME) *see* Chronic fatigue syndrome
myb oncogene 3:1509–10
myc oncogene 3:1510
Myc proteins 3:1510
Mycoplasmas, viruses *see* Plasmaviruses
Mycoviruses
characteristics 2:1147
discovery 2:1147
see also Partitiviruses
Myelin, breakdown *see* Demyelination
Myelin basic protein, in recombinant vaccinia virus 1:111
Myelo-proliferative sarcoma virus 2:995
Myelopathy
HTLV-1-associated 2:792–3, 2:795

Myelopathy (continued)
progressive spastic and HTLV-2 causing 2:802
Myelosuppression, murine CMV causing 1:368
Myocarditis
acute 2:1075
coxsackievirus B3 causing 2:756
coxsackievirus infection 1:308, 1:309
focal 2:1074
neonatal, echoviruses causing 1:416
parvovirus infection 2:1166
virus infections 2:1074
West Nile virus causing 1:429
Myopericarditis
acute 2:1075
clinical features 2:1077
laboratory diagnosis 2:1078
chronic relapsing 2:1076
coxsackievirus infection 1:308
echoviruses causing 1:415
Myositis
coxsackievirus infections 1:308, 2:734
inclusion body 2:994
Myoviridae 1:77, 1:82, 1:83, 1:325, 2:1087, 2:1223, 2:1224
bacteriophage P1 1:455
characteristics 2:1224
mu-like phage 2:981–8
phage included in 2:1224
Synechococcus cyanophage 1:328, 1:330
T4-like phage *see* T4-like phage
see also Halophage φH
Myristic acid, attached to bovine enterovirus proteins 1:462, 1:463
Myristylation
African swine fever virus (AFSV) proteins 1:34
c-Akt protein 3:1516
feline immunodeficiency virus (FIV) 1:536
v-Abl protein 3:1511
Myrobalan latent ringspot virus 2:1008(Table)
Mystery swine disease (MSD) 1:89
Myxoma cells 3:1386
Myxoma virus (MYX)
antigen presentation interference 3:1384
apoptosis inhibition 1:73
clinical features 3:1386
evolution 3:1385
genetic resistance 2:753
genome 3:1383
geographic distribution 3:1384
history 3:1381
immune evasion 3:1386
immunization 3:1387
infection
clinical features 3:1385, 3:1387
immune response 3:1387
pathology/histopathology 3:1386–7
skin tumors 3:1387
see also Myxomatosis
M-T2 gene 1:73
pathogenicity 3:1385–6
replication, sites (lymphocytes) 3:1385, 3:1387
tissue tropism 3:1385
virulence 3:1385, 3:1386
Myxomatosis 3:1384
clinical features 3:1386
history 3:1381
see also Myxoma virus (MYX)
Myxovirus infections 1:63
therapy 1:56, 1:63–4

Myxovirus infections (continued)
vaccine 1:63
Myxoviruses 1:63–4

N

N4 phage *see* Coliphage N4
Nairobi sheep disease 1:211
Nairovirus 1:204, 1:211
infections 1:209
proteins 1:207
serogroups and viruses 1:206(Table)
transmission and epidemiology 1:208, 1:211
see also Bunyaviruses
Nanovirus, geminiviruses similarities 1:606
Naples virus 3:1990
Narcissus tip necrosis virus (NTNV) 1:243
Nasopharyngeal carcinoma (NPC) 1:488, 1:488(Table), 3:1844–5
clinical features 1:492
diagnosis and monitoring 1:490
early diagnosis 1:494
EBV and 3:1845
EBV latent protein expression 1:492
epidemiology 1:490
pathology/histopathology 1:493
treatment 1:494
undifferentiated 1:490
Nasturtium ringspot virus (NRSV) 1:531
genome 1:532
see also Fabaviruses
National Foundation for Infantile Paralysis (NFIP) 2:736
Natronobacterium magadii 1:83
Natural killer (NK) cells 1:69–70, 2:1202
HHV-6 infection 2:702
HSV-1 infections 2:684
LCMV infection 2:919
murine CMV infection 1:367
nonadaptive immune response 2:812
Navarro virus 3:1541
Ndelle virus (NDEV) 2:1045(Table)
Neckar river virus (NRV) 3:1790(Table)
Necrosis, in plant virus disease 2:1190, 2:1318, 2:1323
Necrotizing enterocolitis 1:447
coronaviruses causing 1:296
Necrovirus 1:243, 2:1003
Necroviruses 2:1003–7
genome 2:1004–5, 2:1004(Fig)
geographic distribution 2:1003
history 2:1003
infection, symptoms 2:1003
replication strategy 2:1005–6
structure and properties 2:1004
taxonomy and classification 2:1003
transmission 2:1003
see also Tobacco necrosis virus (TNV)
Negri bodies 3:1438, 3:1440, 3:1960
Nelfinavir (Viracept) 1:60, 2:784
structure 2:784(Fig)
Nematode transmitted viruses with polyhedral particles *see* Nepoviruses

Nematodes
  activity determinants 3:1788–9
  control 3:1788–9
  feeding mechanics/
    behavior 3:1900–1
  spread 3:1789
  vertical/horizontal
    distribution 3:1789
  virus transmission
    bromoviruses 1:203
    dianthoviruses 1:407
    nepoviruses 2:1010, 2:1012
    plant virus
      mechanisms 3:1899–900
    tobraviruses 3:1788
Neoantigens, autoimmunity
  mechanism 1:109
Neodiprion sertifer SNPV 1:149
Neonates
  cardiac disease and viruses
    associated 2:1074–5
  coxsackievirus infection 1:309
  diarrhea *see* Diarrhea
  HSV infections 2:683
  immune response, to HSV 2:684
Neoplasia
  reticuloendotheliosis (RE) viruses
    see also Cancer, tumors;
    Reticuloendotheliosis (RE)
    viruses
Nephropathia epidemica 2:1084
  see also Hemorrhagic fever with
    renal syndrome (HFRS)
Nephropathy, HIV-
  associated 2:1082
Nephrosis, in hepatitis B 2:1082
Nepovirus 2:1007
Nepoviruses 2:1007–13
  coat proteins 2:1010
    sequence comparisons 2:1011
  comoviruses and fabaviruses
    differences 2:1010
  components (top/middle/
    bottom) 2:1010
  cytopathology 2:1012
  effect on host plants 2:1012
  epidemiology 2:1012
  genetic map 2:1010
  genetics 2:1011
  genome 2:1007, 2:1010–11
    organization 2:1010–11
  geographic range 2:1011
  history 2:1007
  host range and
    propagation 2:1011–12
  infections, symptoms 2:1012
  pathogen-derived engineered
    resistance 2:1308(Table)
  pathogenicity 2:1012
  physical properties 2:1011–12
  polyproteins 2:1010, 2:1010(Fig)
    dipeptides cleaved 2:1010,
      2:1011(Table)
  prevention and control 2:1012
  RNA-1 2:1007, 2:1010
  RNA-2 2:1007, 2:1010
  satellite RNAs 2:1011,
    3:1554(Table)
  structure and properties 2:1007,
    2:1008(Table), 2:1010
  taxonomy and
    classification 2:1007–10
  transmission 2:1010, 2:1012
  viruses included 2:1007,
    2:1008(Table)
  VPg 2:1010, 2:1011
Nerves
  virus invasion pathway 2:1014,
    2:1015(Fig)
  virus spread by 2:1179–80
    tropism and 2:1182

Nerves (*continued*)
  see also Neurons; Peripheral
    nerves
Nervous system viruses 2:1013–20
  anatomic considerations 2:1013–
    14
  autoimmunity 2:1017
  cell-to-cell spread 2:1016–17
  CNS invasion pathways 2:1014–
    15, 2:1015(Fig), 2:1016(Fig)
  infections
    acute 2:1018
    clinical features 2:1018–20
    coxsackieviruses 1:308
    slow 2:1018–20
  mechanisms of cell
    damage 2:1017
    apoptosis 2:1017
    cell lysis 2:1017
    host cell growth rate
      change 2:1017
    indirect by immune
      response 2:1017
  neural cell infections 2:1015–17
  see also Central nervous system
neu, transformation, suppression
  by adenovirus E1A 1:29
Neural cell infections 2:1015–17
  noncytopathic 2:1017
  see also Neurons
Neuraminidase (NA) 1:249
  atomic structure 3:1944
  influenza virus *see* Influenza
    viruses
Neuro-ophthalmic lesions,
  AIDS 1:529
Neurodegeneration, prion protein
  (PrP) gene mutations 3:1392
Neuroinvasive, definition 2:1013
Neuroinvasiveness 2:1013
  Japanese encephalitis (JE)
    virus 2:873
Neurologic disorders, in dengue
  virus infection 1:382
Neurological features
  Borna disease virus
    infection 1:171–2
  HIV infection 2:772
  rabies 3:1440
Neurolymphomatosis 2:945
Neuronotropic, definition 2:1013
Neurons
  latent varicella-zoster virus
    infection 3:1884
  membranes 2:1014
  virus spread 2:1180
  see also Nerves; Neural cell
    infections
Neuropil, compact 2:1015–16
Neurospora
  RNA self-cleavage 3:1552
  VS RNA self-
    cleavage 3:1553(Fig),
    3:1554(Fig), 3:1555
Neurospora crassa, TAD
  element 3:1504
Neurotactin 1:343
Neurotropic viruses 2:1013, 2:1180
Neurotropism
  Borna disease virus 1:170
  definition 2:1013
  Kuru 3:1400
Neurovirulence 2:1013
  definition 2:1013
  TMEV *see* Theiler's murine
    encephalomyelitis viruses
    (TMEV)
Neutralization test
  antiviral antibody detection 1:390
  rabies-like viruses 3:1444
  virus identification 1:400

Neutrophils, chemotactic
  cytokines 1:343
Nevirapine (Viramune) 1:59
NeVTA virus 1:553
New World primates
  betaherpesviruses 1:358(Table)
  phylogeny of herpesviruses 2:715,
    2:716(Fig)
New York virus (NYV) 1:621,
  3:1988
New Zealand virus (NZV) 2:1026
Newcastle disease 2:1020
  clinical features 2:1025
  distribution 2:1023
  economic significance 2:1025
  fowlpox virus as vaccine
    vector 1:581–2
  history 2:1020–1
  immune response 2:1025
  panzootics 2:1024
  pathology/histopathology 2:1025
  prevention and control 2:1025
Newcastle disease virus
  (NDV) 2:1020–6, 2:1134
  antigenic variation 2:1024
  antigenome formation 2:1022–3
  apoptosis promotion 1:75
  assembly 2:1023
  epidemiology 2:1024, 2:1139
  evolution 2:1024
  future perspectives 2:1025
  gene order 2:1021
  genetics 2:1024
  genome 2:1021–2
    inverse termini 2:1022
    leader sequence (3′) 2:1021
    trailer sequence (5′) 2:1021–2
  geographic/seasonal
    distribution 2:1023
  history 2:1020–1
  host cytoskeleton damage 3:1960
  host range and
    propagation 2:1023–4
  infection *see* Newcastle disease
  ocular target 1:525(Table)
  pathogenicity 2:1024
  polymerase 2:1022
  post-translational
    processing 2:1023
  promoter 2:1022
  propagation 2:740
  proteins 2:1022
    fusion 2:1022
    hemagglutinin-
      neuraminidase 2:1022
    large 2:1022
    matrix 2:1022
    nucleocapsid 2:1022
    phosphoprotein 2:1022
  replication 2:1022
    'rule of six' 2:1023
    site 2:1024
  RNA replication 2:1022
  serologic relationship and
    variability 2:1024
  structure and properties 2:1021,
    2:1021(Fig)
  taxonomy and
    classification 2:1021
  transcription 2:1022–3
    primary 2:1022
    translation 2:1023
  transmission and tissue
    tropism 2:1024
  transmission by smuggled
    birds 3:1996
  vaccines 2:1023, 2:1025, 2:1139
    recombinant 2:1025
  velogenic strains 2:1024
    distribution 2:1023

NF-1, mouse mammary tumor
  virus (MMTV)
  transcription 2:971
NF-κB transcription factor 3:1820–
  1
  adenovirus E1B19K
    interaction 1:22
  bovine leukemia virus
    (BLV) 1:193
  HIV transcription 2:765
  inhibition proteolysis by
    interferons 2:856
  murine CMV inducing 1:367
  trans-activation in HTLV-1
    and 2:793
Niche, ecological *see* Ecological
  niche
Nicotiana glutinosa, N gene 2:1187
Nicotiana glutinosa stunt
  viroid 3:1930(Table)
Nicotiana velutina mosaic virus
  (NVMV) 1:588
  transmission 1:595
Nidovirales 1:90, 3:1731
  Arteriviridae 1:291, 3:1798
  Coronaviridae 1:291, 3:1798
Nilaparvata lugens reovirus
  (NLRV) 2:1263
  genome 2:1263
  see also Phytoreoviruses
NK cells *see* Natural killer (NK)
  cells
NM23, induction by adenovirus
  E1A 1:29
Noctuid pests, ascovirus
  prevalence 1:100
Nodamura virus (NOV) 2:1026
  coat protein 2:1027
  host range 2:1027
  infection 2:1031
  propagation 2:1027
  RNA replication 2:1028(Fig)
  see also Nodaviruses
Nodaviridae 2:1026–31
  alpha nodaviruses 2:1026
  beta nodaviruses 2:1026
  biological control by 2:843
  characteristics 2:1026
  genera 2:1026
Nodaviruses 2:1026–31
  alpha nodaviruses 2:1026
    genome 2:1028
    host range 2:1026
    members 2:1026
  assembly and packaging 2:1030
  β-barrel structure 2:1027, 2:1028
  beta nodaviruses 2:1026
    host range 2:1026
    members 2:1026
  cDNA clones 2:1029–30
  coat protein 2:1027
    amino acid sequences 2:1027
  composition and
    properties 2:1027
  cytopathic effects 2:1030
  economic significance 2:1031
  epidemiology 2:1031
  gene expression regulation 2:1029
  genome structure 2:1028–9,
    2:1028(Fig)
    coding potential 2:1028–9
    ORFs 2:1028–9
  host cell interactions 2:1030–1
  host range 2:1026–7
  infections 2:1031
  pathogenesis 2:1031
  persistent infections 2:1031
  protein α 2:1028–9
  protein A 2:1029
  protein α 2:1029, 2:1030
  protein B2 2:1029
  protein β 2:1027, 2:1030

Nodaviruses (continued)
  protein γ 2:1028, 2:1030
  protein shell 2:1027
  protomers 2:1027, 2:1028
  recombination 3:1451
  RNA1 and RNA2 2:1026, 2:1027, 2:1028, 2:1029
    control mechanisms 2:1029
    lack of reactivity with RNA ligase 2:1028
    packaging 2:1030
    synthesis 2:1029
  RNA3 2:1029
    synthesis 2:1030
  RNA replication 2:1029–30
    unequal positive/negative strand number 2:1030
  RNA-dependent RNA polymerase 2:1029
  three-dimensional structure 2:1027–8
  translation 2:1029
  see also Nodamura virus (NOV)
Nodavirales 3:1750
  families included 3:1750
Nomenclature of viruses 3:1730–56
  history 3:1730–1
  universal 3:1752–5
  see also Taxonomy of viruses
Non-A non-B hepatitis see Hepatitis
Noncytopathic infections, of neural cells 2:1017
Non-nucleoside reverse transcriptase inhibitors see Reverse transcriptase inhibitors
Nonoccluded baculoviruses (NOB) 2:1031–4, 3:1632
  assembly 2:1032
  genome 2:1032
  history 2:1031–2
  pathology and transmission 2:1033–4
  persistence 2:1034
  properties 2:1032
  proteins 2:1032
  replication 2:1032–3
  see also Hz-1V; Hz-2V; Oryctes virus (Or-1V)
'Non-paralytic polio' 2:734
  see also Coxsackievirus B
Nonpersistent viruses 1:1900
Northern cereal mosaic virus (NCMV) 3:1531
  morphology and composition 3:1534
  see also Plant rhabdoviruses
Norvir see Ritonavir (Norvir)
Norwalk virus 1:218, 1:445, 2:1035–41, 2:1037, 3:1576
  antibodies 2:1038–9, 2:1040
  cloning 2:1040
  detection and diagnosis 2:1040
  emerging/re-emerging virus 1:419(Table)
  genome, comparison with picornaviruses 2:1037(Fig)
  genome organization 2:1037(Fig)
  history/discovery 1:442, 2:1035
  immunity mechanisms 2:1040
  infection
    clinical features 2:1039, 2:1039(Table)
    diarrhea outbreaks 1:445
    immune response 1:449, 2:1039–40
    prevention and control 2:1040
    treatment 2:1040
  pathogenicity 2:1039
  recombinant VLPs 2:1036(Fig), 2:1040

Norwalk virus (continued)
  serologic relationships 2:1038
  structure 2:1036(Fig)
  taxonomy and classification 2:1035–6
  transmission 1:485(Table)
  vaccine 2:1040
  virus-like particles 2:1040
  volunteer studies 2:1035, 2:1039(Table)
Norwalk-like viruses 2:1035
  antigenic relationships 2:1036(Table)
  capsid protein 2:1036
  classification 2:1036(Table)
  detection 2:1040
  epidemiology 2:1038–9
  future perspectives 2:1041
  genome 2:1036
  genome organization 2:1037–8, 2:1037(Fig)
    ORFs 2:1037–8
  host range and propagation 2:1038
  infection
    clinical features 2:1039
    diagnosis 2:1040
    immune response 2:1039–40
    prevention and control 2:1040
    treatment 2:1040
  pathogenicity 2:1039
  properties 2:1036
  serologic/phylogenetic relationships 2:1038
  serotypes 2:1038
  transmission 2:1039
  virus-like particles 2:1036
  see also Norwalk virus
Nosema apis 2:747
Nosocomial infections/transmission 1:484
  Ebola and Marburg viruses 2:943, 3:1993
  echoviruses 1:414
  emerging viral diseases 1:423
  hepatitis A 1:637
  Lassa fever 2:890, 2:892
  zoonotic viruses 3:1987
Nostoc muscorum ISU, cyanophages 1:331
Nostocales 1:325, 1:325(Table)
Notch signaling pathway 1:498
Novirhabdovirus 1:560
Novirhabdoviruses 1:558
Ntaya virus group 1:433(Table)
NUC1 3:1977(Table), 3:1978
Nuclear compartmentalization, HSV-induced modification 2:695
Nuclear export signals, HIV 2:766
Nuclear factor 1 (NF1), cytomegalovirus 1:361, 1:362(Fig)
Nuclear lamins 1:253
Nuclear localizing signal (NLS) 1:28
Nuclear oncogenes 3:1507–11
Nuclear 'pod' structures, HSV-induced disruption of ND10 2:695
Nuclear polyhedrosis viruses (NPVs) 1:140, 1:146–52
  assembly 1:149
  budded virus (BV; extracellular virus) 1:147(Fig), 1:148
    envelope proteins 1:151
    proteins 1:150
  dna polymerase gene 1:148
  DNA replication 1:148
  ecology 1:151
  economic importance 1:151–2
  expression vectors 1:152

Nuclear polyhedrosis viruses (NPVs) (continued)
  gene expression 1:143
    regulation 1:148
  genes 1:141
    clustering 1:148
  genome 1:146, 1:147–8
    packaging 1:150
  gp64 protein 1:151
    anchor domain 1:151
    signal peptide sequence 1:151
  history 1:146
  host distribution 1:146–7
  host range 1:147
  hr-containing plasmids 1:148
  hr-enhancer sequences 1:148
  infection duration 1:149
  infection initiation 1:149
  as insecticides 1:151–2
  late expression factor-3 (lef-3) gene 1:148
  life cycle 1:148–50, 1:149(Fig)
  nucleocapsid, structural proteins 1:150
  occlusion body 1:146, 1:150
  occlusion-derived virion (ODV; polyhedron-derived virus/occluded virus) 1:147(Fig), 1:149
    envelope 1:151
    infection process 1:149–50
    proteins 1:150
    transmission 1:151
  p10 protein 1:150
  p74 gene 1:151
  p143 (helicase) gene 1:148
  pathogenesis 1:148–50
  polyhedra 1:149
    structural proteins 1:150
  polyhedrin 1:146, 1:150, 1:152
  polyhedron envelope protein 1:150
  replication 1:146, 1:148
  RNA polymerase 1:148
  structure and composition 1:150–1
  taxonomy 1:146–7
  transactivating factors 1:148
  transactivator (ie-1) 1:148
  transcription
    early 1:148
    late 1:148
  transposable elements 1:148
  UDP-glucosyltransferase 1:150
  virogenic stroma 1:149
  viruses included 1:146–7
  vp39 protein 1:150
  see also Autographa californica nuclear polyhedrosis virus (AcMNPV)
Nuclei, densoviruses in 1:387
Nucleic acid
  amplification 1:392–4, 1:392(Table)
    false-negative 1:395
    false-positive 1:394–5
    probe 1:392(Table), 1:393–4
    quality control 1:395
    signal 1:392(Table), 1:394
    significance in diagnostic virology 1:395
    target 1:392–3, 1:392(Table)
    see also DNA; Polymerase chain reaction (PCR)
  contamination, in amplification methods 1:394–5
  extraction from clinical sample 1:395
  hybridization see Hybridization
  viral, detection see Diagnostic techniques
  see also DNA; RNA

Nucleic acid sequence-based amplification (NASBA) 1:392, 1:393, 1:393(Fig)
Nucleic acid-mediated resistance, in plants see Plant resistance to viruses
Nucleocapsids
  assembly 3:1478
  complex 3:1478
  helical 3:1478
  icosahedral 3:1478
  types 3:1478
Nucleolus 1:255
Nucleopolyhedrovirus 1:140, 1:146, 2:846
  genetic manipulation 2:848, 2:848(Table)
  see also Baculoviruses; Nuclear polyhedrosis viruses (NPVs)
Nucleoprotein helix, structure 3:1946–7
Nucleorhabdovirus 3:1531
  see also Plant rhabdoviruses
Nucleorhabdoviruses
  polymerases 3:1536
  replication cycle 3:1537(Fig)
  see also Plant rhabdoviruses
Nucleoside analogues, human CMV infections 1:350
Nucleoside reverse transcriptase inhibitors (NRTIs) see Reverse transcriptase inhibitors
Nucleosomes 1:255
Nucleotide decoys, HIV infection therapy 1:61
Nucleotypes 2:1054, 2:1061
  coltiviruses see Coltiviruses
Nucleus 1:254–5
  cytoplasmic exchanges 1:255–6
  hypertrophy, in ascovirus-infected cells 1:101
Nudaurelia 3:1771
  β-virus 3:1765
  Ω-virus 3:1765
  see also Tetraviruses
Nudaurelia capensis cynthera 3:1764
  tetraviruses 3:1764
Nudaurelia Ω capensis virus, protein subunit structure 3:1949(Fig)

O

Oat blue dwarf virus (OBDV) 3:1852–3
Oat golden stripe virus (OGSV) 1:588
  genetics and replication 1:593
  genome structure/expression 1:591
Oat sterile dwarf virus (OSDV) 2:1263
Oats
  economic significance of virus infections 2:1323
  luteovirus resistant crops 2:907
Obodhiang virus 3:1442
Occlusion bodies
  Baculoviridae 2:846
  Cypovirus 2:844
  granuloviruses (GV) 1:141, 1:142(Fig), 1:144–5
  Spodoptera ascovirus 1:102
Ocr protein 2:760
Ocular disease, in AIDS 1:528–9
Ocular infections see Eye infections

Oita rhabdovirus 3:1541
Okazaki fragments 2:729
  synthesis, bacteriophage φX174 as model 1:280–1
Okra mosaic virus 3:1850
Old World primates, betaherpesviruses 1:358(Table)
Oleavirus 1:39
Olfactory spread, of viruses 2:1014–15
2-5 Oligoadenylate synthetase/2-5(A)RNase L system 2:858
Oligodendrocytes
  progressive multifocal leukoencephalopathy (PML) 2:882
  Theiler's murine encephalomyelitis virus infection 3:1777
  virus infection 2:1017
Oligonucleotides, novel antiretroviral drugs 1:61
Oligosaccharides, glycosylation 1:252
Olive latent ringspot virus 2:1008(Table)
Olive latent virus 1 (OLV-1) 2:1003
  genome 2:1004
  infection 2:1003
  see also Necroviruses
Olive latent virus 2 (OLV-2), proteins, comparisons 2:810(Fig)
Oliveros virus 2:887, 2:888(Table)
Olpidium, plant virus transmission 3:1907, 3:1908, 3:1909
Olpidium bornovanus 1:244
Omegatetravirus (Ω-type viruses) 3:1765, 3:1767(Table)
  see also Tetraviruses
Omsk hemorrhagic fever (OHF) 1:429, 1:430
Omsk hemorrhagic fever virus (OHFV) 3:1992
  epidemiology 1:428
  features 1:425(Table)
  geographic/seasonal distribution 1:426
  history/discovery 1:426
  host range 1:434
  tissue tropism 1:435
Oncogenes 1:22, 1:115, 3:1507–18, 3:1843
  adapter proteins 3:1515–16
  cbl 3:1515–16
  crk 3:1516
  adenoviruses 1:22
  avian leukosis virus (ALV) 1:115, 1:116
  cooperation v-*erbA* and v-*erbB* 3:1821
  cytokine receptors 3:1515
  mpl oncogene 3:1515
  discovery 2:723
  feline leukemia viruses (FeLVs) 1:545
  growth factors 3:1511
    sis 3:1511
  novel 1:116
  nuclear 3:1507–11
    erbA 3:1507–8
    ets 3:1508
    fos 3:1508–9
    jun 3:1509
    maf 3:1509
    myb 3:1509–10
    myc 3:1510
    qin 3:1510–11
    rel 3:1510
    ski 3:1511

Oncogenes (continued)
  protein tyrosine kinases 3:1511–15
    see also Protein tyrosine kinases
  role in carcinogenesis 3:1507
  serine/threonine kinases 3:1516–17
    akt 3:1516
    raf 3:1516–17
    ras 3:1517
  viral
    v-*fos* 3:1820
    v-*jun* 3:1820
    v-*onc* 3:1507
    v-*rel* 3:1821
    v-*sis* 3:1819
    v-*src* 3:1819–20
  see also individual oncogenes; Transformation, by animal viruses
Oncogenesis 2:1175
  adenoviruses 1:7
    see also Adenovirus
  feline leukemia viruses see Feline leukemia viruses (FeLVs)
  'hit and run' mechanism 3:1842
  Lucké tumor herpesvirus (LTHV) 1:52
  mechanisms 3:1842–3
  multistep process 2:998, 3:1842–3
  viral 3:1842–3
  see also Carcinogenesis; Tumor viruses
Oncogenic viruses see Tumor viruses
Onconvirinae 1:535
Oncoproteins 1:22
Oncorhynchus masou virus 1:553
Ononis yellow mosaic virus 3:1850, 3:1851
O'Nyong nyong (ONN) virus 1:261–5, 3:1994
  antibodies 1:262
  cell culture 1:262
  classification 1:261
  epidemiology 1:263
  evolution 1:262
  genetics 1:262
  genome structure 1:262
  geographic/seasonal distribution 1:261
  history 1:261
  host range and propagation 1:262
  infection 1:261–2
    clinical features 1:264
    epidemic 1:261
    pathology/histology 1:264
    prevention and control 1:265
  pathogenicity 1:264
  serodiagnosis 1:263
  serologic relationships and variability 1:263
  tissue tropism 1:263–4
  transcription and translation 1:262
  transmission 1:263–4
Open reading frames (ORFs) 1:612
Opportunistic infections, AIDS/HIV infection 2:771, 2:773, 2:823
Oral cavity
  cancers, HPV associated 3:1846
  Orf virus infections 2:1144
  vesicular lesions, VSV causing 3:1918
Oral focal epithelial hyperplasia 2:1112
  HPV causing 2:1109, 2:1111(Table)

Oral rehydration
  Norwalk-like virus infection 2:1040
  rotavirus infections 3:1582
Oran virus 3:1988
Orbivirus 2:1044, 2:1062
  serotype and evolution 2:1052
  viruses included 2:1045(Table)
Orbiviruses 2:1043–61
  assembly 2:1062
  classification 2:1044–8
  cytopathic effect 2:1056
  epidemiology 2:1054–5
  evolution 2:1051–2
  future perspectives 2:1060–1
  genetic reassortment 2:1046, 2:1050, 2:1054, 2:1058
  genetics 2:1050
  genome segments 2:1046, 2:1052, 2:1062–3
    coding relationships 2:1050, 2:1063
    conserved features 2:1063
    ORFs 2:1063
    sequence 2:1061
  geographic/seasonal distribution 2:1048
  history 2:1043–4
  host range 2:1049–50, 2:1054
  infection
    clinical features 2:1057–8
    immune response 2:1058–9
    mortality 2:1044
    pathology/histopathology 2:1058
    prevention and control 2:1059–60
  molecular biology 2:1062–74
  pathogenicity 2:1056–7
  phylogenetic associations 2:1051(Fig)
  propagation 2:1049–50
  proteins 2:1052, 2:1063–7
    crystallographic structure 2:1068–72
    NS1 2:1053
    NS3 2:1052, 2:1056
    types and abbreviations 2:1052
    VP7 2:1053
    see also Bluetongue virus (BTV)
  replication 2:1046, 2:1056, 2:1072–3
  serogroups 2:1046, 2:1052
    crossreactions 2:1047
  serologic relationships and variability 2:1052–4, 2:1052(Fig)
  serotypes 2:1052
  structure and properties 2:1044–6, 2:1062
    aqueous channels 2:1062
    capsid and spikes 2:1062
    core 2:1062
  tissue tropism 2:1055–6
  transcription 2:1072
  transmission 2:1048, 2:1054, 2:1055–6
  vaccinated vs infected animal differentiation 2:1060
  vaccines, attenuated 2:1057
  vector range 2:1049
  vectors 2:1054
    activity and distribution 2:1054
  viral inclusion bodies (VIBs) 2:1046, 2:1058
  virulence 2:1057
  see also African horse sickness virus (AHSV); Bluetongue virus (BTV); Epizootic hemorrhagic disease virus (EHDV)

Orchids, economic significance of virus diseases 2:1324
Orchitis 2:988, 2:992
Orders, virus 2:1223
  see also Taxonomy of viruses
Oregon sockeye salmon disease virus (OSDV) 3:1542
Orf virus 2:1140
  cell culture 2:1143, 2:1144
  epidemiology 2:1144
  genes and vaccinia virus homolog 2:1142
  genetic profile 2:1142
  genome 2:1143
  genomic rearrangements 2:1143
  history 2:1140
  host range 2:1143–4
  infection
    clinical features 2:1144, 2:1144(Fig)
    histopathology 2:1145
    immune response 2:1145
    prevention and control 2:1146
  interleukin-10 (IL-10) homolog 2:1146
  ocular target 1:527(Table)
  proteins 2:1141
  structure and properties 2:1141(Fig)
  transcription 2:1143
  vaccines 2:1146
  vascular endothelial growth factor (VEGF) homolog 2:1145–6
  virulence genes 2:1145
  see also Parapoxviruses
Organ system infections 2:1074–86
  heart 2:1074–8, 2:1075(Table)
  kidney 2:1081–5, 2:1081(Table)
  pancreas 2:1078–81
  thyroid 2:1085
Organotypic cultures (three-dimensional cell culture) 3:1412
Orgyria pseudotsugata MNPV (OpMNPV) 1:147
  genome 1:147–8
Original antigenic sin reactions 1:383
Oropharynx, echovirus replication 1:414
Oropouche disease, outbreaks 1:209
Oropouche virus 3:1992
  transmission 1:209
Orphan viruses 2:736
Orthohepadnavirus 1:650
Orthohepadnvirus 1:645–50
  see also Hepatitis B virus (HBV)
Orthomyxoviridae
  apoptosis promotion 1:75
  characteristics 2:824–5
  fish viruses 1:564–5
  genera 2:824
  influenza viruses 2:824–9
  Influenzavirus A 2:824
  Influenzavirus B 2:824
  Influenzavirus C 2:825
Orthomyxoviruses
  receptors 3:1921
  see also Influenza viruses
Orthopoxvirus 1:298, 3:1668, 3:1865
  characteristics 3:1668–9
  ectromelia (mousepox) virus 2:973
Orthopoxviruses
  apoptosis inhibition 1:74
  cowpox virus comparison 1:298
  horse infections 1:304
  see also Cowpox virus; Monkeypox virus; Smallpox (variola) virus

Orthoptera, entomopoxviruses
  (EPVs) 1:478, 1:479
Orthoreovirus 3:1455, 3:1464
  characteristics 3:1455
  members 3:1455
  see also Reoviruses
Orthoreoviruses *see* Reoviruses
Orungo virus
  (ORUV) 2:1045(Table), 3:1994
Oryctes rhinoceros 2:845,
  2:845(Fig), 2:846, 2:846(Fig),
  2:1031, 2:1033
Oryctes virus (Or-1V) 2:845–6,
  2:1031
  biological control agent 2:846,
    2:1031, 2:1033–4, 2:1034
  cytopathic effects 2:1032
  genome 2:1032
  pathology 2:1033–4
  proteins 2:1032
  replication 2:1032, 2:1033
  transmission 2:1034
Oryzavirus 2:1262
  characteristics 2:1263
  conserved sequences 2:1263
  genome, sequence 2:1264
  members 2:1263
Oscillatoriales 1:325, 1:325(Table)
Otitis media 3:1492
Overwintering
  eastern equine encephalitis
    (EEE) 1:504
  Japanese encephalitis (JE)
    virus 2:875
  pea enation mosaic virus
    (PEMV) 2:1194
Ovine adenovirus isolate 3
  (OAV3), genetics and
  evolution 1:19
Ovine adenovirus isolate 287
  (OAV287) 1:14
  as gene expression vector 1:21
  genetics and evolution 1:19
  genome, E3 region 1:21
  proteins 1:16
  replication 1:18
Ovine herpesvirus 1 1:181(Table)
Ovine herpesvirus 2 1:181(Table)
Ovine pulmonary
  carcinoma 3:1524
Ovine respiratory syncytial virus
  (ORSV) 3:1479
Owls-eye nuclei 3:1827(Fig)
Oyster virus (OV) 1:161

P

P1 bacteriophage 1:455–61
  antirestriction systems (DarA and
    DarB) 1:459, 1:459–60
  applications in genetic
    engineering 1:460
  attachment and infection
    process 1:456
  B particles 1:455
  c4, *icd* and *ant* genes 1:457–8
  C-loop 2:986
  cI repressor 1:457, 1:459
  cin and *cix* genes 1:459(Fig),
    1:460
  classification 1:455
  cloning system 1:460
  as cloning vector 2:1242
  coi inactivator 1:457
  Cre recombinase 1:456, 1:2142
  dam methylation sites 1:457
  DNA
    C-segment 1:456, 1:460

P1 bacteriophage (*continued*)
  DNA (*continued*)
    circularization 1:456
    replication 1:458
    restriction-modification 1:455,
      1:459–60
  extrachromosomal
    prophage 1:455
    replication 1:458
  gene expression 1:459
  generalized transduction, fate of
    DNA 1:1238
  genetic map 1:455, 1:456(Fig)
  genome 1:1242
    sequencing 1:457
    structure and
      organization 1:455–6
    transposon insertion 2:1237–8
  history 1:455
  host cell lysis and genes
    involved 1:457
  host range, control by DNA
    inversion 1:460
  immunity system 1:455, 1:456,
    1:457–8
  immC and *immI* regions 1:457
  incompatibility determinants
    (*incA* and *incB*) 1:458
  induction by UV 1:458
  integration into host
    chromosome 1:460
  inversion system 1:459(Fig),
    1:460
  IS1 element 1:460
  lox site 2:1242
  lox-cre recombination
    system 1:455, 1:456, 1:458,
    1:460, 2:1242
  in gene transfer vector 1:13
  Lxc protein (Bof) 1:457
  lysogeny 1:457–8
  lytic cycle 1:456, 1:458
  mod and *res* genes 1:457, 1:459
  as model system 1:455
  morphogenesis 1:457
  mutants/mutations 1:456, 1:457
  P1*kc* mutant 1:455
  pac endonuclease 1:457
  pac site 1:456, 1:457, 2:762
  packaging 1:456, 1:460, 2:762
    headful 1:457, 2:1235–6
  plasmid partition (*par*) 1:458–9,
    1:458(Fig)
  plasmid replication 1:458–9,
    1:458(Fig)
  promoters 1:457
  proteins 1:455
  R-replicon (*oriR* and *repA*) 1:458
  receptors 1:460
  replication
    initiation/origin (*oriL*) 1:456
    σ form 1:456
    Θ form 1:456
  replication cycle 1:456–7
  S particles 1:455
  site-specific recombinases 2:1236
  structure and morphology 1:455,
    1:456(Fig)
  tail genes 1:457
  transcription 1:459
  transduction 1:460
P1-like viruses 1:455, 2:1224
P2 bacteriophage 1:455, 2:1087–94,
  2:1094
  assembly 2:1103(Table)
  *att*P sites 2:1092(Fig)
  CI protein 2:1090
  Cox and Apl proteins 2:1090
  derepression 2:1102–3
  diversity 2:1094
  excisionase (Cox/Apl) 2:1090,
    2:1091

P2 bacteriophage (*continued*)
  genes, functions 2:1088(Table)
  genome organization 2:1089(Fig)
  genome structure 2:1087
  helix-turn-helix DNA binding
    (HTH) motif 2:1090
  as helper for P4 phage 2:1087,
    2:1102, 2:1102–4
  host lysis 2:1094
  immunity repressors 2:1090
  Int proteins 2:1091
  integrase 2:1090
  late genes 2:1093–4
    function 2:1093–4
    promoter
      structure 2:1101(Table)
    regulation 2:1102(Table)
  lysogenic promoters 2:1089
  repression 2:1091
  lysogeny 2:1087, 2:1090–2
    establishment 2:1090–1
    maintenance 2:1090
    transition to lytic cycle 2:1091
  lytic cycle 2:1087, 2:1092–4
    early transcription 2:1092–3
    late gene transcription 2:1093
  promoters 2:1093
  repression 2:1090
  lytic *vs* lysogenic
    development 2:1087–90
  lytic–lysogenic control
    features 2:1090(Fig)
  lytic–lysogenic
    promoters 2:1090(Fig)
  molecular biology 2:1087–94
  morphogenesis 2:1093–4
    capsid/packaging 2:1093–4
    tail 2:1094
  Ogr transcriptional
    activator 2:1101
  org and *B* genes 2:1093
  Org and B proteins 2:1093
  prophage induction 2:1091
  recombination, site-
    specific 2:1091–2
  replication 2:1093
  structure 2:1095(Table)
  T4 exclusion 3:1715
  taxonomy and
    classification 2:1087
  temperate lifestyle 2:1087
  transactivating factors, amino
    acid sequence 2:1101(Table)
  see also Coliphage lambda
P2-like bacteriophage 2:1087,
  2:1224
  diversity 2:1094
  genome structure 2:1087
  see also P2 bacteriophage
P3 bacteriophage 1:455
P4 bacteriophage 2:1094–104
  α operon 2:1095, 2:1099
  alpha protein 2:1097
    functional
      domains 2:1098(Table)
  assembly 2:1103(Table)
  CI immunity factor 2:1099
  CI RNA 2:1099, 2:1100(Table)
  CP4 sequences 2:1104
  coat protein 2:1095, 2:1101
  DNA replication 2:1095–8,
    2:1101
    origin 2:1095
  genes, functions 2:1096(Table)
  genetic map 2:1097(Table)
  genome, as plasmid 2:1094–5,
    2:1101–2
  genome organization 2:1095
  helper gene requirement 2:1094,
    2:1102
  helper phage *see* P2
    bacteriophage

P4 bacteriophage (*continued*)
  host-encoded functions 2:1097
  immunity 2:1099–100
    establishment/
      maintenance 2:1099
    mutations 2:1099
    prophage immunity 2:1099–100
    uncommitted phase 2:1099
  immunity factor 2:1099
  immunity region 2:1097(Table)
  int gene 2:1104
  late genes,
    regulation 2:1102(Table)
  life cycle 2:1096(Table)
  lysis or lysogeny 2:1100
  lysogeny 2:1098–100
    integration into host
      genome 2:1098–9
  lytic cycle 2:1100–4, 2:1102–4
    morphogenesis 2:1104
    satellite–helper regulatory
      interactions 2:1102–4
  multicopy plasmid state 2:1100–4
  natural history 2:1104
  Ogr transcriptional
    activator 2:1101
  ori1 and *crr* 2:1097–8
  promoters
    late 2:1100–1, 2:1101(Table)
    P_{LE} 2:1095, 2:1100
    P_{sid} and P_{LL} 2:1100
  proteins 2:1095
  replication, model 2:1098(Table)
  as satellite phage 2:1094–5
  seq genes 2:1099
  seqC 2:1099
  sid gene 2:1104
  sid operon 2:1095
  site-specific recombination 2:1098
    in tRNA genes 2:1098–9
  structure 2:1095(Table)
  transactivating factors, amino
    acid sequence 2:1101(Table)
  transcription
    early pattern 2:1099
    late pattern 2:1100
    promoters 2:1099
    termination 2:1099
  transcriptional activators 2:1100–
    1
P7 bacteriophage
  integration into host
    chromosome 1:460
  plasmid replication of phage P1
    and 1:459
  postsegregational host killing
    system 1:459
  toxin 1:459
p21, adenovirus E1A effect on 1:27
$p21^{ras}$ 3:1517
P22 bacteriophage 3:1603–7
  as antibacterial therapeutic
    agent 3:1607
  antirepressor (*ant*) 3:1605, 3:1606
  assembly 3:1605, 3:1607
  c2 protein 3:1605
  chromosome 3:1603
  cI repressor 3:1605
  cloning system 3:1606
  coat protein 3:1603, 3:1605
  Cro protein 3:1604
  DNA
    concatemers 3:1603, 3:1605
    packaging 3:1603–4, 3:1605,
      3:1606
    replication 3:1605
  gene clusters 3:1604
  gene expression 3:1605
  as generalized transducing
    phage 3:1607
  genome 3:1604
    map 3:1604, 3:1604(Fig)

P22 bacteriophage (continued)
    homologous
        recombination 3:1606
    host cell lysis 3:1605
    integration into host
        chromosome 3:1605
    LexA protein 3:1605
    lysogeny 3:1605–6
        homeostatic 3:1605–6
    lytic cycle 3:1604–5
    mutants (HT) 3:1605
    in novel settings 3:1607
    pac site 3:1603, 3:1606
    packaging 3:1605
        'headful' 2:1235–6, 3:1603–4
    promoters 3:1604, 3:1605
    proteins 3:1603
    Red system 3:1606
    research directions 3:1606–7
    structure 3:1603–4, 3:1603(Fig)
    tailspike protein 3:1603, 3:1604, 3:1604(Fig), 3:1606–7
    taxonomy and
        classification 1:450
    transcription 3:1604–5
P22-like viruses 2:1225
p53 gene 3:1821
    adenovirus E1A effect on 1:27
    adenovirus E4ORF6 protein
        interaction 1:22
    adenoviruses replicating in cells
        lacking 3:1887
    apoptosis activation 1:71
    apoptosis inhibition 1:71(Table), 1:72(Table)
    blocked by Autographa
        californica MNPV
        (AcMNPV) 1:150
    HPV E5 protein effect 2:1120
    HPV E6 and E7 gene
        interaction 3:1846
    inhibition of binding to
        TAF$_{II}$31 1:22
    inhibition/inactivation by
        viruses 1:71, 1:72
        adenovirus 1:72
    missense mutations, BLV
        infection 1:197
    pX of HBV interaction 1:72
    repression 1:22
        adenovirus E1B19K
        alleviation 1:22
    upregulation by adenovirus
        E1A13S 1:72
p58 activation, influenza
    virus 2:860
p300, adenovirus E1A effect
    on 1:26(Fig), 1:27
P elements 3:1503
P-loop motifs, benyviruses 1:157
pac site 2:1235
Packaging of viruses 1:252–3, 3:1409
Palm oil trees, insect control by
    viruses 2:844, 2:846, 2:846(Fig)
Palyam virus
    (PALV) 2:1045(Table)
Pancreas
    coxsackievirus infection 1:308
    duck hepatitis B virus (DHBV)
        infection 1:654, 1:655
    mumps virus tropism 2:992
    viruses affecting 2:1078–81
Pancreatic β cells, damage in
    IDDM development 2:1080
Pancreatitis
    after mumps 2:1079
    enteroviruses causing 2:1079
Pandemic, definition 1:482
Pangola stunt virus (PSV) 2:1263
Panhandle structures, hantavirus
    genome 1:623, 1:624(Fig)

Panicovirus 3:1791
Panicum mosaic virus
    (PMV) 2:935, 3:1675
    as helper for SPMV 3:1610
Panicum streak virus (PanSV),
    genome structure 1:597, 1:600
Papillomas see Warts
Papillomavirus 2:1121, 2:1352
Papillomaviruses 2:1105–14
    antivirals 1:57(Table), 1:66–7
    human see Human
        papillomavirus (HPV)
    phylogenetic tree 2:1107(Fig)
    taxonomy and
        classification 2:1121
    types and sequences 2:1121
    three-dimensional cell
        culture 3:1411–12
Papillomaviruses, animal 2:1121–30
    attachment and entry 2:1126
    evolution 2:1124, 2:1125(Fig)
    future perspectives 2:1129–30
    genetics 2:1123–4
        ORFs 2:1123
    geographic distribution 2:1121–2
    history 2:1121
    host range 2:1122–3
    infection
        carcinoma 2:1126–7
        clinical features 2:1127
        immune response 2:1128–9
        pathology/
            histopathology 2:1127–8
        prevention and control 2:1129
        warts see Warts
    life cycle 2:1127(Fig)
    pathogenicity 2:1126–7
    propagation 2:1123
    proteins
        E1 2:1124
        E2 2:1123–4
        E2TA protein 2:1123–4, 2:1124
        E4 2:1124
        E5 2:1124
        E6 2:1124
        E7 2:1124
    replication 2:1126
    serologic relationships and
        variability 2:1124–5
    taxonomy and
        classification 2:1121
    tissue tropism 2:1125–6
    transcription 2:1126
    transcriptional
        promoters 2:1123–4
    transmission 2:1125–6
    vaccination 2:1129
    vaccine, naked DNA 2:1129
    virus-like particles (VLPs) 2:1125, 2:1129, 2:1130
    viruses and hosts 2:1122(Table)
    see also Bovine papillomavirus 1
        (BPV-1); Bovine
        papillomavirus (BPV);
        Cottontail rabbit
        papillomavirus (CRPV)
Papovaviridae
    apoptosis inhibition 1:73
    apoptosis promotion 1:75
    characteristics 2:1121
    genera 2:1352
    human papillomaviruses
        (HPVs) 2:1105
    JC and BK viruses 2:876–83
Papillomavirus 2:1121, 2:1352
Polyomavirus 2:876, 2:1352, 3:1647
    see also individual viruses;
        Papovaviruses;
        Polyomaviruses

Papovaviruses
    replication 1:255
    as vectors 3:1892
Papules, capripoxvirus
    infections 3:1379
Parainfluenza viruses (PIVs),
    animal 2:1134–40
    assembly 2:1137–8
    attachment and entry 2:1137
    budding 2:1138
    cell culture 2:1134
    cell-to-cell spread 2:1139
    defective interfering
        particles 2:1137
    epidemiology 2:1139
    evolution 2:1139
    furin 2:1135
    future perspectives 2:1139–40
    genetic manipulation 2:1138–9
    genetics 2:1139
    genome 2:1137
        nucleotide in multiples of
            6 2:1137
    hemagglutinin (HN) 2:1135
    history 2:1134
    host range and
        propagation 2:1134
    infection
        immune response 2:1139
        prevention and control 2:1139
    intergenic regions 2:1137
    neuraminidase activity 2:1135
    nucleocapsid 2:1135, 2:1137, 2:1138
    pathogenicity 2:1139
    proteins 2:1134–7, 2:1135
        F protein 2:1135
        F protein cleavage 2:1135
        M 2:1135
        NP 2:1138
        P and L 2:1135, 2:1137
        V and C 2:1136–7
    receptors 2:1137, 2:1139
    replication 2:1137–8, 2:1138(Fig)
    RNA minigenomes 2:1138
    serologic relationships and
        variability 2:1139
    structure and properties 2:1134–7, 2:1137(Fig)
    taxonomy and
        classification 2:1134
    transcription 2:1137–8
    transmission and tissue
        tropism 2:1139
    vaccines 2:1139
Parainfluenza viruses (PIVs),
    human 1:65, 2:1130-4
    attachment 2:1131
    cell culture 2:1132
    epidemiology 2:1133
    evolution 2:1132–3
    fusion (with host cell
        membrane) 2:1131
    future perspectives 2:1134
    genetics 2:1132–3
    genome organization 2:1131
    geographic/seasonal
        distribution 2:1132
    hemagglutinin–
        neuraminidase 2:1131
    vaccinia virus
        recombinants 2:1134
    history 2:1130
    host range and
        propagation 2:1132
    infection
        bronchiolitis 3:1493
        clinical features 2:1133
        immune response 2:1133
        pathology 2:1133
        pharyngitis 3:1492
        pneumonia 3:1493

Parainfluenza viruses (PIVs),
    human (continued)
    infection (continued)
        prevention and control 2:1133
        respiratory tract 2:1133
    isolation/identification,
        hemadsorption 1:397
    ocular target 1:525(Table)
    pathogenicity 2:1133
    PIV-1 2:1130
        immune response 2:1133
        infection 2:1133
        Sendai virus relationship 2:1132
    PIV-2 2:1130
        immune response 2:1133
        infection 2:1133
    PIV-3 2:1130
        apoptosis promotion 1:75
        immune response 2:1133
        infection 2:1133
    PIV-4 2:1130, 2:1132
    proteins 2:1131–2
        attachment 2:1131
        F (fusion) 2:1131, 2:1131–2
        F precursors and
            cleavage 2:1131–2
        glycoproteins 2:1131
        M (matrix) 2:1132
        molecular weights 2:1131
        P protein 2:1131
    replication 2:1132
    serologic relationships and
        variability 2:1133
    structure and properties 2:1131
    taxonomy and
        classification 2:1130–1
    transcription 2:1132
    translation 2:1132
    transmission 2:1133
    types 2:1130
    vaccine development 2:1134
Paralysis
    coxsackievirus infection 1:308
    echovirus type 9 causing 1:415
    flaccid, enterovirus 70 (EV70)
        causing 1:472
    honey bees 2:743
    poliomyelitis see Poliomyelitis
    Theiler's murine
        encephalomyelitis viruses
        causing 3:1773
Paramecium, Chlorella algae
    symbiosis 1:44, 1:50
Paramecium bursaria
    algae from 1:44
    Chlorella virus see PBCV-1
        (Paramecium bursaria
        Chlorella virus 1)
Paramural bodies, in viroid
    infections 3:1932
Paramyxoviridae
    apoptosis promotion 1:75
    classification 2:1021
    measles virus 2:952–60
    Morbillivirus 3:1560
    Paramyxovirinae 2:953, 2:988, 2:1130, 2:1134, 3:1616
    Pneumovirinae 2:1131, 3:1479
    Rubulavirus 2:1021
Paramyxovirinae 2:1021, 2:1134
    genera 2:1130, 2:1134, 2:1135(Fig)
    genome comparisons 3:1483(Fig)
    members 2:1135(Fig)
    Morbillivirus 2:953, 2:1130
    Respirovirus 2:1130, 3:1616
    Rubulavirus 2:988, 2:1130
    see also Morbilliviruses;
        Paramyxoviruses
Paramyxovirus 2:1021
    genome 2:1132
    members 2:1021

Paramyxoviruses
  characteristics 2:988
  fusion proteins 3:1922
  fusogens 1:251
  penetration and
    uncoating 3:1922(Fig)
  pneumonia in horses 3:1494
  receptors 3:1921
  RNA editing 3:1473
  structure 3:1956
  therapy 1:57, 1:64–5
  see also Mumps virus (MuV);
    Parainfluenza viruses (PIVs)
Parana virus 2:887, 2:888(Table)
Parapoxvirus 2:1140
  type species see Orf virus
  viruses included and
    synonyms 2:1140–1
Parapoxvirus of red deer 2:1140,
  2:1141
  host range 2:1144
  transmission to humans 2:1144
Parapoxviruses 2:1140–6
  DNA replication 2:1143
  epidemiology 2:1144
  future perspectives 2:1146
  genome 2:1143
    sequence and genes 2:1141,
      2:1143
  genomic rearrangements 2:1143
  history 2:1140
  host range and
    propagation 2:1143–4
  infection
    clinical features 2:1144–5
    histopathology 2:1145
    immune response 2:1145
    prevention and control 2:1146
    repeated 2:1145
  pathogenic determinants 2:1145–
    6
  physical properties 2:1143
  proteins 2:1141
    structural 2:1141
  replication 2:1143
    early–late cascade 2:1143
  serologic relationships 2:1144
  structure and properties 2:1141
  taxonomy and
    classification 2:1140–1
  transcription 2:1143
    regulation 2:1143
  vaccine development 2:1146
  virulence genes 2:1145
  see also Orf virus; Pseudocowpox
    virus
Pararetroviruses
  DNA 3:1894
  origin of name 2:1276
  plant see Plant pararetroviruses
  retroviruses
    differentiation 2:1277
  as vectors 3:1894
Pararotaviruses (nongroup A
  rotaviruses) 1:444
Parasitic infections, in caprine
  arthritis encephalitis (CAE)
  syndrome 1:228
Parasitic wasps, aphid
  control 2:907
Parasitoids
  granulovirus interaction 1:145
  polydnavirus
    morphogenesis 2:1349
Paravaccinia virus see
  Pseudocowpox virus
Parechovirus 1:411, 2:1326
  see also Echovirus type 22;
    Echovirus type 23
Parietaria mottle virus
  (PMoV) 1:39
Parodi–Irgrens (PI) FSV 3:1511

Parotitis 2:992
PARP (poly(ADP-ribose)
  polymerase) 1:71
Parry Creek virus 3:1637
Parsnip yellow fleck virus
  (PYFV) 3:1622, 3:1967(Table),
  3:1969
  comparisons with other
    viruses 3:1623(Table)
  genome 3:1622–3, 3:1623(Fig)
  geographic distribution 3:1623
  helper virus 3:1624, 3:1965,
    3:1968
  host range and
    propagation 3:1624
  prevention and control 3:1624–5
  properties 3:1622
  sequence comparisons 3:1965
  serology 3:1623
  symptoms of infections 3:1624
  transmission 3:1624
  see also Sequiviruses
Particle agglutination
  antiviral antibody detection 1:391
  viral antigen detection 1:389
Partitiviridae 1:312, 2:1147
  characteristics 2:1147
  fungal viruses 1:313
  genera 2:1147
  phenogram 2:1148(Fig)
  RNA-dependent RNA
    polymerases (RDRPs) 1:314
  see also Cryptoviruses;
    Partitiviruses, fungal
Partitivirus 2:1147
  members 2:1148(Table)
Partitiviruses, fungal 2:1147–51
  accumulation in cytoplasm of
    hyphae 2:1149
  antigenic properties 2:1149
  dsRNA segments 2:1149
  genome 2:1149
  history 2:1147
  host range 2:1147, 2:1148–9
  host–virus relationships 2:1149
  infectivity assay lacking 2:1148
  latency 2:1149
  mixed infections of fungi 2:1149
  physical properties 2:1149
  protein shell 2:1149
  replication 2:1150–1
  RNA-dependent RNA
    polymerase (RDRP) 2:1147,
    2:1150
  phenogram of
    relationships 2:1148(Fig)
  structure and composition 2:1149
  taxonomy and
    classification 2:1147
  transcription and
    translation 2:1150
  transmission 2:1147–8
Partitiviruses, plant see
  Cryptoviruses
Parvoviridae 1:446, 2:1151–2,
  2:1159–67, 2:1168
  characteristics 2:1155
  Densovirinae 1:384, 2:1152,
    2:1168
  Parvovirinae 2:1151, 2:1160,
    2:1168
  subfamilies 2:1151
Parvovirinae 2:1151, 2:1168
  Dependovirus 2:1152
  Erythrovirus 2:1152
  genera 2:1168
  Parvovirus 2:1152, 2:1160
Parvovirus 1:385, 2:1152, 2:1160,
  2:1168
  defective particles 3:1411
  genetics 2:1152–3
  members 2:1152

Parvovirus (continued)
  see also Parvoviruses
Parvovirus B19 2:1152
  apoptosis promotion 1:75
  cell culture 2:1152
  fastidious virus 2:1152
  genome packaging
    strategies 2:1152
  in hemolytic anemias 2:1154
  infection 2:1153
    clinical features 2:1154
    see also Parvoviruses
  proteins, small 2:1158–9
  receptor 2:1153
  transcription 2:1157, 2:1157(Fig)
  transmission 2:1152
  vaccine 2:1155
Parvovirus-like particles 1:446
  as endemic 'intestinal'
    viruses 1:446
Parvoviruses 2:1151–5, 2:1159–67
  adsorption and entry 2:1171
  animal infections 1:446
  attenuation 2:1165
  autonomously replicating 1:385
  capsid 2:1156, 2:1168
  capsid proteins 2:1169(Table)
  carcinogenicity 2:1173
  of cattle 2:1167–75
    see also Bovine parvovirus
      (BPV)
  densoviruses similarity 1:387
  DNA integration 2:1159
  DNA replication
    models 2:1156, 2:1156(Fig)
    nonstructural proteins
      binding 2:1157
  epidemiology 2:1153, 2:1164–5,
    2:1172–3
  evolution 2:1152–3, 2:1163,
    2:1172
  future perspectives 2:1155,
    2:1159, 2:1167, 2:1174–5
  GenBank Accession
    numbers 2:1169(Table)
  gene expression 2:1157–8
  gene therapy 2:1159
  genetics 2:1152–3, 2:1161–3,
    2:1172
  genome 2:1152–3, 2:1156–7,
    2:1167, 2:1169
    hairpin termini 2:1156, 2:1169
    internal replication
      sequence 2:1157
    lengths 2:1169
    ORFs 2:1153, 2:1157
    packaging 2:1155, 2:1171
    geographic/seasonal
      distribution 2:1152, 2:1160,
      2:1171–2
  history 2:1159–60, 2:1167–8
  host nucleoli interaction 2:1171
  host range and
    propagation 2:1152, 2:1160–
    1, 2:1161, 2:1172
  immunity
    active 2:1174
    passive 2:1174
  infection
    clinical features 2:1154–5,
      2:1165–6, 2:1174
    detection 2:1155
    gastroenteritis 1:446
    immune response 2:1166,
      2:1174
    latent 2:1172
    morbidity/mortality 2:1173
    pathogenesis 2:1153
    pathology/
      histopathology 2:1166, 2:1174
    prevention and control 2:1155,
      2:1167, 2:1174

Parvoviruses (continued)
  infection (continued)
    temporary 2:1172
    see also Parvovirus B19
  infection process 2:1171
  molecular biology 2:1155–9
  monoclonal antibodies 2:1163
  morphogenesis 2:1171
  NS proteins 2:1157, 2:1158,
    2:1169, 2:1171
  NS1 1:387
  NS2 and pathogenicity 2:1173
  properties and roles 2:1170(Fig)
  packaging strategies 2:1152
  pathogenicity 2:1165, 2:1173–4
  physical properties 2:1168
  of pigs 2:1167–75
    see also Porcine parvovirus
      (PPV)
  promoters 2:1169
  proteins 2:1158–9, 2:1169(Table)
    nonstructural see NS proteins
      (above)
    small 2:1158–9
    structural 2:1158
  receptors 2:1153
  replication 1:446, 2:1153, 2:1159,
    2:1169
    cellular function
      requirement 2:1173
    model 2:1156–7, 2:1156(Fig)
    replicative form DNA 2:1171
  of rodents 2:1167–75
    infections 2:1174
    see also Minute virus of mice
      (MVM); Rat virus
  serologic relationships and
    variability 2:1163–4
  structure and properties 2:1155–
    6, 2:1161, 2:1168–9
  taxonomy and
    classification 2:1151–2,
    2:1160, 2:1168
  tissue tropism 2:1153, 2:1173–4
  transcription and
    translation 2:1157–8,
    2:1157(Fig), 2:1169–71
    attenuation site 2:1171
    cellular transactivators 2:1158
    NS transcripts 2:1169–70,
      2:1170(Fig)
    splicing 2:1170
    start codon 2:1170
    transcript processing 2:1157–8
  transmission 2:1153, 2:1172–3
    aerosol 2:1152
    horizontal 2:1173
  vaccines 2:1174
  of waterfowl 2:1167–75
    see also Goose parvovirus
      (GPV); Waterfowl
      parvoviruses (WEPs)
  see also Canine parvovirus
    (CPV); Feline panleukopenia
    virus (FPV); Mink enteritis
    virus (MEV); Parvovirus B19
Passiflora latent virus (PLV) 1:240
*Passiflora yellow mosaic
  virus* 3:1850
Pasteur, Louis 3:1861
Pasteurization of milk, bovine
  leukemia virus sensitivity 1:191
Pathogen-derived resistance see
  under Plant resistance to
  viruses
Pathogenesis of viral
  infections 2:1175–84
  animal viruses 2:1175–84
  assembly and release of
    viruses 3:1409
  attachment and entry 3:1408
  clearance 2:1179

Pathogenesis of viral infections (continued)
  entry of viruses 2:1175
    tropism and 2:1182
    see also Entry of viruses; Receptors for viruses
  penetration of virus see Penetration of viruses
  respiratory tract 3:1490–1
  spread in host see Spread of viruses
  terminology 2:1175
  transmission and shedding 2:1183–4
  'Trojan Horse' mechanism of entry 2:1179
  tropism see Tissue tropism
  uncoating of virus 3:1408
  virus release 2:1178
Pathogenicity, plant viruses 2:1303
PBCV-1 (Paramecium bursaria Chlorella virus 1) 1:44
  African swine fever virus relationship 1:45
  assembly and release 1:46
  DNA polymerase 1:46
  enzymes 1:50
  genes 1:47(Fig), 1:48
  genome 1:45, 1:46
    methylated bases 1:46
    sequencing 1:45
  proteins 1:45
    Vp54 1:45
  replication 1:46
  structure 1:45
  transcription 1:46
  translation 1:46
PCR see Polymerase chain reaction (PCR)
PDZ domains 1:22
Pea early browning virus (PEBV) 3:1784
  genome 3:1785(Fig)
  symptoms of diseases 3:1787
  see also Tobraviruses
Pea enation mosaic disease 3:1858, 3:1859
Pea enation mosaic virus 1 (PEMV 1) 3:1855, 3:1856(Table), 3:1857
Pea enation mosaic virus 2 (PEMV 2) 3:1855, 3:1856(Table), 3:1857
  genome 3:1856, 3:1857(Fig)
Pea enation mosaic virus (PEMV) 2:904, 2:905, 2:1191–6
  acquisition by vector (aphid) 3:1904
  aphid-nontransmissible strains 2:1191, 2:1194
  in aphids, distribution 2:1195
  bean yellow vein banding complex virus (BYVBV) as dependent 2:1194
  binding to E. coli GroEL 3:1905
  coat protein 3:1904
    deletion mutants 2:1192
    ORF encoding 2:1192
    readthrough 3:1904, 3:1905
    virus uptake regulation by 3:1904
  components (top and bottom) 2:1191
  crystalline inclusions 2:1195
  cytopathology 2:1195, 2:1195(Fig)
    vesicular structures 2:1195, 2:1195(Fig)
  distinguishing features 2:1191
  economic significance 2:1194
  epidemiology 2:1194
  future perspectives 2:1196

Pea enation mosaic virus (PEMV) (continued)
  genome structure 2:1191–3, 2:1192(Fig)
    RNA1/RNA2 and component encapsidating 2:1191
    VPg 2:1192
    see also specific RNAs (below)
  helper dependence 2:1194
  host range 2:1193
  infection
    prevention and control 2:1194
    symptomatology 2:1194
  overwintering reservoirs 2:1194
  resistance 2:1194
  RNA1 (luteovirus component) 2:1192–3, 2:1192(Fig)
    ORFs 2:1192
    replication in protoplasts 2:1193
  RNA2 (umbravirus component) 2:1192(Fig), 2:1193
    infection spread 2:1193, 2:1196
    ORFs 2:1193
  RNA3 (satellite component) 2:1193
  serology 2:1191
  structure and composition 2:1191
  systemic spread 2:1195
  taxonomy and classification 2:1191
  transmission 2:1191, 2:1193–4, 3:1904–5
Pea enation mosaic virus (PEMV) complex 3:1855, 3:1857, 3:1858
Pea green mottle virus (PGMV) 1:285
Pea mild mosaic virus (PMiMv) 1:285, 1:290
Pea seed-borne mosaic virus (PSbMV), replication 3:1373
Pea streak virus (PeSV) 1:240, 1:241
Peach dapple viroid 3:1930(Table)
Peach latent mosaic viroid 3:1930(Table), 3:1931(Fig)
Peach rosette mosaic virus 2:1008(Table)
Peanut chlorotic streak virus (PClSV) 2:1285
  'Chlorotic Vein-banding' strain (PClSV-CVB) 2:1289
  cladogram 2:1291, 2:1291(Fig)
  gene products 2:1291
  genome 2:1290
  geographic distribution 2:1276, 2:1289
  history 2:1289
  host range 2:1290(Table)
  symptoms 2:1289
  transactivation 2:1291–2
  transcription 2:1290–1
  transmission 2:1289
  see also Legume caulimoviruses
Peanut clump virus (PCV) 1:154, 1:588, 2:1196
  coat protein 2:1199
  genetics and replication 1:593
  genome 2:1197, 2:1198(Fig)
  genome structure/ expression 1:590(Fig), 1:591
  host range 2:1197
  isolates and groups 2:1197
  life cycle 2:1198(Fig)
  RNA1 and RNA2 1:591, 1:593
  transmission 2:1197
  see also Pecluviruses
Peanut stunt virus (PSV) 1:315
  classification 1:316

Peanut stunt virus (PSV) (continued)
  geographic/seasonal distribution 1:316
  host range and propagation 1:316
  proteins 1:321(Table)
  replication 1:323
  RNA sequences 1:317(Table)
  RNAs 1:321, 1:321(Table)
  satellite RNAs 1:317, 1:323
    replication 3:1614
  serologic relationships and variability 1:318
  symptoms of infection 1:319
  transmission 1:319
  see also Cucumoviruses
Pear blister canker viroid (PBCVd) 3:1930(Table)
Pear rusty skin viroid 3:1930(Table)
Pecluvirus 1:154, 1:588, 2:1196
  genetics and replication 1:593
  genome structure/ expression 1:589(Table), 1:591
  species included 2:1196
  see also Furoviruses; Peanut clump virus (PCV); Pecluviruses
Pecluviruses 2:1196–200
  economic significance 2:1197
  genome 2:1197, 2:1198(Fig)
    coding sequences 2:1198–9
    ORFs 2:1198–9
    RNA-1 and RNA-2 2:1198–9
    sequence comparisons 2:1199
    terminal noncoding sequences 2:1199
    triple gene block 2:1197
  geographic distribution 2:1197
  history 2:1196
  host range 2:1197
  infections
    prevention and control 2:1199
    symptoms 2:1197
  life cycle 2:1197–8, 2:1198(Fig)
  molecular biology 2:1198–9
  serologic relationships 2:1197
  structure and properties 2:1197
  taxonomy and classification 2:1196–7
  transmission 2:1197
Pelargonium flower break virus (PFBV) 1:243
Pelargonium leaf curl virus (PLCV) 3:1790(Table)
  host range 3:1792
Pelargoniums, economic significance of virus diseases 2:1324
Penaeid hemocytic rod-shaped virus (PHRV) 3:1633
Penaeid rod-shaped DNA virus (PRDV) 3:1633
Penaeid shrimps 3:1625
  farms, rhabdovirus infections see Rhabdovirus of penaeid shrimps (RPS)
  species 3:1625
  viruses see Shrimp viruses
  see also Shrimps
Penaeus japonicus nonoccluded type C baculovirus 3:1632
Penaeus monodon
  baculovirus 3:1630, 3:1631
  diagnosis 3:1631, 3:1632
  genome 3:1632
  infections 3:1631
  replication 3:1631
Penaeus monodon single nuclear polyhedrosis virus (PMSNPV) 3:1630

Penaeus vannamei single nuclear polyhedrosis virus (PVSNPV) see Baculovirus penaei (BP)
Penciclovir, herpesvirus infections 1:62
Penetration of viruses 3:1408, 3:1472
  pathways 3:1922(Fig)
  see also Entry of viruses
Penicillium stoloniferum virus S (PsV-S)
  replication 2:1150(Fig), 2:1151
  see also Partitiviruses, fungal
Penile cancer, HPV association 2:1119
Pentamers 3:1945, 3:1947(Fig)
Pentons 1:16
Peplomers, bovine torovirus (BTV) 3:1799
Pepper huasteco virus (PHV) 1:600
Pepper ringspot virus (PRV) 3:1784
  see also Tobraviruses
Peptide decoys, HIV infection therapy 1:61
PERE binding proteins 1:27
Perforin 2:818, 2:1201
  mRNA synthesis, Borna disease virus 1:171
Perforin/granzyme pathway 1:70
Pericarditis
  in AIDS 2:1077–8
  clinical features 2:1077–8
  coxsackievirus infection 1:308
Perinatal infections, cardiac disease due to 2:1074–5
Perinet virus 1:257
Peripheral blood mononuclear cells (PBMCs), HHV-6 and HHV-7 infection 2:702
Peripheral nerves, Marek's disease 2:946(Fig), 2:948–9, 2:949(Fig)
Permissive host cells 3:1409
Persistence of viruses 3:1410
Persistent infections 1:485, 2:897, 2:1200–5, 3:1843, 3:1957
  adenovirus 2:1082
  antiviral immune response 2:1200–2, 2:1202(Table)
  Borna disease virus 1:170, 1:171
  bovine leukemia virus (BLV) 1:196
  Bunyaviridae 1:204, 1:216
  chronic 2:1200
  coronaviruses 1:296, 1:297
  coxsackieviruses 1:307, 1:308, 1:311
  echoviruses 1:415, 1:416
  emerging viral diseases associated 1:421
  equine herpesviruses 1:511–12
  foot-and-mouth disease viruses (FMDVs) 1:572
  future challenges 2:1204
  Hepadnaviridae 1:640
  hepatitis B virus (HBV) 1:643
  hypoviruses 2:804
  Hz-1V and Hz-2V as models 2:1034
  IDDM pathogenesis 2:1080–1
  immune evasion 2:1202–4, 2:1203(Table)
  importance and health problems due to 2:1200
  influence on population size 1:486
  latent 2:1200
  LCMV see Lymphocytic choriomeningitis virus (LCMV)
  Lentiviruses 1:223

Persistent infections (continued)
  measles virus 2:952, 2:958(Fig)
  model, LCMV as 2:915
  mumps virus (MuV) 2:992
  murine cytomegalovirus
    (MCMV) 1:366
  nodaviruses 2:1031
  shedding of viruses 1:484
  sigma rhabdoviruses 3:1637
  SV40 3:1655
  viruses causing 2:1200,
    2:1201(Table)
  see also Chronic infections;
    Immune evasion;
    Immune
    response/system; Latent
    infections
Persistent viruses,
  terminology 3:1900
Peste des petits ruminants virus
  (PPRV) 2:953, 3:1559–60
  clinical features 3:1566
  geographic distribution 3:1560,
    3:1561(Fig)
  host range 3:1561–2
  pathology 3:1567
  transmission 3:1564–5
  vaccination 3:1569
  see also Distemper viruses;
    Morbilliviruses; Rinderpest
    virus
Pesticides 2:842
  biological see Biological control
  see also Insecticides
Pestivirus 1:174
  hepatitis C virus similarity 1:657
  hog cholera virus 2:738
Pestiviruses
  assembly 1:176
  DI particles 1:374
  evolution 1:177
  genome 1:174–5
    untranslated region
      (UTR) 1:177
  internal ribosome entry site
    (IRES) 1:174
  serologic relationships and
    variability 1:177–8
  taxonomy 1:174
  see also Border disease virus
    (BDV); Bovine viral diarrhea
    virus (BVDV); Classical
    swine fever virus (CSFV)
Petechiae
  Argentine hemorrhagic fever
    (AHF) 2:893
  Bolivian hemorrhagic fever
    (BHF) 2:893
Petunia asteroid mosaic virus
  (PAMV) 3:1790(Table)
Petunia vein clearing virus (PVCV),
  genome 2:1282
Peyer's patches 1:179, 2:1177
PG13 gene delivery vector
  system 1:619
pH, soil 2:1250
Phage see Bacteriophage
Phage, Archaea see Archaea phages
  and viruses
Phage φ6 see Bacteriophage φ6
Phage Group 2:720–1, 2:728
Phage P22 see P22 bacteriophage
Phage PRD1 see Bacteriophage
  PRD1
Phage therapy see under
  Bacteriophage
Phage toxins see Bacteriophage
Phage transduction see
  Transduction
Phage typing 1:137–9
  adapted phage 1:138
  advantages 1:137
  automation 1:137, 1:138, 1:139

Phage typing (continued)
  bacterial strains identified 1:137
  cluster analysis 1:138
  history 1:137–8
  host characteristics 1:137, 1:139
  isolation of phages for 1:138–9
  lambda prophage 1:139
  lytic phage 1:138, 1:139
  phage characteristics 1:138, 1:139
  rapid tests 1:139
  routine test dilution (RTD)
    concept 1:138
  schemes 1:138
  technique 1:138
  temperate phage 1:138, 1:139
Phagemids 1:552, 2:1243
Phagocytes
  cytokines produced 1:339
  virus uptake/entry 2:1179
Pharyngitis 3:1492, 3:1493(Table)
  echoviruses causing 1:415
  Lassa fever 2:893
Pharyngoconjuctival fever 1:526
Phasmids 1:1095
Phenotypic mixing 1:609
  animal viruses 1:609
φX174 see Bacteriophage φX174
Phlebotomus fever 1:211
Phlebotomus fever virus 1:210
  transmission 1:211
Phlebovirus 1:204, 1:210–11,
  3:1990, 3:1993
  proteins 1:207
  serogroups and
    viruses 1:206(Table)
  transmission and
    epidemiology 1:208
Phleboviruses
  genome coding strategy 1:204
  infections 1:209
  RNAs, terminal
    structures 3:1760(Fig)
  tenuivirus relationships 3:1763
Phloem
  BYV-type inclusion bodies 1:271
  necrosis 1:272
Phocid distemper
  clinical features 3:1567
  pathology 3:1567
Phocid distemper virus
  (PDV) 2:953, 3:1560
  epizootiology 3:1565–6
  geographic distribution 3:1560
  host range 3:1562
  see also Morbilliviruses
Phocine (seal)
  morbillivirus 1:420(Table)
Phosphate, effect on
  cyanophages 1:330–1
Phosphate buffer, propagation of
  plant viruses 3:1419
Phosphonoacetate 1:557
Phosphonoformate see Foscarnet
Phosphorylation
  African swine fever virus (AFSV)
    proteins 1:34
  cell signaling 3:1819
  human CMV 1:356
  polyomavirus proteins 2:1360
Phosphotungstic acid (PTA) 1:402
Photyrosine-binding (PTB),
  polyomavirus T protein 2:1358
Phycodnaviridae 1:44–50, 1:45
Phycoerythrin 1:330
Phylogenetic trees 3:1750
Physalis mosaic virus 3:1850
Phytoarboviruses
  continuous serial passage 3:1907
  transmission 3:1906
    barriers 3:1906
    control by virus 3:1906
    mutants 3:1907

Phytoarboviruses (continued)
  transmission (continued)
    pathway 3:1903(Fig), 3:1906
    virus genes involved 3:1906
    virus–vector interactions 3:1906
    mutants 3:1907
Phytohemagglutinin (PHA) 1:196
Phytoreovirus 2:1262
  conserved sequences 2:1263
  gene expression 2:1264
  genome, sequence 2:1263–4
  members 2:1262–3
  transmission 2:1266
  see also Phytoreoviruses
Phytoreoviruses 2:1262–7
  cell lines 2:1264
  defective-interfering (DI)
    RNAs 2:1264
  enzymatic activities 2:1263
  epidemiology 2:1265
  future perspectives 2:1267
  gene expression 2:1264–5
    post-translational
      regulation 2:1265
  gene structure 2:1265
  genome 2:1263–4
    copy number 2:1264
    in vitro expression 2:1264
    packaging 2:1264
    sequences 2:1263–4
  geographic/seasonal
    distribution 2:1265–6
  history 2:1262
  host range (plants) 2:1266
  maintenance in host 2:1266
  multiplication in insect
    vectors 2:1266
  prevention and control 2:1265
  resistance 2:1265
  structure and properties 2:1263
  symptoms of infection 2:1266
  taxonomy and
    classification 2:1262–3
  tissue tropism 2:1266–7
  transmissibility loss 2:1266
  transmission 2:1266–7
  viruses included 2:1262
  see also Fijivirus; Oryzavirus;
    Phytoreovirus
Phytoviruses, Sindbis-like 1:242
Pichinde virus 2:887, 2:888(Table)
'Picobirnaviruses' 1:161, 1:447
Picorna-like viruses 2:1267,
  2:1268(Table)
  comoviruses 1:290
  see also Insect picorna-like
    viruses
Picornaviridae 1:229, 1:468
  animal enteroviruses 1:461
    see also Enteroviruses, animal
  Aphthovirus 1:568
  apoptosis promotion 1:75
  Cardiovirus 3:1773
  cardioviruses 1:229–38
  classification 1:568,
    3:1773(Table)
  coxsackieviruses 1:305–11
  Enterovirus 1:305, 1:411, 2:1326,
    2:1330
  genera 2:1326, 2:1330
  Hepatovirus 1:631
  insect picornaviruses 2:1267
  Parechovirus 1:411, 1:413
  properties 1:462
  rhinoviruses 3:1545
  shrimp viruses 3:1629
  see also Cardioviruses;
    Picornaviruses; Poliovirus;
    Rhinoviruses

Picornaviruses 1:66
  caliciviruses
    relationship 2:1037(Fig),
    2:1038
  capsid, structure 3:1954(Fig)
  characteristics 2:1330
  classification 2:733, 2:734
  infections
    ocular, interferon use 2:861
    therapy 1:57(Table), 1:66
  insect see Insect picornaviruses
  pancreatic infections 2:1079
  structure 3:1953
    three-dimensional 3:1774
  VPg 3:1475
  waikaviruses vs 3:1966–7, 3:1967
  see also Coxsackieviruses;
    Echoviruses; Enteroviruses;
    Poliovirus
Pig polioencephalomyelitis see
  Teschen disease
Pig-tailed macaque virus
  (PTMV) 2:1152
Pigeon pea mosaic mottle
  viroid 3:1930(Table)
Pigeonpox viruses 1:578
Pigs
  African swine fever virus 1:35
    see also African swine fever
      virus (ASFV)
  calicivirus discovery 1:217
  cardiovirus infections 1:235
  hog cholera see Hog cholera
  immunity to vesicular exanthema
    virus 1:220
  influenza virus infection 2:826–7
    clinical features 2:828
  Japanese encephalitis (JE) virus
    infection 2:874–5, 2:875
  nodavirus isolation 2:1027
  Sendai virus infection 3:1619
  stillborn, hog cholera 2:741
  vesicular exanthema 1:217, 1:219
  see also entries beginning
    Porcine, Swine; Pseudorabies
    virus (PRV)
Pike fry virus (PFV) 3:1544
Pili 3:1664
  F, filamentous phage
    infection 1:550
Pilin 1:550
Pineapple bacilliform virus
  (PBV) 2:1296
Pinocytosis 1:250
Piper yellow mottle virus
  (PYMV) 2:1296
  geographic distribution 2:1298
  structure and composition 2:1296
  see also Badnaviruses
Pirital virus 2:888(Table)
Piry virus 1:257–60
  agD and rgD mutants 1:260
  antibodies 1:259
  classification 1:257
  crossreactivity with vesicular
    stomatitis virus 1:257
  genome organization 1:257–9,
    1:259(Table)
  genome sequence 1:258–9
  history 1:257
  host range 1:259
  mutants 1:260
  human infections 1:259
  mRNAs 1:258, 1:259(Table)
  proteins 1:257, 1:258,
    1:259(Table)
  replication 1:260
  structure 1:258(Fig)
  ts mutants 1:260
Piscine erythrocytic necrosis virus
  (PENV) see Viral erythrocytic
  necrosis virus (VENV)

'Pits,' cardiovirus capsid **1**:231, **1**:234
PL/J mice
  experimental autoimmune encephalomyelitis (EAE) **1**:111
  MBP recombinant vaccinia virus **1**:111
Placenta, rubella virus infection **3**:1597
Plant(s)
  breeding, use of resistance to viruses **2**:1306–7
  DI particles **1**:374
  evolution, retrotransposon significance **2**:1317
  inoculation with viruses and vectors **3**:1893–4
  resistant varieties **2**:1325
  transgenic **2**:1325
  virus families/genera infecting **3**:1753(Fig)
  virus-free **3**:1841
  see also Plant virus disease
Plant pararetroviruses **2**:1275–81, **2**:1281–5, **2**:1285–9, **2**:1289–92, **2**:1296–300, **2**:1314–15
  see also Badnaviruses; Cassava vein mosaic virus; Caulimoviruses; Legume caulimoviruses; Rice tungro bacilliform viruses
Plant picornaviruses **3**:1623
Plant resistance to viruses, engineered **2**:1300–7, **2**:1307–9
  new and combined strategies **2**:1313
  nonplant-nonpathogen-derived **2**:1312–13
    interferon-induced 2-5A system **2**:1312
    plantibodies **2**:1312–13
    see also Plantibodies
  nucleic acid-mediated (homology-dependent) **2**:1310–11
    antisense RNAs **2**:1310, **2**:1310–11
    defective interfering nucleic acids **2**:1311
    mechanisms **2**:1310
    other strategies **2**:1310–11
    satellite RNAs **2**:1311
  pathogen-derived **2**:1307–11
    coat protein (CPMR) **2**:1309
    examples by virus and host **2**:1308(Table)
    mechanisms **2**:1309
    nucleic acid-mediated *see above*
    protein-mediated **2**:1309–10
    replicase-mediated **2**:1309
    viral movement proteins **2**:1309–10
  plant-derived genes **2**:1311–12
    monogenic resistance **2**:1311
    naturally occurring genes **2**:1311–12
    ribosome-inactivating proteins **2**:1312
    virus types **2**:1311
Plant resistance to viruses, natural **2**:1300–7
  acquired/induced **2**:1306
    crossprotection **2**:1306
    local and systemic **2**:1306
  active and passive **2**:1301
  cell-to-cell movement importance **2**:1301, **2**:1303
  cowpea mosaic virus (CPMV) **2**:1305
  cultivar **2**:1304–5

Plant resistance to viruses, natural *(continued)*
cultivar *(continued)*
    dominant **2**:1304
    local **2**:1305
    protease inhibitors **2**:1305
    recessive **2**:1305
    ribosome-inactivating proteins **2**:1305
    single gene locus **2**:1304–5
  diversity **2**:1300–1
  importance **2**:1300
  nonhost **2**:1303
    cell-to-cell movement **2**:1303
    chemicals/inhibitors **2**:1303
    subliminal infections **2**:1303
  plant population complexity and **2**:1301, **2**:1301(Table)
  positive and negative **2**:1301
  rice tungro **3**:1970
  targets **2**:1301–3
  tobacco mosaic virus *N* gene **2**:1304–5
  tomato mosaic virus (ToMV) **2**:1305
  types **2**:1300–3
  umbraviruses **3**:1859
  use in plant breeding **2**:1306–7
  see also other specific viruses
Plant retroelements **2**:1314–17
  evolutionary significance **2**:1317
  see also Plant pararetroviruses; Plant retroposons; Plant retrotransposons
Plant retroposons **2**:1316–17
  genomes **2**:1316–17
  LINEs (long interspersed nuclear elements) **2**:1316–17, **2**:1316(Fig)
Plant retrotransposons **2**:1315–16
  copia-like **2**:1315–16, **2**:1316(Fig)
  gypsy-like **2**:1316, **2**:1316(Fig)
  long terminal repeat (LTR) **2**:1315
  replication **2**:1316
Plant retroviruses **2**:1292–6
Plant rhabdoviruses **3**:1531–41
  acquisition by vectors **3**:1539
  budding **3**:1537
  characteristics **2**:1296
  cytopathology **3**:1536–8
  defective interfering RNAs **3**:1536
  diseases **3**:1531
    control **3**:1539–40
  distribution **3**:1538–9
  economic significance **3**:1531
  epidemiology **3**:1539–40
  evolution **3**:1538–9
  future perspectives **3**:1540
  gene order **3**:1534
  genome **3**:1534
    leader and trailer genes **3**:1534
  infection of plants and insects **3**:1539
  morphogenesis **3**:1536–8
  morphology and composition **3**:1533–4, **3**:1533(Fig)
    layers **3**:1533–4
  polymerase **3**:1536
    activity **3**:1536
  potyviruses interactions **3**:1539
  proteins **3**:1533–4, **3**:1534–6
    glycoprotein (G) **3**:1535–6
    matrix (M) **3**:1535
    nucleocapsid (N) **3**:1535
    phosphoprotein **3**:1535
    polymerase (L) **3**:1536
    sc4 **3**:1535
  replication **3**:1536–8
    cycle **3**:1537(Fig)

Plant rhabdoviruses *(continued)*
  resistance to **3**:1540
  RNA-dependent RNA polymerase **3**:1536
  taxonomy and classification **3**:1531–3
  transcription **3**:1537
  transmission **3**:1531, **3**:1538
  vector relationships **3**:1538–9, **3**:1539
  vectorless, evolution **3**:1538–9
  viruses included **3**:1531, **3**:1532(Table)
  see also Sonchus yellow net virus (SYNV)
Plant virus disease **2**:1318–26
  abnormal leaf morphology **2**:1318–19
  'beneficial' **2**:1324
  color changes **2**:1318
  damage **2**:1319(Fig), **2**:1321–4
    assessment **2**:1324–5
    direct **2**:1321
    indirect **2**:1321
    market value reductions **2**:1323–4
    plant growth reductions **2**:1318, **2**:1321–3
    quality reductions **2**:1323–4
    vigor reductions **2**:1323
  'degeneration'/'running out' and 'senility' **2**:1323
  economic aspects **2**:1318–26
    costs of maintaining plant health **2**:1324
    definition **2**:1318
    future perspectives **2**:1325
    indirect costs **2**:1324
    see also Plant virus disease, damage
  economic significance *see* Economic significance
  fungal infections after **2**:1323
  host response **2**:1184
    induction **2**:1185
  latent (inapparent) infections **2**:1318
  necrosis **2**:1318
  pathogenesis **2**:1184–90
    determinants **2**:1184
    immune interactions **2**:1185
  percentage infection in clinic samples **2**:1325(Table)
  resistance interactions **2**:1185–8
    genes involved **2**:1186(Table)
    hypersensitivity **2**:1186–8
    localized infections **2**:1186
    single cell/subliminal infections **2**:1185
  susceptible responses **2**:1188–90
    chlorosis *see* Chlorosis sensitive **2**:1188
    systemic necrosis **2**:1190
    tolerance **2**:1190
  symptom syndrome **2**:1319
  symptoms **2**:1301–3, **2**:1306, **2**:1318–21
    systemic **2**:1321
  wilting and desiccation **2**:1318
Plant viruses
  avirulent **2**:1304
  biological assay using TMV **3**:1780
  cell-to-cell spread *see* Cell-to-cell movement
  classification
    in groups **3**:1749–50
    history **3**:1730
  co-infections **3**:1694
  control strategies **2**:1300
  economic significance *see* Economic significance

Plant viruses *(continued)*
  extraction, buffers for **3**:1420
  'floating genera' **3**:1750
  fungal vectors *see* Fungi
  gene-for-gene relationship with plants **2**:1304, **2**:1304(Table)
  host range and determinants **2**:1303
  infection initiation **2**:1301
  infections *see* Plant virus disease
  inoculation *see* Inoculation; Mechanical transmission
  insect transmission *see* Insect transmission, of plant viruses
  isolation from propagative hosts **3**:1420–1
  local lesion hosts **3**:1418
  long-distance movement **2**:1301
  mixed infections **3**:1694
  nonpersistent **3**:1901
  nontransmissible **3**:1901
  pathogenicity **2**:1303
  persistent **3**:1900
  propagation **3**:1418–21
    buffers/conditions used **3**:1419
    choice of host **3**:1418
    conditions **3**:1418
    criteria for host choice **3**:1418
    cycling **3**:1418
    preserving infectivity during transmission **3**:1419–20
    transmission methods **3**:1418–19
    transmission by vectors **3**:1419
  purification **3**:1420
  recombination **3**:1450
  release **2**:1303
  replication **2**:1301
  replicative cycle (model) **2**:1302(Fig)
  resistance to *see* Plant resistance to viruses, natural
  satellites **3**:1610
  semipersistent **3**:1900, **3**:1901, **3**:1903–4
  spread and movement **2**:1301
  'subliminal' infection **2**:1303
  synergism **3**:1694–8
    model form **3**:1694–5
    nonpotyviral **3**:1698, **3**:1698(Table)
    potyvirus-associated **3**:1694, **3**:1694(Table)
    symptoms **3**:1695(Fig), **3**:1696
    see also Potato virus Y (PVY); Potyviruses
  transmission
    arthropods *see* Arthropods; Phytoarboviruses
    mechanisms of specific viruses **3**:1902(Table)
    see also Mechanical transmission
  vector transmission *see* Insect transmission, of plant viruses
Plant-to-plant transmission, dianthoviruses **1**:407
Plantago mottle virus **3**:1850
Plantain 6 virus (PIV-6) **1**:245
Planthoppers **3**:1757(Table)
  morphology **3**:1758(Fig)
  population fluctuations **3**:1764
  tenuiviruses transmission **3**:1756, **3**:1757(Table), **3**:1763
Plantibodies **2**:1312–13
  monoclonal **2**:1313
  scFv antibodies **2**:1313
  targeting to subcellular compartments **2**:1313

Plaque 3:1412
  bacteriophage 2:925–6
  formation, virus isolation/
    identification 1:397
  halos 3:1416
  morphology 3:1416
  purification 3:1416
  turbid 3:1416
Plaque assay 3:1413(Fig), 3:1416
  method development 2:722
Plaque-forming units (PFUs) 1:397,
    3:1412, 3:1416
Plasma cells 2:814
Plasma membrane 1:249–51
  bilayer organization 1:249
  envelope fusion 2:1181, 2:1182
  functions 1:250
  internalization of extracellular
    material 1:250
  ion transfer and ion pumps 1:250
  as mosaic of domains 1:250
  receptors 1:250
  signal transduction 1:250
  trafficking of molecules 1:250
  virus entry and uncoating 1:251
  see also Host, membrane;
    Membranes
Plasmalemmasomes, in viroid
    infections 3:1932
Plasmaviridae 2:1226
  characteristics 2:1226
  phage included 2:1226
Plasmaviruses 3:1416
  assembly and release 3:1416
  genome integration 3:1416
  nonlytic multiplication 3:1416
  plaque morphology 3:1416
  release 3:1415
Plasmid pCV1 1:136
Plasmid pϕH1 1:82
Plasmid pME2001 1:83
Plasmid/phage cloning
    vectors 2:1243
Plasmids 1:139
  addiction (postsegregational host
    killing) 1:455, 1:459
  adenovirus vector
    construction 3:1886
  baculovirus vectors 1:152
  coliphage lambda 1:284
  expression vectors 2:1243
  P4 bacteriophage 2:1094–5
  promiscuous 2:1243
  shuttle 2:1243
Plasmodesmata
  cell-to-cell movement of plant
    viruses 2:1185, 2:1186, 3:1892
  enlargement, caulimoviruses
    causing 2:1280
  movement protein action 2:1310
  plant rhabdovirus
    movement 3:1539
  tobamoviruses movement 3:1783
Plasmodiophorales 1:154
Plasmodiophoromycetes
  furovirus vectors 1:594
  life cycle 1:594
  plant virus transmission 3:1907
  zoospores 1:594
    encysted and 'stachels' 1:594
Platelet factor 4 (PF4) 1:343
Platelet-derived growth factor
    (PDGF)
  gene 1:1819
  v-sis product homology 3:1511
Platelets, in Lassa fever 2:892
Plautia stali intestinal virus
    (PsIV) 2:1268, 2:1273
Plebejus baculovirus (PBV) 3:1631
Pleckstrin, expression induced by
    EBNA-3 of EBV 1:499
Pleconaril (ViroPharma) 1:66

Plectonema boryanum 1:331
Plectrovirus 2:1227
Pleurocapsales 1:325(Table)
Pleurodynia 1:308
  echoviruses causing 1:415
Plum dapple viroid 3:1930(Table)
Plum pox virus (PPV) 3:1369
PMEA (2-
    phosphonylmethoxyethyl)-
    adenine 2:781
PMPA (9′(2-phosphonylmethoxy-
    propyl)adenine 2:779, 2:781
Pneumoencephalitis, Newcastle
    disease virus 2:1021
Pneumonia 1:493–4,
    3:1493(Table)
  adenovirus 1:6
  Aleutian mink disease 2:1166
  causative agents 3:1493
  echoviruses causing 1:416
  giant cell 2:956
  influenza viruses causing 2:828
  interstitial
    caprine arthritis encephalitis
      virus (CAEV) 1:227
    human CMV 1:349
  in measles 2:956, 2:957
  myxoviruses causing 1:63
  progressive 3:1962
  respiratory syncytial virus
    causing 1:64, 1:65, 3:1832
Pneumonia virus of mice
    (PVM) 3:1479
Pneumonitis
  CMV 3:1824
  features 1:493
  HSV 2:681
  Sendai virus causing 3:1616
Pneumovirinae 2:1131, 2:1134
  genome comparisons 3:1483(Fig)
Pneumovirus 3:1479
Pneumovirus 2:1131, 3:1479
  members 2:1021
  see also Respiratory syncytial
    virus (RSV)
Poa semilatent virus (PSLV) 2:749
  host range 2:750
Poaceae, tenuiviruses
    infection 3:1756
Podospora 3:1406
  het genes 3:1406
  [HET-S] as prion form of het-s
    protein 3:1406
  het-s strain 3:1406
Podoviridae 1:325, 2:1223, 2:1225
  characteristics 2:1225
  coliphage N4 1:450
  phage ϕ29 1:119–30
  phage included 2:1225
  T7-like phage 3:1722–9
  see also Coliphage N4; T7-like
    phage
Poinsettia mosaic virus 3:1850
Pokeweed antiviral proteins
    (PAP) 1:1312
pol gene
  caprine arthritis encephalitis
    virus (CAEV) 1:223, 1:225–6
  caulimoviruses 2:1277–8
  equine infectious anemia virus
    (EIAV) 1:516
  lymphoproliferative disease virus
    (LPDV) 2:913
  see also other specific
    retroviruses
pol II 3:1472
Pol protein, Ty elements 3:1505
Polerovirus 2:901, 2:902(Table)
Poleroviruses 2:902
  cytopathology 2:906–7
  economic significance 2:907–8
  evolution 2:905

Poleroviruses (continued)
  genome organization 2:903,
    2:903(Fig)
  geographic distribution 2:902–3
  host range 2:903
  prevention and control 2:907
  protein functions 2:903–4
  replication 2:903–4
  structure and composition 2:903
  subgenomic (sg) RNAs 2:904
  taxonomy 2:902, 2:902(Table)
  transcription 2:904
  translation 2:904
  transmission 2:906
  viruses included 2:901–2
Polioencephalomyelitis, pigs see
    Teschen disease
Poliomeningitis, bulbospinal,
    echovirus infection
    mimicking 1:416
Poliomyelitis
  abortive 2:1328
  children 1:421
  clinical features 2:1018, 2:1328
  coxsackievirus A (CA)
    infection 1:309
  epidemic, host ecology
    influencing virus
    emergence 1:421
  eradication 1:417, 3:1861
  history 2:1326, 2:1330, 2:1347
  immunization strategy 2:1329
  nonparalytic 2:1328
  paralytic 2:1328
  pathology/histopathology 2:1328
  prevention and control 2:1329
  'provoking effects' 2:1182
  Theiler's viruses causing 3:1773,
    3:1776
  vaccines see under Polioviruses
  see also Poliovirus, infection
Poliomyelitis virus see Poliovirus
Poliovirus 2:1326–9, 2:1330–48
  'A-particle' 2:1335
  antiviral mechanisms 2:860
  antibodies, historical
    aspects 2:732
  antigenic drift 2:1327
  attachment and entry 2:1333–4
  capsid structure and
    antigenicity 2:1330–3
    β cylinder 2:1331, 2:1333(Fig)
    'canyon' and drug
      binding 2:1331
    'escape' mutants 2:1332–3
    myristate action 2:1331
    neutralization antigenic
      sites 2:1332–3
    proteins 2:1333(Fig)
    protrusions 2:1331
    tertiary structures 2:1330–1
    VP1/VP2/VP3 2:1330
    VP4 2:1330
  cDNA 2:1330, 2:1347
  cell-free de novo synthesis 2:1347
  'chemical' 2:1347–8
  classification, historical
    aspects 2:733–4
  conferences on 2:733
  cytopathic effects 1:397(Fig),
    2:1344–5
  emerging/re-emerging
    virus 1:419(Table)
  empty capsids
    (procapsids) 2:1344
  epidemiology 2:1327
  future perspectives 2:1329,
    2:1347–8
  gene expression
    regulation 2:1337–41
  genetic 'plasticity' 2:1347

Poliovirus (continued)
  genetic recombination 2:1327,
    2:1347
  genetics 2:1327
  genome 2:1335–6
    5′NTR 2:1336, 2:1336–7,
      2:1342
    characteristics 2:1330
    cis-acting signal for
      replication 2:1335–6
    comparison with
      caliciviruses 2:1037(Fig)
    compression by error
      frequency 2:1346–7
    dicistronic 2:1337, 2:1340–1
    monocistronic 2:1337
    organization 2:1336(Fig)
    sequence 2:1326
    size 2:1346
    Vpg 2:1335, 2:1342
  geographic/seasonal
    distribution 2:1326–7
  H (C) form 2:1328
  history 2:722, 2:730–4, 2:1326,
    2:1330, 2:1347
    antibody development and
      protection 2:732
    chimpanzee infections 2:732
    classification 2:733–4
    early developments 2:730–2
    fecal contamination 2:731
    growth in tissue culture 2:731,
      2:735
    isolation from blood 2:732
    laboratory animals 2:731–2
    laboratory findings
      applications 2:732–3
    olfactory lesions 2:730
    oral–alimentary route of
      infection 2:730–1
    research using Rhesus
      monkeys 2:730
    transmission 2:731
    vaccines see below
  host cell structure 1:255(Fig)
  host protein synthesis
    shutoff 2:1344
  host range and
    propagation 2:1327
  host translational damage 3:1959
  inactivated (IPV) 3:1864
  infection 2:1330
    cellular response 2:1344–5
    clinical features 2:1328
    enteric 2:731
    immune response 2:1328–9
    outbreaks 2:732
    pathology/
      histopathology 2:1328
    prevention and control 2:1329
    see also Poliomyelitis
  infection initiation 1:234
  internal ribosome entry site
    (IRES) 2:1335, 2:1336–7,
    3:1474
    dicistronic poliovirus 2:1341
    hybrid virus (PV1
      (RIPO)) 2:1334, 2:1337
    mechanisms 2:1337
    point mutations 2:1337
    structure 2:1338(Fig)
  isolation, history 2:730
  live (OPV) 3:1861, 3:1864
  maize chlorotic dwarf virus strain
    TN vs 3:1967(Table)
  molecular biology 2:1330–48
  molecular genetics 2:1346–7
  morphogenesis 2:1346
  mRNA structure 2:1336
  mutants, 'escape' 2:1332–3
  mutations
    point 2:1327

Poliovirus (continued)
  mutations (continued)
    rates 2:1327, 2:1335, 2:1346
    suppressor 2:1342
  N (D) form 2:1328
  passive immunoglobulin 2:1329
  pathogenicity 2:1328
  PKR degradation 2:860
  polypeptide 3CD^{pro} 2:1339–40, 2:1340, 2:1342
  polypeptide 3C^{pro} 2:1340, 2:1342
  polyprotein processing 2:1331, 2:1337–41, 2:1339(Fig)
    steps and cleavage sites 2:1339–40, 2:1339(Fig)
  polyproteins 2:1346
  prophylaxis, historical reports 2:730
  proteinase 2A^{pro} 2:1340
  proteins 1:462, 2:738
    genes encoding 2:1337–9
    morphogenesis 2:1344
    P2-encoded 2:1341
    structural 2:1330, 2:1333(Fig)
    VP3 structure 3:1949(Fig)
  protomer structure 2:1332(Fig)
  quasi-species and 2:1346
  receptor (CD155; PVR) 2:1333–5, 2:1348
    cDNAs 2:1334
    destabilization of virus 2:1335
    genetic organization of isoforms 2:1334(Fig)
    role in docking of virus 2:1335
    structure 2:1334(Fig)
    see also CD155
  replication 2:1348, 3:1474–5
    overview 2:1345–6, 2:1346(Fig)
  replicative cycle 2:1345–6, 2:1346(Fig)
  resistance 2:1335
  RNA replication 2:1341–4
    cloverleaf model 2:1342, 2:1343(Fig), 2:1348
    dsRNA formation 2:1342
    in vivo 2:1345
    initiation 2:1342, 2:1342–3
    model overview 2:1343(Fig), 2:1344, 2:1345–6
    origin 2:1342
    P2-encoded polypeptide role 2:1341
    P3 polypeptide role 2:1341–2
    replicative form (RF) 2:1342, 2:1343–4
    replicative intermediates (RI) 2:1340, 2:1344
    semiconservative 2:1342
    site 2:1344
  RNA-dependent RNA polymerase 3:1475
  Sabin strains 2:1328, 2:1329
    point mutations in IRES 2:1337
  serologic relationships and variability 2:1327
  serotype 1 strain Mahoney (PV1(M)) 2:1330
    properties 2:1331(Table)
  serotype 2
    immune response 2:1328
    infection 2:1327
  serotypes 2:1326, 2:1327, 2:1330
    pathogenicity 2:1328
    receptor 2:1334
    relationships 2:1327
  structure and properties 2:1330, 2:1332(Fig)
  taxonomy and classification 2:1326, 2:1330
  tissue culture 2:735
    history 2:731

Poliovirus (continued)
  tissue tropism 2:1327–8, 2:1328, 2:1330, 2:1334–5, 2:1348
  transcription 3:1474–5
  transgenic mice 2:1327, 2:1335
  translation 2:1336–7, 3:1474–5
    cap-independent 2:1336
    efficiency and mutation effect 2:1337
    mechanisms 2:1337
    start codons 2:1336, 2:1337
    unique features 2:1336
  transmission 1:485(Table), 2:1327–8
    oral 2:1327
  types 2:732, 2:733
  uncoating 3:1472
  vaccines
    adverse effects 2:1329
    'Cutter incident' 2:1182, 2:1329
    development 2:735
    history 2:723, 3:1861
    Sabin 2:1329
    safety 3:1861
    Salk 2:1329
    SV40 contamination 3:1647, 3:1655–6
    as vectors 3:1891
  vesicle, structure 2:1345
  vesiculation 2:1344–5
  VSV interference 2:850
  see also Picornaviruses
Poliovirus receptor-related proteins (PRR1 and PRR2) 2:1334
Pollen transmission
  ilarviruses 1:43
  nepoviruses 2:1012
  raspberry bushy dwarf virus (RBDV) 2:811
Pollution, emergence and re-emergence of diseases 1:422
Poly(A)-type retrotransposons 3:1503, 3:1504(Fig), 3:1505
Polyamines, in comoviruses 1:286
Polyarthralgia
  Chikungunya (CHIK) fever 1:264
  rubella 3:1598
Polyarthritis
  Barmah Forest virus (BFV) causing 3:1570
  epidemic see Epidemic polyarthritis
  see also Arthritis
Polydnaviridae 2:1349–51
Polydnaviruses 2:1349–51
  biological control 2:1351
  DNA replication 2:1350
  economic significance 2:1351
  genera 2:1349
  genetic colonization of host 2:1350
  genome 2:1349, 2:1349–50
  life cycle 2:1350
  morphogenesis 2:1349
  origin 2:1350, 2:1350–1
  packaging 2:1350
  structure and properties 2:1349
  taxonomy and classification 2:1349
  transmission 2:1350
  see also Bracoviruses; Ichnoviruses
Polyethylene glycol (PEG), precipitation of phage 3:1417
Polyhedra 1:332, 1:334(Fig)
  properties 1:333
  shape 1:335
  transmission 1:334
  see also Cypoviruses
Polyhedrin 1:141, 1:333
  crystallization 1:335

Polyhedrin (continued)
  formation 1:336
  gene 1:333, 3:1888
    shuttle vectors 3:1888
  location 1:335
  nuclear polyhedrosis viruses (NPVs) 1:146, 1:150, 1:152
Polyhedrosis disease 1:146
  viruses causing see Nuclear polyhedrosis viruses (NPVs)
Polymerase, measles virus (MV) 2:953
Polymerase chain reaction (PCR) 1:139, 1:392
  badnavirus detection 2:1299
  birnavirus detection 1:166
  bovine leukemia virus (BLV) detection 1:197
  carlavirus detection 1:242
  closterovirus detection 1:273
  cytomegaloviruses 1:345
  dengue viruses 1:379
  DNA amplification technique 1:392–3, 1:392(Fig)
  hepatitis E virus 1:675
  human papillomavirus detection 2:1106, 2:1108
  Iridovirus classification 2:864
  lymphoproliferative disease virus of turkeys 2:914
  Marek's disease virus 2:948
  morbilliviruses infection 3:1568, 3:1568(Fig)
  nested 1:393
  post-PCR photochemical method 1:395
  rabies virus studies 3:1439
  respiratory viruses 3:1494
  specificity and sensitivity 1:393
  see also Reverse transcriptase PCR (RT-PCR)
Polymyositis 2:802
  coxsackievirus A (CA) infection 1:309
Polymyxa
  pecluvirus vector 2:1197, 2:1198(Fig)
  plant virus transmission 3:1908
Polymyxa beta
  benyvirus transmission 1:159
  requirements for zoospores 1:159
  symbiotic reaction with BNYVV 1:159
  zoospores and life cycle 1:159
Polymyxa betae 1:155
Polyomavirus 2:1352, 3:1647
  JC and BK viruses 2:876
  members 2:1352
  SV40 see Simian virus 40 (SV40)
  see also BK virus; JC virus
Polyomaviruses
  characteristics 3:1647
  culture 2:878
  enhancer elements 2:1182
  infections, post-transplant 3:1831
  structure 3:1951
Polyomaviruses, murine 2:1352–6
  abortive transformation 2:1354, 2:1355
  assembly site 2:1360
  attachment and entry 2:1354, 2:1360
  cell cultures 2:1354
  classification 2:1352
  cytopathic effects 2:1354, 2:1360
  DNA replication 2:1353, 2:1354, 2:1359
    enhancer 2:1359
    initiation 2:1359
    LT role 2:1356–7, 2:1359
    origin 2:1352, 2:1356, 2:1359
  genetics 2:1355

Polyomaviruses, murine (continued)
  genome 2:1352–3, 2:1356
    additional ORFs 2:1353
    early region 2:1353, 2:1356
    late region 2:1353, 2:1356
    organization 2:1357(Fig)
    regulatory region 2:1352–3
  history 2:1352
  in vitro mutagenesis 2:1355
  large T (LT) 2:1352, 2:1353, 2:1355, 2:1356, 2:1356–7
    complex with Rb 2:1357
    mutations 2:1357
    phosphorylation 2:1360
  middle T (MT) 2:1353, 2:1355, 2:1356, 2:1357–8
    binding 2:1357–8, 2:1358(Table)
    binding to pp60$^{c\text{-}src}$ 2:1357–8
    mutations 2:1358
    phosphorylation 2:1360
  molecular biology 2:1356–60
  mRNA 2:1359
    early region 2:1353
  mutants 2:1355, 2:1357, 2:1358
    host-range phenotype 2:1355
    ts-a 2:1355
  permissive/nonpermissive cells 2:1354
  physical properties 2:1358
  post-translational processing 2:1360
  productive infection 2:1354, 2:1359
  proteins 2:1352–3, 2:1356–8
    PTB domain 2:1358
    roles 2:1353, 2:1356–8
    tiny T (TT) 2:1353
    VP1, VP2 and VP3 2:1353, 2:1356, 2:1358, 2:1360
    VP1 acylation 2:1360
    VP1 structure 2:1360
    see also specific T proteins (above/below)
  receptor 2:1354
  relations to polyomavirus group 2:1356
  release 2:1360
  small T (ST) 2:1353, 2:1355, 2:1356
    function 2:1358
  structure and properties 2:1352, 2:1356
  transcription
    antisense transcripts 2:1359
    characterization 2:1359
    early 2:1352–3, 2:1354, 2:1359
    late 2:1359
  transformation 2:1354–5
    rate-limiting step 2:1355
  translation, characterization 2:1359–60
  tumor antigens 2:1355
Polyploidy, animal viruses 1:610–11
Polyproteins 3:1955
  synthesis 3:1473
Polyribonucleotides, inducers of interferons 2:861
Polythetic classes 3:1734
Pomovirus 1:155, 1:588, 3:1361
  genetics and replication 1:593
  genome structure/expression 1:589(Table), 1:591–2
  see also Furoviruses; Potato mop-top virus (PMTV)
Pomoviruses 3:1361–3
  control 3:1363
  cytopathology 3:1362
  ecology 3:1363

Pomoviruses (continued)
  genome 3:1361–2
    ORFs 3:1361
  geographic distribution 3:1362
  history 3:1361
  host range 3:1362
  physical properties 3:1361
  resistance to 3:1363
  RNA1 3:1361
  RNA2 3:1361
  RNA3 3:1361
  serological relationship 3:1362
  taxonomy and
    classification 3:1361
  transmission 3:1361, 3:1362–3
  see also Potato mop-top virus
    (PMTV)
Pongine herpesvirus 1 see
  Herpesvirus pan
Pongine herpesviruses 2:708
Poplar mosaic virus (POPMV),
  genome 1:239
Population biology,
  bacteriophage 2:1209
Population genetics, quasispecies
  connections 3:1435–6
Population movements, emergence
  and re-emergence of
  diseases 1:422
Population number,
  definition 3:1433(Table)
Population size
  critical 1:486
  effect on perpetuation of
    viruses 1:486
Porcine enteroviruses (PEVs) 1:461
  host range 1:464
  immune response to 1:467
  PEV-1, clinical features 1:466
  propagation 1:464
  serotypes 1:462, 1:464, 1:465
  see also Enteroviruses, animal;
    Teschen disease
Porcine epidemic abortion and
  respiratory syndrome
  (PEARS) 1:89
Porcine hemagglutinating
  encephalomyelitis virus
  (HEV) 1:294
  infection 1:297
Porcine parvovirus (PPV) 2:1152
  cell cultures and isolates 2:1172
  geographic distribution 2:1171
  history 2:1168
  infection 2:1153, 2:1173
    clinical features 2:1174
  pathogenicity 2:1173
  SMEDI syndrome due to 2:1168,
    2:1171
  structure 2:1168
  tissue tropism 2:1173
  transcription 2:1170(Fig)
  vaccine 2:1174
  see also Parvoviruses
Porcine respiratory coronavirus
  (PRCV) 1:294, 1:295
  epidemiology 1:296
Porcine respiratory and
  reproductive syndrome 1:89
  immune response 1:96
  pathogenicity and clinical
    features 1:95
Porcine respiratory and
  reproductive syndrome virus
  (PRRSV) 1:89–90, 1:420(Table)
  apoptosis promotion 1:75
  evolution 1:93
  genome 1:90(Fig), 1:91, 1:93
  geographic/seasonal
    distribution 1:92
  host range and propagation 1:93
  macrophage infection 1:92

Porcine respiratory and
  reproductive syndrome virus
  (PRRSV) (continued)
  receptor 1:92
  taxonomy and classification 1:90
  tissue tropism 1:94
  transmission 1:94
  vaccine 1:94, 1:96
  virulent and avirulent strains 1:94
Porin, yeast 3:1977, 3:1977(Table)
Pork, hog cholera virus
  transmission 2:740, 2:743
Porpoise morbillivirus
  (PMV) 1:420(Table), 2:953
Pospiviroidae 3:1930,
  3:1930(Table)
Post-transcriptional silencing,
  genes 2:1310
Post-translational processing
  African swine fever virus
    (AFSV) 1:34–5
  animal enteroviruses 1:463–4
  cardiovirus proteins 1:232–3
  Drosophila melanogaster gypsy
    virus 3:1528
  equine torovirus (ETV) 3:1800
  foot-and-mouth disease viruses
    (FMDVs) 1:571
  hantaviruses 1:625
  herpes simplex viruses
    (HSV) 2:695
  human CMV 1:356
  influenza viruses 2:834–5
  Newcastle disease virus 2:1023
  polyomaviruses 2:1360
  retroviruses, type D 3:1522
  rhinoviruses 1:1547
  sendai virus 3:1617–18
  simian virus 40 (SV40) 3:1653
  spumaviruses 3:1690
  Theiler's viruses 3:1774–5
  vaccinia virus 3:1867–8
  varicella-zoster virus 3:1882–3
  see also Proteolytic processing
Post-viral fatigue syndrome see
  Chronic fatigue syndrome
Postherpetic neuralgia 3:1876,
  3:1877
Postinfectious
  encephalomyelitis 2:1018
Postperfusion syndrome 1:349
Postsegregational host killing
  (plasmid addiction) 1:455,
  1:459
Potato black ringspot
  virus 2:1008(Table)
Potato leafroll virus (PLRV) 2:901
  economic significance 2:907,
    2:907–8
  geographic distribution 2:902
  homology-dependent
    resistance 2:1310
  movement protein-mediated
    resistance 2:1310
  structure and composition 2:903
  transcription 2:904
  in viroid transmission 3:1932
  see also Poleroviruses
Potato mop-top virus
  (PMTV) 1:155, 1:588, 3:1361
  control 1:595
  ecology and control 3:1363
  genetics and replication 1:593
  genome 3:1361
    structure/expression 1:591
  host range and
    distribution 3:1362
  infection features 1:594
  physical properties 3:1361
  serologic relationships 3:1362
  structure 3:1362(Fig)

Potato mop-top virus (PMTV)
  (continued)
  symptoms of infection 3:1363,
    3:1363(Fig)
  transmission 1:595, 3:1363
  see also Pomoviruses
Potato potexvirus X (PVX) see
  Potato virus X (PVX)
Potato potyvirus Y (PVY) see
  Potato virus Y (PVY)
Potato spindle tuber
  disease 3:1928–9
Potato spindle tuber viroid
  (PSTVd) 3:1929, 3:1930(Table)
  control 3:1933
  cytopathic effects 3:1932
  epidemiology 3:1932
  genome structure 3:1929,
    3:1931(Fig)
  geographic distribution 3:1932
  host range and
    transmission 3:1930, 3:1932,
    3:1936
  pathogenicity 3:1936
  replication 3:1935, 3:1936(Fig)
Potato sunken vein virus
  (SPSVV) 1:270
Potato U virus 2:1008(Table)
Potato virus M (PVM)
  disease 1:242
  economic significance 2:1321
  genome 1:239
  translation 1:240
Potato virus S (PVS) 1:238
  resistance in transgenic
    plants 1:242
  testing 1:242
  translation 1:240
Potato virus T (PVT) 1:222,
  3:1838(Table)
  classification 3:1837, 3:1842
  coat protein 3:1838
  disease 3:1841
  genome 3:1839, 3:1839(Fig)
  geographic distribution 3:1838
  host range 3:1838
  host relations 3:1840
  particle structure 3:1838
  transmission 3:1840
Potato virus X (PVX) 3:1364
  accumulation 3:1695
  co-infections 3:1695
  coat protein and hypersensitive
    response 2:1187
  coat protein-mediated
    resistance 2:1309
  economic significance 2:1321
  genome 3:1366, 3:1366(Fig)
  homology-dependent
    resistance 2:1310
  mixed infections 3:1368
  potato virus Y interaction see
    Potato virus Y (PVY)
  replication 3:1367, 3:1695
  resistance 3:1368
    breaking strains 3:1368
  Rx resistance 2:1185,
    2:1186(Table)
  TBSV-Ch gene expression 3:1796
  see also Potexviruses
Potato virus Y (PVY) 3:1369
  coat protein, severity of disease
    and 2:1188, 2:1189
  homology-dependent
    resistance 2:1310
  PVX interaction 3:1368, 3:1694–8
    induction 3:1695
    mediated by P1/Hc-Pro
      sequence 3:1695–6
    as model of synergism 3:1694–5
    symptoms 3:1695, 3:1698
  transgenic plant resistance 2:1312

Potato virus Y (PVY) (continued)
  transmission reduction 2:1303
Potato yellow dwarf virus
  (PYDV) 3:1531
  control 3:1540
  defective interfering
    particles 3:1536
  morphology and
    composition 3:1534
  transmission 3:1538
Potato yellow mosaic virus
  (PYMV) 1:600
Potatoes
  control and costs of
    viruses 2:1324
  luteovirus resistant crops 2:907
  seed, potato virus S testing 1:242
  value of crops and virus
    infections 2:1321
Potexvirus X (PVX) see Potato
  virus X (PVX)
Potexviruses 3:1364–8
  assembly 3:1364–5
    elongation 3:1365
    initiation 3:1364–5
  characteristics 3:1364
  coat protein 3:1364, 3:1365
  defective-interfering-like
    RNA 3:1366
  gene silencing 3:1368
  genome 3:1365–6
    5' cap structure 3:1367
    carlavirus similarity 1:239
    ORFs 3:1365–6
    organization 3:1366(Fig)
    sequences 3:1365(Table)
    triple gene block 3:1366, 3:1367
  host range 3:1365(Table)
  host resistance 3:1368
  infection
    inclusion bodies 3:1367–8
    pathology 3:1367–8
    symptoms 3:1367
  members 3:1364
  mixed infections 3:1368
  pathogen-derived engineered
    resistance 2:1308(Table)
  replication 3:1366–7
    RNA intermediate 3:1366–7
  reporter gene fusion 3:1367
  RNA-dependent RNA
    polymerase 3:1367
  structure and properties 3:1364–5
  subgenomic RNA
    (sgRNA) 3:1366, 3:1366–7
  translation 3:1367
  transmission 3:1364
  as vectors 3:1367
Pothos latent virus (PoLV) 3:1790,
  3:1790(Table)
  genome 3:1791(Fig)
  host range 3:1792
  proteins 3:1791(Table)
Potyviridae
  characteristics 3:1369
  classification and taxonomic
    standards 3:1369
  corn lethal necrosis (CLN) 2:935
  diagnostic criteria 3:1942,
    3:1942(Table)
  evolution 3:1374
  genera 3:1369
  members 3:1370(Table)
  Potyvirus 3:1369
  serologic relationships 3:1370
Potyvirus 3:1369
  members 3:1369
Potyviruses 3:1369–75
  aphid-transmitted,
    numbers 3:1374
  biotechnological uses 3:1375
  characteristics 3:1369

Potyviruses (continued)
    coat protein (CP) 3:1369–70, 3:1371(Fig), 3:1372–3
        DAG motif 3:1374, 3:1901
        N-terminus 3:1903
        role in transmission 3:1374
    cytopathology 3:1370(Fig)
    economic significance 3:1369
    epidemiology 3:1369
    evolution 3:1374
    future perspectives 3:1375
    gene expression strategy 3:1373
    genome 3:1370–2
        map 3:1371(Fig)
        noncoding region (NCR) 3:1371–2
        ORF 3:1370
        synergism mediation 3:1696
    geographic distribution 3:1369
    HC-Pro 3:1696
        functional domains 3:1696, 3:1697
    helper component (HC) 3:1372
        pathogenicity enhancer 3:1374
        role in transmission 3:1374
    helper viruses 3:1901
        KITC box and PTK box 3:1901
    history 3:1369
    host range and propagation 3:1369
    infection
        process and events 3:1373(Fig)
        symptoms 3:1374
    maize chlorotic mottle virus (MCMV) co-infection 2:937–8
    P1 protease 3:1372, 3:1696
        functional domains 3:1697
    P1/Hc-Pro sequence 3.1696(Fig), 3.1697
    P1/Hc-Pro sequence
        functional domains 3:1697
    PVY/PVX 3:1695–6
        synergism mediated by 3:1696–7
    packaging 3:1373
    pathogen-derived engineered resistance 2:1308(Table)
    pathogenicity 3:1374–5
    plant rhabdovirus interactions 3:1539
    polyprotein 3:1372
    prevention and control 3:1375
    proteinases 3:1371
    proteins 3:1372–3
        6K$_2$ 3:1372
        C1 3:1372
        NIa 3:1372
        NIb 3:1372
        P3 3:1372
        proteolytic cleavage 3:1371
    replication 3:1373–4, 3:1695
        sites 3:1373
    resistance to 3:1375
    RNA-dependent RNA polymerase 3:1372
    serologic relationships 3:1370
    structure and properties 3:1369–70, 3:1371(Fig)
    synergisms 3:1694
        examples 3:1697(Fig), 3:1698
        possible mechanisms 3:1698
        see also Potato virus Y (PVY)
    taxonomy and classification 3:1369
    transgenic plants 3:1375
    transmission 3:1369, 3:1374, 3:1901–3
    VPg 3:1372
        pathogenicity determinant 3:1374

Poultry
    fowlpox virus infection 1:576, 1:578
        transmission 1:578–9
        vaccination 1:581
        see also Fowlpox
    Newcastle disease 2:1023, 2:1023–4
    see also Chicken(s); Duck(s)
Powassan (POW) virus 3:1991
    transmission 1:435
Poxviridae 3:1865
    apoptosis inhibition 1:73–4
    Avipoxvirus 1:576
    Chordopoxvirinae 1:475, 2:960, 3:1376, 3:1383, 3:1668
    Chordopoxvirinae subfamily 1:298
    classification 1:475
    cowpox virus 1:298–304
    Entomopoxvirinae 1:475
    Molluscipoxvirus 2:960
    molluscum contagiosum virus 2:960–5
    Orthopoxvirus 2:973
    Parapoxvirus 2:1140
    yatapoxviruses 3:1971
    see also genera listed above and viruses; Poxviruses
Poxviruses 3:1887
    antiantiviral mechanisms 2:860
    apoptosis inhibition 1:74
    capripoxviruses see Capripoxviruses
    DNA 2:962
    genome 3:1887
    leporipoxviruses see Leporipoxviruses
    promoters 3:1887
    rabbits see Leporipoxviruses
    recombinants 3:1887
    replication 3:1478
    sheep and goats see Capripoxviruses
    structure and properties 3:1887
    swine (suipoxvirus) see Suipoxvirus
    as vectors 3:1887–8
        construction and selection 3:1887
    vertebrate 1:474
        entomopoxviruses (EPVs) similarity 1:474–5
    genome 1:474
    'viral factories' 1:478
pp60^{c-src}, polyomavirus T protein binding 2:1357–8
pRb see Retinoblastoma protein (pRb)
PRD1 phage see Bacteriophage PRD1
Predator–prey relationships 2:1253
Pregnancy
    azidothymidine (AZT) in 1:58
    coxsackievirus infection 1:309
    fulminant hepatitis E 1:674, 1:676
    HSV infections 2:683
    rubella vaccine contraindicated 1:1600
    zidovudine 2:787
Prelysosomes 1:250
Prenylation, hepatitis delta virus 1:666
Presbytis obscurus (PO-1-Lu) 3:1518, 3:1519(Table), 3:1523
Prevalence rates 1:482
Primary human fetal glial (PHFG) cells, JC virus culture 2:878
Primates, non-human
    dengue virus infection 1:377
    Ebola virus 3:1993

Primates, non-human (continued)
    herpesviruses see Herpesviruses, baboon and chimpanzee
    Marburg virus 3:1993
    Simian hemorrhagic fever virus (SHFV) 1:93
    simian retroviruses 3:1523(Table)
    yellow fever virus 3:1979, 3:1984, 3:1989
    see also Chimpanzees; Monkey(s)
Prion diseases 3:1389(Table), 3:1390–2
    animal 3:1388, 3:1389(Table), 3:1396–7
    classification 3:1388, 3:1398
    human 3:1388, 3:1389(Table)
        clinical features 3:1390
        infectious 3:1392
        see also Creutzfeldt–Jakob disease (CJD); Gerstmann–Sträussler–Scheinker disease; Kuru
    incubation times 3:1393(Table)
        rates of PrP^{Sc} clearance and 3:1394–5
    inherited 3:1392
        PrP gene mutations 3:1389
    neuropathology 3:1391(Fig)
    regional distribution of PrP^{Sc} 3:1395(Fig)
    see also Kuru
Prion proteins (PrP) 3:1388, 3:1402
    aberrant metabolism in disease 3:1389
    amino acid sequence 3:1389, 3:1393
    amyloid plaques 3:1390
    bovine 3:1396
        origin 3:1396–7
        PrP^{Sc} selection 3:1397
        transmission to humans 3:1397
    gene (PRNP) 3:1389, 3:1399
        sequence 3:1389
    gene (PRNP) mutations 3:1389, 3:1392, 3:1392(Fig), 3:1398, 3:1399
        P102L 3:1392
        transgenic mice 3:1392, 3:1395–6
    gene (PRNP) polymorphisms 3:1392(Fig)
        sheep/cattle 3:1392(Fig), 3:1396
    implications 3:1398
    isoforms 3:1389–90
        Western immunoblot 3:1390(Fig)
    modified see PrP^{Sc} (below)
    neuronal targeting 3:1395–6
    normal cellular (PrP^C) 3:1389, 3:1389–90
        conversion to PrP^{Sc} 3:1389
        structure 3:1389
    proteinase K digestion 3:1393
    sensitivity 3:1395
    PrP* 3:1394
    PrPres 3:1400, 3:1401
    PrP^{Sc} 3:1389, 3:1389–90
        accumulation in disease 3:1390
        clearance rates 3:1394–5
        conformation-dependent immunoassay 3:1394
        distribution in prion disease 3:1395(Fig)
        evidence for different conformations 3:1394–5
        formation and Asn-linked glycosylation 3:1395
        immunoassays 3:1397
        neuronal targeting 3:1395
        in new variant CJD 3:1397

Prion proteins (PrP) (continued)
    PrP^{Sc} (continued)
        number of conformations 3:1394
        protease-resistant fragment 3:1393
        protease-sensitive fraction 3:1394
        strain-specific information 3:1393
        as template for PrP^C conversion 3:1389, 3:1393
        tertiary structure 3:1393, 3:1394
    in sporadic CJD 3:1390–2
    summary of information 3:1397–8
Prions 2:1018, 2:1020, 3:1388–98, 3:1744(Table)
    comparisons 3:1407(Table)
    concept 3:1389
    de novo generation by PrP mutations 3:1392
    definitions 3:1388, 3:1389, 3:1402
    discovery 2:722
    diversity 3:1394
    DY strain 3:1393
    genetic properties 3:1403(Fig)
    history 3:1402
    monitoring BSE cattle 3:1397
    origin of concept 3:1402
    propagation and chaperone role 3:1407
    reversible curability 3:1402, 3:1404, 3:1406
    strains 3:1392–6
        Asn-linked carbohydrates 3:1395
        conformation-dependent immunoassays 3:1394, 3:1394(Fig)
        different conformations of PrP^{Sc} 3:1394–5
        in human prion diseases 3:1393(Table)
        interplay with species 3:1393–4
        neuronal targeting 3:1395–6
        PrP^{Sc} conformations and 3:1395
        typing 3:1393
    yeast and fungi 3:1402–7
        comparisons 3:1407, 3:1407(Table)
        expected properties 3:1402
        [HET-S] see [HET-S]
        [PSI] see [PSI]
        [URE3] see [URE3]
Pro-opiomelanocortin processing 3:1978, 3:1978(Fig)
Productive infections 3:1957
Programmed cell death (PCD) see Apoptosis
Progressive multifocal leukoencephalopathy (PML) 2:876, 2:1019
    at-risk groups 2:881
    clinical features 2:881–2
    development 2:881
    HIV infection with 2:882
    immune response 2:882
    JC virus DNA from 2:878–9
    long-term survivors 2:882
    pathogenesis 2:881
    pathology/histopathology 2:882
    prevention and control 2:882–3
    prognosis 2:882
    reactivation 2:881, 2:882
    therapy 2:882
    see also JC virus
Progressive rubella panencephalitis (PRP) 3:1598
Prohormone processing, mammalian 3:1978, 3:1978(Fig)

Proliferating nuclear antigen
    (PCNA) 1:27
Promoters
    Hz-1V 2:1033
    methylation 2:762
    TATAAT sequence 1:126
    tissue-specific 2:1182
    transgenes 2:1307
    tropism affected by 2:1182
    see also individual viruses
Promyelocytic leukemia (PML)
    protein, adenovirus Ad12-
    infected cells 1:10
Propagation of viruses 3:1408–13
    animal viruses 3:1408–13
        blocking infection 3:1410
        in cell culture see Cell culture
        concentration of viruses 3:1412
        cytopathic effects 3:1409
        host range 3:1409–10
        multiplication cycle 3:1408–9
        permissiveness and
            susceptibility 3:1409–10
        purification 3:1412
        titration 3:1412–13
        in whole organisms 3:1410
    applications/uses 3:1408
    in bacteria see Bacteriophage
    plant viruses see Plant viruses
    see also Multiplication cycle of
        viruses
Prophage 2:925–33, 2:1209, 3:1415
    bacterial survival and 2:1209
    defective 1:134–5
        benefits to host 1:135
    induction 3:1415
    loss 3:1415
    origin of term 2:721
    transposon insertion 2:1237
    see also Coliphage lambda;
        Lysogeny
Prophage PBSX 1:134
Prospect Hill virus,
    infection 2:1083(Table), 2:1084
Prospective studies 1:483
Protease inhibitors 1:57, 1:60,
    2:783–5
    activity and
        pharmacokinetics 2:785
    design 3:1946
    HIV infection 2:772
    HIV resistance 2:785, 2:785(Fig)
    in HAART 1:58
    licensed drugs 2:783
    mechanisms of action 2:783–5
    metabolism 2:785
    new agents 1:60–1
    recommendations 2:787
    resistance 1:60
    side effects 1:60
    structures 2:784(Fig)
Protease-resistant protein see Prion
    proteins (PrP)
Proteasomes 2:841
Protein(s)
    encoded by same nucleotide
        sequence 3:1473
    'free' in cytosol 1:253
    infectious see Prion proteins
        (PrP); Prions
    membrane see Membranes, viral
    modification in endoplasmic
        reticulum 1:251
    nuclear–cytoplasmic
        exchange 1:256
    plant resistance to
        viruses 2:1309–10
    synthesis
        endoplasmic reticulum 1:251
        host see Host
        viral 3:1473

Protein(s) (continued)
    viral
        atomic structure 3:1944–5
        nucleic acid interaction 3:1945
    virus-specific, synthesis 1:253
Protein kinase
    dsRNA-dependent see Protein
        kinase RNA (PKR)
    induced by interferons 3:1961
    Tupaia herpesvirus 3:1835
Protein kinase RNA (PKR) 2:856,
    2:858
    phosphorylation
        inactivation 2:860
    as target for antiantiviral
        mechanisms 2:860
Protein tyrosine kinases
    abl oncogene 3:1511–12
    erbB 3:1512
    eyk (ryk) 3:1512
    fes/fps oncogene 3:1512–13
    Fgr 3:1513
    fms 3:1513
    kit 3:1513–14
    oncogenes 3:1511–15
    ros 3:1514
    sea 3:1514–15
    src oncogene 3:1514
    yes 3:1515
Protein–protein crosslinking 1:452
Proteinase K, prion digestion see
    Prion proteins (PrP)
Proteinuria
    Argentine hemorrhagic fever
        (AHF) 2:894
    Bolivian hemorrhagic fever
        (BHF) 2:894
    Lassa fever 2:893
Proteoglycans 1:249
Proteolipid protein (PLP), in
    autoimmunity model 1:111–12
Proteolytic enzymes, in
    gastrointestinal tract 2:1177
Proteolytic processing
    African swine fever virus
        (AFSV) 1:34
    human CMV 1:356
    polioviruses 2:1331, 2:1337–41
    see also Post-translational
        processing
Proto-oncogenes 3:1818, 3:1821
    activation by murine leukemia
        viruses 2:998, 2:998(Fig),
        2:998(Table)
    see also Oncogenes
Protomers 1:230, 3:1945
Proton motive force (PMF) 3:1701
Protozoa
    dsRNA viruses infecting 3:1808
    pomovirus vectors 3:1362
    virus families/genera
        infecting 3:1754(Fig)
    viruses from 1:613
'Provoking effects,'
    poliomyelitis 2:1182
PrP see Prion proteins (PrP)
Prune dwarf virus (PDV) 1:39
    genome 1:39
    host range and distribution 1:40
    replication 1:42
    virus–host relationships 1:42
Prunus necrotic ringspot virus
    (PNRSV) 1:38
    host range and distribution 1:40
    replication 1:42
    virus–host relationships 1:42
Pseudaletia separata
    entomopoxvirus (PsEPV) 1:477
Pseudocholera infantum 1:442
Pseudocowpox virus 2:1140
    epidemiology 2:1144
    history 2:1140

Pseudocowpox virus (continued)
    host range 2:1144
    transmission 2:1144
    see also Parapoxviruses
Pseudoknot ribozyme 3:1552,
    3:1558
Pseudoknot structure
    echovirus genome 1:412
    mouse hepatitis virus (MHV)
        polymerase gene 1:295
Pseudolumpy skin disease 1:181,
    1:183
Pseudolysogeny 1:133
    algal viruses 1:50
Pseudomonas
    filamentous phage 1:547
    phage D3112 see Bacteriophage
        D3112
    transposable phage 2:981, 2:986–
        7
Pseudomonas aeruginosa
    exotoxin A 2:1229
    ssRNA phage 3:1664
Pseudomonas pseudoalcaligenes,
    bacteriophage φ6 2:1206
Pseudoplusia includens, cricket
    paralysis virus (CrPV)
    isolate 2:1271
Pseudorabies 3:1421
    see also Pseudorabies virus
        (PRV), infection
Pseudorabies virus (PRV) 3:1421–9
    antibodies 3:1427
    characteristics 3:1421–3
    deletion mutants 3:1423, 3:1428
    DNA replication phases 3:1424
    economic significance 3:1424
    epidemiology 3:1424–5
    future perspectives 3:1428
    genes 3:1422(Table), 3:1423–4
        early 3:1423, 3:1424
        immediate early (IE) 3:1423
        late 3:1423
        latency-associated transcripts
            (LAT) 3:1423–4
    genome 3:1421, 3:1423–4
        inversion of U_L 3:1423
        IRS/TRS and US
            segments 3:1423(Table)
        UL segment 3:1422(Table)
    geographic distribution 3:1424
    glycoproteins 3:1426–7
        gB 3:1426
        gC 3:1426–7
        gK 3:1427
        immune response 3:1427
    history 3:1421
    host range 3:1424
    infection
        clinical features 3:1425–6
        diagnosis 3:1428
        epidemiology and
            outbreaks 3:1424
        iatrogenic 3:1425
        immune response 3:1426–7
        increase and spread 3:1424–5
        pathology/
            histopathology 3:1426
        prevention and control 3:1427–
            8
    latent infections 3:1425, 3:1426
    molecular biology 3:1423–4
    pathogenesis 3:1425
    physical properties 3:1425
    replication 3:1426
        sites 3:1425
    shedding 3:1426
    taxonomy and
        classification 3:1421–3
    transmission 3:1425
    vaccination 3:1427–8

Pseudorabies virus (PRV)
    (continued)
    vaccines
        Bucharest strain 3:1428
        gene-deleted marker 3:1428
        modified-live virus
            (MLV) 3:1427
        OMNIMARK 3:1428
        TK-deleted recombinant 3:1428
    variants 3:1424
    VSV interference 2:850
Pseudorecombination,
    dianthoviruses 1:407
Pseudotemperate phage 1:133
    host–phage relationship 1:133
[PSI] 3:1404–5, 3:1405(Fig)
    in vitro propagation 3:1405
    as infectious form of
        Sup35p 3:1404–5
    as prion, evidence 3:1405
    prion domains 3:1405
    propagation and loss by
        Hsp104 3:1405
    reverse curability 3:1404
ψM phage see Bacteriophage ψM1
PTK box, potyvirus helper
    factors 3:1901
PU.1, as oncoprotein 1:498
Public health, seroepidemiologic
    studies 1:483
Pulmonary disease, in visna-maedi
    virus infections 3:1962
Pulmonary edema
    Argentine hemorrhagic fever
        (AHF) 2:894
    Bolivian hemorrhagic fever
        (BHF) 2:894
    Hantavirus pulmonary syndrome
        (HPS) 1:628
    Lassa fever 2:892
Pulmonary syndrome,
    hantavirus 3:1988
Purification of viruses 3:1412
    plant viruses 3:1420
    see also Diagnostic techniques
Puumala virus (PUUV) 1:210,
    1:621, 2:1083(Table), 3:1988
    geographic/seasonal
        distribution 1:626
    see also Hantaviruses
Pyrogenic toxins 2:1230–2
    Staphylococcus aureus 2:1230,
        2:1231
        production 2:1231
        types 2:1231
    Streptococcus pyogenes 2:1230
        formation 2:1231
        SpeA converting phage 2:1231
    as superantigens 2:1231–2

Q

Qβ phage see Bacteriophage Qβ
Q-β replicase, amplification
    method 1:392, 1:394
qin oncogene 3:1510–11
Quail pea mosaic virus
    (QPMV) 1:285, 1:290
Quailpox virus 1:578
    vaccine 1:581
Quantitative taxonomy 3:1750
Quarantine, vesicular stomatitis
    virus (VSV) infections 3:1919
Quasi-equivalent theory 3:1948–51,
    3:1951(Fig)
    rules 3:1948

Quasispecies 1:660, 3:1431–6, 3:1449, 3:1915, 3:1941
　aims of theory 3:1432
　chemical definition 3:1431
　complexity concepts
　　connections 3:1435–6
　definition 3:1431
　definition of terms
　　related 3:1433(Table)
　disease prevention/control
　　strategies 3:1436
　environmental
　　perturbations 3:1434
　　adaptability 3:1434
　　compartmentalization of
　　　replication 3:1434
　　competition 3:1434
　equations 3:1432(Table)
　generalized concept 3:1433
　HIV 2:770
　implications 3:1434–5,
　　3:1435(Table)
　　practical 3:1436(Table)
　occupation of sequence
　　space 3:1434
　origin of concept 3:1431–2
　physical definition 3:1431
　polioviruses 2:1346
　population genetic
　　connections 3:1435–6
　real virus 3:1432–4
　representation and outcome of
　　evolution 3:1433(Fig)
　selection equilibria and 3:1431
Queensland fruit fly virus
　(QFFV) 2:1273

R

RA1 parvovirus 2:1154–5
Rabbit
　myxomatosis 3:1384
　papillomas 2:1105
Rabbit coronavirus (RbCV) 1:294,
　1:297
Rabbit hemorrhagic disease 1:217
　clinical features 1:220
　pathogenesis 1:219
　prevention and control 1:220
Rabbit hemorrhagic disease virus
　(RHDV) 1:218, 1:420(Table)
　antigenic variation 1:219
　in Australia 1:217–18, 1:221
　as biocontrol agent 1:217, 1:221
　culture 1:221
　genome 1:218, 2:1038
　　comparison with
　　　picornaviruses 2:1037(Fig)
　　sequence 1:221
　geographic distribution 1:219
　smooth variant 1:221
　transmission 1:219
　vaccines 1:220, 1:221
Rabbit oral papilloma virus
　(ROPV), infection 2:1127
Rabbit papillomavirus 2:1105
　discovery 2:722
Rabbitpox 3:1870
　clinical features 2:979(Fig), 2:980
　history 2:978
　immune response 2:980
　pathology/
　　histopathology 2:979(Fig),
　　2:980
　'pockless' 2:980
　prevention and control 2:980

Rabbitpox virus (RPV) 2:973–80,
　2:978–80, 3:1869, 3:1871
　apoptosis inhibition 1:74
　classification 2:978
　epidemiology 2:978–9
　genetics 2:980
　history 2:978
　as laboratory artifact 2:980
　as model of smallpox 2:980
　pathogenesis 2:980
　Utrecht strain 2:978, 2:980
Rabies
　canine 3:1437, 3:1438, 3:1440
　　epidemiology 3:1439
　clinical features 2:1018, 3:1440
　diagnosis 3:1988
　dumb (passive) 2:1018
　epidemiology 3:1439
　'furious' 3:1440
　history 3:1437
　immune response 3:1441
　incubation period 3:1439
　mortality 3:1440
　'paralytic' 3:1440
　pathogenesis 3:1440
　pathology/histopathology 3:1440
　postexposure treatment 3:1988
　prevention and control 3:1441,
　　3:1995
　vaccination
　　programs 3:1441
　　rates 3:1439
　vaccines 3:1441, 3:1988
　　history 3:1861
　　reservoir animal hosts 3:1995
　in wild canid
　　species 1:420(Table)
Rabies virus 3:1437–41, 3:1987–8
　antibodies to 3:1441
　apoptosis promotion 1:76
　attenuated 3:1441
　emerging/re-emerging
　　virus 1:419(Table)
　epidemiology 3:1439
　evolution 3:1438–9, 3:1444
　future perspectives 3:1441
　G glycoprotein, in
　　canarypoxvirus vector 3:1888
　G–L intergene 3:1438
　gene expression,
　　regulation 3:1438
　genetics 3:1438
　geographic/seasonal
　　distribution 3:1438, 3:1440
　ψ pseudogene 3:1438–9
　history 3:1437–8
　　outbreaks 3:1437
　host range 3:1439, 3:1440–1
　infection see Rabies
　isolates 3:1439
　isolation 1:399
　ocular target 1:525(Table)
　pathogenicity 3:1440
　PCR studies 3:1439
　propagation 3:1440–1
　proteins
　　L protein 3:1438
　　N protein 3:1438
　　PV strain 3:1438
　　receptors 1:250
　replication, conservation of
　　elements involved 3:1438
　SAD strain 3:1438
　serologic relationships and
　　variability 3:1439
　'street' isolates 3:1440
　taxonomy and
　　classification 3:1438
　tissue tropism 3:1439–40
　transcription, conservation of
　　elements 3:1438

Rabies virus (continued)
　transmission 1:485(Table),
　　3:1439, 3:1440, 3:1987
　　ecological change and 3:1996
Rabies-like viruses 3:1439, 3:1442–
　5, 3:1987
　characteristics 3:1442–3
　epidemiology 3:1444
　evolution 3:1444
　future perspectives 3:1445
　genetics 3:1443–4
　geographic/seasonal
　　distribution 3:1443
　history 3:1442
　host range 3:1443
　infection
　　clinical features 3:1445
　　immune response 3:1445
　　pathology/
　　　histopathology 3:1445
　　prevention and control 3:1445
　monoclonal antibodies 3:1444
　pathogenicity 3:1445
　propagation 3:1443
　serologic relationships and
　　variability 3:1444
　taxonomy and
　　classification 3:1442–3
　tissue tropism 3:1444–5
　transmission 3:1444–5
Raccoon parvovirus (RPV) 2:1159
　clinical features of
　　infection 2:1165
　host range 2:1160
　pathogenicity 2:1165
　phylogeny 2:1164(Fig)
　propagation 2:1161
Raccoonpox virus 1:304
Raccoons
　rabies transmission 3:1996
　rabies vaccination 3:1988, 3:1995
Radiculomyelitis, enterovirus 70
　(EV70) causing 1:472
Radioimmunoassays (RIA)
　antiviral antibody detection 1:391
　viral antigen detection 1:389
Radish mosaic virus
　(RaMV) 1:285, 1:290
raf oncogene 3:1516–17
Raft cultures (three-dimensional
　cell culture) 3:1412
Rainbow trout, viral hemorrhagic
　septicemia virus (VHSV)
　infection 3:1543
Rainfall, dengue virus
　transmission 1:377
Ramsay Hunt syndrome 3:1876
Rana pipiens
　kidney tumors 1:51
　Lucké tumors 1:52
　renal adenocarcinoma 1:582
Ranavirus 1:582
　see also Frog virus 3 (FV3)
Range paralysis 2:948
　see also Marek's disease
ras oncogene 3:1517
　HCV-associated hepatocellular
　　carcinoma 3:1847
　transformation, suppression by
　　adenovirus E1A 1:29
Ras proteins 1:517, 3:1820
　GTPase activity 3:1820
RAS signaling pathway, activation
　by HSV-2 RR1 PK 2:682,
　2:683(Fig)
Ras superfamily 3:1517
rasGAP complex, immortalization
　of cells 1:28
Rash
　coxsackievirus infection 1:308

Rash (continued)
　maculopapular
　　Chikungunya (CHIK)
　　　fever 1:264
　　measles 2:957
　　Ross River virus (RRV) 3:1574,
　　　3:1575
　　rubella 3:1597, 3:1598
　　smallpox 3:1671
　　VZV infections 3:1875, 3:1876
Raspberry, yellows disease 2:809
Raspberry bushy dwarf virus
　(RBDV) 2:809
　proteins, comparisons 2:810(Fig)
　taxonomy 2:809
　see also Idaeovirus
Raspberry ringspot virus
　(RpRSV) 2:1009(Table)
　RNA 2:1011
Raspberry veinal chlorosis
　virus 3:1540
Rat(s)
　Borna disease virus
　　infection 1:169, 1:170–1,
　　1:172
　hantavirus transmission 3:1988
　see also Rodents
Rat coronaviruses 1:297
Rat cytomegalovirus
　(RCMV) 1:357
　genome structure 1:359
　MIE enhancer 1:361
　see also Cytomegalovirus
　　(CMV)
Rat virus (RV)
　clinical features of
　　infection 2:1174
　history 2:1167
　host range 2:1172
RAV-0 1:116
Rb gene see Retinoblastoma gene
　(Rb)
RBC-CD4 1:61
RE viruses see
　Reticuloendotheliosis (RE)
　viruses
Re-emerging viral diseases 1:418–
　23
　childhood 1:423
　ecological and zoonotic factors
　　affecting 1:422
　influenza 1:421
　see also Emerging viral diseases
Reactivation of viruses
　animal CMVs as model 1:361
　cross-reactivation 1:609
　latent infections 2:1200
　multiplicity reactivation 1:609
Rec proteins 3:1446, 3:1447(Fig)
RecBCD enzymes
　phage lambda
　　recombination 2:1215
　in recombination, ssDNA
　　phage 2:1213
Receptor-mediated
　endocytosis 1:250, 2:1180,
　3:1472
　rotavirus infection
　　mechanism 3:1589
　SV40 3:1653
Receptors for viruses 1:250, 2:754,
　2:1180–1, 3:1408, 3:1471,
　3:1921, 3:1926–8
　atomic structure 3:1945
　binding sites on viruses 2:1181–2
　controversies over 2:1181
　functions 3:1818
　'restrictive' systems and 3:1472
　for specific viruses 1:250
　types 2:1180–1, 3:1471–2, 3:1926,
　　3:1926(Table)
　viruses sharing 2:1181

Receptors for viruses (continued)
see also individual viruses
Recombinant DNA technology
  animal viruses 1:612
  see also Genetic engineering
Recombinant viruses 1:3
Recombination of viruses 1:608,
  2:1213, 3:1446–54
  animal viruses 1:608
  bacteriophage see Genetic
    recombination,
    bacteriophage
  bromoviruses 1:202
  cauliflower mosaic virus
    (CaMV) 3:1894
  caulimoviruses 2:1277
  copy-choice 1:246
  coronaviruses 1:294, 1:295
  defective-interfering (DI) particle
    generation 1:371
  defective-interfering
    RNAs 3:1453–4
  carmoviruses 1:246
  definition 3:1446
  DNA viruses 3:1446–9
    analyses of mutants 3:1446–8
    bacteriophage 3:1446,
      3:1448(Fig)
    cauliflower mosaic virus
      (CaMV) 3:1449
    frequency 3:1448
    geminiviruses 3:1449
    with host genes 3:1446
    proteins encoded 3:1446
    in somatic cells 3:1449
    see also DNA, recombination
  emerging viral diseases
    associated 1:419
  Epstein–Barr virus (EBV) 3:1449
  foot-and-mouth disease viruses
    (FMDVs) 1:572
  frequency, frog virus 3
    (FV3) 1:586
  genetic mapping by see Genetic
    mapping
  high frequency 1:606
  homologous 2:1213, 3:1449
    adenoviruses 3:1886
    bromoviruses 1:202
  initiation, model 3:1447(Fig)
  integrase pathway 1:284
  intramolecular 1:606, 1:609
    unrelated viruses 1:609
  nodaviruses 3:1451
  plant virus vectors 3:1898
  polioviruses 2:1327, 2:1347
  recABCD genes 1:284
  redX and redB pathway 1:284
  rhinoviruses 3:1548
  RNA viruses 3:1449–53
    aberrant homologous
      recombination 3:1450
    brome mosaic virus 3:1450,
      3:1451(Fig)
    copy-choice template
      mechanism 3:1451
    coronaviruses 3:1451
    homologous 3:1450
    nonhomologous 3:1450
    phage Qβ 3:1451
    plant 3:1450
    positive-stranded 3:1449–50
    by reassortment 3:1450
    replicase role 3:1451,
      3:1453(Fig)
    retroviruses 3:1451–3
    sequence
      rearrangements 3:1450
    template switching
      model 3:1452(Fig)
  Semliki Forest virus (SFV) 3:1662
  Sindbis (SIN) virus 3:1662

Recombination of viruses
  (continued)
  site-specific, bacteriophage P1 as
    model system 1:455
  smallpox (variola) virus 3:1669
  transduced donor DNA 2:1238
  transgenic plants 3:1450
Recombinosome 1:1451,
  3:1452(Fig)
Recurrent respiratory
  papillomatosis (RRP) 1:67
Red cells see Erythrocytes
Red clover cryptic virus 2 1:314
Red clover mottle virus
  (RCMV) 1:285, 1:290
  economic importance 1:291
  genome structure 1:287
Red clover necrotic mosaic virus
  (RCNMV) 1:243, 1:403, 1:409
  amino acid sequence
    homologies 1:403
  capsid protein 1:406
    domains 1:404
    homology with other
      species 1:404(Table)
  coat protein, long-distance
    movement and 2:1186
  features of infection 1:406
  genetics 1:406–7
  genome structure 1:404(Fig),
    1:405
  RNA-1 and RNA-2 1:406
  geographic/seasonal
    distribution 1:403
  host range and propagation 1:406
  as model system 1:409
  movement proteins 1:406–7
    homology with other
      species 1:407(Table)
  pathogenicity 1:408
  pathology and
    histopathology 1:408
  prevention and control 1:408
  replicase, homology with other
    species 1:406(Table)
  replication 1:405–6
  strains and serologic
    relationship 1:407
  transmission and tissue
    tropism 1:407–8
  see also Dianthoviruses
Red clover vein mosaic virus
  (RCVMV) 1:239, 1:240
Red deer, herpesvirus disease 1:183
'Red disease' 3:1544
Red pathway, recombination see
  Coliphage lambda
Redspotted grouper nervous
  necrosis virus
  (RGNNV) 2:1026
Reed–Sternberg cells 1:491, 1:493
Reindeer, herpesvirus disease 1:183
rel oncogene 3:1510
Release of viruses 2:1178, 3:1409
  polarized 2:1178
  see also Budding (of viruses)
Renal failure
  acute, echoviruses causing 1:416
  adenovirus infection
    causing 1:1832
  hemorrhagic fever with renal
    syndrome (HFRS) 1:629
Renal transplantation
  BK virus and JC virus
    infections 2:1083, 3:1831
  CMV infection after 2:1082
  HBV infection 3:1830
Rendering, offal, BSE
  epidemic 3:1396, 3:1397
Reoviridae 3:1464
  apoptosis promotion 1:75
  biological control by 2:844

Reoviridae (continued)
  characteristics 2:1044–6, 3:1455
  Coltivirus 2:1044
  Cypovirus 1:332, 1:332–9
  fish viruses 1:564
  genera 2:1044, 3:1464
  genetic reassortment 2:1046
  Orbivirus 2:1044, 2:1062
  Orthoreovirus 3:1455, 3:1464
  Phytoreovirus 2:1262
  plant-associated reoviruses see
    Phytoreoviruses
  reverse genetics 2:1061
  Rotavirus 1:442–4, 3:1577
  see also individual genera/
    viruses
Reoviruses 3:1454–64
  antibodies 3:1462
  apoptosis promotion 1:75, 3:1461
  attachment and entry 3:1459–60,
    3:1468
  avian 3:1464
  binding to murine cell
    lines 3:1926(Table)
  capsid, degradation on
    infection 3:1468
  capsomers 3:1464, 3:1465(Fig)
  cell attachment protein
    (σ1) 3:1468
  characteristics 3:1454,
    3:1456(Table)
  core particles 3:1464, 3:1465(Fig)
  cytopathic effects 3:1456, 3:1470–
    1
  dsRNA-containing complexes
    (dsRCCs) 3:1468–9, 3:1470
  effect on infected cells 3:1470–1
  enzymes 3:1466, 3:1469
  epidemiology 3:1458–9
  evolution 3:1458
  experimental infections in
    mice 3:1458, 3:1461
  future perspectives 3:1463–4
  genetics 3:1456–8
  genome 3:1456, 3:1465
    acceptance signals 3:1470
    assortment of segments 3:1470
    RNA classes 3:1465
    segments 3:1456, 3:1457,
      3:1457(Fig), 3:1465,
      3:1466(Fig)
    sequences 3:1457
  geographic/seasonal
    distribution 3:1455–6
  history 3:1454–5
  host range and
    propagation 3:1456, 3:1464
  immunity
    cell-mediated 3:1462
    passive 3:1462
  inclusions ('viral
    factories') 3:1470
  infection
    clinical features 3:1460–1
    enteric 1:447
    immune response 3:1462–3
    pancreas 2:1079
    pathogenesis 3:1459
    pathology/
      histopathology 3:1461–2
    prevention and control 3:1463
  infectious RNA 3:1470
  infectious subviral particles
    (SIVPs) 2:1177
  intermediate subviral particles
    (ISVPs) 3:1459, 3:1463
  molecular biology 3:1464–71
  monoclonal antibodies 3:1462
  mRNAs 3:1468
    capping 3:1469–70
    transcription 3:1469–70

Reoviruses (continued)
  mutants 3:1457
  ts 3:1457
  oligonucleotides 3:1465–6
  phylogenetic trees 3:1455,
    3:1457(Fig)
  physical properties 3:1464
  plant-associated see
    Phytoreoviruses
  as possible human
    pathogen 3:1460–1,
    3:1461(Table)
  proteins 3:1466–7
    core shell components λ1 and
      σ2 3:1466
    genome segments
      encoding 3:1466(Table)
    involvement in neural
      spread 2:1180
    minor core components λ3 and
      μ2 3:1467
    μ1C 3:1467
    μNS 3:1468
    μNSC 3:1468
    nonstructural 3:1468
    outer capsid shell 3:1467
    σ1 3:1467–8, 3:1469
    σ1S 3:1468
    σ3 3:1467
    σNS 3:1468
    spike component λ2 3:1466–7
  reassortment of dsRNA 3:1458
  receptors 3:1460, 3:1469
  release 3:1470
  replication 3:1468–71,
    3:1468(Fig)
    strategy 3:1468–9
  RNA triphosphatase 3:1466
  in SCID mice 3:1458
  sensitivity to interferon γ 3:1463
  seroepidemiology 3:1458
  serologic relationship and
    variability 3:1458
  serotype 1 Lang (T1L) 3:1455
    spread 2:1180
  serotype 2 Jones (T2J) 3:1455
  serotype 3, infectious
    RNA 3:1470
  serotype 3 Abney (T3A) 3:1455
  serotype 3 Dearing (T3D) 3:1455,
    3:1463
  serotype 3 receptor 3:1926–7
    β-adrenergic receptors 1:250
    CNS 3:1928
    functional studies 3:1927–8
    lymphoid cells 3:1927–8
    monoclonals 3:1927,
      3:1927(Table)
  serotypes 3:1455, 3:1458, 3:1464
  serotyping 3:1455
  shedding 3:1460
  sigma 1 1:75
  small viral particles
    (SVPs) 3:1468, 3:1469
  spread 3:1460
  ssRNA-containing complexes
    (ssRCCs) 3:1470
  structure and properties 3:1464,
    3:1465(Fig)
  spikes 3:1464
  survival in environment 3:1459
  taxonomy and
    classification 3:1455
  tissue tropism 3:1460
    factors affecting 3:1460
  transcriptase (RNA
    polymerase) 3:1466, 3:1467
    activation 3:1469
  transcription 3:1469–70
    frequencies and lengths 3:1469
  translation 3:1469–70

Reoviruses (continued)
  transmission 3:1459–60
    efficiency 3:1459
    fecal–oral 3:1459
  vaccines 3:1463
  virulence 3:1459(Fig)
REP protein, human herpesvirus 6 encoding 1:359
Replacement vectors 2:1241, 2:1241–2
  screening 2:1242
Replicase
  dominant-negative mutations 2:1309
  'leaping' 1:371
  pathogen-derived resistance in plants 2:1309
  role in RNA recombination 3:1451, 3:1453(Fig)
  supergroup II type 1:408
Replication enhancer, geminiviruses 1:599
Replication of viruses 3:1471–8
  animal viruses 1:607
  assembly of viruses 3:1478
    see also Assembly of viruses
  blocked by interferons 2:859
  blocked in 'restrictive' systems 3:1472
  compartmentalization 3:1434
  DNA viruses see DNA viruses
  early events 3:1471–2
    attachment 3:1471–2
    penetration and uncoating 3:1472
  interference by heterologous viruses 2:850
  RNA viruses see RNA viruses
  synthesis of virus-specific macromolecules 3:1472–3
    cytoskeleton 3:1473
    gene regulation 3:1472–3
    genome replication 3:1472
    protein synthesis 3:1473
    transcription see Transcription
Replicative forms
  animal enteroviruses 1:463
  foot-and-mouth disease viruses (FMDVs) 1:570–1
Replicative intermediates
  animal enteroviruses 1:463
  bovine immunodeficiency virus (BIV) 1:185
  cardioviruses 1:234
  cucumoviruses 1:322
Reporter genes, enzyme-linked virus inducible system (ELVIS) 1:398
Repressor
  bacteriophage P1 1:457, 1:459
  bacteriophage P22 1:1605
  DNA, replication 1:459
  see also Coliphage lambda
Rescriptor (delavirdine) 1:60
Reservoir hosts
  control measures 3:1995
  immunization 3:1995
  rabies virus 3:1987
Resistance
  to disease, genetic regulation see Host genetic resistance
  genes see under Host genetic resistance
  by plants see Plant resistance to viruses
  response, plant viruses 2:1185–8
RespiGam 1:65
Respiratory cycle 1:484
Respiratory disease
  in children, adenoviruses causing 1:5

Respiratory disease (continued)
  enterovirus-associated 2:736
  see also Respiratory tract infections
Respiratory distress, Lassa fever 2:893
Respiratory enteric orphan virus see Reoviruses
Respiratory mucosa, virus replication 2:1176
Respiratory papillomatosis 2:1112
Respiratory syncytial virus (RSV) 1:64, 3:1479–87, 3:1488
  antibodies 3:1484, 3:1486
    neutralizing 3:1487
  antigenic subgroups 3:1484
  antigenic variation 3:1486
  antigenic/sequence relatedness 3:1484–5
  antigens 3:1484
  cDNA 3:1484
  cell culture 3:1485
  cytopathic effects 1:397(Fig), 3:1485
  cytotoxic T lymphocyte-induced resistance 3:1486
  epidemiology 3:1485–6
  epitopes 3:1484
  F glycoprotein, monoclonal antibodies 1:65
  gene order 3:1482, 3:1482(Fig)
  genetics 3:1483(Fig), 3:1484
  genome 3:1482–4
    comparisons 3:1483(Fig)
    intergenic regions 3:1483
    leader and trailer sequences 3:1482–3
  history 3:1479
  host range 3:1485
  immunization 3:1487
    intranasal infection 3:1487
  immunoglobulin (RSVIg) 1:65
  infection 3:1492
    animals 3:1485
    bronchiolitis 3:1491
    children 3:1485
    clinical features 3:1485–6
    diagnosis 3:1486
    diagnosis (immunofluorescence) 1:389
    epidemics 3:1485, 3:1489(Fig)
    immunity 3:1486
    immunoprophylaxis 3:1487
    incubation period 3:1486
    infants 3:1486
    mortality 3:1485–6
    pathogenesis 3:1486
    pneumonia 1:64, 1:65, 3:1493, 3:1832
    post-transplant 3:1831–2
    therapy 1:64–5, 3:1487
  isolates and strains 3:1484
  minireplicons 3:1483, 3:1484
  monoclonal antibodies 3:1487
  mRNAs 3:1483
  ocular target 1:525(Table)
  proteins 3:1479–82, 3:1481(Table)
    amino acid sequences 3:1484
    F protein 3:1479, 3:1484, 3:1485
    functions 3:1481(Table)
    G glycoprotein 3:1479–80, 3:1484, 3:1486
    L 3:1485
    locations 3:1480(Fig)
    M (matrix) 3:1481
    NS1 and NS2 3:1481–2
    nucleocapsid 3:1479
    SH 3:1480–1
    transmembrane 3:1479–81
    recombinant 3:1484
    lacking G protein gene 3:1480

Respiratory syncytial virus (RSV) (continued)
  reinfection 3:1486
  replication 3:1482–4
  seasonal distribution 3:1488
  shedding 3:1485
  structure and properties 3:1479–82
  taxonomy and classification 3:1479
  transcription 3:1482–4
    polarity 3:1483
  vaccine safety 3:1487
Respiratory tract
  host defense mechanisms 2:1176, 3:1490(Fig)
  immune system in 2:1176
  infection route 3:1488, 3:1490(Fig)
  virus entry 2:1176
Respiratory tract infections 3:1493(Table)
  animal parainfluenza viruses 2:1139
  animals 3:1494(Table)
  bronchiolitis 3:1493, 3:1493(Table)
  bronchitis 3:1492
  common cold see Common cold
  coxsackieviruses 1:309
  croup (laryngotracheobronchitis) 3:1492, 3:1493(Table)
  frequencies 3:1492(Fig)
  immune response 3:1491
  incubation period 3:1489
  laboratory diagnosis 3:1494
  lower tract, rhinoviruses 3:1549
  memory response 3:1491
  parainfluenza viruses (PIVs) 2:1133
  pathogenesis 3:1490–1
  pharyngitis 3:1492, 3:1493(Table)
  pneumonia 3:1493–4, 3:1493(Table)
  rhinitis 3:1492, 3:1493(Table)
  rhinoviruses 3:1549
  seasonal distribution 3:1488
  Sendai virus 3:1620
  superinfection (bacterial) 3:1491
  therapy 3:1494–5
  transmission 1:484, 3:1488, 3:1490–1
  types 3:1491–4
  upper tract 3:1492
    echoviruses 1:415
  vaccines 3:1494–5
  veterinary 3:1493–4
  see also specific infections/viruses
Respiratory viruses 3:1488–96, 3:1493(Table)
  animals 3:1494(Table)
  control 3:1491
  culture 3:1494
  detection/diagnosis 3:1494
  dissemination/spread 3:1488, 3:1489, 3:1490–1
  epidemiology 3:1488–90
  evolution 3:1489
  families 3:1488
  frequency of infections 3:1492(Fig)
  immunity 3:1490–1
  multiplication cycle 3:1490
  neutralizing antibodies 3:1491
  pathogenicity 3:1490–1
  post-transplant infections 3:1831–2
  superinfection after 3:1491
  transmission 3:1488
  vaccines
    live 'cold adapted' 3:1495

Respiratory viruses (continued)
  vaccines (continued)
    mucosal adjuvants 3:1495
    recombinant 3:1495
    see also Influenza viruses; Respiratory syncytial virus (RSV)
Respirovirus 2:1130, 2:1134, 2:1135(Fig), 3:1616
Reston viruses
  evolution 2:942
  see also Ebola-Reston virus
Restriction endonucleases 1:611
  algal viruses 1:49, 1:49(Table)
  applications 2:758
  coliphage N4 resistance 1:454
  history 2:720, 2:729
  inactivation by T5-like phage 3:1719
  maps, granuloviruses 1:141
Restriction-modification systems see Host-controlled modification and restriction
Restrictive infections 3:1410
'Restrictive' systems 3:1472
Reticuloendothelial system 2:1015
Reticuloendotheliosis associated virus (REV-A) 3:1496, 3:1499
  retroviral vectors 3:1502–3
Reticuloendotheliosis (RE) viruses 3:1496–503
  attachment and entry 3:1497
  cytopathic effect 3:1499
  detection 3:1499
  env gene 3:1497, 3:1499
  evolution 3:1496, 3:1497(Fig)
  gag gene 3:1497, 3:1499
  genome 3:1496–7, 3:1498(Fig)
  glycoproteins 3:1497
  host range 3:1497
  immune tolerance 3:1497
  immunosuppressive peptide (ISP) 3:1499
  infection
    diagnosis 3:1498–9
    epidemics 3:1498
    immune response 3:1497–8
    prevention and control 3:1498–9
  integration, c-myc activation 3:1500
  mammalian retrovirus relationship 3:1496
  members 3:1496
  packaging 3:1502
  pathogenesis 3:1499–500
    chronic neoplasia 3:1499–500
    herpesvirus interaction 3:1500
    nonneoplastic disease 3:1499
  pol gene 3:1497
  proteins 3:1496–7
  receptors 3:1497, 3:1522–3
  recombination with Marek's disease virus 3:1500
  replication 3:1497
  retroviral vectors 3:1502–3
  REV-T 3:1496, 3:1501(Fig), 3:1820
    disease induced by 3:1510
    helper virus 3:1496
    oncogene 3:1510
  REV-T induced neoplasia 3:1500–2
    altered gene expression in v-rel cells 3:1501–2, 3:1502(Table)
    v-rel mutations role 3:1500–1
  RNA classes
    genomic length 3:1497
    subgenomic 3:1497
  strain T see REV-T (above)
  structure and properties 3:1496–7
  syncytia formation 3:1499

Reticuloendotheliosis (RE) viruses (*continued*)
 taxonomy and classification 3:1496
 tissue tropism 3:1497
 transmission 3:1498–9
 vaccine unavailability 3:1499
Retinal degeneration, Borna disease virus infection 1:172
Retinal infections 1:523
Retinal necrosis, acute 1:529
Retinitis
 CMV 1:62, 1:63, 1:349, 1:528, 1:529, 1:529(Fig)
Retinoblastoma gene (Rb) 3:1821
 HPV E6 and E7 gene interaction 3:1846
Retinoblastoma protein (pRb)
 activation by adenovirus E1A 1:26(Fig)
 binding proteins 1:25
 degradation by E7 protein from HPV 2:1119
 function as master regulator 2:1119
 large T protein of polyomavirus and 2:1357
 mutational loss 2:1117, 2:1119
 phosphorylation 1:24
 role in immortalization/co-transformation 1:24
Retinoic acid receptor (RAR), adenovirus E1A interaction 1:26
Retinopathy, HIV 1:528–9
Retroelements 1:437
 bacterial 2:1314, 2:1315(Table)
 characteristics 1:438(Table)
 classes 2:1315(Table)
 definition 2:1314
 features 2:1314
 groups 2:1314
 long terminal repeats *see* Long terminal repeat (LTR)
 nonviral 2:1314, 2:1315(Table)
 plant *see* Plant retroelements
 retroposons 2:1314
 retrotransposons 2:1314
 viral 2:1314, 2:1315(Table)
 see also Retrotransposons
Retrolentiviruses 2:764
Retrons (reverse transcriptase-producing elements) 2:1087, 2:1104
Retroperitoneal fibromatosis (RF) 3:1518, 3:1525
Retroposons 2:1314
Retroregulation, transcription 1:284
Retrosequences 2:1314
Retrotransposons 2:1314, 3:1503
 distribution 2:1317
 long terminal repeat (LTR) 3:1503
 plant *see* Plant retrotransposons
 poly(A)-type 3:1503
Retrotransposons of fungi 3:1503–7
 history 3:1503
 host functions 3:1507
 during retrotransposition 3:1506(Table)
 list of types 3:1504(Table)
 LTR-sequences 3:1503–4, 3:1504(Fig)
 see also Ty elements
 poly(A)-type 3:1504(Fig), 3:1505
 structural features 3:1503–4
 TAD element 3:1504
 transposition mechanism 3:1504–6

Retrotransposons of fungi (*continued*)
 virus-like particles relationship 3:1506–7
Retrovir *see* Zidovudine
Retroviral oncogenes *see* Oncogenes
Retroviral vectors 3:1889–91
 advantages/disadvantages 2:1000–1, 3:1891
 delivery into cells 3:1503
 generation, principles and method 2:1000
 MuLV-based 2:1000–1, 2:1000(Fig)
 modification 2:1001
 packaging cell lines 3:1889, 3:1890(Fig)
 packaging proteins 3:1889
 reticuloendotheliosis (RE) viruses 3:1502–3
 REV-A 3:1502–3
 spleen necrosis virus (SNV)-based 3:1502–3
 transgenes 3:1890–1
Retroviridae 1:184, 1:191–8, 1:223
 apoptosis inhibition 1:74
 apoptosis promotion 1:75–6
 avian type C retroviruses 1:112–17
 Betaretrovirus 3:1496, 3:1518
 caprine arthritis encephalitis virus 1:223–9
 characteristics 3:1640
 classification 1:438
 Deltaretrovirus 1:191, 2:795
 DNA integration 1:641–2
 Epsilonvirus 1:541
 fish viruses 1:565
 Gammaretrovirus 2:966, 2:995
 genera 1:438, 2:795
 gibbon ape leukemia virus (GaLV) 1:617–19
 Hepadnaviridae relationship 1:641
 human immunodeficiency viruses 2:763–73
 Lentivirus 1:535, 2:774, 2:789, 3:1640
 equine infectious anemia virus (EIAV) 1:515–22
 lymphoproliferative disease virus (LPDV) of turkeys 2:911–15
 mouse mammary tumor virus (MMTV) 2:965–72
 proviral DNA 1:191
 provirus DNA 1:642
 Spumavirus 3:1686
 see also individual genera/viruses; Retroviruses
Retroviruses 1:184, 2:1314
 animal 1:184
 avian 3:1496
 C-type 1:112, 1:113, 2:713
 avian *see* Avian type C retroviruses
 gibbon ape leukemia virus (GaLV) 1:617
 morphology 1:496–7
 properties 2:789
 characteristics 1:184–5, 2:789
 classification 1:184–5
 complete, LINEs and SINEs vs 1:438
 discovery 1:184
 Drosophila see Drosophila melanogaster gypsy virus
 endogenous
 distribution 1:437
 insects 3:1530, 3:1530(Table)

Retroviruses (*continued*)
 endogenous (*continued*)
 see also Drosophila melanogaster gypsy virus; Endogenous proviruses
 env proteins, expression in vectors 3:1890
 evolution 1:188
 genome 2:765, 3:1889
 conserved 1:188
 glycoproteins, translation 3:1477
 importance 3:1818
 lenti- 3:1963
 long terminal repeat (LTR) 3:1476
 mammalian, RE viruses relationship 3:1496
 packaging 3:1889
 pararetroviruses differentiation 2:1277
 pathogenicity 1:618(Table)
 phenotypic mixing 1:609
 phylogeny 1:188, 1:189(Fig)
 plasmids 3:1889
 provirus 3:1477
 recombination 3:1451–3
 replication 2:995–6, 3:1409, 3:1476–7, 3:1476(Fig)
 Rev protein 3:1477
 reverse transcription 3:1476–7
 ribosomal frameshifting 3:1977
 serological relationships 1:188, 1:190(Fig)
 spuma 3:1963
 Tat protein 3:1477
 taxonomy and classification 1:437
 transcription 3:1472
 transformation by *see* Transformation
 translation 3:1477
 tumorigenicity, discovery 2:723
 as vectors *see* Retroviral vectors
 visna-maedi viruses 3:1963
 yeast 3:1974
 see also Reticuloendotheliosis (RE) viruses
Retroviruses, type D 3:1518–26
 assembly 3:1522
 budding 3:1522
 cell fusion 3:1522
 constitutive transport element (CTE) 3:1521
 crossreactivity 3:1523–4
 cytopathology 3:1522
 endogenous viruses 3:1523
 epidemiology 3:1524
 evolution 3:1523–4
 future perspectives 3:1526
 gene order 3:1519–20, 3:1523
 genetics 3:1523
 genome 3:1519, 3:1523
 long terminal repeat 3:1521
 geographic distribution 3:1522
 history 3:1518
 host range and propagation 3:1522–3
 infection
 clinical features 3:1525
 immune response 3:1525
 pathology/histopathology 3:1525
 prevention and control 3:1525–6
 intracytoplasmic A-type particles (ICAPs) 3:1518, 3:1520, 3:1522
 maturation 3:1519, 3:1520
 pathogenicity 3:1524–5
 physical properties 3:1521
 post-translational processing 3:1522

Retroviruses, type D (*continued*)
 proteins 3:1519–21
 receptors 3:1522–3
 release 3:1522
 resistance to 3:1525
 reverse transcriptase 3:1521
 reverse transcription 3:1521
 RNA replication 3:1521
 serologic relationships and variability 3:1524
 structure and properties 3:1519
 taxonomy and classification 3:1518–19
 tissue tropism 3:1524
 transcription 3:1521
 translation 3:1521–2
 transmission 3:1524
 vaccines 3:1525–6
 viruses included 3:1519(Table)
 see also Mason Pfizer monkey virus (M-PMV); Simian retrovirus (SRV)
rev gene
 caprine arthritis encephalitis virus (CAEV) 1:224–5
 equine infectious anemia virus (EIAV) 1:516
 see also other specific viruses
Rev responsive element (RRE) 1:225
REV-T *see* Reticuloendotheliosis (RE) viruses
Reverse genetics 2:754
 parainfluenza virus 3 (PIV-3) 2:1132
Reoviridae 2:1061
Reverse gyrase, in SSV1 virus 1:86
Reverse transcribing viruses 3:1738–9(Table)
Reverse transcriptase 3:1476
 amino acid sequences 1:189(Fig)
 assay, lymphoproliferative disease virus of turkeys 2:914
 badnaviruses 2:1297
 bovine leukemia virus (BLV) 1:192
 cassava vein mosaic virus (CsVMV) 2:1287
 caulimoviruses 2:1283
 discovery 2:722
 equine infectious anemia virus (EIAV) 1:517, 1:518
 error rates 2:776
 hepatitis B virus (HBV) 1:647
 HIV *see* HIV
 magnesium requirement 1:192
 Mg^{2+} required 1:188
 murine leukemia viruses (MuLVs) 2:996
 ssDNA viruses 3:1477
 type D retroviruses 3:1521
Reverse transcriptase inhibitors 1:54, 2:779–83
 in combination therapy 2:783
 in HAART 1:58
 HIV resistance 2:781–3, 2:782(Fig)
 non-nucleoside (NNRTI) 1:59–60, 2:779, 2:781
 approved drugs 2:781, 2:786
 mechanism of action 2:781
 mutations and resistance 2:782(Fig)
 new developments 1:60, 2:782–3
 recommendations 2:787
 resistance 1:59
 resistance mechanism 2:782
 specificity 2:781
 structures 2:780(Fig)
 nucleoside (NRTI) 1:58–9, 2:779, 2:779–81

INDEX I lxxxv

Reverse transcriptase inhibitors (*continued*)
  nucleoside (NRTI) (*continued*)
    approved drugs 2:786
    azidothymidine *see* Zidovudine
    indications 2:781
    kinase and activation 2:780–1
    mechanisms of action 2:780–1
    mutations and resistance 2:782(Fig)
    recommendations 2:787
    resistance mechanism 2:781–2
    structure 2:780(Fig)
  target 2:779
Reverse transcriptase-PCR (RT-PCR)
  astroviruses 1:107
  benyviruses 1:158
  caliciviruses 1:445
Reverse transcription 2:765, 3:1472, 3:1476–7
  antiviral drug target 1:54
  avian hepatitis B viruses 1:650
  avian leukosis virus (ALV) 1:113, 1:114, 1:115
  badnaviruses 2:1297
  caprine arthritis encephalitis virus (CAEV) 1:225
  Drosophila melanogaster gypsy virus 3:1528–9
  Hepadnaviridae 1:641
  HIV *see* HIV
  'jumping' 1:114, 1:115
  murine leukemia viruses (MuLVs) 2:996
  in plants, cauliflower mosaic virus (CaMV) 2:1275
  priming
    in Tf elements 3:1505
    in Ty elements 3:1505
  Ty elements 3:1505
  type D retroviruses 3:1521
  virus replication strategy 3:1476–7
Rex protein, HTLV-1 *see* Human T-cell leukemia virus type 1 (HTLV-1)
Rex-responsive element (RxRE), HTLV-2 2:801
Reye's syndrome 2:828
  in varicella 3:1876
RGD motif, bacteriophage φ29 terminal protein 1:123
Rgl system 2:761, 2:762(Table)
Rhabdomyolysis, coxsackievirus infection 1:308
Rhabdoviridae
  apoptosis promotion 1:76
  characteristics 1:257, 3:1438
  fish viruses 1:558
  genera 3:1541
  IHNV-like viruses 1:558
  Lyssavirus 3:1442
  rabies viruses 3:1437–41
  shrimp viruses 3:1627
  sigma rhabdoviruses 3:1636
  Vesiculovirus 1:257, 3:1911
  see also Lyssaviruses; Rabies virus; Vesicular stomatitis virus (VSV); *Vesiculovirus*
Rhabdovirus of penaeid shrimps (RPS) 3:1627–8
  diagnosis and detection 3:1628
  genome 3:1628
  replication 3:1627
  structural proteins 3:1628
  susceptibility studies 3:1627
Rhabdoviruses
  animal, *see also* Vesicular stomatitis virus (VSV)
  characteristics 3:1531

Rhabdoviruses (*continued*)
  fish *see* Fish rhabdoviruses
  plant *see* Plant rhabdoviruses
  sigma *see* Sigma rhabdoviruses
  ungrouped 3:1541–4
Rhadinovirus 2:714, 2:715, 2:717
  future perspectives 2:718
  Lymphocryptovirus comparison 2:704(Table)
  see also Herpesvirus ateles 2 (HVA-2); Herpesvirus saimiri 2 (HVS-2)
Rhesus macaque monkeys, specific-pathogen-free (SPF) 3:1524
Rhesus macaque virus (RMV) 2:1152
Rhesus monkey kidney cells (RhMK), normal 1:397(Fig)
Rhesus monkeys, poliovirus research 2:730
Rheumatoid arthritis, RA1 parvovirus association 2:1154–5
Rhinitis 3:1492, 3:1493(Table)
  acute, HSV-1 causing 2:681
Rhinoceros beetle *see* Oryctes rhinoceros
Rhinopneumonitis, equine 1:508
  epidemiology 1:512
Rhinotracheitis, infectious bovine *see* Infectious bovine rhinotracheitis (IBR)
Rhinovirus 2:1326
Rhinoviruses 3:1545–51
  acid lability 2:1177
  antibodies 3:1550
  assembly and release 3:1547
  attachment and entry 3:1547
  bovine 3:1545
  cytopathic effect 1:397(Fig)
  cytopathology 3:1547
  detection 3:1548, 3:1550
  drug binding groups 3:1545(Table)
  drug design 3:1495, 3:1551, 3:1551(Fig), 3:1946
  economic significance 3:1549
  epidemiology 3:1549
  equine 3:1545
  evolution 3:1548, 3:1548(Fig)
  future perspectives 3:1550–1
  genetics 3:1548
  genome 3:1546, 3:1546(Fig)
    untranslated region (UTR) 3:1546, 3:1547
  geographic/seasonal distribution 3:1548
  history 3:1545
  host range and propagation 3:1548
  infection 3:1492
    clinical features 3:1549
    epidemiology 3:1549
    immune response 3:1550
    pathology/histopathology 3:1550
    pharyngitis 3:1492
    prevention and control 3:1550, 3:1551(Fig)
    site 3:1549
    treatment 1:66, 3:1550
    see also Common cold
  infection initiation 1:234
  intertypes 3:1548
  ocular target 1:525(Table)
  pathogenicity 3:1549
  physical properties 3:1547
  polymerase, inhibitors 1:66
  polyprotein 3:1546(Fig), 3:1547
  post-translational processing 3:1547
  proteins 2:738, 3:1546–7

Rhinoviruses (*continued*)
  proteins (*continued*)
    2C and 2C 3:1546–7, 3:1548(Fig)
    3C and 3D 3:1546–7
    nonstructural 3:1546–7
    processing 1:233
    VP1-4 3:1545–6, 3:1546
  receptors 3:1545, 3:1545(Table)
    blocking 3:1551
    ICAM-1 1:66
  recombination 3:1548
  replication 3:1547
    strategy and early events 3:1547
  RNA synthesis 3:1547
  RNA-dependent RNA polymerase 3:1547
  serologic relationships and variability 3:1548–9, 3:1548(Fig)
  serotypes 3:1545, 3:1548–9, 3:1548(Fig)
  structure and properties 3:1545–6
    canyons 3:1547
    three-dimensional 3:1546
  taxonomy and classification 3:1545
  tissue tropism 3:1549
  translation 3:1547
  transmission 1:485(Table), 3:1549
    prevention 3:1550
  VPg 3:1546
Rhizomania
  furoviruses causing 1:594
  occurrences 1:155(Table)
  sugarbeet 1:155, 1:158
Rhopalosiphum padi virus (RhpV) 2:1268, 2:1273
Rhubarb, economic significance of plant virus diseases 2:1324
Ribavirin
  hantavirus infection 1:68
  HPV infections 1:67
  for infants 1:65
  influenza 1:64
  Intron A with 1:66
  Lassa fever prophylaxis 2:895
  Lassa fever therapy 2:895, 2:895–6
  mechanism of action 1:64
  resistance 1:64
  respiratory virus infections 3:1495
  RSV infection 1:64, 3:1487
Ribonuclease P (RNaseP) 3:1552, 3:1554(Fig)
  reaction 3:1553, 3:1553(Fig)
Ribonucleotide reductase
  HSV 2:693
  inhibitor (348U87) 1:62
Ribosomal frameshifting 3:1473
  astroviruses 1:104
  bacteriophage φX174 1:278
  bovine leukemia virus (BLV) 1:194
  closteroviruses 1:270
  dianthoviruses 1:405
  HIV 2:777
  L-A virus 3:1975–7, 3:1976(Fig)
  luteoviruses 2:904
  mouse mammary tumor virus (MMTV) 2:967
  retroviruses 3:1977
  'slippery site' mechanism 3:1505
  spumaviruses 3:1688
  totiviruses 3:1809
  Ty elements translation 3:1505
Ribosomal proteins, arenaviruses 2:888

Ribosomal RNA (rRNA), ribosome-inactivating proteins action 2:1312
Ribosome
  60S subunit, in yeast RNA virus replication 3:1977
  membrane protein synthesis 3:1923
  modification by cardioviruses 1:235
Ribosome shunt mechanism
  caulimoviruses 1:1284
  rice tungro bacilliform virus (RTBV) 2:1295
Ribosome-inactivating proteins (RIPs) 2:1305, 2:1312
  type I (single-chain proteins) 2:1312
  type II 2:1312
Ribozymes 1:61, 3:1551–9
  definition 3:1551
  hepatitis delta virus (HDV) RNA 1:665, 1:667
  history 3:1551–2
  HIV therapy approach 1:61
  in HPV infections 1:67
  of non-viral origin 3:1552–5, 3:1554(Table)
    group I introns 3:1553–4, 3:1553(Fig)
    group II introns 3:1553(Fig), 3:1554–5
    Neurospora VS RNA 3:1553(Fig), 3:1554(Fig), 3:1555
    RNase P 3:1553, 3:1553(Fig), 3:1554(Fig)
    plant and animal RNAs 3:1554(Table)
  in satellite RNA 3:1615
  trans systems 3:1555, 3:1557, 3:1558
  types 3:1552(Table)
  of viral origin 3:1555–8, 3:1555(Fig)
    hairpin 3:1557–8, 3:1557(Fig)
    hammerhead *see* Hammerhead ribozyme
    pseudoknot of HDV 3:1558
Rice, tungro virus infections *see* Rice tungro bacilliform virus (RTBV); Rice tungro disease
Rice black streaked dwarf virus (RBSDV) 2:1263
  genome 2:1264
Rice dwarf virus (RDV) 2:1262
  genome 2:1263
  in vitro expression 2:1264
  transmissibility loss 2:1266
  see also Phytoreoviruses
Rice gall dwarf virus (RGDV) 2:1262
Rice grassy stunt virus (RGSV) 3:1756
  transmission 3:1907
  see also Tenuiviruses
Rice hoja blanca virus (RHBV) 3:1756, 3:1759(Fig)
  replication, in planthoppers 3:1757
  transmitters and nontransmitters 3:1758
  see also Tenuiviruses
Rice ragged stunt virus (RRSV) 2:1263
Rice stripe necrosis virus (RSNV) 1:588
Rice stripe virus (RSV) 3:1756
  genomic RNAs 3:1759
  serologic relationships 3:1763
  see also Tenuiviruses

Rice transitory yellowing virus (RTYV) 3:1531
Rice tungro bacilliform virus (RTBV) 2:1292–6, 2:1296, 3:1965
  classification 2:1293
  control 2:1293
  disease induced by 2:1299, 3:1969
    see also Rice tungro disease
  epidemiology 2:1299
  gene expression 2:1295
  general features 2:1292–3
  genome 2:1294, 2:1297
    gag and pol 2:1295
    ORF1 and ORF2 2:1294, 2:1295
    ORF3 2:1294–5, 2:1295
    ORF4 2:1295
    organization 2:1294–5, 2:1294(Fig)
  genomic map 2:1287(Fig)
  geographic distribution 2:1293(Fig)
  history 2:1292–3
  host range 2:1293
  host relationship 2:1298
  Indian strain 2:1295
  pathogenicity 3:1969
  promoters 2:1295
  proteins 2:1297
  replication 2:1295
  ribosome shunt mechanism 2:1295
  rice tungro spherical virus (RTSV) relationship 2:1292, 2:1299
  southeast Asian strain 2:1295
  structure and properties 2:1293, 2:1294(Fig), 2:1296
  symptomatology 2:1293
  tolerance and resistance to 2:1293
  transcription 2:1295
  transmission 2:1293, 2:1299, 3:1968
    control 2:1293
  variation and variants 2:1295
  see also Badnaviruses
Rice tungro disease 2:1292, 3:1965, 3:1968, 3:1969
  causative agents 2:1292–3
  clinical features 3:1969
  economic significance 2:1292
  history 2:1292
  prevention and control 3:1969–70
  see also Rice tungro bacilliform virus (RTBV)
Rice tungro spherical virus (RTSV) 2:1292, 3:1965
  epidemiology 3:1968
  genome 3:1966
  geographic distribution 3:1965
  as helper virus 3:1968
  host range 3:1966
  infections
    clinical features 3:1969
    pathology and histopathology 3:1969
    prevention and control 3:1969–70
  pathogenicity 3:1969
  rice tungro bacilliform virus (RTBV) transmission 2:1293, 2:1299
  seasonal distribution 3:1966
  sequence comparisons 3:1967(Table)
  serologic relationships and variability 3:1967–8
  transmission 2:1293, 2:1299, 3:1968
Rice tungro virus (RTV) 3:1965

Rice tungro waikavirus see Rice tungro spherical virus (RTSV)
Rice waika virus (RWV) 3:1965
  epidemiology 3:1968
  genome 3:1970
  geographic distribution 3:1966
  host range 3:1966
  infections 3:1965
    clinical features 3:1969
    pathology and histopathology 3:1969
    prevention and control 3:1969, 3:1970
    seasonal distribution 3:1966
    serologic relationships and variability 3:1968
    transmission 3:1968
Rice yellow mottle virus (RYMV) 3:1674
  epidemiology and control 3:1680
Rice yellow stunt virus (RYSV) 3:1531
Rift Valley fever (RVF) 1:209, 3:1993
  clinical features 3:1993
  epidemiology 3:1993
  outbreaks 1:209, 1:210
  prevention and control 3:1993
Rift Valley fever (RVF) virus 1:210, 3:1993
  budding 1:216
  emerging/re-emerging virus 1:419(Table)
  epizootics 1:210
  ocular target 1:525(Table)
  transmission 1:210, 3:1993
    ecological change and 3:1996
  vaccines 1:211, 3:1993
Rimantadine (Flumadine) 1:63
  disadvantages of use 1:64
  prophylaxis 1:64
  respiratory virus infections 3:1495
Rinderpest
  clinical features 3:1566
  diagnosis 3:1568
  eradication campaigns 3:1568–9
  history 3:1559
  immune response 3:1567
  outbreaks 3:1564
  panzootic spread 3:1559
  pathology/histopathology 3:1567
  prevention and control 3:1567
Rinderpest virus 1:420(Table), 3:1559–69
  epizootiology 3:1564–5
  evolution 3:1563–4, 3:1565(Fig)
  future perspectives 3:1569
  genome 3:1562
  geographic distribution 3:1560, 3:1561(Fig)
  history 3:1559–60
  host range and propagation 3:1561–2
  infection see Rinderpest
  monoclonal antibodies 3:1563
  pathogenicity 3:1566
  replication 3:1562–3
  serologic relationships and variability 3:1564
  structure and properties 3:1562
  taxonomy and classification 3:1560
  transmission and tissue tropism 3:1564–5, 3:1566
  vaccination 3:1568–9
  vaccines 3:1564, 3:1568
    Plowright tissue culture attenuated 3:1568
  in wild ruminant species 1:420(Table)
  see also Morbilliviruses

RING zinc finger motif, IAP (inhibitor of apoptosis) 1:73
Rio Bravo virus group 1:433(Table)
RIP 1:71
Risk assessment, emerging viral diseases 1:418
Ritonavir (Norvir) 1:60, 2:783–4
  structure 2:784(Fig)
RIZ (pRB binding protein) 1:25
RNA
  5′ cap, in furoviruses 1:590
  ambisense see Ambisense RNA
  amplification 1:393
    techniques 1:392
  antisense
    homology-dependent resistance in plants 2:1310
    mRNA, phage development prevention 2:1248
    plant resistance to viruses 2:1310–11
  antisense genome see RNA, negative-strand
  bipartite, nepoviruses 2:1007
  catalytic see Ribozymes
  defective-interfering see Defective interfering (DI) viruses/RNAs
  double-stranded (dsRNA) 3:1739, 3:1746(Table)
    apoptosis trigger 1:74
    bacteriophage φ6 2:1205
    bisegmented 1:160
    chloroplasts of marine green alga 1:312
    cryptoviruses 1:312, 1:313
    cypoviruses 1:332
    fungal partitiviruses 2:1147
    interferon action 2:859
    interferon induction 2:856
    L-A virus 3:1975
    phytoreoviruses 2:1262, 2:1263
    reoviruses 3:1456
    replication 1:322–3, 3:1476
    ribosomal frameshifting 3:1975–7
    rotaviruses 3:1577, 3:1583
    totiviruses 3:1808, 3:1813
    in umbravirus-infected plants 3:1856–7, 3:1857
  double-stranded (dsRNA) linear, giardiavirus (GLV) 1:614
  double-stranded (dsRNA) segmented
    coltiviruses 2:1047
    orbiviruses 2:1046, 2:1062
    reoviruses 3:1465
  editing 3:1473, 3:1563
    hepatitis delta virus (HDV) 1:666–7
  homologous recombination 3:1449–50
  messenger see mRNA
  negative-strand 3:1474
    Borna disease virus 1:168
    Bunyaviridae 1:207
    Chandipura and Piry viruses 1:257
    filoviruses 2:940
    influenza viruses 2:830
    Morbillivirus 2:953
    mumps virus (MuV) 2:989
    Newcastle disease virus 2:1021
    parainfluenza viruses 2:1131
    rabies-like viruses 3:1442
    respiratory syncytial virus (RSV) 3:1482
    Sendai virus 3:1616
    tospoviruses 3:1805
    tripartite in hantaviruses 1:623

RNA (continued)
  negative-strand (continued)
    vesicular stomatitis virus (VSV) 3:1911
  nonhomologous recombination 3:1450
  plant resistance to viruses mediated by 2:1310
  positive-strand 3:1474
    alphaviruses 1:262, 3:1657
    animal enteroviruses 1:462
    arteriviruses 1:91
    avian leukosis virus (ALV) 1:113
    barnaviruses 1:153
    benyviruses 1:156
    bovine immunodeficiency virus (BIV) 1:185
    bovine leukemia virus 1:191
    bromoviruses 1:199
    caliciviruses 1:218, 2:1036
    caprine arthritis encephalitis virus (CAEV) 1:223
    cardioviruses 1:230, 1:231
    carlaviruses 1:239
    carmoviruses 1:243
    closteroviruses 1:267
    coronaviruses 1:292
    dianthoviruses 1:403, 1:405
    encephalitis viruses 1:426
    enterovirus 70 (EV70) 1:470
    equine encephalitis viruses 1:502
    equine infectious anemia virus (EIAV) 1:516
    feline leukemia viruses (FeLVs) 1:541
    foot-and-mouth disease viruses (FMDVs) 1:569
    hepatitis A virus (HAV) 1:631
    hepatitis C virus (HCV) 1:657
    hepatitis E virus (HEV) 1:671
    hog cholera virus (HCV) 2:739
    hypoviruses 2:805
    Japanese encephalitis (JE) virus 2:871
    lymphoproliferative disease virus (LPDV) 2:912
    machlomoviruses 2:935
    murine leukemia viruses (MuLVs) 2:995
    necroviruses 2:1004
    nodaviruses 2:1026
    pea enation mosaic virus (PEMV) 2:1191
    polioviruses 2:1330
    pomoviruses 3:1361
    potexviruses 3:1364, 3:1365
    potyviruses 3:1370
    rhinoviruses 3:1546
    RNA phage 3:1663
    rubella virus 3:1594
    sequiviruses 3:1622
    sobemoviruses 3:1676
    spumaviruses 3:1687
    tetraviruses 3:1764
    tobamoviruses 3:1781
    tobraviruses 3:1784
    tombusviruses 3:1794
    trichoviruses 3:1839
    tombusviruses 3:1794
    trichoviruses 3:1839
    umbraviruses 3:1856
    waikaviruses 3:1966
    yellow fever virus 3:1980
  probes 1:391
  processing reactions 3:1553(Fig)
  replication see RNA replication
  satellite see Satellite RNAs
  self-cleavage reactions 3:1552(Table)
  sequencing, history 2:720

RNA (continued)
　single-stranded (ssRNA)
　　ambisense see Ambisense
　　　RNA
　　animal viruses 2:722
　　arenaviruses 2:887
　　chronic paralysis virus 2:745
　　fabaviruses 1:532
　　hepatitis delta virus 1:665,
　　　1:665(Fig)
　　messenger sense see RNA,
　　　positive-strand
　　mouse mammary tumor virus
　　　(MMTV) 2:966
　　pecluviruses 2:1198
　　simian immunodeficiency
　　　viruses (SIV) 3:1642
　　tenuiviruses 3:1759
　　tymoviruses 3:1851
　　viroids 3:1929
　splicing 1:255
　　Borna disease virus 1:169
　　bovine leukemia virus
　　　(BLV) 1:193
　subgenomic messenger (sgRNA),
　　apple chlorotic leaf spot virus
　　(ACLSV) 3:1840
　synthesis, host see Host
　tRNA see tRNA
　types
　　in animal viruses,
　　　discovery 2:722
　　in plant viruses,
　　　discovery 2:724
RNA bacteriophage
　history 2:721
　release 3:1415
RNA bacteriophage, single-
　stranded 3:1663–8
　6SRNA 3:1667
　assembly 3:1415
　attachment process 3:1664,
　　3:1665(Fig)
　coat protein 3:1666
　ecology 3:1665
　gene expression control 3:1666
　genetic map 3:1664(Fig), 3:1666
　genome, rigidity and
　　plasticity 3:1667–8
　geographic distribution 3:1665
　Group B, lysing protein 3:1666
　Group I 3:1663, 3:1664(Fig)
　Group II 3:1663, 3:1664(Fig)
　Group III 3:1663, 3:1664(Fig)
　Group IV 3:1663, 3:1664(Fig)
　history 3:1663
　host range 3:1664–5
　as index organisms 3:1665–6
　infection process 3:1664
　lysis (L) gene 3:1666
　maturation (A) protein 3:1664
　　cleavage 3:1664
　　expression control 3:1666
　natural hosts 3:1665
　phylogeny 3:1668
　Qβ RNA variants 3:1667
　replicase 3:1666
　　expression control 3:1666
　replication 3:1666–7
　structure and properties 3:1663–
　　4, 3:1665(Fig)
　supergroup A 3:1663
　　genome 3:1664(Fig), 3:1666
　supergroup B 3:1663
　　genome 3:1664(Fig), 3:1666
　taxonomy and
　　classification 3:1663
　therapeutic uses 3:1668
　see also Bacteriophage MS2;
　　Bacteriophage Qβ
RNA coliphage see RNA
　bacteriophage, single-stranded

RNA helicase, tick-borne
　encephalitis (TBE) virus
　complex 1:431
RNA polymerase
　arteriviruses 1:91
　bacteriophage φX174
　　replication 1:278
　bacteriophage P1 1:459
　domains, in furoviruses 1:590
　host
　　bacteriophage
　　　transcription 3:1414
　　modification by bacteriophage
　　　PBS1 1:133
　host σ70-, coliphage N4
　　transcription 1:451, 1:452
　L-A virus see L-A virus, Gag-Pol
　　protein
　'leading' 1:371
　modification by T5-like
　　phage 3:1720
　promoter recognition,
　　model 1:451
　RNA-dependent see RNA-
　　dependent RNA polymerase
　σ^A
　　bacteriophage SPO1 1:131
　　see also Bacteriophage φ29
　slippage, in hantavirus
　　transcription 1:625
　for T4-like phages
　　replication 3:1706
　umbraviruses 3:1855
　vaccinia virus as vector 3:1887
RNA polymerase II
　avian leukosis virus (ALV)
　　transcription 1:114
　frog virus 3 (FV3)
　　transcription 1:585
　polyomavirus
　　transcription 2:1359
　type D retrovirus
　　transcription 3:1521
　in viroid replication 3:1935
RNA polymerase III,
　adenoviruses 1:18
RNA replicase
　carlaviruses 1:239, 1:240
　furoviruses 1:590
RNA replication
　dsRNA viruses 3:1815
　error rate 1:607
　hepatitis delta virus 1:666,
　　1:666(Fig)
　LCMV 2:922
　machlomoviruses 2:936
　rolling circle model 1:666,
　　1:666(Fig), 3:1555,
　　3:1555(Fig)
　satellite RNA 3:1614–15
　sobemovirus satellites 3:1679
　self-cleavage reactions 3:1555,
　　3:1555(Fig)
　see also individual viruses
RNA satellite virus
　hepatitis delta virus 1:664
　see also Satellite RNAs
RNA virus core (RVC) motif 1:230
RNA viruses 3:1739–44(Table)
　animal viruses 1:607
　antibody-resistant
　　mutants 3:1434
　antigenic variation 2:812, 2:816
　apoptosis inhibition 1:74
　apoptosis promotion 1:75–6
　capsid functions 3:1946(Table)
　defective-interfering (DI)
　　mutants 1:608
　DNA virus recombination 3:1500
　double-stranded
　　algae/fungi and
　　　protozoa 3:1754

RNA viruses (continued)
　double-stranded (continued)
　　bacterial 3:1755
　　invertebrates 3:1752
　　plants 3:1753
　　vertebrates 3:1751
　evolution 3:1435, 3:1489–90
　　satellite RNAs as model 1:318,
　　　1:322
　eye infections 1:524–6,
　　1:525(Table)
　　see also Eye infections; specific
　　　viruses
　fish viruses see Fish viruses
　fitness concept 3:1435
　genome features 2:1335
　infecting cucurbits 1:244
　insect pest control by 2:843–4
　　see also Biological control
　interferon induction 2:856
　light microscopy 1:400
　multiplication cycle 3:1408–9
　mutation frequency 1:419
　mutation rates 2:1335, 3:1449,
　　3:1489
　negative-stranded 3:1475–6,
　　3:1739–41(Table), 3:1746–
　　7(Table)
　　ambisense gRNA 3:1476
　　classes 3:1475
　　copy-back DI RNAs 3:1373
　　defective-interfering
　　　RNAs 3:1454
　　genome replication 3:1475–6
　　invertebrates 3:1752
　　monopartite
　　　(unsegmented) 3:1475
　　plants 3:1753
　　replication 3:1474(Fig), 3:1475–
　　　6, 3:1475(Fig)
　　segmented (multipartite) 3:1476
　　unsegmented, evolution 3:1438
　　vertebrates 3:1751
　　see also RNA, negative-strand
　plant viruses
　　structure 3:1948
　　as vectors 3:1895–7
　positive-stranded 3:1474–5,
　　3:1474(Fig), 3:1741–4(Table),
　　3:1747–8(Table)
　　invertebrates 3:1752
　　plants 3:1753
　　vertebrates 3:1751
　　see also RNA, positive-strand
　quasispecies 3:1434
　　see also Quasispecies
　recombination 3:1449–53
　replication 3:1472, 3:1474–7
　　double-stranded viruses 3:1476
　　negative-strand
　　　viruses 3:1474(Fig), 3:1475–6,
　　　3:1476(Fig)
　　positive-strand viruses 3:1474–
　　　5, 3:1475(Fig)
　　reverse transcription
　　　strategy 3:1476–7
　　reverse transcribing 3:1738–
　　　9(Table), 3:1746(Table)
　　reverse transcription 3:1476–7
　shrimp viruses 3:1627–30
　single-stranded
　　algae/fungi and
　　　protozoa 1:754
　　bacterial 3:1755
　　ribosomal frameshifting 3:1977
　single-stranded RT
　　algae/fungi and
　　　protozoa 3:1754
　　plants 3:1753
　small, insect 2:1267,
　　2:1268(Table)
　supergroups 1:243

RNA viruses (continued)
　in thin-sectioned cells 1:400(Fig)
　transcription 3:1472, 3:1474(Fig)
　transformation by 3:1818
　vector systems 3:1891
　as vectors 3:1891, 3:1895–7
　　coat protein genes 3:1897,
　　　3:1897(Table)
　　genes encoding proteins for
　　　RNA replication 3:1896
　　heterologous gene
　　　expression 3:1897(Table)
　　in vitro transcription
　　　systems 3:1896
　　independent vs
　　　'disarmed' 3:1897
　　infectivity approaches 3:1895–6
　　infectivity of cloned
　　　DNA 3:1895–6,
　　　3:1896(Table)
　　insertion/expression of foreign
　　　genes 3:1896
　　miscellaneous genes 3:1897
　　movement protein genes 3:1896
RNA-dependent DNA polymerase
　see Reverse transcriptase
RNA-dependent RNA polymerase
　(RDRP) 3:1472
　animal enteroviruses 1:463
　cryptoviruses 1:314
　cucumoviruses 1:323
　discovery 2:722
　fungal partitiviruses 2:1147,
　　2:1148(Fig), 2:1150
　giardiavirus (GLV) 1:614
　hantaviruses 1:622
　hepatitis E virus 1:675
　insect picorna-like viruses 2:1268
　luteoviruses and
　　poleroviruses 2:903, 2:905
　nodaviruses 2:1029
　plant rhabdoviruses 3:1536
　poliovirus 3:1475
　potexviruses 3:1367
　potyviruses 3:1372
　rhinoviruses 3:1547
　rotaviruses 3:1577
　tick-borne encephalitis (TBE)
　　virus complex 1:431
　totiviruses 3:1809, 3:1811,
　　3:1811(Fig), 3:1816
　see also Transcriptase
RNase, sensitivity of trichovirus
　genomic RNA 3:1839
RNase L 2:1312
　interferon antiviral system 2:858
RNase P 3:1553, 3:1554(Fig)
　reaction 3:1553, 3:1553(Fig)
'Road block' hypothesis,
　interference by dominant-
　negative mutants 2:852
Robinia mosaic virus
　(RoMV) 1:315
Rocio virus 3:1992
Rocky Mountain wood
　ticks 2:1044
Rod-shaped nuclear virus of
　Penaeus japonicus 3:1633
Rodents
　betaherpesviruses 1:358(Table)
　see also Rat cytomegalovirus
　　(RCMV)
　Colorado tick fever (CTF)
　　virus 3:1991
　control 2:895, 3:1995
　Cricetid and arenavirus
　　infection 2:889–90
　evolution, relationship to
　　hantaviruses 1:626, 1:627(Fig)
　exposure to, prevention and
　　control 1:630

Rodents (continued)
geographic/seasonal distribution 1:626
human interactions and dynamics 2:890, 2:895
parvoviruses, see also Minute virus of mice (MVM); Parvoviruses; rat virus (RV)
vesicular stomatitis virus 3:1992
virus transmission
arenaviruses 2:890, 2:891
hantaviruses 1:210, 1:621, 1:626, 1:627, 3:1988
Omsk hemorrhagic fever virus 3:1992
Roferon-A, hepatitis C therapy 1:65
ros oncogene 3:1514
Rosai–Dorfman disease, HHV-6 infection associated 2:702
Rose mosaic virus 1:38
Roseola infantum 2:701
Roseolovirus 1:357, 2:698
see also Human herpesvirus 6 (HHV-6); Human herpesvirus 7 (HHV-7)
Roses, economic significance of virus diseases 2:1324
Ross River fever, misuse of term 3:1570
Ross River virus (RRV) 3:1570–6, 3:1995
antibodies 3:1575
antigenic variants 3:1574
assembly 3:1572
culture 3:1572
emerging/re-emerging virus 1:419(Table)
epidemiology 3:1574
genetics and evolution 3:1573–4
genome 3:1571
comparison of sequences 3:1573
conserved regions 3:1571
geographic/seasonal distribution 3:1572–3
history 3:1570
host range and propagation 3:1573
infection
clinical features 3:1574
immune response 3:1575
incubation period 3:1575
pathology/ histopathology 3:1575
prevention and control 3:1576
'island-hopping' 1:422
man-mosquito-man cycle 3:1574
Nelson Bay strain 3:1575
pathogenicity 3:1575
phylogenetic tree 3:1574
polyprotein 3:1571
proteins 3:1571–2
prototype (T48)
genome 3:1571, 3:1573
isolation 3:1572
replication 3:1572
serologic relationships and variability 3:1574
structure and properties 3:1570–1
taxonomy and classification 3:1570
transmission and vectors 3:1574
vaccination 3:1576
'virgin soil' epidemic 3:1573, 3:1575
virulence 3:1575
Rotamase 1:279
Rotavirus 1:1577
Rotaviruses 1:442–4, 3:1576–83
antibodies 3:1581–2
antigen processing 3:1582

Rotaviruses (continued)
apoptosis promotion 1:75
assembly 3:1591
transient envelope 3:1591–2
double-layered particles 3:1585(Fig), 3:1588, 3:1591
electropherotype classification 3:1577
emerging/re-emerging virus 1:419(Table)
epidemiology 3:1579–80
evolution 3:1579
future perspectives 3:1583, 3:1592
gene-coding assignments 3:1578–9
genes 3:1584(Fig)
genetic reassortment 3:1578
genetics 3:1577–9
genome 1:442, 3:1583, 3:1584–7
RNA segments 3:1584–7, 3:1586(Table)
sequence 3:1584
terminal consensus sequences 3:1587
geographic/seasonal distribution 3:1577
group A 1:443–4, 3:1577
antigenic variation 1:443
epidemics 1:443
G1P1A[8] 1:444
genes 3:1578–9
genetic variation 1:443
geographic distribution 1:443
proteins 3:1579
reinfections 1:443
serotypes 1:444, 3:1580
group B and C 1:444, 3:1577
genes 3:1579
intestinal lesions 3:1581
group D, F and G 1:444
group E 1:444
guanyltransferase 3:1583, 3:1587
history/discovery 1:442, 2:1035, 3:1576
host range and propagation 3:1577
infection
cell-mediated immunity 1:449
clinical features 3:1580, 3:1581(Table)
epidemics 3:1580
immune response 3:1581–2
immunity 1:448
pathology/ histopathology 1:448(Fig), 3:1580–1
prevention and control 3:1582–3
surveillance 1:449(Fig)
therapy 3:1582
infection by receptor-mediated endocytosis 3:1589
in M cells 3:1582
maturation 3:1591
molecular biology 3:1583–92
mRNAs 3:1588
nongroup A (atypical/ 'novel') 1:444, 3:1579
cell culture difficulties 1:444
genome 1:444
see also groups above
pathogenicity 3:1580
physical properties 3:1588
poly(A) binding protein (PABP) 3:1587
proteins 3:1579, 3:1583, 3:1584(Fig), 3:1586(Table)
antibodies to 3:1581–2
capsid 3:1587
G and P types 3:1587
glycoproteins 3:1579

Rotaviruses (continued)
proteins (continued)
nonstructural 3:1578–9, 3:1587, 3:1588
NSP3 3:1587
NSP4 3:1581, 3:1587, 3:1591
properties 3:1587
RNA segments encoding 3:1586(Table)
structural 3:1588
synthesis 3:1591
VP1 3:1583, 3:1587, 3:1590
VP2 3:1587
VP2 shells 3:1583
VP3 3:1583, 3:1587, 3:1590
VP4 3:1581–2, 3:1587, 3:1591
VP4 cleavage 3:1584, 3:1589
VP4 spikes 3:1583, 3:1588
VP5* 3:1589
VP6 3:1579, 3:1583, 3:1587
VP7 3:1579, 3:1581–2, 3:1583, 3:1587, 3:1591
VP7 serotypes (G) 3:1587
VP7 synthesis 3:1591
VP8* 3:1589
receptor 3:1588
release by cell lysis 3:1591–2
replication 3:1588
adsorption and penetration 3:1588–9
dsRNA 3:1590
in vitro system 3:1590–1
minus-strand RNA 3:1590
plus-strand RNA 3:1590
process 3:1589–91
sites 3:1580, 3:1591
uncoating and internalization 3:1589
RNA-binding protein (VP2) 3:1587
RNA-dependent RNA polymerase 3:1577
serologic relationships and variability 3:1579
serotypes 3:1580
shedding 3:1580
single-layered 3:1583
stability 3:1588
structure and properties 3:1577, 3:1578(Table), 3:1583–4, 3:1584(Fig)
channels 3:1584
EM structure 1:443(Fig)
outer shell 3:1583, 3:1588
spikes 3:1577, 3:1583, 3:1588
triple layered 3:1577
taxonomy and classification 3:1577
tissue tropism 3:1580
transcriptase 3:1583, 3:1587, 3:1589
activation 3:1590
transcription 3:1578, 3:1585(Fig), 3:1589–91
apparatus 3:1585(Fig)
transmission 1:485(Table), 3:1580
triple-shelled 3:1583, 3:1588
assembly 3:1591
transcriptase activation 3:1590
trypsin effect 3:1589
vaccines 3:1582
live attenuated 3:1582–3
new strategies 3:1583
VP6 3:1579
Rottboellia yellow mottle virus (RoYMV) 3:1674
host range 3:1677
see also Sobemoviruses
'Rotten apple' hypothesis, interference by dominant-negative mutants 2:852

Rous sarcoma virus (RSV) 1:112, 1:113, 3:1507
apoptosis inhibition 1:74
history 2:721
NR-13 1:74
oncogenes 1:115, 1:514
reverse transcriptase discovery 2:722
v-Src protein 3:1819
RT-PCR see Reverse transcriptase-PCR (RT-PCR)
RTG-2 cell line, infectious pancreatic necrosis virus of fish replication 1:163
Rubarth's disease (infectious canine hepatitis) 1:20
Rubella
clinical features 3:1598
complications 3:1598
congenital see Congenital rubella syndrome (CRS)
epidemic 3:1593, 3:1597
epidemiology 3:1597
eye infection 1:524
fetal see Congenital rubella syndrome (CRS)
future perspectives 3:1600–1
history 3:1592–3
immune response 3:1599
detection 3:1599
incidence 3:1600
maternal 2:1074
pathogenesis 3:1598–9
pathology/ histopathology 3:1598–9
in pregnancy 3:1597–8
prevention and control 3:1599–600
rash 3:1597, 3:1598
seroconversion after vaccine 3:1599
vaccination program 3:1593, 3:1597
at-risk 3:1600
Japan and Europe 3:1600
underdeveloped countries 3:1600
US 3:1600
vaccines
adverse effects 3:1600
contraindication during pregnancy 3:1600
live attenuated 3:1593, 3:1599
RA 27/3 3:1599
Rubella virus 3:1592–601
alphaviruses relationship 3:1596–7
antibodies 3:1599
attachment and entry 3:1594
budding 3:1596
capsid morphogenesis 3:1596
cDNA 3:1594
in cell lines 3:1593
cytopathic effects 3:1593
economic significance 3:1600
eradication possibility 3:1600
evolution 3:1596–7
genetics 3:1596–7
genome 3:1594
coding strategy 3:1594(Fig)
ORFs 3:1594
genotypes 3:1597
history 3:1592–3
host range and propagation 3:1593
infection see Rubella
intracellular replication cycle 3:1594–6
intrinsic interference 2:851
ocular target 1:525(Table)
persistence 3:1598
persistent culture 3:1593

Rubella virus (continued)
  physical properties 3:1594
  proteins
    E1 and E2 3:1593–4, 3:1595–6
    E2 Golgi retention
      signal 3:1596
    receptor 3:1594
  reinfection 3:1597
  replication 3:1594, 3:1595(Fig)
    site 3:1596, 3:1597
  serologic relationships and
    variability 3:1597
  spread 3:1597
  strains 3:1596
  structure and properties 3:1593–4
    spikes 3:1593–4
  subgenomic RNA
    synthesis 3:1595, 3:1595(Fig)
  taxonomy and
    classification 3:1593
  in thyroid 2:1085
  tissue tropism 3:1597–8
  translation 3:1594–6
  transmission 1:485(Table),
    3:1597–8
Rubeola virus *see* Measles virus
  (MV)
Rubivirus 1:261, 3:1593
  characteristics 3:1593
Rubulavirus 2:1021, 2:1130, 2:1134,
  2:1135(Fig)
  genome 2:1132
  members 2:1021
  mumps virus (MuV) 2:988
  see also Mumps virus (MuV);
    Newcastle disease virus
Rubus
  'crumbly fruit' 2:809
  raspberry bushy dwarf virus
    (RBDV) 2:811
Rubus Chinese seed-borne
  virus 2:1009(Table)
Rudiviridae 1:86, 2:1226
  characteristics 2:1226
  phage included 2:1226
Rudivirus 1:88
Rugose wood diseases,
  grapevines 3:1841
'Rule of six,' Newcastle disease
  virus replication 2:1023
Runt-deformity syndrome
  (RPS) 3:1634
Runting disease syndrome 3:1499
Rupestris stem pitting,
  grapevines 3:1841
Russian spring summer
  encephalitis 1:426, 1:429
  prevention and control 1:429
Russian spring summer encephalitis
  virus (RSSEV)
  epidemiology 1:428
  features 1:425(Table)
  genetic stability 1:427
  geographic/seasonal
    distribution 1:426
  history/discovery 1:424–6
  pathogenicity 1:428
  transmission 1:485(Table)
Ruv proteins, mechanism of
  action 3:1447(Fig)
Ryegrass cryptic virus
  (RGCV) 1:312
Ryegrass mottle virus
  (RgMV) 3:1675
Ryegrass spherical virus 1:312
ryk oncogene 3:1512
Rymoviruses, transmission and
  characteristics 3:1369, 3:1374

S

SA6 virus 2:708
SA8 *see* Herpesvirus cercopithecus
  2 (SA8)
Sabia virus 2:888(Table), 3:1988
  classification 2:887
  emerging/re-emerging
    virus 1:419(Table)
  history 2:887
Sacbrood 2:743, 2:746, 2:1272
  outbreaks 2:746
  pathology and
    epizootiology 2:746
  symptoms 2:746
Sacbrood virus (SBV) 2:744(Table),
  2:746, 2:1271–2
  vectors 2:746
Saccharomyces cerevisiae
  bromovirus mRNA
    synthesis 1:201
  killer phenomenon 3:1808, 3:1812
  killer toxin 3:1611
  RNA viruses *see* Yeast RNA
    viruses
  satellite dsRNAs 3:1611
  Ty1 and Ty3 elements *see* Ty1
    elements; Ty3 elements
Saccharomyces cerevisiae virus L
  (ScV-L) 1:616(Table)
Saccharomyces cerevisiae virus L-A
  (ScV-L-A) 3:1812
  genome 3:1809–10
  RNA replication 3:1810
Saccharomyces cerevisiae virus La
  (ScV-La) 3:1809–10
Saccharomyces cerevisiae virus
  (ScV)
  killer toxins 3:1813
  structure and composition 3:1813
Sacramento River Chinook disease
  virus (SRCDV) 3:1542
Saguaro cactus virus (SCV) 1:245
  genome 1:245
Saimiriine herpesvirus 2 *see*
  Herpesvirus saimiri 2 (HVS-2)
Saint Augustine decline 2:935
St Louis encephalitis (SLE) 1:428–9,
  3:1991
  pathology/histopathology 1:429
St Louis encephalitis virus
  (SLEV) 3:1991
  epidemiology 1:428
  features 1:425(Table)
  genetic drift 1:427
  geographic/seasonal
    distribution 1:426
  history/discovery 1:424
  host range 1:427
  topotypes 1:427
St particles 1:371
St viruses 1:373
Salinity, phage HS1 infection 1:83
Salivary gland virus *see* Human
  cytomegalovirus (HCMV)
Salivary glands
  CMV in 1:350
  mumps virus infection 2:992,
    2:993
Salmon
  Atlantic, infectious salmon
    anemia 1:564
  infectious hematopoietic necrosis
    virus (IHNV) 1:560, 3:1542
  infectious pancreatic necrosis
    virus of fish (IPNV) 1:161
  viral hemorrhagic septicemia
    virus (VHSV) 1:561
Salmonella
  ε-prophage 2:1209

Salmonella (continued)
  filamentous phage 1:547
Salmonella typhi, Vi antigen 1:138
Salmonella typhimurium
  P22 phage 3:1603
  see also P22 bacteriophage
Salmonid herpesvirus 1 (SalHV-
  1) 1:553
  genome 1:555
Salmonid herpesvirus 2 (SalHV-
  2) 1:553
Salmonid herpesviruses 1:553
San Miguel sea lion virus 1:217,
  1:218
Sanctuary sites, immune evasion
  mechanism 2:816
Sandflies
  Phlebotomus fever virus
    transmission 1:211
  vesicular stomatitis virus
    transmission 3:1992
Sandfly fever 3:1990
Sandfly fever viruses 1:211
Sap inoculation,
  closteroviruses 1:271
Sapporo virus 1:218, 1:445, 1:448,
  2:1038
  detection 2:1040
Sapporo-like viruses 2:1035
  antigenic
    relationships 2:1036(Table)
  capsid protein 2:1036
  classification 2:1036(Table)
  genome 2:1036
  genome organization 2:1038
  host range and
    propagation 2:1038
  properties 2:1036
  serologic/phylogenetic
    relationships 2:1038
  single serotype 2:1038
  see also Caliciviruses;
    Manchester virus; Norwalk-
    like viruses
Saquinavir (invirase) 1:60, 2:783,
  2:785
  structure 2:784(Fig)
α-Sarcin, rotavirus infection
  with 3:1589
Satellite cells, latent varicella-zoster
  virus infection 3:1884
Satellite maize white line mosaic
  virus (SMWLMV) 3:1610
Satellite molecules,
  nepoviruses 2:1011
Satellite nucleic acids 3:1609(Table)
  RNAs *see* Satellite RNAs
  ssDNA 3:1609(Table), 3:1611
Satellite panicum mosaic virus
  (SPMV) 3:1610
  PMV as helper 3:1610
Satellite phage 2:1094–5
Satellite RNAs 2:1311, 3:1607–15,
  3:1609(Table)
  B-type 2:1193
  categories 3:1608, 3:1609(Table)
  cucumber mosaic virus
    (CMV) 3:1612
  cucumoviruses *see*
    Cucumoviruses
  dependence on helper
    viruses 3:1614
  dsRNA 3:1611
  encoding killer toxin 3:1808,
    3:1812
  in killer systems, M-
    dsRNA 3:1812
  Saccharomyces
    cerevisiae 3:1611
  T. vaginalis 3:1611
  totivirus requirement 3:1808

Satellite RNAs (continued)
  effects on helper virus and
    host 3:1611–13
  general properties 3:1611–13
  grapevine fanleaf virus
    (GFLV) 3:1611
  hammerhead ribozymes 3:1556
  hepatitis delta virus 1:664
  history 3:1608
  L-A virus *see* M satellite viruses
  luteoviruses and
    poleroviruses 2:904
  origin 3:1615
  pea enation mosaic virus
    (PEMV) 2:1193
  plant disease severity reduced
    by 2:1306
  replication 3:1555–6, 3:1614–15,
    3:1679
  rolling circle
    mechanism 3:1614–15
  ribozyme structures 3:1615
  self-cleavage 3:1554(Table),
    3:1615
  sobemoviruses 3:1676–7
  ssRNAs 3:1608, 3:1611–13
    effect on symptoms by helper
      virus 3:1612
    ORFs 3:1611
    subgroup I
      (large) 3:1609(Table),
      3:1611–12
    subgroup II (small
      linear) 3:1609(Table), 3:1612
    subgroup III (small
      circular) 3:1609(Table),
      3:1612–13
  structure 3:1614–15
    secondary 3:1614
  tobacco ringspot virus (TRSV)
    see Tobacco ringspot virus
    (TRSV)
  tombusviruses 3:1797
  transgenic plant resistance 2:1311
  tRNA-like structure 3:1614
  turnip crinkle virus (TCV) 3:1607
  types/examples 3:1608,
    3:1609(Table), 3:1611–14
  umbraviruses 3:1857
  viroid-like 3:1930, 3:1931(Fig),
    3:1937
  see also Satellite viruses
Satellite St Augustine decline virus
  (SSADV) 3:1610
Satellite tobacco mosaic virus
  (STMV) 3:1783
Satellite tobacco necrosis virus
  (STNV) *see* Tobacco necrosis
  virus (TNV)
Satellite tobacco ringspot virus
  (sTRSV) 3:1556, 3:1557–8
Satellite viruses 3:1607–8, 3:1607–
  15, 3:1744(Table)
  categories 3:1608
  classification 3:1608
  control strategies 3:1615
  effects on helper virus and
    host 3:1610
  evolution and origins 3:1615
  general properties 3:1610
  history 3:1608
  P4 bacteriophage as
    prototype 2:1094
  RNA sizes 3:1608(Table)
  sequence variation 3:1615
  subgroup I 3:1610
  subgroup II 3:1610
  tobacco necrosis virus (TNV) *see*
    Tobacco necrosis virus
    (TNV)
  viruses included 3:1608(Table),
    3:1610

Satellite-related agents 3:1608, 3:1610(Table), 3:1613–14
  hepatitis delta virus 3:1613–14
  satellite-like ssRNAs 3:1613
Satsuma dwarf virus (SDV) 2:1009(Table)
Scab *see* Parapoxviruses, infection
Scabby mouth *see* Orf virus
Scale mites 3:1840
Scarab beetle pests, biological control by *Entomopoxvirinae* 2:845
Schefflera ringspot virus (SRV) 2:1296
Schizophrenia, Borna disease virus association 1:169
Sciatic nerves, Marek's disease 2:946(Fig)
SCID mice, reovirus infection 3:1458
Scorpion toxins, similarity to KP4 killer toxins 3:1814
Scrapie 2:1018, 3:1388
  background 3:1402
  development 3:1396
  incidence (UK) 3:1396
  prion causing 3:1402
  prion concept 3:1402
  see also Prion diseases
Scrophularia mottle virus 3:1850
Sea lions, San Miguel virus 1:217, 1:218
sea oncogene 3:1514–15
Seabirds, tick-borne encephalitis viruses 1:431, 1:433(Table), 1:434
Sealpox virus 2:1141
Seals
  distemper-like disease 3:1560
  phocid distemper virus 3:1562, 3:1565–6
Seasonal distribution, respiratory tract infections 3:1488
Seed transmission
  alfalfa mosaic virus (AMV) 1:43
  badnaviruses 2:1299
  ilarviruses 1:43
  nepoviruses 2:1012
  pecluviruses 2:1197
  potexviruses 3:1364
  potyviruses 3:1369
  tobraviruses 3:1788
  tombusviruses 3:1792
Selection equilibria, quasispecies and 3:1431
Self proteins, autoimmunity mechanism 1:109
Self-cleavage reactions
  in RNA replication 3:1555
  RNAs involved 3:1552(Table)
  satellite RNAs 3:1554(Table)
  types *see* Ribozymes
  viroids 3:1554(Table), 3:1556
Self-sustaining sequence replication (3SR) 1:392, 1:393
Semipersistent viruses 3:1900
Semliki Forest virus (SFV) 3:1570, 3:1656–63, 3:1994
  apoptosis promotion 1:76
  assembly 3:1661
  capsid, RNA encoding 3:1660–1
  CNS infection and viremia 2:1179
  defective interfering particles 3:1662
  E2 protein 3:1661
  epitopes 3:1662
  evolution 3:1662
  genetics 3:1662
  genome 3:1657, 3:1660(Fig)
  geographic/seasonal distribution 3:1657

Semliki Forest virus (SFV) (*continued*)
  history 3:1656–7
  host range and propagation 3:1657
  infection
    immune response 3:1662
    pathology/histopathology 3:1661–2
  molecular biology 3:1658–61
  mutants 3:1662
  mutation frequency 3:1662
  nsP1-3 polyprotein 3:1659–60
  proteins 3:1657–8, 3:1659(Table)
    sizes and functions 3:1659(Table)
  recombination 3:1662
  replication 3:1658–61
    in mosquito 3:1662
  structure and properties 3:1657–8, 3:1661
    spikes 3:1657
  taxonomy and classification 3:1657
  tissue culture 3:1661–2
  transcription 3:1659–60
  translation 3:1659
  as vectors 3:1662, 3:1891
Sendai virus 2:1130, 2:1139, 3:1616–21
  assembly and release 3:1618
  attachment and entry 3:1617
  budding 3:1618, 3:1620
  cDNA 3:1616
  cell fusion 3:1619
  cytopathology 3:1618–19
  epidemiology 3:1619
  F glycoprotein 3:1617
    cleavage 3:1617–18, 3:1618(Fig), 3:1620
    pathogenicity 3:1620
    precursor 3:1617–18
  genome 3:1616–17, 3:1617(Fig)
  geographic distribution 3:1619
  history 3:1616
  HN glycoprotein 2:1131, 3:1616, 3:1617
    antigenic epitopes 3:1621
    precursor 3:1617
  host range and propagation 3:1619
  infection
    clinical features 3:1620
    immune response 3:1621
    mice 3:1620
    newborn/suckling mice 3:1619
    pathology/histopathology 3:1620
    prevention and control 3:1621
  infection-free mice 3:1621
  interferon induction 3:1621
  mRNA 3:1617
  pantropic mutant 3:1620
  parainfluenza virus 1 (PIV-1) relationship 2:1132
  pathogenicity 3:1620
  pneumotropism 3:1619, 3:1620
  post-translational processing 3:1617–18
  proteins 3:1616
    NP 3:1616, 3:1619
  replication 3:1617
    site 3:1619
  RNA replication 3:1618
  serologic relationship and variability 3:1619
  structure and properties 2:1136(Fig), 3:1616–17
  taxonomy and classification 3:1616
  transcription 3:1617

Sendai virus (*continued*)
  translation 3:1617
  transmission and tissue tropism 3:1619–20
  V protein deletion mutant 3:1620
  vaccines 3:1621
Sentinel studies 1:483
Seoul virus (SEOV) 1:210, 1:621, 3:1988
  geographic/seasonal distribution 1:626
  infection, renal involvement 2:1083(Table), 2:1084
  see also Hantaviruses
Sequence space, definition 3:1431, 3:1433(Table)
Sequiviridae 3:1622, 3:1965
  characteristics 3:1622
Sequivirus 3:1622, 3:1965
Sequiviruses 3:1622–5, 3:1623(Table)
  coat proteins 3:1623
  components (top and bottom) 3:1622
  evolution 3:1623
  genome 3:1622–3
    comparisons 3:1623(Table)
  geographic distribution 3:1623–4
  history 3:1622
  host range and propagation 3:1624
  pathogenicity 3:1624
  physical properties 3:1622
  polyprotein translation 3:1622–3
  prevention and control 3:1624–5
  proteins, sequence comparisons 3:1623
  serology 3:1623
  structure and properties 3:1622
  symptoms of infections 3:1624
  taxonomy and classification 3:1622
  transmission and tissue tropism 3:1624
  virus yields 3:1622
  viruses included 3:1622
  see also Dandelion yellow mosaic virus (DYMV); Parsnip yellow fleck virus (PYFV)
Serine proteases (granzymes) 2:818, 2:1201
Serine/threonine kinases
  akt 3:1516
  raf 3:1516–17
  ras 3:1517
Serodiagnosis
  Chikungunya (CHIK) virus 1:263
  O'Nyong nyong (ONN) virus 1:263
Seroepidemiologic studies 1:483
Serology, respiratory virus 3:1494
Seroprevalence rates 1:482
Serpins 1:74
  CmrA (cowpox virus) similarity 1:300
Serum hepatitis *see* Hepatitis B
Serum response elements (SREs), lymphoproliferative disease virus (LPDV) 2:912
Sesbania mosaic virus (SsbMV) 3:1675
Seven-membrane spanning receptors (GCR), human CMV 1:359
Sex, effect on viral infection outcome 2:1183
Sexually transmitted diseases
  emerging diseases 1:423
  hepatitis C 1:662
  molluscum contagiosum virus (MCV) 2:963

SH2 domain 3:1820
  polyomavirus T protein binding 1:1357–8
SH3 domain 3:1820
Shallot latent virus (SLV), genome 1:239
Shallot virus X (ShVX), genome 1:239
Shedding of viruses 1:483–4, 2:1183–4
  continuous 2:1175
  gastrointestinal tract 2:1177
  persistent infections 1:485
Sheep
  bluetongue 2:1056, 2:1057
  bovine leukemia virus (BLV) infection 1:196
  louping ill 1:432, 1:434
  parapoxviruses 2:1144
  pox disease *see* Sheeppox
  prion protein (PrP) gene polymorphisms 3:1392(Fig), 3:1396
  Rift Valley fever virus infection 1:210
  visna virus 1:223
Sheeppox 3:1376
  clinical features 3:1379, 3:1379(Fig)
  epidemiology 3:1378
  pathology 3:1379(Fig)
  transmission 3:1378
  see also Capripoxviruses
Shell vial centrifugation culture 1:397–8, 1:398(Fig)
Shellfish
  coxsackievirus infection prevention 1:310
  echovirus transmission 1:414
  hepatitis A virus infection 1:637
  human astrovirus (HAstV) transmission 1:107
Shiga toxins, of *E. coli see* Shiga-like toxins
Shiga-like toxins 2:1229, 2:1229–30
  classification 2:1229
  operons encoding 2:1229–30
  Stx1 and Stx2 2:1229–30
  pathogenic roles 2:1230
  prototype converting phage 2:1230
  SLT 2:1229
  structure 2:1230
  uptake and mechanism of action 2:1230
Shigella, D20 phage 3:1701
Shigella dysenteriae, Shiga toxin (Stx) 2:1229
Shine–Dalgarno sequences
  bacteriophage φ29 1:120
  Halophage φH 1:82
Shinga toxin, dysentery pathogenesis 2:1230
Shingles *see* Herpes zoster
'Shipping fever' 2:1134
Shock
  endotoxin-induced 1:341
  hypovolemic *see* Hypovolemic shock
Shope fibroma virus (SFV)
  genome 3:1383
  history 3:1381
  symptoms of infection 3:1385
Shope papillomavirus 2:1121
Short interspersed elements (SINEs) 1:437, 1:438(Table)
Shrimp viruses 3:1625–35
  baculoviruses
    non-occluded 3:1632
    occluded 3:1630–2
  control and prevention 3:1626–7
  detection and diagnosis 3:1627

Shrimp viruses (continued)
  economic significance 3:1632
  general features 3:1625–7
  growth and assay 3:1627
  host range 3:1625–6
  infection, severity 3:1626
  Picornaviridae 3:1629–30
  properties 3:1627–35
    DNA viruses 3:1630–5
    RNA viruses 3:1627–30
  rhabdoviruses 3:1626(Table),
    3:1627–9
  transmission 3:1626
  virus families 3:1625
  viruses included and
    properties 3:1626(Table)
  see also Rhabdovirus of penaeid
    shrimps (RPS); *specific
    viruses*
Shrimps 3:1625
  bioassay system 3:1627
  specific-pathogen free
    (SPF) 3:1626
  see also Penaeid shrimps
Shuttle vectors 3:1888
  entomopoxviruses (EPVs)
    as 1:481
Sialic acid 1:249, 3:1921
  binding in influenza viruses 2:838
  of glycophorin A 1:231
  hemagglutinin 1:1589
  rotavirus receptor 3:1588
  as virus receptor 2:1181
Sialodacryadenitis virus of rats
  (SDAV) 1:294
Sibine fusca, biological control by
  densoviruses 1:387
Sibine fusca virus (SfDNV) 1:387,
  2:844
Sicilian virus 3:1990
Sigma factors, bacteriophage SPO1
  transcription 1:131, 3:1682
Sigma rhabdoviruses 3:1635–9
  carbon dioxide sensitivity 3:1636,
    3:1639
  culture 3:1636
  ecology 3:1639
  genome 3:1636
  history 3:1635–6
  intergenic sequences 3:1636
  morphogenesis 3:1639
  pathology 3:1636
  persistent infection 3:1637
  replication 3:1638
  resistance 3:1637
  restrictive effects of
    infections 3:1637
  in rho lines 3:1637
  serology 3:1636–7
  structure and properties 3:1636
  taxonomy and
    classification 3:1636–7
  temperature sensitive
    mutants 3:1638
  transmission 3:1637
  virus–host interactions 3:1637–9
  X protein 3:1636, 3:1639
Sigma virus of *Drosophila* 3:1635
  see also Sigma rhabdoviruses
Signal transduction
  cascade 3:1819
  hypovirus-mediated changes in
    host 2:806
  interferon–receptor
    binding 2:857–8
  intracellular molecules 3:1819–20
    see also Oncogenes
  mechanisms 3:1818–19
  plasma membrane 1:250
  Ras proteins 3:1820

Signal transduction (continued)
  through transcription
    factors 3:1820–1
    AP1 3:1820
    NF-κB 3:1820–1
  see also Transformation
Sikte waterborne virus
  (SWBV) 3:1790(Table)
  host range 3:1792
  serologic relationships 3:1792
Silkworm see *Bombyx mori*
Silkworm diseases 1:146
Simian acquired immune deficiency
  disease (SAIDS) 3:1518,
    3:1524–5, 3:1525
  clinical features 3:1525(Table)
  D type (SAIDS-D) 3:1518
  see also Retroviruses, type D
Simian adenoviruses
  phylogeny 1:19
  type 7, E1A proteins 1:28
Simian cytomegalovirus see
  Cytomegalovirus (CMV),
  animal
Simian endogenous retrovirus
  (SERV) 3:1519(Table), 3:1523
Simian enteroviruses (SEVs) 1:461
Simian foamy virus (SFV)
  env glycoprotein 3:1689
  genome 3:1687, 3:1687(Fig)
  isolates 3:1686(Table)
  propagation 3:1691
  serologic
    relationships 3:1688(Table),
    3:1691
  serotypes 3:1691
  transmission and tropism 3:1692
  see also Spumaviruses
Simian hemorrhagic fever virus
  (SHFV) 1:89
  evolution 1:93
  genome 1:90(Fig), 1:91, 1:93
  geographic/seasonal
    distribution 1:92
  host range and propagation 1:93
  immune response 1:96
  macrophage infection 1:92
  pathogenicity and clinical
    features 1:95
  taxonomy and classification 1:90
  transmission 1:94
  virulence mutants 1:93
Simian immunodeficiency viruses
  (SIV) 3:1640–6
  apoptosis promotion 1:75–6
  cell lines 3:1642
  cross-reactions 1:188
  epidemiology 3:1643
  evolution 3:1643
  future perspectives 3:1646
  genes,
    nonstructural 3:1641(Table)
  genetics 3:1642–3
  genome
    gag, *pol* and *env* genes 3:1642,
      3:1643
    long terminal repeats 3:1642
    ORFs 3:1644(Fig)
  geographic/seasonal
    distribution 3:1640–1
  history 3:1640
  host range and
    propagation 3:1640, 3:1641–2
  infection
    clinical features 3:1645
    course 3:1645
    diarrhea 3:1646
    diseases associated 3:1645
    encephalitis 3:1645, 3:1645–6
    end-stage 3:1645
    immune response 3:1646

Simian immunodeficiency viruses
  (SIV) (continued)
  infection (continued)
    opportunistic infections 3:1645,
      3:1646
    pathology/
      histopathology 3:1645–6
    prevention and control 3:1646
  inflammatory lesions 3:1646
  mutation rate 3:1643
  neoplastic diseases due to 3:1645
  nomenclature 3:1640
  pathogenicity 3:1644–5
  PBJ14 mutant 2:769
  proteins 3:1643
  provirus 3:1642
  receptor 3:1642, 3:1644
  relevance to AIDS
    research 3:1646
  replication 3:1642
  serologic relationship and
    variability 3:1643
  taxonomy and
    classification 3:1640
  tissue tropism 3:1643–4, 3:1645
  transmission 3:1641, 3:1643–4
  viremia 3:1646
Simian parvovirus (SPV) 2:1152,
  2:1154
Simian retrovirus (SRV) 3:1518
  crossreactivity and
    evolution 3:1524
  genome 3:1523
  host range 3:1523
    primates 3:1523(Table)
  infection
    clinical features 3:1525
    pathology/
      histopathology 3:1525
  serotypes 3:1518, 3:1519(Table),
    3:1524
  SRV-2, clinical features 3:1525
  transmission 3:1524
  vaccine 3:1525–6
  see also Retroviruses, type D
Simian sarcoma associated virus
  (SSAV), gibbon ape leukemia
  virus (GaLV) relationship 1:618
Simian sarcoma virus (SSV)
  fusion protein with *env* and *c-sis*
    gene products 3:1819
  gibbon ape leukemia virus
    (GaLV) relationship 1:617,
    1:618
  v-Sis protein 3:1819
Simian T-cell leukemia virus
  (STLV-1) 2:710–11
  future perspectives 2:713
  HTLV-1 relationship 2:713,
    2:789
  infection 2:712
  pathogenicity 2:711
  taxonomy and
    classification 1:191
  transmission 2:710
Simian virus 5 (SV5) 2:1130
  parainfluenza virus
    relationships 2:1132
Simian virus 40 (SV40) 2:1352,
  3:1647–56
  antigenic determinant 3:1655
  apoptosis inhibition 1:73
  assembly and release 3:1653
  attachment and entry 3:1653
  DNA, histone association 3:1648
  DNA replication 3:1652
    mechanism 3:1652
    onset 3:1652
    T-ag role 3:1652
  epidemiology 3:1655
  evolution and origin 3:1654,
    3:1654(Table)

Simian virus 40 (SV40) (continued)
  future perspectives 3:1656
  genetic map 3:1648–9,
    3:1649(Fig)
  genetics 3:1654
  genome 3:1648–9
    early and late regions 3:1649
    JC and BK viruses
      similarity 2:876
    supercoiled DNA 3:1648
  geographic/seasonal
    distribution 3:1653
  history 3:1647
  host range and
    propagation 3:1653–4
  human exposure 3:1655
  infection
    clinical features 3:1655
    immune response 3:1655–6
    pathology 3:1655
    prevention and control 3:1656
  interferon induction 3:1656
  intramolecular recombination,
    with adenovirus 1:609
  large T-ag 2:877, 3:1649, 3:1649–
    51, 3:1821
    functional domains 3:1651(Fig)
    functions 3:1649–51,
      3:1650(Table), 3:1652
    modification 3:1649
    p53 and Rb association 3:1821
    properties 3:1650(Table)
    protein complexes 3:1651
    role in transformation 3:1821
  large T-*ag* gene 3:1649
    evolution 3:1654
    sequence variation 3:1654
  as model for
    carcinogenesis 3:1647
  mRNAs 3:1652
  pathogenicity 3:1655
  persistent infections 3:1655
  physical properties 3:1647–8,
    3:1648
  plaque assay 3:1413(Fig)
  poliovirus vaccine
    contamination 3:1647,
    3:1655–6
  post-translational
    processing 3:1653
  proteins 3:1649–52
    agnoprotein LP1 3:1652, 3:1653
    capsid 3:1651
    late 3:1651–2
    nonstructural 3:1649–51
    VP1 3:1648, 3:1651
    VP1 structure 3:1949(Fig)
    VP2 and VP3 3:1652
  public health risks 3:1647
  receptors 3:1653
  replication 3:1652
    as minichromosome 3:1652
    overview 3:1652
    T-ag role 3:1652
  SELP (SV40 early leader
    protein) 2:877
  serologic relationships and
    variability 3:1655
  single serotype 3:1655
  small t-ag 3:1649
  structure and properties 3:1647–
    8, 3:1648(Table)
    icosahedral symmetry 3:1647–8
  taxonomy and
    classification 3:1647
  tissue culture 3:1654
  transcription 3:1652, 3:1652–3
    early 3:1652–3
    late 3:1653
  transformation by 3:1821
  translation 3:1653

Simian virus 40 (SV40) (continued)
  transmission and tissue
    tropism 3:1655
  tumorigenic potential 3:1654
  tumors 3:1655, 3:1656
Simian viruses, varicella-zoster
  virus (VSV)-related 3:1873
Simplexvirus 2:677, 2:714
Sin Nombre virus 1:210, 1:621,
  3:1988
  related viruses 1:210
  transmission 1:485(Table)
Sinc gene 3:1402
Sindbis (SIN) virus 1:502, 1:503,
  3:1656–63, 3:1989–90
  apoptosis promotion 1:76
  assembly 3:1661
  attachment and entry 3:1658–9
  capsid, RNA encoding 3:1660–1
  core protein, tertiary
    structure 3:1955–6,
    3:1955(Fig)
  defective interfering
    particles 3:1662
  E2 protein 3:1662
  epitopes 3:1662
  evolution 3:1662
  genetics 3:1662
  genome 3:1657, 3:1660(Fig)
  geographic/seasonal
    distribution 3:1657
  history 3:1656–7
  host range and
    propagation 3:1657
  infection
    immune response 3:1662
    pathology/
      histopathology 3:1661–2
  molecular biology 3:1658–61
  mutants 3:1662
  mutation frequency 3:1662
  Nsp1 protein 3:323
  nsP1-3 polyprotein 3:1659–60
  pathogenicity 3:1661
  proteins 1:262, 1:322, 3:1657–8,
    3:1659(Table)
    sizes and
      functions 3:1659(Table)
  receptor 3:1658
  recombination 3:1662
  replication 3:1658–61
    in mosquito 3:1662
  structure and properties 3:1657–
    8, 3:1658(Fig), 3:1661
  spikes 3:1657, 3:1658(Fig)
  taxonomy and
    classification 3:1657
  tissue culture 3:1661–2
  transcription 3:1659–60
  translation 3:1659
  as vectors 3:1662, 3:1891
Sindbis-like phytoviruses 1:242
SINEs (Short interspersed
  elements) 1:437, 1:438(Table)
Sinus histiocytosis with massive
  lymphadenopathy
  (SHML) 2:702
Sinusitis 3:1492
Siphoviridae 1:82, 1:83, 1:281–5,
  1:325, 2:1223, 2:1224–5
  characteristics 2:1224–5, 3:1716–
    17
  phage included 2:1224–5
  T5-like phage 3:1716–22
SIRV (*Sulfolobus islandicus* rod
  shaped virus) 1:78(Fig), 1:88
sis oncogene 3:1511
Sixth disease 2:701
SJL mice, Theiler's mouse
  encephalomyelitis virus
  (TMEV) susceptibility 2:756

SJL/J mice
  autoimmunity model 1:111
  experimental autoimmune
    encephalomyelitis
    (EAE) 1:111
SKI genes 3:1812
  yeast 3:1977
ski oncogene 3:1511
Skin
  barrier to viruses 2:1176
  capripoxvirus infections 3:1380
  coxsackievirus infection 1:308
  hemorrhage, dengue viruses
    causing 1:381
  HSV-1 infection 2:678, 2:680–1
  infections 2:1176
  murine CMV infection 1:367
  rash *see* Rash
  virus entry 2:1176
Skin cancer 3:1846–7
  HPVs causing 2:1110
  molluscum contagiosum virus
    causing 2:960
  see also Squamous cell
    carcinoma
'Slapped cheek' rash 2:1153, 2:1154
'Slippery sequence,'
  heptanucleotide,
  astroviruses 1:105
Sloan–Kettering virus (SKV),
  oncogene 3:1511
Slow paralysis virus
  (SPV) 2:744(Table), 2:747,
  2:1272
Slow virus infections 2:1018–20
Small round structureless viruses
  (SRSV) 1:445
Small round-structured viruses
  (SRSVs) 2:1035
Smallpox
  antibody response 3:1671
  clinical features 3:1671
  deaths 1:298
  eradication 2:723, 3:1861, 3:1865
  eradication campaign 3:1669
    success 3:1671
  immune response 3:1671
  incubation period 3:1670, 3:1671
  last case 3:1669
  natural infections 3:1670
  outbreaks 3:1670
    control 3:1671
  pathology/histopathology 3:1671
  prevention/control 3:1671
  prognosis 3:1671
  rabbitpox virus as animal
    model 2:980
  routine 3:1671
  vaccination 1:528, 3:1671
  vaccine 1:298, 2:823, 3:1869
    administration
      techniques 3:1870
    clinical effects 3:1871
    complications 3:1871
    future 3:1871–2, 3:1872
    history 3:1861, 3:1865
    immune response 3:1871
    pathology and
      histopathology 3:1871
    safety 3:1861, 3:1870–1
    see also Vaccinia virus
Smallpox (variola) virus 3:1668–72,
  3:1865, 3:1870
  alastrim strain 3:1669
  epidemiology 3:1670
  evolution 3:1670
  eye infections 1:528
  future perspectives 3:1671–2
  genetics 3:1669
  genome
    sequence 3:1669

Smallpox (variola) virus
  (continued)
  genome (continued)
    vaccinia virus
      comparisons 3:1669
  geographic/seasonal
    distribution 3:1669
  history 3:1668
  host range and
    propagation 3:1669
  infection *see* Smallpox
  laboratory stocks 3:1669, 3:1672
  monkeypox virus as
    progenitor 3:1673
  ocular target 1:527(Table)
  recombination 3:1669
  serologic relationships and
    variability 3:1670
  structure and properties 3:1669
  taxonomy and
    classification 3:1668–9
  transmission 3:1669, 3:1670
  variola major 1:419, 3:1669,
    3:1670
  variola minor 1:419, 3:1670,
    3:1671
SMEDI enteroviruses 1:467
SMEDI (stillbirths, mummification,
  embryonic death and infertility)
  syndrome 1:466, 2:1168
  clinical features 1:466
  geographic distribution 2:1171
Smith, W.H. 2:729
SNDV (*Sulfolobus newzealandicus*
  droplet-formed
  virus) 1:78(Fig), 1:88
Sneeze, aerosol transmission of
  viruses 3:1488
Snow Mountain agent (SMA) 1:445
  diarrhea outbreaks 1:445
Snow Mountain virus 2:1038
  detection 2:1040
Snowshoe hare (SSH) virus 3:1991
Sobemovirus 3:1674
Sobemoviruses 3:1674–80
  assembly 3:1679
  capsid organization 3:1676
  coat protein,
    relationships 3:1678(Fig)
  control 3:1680
  epidemiology 3:1680
  evolution 2:938
  experimental host range 3:1677
  future perspectives 3:1680
  gene expression
    strategies 3:1678–9
  genome 3:1676
    ORFs 3:1678
    organization 3:1678(Fig)
  geographic distribution 3:1675,
    3:1675(Table)
  history 3:1674
  in vivo distribution and
    cytopathology 3:1679
  infection process 3:1677–8
  natural hosts and vectors 3:1675,
    3:1675(Table)
  replication 3:1678–9
  satellite RNAs 3:1554(Table),
    3:1676–7
  serology 3:1679–80
  stabilizing interactions 3:1676
  structure and properties 3:1675–6
  subgenomic RNAs
    (encapsidated) 3:1676–7
  symptomatology 3:1677
  taxonomy and
    classification 3:1674–5
  transmission 3:1677
  vectors 3:1675(Table), 3:1677
  viruses included 3:1674–5

Sobemoviruses (continued)
  see also Southern bean mosaic
    virus (SBMV)
Social change, zoonotic disease
  spread and 3:1997
Soil
  bacterial counts 2:1248
  dianthovirus transmission 1:407
  energy-rich, phage counts 2:1250
  enrichment method for phage
    isolation 2:1249
  macroenvironment 2:1248
  as microbial environment 2:1248
  microenvironment 2:1248
  moisture content 2:1251
  pH 2:1250
  phage in *see* Bacteriophage
  solarization, pecluvirus
    control 2:1199
  sterilants, furoviruses
    control 1:595
  temperature 2:1250–1
  tombusviruses
    transmission 3:1792–3
Soil biocides, pecluvirus
  control 2:1199
Soil fumigants
  benyvirus control 1:159–60
  pomovirus transmission
    control 3:1363
Soil-borne wheat mosaic virus
  (SBWMV) 1:154, 1:588
  control measures 1:595
  deletion mutants 1:592
  economic significance 1:595
  genetics and replication 1:592–3
  genome structure/
    expression 1:590(Fig), 1:591
  resistant cultivars 1:595
  RNA1 and RNA2 1:591, 1:592
  transmission 3:1909
Solanaceae, cauliflower mosaic
  virus (CaMV) infection 2:1277
Solanum dulcamare yellow fleck
  virus, resistance
  mechanism 2:1305
Solanum nodiflorum mottle virus
  (SNMV) 3:1674
  host range 3:1677
Sonchus virus (SV) 3:1531
Sonchus yellow net virus
  (SYNV) 3:1531
  defective interfering
    particles 3:1536
  gene order 3:1534
  genome 3:1533(Fig), 3:1534
  intergenic 'gene-junction'
    sequences 3:1534, 3:1534(Fig)
  morphology and
    composition 3:1533(Fig),
    3:1534
  proteins 3:1534–6
    glycoprotein (G) 3:1535–6
    matrix (M) 3:1535
    nucleocapsid (N) 3:1535
    phosphoprotein (P) 3:1535
    polymerase (L) 3:1536
    sc4 3:1535
  replication 3:1537
  RNA-dependent RNA
    polymerase 3:1536
  transmission and infection 3:1539
  see also Plant rhabdoviruses
Sorghum chlorotic spot virus
  (SCSV) 1:588
SOS response 1:283
Southampton virus 2:1037
Southern bean mosaic virus
  (SBMV) 3:1674
  assembly 3:1679
  capsid 3:1676
  epidemiology and control 3:1680

Southern bean mosaic virus
(SBMV) (continued)
genome 3:1676
ORFs 3:1678
host range 3:1677
infection process 3:1677–8
properties 3:1675–6
protein subunit
structure 3:1949(Fig)
structure and
properties 3:1676(Fig), 3:1948
vectors 3:1677
see also Sobemoviruses
Sowbane mosaic virus
(SoMV) 3:1674
Sowthistle yellow vein virus
(SYVV) 3:1531
epidemiology 3:1539
transmission 3:1538, 3:1907
Soybean chlorotic mottle virus
(SoyCMV) 2:1285, 2:1289
cladogram 2:1291, 2:1291(Fig)
gene products 2:1291
genome 2:1290
geographic distribution 2:1276,
2:1289
host range 2:1290(Table)
symptoms of infections 2:1276,
2:1289
transcription 2:1290
transmission 2:1289
see also Legume caulimoviruses
Soybean dwarf virus (SBDV) 2:902
genome organization 2:903
geographic distribution 2:903
see also Luteoviruses
Soybeans, nucleopolyhedrovirus
control of caterpillars 1:151
Sp1, MVM nonstructural protein
interaction 2:1158
Spanish influenza pandemic 2:824,
2:826
SpeA converting phage 2:1231
Special AT-rich binding protein 1
(SATB1) 2:971
Species
biological 3:1938, 3:1940
as classes 3:1938–9
concepts 3:1938–40
definitions 2:1210, 3:1940
evolutionary 3:1940
as fuzzy sets 3:1939–40
phenetic 3:1940
polythetic 3:1939
type 3:1943
virus 2:1222–3, 3:1734–49,
3:1937–43
concept 2:1051, 3:1732–4
definition 2:1222–3, 3:1938,
3:1940
demarcating criteria 3:1734
demarcation 3:1941–3,
3:1942(Table)
ecological niche
occupancy 3:1941
as polythetic class 3:1940–1
as replicating lineage 3:1941
versus quasi-species 3:1941
Species barriers, viruses
crossing 2:707
Spherical viruses see Icosahedral
viruses
Spheroidin 1:475, 1:476
gene 1:476
propagation 1:475
Spheroplasts, transfection by T5-
like phage 3:1721
Spi-1 factor 1:498
Spi-B factor 1:498
Spider monkey virus see
Herpesvirus ateles 2 (HVA-2)

Spider monkeys, herpesvirus
ateles 2:714, 2:715
Spinach, closterovirus
infection 1:272
Spinach latent virus (SPLV) 1:38
genome 1:39, 1:41
structure 1:40
Spinal fluid 2:1014
Spiromicrovirus 2:1227
Spleen, Tupaia herpesvirus
tropism 3:1836
Spleen focus-forming virus
(SFFV) 2:995, 2:998
Spleen necrosis virus (SNV) 3:1496
retroviral vectors 3:1502–3
Splenic hemorrhage 2:894
Splenic necrosis, Lassa fever 2:894
Splenomegaly
LDV infection 1:95
lymphoproliferative disease of
turkeys 2:913–14, 2:913(Fig)
Spliceosomes 1:255
Splicing
plant virus vectors 3:1898
see also RNA, splicing
SPO1 phage 3:1681–5
burst size 3:1681
as cloning vehicle 3:1685
DNA replication 3:1683–4
origins 3:1683
process 3:1684
effect on host cell 3:1684
evolution 3:1681
gene action regulation 3:1682–3
sigma cascade 3:1683
sigma factors 3:1682
TF1 3:1683, 3:1684
genes 3:1681
functions 3:1681
middle 3:1682
genome 3:1681
map 3:1682(Fig)
terminal redundancy 3:1681
growth cycle 3:1681–2
history 3:1681
host shutoff 3:1684
hydroxymethyluracil in 3:1681
morphogenesis 3:1684
mutagenesis 3:1684–5
mutations
conditional lethal 3:1683
gene 28 3:1682
genes 22 and 27 3:1683
proteins 3:1681
recombination 3:1684–5
self-splicing intron 3:1681
structure and properties 3:1681
taxonomy and
classification 3:1681
transcription 3:1683
early 3:1683
late 3:1683
middle 3:1683
SPO1-like phage 2:1224
SPOD-X LC™ 2:847
Spodoptera ascovirus 1:98
genome 1:98
host range and propagation 1:100
occlusion bodies 1:102
replication 1:102
structure 1:99(Fig)
tissue tropism 1:102,
1:102(Table)
Spodoptera exigua, biological
control 2:847
Spondweni virus
group 1:433(Table)
Spongiform degeneration
Kuru 3:1401
mechanism 3:1395
Spongiform encephalopathy
diseases included 3:1398

Spongiform encephalopathy
(continued)
subacute see Kuru
see also Prion diseases
Spongospora, plant virus
transmission 3:1908
Spores
fungal partitiviruses
transmission 2:1147
furoviruses transmission 1:594–5,
1:595
hypovirus transmission 2:806–7
plant virus transmission 3:1908,
3:1909
pomovirus transmission 3:1363
resting, virus transmission 3:1908
Sporogenesis, fungal partitiviruses
transmission 2:1147
Sporulation, bacteria 2:1251
phage abundance 2:1252
'Spraing' disease 1:594
Spread of viruses 2:1178–80
factors restricting 2:1178
hematogenous 2:1014,
2:1016(Fig), 2:1178–9
local cell-to-cell 2:1178
neural 2:1014, 2:1015(Fig)
olfactory 2:1014–15
respiratory viruses 3:1488, 3:1489
through nerves 2:1179–80
tropism and 2:1182
see also Cell-to-cell movement
Spring beauty latent virus 1:198
Spring viremia of carp
(SVC) 1:562–3
Spring viremia of carp virus
(SVCV) 1:562, 3:1543–4
disease 3:1543–4
genome 1:562
geographic/seasonal
distribution 1:562
history 1:562
host range and propagation 1:562
immune response 1:563
taxonomy and
classification 1:562
transmission and tissue
tropism 1:562
SPT genes 3:1506(Table), 3:1507
Spuma retroviruses 3:1963
Spumavirus 3:1686
characteristics 3:1686–7
Spumaviruses 3:1685–93
assembly and release 3:1690
attachment and entry 3:1690
bel-2 and bel-3 genes 3:1690
cytopathology 3:1685, 3:1690
epidemiology 3:1691
evolution 3:1691
future perspectives 3:1692–3
gag gene 3:1688, 3:1690
Gag precursor protein 3:1688
genetics 3:1691
genome 3:1687–8
prt-pol gene 3:1688
sequences 3:1687
geographic/seasonal
distribution 3:1690–1
history 3:1685–6
host range and
propagation 3:1691
in vitro cell cultures 3:1689
infection
clinical features 3:1692
immune response 3:1692
pathology/
histopathology 3:1692
prevention and control 3:1692
long terminal repeats 3:1689
natural hosts,
seronegative 3:1692
pathogenicity 3:1692

Spumaviruses (continued)
physical properties 3:1689
post-translational
processing 3:1690
proteins 3:1688–9
MA 3:1690
receptor 3:1690, 3:1693
replication 3:1693
host cell division and 3:1689
initiation 3:1689
strategy 3:1689
ribosomal frameshifting 3:1688
serologic relationship and
variability 3:1688(Table),
3:1691
structure and properties 3:1686–7
taxonomy and
classification 3:1686
transcription 3:1689–90
internal promoters (IPs) 3:1689
transactivation 3:1690, 3:1693
transgenic mice 3:1692
translation 3:1690
transmission and tissue
tropism 3:1691–2
viruses included 3:1686,
3:1686(Table)
see also Simian foamy virus
(SFV)
Squamous cell carcinoma, HPVs
causing 2:1110, 3:1845
Squamous intraepithelial lesions
(SIL), HPVs causing 2:1111,
2:1112
Squash leaf curl virus (SLCV) 1:600
transmission 3:1905
Squash mosaic virus (SqMV) 1:285,
1:290
economic importance 1:291
Squirrel fibroma virus
(SqFV) 3:1383
Squirrel monkey retrovirus
(SMRV) 3:1518, 3:1519(Table),
3:1523
proteins 3:1520
Squirrel monkeys, herpesvirus
saimiri 2:714
Squirrels, subcutaneous
fibromatosis 3:1383
src oncogene 3:1514
Src protein 3:1819–20
SH2 and SH3 domains 3:1820
Src superfamily 3:1514
polyomavirus T protein
binding 2:1357–8
SSV1 virus 1:77, 1:86–8, 1:88
coat proteins 1:86, 1:88
genome 1:86, 1:87(Fig), 1:88
integration and integrase 1:86
map 1:87(Fig)
organization 1:86–7, 1:87(Fig)
hosts 1:86
lambdoid phage similarity 1:88
morphology 1:78(Fig)
spindle-shaped virus 1:86
'sunflowers' and 'virus-
rosettes' 1:86
transcript T_{ind} 1:87–8, 1:88
transcription and
transcripts 1:87–8
'virus membrane islands' 1:88
Staining techniques
electron microscopy 1:402
viruses, light microscopy 1:400
Staphylococcus aureus
enterotoxins SEA and SEE 2:1231
phage conversion 2:1231
pyrogenic exotoxins see
Pyrogenic toxins
STAT1 and STAT2 2:860
Stavudine (d4T) 1:59, 2:779
'Stealth virus' 1:357

Stem cells, genetic alteration in HIV therapy 1:61
Stem pitting 1:272
Stigonematales 1:325(Table)
Stillbirth
  animal enteroviruses causing 1:466
  echoviruses causing 1:416
STLV-III *see* Simian immunodeficiency viruses (SIV)
Stomach, acidity 2:1177
Strain, virus 2:1221
  definition 1:3
Strand displacement amplification (SDA) 1:392, 1:393
Stratum germinativum, lesions due to VSV 3:1918
Strawberry crinkle virus (SCV) 3:1531
  control 3:1540
  transmission 3:1538–9
Strawberry latent ringspot virus (SLRV) 1:534, 2:1009(Table)
  satellite RNA 3:1611
Strawberry mild yellow edge-associated potexvirus (SMYEAV), genome 3:1366
Strawberry vein banding virus (SVBV) 2:1276
  economic significance 2:1280
  transmission 2:1278
Streptavidin 1:392
Streptococcus pneumoniae, DpnI 2:761
Streptococcus pyogenes
  phage conversion for exotoxin A (SpeA) 2:1231
  pyrogenic exotoxins *see* Pyrogenic toxins
Streptococcus thermophilus 2:1253
Streptococcus thermophilus, phage 2:1253–62
  characteristics 2:1256(Table)
  deletions 2:1261
  diversity 2:1260–1
  ecology 2:1254
  evolution 2:1261
  genes 2:1256(Table)
  industrial background 2:1253–4
  lysis cassette 2:1259
  lysogeny module 2:1258–9
  mutations 2:1260
  replication origin 2:1260
  resistance mechanisms 2:1260
  structural gene cluster 2:1260
  temperate phage 2:1258
    cos-site phage φSfi21 2:1258
      genomics 2:1258
    pac-site ψO1205 2:1258
  virulent phage
    classification 2:1254–6
    genomics 2:1256–8
    lytic group I *cos*-site phage 2:1256
    lytic group II *pac*-site phage 2:1256
    lytic groups I and II 2:1254
Streptomycete phage
  half-life in soil 2:1250
  phage–host interactions 2:1251
Streptomycetes, phage interactions in soil 2:1252–3
Streptozotocin 2:1080
Stress, abiotic/biotic, economic significance of virus diseases 2:1323
Stress fibers *see* Microfilaments
Striped jack nervous necrosis virus (SJNNV) 2:1026
  economic significance 2:1031

Structure of viruses 3:1943–6, 3:1946–56
  architecture 3:1943
  atomic *see* Atomic structure
  determination methods 3:1943–4
  dimensions 3:1956
  helical 3:1943
  icosahedral 3:1943
  principles
    complex structures 3:1956
    helical rods 3:1946–7
    icosahedral capsids 3:1947–55
    quasi-equivalence 3:1948–51, 3:1951(Fig)
    spherical viruses 3:1947–55
    subunit tertiary structure 3:1949(Fig), 3:1955–6
  symmetric virions 3:1946
  see also Icosahedral symmetry
Stunting
  phytoreoviruses causing 2:1266
  in viroid infections 3:1932, 3:1933(Fig)
Sturgeon adenovirus 1:567–8
'Stuttering,' VSV replication 3:1475
Styloviridae 1:330
Subacute sclerosing panencephalitis (SSPE) 1:374, 2:955, 2:957, 2:1018–19
  clinical features 2:1018–19
  course 2:957
  ocular abnormalities 1:524
  pathology 2:957
Subclinical infections 1:484
Subconjunctival hemorrhage 1:472
Subterranean clover mottle virus (SCMoV) 3:1674
  host range 3:1677
  see also Sobemoviruses
Subterranean clover red leaf virus (SCRLV) 2:902
  geographic distribution 2:903
Sudan, sheeppox and goatpox 3:1378
Sudden infant death syndrome (SIDS) 3:1493
Sugarbeet
  beet necrotic yellow vein virus (BNYVV) infection 1:158
    importance 1:155–6
  crop failure due to virus disease 2:1321
  rhizomania 1:155, 1:158
    occurrences 1:155(Table)
  virus vector control 2:1325
Sugarcane, crop growth reduction 2:1321
Sugarcane bacilliform virus (ScBV) 2:1296
  geographic distribution 2:1298
  structure 2:1296(Fig)
  see also Badnaviruses
Sugarcane streak virus (SSV), genome structure 1:597
Suipoxvirus 3:1381–8
  characteristics 3:1383
  members 3:1382(Table)
  pathogenic mechanisms 3:1384
  taxonomy and classification 3:1383
Suipoxvirus 3:1383
  DNA replication 3:1384
  evolution 3:1385
  future perspectives 3:1387–8
  genetic variability 3:1385
  genome 3:1383–4
    terminal inverted repeat (TIR) 3:1383
  geographic/seasonal distribution 3:1384
  history 3:1381–3

Suipoxvirus (*continued*)
  host range and propagation 3:1384–5
  infection
    clinical features 3:1386
    immune response 3:1387
    pathology/histopathology 3:1386–7
    prevention and control 3:1387
  pathogenicity 3:1385–6
  proteins 3:1383–4
  structure and properties 3:1383
  transcription and translation 3:1384
  transmission and tissue tropism 3:1385
  see also Swinepox virus (SPV)
Sulfolobus 1:86
  transformation system absence 1:89
  viruses 1:86–8, 1:88
Sulfolobus islandicus rod shaped virus (SIRV) 1:78(Fig), 1:88
Sulfolobus newzealandicus droplet-formed virus (SNDV) 1:78(Fig), 1:88
Sulfolobus shibatae strain B12 1:86
Sulfolobus virus (SNDV) 2:1226
Sulfolobus virus SSV1 *see* SSV1
Summer grippe 1:309
Sunflower crinkle virus (SCV) 3:1856(Table)
Sunflower rugose mosaic virus 3:1856(Table)
Sunflower yellow blotch virus (SYBV) 3:1856(Table)
Sunflower yellow ringspot virus 3:1856(Table)
Sunn-hemp mosaic virus (SHMV), structure 3:1781
Sup35p 3:1405
  deletion mutants 3:1404
  in vitro propagation of [PSI] 3:1405
  overproduction 3:1405
  [PSI] as infectious form 3:1404–5
  see also [PSI]
  as translation release factor 3:1405
Superantigens
  pyrogenic toxins as 2:1231–2
  T cell activation 1:108
Superinfecting bacteriophage, immunity in lysogenic state 2:925
Superinfection 2:851
  exclusion by 2:851
  phage immunity 3:1415
Superkiller genes 3:1812
Susan McDonough feline sarcoma virus (SM-FSV) 3:1513
Susceptibility, host 3:1409
Susceptible responses, plant viruses 2:1188–90
SV40 *see* Simian virus 40 (SV40)
Swamp fever *see* Equine infectious anemia (EIA)
Sweet clover necrotic mosaic virus (SCNMV) 1:403
  capsid proteins, species homology 1:404(Table)
  features of infection 1:406
  genome properties 1:405
  geographic/seasonal distribution 1:403
  host range and propagation 1:406
  movement protein 1:407(Table)
  pathogenicity 1:408
  replicase, species homology 1:406(Table)
  strains and serologic relationship 1:407

Sweet potato sunken vein virus (SPSVV), transmission 1:272
Swimming pools, adenovirus transmission 1:5
Swine
  pseudorabies *see* Pseudorabies virus (PRV)
  vesicular stomatitis 3:1918
Swine fever *see* Hog cholera
Swine herpesvirus-1 *see* Pseudorabies virus (PRV)
Swine infertility and respiratory syndrome (SIRS) 1:89
Swine vesicular disease
  clinical features 1:467
  geographic/seasonal distribution 1:464
  pathology/histopathology 1:467
  spread and epidemiology 1:465
Swine vesicular disease virus (SVDV) 1:461
  coxsackievirus B5 similarity 1:464, 1:465
  cytopathic effects 1:464
  evolution 1:465
  genome 1:462
  immune response to 1:467
  pathogenicity 1:466
  serotype 1:465
  transmission and tissue tropism 1:466
  vaccines 1:468
  see also Enteroviruses, animal
Swinepox virus (SPV) 3:1383
  antigenic crossreactivity 3:1385
  genome 3:1383
  geographic distribution 3:1384
  immune response 3:1387
  infection
    clinical features 3:1386
    pathogenesis 3:1386, 3:1387
    replication, sites 3:1385
  see also Suipoxvirus
Sylvilagus rabbits, myxomatosis *see* Myxoma virus (MYX); Myxomatosis
Symbionin 2:906, 3:1905
Syncytium formation
  bovine immunodeficiency virus 1:187
  mumps virus (MuV) 2:991
  reticuloendotheliosis (RE) viruses 3:1499
Syncytium-forming viruses 2:775, 3:1685
  see also Spumaviruses
Synechococcus 1:325
  annual cycle in marine water 1:328, 1:328(Fig)
  carbon fixation role 1:325–30, 1:330
  cyanophage *see* Cyanophages
  resistance to cyanophage 1:328–9
  strains 1:329
Synergism, plant viruses *see* Plant viruses
Syrian hamster cells
  Ad12 abortive infection 1:7–9, 1:9
  transfection by adenovirus AD12 1:9
Systemic acquired resistance (SAR), in plants 2:1306
Systemic ectodermal and mesodermal baculovirus (SEMBV) 3:1633

T

T1-like phages 3:1701–5
  adsorption 3:1701
  capsid assembly 3:1703
  co-infection 3:1705
  complementation 3:1705
  DNA methyltransferase 3:1702
  DNA synthesis 3:1702–3
    phage genes required 3:1702
    products 3:1702
  early events in infection 3:1701–2
    resealing and proton motive force 3:1701–2
  FhuA, functions 3:1701
  fhuA gene 3:1701
  as generalized transducing phages 3:1705
  genes 3:1703
  genetic map 3:1703–4, 3:1704(Fig)
  genome 3:1701
  Grn function 3:1702
  'head-to-tail' recombination 3:1704
  host DNA degradation 3:1702, 3:1705
  host range 3:1701
  host shutoff 3:1701
  infection of lysogens 3:1705
  morphogenesis 3:1703
  mutants 3:1703–4
    head production 3:1703
    pip 3:1703
  natural history 3:1701
  pac site 3:1703, 3:1704, 3:1705
  packaging 3:1703
    heterologous DNA 3:1703
    homologous DNA 3:1703
  protein synthesis 3:1702
  receptor 3:1414
  restriction and modification 3:1704–5
  structure and properties 3:1701
  transcription 3:1702
  transduction 3:1705
    plasmids 3:1705
T1-like viruses 2:1224–5
T2 phage 3:1706
T3 phage
  AdoMet hydrolase 2:761
  discovery 3:1722
  similarity to halophage HF1 and HF2 1:82
T4-like phage 3:1706, 3:1706–16
  assembly 3:1708–10
    chaperonins 3:1709
    head 3:1709
    tail fibers 3:1709–10
    tails 3:1709
  chromosomes 3:1707
  concatemers 3:1707
  Dam methylase 3:1715
  DNA packaging 3:1706, 3:1711(Fig), 3:1714
  DNA replication 2:1218, 3:1711(Fig)
    'DNA-arrest' type 2:1218
    host functions for 3:1706
    in vitro 3:1714
    in vivo 3:1713–14
    origins and initiation 3:1706, 3:1713
    recombination-dependent 2:1218, 2:1219, 2:1220, 3:1713–14
    σ^{70}-dependent 3:1713
  DNA replication fork 2:1218
  evolution 3:1715–16

T4-like phage (*continued*)
  exclusion 3:1714–15
    phage P2 3:1715
    prr 3:1715
  future perspectives 3:1716
  gene 46/47 2:1219
  gene 59 2:1219
  gene expression, temporal control 3:1710
  genes 3:1707(Fig)
    classes 3:1710
    early (prereplicative) 3:1710
    essential 3:1715
    immediate early (IE) 3:1710
    late (post-replicative) 3:1710
    proteins encoded 3:1710
    redundant (nonessential) 3:1708, 3:1715
  genetic map 3:1707–8, 3:1707(Fig)
  genome 3:1707–8
    circular permutation 2:1218
    ORFs 3:1707–8
  heads 3:1706, 3:1709
    'giants' 3:1709
    size 3:1709
    small ('petites') 3:1709
  history 3:1706
  host DNA/mRNA degradation 3:1706
  host functions for 3:1706
  host gene acquisition 3:1446, 3:1448(Fig)
  host range 3:1708–10
  hydroxymethylcytosine (HMC) in 3:1706, 3:1715
  infection 3:1708–10
  integration of plasmid into genome 2:1219
  life cycle 3:1448(Fig)
  overview 3:1706–7
  proteins
    gp32 2:1219
    gp46/47 2:1219
  recombination 2:1218–19, 3:1711(Fig), 3:1713–14
    double-stranded breaks 2:1219
    illegitimate 3:1715–16
    in vitro 2:1218–19
    intermediates 2:1218, 3:1714
    join-copy mechanism 3:1714
    join-cut-copy mechanism 3:1714
    model 2:1218
    mutations reducing 2:1218, 2:1219
    pathways 2:1219
    replication dependence 3:1713–14
    ssDNA annealing 2:1219, 2:1220
    UvsX and UvsY proteins 2:1218–19
  restriction-modification 3:1714–15
  rho mutations 3:1712
  sigma factor gp55 3:1710
  structure 3:1706, 3:1708–10, 3:1708(Fig)
  tail fibers 3:1709–10, 3:1715
  tails 3:1706, 3:1709
  transcription 3:1710–13, 3:1711(Fig), 3:1712(Fig)
    introns 3:1713
    MotA protein 3:1711–12
    promoters 3:1710, 3:1712, 3:1712(Fig)
    RNA polymerase 3:1710, 3:1712
    timing 3:1712–13
  translation control 3:1706, 3:1713
  uvsX gene mutations 2:1220

T4-like phage (*continued*)
  UvsX protein 2:1219
  UvsY protein 2:1218, 2:1219
  UvxX protein 2:1218
T4-like viruses, characteristics 2:1224
T5-like phage 3:1716–22
  abortive infection in ColIb host 3:1720–1
  attachment 3:1718
  classification 3:1716–17
  cloning genes 3:1721
  DNA composition/structure 3:1717
  DNA replication 3:1720
    rolling circle model 3:1720
  early genes 3:1719
    proteins 3:1719
  eclipse period 3:1719
  effect on host cell metabolism 3:1719
  future perspectives 3:1721
  genetic map 3:1717(Fig), 3:1718
  genome 3:1717–18
    deletions 3:1717–18
    nicks and sequences for 3:1717
    sequences 3:1718
    terminal repetitions 3:1717, 3:1718
  head, packaging 3:1720
  host DNA degradation 3:1719
  host RNA polymerase modification 3:1720
  infection process 3:1718
    DNA transfer 3:1718
  late genes 3:1719–20
  morphogenesis 3:1720
  morphology 3:1716–17
  pre-early genes 3:1718–19
  receptor 3:1717, 3:1718
  restriction map 3:1718
  structure 3:1716–17
  tail and tail fibers 3:1716–17, 3:1718
    formation 3:1720
  transcription regulation 3:1720
  transfection 3:1721
T5-like viruses 2:1225
T6 phage 3:1706
T7-like phage 3:1722–9
  attachment 3:1722
  capsid assembly 3:1727–8
  DNA
    copy number 2:1216
    metabolism, class II genes role 3:1723
    nicks 3:1728
    terminal repeats 2:1217
  DNA ejection 3:1724, 3:1725(Fig)
    channel assembly 3:1724
  DNA replication 3:1726–7
    bidirectional 3:1727
    in vitro 3:1727
    in vivo 3:1726–7
    origins 3:1727, 3:1727(Fig)
    requirements 3:1726
    terminal repeat duplication 3:1728(Fig)
  ecology 3:1722
  endonuclease I 3:1217
  evolution 3:1722
  exclusion 3:1729
  exonuclease (gene 6) 2:1217, 2:1218
  future perspectives 3:1729
  gene 4 helicase 2:1216, 2:1217, 2:1218
  gene 6 mutation 2:1217
  gene products
    class I 3:1723
    class II 3:1723–4
    class III 3:1723–4

T7-like phage (*continued*)
  general properties 3:1722
  genes 3:1722–4
    class I 3:1722, 3:1723
    class II 3:1722, 3:1723–4
    class III 3:1722, 3:1723–4
  genetic map 3:1722–4, 3:1723(Fig)
  gp14 and gp16 functions 3:1724
  helicase/primase 2:1217
  host functions in development of 3:1728–9
  infection cycle 3:1724, 3:1725(Fig)
  lysis of host cell 3:1728
  nonpermissive hosts 3:1728
  packaging of genome 2:1217, 3:1727–8
  phage inhibiting growth of 3:1729
  procapsid 3:1727–8
  promoters 3:1722–3, 3:1724, 3:1725, 3:1726(Fig)
    class II and III 3:1725, 3:1726
    specificities 3:1726, 3:1729
  proteins 3:1724
  receptor 3:1722
  recombination 2:1216–18
    gene 6 protein 2:1217
    in vitro 2:1216
    models 2:1216, 2:1217–18
    replication coupling 2:1216
    ssDNA annealing reaction 2:1217
  RNA polymerase 3:1722
    expression systems based on 3:1729
  similarity to halophage HF1 and HF2 1:82
  ssDNA-binding protein 2:1216, 2:1217, 2:1218
  structure 3:1724
  taxonomy 3:1722
  terminators 3:1722–3
  transcription 3:1724–6
    class II and III genes 3:1725–6
    direction 3:1724
    termination 3:1724
    transcript processing 3:1725
T7-like viruses 1:450, 2:1225
T=3 viruses *see* Icosahedral symmetry
T cell leukemia *see* Adult T-cell leukemia (ATL)
T cell leukemia/lymphoma, gibbon ape leukemia virus (GaLV) causing 1:617
T cell lymphomas
  EBV-associated 1:488(Table), 1:490
  HTLV-1 discovery 2:788
  mouse mammary tumor virus (MMTV) 2:970
  reticuloendotheliosis (RE) viruses inducing 3:1500
T cell receptor (TCR) 2:814, 2:818, 2:1201
  $\alpha\beta$ 2:818
  antagonism by viruses 2:1204
  autoimmune disease association 2:756
  in autoimmunity pathogenesis 1:108
  class I molecule interaction 2:840
  cytotoxic T cells 1:69
  $\gamma\sigma$ 2:818
  peptide and MHC interactions 1:108, 1:109(Fig)
  Sag protein of mouse mammary tumor virus and 2:972, 2:972(Fig)
  superantigen binding 2:1231

T cells 2:813, 2:818, 2:840, 2:1201
  activation 2:813, 2:813–14, 2:839–40
    heat shock proteins 1:109
    by superantigens 1:108, 2:1231
  anergy, superantigens inducing 2:1231
  antigen-presenting cell interaction 1:109(Fig)
  apoptosis, HIV causing 1:75–6
  B cell activation 2:814
  Borna disease virus infection 1:171, 1:172
  CD4 and CD8 molecule expression 2:840
  CD4 cells see CD4 T cells; T cells, helper
  CD8 cells see CD8 T cells
  circulation 2:821
  congenital deficiency, respiratory virus infections 3:1491
  cytokines released 2:813, 2:819, 2:840
  cytotoxic see Cytotoxic T lymphocytes
  development 2:818
  effector 3:1862–3
  epitopes 2:838–9, 3:1863
  in feline immunodeficiency virus (FIV) infection 1:538
  helper (CD4 cells) 1:340, 2:813, 2:819, 2:840
    cytokines produced 1:340
    functions 2:819
    lymphokines released 2:819
    MHC class II restriction 2:819, 2:820, 2:841
    properties 2:813(Table)
    response to HIV 2:772
  Th1 and autoimmunity mechanism 1:110
  Th1 in caprine arthritis encephalitis syndrome 1:228
  Th1 cell protective function 3:1863
  Th1 cells 3:1862
  Th1 and Th2 1:340, 2:813–14
  Th2 cells 3:1862
  see also CD4 T cells
  immunopathology mediated by 2:821–2
  influenza virus antigenic determinants 2:839–40
  LCMV infection 2:917, 2:919
  lymphotoxic production 1:340
  memory 2:815, 2:822
    lag phase 2:822
  MHC molecule recognition 2:841
  MHC restriction see Major histocompatibility complex (MHC)
  mouse mammary tumor virus (MMTV) infection 2:968
  mumps virus tropism 2:994
  numbers 2:822
  polyclonal activation by viruses 1:108
  primary response 2:821(Fig)
  properties 2:813(Table)
  receptors 2:814
  stimulation by HTLV-2 and HTLV-1 2:803
  subclasses 2:818
  surveillance by 2:819(Fig)
  Tc1 and Tc2 cells 2:813–14, 3:1862
  transformation by HTLV-2 see Human T-cell leukemia virus type 2 (HTLV-2)
  type 1 and type 2 responses 2:813–14

T cells (continued)
  see also Cell-mediated immune response
T dsRNA 3:1978–9
T even phage 3:1706
  see also T4-like phage
T lymphocytes see T cells
'T' tropic viruses 2:775, 2:786
TAAAT transcription initiator, molluscum contagiosum virus (MCV) 2:962
Tabasco pepper, virus infections 2:1318
Tacaribe complex viruses 2:888(Table)
  classification 2:887
  evolution 2:889
  serologic relationships 2:917
Tacaribe virus 2:887, 2:888(Table)
  host range 2:889
Tamiami virus 2:887, 2:888(Table)
TAD element 3:1504
Tahyna (TAH) virus 3:1992
Talfan disease 1:466
  clinical features 1:466
  pathology/histopathology 1:467
Tamiami virus 2:887, 2:888(Table)
Tanapox virus
  epidemiology 3:1972
  evolution 3:1971
  future perspectives 3:1973
  genome 3:1971
  history 3:1971
  immune response 3:1973
  infections
    clinical features 3:1973
    pathology and histopathology 3:1973
    prevention and control 3:1973
  pathogenicity 3:1973
  proteins 3:1971
  serological relationships and variability 3:1972
  taxonomy and classification 3:1971
  transmission and tissue tropism 3:1973
  virions 3:1971
TAP molecules 2:819
TAP system 2:841
  peptide loading 2:841
Tapasin 2:819, 2:841
tat gene
  caprine arthritis encephalitis virus (CAEV) 1:224
  equine infectious anemia virus (EIAV) 1:516
TATA box 1:192
  Densovirus (Densovirinae) 1:386
  HSV promoter homology 2:688
  lymphoproliferative disease virus (LPDV) 2:912
TATAA sites in promoters 1:24
Tau protein, N protein of coronavirus JHM interaction 1:254, 1:256(Fig)
Taunton virus 2:1038
Taura syndrome (TS) 3:1629
Taura syndrome virus (TSV) 3:1629
  host range 3:1629
  structure and properties 3:1630
Tax protein see individual viruses
Taxonomy of viruses 3:1730–56, 3:1735(Table), 3:1751(Fig), 3:1937–8, 3:1939
  bacteriophage see Bacteriophage
  criteria demarcating virus taxa 3:1749(Table)
  descending hierarchies 3:1730

Taxonomy of viruses (continued)
  families and genera 2:1223, 3:1732, 3:1734, 3:1749–50, 3:1752(Fig), 3:1753(Fig), 3:1754(Fig), 3:1755(Fig)
  history 3:1730–1
  order of presentation 3:1732, 3:1735(Table)
  orders 2:1223, 3:1750
  reports 3:1731
  species see Species
  strains 2:1221
  taxa 2:1221
    descriptions 3:1750–2
  universal classification systems 3:1731, 3:1731–2, 3:1734–50
  virus descriptors 3:1733(Table)
  see also International Committee on Taxonomy of Viruses (ICTV)
TBE virus complex see Tick-borne encephalitis (TBE) virus complex
TBP (TATA binding protein) 1:26
Tc1 cells see T cells
3TC (lamivudine) 1:59
Tears and tear film, immune defense system 1:524
Teat, Orf virus infections 2:1144
Tectiviridae 2:1225
  characteristics 2:1210, 2:1225
  phage included 2:1225
  Tectivirus 2:1210
  see also Bacteriophage PRD1
Tectivirus 2:1210
  see also Bacteriophage PRD1
Tectiviruses 2:1225
Tellina virus (TV) 1:161
Tembe virus (TMEV) 2:1045(Table)
Temperate phage see Bacteriophage
Temperature, soil 2:1250–1
Tenangaja, economic significance 2:1323
Tenuivirus 3:1756
  members 3:1756
Tenuiviruses 3:1756–64
  biology 3:1756–8
  control 3:1763–4
  economic significance 3:1758
  epidemiology 3:1763–4
  gene expression strategies 3:1761–2
  genome 3:1760–1
    composition and structure 3:1760–1
    map 3:1761(Fig)
    genomic RNAs 3:1759
    organizations and proteins encoded 3:1760
    RNA1 3:1761(Fig)
    RNA2, 3 and 4 3:1761, 3:1761(Fig)
    RNA5 3:1760, 3:1761(Fig)
    sequences 3:1760
    terminal structures 3:1760, 3:1760(Fig)
  geographic/seasonal distribution 3:1757(Table), 3:1758, 3:1764
  history 3:1756
  host range 3:1756–8
  nucleic acid-based relationships 3:1762–3
  pathogen-derived engineered resistance 2:1308(Table)
  proteins
    functions 3:1761
    N (nucleocapsid) 3:1759
    noncapsid 3:1762

Tenuiviruses (continued)
  proteins (continued)
    p3 and pc4 3:1761
    p4 3:1761, 3:1762
    pc1 and pc2 3:1761
  replication, in planthoppers 3:1757
  resistance 3:1764
  ribonucleoprotein particles (RNPs) 3:1758, 3:1761(Fig)
    circular 3:1760
  serologic relationships 3:1762–3
  structure and composition 3:1758–60
  subgenomic mRNAs 3:1761
    cap snatching 3:1762
  symptomatology 3:1757(Fig)
  taxonomy and classification 3:1756
  vector transmission 3:1756–8, 3:1757(Table)
  virus–host relationships 3:1762
  see also Maize stripe virus (MSpV); Rice hoja blanca virus (RHBV); Rice stripe virus (RSV)
Tephrosia symptomless virus (TeSV) 1:245
Terminal consensus sequence, Tupaia herpesvirus 2 (THV-2) 3:1835
Terminal inverted repeats (TIRs)
  adeno-associated viruses (AAV) 3:1885
  adenoviruses 1:10, 1:13, 1:17, 1:19
  African swine fever virus (AFSV) 1:31, 1:32(Fig)
  Densovirus (Densovirinae) 1:386
  Iteravirus (Densovirinae) 1:385
  leporipoxviruses and suipoxvirus 3:1383
  molluscum contagiosum virus (MCV) 2:961
  vaccinia virus 3:1866
  see also Terminal repeats
Terminal redundancy
  badnaviruses genome 2:1297
  caulimoviruses 2:1281, 2:1284
  headful packing of phage 2:1236
  Iridoviridae genome 2:864, 2:868
  rice tungro bacilliform virus (RTBV) 2:1295
  SPO1 phage 3:1681
Terminal repeats
  HHV-6 and HHV-7 2:698
  long see Long terminal repeat (LTR)
  see also Terminal inverted repeats (TIRs)
Tertiary structure, virus subunits 3:1949(Fig), 3:1955–6
Teschen disease 1:461, 1:466
  clinical features 1:466
  geographic/seasonal distribution 1:464
  pathology/histopathology 1:467
  vaccines 1:467–8
Tetragonia expansa 1:158
  benyviruses infection 1:157
Tetrahydroimidazoles 2:781
Tetrahymena
  introns 3:1552, 3:1553–5
  self-splicing intervening sequences 3:1552, 3:1553–5
Tetraviridae 3:1764
  Betatetravirus 3:1765, 3:1765(Table)
  biological control by 2:843
  members 3:1765(Table)
  Omegatetravirus 3:1765, 3:1765(Table)

INDEX I xcvii

Tetraviridae (continued)
  Sobemovirus 3:1674
Tetraviruses 3:1764–72
  β-type 3:1765
  biological control use 3:1771
    obstacles 3:1771
  biophysical
    properties 3:1767(Table)
  capsid structure 3:1766
    Ig-like structure 3:1766
  cell culture system lacking 3:1769
  coat proteins
    assembly 3:1770
    functions 3:1770
    structure 3:1768(Fig)
  ecology 3:1771
  economic uses 3:1771–2
  future perspectives 3:1771–2
  genetic manipulation 3:1769
  genome 3:1766, 3:1768(Fig)
    β-like organization 3:1769,
      3:1769(Fig)
    RNA1 and RNA2 3:1768
    sequences 3:1768
    Ω-like organization 3:1768–9,
      3:1768(Fig)
  history 3:1764
  host range 3:1764, 3:1770
  infection
    histopathology 3:1771
    symptoms 3:1770–1
  molecular biology 3:1768–70
  mutants 3:1769
  pathobiology 3:1770–1
  physical properties 3:1765–6
  plasmid construction 3:1769
  proteins, structural 3:1765–6
  replication 3:1769–70
  serology 3:1765
  structure and properties 3:1766,
    3:1766(Fig)
  subgenomic RNA 3:1765
  taxonomy and
    classification 3:1764–5
  transgenic tobacco 3:1772,
    3:1772(Fig)
  translation, leaky scanning
    mechanism 3:1768
  transmission 3:1770–1
    vertical 3:1770
  tRNA-like structures 3:1766
  tropism 3:1771
  as viral vectors 3:1772
  virus-like particles (VLPs) 3:1770
  viruses included 3:1765(Table)
  Ω-type 3:1765
  see also *Helicoverpa armigera*
    stunt virus (HaSV)
Tf1 elements 3:1504
Tf elements 3:1505
Th1 cells see T cells, helper
Th2 cells see T cells, helper
Thailand Sacbrood virus
  (TSBV) 2:746
Theilen–Petersen feline sarcoma
  virus (TP1-FSV),
  oncogene 1:1513
Theiler's murine encephalomyelitis
  viruses (TMEV)
  apoptosis promotion 1:75
  BeAn strain 3:1774
    polyprotein 3:1774
  DA strain 3:1774
  demyelination 3:1773, 3:1778(Fig)
    DTH-mediated 3:1778(Fig),
      3:1779
    mechanisms 3:1773, 3:1778–9
  GDVII strain 3:1774
  genome 3:1774
    determinants important in
      pathogenesis 3:1775–6
  geographic distribution 3:1773

Theiler's murine encephalomyelitis
  viruses (TMEV) (continued)
  history 3:1773
  host range 3:1773
  infection 2:756
    clinical features 3:1776–7
    histopathology 3:1777
    immune response 3:1777–8
    paralytic 2:756
    pathogenesis 3:1777
  internal ribosome entry site
    (IRES) 3:1774
  lytic infection of
    oligodendrocytes 3:1777
  as multiple sclerosis
    model 3:1773, 3:1776
  neuronophagia 3:1777
  neurovirulence 3:1776
    groups 3:1776, 3:1776(Table)
    pathogenesis 3:1776
  pathogenesis 3:1776
    mapping of genomic
      determinants 3:1775–6
  persistence
    genomic determinants 3:1776
    sites 3:1777
  physical properties 3:1775
  polyprotein 3:1774–5
    cleavage 3:1775, 3:1775(Fig)
    post-translational
      processing 3:1774–5
  replication 3:1775
    in CNS cells 3:1777
  resistance genes 2:756
  serologic relationships 3:1773
  stability 3:1775
  structure
    Mengo virus
      comparisons 3:1774
    three-dimensional 3:1774
  taxonomy and
    classification 3:1773,
    3:1773(Table)
  transmission and tissue
    tropism 3:1776
Theiler's viruses 3:1773–9
  history 3:1773
  polyprotein organization 1:233
  taxonomy and
    classification 3:1773
  see also Theiler's murine
    encephalomyelitis viruses
    (TMEV)
Theiler's-like viruses 1:230
Thermophilic *Archaea* 1:76
Thermoproteus tenax 1:85, 1:88
  viruses 1:85–6, 1:85(Table)
  TTV1 1:78(Fig), 1:85–6
  TTV2 1:78(Fig)
  TTV2 and TTV3 1:85
  TTV4 1:78(Fig), 1:85–6
Thermus aquaticus (Taq) DNA
  polymerase 1:393, 1:395
3′Thiacytidine (lamivudine) 1:59
Thin sectioning 1:400(Fig)
Thioredoxin, filamentous phage
  assembly 1:551
Thistle mottle virus
  (ThMV) 2:1276
Thogovirus 2:825
Thottapalayam virus 1:621
Three-factor crosses 3:1448, 3:1449
Thrips
  control 3:1807
  Tospovirus transmission 1:211
  tospoviruses transmission 3:1806
Thrombocytopenia
  dengue virus infection 1:382
  equine infectious anemia
    (EIA) 1:520
Thymic humoral factor, in murine
  CMV infection 1:368

Thymic involution, murine CMV
  causing 1:368
Thymic tumors, feline leukemia
  viruses (FeLVs) causing 1:544,
  1:545
Thymidine kinase
  entomopoxviruses (EPVs) 1:480
  fowlpox virus 1:577
  HSV 2:693
Thymosin α₁, interferons with 1:66
Thymus, *Tupaia* herpesvirus-
  induced hyperplasia 3:1836
Thyroid, viruses affecting 2:1085
Thyroid hormone receptor α
  (THRA1) 3:1508
  as zinc-finger transcription
    factor 3:1508
Thyroiditis, acute and
  subacute 2:1085
Tibrogagan virus 3:1636
Tick(s)
  avoidance of exposure 1:436
  control 2:1060
  susceptibility to encephalitis
    viruses 1:427
  virus transmission
    African swine fever virus
      (AFSV) 1:35, 1:36
    Colorado tick fever (CTF)
      virus 3:1992
    Crimean-Congo hemorrhagic
      fever (CCHF) virus 3:1990
    emergence/re-emergence of
      diseases 1:422
    encephalitis viruses see
      Encephalitis viruses
    Nairovirus 1:211
    orbiviruses and
      coltiviruses 2:1048, 2:1054
Tick-borne encephalitis (TBE)
  viruses 1:430
  antibodies 1:436
  antigenic relationships 1:430
  antigenic variability 1:434
  capsid protein 1:430
  Central European tick-borne
    encephalitis virus 3:1992
  closely related viruses 1:434
  Eastern 1:426
  envelope E gene
    domains 1:434
    variability 1:432, 1:434
  envelope E protein 1:430, 1:431
  epidemiology 1:434–5
  evolution 1:431, 1:432(Fig)
  future perspectives 1:436–7
  genetic marker sequences 1:434
  genetics 1:432–4
  genome 1:430
    organization 1:431
  geographic distribution 1:431,
    1:432(Fig)
  host range and propagation 1:432
  infections 1:435
    clinical features 1:435–6
    epidemics 1:434
    immune response 1:436
    pathology/
      histopathology 1:436
    prevention and control 1:436
    Kyasanur Forest disease
      virus 3:1994
  nonstructural proteins 1:431
  Omsk hemorrhagic fever
    virus 3:1992
  pathogenicity 1:435
  persistence 1:436
  physical properties 1:430
  properties 1:430–1
  replication 1:431
  in seabirds 1:431, 1:434
  serologic relationships 1:434

Tick-borne encephalitis (TBE)
  viruses (continued)
  tissue tropism 1:435
  transmission 1:435
  vaccines 1:436
  viruses included 1:433(Table)
  Western 1:426
  see also Encephalitis viruses
Tick-borne viruses see Tick(s),
  virus transmission
Tiger puffer nervous necrosis virus
  (TPNNV) 2:1026
Tight junctions (zona
  occludens) 1:249, 2:1013,
  2:1179
Tipula iridescent virus
  (TIV) 2:862–3
  evolution 2:868
  genes 2:865
  inclusion bodies 2:866
  pathology 2:866(Fig)
  serology 2:866
  structure and
    properties 2:865(Fig)
  viroplasmic centers 2:867
  see also Iridoviruses
Tissue culture
  coxsackieviruses 1:305, 2:735–6
  cypoviruses 1:336
  echoviruses 1:411
  equine herpesviruses 1:509
  hepatitis E virus (HEV) 1:672
  history 2:721–2, 2:735–6
  poliovirus see Poliovirus
  vesicular stomatitis virus
    (VSV) 3:1914
Tissue tropism, of viruses 2:1180–
  3, 3:1471
  enhancers and transcriptional
    activators 2:1182
  host factors 2:1182–3
  receptors 2:1180–1
  site of entry and spread
    route 2:1182
  tissue-specific promoters and
    enhancers 2:1182
  viral attachment proteins 2:1181–
    2
Titration of viruses 3:1412–13
  infectivity assays 3:1412
  particle assays 3:1412, 3:1413
Tnt1 gene 2:1316
Tobacco
  crop losses due to TMV
    infection 2:1320(Fig), 2:1321
  hypersensitive response 2:1311
  N gene 2:1311–12
  resistance to alfalfa mosaic
    virus 1:43
  resistance to tobacco streak
    virus 1:43
  tolerance to TMV 2:1190
  transgenic 2:1312
    KP4 and KP6 killer
      toxin 3:1817
    tetravirus genes 3:1772,
      3:1772(Fig)
Tobacco bushy-top virus
  (TBTV) 3:1856(Table)
Tobacco etch virus (TEV) 2:1318,
  3:1368
  genome 3:1372, 3:1695
  homology-dependent
    resistance 2:1310
  P1/HC-Pro sequence 3:1697
  polyprotein 3:1372
  structure and
    properties 3:1370(Fig)
  see also Potyviruses
Tobacco leaf enation virus
  (TLEV) 2:1262

Tobacco mild green mosaic
     tobamovirus
     (TMGMV) 3:1783
Tobacco mosaic virus (TMV)
  antibodies expressed in 2:1313
  assembly, discovery 2:724
  atomic structure 3:1944
  biological assay for plant
     viruses 3:1780
  coat protein 2:1186
     elicitor of hypersensitive
        response 2:1186–7,
        2:1187(Fig)
     mutants and symptom
        variation 2:1188–9,
        2:1189(Fig)
  coat protein bodies 2:1189
  coat protein-mediated
     resistance 2:1309
  discovery/history 3:1780
  economic
     significance 2:1320(Fig),
     2:1321
  genes involved in
     resistance 2:1186(Table)
  history 2:719, 2:723–4
     composition/structure 2:720
  long distance movement 2:1186,
     2:1186(Table)
  mosaic response 2:1188–9
  mutants, necrosis induced
     by 2:1190
  N6 gene 2:1304, 2:1304–5
     cDNA 2:1305
  naturally occurring resistance
     gene 2:1311–12
  P1/HC-Pro region and
     synergism 3:1696, 3:1698
  replicase, elicitors of
     hypersensitive
     response 2:1187
  resistance mechanism 2:1304–5
  RNA 3:1782(Fig)
  satellite TMV (STMV) 3:1783
  strains 3:1780, 3:1782(Fig)
  structure 3:1946–7
     discovery 2:723–4
  symptoms of infection 2:1306,
     2:1306(Fig)
     development 2:1188–9
  $Tm2$ and $Tm2^2$ genes in
     resistance
     against 2:1186(Table), 2:1187
  tolerance to 2:1190
  see also Tobamoviruses
Tobacco mottle virus
     (TMoV) 3:1855, 3:1856(Table)
Tobacco necrosis virus
     (TNV) 2:1003, 3:1908(Fig)
  cell-to-cell movement 2:1005
  coat protein 2:1003, 2:1004
     deletion mutant 2:1005
     gene 2:1004, 2:1005
     synthesis 2:1005
  future perspectives 2:1007
  gene function 2:1005
  genome 2:1004–5
     absence of 5′ cap and 3′ poly(A)
        tail 2:1005
     expression 2:1005
     homologies 2:1004–5
     ORFs 2:1004
     organization 2:1004(Fig)
  genotypes 2:1003
  geographic distribution 2:1003
  as helper virus 2:1003
  history 2:724
  host range 2:1003
  infection, symptoms 2:1003
  isolates 2:1003
  proteins 2:1004
  replication strategy 2:1005–6

Tobacco necrosis virus (TNV)
     (continued)
  RNA polymerase 2:1005
  satellite viruses (STNV) 2:1003,
     2:1005, 2:1006–7, 3:1608,
     3:1610
     cap-independent
        translation 2:1006
     coat protein 3:1610
     coat protein coding
        region 2:1006
     leader and trailer 2:1007
     RNA 2:1006
     serotypes 2:1006
     stem-loop structure 2:1006
     STNV-1 2:1006
     STNV-2 2:1006
     STNV-C 2:1006
     STNV-C leader and
        trailer 2:1007
     structure and
        properties 2:1004, 3:1948
     translational enhancer domain
        (TED) 2:1006
     in STNV replication 3:1948
  structure and properties 2:1004
  subgenomic RNAs 2:1005
  TNV-A 2:1003
     proteins 2:1005
     RNA 2:1005–6
     subgenomic RNAs 2:1005
  TNV-D 2:1003, 2:1004, 2:1005
     mutants 2:1005
     replication prevention 2:1005
  translation, cap-
     independent 2:1005, 2:1006
  transmission 2:1003
     fungal zoospores
        association 2:1003
     by fungi 3:1908(Fig), 3:1909
     in vitro 3:1909
  virulence 2:1003
  see also Necroviruses
Tobacco necrotic dwarf virus
     (TNDV) 2:902
Tobacco rattle virus (TRV) 3:1784
  genome 3:1785(Fig)
  history 2:724
  symptoms of diseases 3:1787
  transmission 3:1903
  see also Tobraviruses
Tobacco ringspot virus
     (TRSV) 2:1009(Table)
  control strategies 3:1615
  economic significance 2:1323
  hairpin ribozyme 3:1557–8,
     3:1557(Fig)
  nucleic acid-mediated
     resistance 2:1311
  satellite RNA 3:1608, 3:1613
     replication 3:1614
  satellite (sTRSV) 3:1556, 3:1557–
     8
Tobacco rosette disease 3:1855,
     3:1859
Tobacco streak virus (TSV) 1:38
  2b protein 1:317
  genome 1:39, 1:41
  host range and distribution 1:39
  replication 1:42
  resistance to 1:43
  structure 1:40
  virus–host relationships 1:42
Tobacco vein distorting virus
     (TVDV) 3:1855, 3:1856(Table)
Tobacco vein mottling virus
     (TVMV) 1:1368
  genome 3:1372
Tobacco yellow dwarf virus
     (TYDV), genome
     structure 1:597

Tobacco yellow vein assistor virus
     (TYVAV) 3:1856(Table)
Tobacco yellow-vein virus
     (TYVV) 3:1856(Table)
Tobamovirus 3:1780
  benyviruses comparison 1:155
  characteristics 3:1780
  see also Tobacco mosaic virus
     (TMV)
Tobamoviruses 3:1780–3
  assembly 3:1781
  cis-acting sequences 3:1783
  coat protein 3:1780, 3:1782
     sg mRNA promoter 3:1783
  furovirus genome
     comparison 1:589(Table)
  gene expression 3:1781,
     3:1781(Fig)
  genome 3:1781–2
     ORFs 3:1781
     organization 3:1781(Fig)
  history 3:1780
  members and
     abbreviations 3:1780(Table)
  movement 3:1783
  movement protein 3:1781, 3:1782
  pathogen-derived engineered
     resistance 2:1308(Table)
  promoters 3:1781
  proteins 3:1782
  replicase complex 3:1782
  replication 3:1782–3
     proteins required 3:1782
     site 3:1783
  resistance mediated by N gene of
     tobacco 2:1311–12
  RNA, stem-loop structure 3:1780
  structure and
     composition 3:1780–1
  subgenomic mRNAs 3:1781
  taxonomy and
     classification 3:1780
  virus–host interactions 3:1782
  see also Tobacco mosaic virus
     (TMV)
Tobravirus 3:1784
  benyviruses comparison 1:155
  members 3:1784
Tobraviruses 3:1784–9
  acquisition and release by
     nematodes 3:1788
  'anomalous' isolates 3:1786
  cDNA 3:1784, 3:1786
  defective interfering (DI)
     RNAs 3:1786–7, 3:1787(Fig)
  detection and
     identification 3:1787–8
  diseases caused 3:1787–8
  economic significance 3:1787
  epidemiology 3:1788–9
  GDD box 3:1785
  genetics 3:1786–7
  genome 3:1784–6, 3:1785(Fig)
     3′ sequence homologies 3:1786
     sequence similarities 3:1785
  geographic distribution 3:1788
  host range 3:1787
  infection cycle 3:1784
  L and S particles 3:1784
  M-type infections 3:1784
  molecular biology 3:1784–6
  NM (non-multiplying)-type
     infections 3:1784
  pathogen-derived engineered
     resistance 2:1308(Table)
  prevention and control 3:1788–9
  proteins 3:1785
  pseudorecombinants 3:1786
  resistant cultivars 3:1789

Tobraviruses (continued)
  RNA1 and RNA2 3:1784,
     3:1784–6
     RNA1-encoded
        proteins 3:1784–5
     RNA2 length
        variations 3:1785–6
     RNA2-encoded
        proteins 3:1785–6
  structure and properties 3:1784
  symptomatology 3:1787
  taxonomy and
     classification 3:1784
  transmission 3:1788
     nematode 3:1788
     prevention 3:1788
     seed 3:1788
     specificity 3:1788
  viruses included 3:1784
  see also Pea early browning virus
     (PEBV); Pepper ringspot
     virus (PRV); Tobacco rattle
     virus (TRV)
Togaviridae 1:90
  Alphavirus 1:261, 1:502, 3:1570,
     3:1657
  apoptosis promotion 1:76
  border disease virus (BDV) 1:174
  bovine viral diarrhea virus
     (BVDV) 1:174
  characteristics 3:1593
  Chikungunya, O'Nyong nyong
     virus and Mayaro
     viruses 1:261–5
  classical swine fever virus
     (CSFV) 1:174
  equine encephalitis viruses 1:501–
     7
  original grouping of Alphavirus
     and Flavivirus 1:424, 1:426
  Rubivirus 3:1593
  see also individual genera/
     viruses
Togavirus 3:1593
  evolution 3:1597
Togaviruses
  detection, suckling mice 1:399
  membrane assembly 3:1925
  nonarthropod-borne 1:174
ToLCV-Aus, satellite DNA 1:601
Tolerance, to plant viruses 2:1190,
     2:1302
TolQ, R and A proteins,
     filamentous phage
     infection 1:550
Toluca-1 virus 1:469
Tomato apical stunt viroid
     (TASVd) 3:1930(Table), 3:1935
Tomato aspermy virus
     (TAV) 1:316
  classification 1:316
  geographic/seasonal
     distribution 1:316
  host range and propagation 1:316
  proteins 1:321(Table)
     comparisons 2:810(Fig)
  RNA sequences 1:317(Table)
  RNAs 1:321, 1:321(Table)
  serologic relationships and
     variability 1:318
  symptoms of infection 1:319
  transmission 1:319
  see also Cucumoviruses
Tomato black ring virus
     (TBRV) 2:1009(Table),
     3:1967(Table)
  RNA 2:1011
  satellite RNA 3:1611–12
Tomato bunchy top
     viroid 3:1930(Table)

Tomato bushy stunt virus
  (TBSV) 1:245, 3:1790(Table)
  genes involved in
    resistance 2:1186(Table)
  high resolution
    crystallography 3:1948–51
  host range 3:1792
  proteins 3:1795–6
    homology with
      dianthoviruses 1:404(Table),
      1:406(Table), 1:407(Table)
    red clover necrotic mosaic virus
      (RCNMV) homology 1:403
  structure 3:1793–4, 3:1794(Fig),
    3:1948, 3:1948–51
  see also Tombusviruses
Tomato bushy stunt virus (TBSV),
  cherry strain (TBSV-Ch) 3:1790
  coat protein 3:1796
Tomato golden mosaic virus
  (TGMV) 1:600
  genome organization/
    expression 1:600
Tomato infectious chlorosis virus
  (TICV) 1:269
  transmission 1:272
Tomato leaf curl virus (TLCV),
  satellite DNA 3:1611
Tomato leaf curl virus-Australia
  (ToLCV-Au) 1:600
Tomato mosaic virus (ToMV)
  gene-for-gene
    relationship 2:1304,
    2:1304(Table)
  replicase, inhibitors 2:1305
  resistance mechanisms
    against 2:1305
  $Tm1$ gene 2:1185, 2:1186(Table)
  Tm-2 and Tm-2^2 genes in
    tomatoes and 2:1305, 2:1306
Tomato mottle virus
  (ToMoV) 1:600
Tomato necrosis 1:319, 1:321
Tomato planta macho viroid
  (TPMVd) 3:1930(Table)
Tomato pseudo-curly top virus
  (TPCTV) 1:598
Tomato ringspot virus
  (ToRSV) 2:1009(Table)
Tomato spotted wilt virus
  (TSWV) 1:211, 3:1803
  genetics and evolution 3:1806
  homology-dependent
    resistance 2:1310
  infection 1:211–12
  serogroup and related
    viruses 3:1804–5
  transmission 3:1906
  see also Tospoviruses
Tomato top necrosis
  virus 2:1009(Table)
Tomato yellow leaf curl virus,
  transmission 3:1905
Tomato yellow leaf curl virus-India
  (TYLCV-In) 1:600
Tomato yellow leaf curl virus-
  Israel (TYLCV-Is) 1:600
Tomato yellow leaf curl virus-
  Sardinia (TYLCV-Sar) 1:600
Tomato yellow leaf curl virus-
  Thailand (TYLCV-Th) 1:600
Tomatoes
  economic significance of virus
    diseases 2:1324
  hypersensitive response and
    resistance 2:1187
  $Tm2$ and $Tm2^2$ genes 2:1187
Tombusvirus 1:243
Tombusviridae 1:243
  carmoviruses 1:243–7
  characteristics 3:1791
  dianthoviruses 1:403–9

Tombusviridae (continued)
  genera 1:243, 3:1790–1
  Machlomovirus 2:935, 2:935–9
  Necrovirus 2:1003
  phylogeny 3:1791
  relationships 1:243
  structure 1:245
  Tombusvirus 3:1789
  transmission by fungi 3:1908
  umbravirus relationships 3:1855,
    3:1857
  see also individual genera/
    viruses; Tombusviruses
Tombusvirus 1:243, 3:1789
  genome 3:1794
Tombusviruses 3:1789–98
  carmoviruses similarity 1:243
  cytopathology 3:1793
  defective interfering (DI)
    RNAs 3:1453, 3:1796–7
    formation 3:1797
    interference 3:1797
    sequences/structures in
      replication 3:1797
    structure 3:1796–7, 3:1797(Fig)
  evolution 2:938
  GDD motif 3:1795
  genome
    comparisons 3:1791(Fig)
    expression 3:1795
    leaky scanning 3:1795
    ORF1 initiation 3:1795
    ORFs 3:1792, 3:1794–5
    sequences 3:1790
    structure 3:1794–5, 3:1794(Fig)
  geographic
    distribution 3:1790(Table),
    3:1792
  host range 3:1790(Table), 3:1792
  molecular biology 3:1794–6
  multivesicular bodies
    (MVB) 3:1793, 3:1793(Fig)
  pathogen-derived engineered
    resistance 2:1308(Table)
  phylogeny 3:1791(Fig)
  proteins 3:1795–6
    coat protein 3:1794, 3:1796
    coat protein
      dendrogram 3:1792(Fig)
    comparisons 3:1791(Table)
    p19 3:1796
    p22 3:1796
    p33 3:1795–6
    p92 3:1795–6
    pX 3:1796
  replication
    minus strand 3:1795
    plus strand 3:1795
    sgRNA 3:1795
  resistant transgenic plants 3:1797
  satellite RNAs 3:1797
  serologic relationship 3:1792
  structure and properties 3:1793–4
  subgenomic RNAs
    (sgRNA) 3:1795
  symptomatology 3:1792
  taxonomy and
    classification 3:1789–91
  transmission 3:1792–3
  viruses included 3:1790,
    3:1790(Table)
  see also Cucumber necrosis virus
    (CNV); Cymbidium ringspot
    virus (CyRSV)
Tonsillar carcinoma, HPVs
  causing 3:1111(Table), 2:1112
Topoisomerase, entomopoxviruses
  (EPVs) 1:477
Topoisomerase II, African swine
  fever virus (AFSV) 1:33, 1:36
Topotypes, orbiviruses 2:1051,
  2:1053, 2:1061

Torovirus 3:1798
Toroviruses 3:1798–803
  assembly and budding 3:1800–1
  classification 3:1801
  coronaviruses relationship 3:1801
  defective interfering (DI) 3:1801
  enteric infections 1:447
  epidemiology 3:1802
  evolution 3:1801–2
  future perspectives 3:1803
  genome 3:1799
  geographic/seasonal
    distribution 3:1801
  history 3:1798
  host range and
    propagation 3:1801
  infection
    children 3:1801
    clinical features 3:1802
    of colon 1:448
    immune response 3:1803
    pathology/
      histopathology 3:1802–3
    pathogenicity 3:1802
    physical properties 3:1800
  post-translational
    processing 3:1800
  properties 3:1798–9
  proteins 3:1799
  replication 3:1800
  serologic relationships and
    variability 3:1802
  structure 3:1798
    model 3:1799(Fig)
  taxonomy and
    classification 3:1798
  transcription 3:1800
  translation 3:1800
  transmission and tissue
    tropism 3:1802
  see also Bovine torovirus (BTV);
    Equine torovirus (ETV)
Toscana virus 1:211, 3:1990
Tospovirus 1:204, 1:211–12, 3:1804
  characteristics 3:1804
  classification 3:1804
  genome 1:211
    coding strategy 1:204
  isolates 3:1804
  serogroups and
    viruses 1:206(Table), 3:1804,
    3:1804(Table)
  transmission and
    epidemiology 1:208, 1:211
  viruses included 3:1804,
    3:1804(Table)
  see also Tospoviruses
Tospoviruses 3:1803–7
  ambisense RNA 1:207
  cell-to-cell movement 3:1805
  cytopathology 3:1807
  defective interfering (DI)
    RNAs 3:1805
  economic significance 3:1807
  as emerging viruses 3:1806
  epidemiology 3:1806–7
  evolution 3:1806
  genetics 3:1806
  genome 3:1805
  geographic distribution 3:1806
  histopathology 3:1807
  history 3:1803–4
  host range and
    propagation 3:1806
  pathogen-derived engineered
    resistance 2:1309(Table)
  pathogenicity 3:1807
  prevention and control 3:1807
  proteins 1:207, 3:1805
    NSm 1:214
  replication 3:1805–6
  resistant cultivars 3:1807

Tospoviruses (continued)
  RNA replication 3:1806
  RNA segments 3:1805
    L RNA 3:1805
    M and S segments 3:1805
  serogroups 3:1804(Table)
  serologic relationships 3:1804–5
  structure and properties 3:1805
  symptomatology 3:1807
  taxonomy and
    classification 3:1804–5
  transmission 1:204, 3:1806,
    3:1806–7
  vectors 3:1806
  viruses included 3:1804(Table)
  see also Impatiens necrotic spot
    virus (INSV); Tomato
    spotted wilt virus (TSWV);
    Tospovirus
Totiviridae 3:1808, 3:1812, 3:1974
  characteristics 1:616(Table),
    3:1812
  genera 3:1808, 3:1812
  Giardiavirus 1:613–16
  members 3:1809(Table)
Totivirus 3:1808, 3:1974
  viruses included 3:1808,
    3:1809(Table)
Totiviruses 3:1808–12
  dsRNA replication 3:1810–11
  evolution 3:1816
  evolutionary
    relationships 3:1811,
    3:1811(Fig)
  fungi 3:1812
  genes 3:1812
  genome 3:1809–10
  dsRNA 3:1808
  ORFs 3:1809–10
  host range 3:1811–12
  physical properties 3:1808
  requirement for satellite dsRNA
    replication 3:1808
  RNA-dependent RNA
    polymerase 3:1809,
    3:1811(Fig), 3:1816
  structure and
    composition 3:1808–9
  taxonomy and
    classification 3:1808
  translational
    frameshifting 3:1809
  transmission 3:1811–12
  virus–host relationships 3:1812
  see also Helminthosporium
    victoriae 190S virus
    (Hv190SV); Ustilago maydis
    viruses
tox gene 2:1229
Toxic shock syndrome
  staphylococcal 2:1230
  streptococcal 2:1231
Toxic shock syndrome toxin 1
  (TSST-1) 2:1231
Toxin converting phage see
  Bacteriophage, conversion
Toxinogenicity,
  determinants 2:1228
Toxins
  diarrhoea due to 2:1177
  erythrogenic (scarlatinal) see
    Pyrogenic toxins
  phage see Bacteriophage
  phage conversion of
    bacteria 2:1228
  see also Bacteriophage
  pyrogenic see Pyrogenic toxins
Toxoplasma gondii, interferon-γ
  action 2:859
TRADD (TNFR associated-death
  protein) 1:71

INDEX

TRAFs (TNFR-associated factors) 1:71
  IAP complex with 1:71
Trans-synaptic transport, of viruses 2:1180
Transactivation
  caulimoviruses 2:1284
  HTLV-1 see Human T-cell leukemia virus type 1 (HTLV-1)
  HTLV-2 see Human T-cell leukemia virus type 2 (HTLV-2)
  legume caulimoviruses 2:1291–2
Transactivators 2:1286
  hepatitis B virus (HBV) 3:1847
Transcapsidation 1:609
Transcriptase
  Bunyaviridae 1:214
  cypoviruses 1:333, 1:336
  rotaviruses see Rotaviruses
  see also Reverse transcriptase; RNA-dependent RNA polymerase
Transcription 3:1472
  African swine fever virus (AFSV) 1:33–4
  alternative 3:1563
  see also RNA, editing
  bacteriophage 3:1414–15
  bacteriophage φ29 see Bacteriophage φ29
  bacteriophage φ6 2:1207
  bacteriophage φX174 1:275(Fig), 1:279–80
  bovine immunodeficiency virus (BIV) 1:186–7
  bovine leukemia virus (BLV) 1:192, 1:192–3
  bromoviruses 1:200
  Bunyaviridae 1:214–15, 1:215(Fig)
  'cap-snatch' mechanism 1:214
  caprine arthritis encephalitis virus (CAEV) 1:225–6
  'cascade' mechanism 1:550
  coliphage lambda 1:282
  coliphage N4 see Coliphage N4
  coronaviruses 1:293–4
  cucumoviruses 1:323
  cypoviruses 1:336
  cytomegaloviruses, animal 1:360–1
  DNA viruses 3:1477
  Drosophila melanogaster gypsy virus see *Drosophila melanogaster* gypsy virus
  entomopoxviruses (EPVs) 1:480
  equine encephalitis viruses 1:503
  equine herpesviruses 1:510–11
  equine infectious anemia virus (EIAV) 1:517
  equine torovirus (ETV) 3:1800
  filamentous phage 1:549–50
  filoviruses 2:941–2
  frog virus 3 (FV3) 1:585
  geminiviruses see Geminiviruses
  granuloviruses 1:143
  hantaviruses 1:624–5, 1:624(Fig)
  hepatitis B virus (HBV) 1:647, 1:648–9
  HIV see HIV
  HPVs see Human papillomavirus (HPV)
  HSV see Herpes simplex virus (HSV)
  HTLV-1 see Human T-cell leukemia virus type 1 (HTLV-1)
  human CMV 1:355
  Hz-1V 2:1033
  influenza viruses 2:833–4

Transcription (continued)
  internal initiation, bromoviruses 1:202
  in latent infections 2:897
  LCMV 2:922–3
  legume caulimoviruses 2:1290–1
  leporipoxviruses and suipoxvirus 3:1384
  luteoviruses 2:904
  measles virus (MV) 2:954(Fig)
  molluscum contagiosum virus (MCV) 2:962
  mouse mammary tumor virus see Mouse mammary tumor virus (MMTV)
  mumps virus (MuV) see Mumps virus (MuV)
  murine CMV 1:364
  murine leukemia viruses (MuLVs) 2:996
  Newcastle disease virus 2:1022–3
  nuclear polyhedrosis viruses (NPVs) see Nuclear polyhedrosis viruses (NPVs)
  orbiviruses 2:1072
  P1 bacteriophage 1:459
  P2 bacteriophage see P2 bacteriophage
  P22 bacteriophage 3:1604–5
  parainfluenza viruses (PIVs) 2:1132
  partitiviruses 2:1150
  parvoviruses 2:1169–71
  poleroviruses 2:904
  polyomaviruses see Polyomaviruses, murine
  primary 1:214
  prime and realign mechanism 1:214, 1:624–5
  rabies virus 3:1438
  reoviruses see Reoviruses
  respiratory syncytial virus (RSV) 3:1482–4
  retroviruses type D 3:1521
  rice tungro bacilliform virus (RTBV) 2:1295
  RNA viruses see RNA viruses
  rotaviruses see Rotaviruses
  secondary 1:214
  Semliki Forest virus (SFV) 3:1659–60
  sendai virus 3:1617
  simian virus 40 (SV40) see Simian virus 40 (SV40)
  Sindbis (SIN) virus 3:1659–60
  splicing 3:1473
    acceptor sequences in parvoviruses 2:1170
  SPO1 phage see SPO1 phage
  spumaviruses 3:1689–90
  T1-like phages 3:1702
  T4-like phages see T4-like phage
  T5-like phage 3:1720
  T7-like phage 3:1724–6
  termination signals, hantaviruses 1:625
  trans-activation by Tax 1:192, 1:194
  Ustilago maydis viruses 3:1816
  vaccinia virus 3:1867
  varicella-zoster virus 3:1882, 3:1884
  vesicular stomatitis virus (VSV) 3:1913, 3:1914
Transcription activators 2:1182
  Ogr family 2:1101
Transcription factors
  AP1 3:1820
  binding to HPV genome 2:1117
  E2F, in HPV-induced carcinogenesis 2:1119
  IκB, V-Rel complex with 3:1510

Transcription factors (continued)
  in latent infection establishment 2:899
  negatively-acting 2:1117
  NF-κB see NF-κB transcription factor
  positively-acting 2:1117
  thyroid hormone receptor α (THRA1) 3:1508
  see also Activating transcription factor (ATF)
Transcription terminators
  bacteriophage φ29 1:126–7, 1:132
  TA1 1:126
  TD1 1:126
Transcription-based amplification system (TAS) 1:392
  method 1:393
Transcription-mediated amplification (TMA) 1:392, 1:393
Transduction 2:1234–40
  abortive 2:1235, 2:1238
  'addition' type 1:135
  applications 2:1239
  bacteriophage 2:1209
  bacteriophage P1 1:460
  definition 2:1234–5
  discovery 2:1234–5
  as element of biological evolution 2:1239–40
  experimental evidence 2:1235
  fate of donor DNA
    autonomous replication 2:1238
    recombination 2:1238
  feline leukemia viruses (FeLVs) 1:544–5, 1:545(Table)
  frequencies 2:1236, 2:1238
  generalized 2:1235, 2:1236
    Bacillus subtilis phage PBS1 1:135
  specialized vs 2:1235
  mechanistic features 2:1235
  'replacement' type 1:135
  restriction-modification systems 2:1238–9
  specialized 2:1235, 2:1237
    applications 2:1239
    Bacillus subtilis phage 1:135
    generalized vs 2:1235
    host–vector studies 2:1239
    transposition as alternative source 2:1237–8
  T1-like phages 3:1705
  uptake of cellular DNA into phage 2:1235–7
    headful packaging 2:1235–6
    packaging of genomes 2:1236–7
Transfection
  Bacillus subtilis phage 1:135–6
  T5-like phage 3:1721
Transformation, by animal viruses 3:1817–22, 3:1843, 3:1960
  abortive, polyomaviruses 2:1354, 2:1355
  'Berry-Dedrick' 3:1383
  DNA tumor viruses 3:1821–2
    adenoviruses 3:1821–2
    Epstein–Barr virus 3:1822
    hepatitis B virus 3:1822
    HPV 3:1822
    SV40 3:1821
  equine herpesviruses 1:511
  future perspectives 3:1822
  herpesvirus saimiri 2 (HVS-2) 2:716
  history 3:1817
  HSV 2:684
  mutations causing 3:1819
  polyomaviruses 2:1354–5

Transformation, by animal viruses (continued)
  reticuloendotheliosis (RE) viruses 3:1500–2
  role of v-*rel* mutations 3:1500–1
  retroviruses 3:1818–21, 3:1960
    acutely transforming 3:1818
    as carcinogen 3:1818
    cell signaling 3:1818–19
    cell signaling by transcription factors 3:1820–1
    growth factors and receptors 3:1819
    human retroviruses 3:1821
    intracellular signal transduction 3:1819–20
    long latency 3:1818
    monoclonal/oligoclonal tumors 3:1818
    oncogene cooperation 3:1821
    polyclonal tumors 3:1818
    proteins involved 3:1818
    proto-oncogene activation 3:1818
    Ras proteins 3:1820
    types/mechanisms 3:1818
    v-*erbB* gene product 3:1819
    v-*sis* gene product 3:1819
    v-Src protein role 3:1819–20
  RNA viruses 3:1818
  viruses associated 3:1817–18
  see also individual viruses; Oncogenes
Transformation-associated genes, herpesviruses saimiri and ateles 2:718
Transforming growth factor β (TGFβ)
  adenovirus E1A protein interaction 1:27
  downregulation 1:27
Transforming proteins 2:897
Transfusion transmitted virus (TTV) 2:1155
Transgenes 2:1307
  post-transcriptional silencing 2:1310
Transgenic animals, papillomaviruses 2:1123
Transgenic mice 1:612–13
  autoimmunity model 1:110–11
  bovine papillomaviruses 1 (BPV-1) 2:1123
  E6 protein from HPVs 2:1120
  E7 protein from HPVs 2:1120
  LCMV genes and LCMV infection 2:925
  pim-1 proto-oncogene 2:998
  polioviruses 2:1327, 2:1335
  PrP gene mutations 3:1392, 3:1395–6
  spumaviruses 3:1692
Transgenic plants 2:1307, 2:1307–9, 2:1325
  Arabidopsis and turnip crinkle virus (TCV) 1:246, 1:247
  cauliflower 2:1280, 2:1281
  cauliflower mosaic caulimovirus 2:1188
  cucumovirus genes 1:319, 1:320
  Heliothis armigera stunt virus (HaSV) expression 2:843
  naturally occurring resistance genes 2:1311–12
  plantibodies 2:1313
  potato virus S (PVS) resistance 1:242
  potyviruses 3:1375
  recombination 3:1450
  resistance by ribosome-inactivating proteins 2:1312

Transgenic plants (continued)
  tobacco, KP4 and KP6 killer toxin 3:1817
  tombusvirus resistance 3:1797
  see also Plant resistance to viruses
Transgenic rabbits, cottontail rabbit papillomavirus (CRPV) 2:1123
Translation
  alterative initiation codons 3:1473
  animal enteroviruses 1:463
  bacteriophage φX174 1:279–80
  bovine immunodeficiency virus (BIV) 1:186–7
  bovine leukemia virus (BLV) 1:193–4
  bromoviruses 1:200
  Bunyaviridae 1:214, 1:215
  caprine arthritis encephalitis virus (CAEV) 1:225–6
  cardioviruses 1:232, 1:232–3, 1:234
  carlaviruses 1:240
  comoviruses 1:287–8
  coronaviruses 1:293–4
  cowpea mosaic virus (CPMV) 1:287–8
  cucumoviruses 1:323
  Drosophila melanogaster gypsy virus 3:1528
  equine encephalitis viruses 1:503
  equine torovirus (ETV) 3:1800
  filamentous phage 1:550
  foot-and-mouth disease viruses (FMDVs) 1:571
  frameshifting and read-through mechanisms 3:1473
  frog virus 3 (FV3) 1:585
  hantaviruses 1:625
  hepatitis A virus (HAV) 1:635
  hepatitis B virus (HBV) 1:646–7, 1:649
  herpes simplex viruses (HSV) 2:695
  host, virus-induced damage 3:1958
  human CMV 1:355–6
  influenza viruses 2:834
  leporipoxviruses and suipoxvirus 3:1384
  luteoviruses 2:904
  mumps virus (MuV) 2:990
  murine CMV 1:364
  Newcastle disease virus 2:1023
  nodaviruses 2:1029
  parainfluenza viruses (PIVs) 2:1132
  partitiviruses 2:1150
  parvoviruses 2:1169–71
  poleroviruses 2:904
  polioviruses 2:1336–7
  polyomaviruses 2:1359–60
  potexviruses 3:1367
  reoviruses see Reoviruses
  retroviruses, type D 3:1521–2
  rhinoviruses 3:1547
  rubella virus 3:1594–6
  satellite tobacco necrosis virus (STNV) 2:1006
  sendai virus 3:1617
  sequiviruses 3:1622–3
  simian virus 40 (SV40) 3:1653
  spumaviruses 3:1690
  T4-like phages 3:1706, 3:1713
  tetravirus Ω-like genome 3:1768
  tobacco necrosis virus (TNV) 2:1005
  transactivation see Transactivation
  Ty elements 3:1505

Translation (continued)
  in umbraviruses 3:1857
  Ustilago maydis viruses 3:1815–16
  vaccinia virus proteins 3:1867
  varicella-zoster virus 3:1882
  vesicular stomatitis virus (VSV) 3:1913
Translation release factor, Sup35p 3:1405
Translational enhancer domain (TED) 2:1006
Translational frameshifting see Ribosomal frameshifting
Transmissible gastroenteritis virus (TGEV) 1:294, 1:295, 1:446
Transmissible mink encephalopathy (TME) 3:1388
Transmissible spongiform encephalopathies 3:1402
  see also Prion diseases
Transmission of viruses 1:483–4, 2:1183–4
  aerosol see Aerosol transmission
  airborne, pseudorabies virus (PRV) 3:1425
  by arthropods 1:486
  biological 3:1899
  blood products 2:1184
  common patterns 1:484
  cycles 1:483
  direct contact, zoonotic viruses 3:1987
  droplet 3:1488, 3:1490
  endemic and epidemic 1:486
  fecal–oral see Fecal–oral transmission
  horizontal 1:484, 1:485(Table), 1:486
  iatrogenic, equine infectious anemia virus (EIAV) 1:519
  indirect contact, zoonotic viruses 3:1987
  mechanical see Mechanical transmission
  modes 1:484
  nosocomial see Nosocomial infections/transmission
  perpetuation of viruses see under Epidemiology of viral diseases
  plant viruses see Insect transmission; Plant viruses
  sexual 2:1183
  shedding of viruses see Shedding of viruses
  specific viruses 1:485(Table)
  'taste-tests' by insects 3:1900
  transovarial see Transovarial transmission
  transplacental see Transmission of viruses, vertical
  vertical (in utero) 1:484
    endogenous proviruses 1:439
    tetraviruses 3:1770
    zoonotic viruses 3:1987
  virus entry 1:483
  zoonotic cycles 1:486
  zoonotic viruses 3:1987
Transneural transport, of viruses 2:1180
Transovarial transmission
  Bunyaviridae 1:208
  Chandipura (CHP) virus 1:259
  cypoviruses 1:336
  iridoviruses 2:866
  St Louis encephalitis virus 1:428
  tomato yellow leaf curl virus 3:1905

Transplantation, virus infections after 3:1823–33
  EBV-associated B cell lymphomas 1:490
  emerging viral diseases associated 1:423
  hepatitis viruses 3:1829–31
    see also Hepatitis B; Hepatitis C
  herpesviruses 3:1823
    CMV see below
    EBV 3:1825–8
    HHV-6 2:702, 3:1829
    HSV 3:1828
    VZV 3:1828
    see also Epstein–barr virus (EBV); Herpes simplex virus (HSV); Human cytomegalovirus (HCMV)
  human CMV infections after 1:347, 1:349, 3:1823–5
    importance 1:344, 1:345
  immunization 3:1833
  polyomavirus 3:1831
  respiratory viruses 3:1831–2
    adenovirus 3:1832–3
    RSV 3:1831–2
Transporter associated with antigen processing (TAP) 2:1204
Transposable elements 2:981, 3:1503
  Drosophila melanogaster, Gypsy see Drosophila melanogaster gypsy virus
Transposition 2:1237
  fate of donor DNA 2:1238
  plant virus vectors 3:1898
  probability and natural limits 2:1238–9
  as sources of specialized transducing phage genome 2:1237–8
  see also Recombination of viruses; Retrotransposons; transposons
Transposition-mediated cointegration 2:1236
Transposons 2:1237, 2:1237–8
  copy, Ty elements 3:1505
  functions/actions 2:1237–8
  insertion into prophages 2:1237
  plants and fungi 3:1503
  Tn917 1:135
Traumatic herpes 2:680
Travel, emergence and re-emergence of diseases 1:422
Tree shrews 3:1834
  evolution 3:1835
  herpesviruses see Tupaia herpesviruses
  other viruses 3:1837
Tremors
  Kuru 3:1400
  Lassa fever 2:893
Triangulation number 3:1943
Triatoma virus 2:1273–4
Trichomonas vaginalis, satellite dsRNA 3:1611
Trichomonas vaginalis virus (TVV) 1:613
  characteristics/properties 1:616(Table)
Trichoplusia ascovirus 1:98
  genome 1:98
  host range and propagation 1:100
  replication 1:102
  structure 1:99(Fig)
  tissue tropism 1:102, 1:102(Table)
  variants 1:98, 1:102

Trichoplusia ni (cabbage looper) 1:98, 1:102
  cypoviruses 1:335
  granuloviruses 1:141
Trichovirus 3:1837
  splitting of genus 3:1842
  taxonomy 3:1837–8
Trichoviruses 3:1837–42
  capsid proteins (CP) 3:1839, 3:1840
  coat proteins 3:1838(Table), 3:1839
  cytopathic effects 3:1840
  diseases 3:1840–1
    control 3:1841–2
    economic significance 3:1840–1
    epidemiology 3:1841–2
  future perspectives 3:1842
  genome
    organization and expression 3:1839–40
    phylogenetic relations 3:1840
    size 3:1838(Table), 3:1839
    structure 3:1839
  geographic distribution/host range 3:1838
  history 3:1837
  host relations 3:1840
  particle structure/composition 3:1838–9
  serological relationships and variability 3:1841
  taxonomy and classification 3:1837–8
  transmission 3:1838(Table), 3:1840
Trigeminal ganglia
  HSV infection 2:682
  HSV re-activation 2:899
Trigeminal nerve, Borna disease virus infection 1:170
Triple gene block 1:239
  benyviruses 1:157
  furoviruses 1:591, 1:593
  hordeiviruses 2:750
  pecluvirus genome 2:1197
  potexviruses 3:1366, 3:1367
Tristeza 1:272, 1:273
  see also Citrus tristeza virus (CTV)
tRNA
  cleavage by RNase P 3:1553
  genes, P4 genome integration 2:1098–9
  mimicry, bromoviruses 1:201
tRNA nucleotidyl transferase, bromoviruses 1:201, 1:202
tRNA-like RNAs
  bromoviruses 1:201
  furoviruses 1:590
  satellite RNAs 3:1614
'Trojan Horse' mechanism of entry 2:1179
Tropical spastic paraparesis (TSP) 1:792–3, 2:1019–20
  clinical features 2:1019–20
Tropism see Tissue tropism
Trout
  infectious pancreatic necrosis 1:563
  viral hemorrhagic septicemia virus infection 1:561
TTV1 virus 1:85
  dsDNA genome 1:85
  genetic variability 1:85
  morphology 1:78(Fig)
  proteins 1:85
  TPX protein 1:85
TTV2 virus 1:85
  morphology 1:78(Fig)
TTV3 virus 1:85

TTV4 virus 1:85–6
  morphology 1:78(Fig)
Tulare apple mosaic virus
    (TAMV) 1:38
  host range and distribution 1:40
  virus–host relationships 1:42
Tulips
  economic significance of virus
      diseases 2:1324
  virus infections 2:1319(Fig)
Tumor necrosis factor 1
    (TNFR1) 1:70
  apoptosis pathway 1:71
  TRADD interaction 1:71
Tumor necrosis factor 2
    (TNFR2) 1:70, 1:71
  apoptosis pathway 1:70(Fig)
Tumor necrosis factor (TNF) 1:339
  interactions and functions 1:341
  leporipoxvirus homologs 1:1387
  production and sources 1:340–1
  receptors 1:341
  virus interference and immune
      evasion 2:1204
Tumor necrosis factor α (TNF-
    α) 1:340
  HHV-6 inducing 2:702
  LCMV infection 2:919
Tumor necrosis factor β (TNF-
    β) 1:340
Tumor necrosis factor (TNF)
    family 1:340–1
Tumor necrosis factor receptor
    (TNFR) 2:1204
  associated death domain protein
      (TRADD) 1:499
  associated factors (TRAFs) 1:499
  LMP-1 of EBV interaction 1:499
Tumor suppressor genes
  adenovirus oncogenesis and 1:11
  see also p53; Retinoblastoma
      gene (Rb)
Tumor vaccines 3:1888
Tumor virology, history 2:722–3
Tumor viruses, human 3:1842–9
  Burkitt's lymphoma 3:1843–4
  criteria for causal relationship
      with cancer 3:1842–3
  EBV-associated
      lymphoproliferative
      syndrome see
      Lymphoproliferative
      syndrome
  future perspectives 3:1848–9
  genital cancer 3:1845–6
  hepatocellular carcinoma 3:1847
  impact on understanding of
      transformation 3:1961
  Kaposi's sarcoma 3:1848
  latency periods 3:1849(Table)
  nasopharyngeal
      carcinoma 3:1844–5
  oncogenesis mechanisms 3:1842–
      3
  skin cancer 3:1846–7
  T-cell leukemia 3:1845
  see also specific tumors and
      viruses
Tumorigenesis
  latent infections and 2:897
  multistep-process 2:794
  see also Carcinogenesis;
      Oncogenesis
Tumors
  as clonal outgrowths of BLV-
      infected cells 1:197
  induction by viruses see
      Transformation, by animal
      viruses
  monoclonal/oligoclonal 3:1818
  polyclonal 3:1818

Tumors (continued)
  in Yabapox virus
      infections 3:1973
  see also Cancer
Tungro see Rice tungro disease
Tupaia 3:1834
Tupaia herpesvirus 1 (THV-1)
  clinical features of
      infection 3:1836
  genome 3:1834–5
  isolation 3:1834
  pathogenicity 3:1836
  proteins 3:1835
Tupaia herpesvirus 2 (THV-2)
  classification 3:1834
  genome 3:1834–5
  infections
    clinical features 3:1836
    pathology/
        histopathology 3:1836
  isolation 3:1834
  pathogenicity 3:1836
  proteins 3:1835
  terminal consensus
      sequence 3:1835
  virions 3:1834
Tupaia herpesvirus 3 (THV-3)
  genome 3:1834–5
  infections
    clinical features 3:1836
    pathology/
        histopathology 3:1836
  isolation 3:1834
  pathogenicity 3:1836
  proteins 3:1835
Tupaia herpesvirus 4 (THV-4)
  clinical features of
      infection 3:1836
  genome 3:1834–5
  pathogenicity 3:1836
Tupaia herpesviruses
    (THV) 3:1834–7
  enzymes 3:1835
  evolution 3:1835–6
  future perspectives 3:1837
  genetics 3:1835
  genome 3:1834–5
  history 3:1834
  infections
    clinical features 3:1836
    epidemiology 3:1836
    geographic/seasonal
        distribution 3:1835
    host range and virus
        propagation 3:1835
    pathology/
        histopathology 3:1836–7
  pathogenicity 3:1836
  proteins 3:1835
  serologic relations and
      variability 3:1836
  taxonomy and
      classification 3:1834
  transmission and tissue
      tropism 3:1836
  virion 3:1834
Tupaia virus 3:1636
Tupaiidae 3:1834
Turbot herpesvirus 1:553
Turkey, lymphoproliferative
    disease see Lymphoproliferative
    disease (LPD)
Turkey bluecomb coronavirus
    (TCV) 1:294
  cell culture 1:294
Turkey hemorrhagic enteritis 1:20
Turkey hepatitis virus
    (THV) 1:461, 1:467
  geographic/seasonal
      distribution 1:464
  transmission and tissue
      tropism 1:466

Turkey hepatitis virus (THV)
    (continued)
  see also Enteroviruses, animal
Turkey herpesvirus see Herpesvirus
    of turkeys (HVT)
Turkey rhinotracheitis virus
    (TRTV) 3:1479
Turnip crinkle virus (TCV) 1:243
  Arabidopsis interactions 1:246
  defective-interfering RNA 1:246
  FaFf element 1:246
  genome 1:245
  in vitro assembly 1:245
  red clover necrotic mosaic virus
      (RCNMV) homology 1:403
  replicase in RNA
      recombination 3:1451,
      3:1453(Fig)
  resistance
    Arabidopsis thaliana ecotype
        Di-0 1:247
    transgenic Arabidopsis 1:247
  satellite RNA 3:1607
  structure 1:245
  in transgenic plants 1:246, 1:247
  transmission 1:244
  see also Carmoviruses
Turnip rosette virus
    (TRoSV) 3:1674
  capsid 1676
  host range 3:1677
  properties 3:1675–6
  see also Sobemoviruses
Turnip yellow mosaic virus
    (TYMV) 3:1850
  effect on chloroplast
      structure 2:1189–90
  geographic distribution 3:1850
  structure 3:1948
  transmission 3:1853
  variability 3:1852
  virion protein 3:1851
20S RNA virus 3:1974,
    3:1974(Table), 3:1978–9
  future perspectives 3:1979
  host functions 3:1977,
      3:1977(Table)
  replication 3:1978
  T dsRNA and 3:1978–9
  W dsRNA and 3:1978–9
23S RNA virus 3:1974,
    3:1974(Table)
Two-factor crosses 3:1448, 3:1448–
    9
Twort 2:1221
  F.W. 2:720, 2:727–8
Ty1 elements 3:1504
  integration site 3:1506
  see also Ty elements
Ty3 elements 3:1504
  integration site 3:1506
  see also Ty elements
Ty5 elements 3:1504
Ty elements
  assembly process 3:1505
  DNA synthesis 3:1506
  host functions during retrotrans-
      position 3:1506(Table),
      3:1507
  reverse transcription 3:1505
  translation 3:1505
  transposition mechanism 3:1504–
      5
  transposon copy 3:1505
  virus-like particles (VLPs) 3:1505,
      3:1505–6
  as evolutionary
      vestiges 3:1506–7
  as transposition
      intermediates 3:1506–7
Ty integrase 3:1506
Tymoboxes 3:1851, 3:1853

Tymovirus 3:1850
Tymoviruses 3:1850–3
  diseases
    epidemiology 3:1853
    symptoms 3:1853
  evolution 3:1852–3, 3:1852(Fig)
  features 3:1850
  genome 3:1851
  geographic distribution 3:1850
  history 3:1850
  host ranges 3:1850
  molecular biology 3:1850–1
  overlapping protein (OP) 3:1851
  pathogen-derived engineered
      resistance 2:1309(Table)
  pathogenicity 3:1853
  prevention/control 3:1853
  proteins 3:1851
  replicase protein (RP) 3:1851,
      3:1852, 3:1853
  replication 3:1851–2
  taxonomy 3:1852–3
  transmission 3:1853
  virion protein (VP) 3:1851,
      3:1852
    phylogenetic
        relationships 3:1852,
        3:1852(Fig)
    structure 3:1851
  virions 3:1850–1
Tyrophostins 2:783
Tyrosine kinase, v-Src
    protein 3:1819–20

U

U90152 (Rescriptor,
    delavirdine) 1:60
UBC9, adenovirus E1A protein
    interaction 1:25
Ubiquitin, insertion in bovine viral
    diarrhea virus gene 1:177
Ubiquitination
  African swine fever virus (AFSV)
      proteins 1:34–5
  p53 by association with E6
      protein of HPV 2:1120
UDP-glucosyltransferase, nuclear
    polyhedrosis viruses
    (NPVs) 1:150
Uganda S virus 1:430
Ullucus C virus (UCV) 1:285, 1:290
Ultracentrifugation
  bacteriophage purification 3:1417
  plant virus isolation 3:1420
Ultraviolet radiation
  densoviruses sensitivity 1:387
  effect on cypoviruses 1:333
  multiplicity reactivation
      after 1:609
  sensitivity of viroids 3:1929
Umatilla virus
    (UMAV) 2:1045(Table)
Umbelliferae, sequiviruses 3:1622
Umbravirus 3:1855
Umbraviruses 3:1855–9
  diseases
    epidemiology 3:1858
    pathology/
        histopathology 3:1858
  evolution 3:1857
  genome 3:1855, 3:1856,
      3:1857(Fig)
  geographic distribution 3:1858
  history 3:1855
  host range/virus
      propagation 3:1858

Umbraviruses (continued)
  prevention and control 3:1859
    avoidance of infection 3:1859
    host plant resistance 3:1859
    vector control 3:1859
  properties 3:1855–6
  replication 3:1856–7
    nucleic acid 3:1856–7
    translation 3:1857
  satellite RNA 3:1857
  serology 3:1858
  taxonomy and
    classification 3:1855
  transmission 3:1858
Uncoating of viruses 1:251, 3:1408, 3:1472
  blocking by transgenic coat
    proteins 2:1309
  enveloped viruses 3:1472
  pathways 3:1922(Fig)
Universal Virus
  Classification 3:1731, 3:1731–2, 3:1734–50
Uracil biosynthesis, yeast 3:1403
Uracil DNA glycosylase
  (UDG) 1:358, 1:394
Urbanization
  emergence/re-emergence of
    diseases 1:422
  increased dengue virus
    infections 1:375, 1:379
Ure2p 3:1403, 3:1404(Fig)
  C-terminal domain 3:1403
  overproduction 3:1403
  prion domain 3:1403
    mechanism of prion
      generation 3:1404
    structure 3:1403
  as transcription regulatory 3:1403
  [URE3] as infectious form 3:1403
  [URE3] 3:1403, 3:1405(Fig)
    as infectious form of
      Ure2p 3:1403
  as prion
    criteria for 3:1403
    evidence for 3:1403
    generation and
      propagation 3:1403
    infectious nature 3:1403
Ureidosuccinate 3:1403, 3:1404(Fig)
Urethritis, HSV-2 causing 2:681
Urochlora hoja blanca virus
  (UHBV) 3:1756
USA
  benyvirus distribution 1:155
  crop losses 2:1320(Fig)
  rubella vaccination
    program 3:1600
Ustilago maydis
  a gene 3:1813
  b gene 3:1813
  characteristics and life
    cycle 3:1813
  killer phenomenon 3:1808
  pathogen 3:1816
  resistance by plants 3:1816
Ustilago maydis virus (UmV-H1),
  RNA replication 3:1810
Ustilago maydis virus (UmV-P1),
  characteristics/
    properties 1:616(Table)
Ustilago maydis viruses 3:1812–17
  characteristics of host
    fungus 1:1813
  economic significance 3:1816–17
  evolution 3:1816
  genes, p1r, p4r, and p6r 3:1813
  genome 3:1815
    dsRNAs 3:1815
    L segments 3:1815
    M segments 3:1815
    P1H1 and P6H1 3:1815

Ustilago maydis viruses (continued)
  genome (continued)
    P1M2 3:1815
    P4M2 3:1815
    P6M2 3:1815
    sequences 3:1815
  geographic distribution 3:1816
  interstrain inhibition (killing
    phenomenon) 3:1813
  killer toxins 3:1813
    economic significance 3:1816
    genes encoding 3:1813
    KP1 3:1813
    KP4 3:1813, 3:1814–15
    KP4 α/β sandwich
      structure 3:1814
    KP4 effect on calcium
      channel 3:1814
    KP4 in transgenic
      tobacco 3:1817
    KP6 3:1813, 3:1814
    KP6 as channel-former 3:1814
    KP6 in transgenic
      tobacco 3:1817
    KP6α structure 3:1814
    KP6β structure 3:1814
    processing 3:1816(Fig)
    structure and function 3:1814–15
    types and specificity 3:1813
    no toxicity for humans 3:1817
  replication 3:1815–16
  structure and composition 3:1813
    T=1 symmetry 3:1813
  taxonomy and
    classification 3:1812–13
  toxin peptides, structures 3:1815
  transcription 3:1815–16
  translation 3:1815–16
  viruses included 3:1813–14
  see also Totiviruses
Uukuvirus 1:210–11

V

v-abl oncogene 3:1511
v-Abl protein 3:1511–12
  location and structure 3:1511–12
v-akt oncogene 3:1516
v-crk oncogene 3:1516, 3:1820
v-Crk protein 3:1516
v-erbA oncogene 3:1507–8
  cooperation with v-erbB 3:1821
v-ErbA protein, disease induced
  by 3:1508
v-erbB oncogene 3:1507–8, 3:1512, 3:1819
  cooperation with v-erbA 3:1821
  epidermal growth factor receptor
    (EGFR) 3:1512
v-ErbB protein 3:1512, 3:1819
  mechanism of action 3:1819
v-Ets protein 3:1508
v-eyk oncogene 3:1512
v-fes/fps oncogene 3:1512–13
v-Fes/Fps proteins 3:1513
v-fgr oncogene 3:1513
v-Fgr protein 3:1513
v-FLIP 1:73
v-fms oncogene 3:1513
v-fos oncogene 3:1820
v-Fos protein 3:1509
v-H-ras oncogene 3:1517
  point mutations 3:1517
v-jun gene 3:1820
v-Jun product 3:1509
  structure 3:1509
  tumors induced by 3:1509

v-K-ras oncogene 3:1517
  point mutations 3:1517
v-kit oncogene 3:1513–14
v-Kit protein 3:1513–14
v-maf oncogene 3:1509
v-mht oncogene 3:1516
v-mpl oncogene 3:1515
v-myb oncogene 3:1509
v-Myb protein 3:1509–10
v-myc oncogene 3:1510
  expression 3:1510
v-Myc protein
  fibroblast immortalization 3:1510
  structure 3:1510
v-Qin, structure 3:1511
v-raf oncogene 3:1516–17
  tumors induced by 3:1517
v-rel oncogene 3:1510, 3:1821
  genes altered by 3:1501–2, 3:1502(Table)
  mutation positions 3:1501(Fig)
  oncogenicity mechanism 3:1500–1
  protein product 3:1510
  structure 3:1510
  in transformation by REV-T
    virus 3:1500
v-Rel protein 3:1510
  complex with transcription factor
    IkB 3:1510
  structure 3:1510
  up/down-regulation of
    genes 3:1502, 3:1502(Table)
v-Ros protein 3:1514
v-ryk oncogene 3:1512
v-sea oncogene 3:1511, 3:1514
v-Sea protein 3:1515
v-sis oncogene 3:1511
v-Sis protein 3:1511, 3:1819
  as peptide mitogen 3:1819
v-ski oncogene 3:1511
v-Ski protein
  functions 3:1511
  structure 3:1511
v-src oncogene 3:1514
v-Src protein 3:1819–20
v-yes oncogene 3:1515
v-Yes protein 3:1515
Vaccination, pre/post
  transplant 3:1833
Vaccine vectors
  adenoviruses as 1:6
  animal adenoviruses 1:21
  HSV 2:697
  see also Vaccinia virus
Vaccines 3:1861–5
  antibody roles 3:1862
  attenuated live 3:1861
  cardioviruses 1:237
  DNA see DNA vaccine
  effector T cell roles 3:1862–3
  efficacy 3:1861–2
  factors affecting
    feasibility 3:1864, 3:1864(Table)
  genetically engineered,
    HSV 2:685
  history 1:298, 2:723, 3:1861
  immunological
    requirements 3:1864
  live, dominant-negative
    mutants 2:854
  main requirements 3:1861–3
  naked DNA animal
    papillomaviruses 2:1129
  recombinant
    dengue virus 1:383
    respiratory viruses 3:1495
  recombinant vaccinia virus-
    based 3:1869, 3:1872
  routes of administration 3:1864
  safety 3:1861

Vaccines (continued)
  secondary responses 3:1863
  trials 1:483
  tumor 3:1888
  viral 3:1862(Table)
  zoonotic infections 3:1995
  see also individual vaccines/
    viruses
Vaccinia
  generalized 3:1871
  progressive 3:1871
  see also Smallpox
Vaccinia growth factor 1:612
Vaccinia virus 3:1865–72
  apoptosis inhibition 1:74
  assembly 3:1868, 3:1868(Fig)
  B13R gene 1:74
  Chlorella virus similarities 1:45
  cowpox virus
    differences 1:299, 1:300
    similarities 1:300
  cytopathology 3:1868
  envelopment and
    release 1:254(Fig)
  evasion of host immune
    response 3:1871
  evolution 3:1870
  future perspectives 3:1872
  genes
    E3L 2:1146
    homologue in Amsacta moorei
      entomopoxvirus
      (AmEPV) 1:477
    Orf virus gene
      homologs 2:1142
    parapoxvirus
      similarities 2:1141
  genetics 3:1869–70
  genome 3:1866
    smallpox virus
      comparison 3:1669
  geographic and seasonal
    distribution 3:1869
  history 3:1865
  homologous genetic
    recombination 3:1449
  host range and
    propagation 3:1869
  infections
    clinical features 3:1871
    epidemiology 3:1870
    immune response 3:1871
    pathology and
      histopathology 3:1871
  intracellular naked/mature virus
    (INV/IMV) 3:1868, 3:1868(Fig)
  molluscum contagiosum virus
    (MCV) homology 2:961
  'neurovaccinia' variants 2:978
  ocular target 1:527(Table)
  pathogenicity 3:1870–1
  phage T7 hybrid system 3:1869
  physical properties 3:1866–7
  post-translational
    processing 3:1867–8
  prevention and control 3:1871–2
  protection against
    monkeypox 3:1993
  proteins 3:1866
    parapoxvirus
      similarities 2:1141
  receptor 3:1926
  recombinant
    as expression vector 3:1868–9
    generation 3:1868–9
    myelin basic protein 1:111
    vaccines based on 3:1869, 3:1872
  release 3:1868
  replication 3:1867

Vaccinia virus (continued)
  serologic relationships and variability 3:1870
  taxonomy and classification 3:1865
  tissue tropism 3:1870
  transcription 3:1867
  translation 3:1867
  transmission 3:1870
  uptake 3:1868
  vaccine, hemorrhagic fever with renal syndrome (HFRS) 1:630
  as vector 3:1887–8
    applications 3:1888
    EBV glycoprotein 3:1888
    HIV-1 infections 3:1888
    RNA polymerase 3:1887
    safety concerns and deletion mutants 3:1888
  virions 3:1865–6, 3:1866(Fig)
  see also Smallpox, vaccine
Vacuolating virus see Simian virus 40 (SV40)
Valacyclovir (Valtrex)
  herpesvirus infections 1:62
  VZV infections 3:1877
Valganciclovir 1:62
Vampire bats
  rabies 3:1437
  rabies virus transmission 3:1439
Varicella see Chickenpox
Varicella-zoster immune globulin (VZIG) 3:1876–7
Varicella-zoster (VZ), simian 2:708, 2:709
  genetics 2:710
  host range and propagation 2:709
  immune response 2:713
  infection, pathology/ histopathology 2:712
  serologic relationship and variability 2:710
Varicella-zoster virus (VZV) 3:1872–7
  animal models 3:1873
  apoptosis promotion 1:74–5
  assembly site uptake, release 3:1883–4, 3:1883(Fig)
  cytopathology 3:1884
  DNA polymerase 3:1879
  early proteins (E) 3:1882
  evolution 3:1873–4
  future investigations 3:1884
  future perspectives 3:1877
  gene 29 DNA binding protein 3:1879, 3:1882
  gene 47 protein 3:1878, 3:1879
  genes 3:1878, 3:1879, 3:1880(Table)
    regulation of expression 3:1884
  genetics 3:1873
  genome 3:1878
    isomeric forms 3:1878
  glycoproteins 3:1879, 3:1884
    gB 3:1879
    gC 3:1879
    gE 3:1879, 3:1882
    gH 3:1879
    gI 3:1879
    gL 3:1879
  history 3:1872
  host range 3:1873
  IE4 protein 3:1879
  IE62 protein 3:1878, 3:1879, 3:1882, 3:1883
  IE63 protein 3:1879
  immediate early proteins (IE) 3:1882
  late proteins (L) 3:1882
  latency 3:1884
  major capsid protein 3:1878, 3:1882

Varicella-zoster virus (VZV) (continued)
  molecular biology 3:1878–84
  nucleocapsid 3:1878
  ocular target 1:527(Table)
  ORF 10 protein 3:1878, 3:1879, 3:1882
  ORF 61 protein 3:1879, 3:1883
  pathogenicity 3:1875
  physical properties 3:1881
  propagation 3:1873
  proteins 3:1878–81
    HSV homologues 3:1878, 3:1879, 3:1880(Table)
    post-translational processing 3:1882–3
    in virion 3:1878
    see also specific proteins
  reactivation 3:1828
  recombinant 3:1873
  replication 3:1881–2
  sensitivity to environment 3:1881
  serologic relationships 3:1874
  spread through nerves 2:1179
  taxonomy and classification 3:1872–3
  terminal consensus sequence 3:1835
  tissue tropism 3:1874–5
  transcription 3:1882, 3:1884
  translation 3:1882
  transmission 3:1874–5
  vaccine (Oka strain) 3:1875, 3:1877, 3:1884
  variability 3:1874
  virions 3:1878
    morphology 3:1878
    proteins 3:1878
Varicella-zoster virus (VZV) infections 1:61, 1:61–2
  clinical features 3:1875–6
  epidemiology 3:1874
  eye 1:526
  geographic and seasonal distribution 3:1873
  immune response 3:1876
  latent 3:1884
  pathology and histology 3:1876
  post-transplant 3:1828
    clinical features 3:1828
    epidemiology 3:1828
    pathogenesis 3:1828
    treatment 3:1828
  prevention and control 3:1876–7, 3:1877
  treatment
    approved agents 1:62
    experimental agents 1:62
  see also Chickenpox; Herpes zoster (shingles)
Varicellovirus 3:1421, 3:1872
  see also Pseudorabies virus (PRV)
Variola see Smallpox
Variola virus see Smallpox virus
Variolation 3:1670
Varroa jacobsoni 2:743, 2:746, 2:749
Vascular endothelial growth factor (VEGF) 2:1145–6
Vascular leak syndrome, in dengue virus infection 1:380, 1:382
Vascular permeability, virus exit from blood and 2:1179
VCAM, receptor for EMC-like cardioviruses 1:231
Vector-borne transmission 1:484
Vectors
  animal viruses 3:1885–92, 3:1892
    adeno-associated viruses 3:1885–6
    adenoviruses 3:1886–7

Vectors (continued)
  animal viruses (continued)
    applications/uses 3:1885
    baculovirus expression vectors 3:1888–9
    future perspectives 3:1891–2
    helper-dependent/helper- independent 3:1889
    herpesviruses 3:1889
    papovavirus 3:1892
    poxvirus-based 3:1887–8
    retroviruses 3:1889–91
    RNA viruses 3:1891
    vaccinia virus 3:1887–8
  cauliflower mosaic virus (CaMV) as 2:1275
  control measures 3:1995
  cytolytic viruses 3:1891
  definition 3:1885
  fowlpox virus as 1:581–2
  giardiavirus (GLV) as 1:615
  gibbon ape leukemia virus (GaLV) 1:619
  habitat changes 3:1995–6
  history 3:1892
  LCMV gene expression 2:924
  passenger genes 3:1892
  plant viruses 3:1892–9
    Agrobacterium T-DNA transfer 3:1898
    for DNA/RNA rearrangement studies 3:1898
    future perspectives 3:1898–9
    geminiviruses 3:1894–5, 3:1895(Table)
    inoculation of plants with 3:1893–4
    pararetrovirus 3:1894
    recombination 3:1898
    RNA viruses 3:1895–7
    splicing 3:1898
    spreading within plant 3:1892–3
    transposition 3:1898
    viruses included 3:1893(Table)
    see also RNA viruses
  potexviruses 3:1367
  Semliki Forest virus (SFV) 3:1662
  shuttle 3:1888
  Sindbis (SIN) virus 3:1662
  Tanapox and Yabapox viruses 3:1973
  tetraviruses 3:1772
  transport/spread 3:1996
  trichoviruses 3:1838(Table), 3:1840
  tymoviruses 3:1853
  umbraviruses 3:1858, 3:1859
  vaccines see Vaccine vectors; Vaccinia virus
  waikaviruses 3:1968
  zoonotic viruses 3:1987
  see also Cloning vectors; Plasmids; specific viruses
Vein clearing diseases 3:1850, 3:1853
Velvet tobacco mottle virus (VTMoV) 3:1674
  host range 3:1677
  RNAs 3:1677(Fig)
  satellite RNA 3:1613
  see also Sobemoviruses
Venezuelan equine encephalitis (VEE) 3:1990
  enzootic 1:502, 1:505
    geographic/seasonal distribution 1:503
    host range 1:504
  epidemiology 1:505
  epizootic 1:502, 1:505
    clinical features of infection 1:506

Venezuelan equine encephalitis (VEE) (continued)
  epizootic (continued)
    host range 1:504
    pathogenicity 1:506
    replication 1:505
  experimental infections 1:506
  history 1:502
  human infections 1:505
  infection, pathology/ histopathology 1:507
  subtypes 1:502
  transmission 1:505
  vaccines 1:505, 1:507
  see also Equine encephalitis viruses
Venezuelan equine encephalitis (VEE) virus 3:1990
  diagnosis 3:1990
  emerging/re-emerging virus 1:419(Table)
  IAB variant 3:1990
  IC variant 3:1990
  as vector 3:1891
  virulence increase 1:420
Venezuelan hemorrhagic fever 2:891
  clinical features 2:894
  epidemiology 2:891
  immune response 2:895
  pathology/histopathology 2:894
  transmission 2:891
  see also Guanarito virus
Ventricles, lateral, dilatation in Borna disease virus infection 1:172
Vero toxins 2:1229
Vertebrate reservoir hosts, arboviruses 1:486
Vertebrates, virus families/genera infecting 3:1751(Fig)
Vertical transmission see Transmission of viruses
Vervet monkeys, CMV 1:357
Vesicles
  foot-and-mouth disease viruses causing 1:574
  formation 1:249
  pea enation mosaic virus (PEMV) 2:1195, 2:1195(Fig)
Vesicular exanthema 1:217
  clinical features 1:220
  pathogenesis 1:219
  prevention and control 1:220
Vesicular exanthema virus
  antigenic variation 1:219
  genome 1:218
  transmission 1:219
Vesicular stomatitis disease 3:1910
  clinical features 3:1918
  epizootics 3:1911, 3:1915, 3:1917
  immune response 3:1918
  pathology/histopathology 3:1918
  prevention and control 3:1919
  quarantine 3:1919
Vesicular stomatitis virus (VSV) 3:1910–19, 3:1992
  antigenic variation 3:1916
  assembly and release 1:249, 3:1914
  cDNA clones 3:1919
    HIV-1 receptor/coreceptor incorporation 3:1919
  Chandipura (CHP) virus protein similarity 1:258
  crossreactivity with Piry virus and Chandipura virus 1:257
  cytopathic effects 3:1914
  defective-interfering (DI) RNAs 1:371, 3:1454
  differential diagnosis 3:1919

Vesicular stomatitis virus (VSV) (*continued*)
  effect on host RNA synthesis 3:1958
  endemic area 3:1917
    Ossabaw Island 3:1915
  epidemiology 3:1917
  evolution 3:1915–16, 3:1916(Fig)
    molecular clock absence 3:1916
  future perspectives 3:1919
  genome 3:1911, 3:1911–12
  geographic/seasonal distribution 3:1914–15, 3:1914(Fig)
  growth in tissue culture 3:1914
  history 3:1910–11
  in HIV therapeutic strategy 1:61
  host range 3:1915
  Indiana serotype 3:1911, 3:1914, 3:1916
    distribution 3:1914(Fig)
    EM structure 3:1911(Fig)
  infection cycle 3:1913
  infections
    animals *see* Vesicular stomatitis disease
    human 3:1911, 3:1917, 3:1918
  as insect viruses 3:1917
  interference
    influenza A virus 2:850
    poliovirus 2:850
    pseudorabies virus 2:850
  natural history 3:1915
  New Jersey serotype 3:1911, 3:1914, 3:1915, 3:1916
    distribution 3:1914(Fig)
  non-endemic area 3:1917
  pathogenicity 3:1918
  pH effect on infectivity 3:1911
  physical properties 3:1911
  productive infection 3:1957
  proteins 3:1911, 3:1912(Table)
    C and C′ proteins 3:1912, 3:1912(Table)
    G (glycoprotein) 3:1912, 3:1912(Table)
    L (large polymerase) 3:1912, 3:1912(Table)
    M (matrix) 3:1912, 3:1912(Table)
    N (nucleocapsid) 3:1912, 3:1912(Table)
    P (phosphoprotein) 3:1912, 3:1912(Table)
    properties 3:1912
  replication 3:1475
  replication cycle 3:1912–14
    model 3:1913–14, 3:1913(Fig)
    switch mechanism 3:1913
  serologic relationships and variability 3:1916–17
  serotypes 1:257, 3:1911
  structure and properties 3:1911
    EM 3:1911(Fig)
  'stuttering' 3:1475
  superinfection prevention 2:851
  taxonomy and classification 3:1911
  tissue tropism 3:1917
  transcription 3:1475, 3:1913, 3:1914
  translation 3:1913
  transmission 3:1917, 3:1919
  vaccines 3:1919
  as vector 3:1891
Vesiculation, polioviruses 2:1344–5
Vesiculovirus 1:218, 1:257, 2:1035, 3:1911
  morphology 1:258(Fig)
  see also Chandipura (CHP) virus; Piry virus; Vesicular stomatitis virus (VSV)

Vi antigen 1:138
Vi phage 1:138
Vibrio cholerae 2:1233
  biotypes 2:1233
  filamentous phage 1:547
  toxin *see* Cholera toxin
  transposable phage 2:987
Vicia cryptic virus (VCV) 1:312
Vidarabine
  herpesvirus infections 1:62
  post-transplant HBV infection 3:1831
  VZV infections 3:1828, 3:1877
Videx *see* ddI (didanosine)
vif gene, caprine arthritis encephalitis virus (CAEV) 1:224
Villi
  atrophy, bovine torovirus (BTV) causing 3:1802
  destruction 2:1177
  enteric virus infection 1:448, 1:448(Fig)
  epithelial cells, virus replication 1:448
  pathological changes in rotavirus infection 3:1580
Vilyuisk viruses 1:230
Vimentin, frog virus 3 (FV3)-infected cells 1:586
Viracept *see* Nelfinavir
Viral diseases
  epidemiology *see* Epidemiology of viral diseases
  prevention, epidemiology role 1:487
  resistance genes *see* Host genetic resistance
Viral erythrocytic necrosis (VEN) 1:566
  clinical features 1:567
  pathology/histopathology 1:567
Viral erythrocytic necrosis virus (VENV) 1:566
  geographic distribution 1:567
  history 1:566
  host range and transmission 1:567
  infection *see* Viral erythrocytic necrosis
  taxonomy and classification 1:566–7
Viral hemorrhagic septicemia (VHS) 1:561
  clinical features and pathology 1:562, 3:1543
  immune response 1:562
  outbreaks 1:561
Viral hemorrhagic septicemia virus (VHSV) 1:561–2, 3:1543
  genome and proteins 1:561, 3:1543
  geographic/seasonal distribution 1:561
  history 1:561, 3:1543
  host range and propagation 1:561
  immunology 3:1543
  interferon production 3:1543
  taxonomy and classification 1:561
  transmission and tissue tropism 1:561–2
Viral inclusion bodies (VIBs) *see* Inclusion bodies
Viral interference *see* Interference, viral
Viral membranes *see* Membranes
Viral oncogenesis *see* Oncogenesis
Viral receptors *see* Receptors for viruses
Viramune (nevirapine) 1:59
Virazole *see* Ribavirin

Viremia
  active 2:1178
  magnitude 2:1179
  passive 2:1178
  persistent, mechanisms 2:1015
  primary 2:1178
  secondary 2:1178
  termination 2:1179
  transit time of virus 2:1179
Virions
  definition 3:1408, 3:1946
  viruses *vs* 3:1938
'Viroceptors,' leporipoxviruses 3:1384
Viroid-like satellite RNAs *see* Satellite RNAs, viroid-like
Viroids 1:664, 2:724, 3:1928–37
  classification 3:1929–30, 3:1930(Table)
  epidemiology and control 3:1932–4
  family and genera 3:1744(Table)
  genome structure 3:1929, 3:1931(Fig)
  geographic distribution 3:1932
  hammerhead ribozymes 3:1556
  history 3:1928–9
  host range 3:1930–2, 3:1936
  molecular biology 3:1935–6
  origin and evolution 3:1931(Fig), 3:1936–7
  pathogenicity 3:1935–6
  replication 3:1935, 3:1936(Fig)
  self-cleavage 3:1554(Table), 3:1556
  symptomatology 3:1932, 3:1933(Fig), 3:1934(Fig)
  transmission 3:1930–2
'Virokines,' leporipoxviruses 3:1384
Virology, history *see* History of virology
Viroplasms 3:1969
  cypoviruses 1:334
  entomopoxviruses (EPVs) 1:479
Virosomes 3:1922
  leporipoxviruses 3:1384
Virulence 2:1304
  increase contributing to emerging viral diseases 1:420
  influence on perpetuation of virus 1:485–6
  quasispecies implications 3:1434–5
Virulence enhancing factor, entomopoxviruses (EPVs) 1:477
Viruria 2:1184
Virus
  Archaea *see* Archaea phages and viruses
  cell attachment proteins 2:1181–2
  definition 3:1471, 3:1938
  emergent properties 3:1938
  'filterable' 2:719
  head and tail evolution 1:88–9
    see also Phage
  history of use of term 2:719
  intrinsic properties 3:1938
  methanogens 1:83
  receptor-binding sites 2:1181–2
  relational properties 3:1938
  resultant properties 3:1938
  self-sufficient, cryptoviruses 1:314
  transgenes derived from 2:1307
  transmission *see* Transmission of viruses
  uncoating *see* Uncoating of viruses

Virus (*continued*)
  variation, emerging viral diseases 1:419–21
  virions *vs* 3:1938
Virus diarrhea (VD) virus 1:173
  see also Bovine viral diarrhea virus (BVDV)
Virus infections
  emerging *see* Emerging viral diseases
  types 3:1957
Virus SSV1 *see* SSV1
Virus structure *see* Structure of viruses
Virus vectors *see* Vectors
Virus–host interactions *see under* Host
Virus–host responses
  hypersensitive *see* Hypersensitive response (HR)
  plant viruses *see* Plant virus disease
Virus-like particles (VLPs)
  isometric, in fir trees 1:312
  in mushrooms 1:152
  in plants 1:312
  tetraviruses 3:1770
  Ty elements *see* Ty elements
Visna 2:1018, 3:1961–2
  clinical/pathological criteria 3:1962
  pathology 3:1962
Visna virus 1:223
Visna-maedi viruses 3:1961–4
  cell biology and pathogenesis 3:1963–4
  future perspectives 3:1964
  history 3:1961–2
  host range and epizootiology 3:1962–3
  immune responses 3:1963
  infections *see* Maedi; Visna
  prevention and control 3:1964
  taxonomy and classification 3:1963
  variability 3:1963
  see also Caprine arthritis encephalitis virus (CAEV)
Vistide *see* Cidofovir
Vitivirus, new genus 3:1842
Vitrasert 1:62
Vitronectin receptor, coxsackievirus receptor 1:306
VLA-2, as receptor for echoviruses 1:411, 1:412(Fig)
Voandezia necrotic mosaic virus 3:1850
Vomiting
  enteric viruses causing 1:448
  Lassa fever 2:893

W

Wad Medani virus (WMV) 2:1045(Table), 2:1047
Waikavirus 1:1622, 1:1965
Waikaviruses 3:1965–70
  capsid proteins (CPs) 3:1966, 3:1967, 3:1970
  epidemiology 3:1968
  evolution 3:1623, 3:1966–7
  future perspectives 3:1970
  genome 3:1966
    non-coding region 3:1966
    unanswered questions 3:1970
  geographic and seasonal distribution 3:1965–6
  history 3:1965

Waikaviruses (continued)
  host range and
    propagation 3:1966
  infections
    clinical features 3:1969
    pathology and
      histopathology 3:1969
  P1 protein 3:1966, 3:1967, 3:1970
  pathogenicity 3:1968–9
  serologic relationships and
    variability 3:1967–8
  taxonomy and
    classification 3:1965
  tissue tropism 3:1968
  transmission 3:1968
Walker nucleotide binding site,
  filamentous phage 1:551
Wallal virus
  (WLAV) 2:1045(Table), 2:1051
Walleye dermal sarcoma 1:565
  clinical features and immune
    response 1:565
Walleye dermal sarcoma retrovirus
  (WDSV) 1:565
  geographic/seasonal
    distribution 1:565
  host range and propagation 1:565
  taxonomy and
    classification 1:565
  transmission 1:565
Walleye discrete epidermal
  hyperplasia (WEH) 1:565
Walleye epidermal hyperplasia
  retrovirus (WEHV) 1:565
  clinical features and immune
    response 1:565
  geographic/seasonal
    distribution 1:565
  host range and propagation 1:565
  taxonomy and
    classification 1:565
  transmission 1:565
Walleye herpesvirus 1:553
Warrego virus
  (WARV) 2:1045(Table), 2:1051
Warthin–Finkeldey cells 2:957
Warthogs, African swine fever
  virus (AFSV) 1:36
Warts 2:1126
  animal papillomaviruses
    causing 2:1121, 2:1126
    malignant potential 2:1126–7
    regression 2:1128, 2:1129
    treatment 2:1129
  anogenital 2:1110
  clinical features 2:1112
  common type 2:1110, 2:1112
  discovery of viruses
    causing 2:1105
  flat 2:1110, 2:1112
  genital see Genital warts
  HPVs causing 2:1108, 2:1110,
    2:1111(Table), 2:1115
  myrmecia 2:1110
  palmoplantar myrmecia 2:1112
  prevalence and geographic
    distribution 2:1106
  types 2:1110
Wasps
  ascovirus transmission 1:100
  picorna-like viruses 2:1271–2
  polydnavirus
    morphogenesis 2:1349
  symbioses with viruses 2:1351
Water
  carmovirus transmission 1:243
  echoviruses transmission 1:414
  hepatitis E virus
    transmission 1:669, 1:673
  tombusviruses
    transmission 3:1792

Water (continued)
  usage, emergence/re-emergence
    of diseases 1:422
Waterfowl parvoviruses (WFPs)
  classification 2:1168
  genome 2:1169
    organization 2:1171
  history 2:1168
  see also Parvoviruses
Watermelon silver mottle virus
  (WSMV) 3:1805
Wesselsbron (WSL) virus 1:430–7
  abortion in sheep 1:435, 1:436
  distribution 1:431
  epidemics 1:434–5
  infections
    clinical features 1:436
    pathology/
      histopathology 1:436
  transmission 1:430, 1:431, 1:432,
    1:435
  yellow fever virus
    relationship 1:431, 3:1986
West Nile virus (WNV) 3:1989
  antigenic types 1:427
  evolution 1:427
  features 1:425(Table)
  geographic/seasonal
    distribution 1:426
  history/discovery 1:424
  host range 1:427
  infections
    clinical features 1:428
    pathology/
      histopathology 1:429
  pathogenicity 1:428
Western equine encephalitis (WEE)
  virus 3:1662, 3:1990–1
  diagnosis 3:1991
  epidemiology 1:505
  epizootic and enzootic
    strains 1:502
  evolution 1:504
  geographic/seasonal
    distribution 1:503
  history 1:502
  host range 1:503–4
  human infections 1:505
    clinical features 1:506
    pathology/
      histopathology 1:506–7
  interseasonal persistence 1:505
  pathogenicity 1:506
  replication 1:505
  subtypes 1:502
  transmission 1:505
  vaccine 1:507
  see also Equine encephalitis
    viruses
Whales, morbillivirus
  infection 3:1560, 3:1564, 3:1566
Wheat, economic significance of
  virus infections 2:1323
Wheat American striate mosaic
  virus (WASMV) 3:1531
Wheat dwarf virus (WDV), genome
  structure 1:597
Wheat germ system, TNV coat
  protein synthesis 2:1005
Wheat yellow leaf virus
  (WYLV) 1:271
White Arroyo virus 2:888(Table)
White cell count
  Argentine hemorrhagic fever
    (AHF) 1:893
  Bolivian hemorrhagic fever
    (BHF) 2:894
  Lassa fever 2:893
White clover
  cryptoviruses 1:312
  economic significance of virus
    infections 2:1323

White clover cryptic virus 1
  (WCCV1) 1:312–13, 1:314
  serologic relationships 1:314
White clover cryptic virus 2
  (WCCV2) 1:313, 1:314
White clover mosaic potexvirus
  (WCMV) 1:239
  RNA 3:1367
White spot baculovirus
  (WSBV) 3:1626, 3:1633
  diagnosis and detection 3:1633
  genome 3:1633
  structure and properties 3:1633
Whitefly
  begomovirus transmission 1:603
  explosion in populations 1:272,
    1:273
  geminivirus transmission 3:1905
  viruses transmitted 1:268(Table),
    1:272
Whitlow, herpetic 2:681
Wild boars, hog cholera
  epidemics 2:739
Wild cucumber mosaic
  virus 3:1850, 3:1851
Wildlife
  cowpox virus reservoir 1:300,
    1:301–2, 1:304
  rinderpest 3:1559(Table), 3:1565
Wilting, plants 2:1318
WIN compounds 2:1331
Wind-borne viruses,
  orbiviruses 2:1054
Winter wheat
  crop losses, furoviruses
    causing 1:595
  furoviruses resistance 1:595
Wiseana iridescent virus (WIV)
  economic importance 2:868
  genome 2:868
  replication 2:867
Wiskott–Aldrich syndrome 1:490
  HPV infections 2:1109
Wongorr virus species
  (WGRV) 2:1045(Table)
Woodchuck hepatitis virus
  (WHV) 1:640, 1:645
  carcinogenic mechanism 1:643
  genome 1:645–6
  geographic/seasonal
    distribution 1:641
  hepatitis delta virus infection
    with 1:664
  host range and propagation 1:641
  transcription 1:649
Woods Hole Harbor water,
  cyanobacteria 1:328–30,
    1:328(Fig)
World Health Organization
  (WHO)
  dengue hemorrhagic fever/dengue
    shock syndrome (DHF/DSS)
    diagnostic criteria 1:382,
    1:382(Table)
  poliomyelitis elimination
    goal 2:1326, 2:1329, 2:1348
  smallpox eradication 3:1865
  viruses associated with cardiac
    disease 2:1074
Wound tumor virus (WTV) 2:1262
  gene expression 2:1265
  host range 2:1266
  in vitro expression 2:1264
  infection, symptoms 2:1266
  transmissibility loss 2:1266
  vegetative propagation 1:1907
  see also Phytoreoviruses
Wounding, animal papillomavirus
  infection 2:1126

X

X-linked lymphoproliferative
  syndrome (XLPS) 3:1844
  EBV association 3:1844
  EBV latent protein
    expression 1:492
  EBV-associated B cell
    lymphomas 1:490
  fatal infectious
    mononucleosis 1:492
  see also Lymphoproliferative
    syndrome
X-ray crystallography 3:1943
  influenza virus proteins 2:838–9
X-ray diffraction 3:1943
X-ray fiber diffraction 3:1943
Xanthomonas, filamentous
  phage 1:547
Xenotransplantation
  baboon herpesvirus
    concerns 2:714
  endogenous proviruses,
    concerns 1:440

Y

Y62-33 virus 1:502, 1:503
Yabapox virus
  cell transformation 3:1972
  epidemiology 3:1972
  evolution 3:1971
  future perspectives 3:1973
  genome 3:1971
  history 3:1971
  immune response 3:1973
  infections
    clinical features 3:1973
    pathology and
      histopathology 3:1973
    prevention and control 3:1973
  pathogenicity 3:1973
  physical properties 3:1971
  proteins 3:1971
  replication 3:1972
    morphogenesis 3:1972
    nucleic acid 3:1972
    protein synthesis 3:1972
    virus synthesis 3:1972
  serological relationships and
    variability 3:1972
  taxonomy and
    classification 3:1971
  transmission and tissue
    tropism 3:1973
  virions 3:1971
Yabavirus-like disease 3:1971
Yamame tumor virus 1:553
Yatapoxviruses 3:1971–4
  see also Tanapox virus; Yabapox
    virus
Yeast
  functions, in RNA virus
    replication 3:1977–8
  killer system 3:1808, 3:1812
  use in industry 3:1812
  prions see Prions
  retroviruses 3:1974
  uracil biosynthesis 3:1403
  Ure2p see Ure2p
Yeast RNA viruses 3:1974–9
  23S RNA 3:1974
  chromosomal genes
    affecting 3:1977(Table)
  classification 3:1974
  future perspectives 3:1979
  history 3:1974

Yeast RNA viruses (continued)
 host functions 3:1977, 3:1977(Table)
 killer toxins
  action 3:1978
  applications 3:1979
  processing 3:1978, 3:1978(Fig)
 replicons 3:1974–5, 3:1974(Table)
 see also L-A virus; L-BC virus; 20S RNA virus
Yellow fever 3:1989
 clinical features 3:1985
 diagnosis 3:1989
 epidemiology 3:1984–5
 genetic resistance 2:753
 history 3:1979–80
 incidence 3:1984, 3:1984(Fig)
 intoxication phase 3:1985
 jungle 3:1984, 3:1985
 pathology and pathogenesis 3:1985–6
 prevention and control 3:1986, 3:1989
 re-emergence 1:422
 urban 3:1984, 3:1984–5, 3:1989
 vaccine 3:1861, 3:1986, 3:1989
  17D 3:1982–3, 3:1982(Table), 3:1986
  French neurotropic (FNV) 3:1983
  history 2:723
 viremic phase 3:1985
Yellow fever virus 3:1979–86, 3:1989
 Asibi strain 3:1982, 3:1982(Table)
 C protein 3:1980
 E glycoprotein 3:1980, 3:1980–1
  in cell attachment 3:1983
  role in virulence 3:1982–3
  structure 3:1980–1
 evolution 3:1982
 French viscerotropic strain 3:1983
 genome 3:1980, 3:1981(Fig)

Yellow fever virus (continued)
 geographic distribution 3:1983–4, 3:1985(Fig)
 history 2:719, 3:1979–80
 host range 3:1983
 immune response 3:1986
 infections see Yellow fever
 M protein 3:1980
 neurotropism 3:1986
  molecular basis 3:1982–3
 NS1 glycoprotein 3:1981
 NS3 protein 3:1981
 NS5 protein 3:1981
 prM protein 3:1980
 propagation 3:1983
 proteins 3:1980–1
 re-emerging virus 1:419(Table)
 replication 3:1981–2
 seasonal distribution 3:1984
 taxonomy and classification 3:1980
 transmission 2:719, 3:1984–5
  ecological change and 3:1996
  forest cycle 3:1984
  urban cycle 3:1984
 variation 3:1982
 virions 3:1980, 3:1981(Fig)
 virulence, molecular basis 3:1982–3
 viscerotropism 3:1986
  molecular basis 3:1983
 Wesselsbron (WSL) virus relationship 1:431
Yellow fever virus group 1:433(Table)
Yellow foliar mottle, badnavirus infections 2:1298
Yellow mosaic diseases 3:1850, 3:1853
Yellow summer squash, economic significance of viruses 2:1323
Yellowhead virus 3:1628
 culture 3:1628
 detection and diagnosis 3:1629
 genome 3:1629
 host range 3:1628

Yellowhead virus (continued)
 purification 3:1629
 recombinant clones 3:1629
 structural proteins 3:1629
 structure and properties 3:1628
Yellowtail ascitic virus (YAV) 1:161
Yemen Arab Republic, sheeppox and goatpox 3:1378
yes oncogene 3:1515
Yoghurt 2:1253, 2:1254
 phage ψO1205 from 2:1258
Yoghurt industry 2:1254
Yokose virus group 1:433(Table)
YPHFMPTNL immune modulator 1:368
Yug Bugdanovac virus 1:257

Z

Zadaxin 1:66
Zalcitabine see ddC (Zalcitabine)
Zanamavir 1:64
Zebra stripes, peste des petits ruminants 3:1567
Zenker's fixing solution 1:400
Zenker's necrosis 1:469
Zerit (d4T) 1:59
Zidovudine (azidothymidine - AZT) 1:58, 2:779
 feline immunodeficiency virus (FIV) infection 1:540
 in HAART 1:58
 HIV resistance 1:58
 mechanism of action 1:58
 in pregnancy 1:58, 2:787
 resistance 2:787
 side effects 1:58
Zika virus, yellow fever virus cross-protection 3:1986
Zinc chelators 2:785–6
Zinc fingers 1:61

Zinc fingers (continued)
 E6 protein of HPV 2:1120
 inhibition 1:61
 reovirus protein $\sigma 3$ 3:1467
Zinc sulfate 2:730
Zinc-binding ring-finger protein, arenaviruses 2:888
Zinc-finger transcription factor, thyroid hormone receptor α (THRA1) 3:1508
Zintevir 1:61, 2:783
Zona occludens see Tight junctions
Zoonoses 1:486, 3:1987–97
 in Africa 3:1993–4
 in Americas 3:1990–2
 in Asia 3:1994
 in Australia 3:1994–5
 control 3:1995
 emerging and re-emerging 3:1995–7
  ecological change and 3:1995–6
  social change and 3:1997
 in Europe 3:1992–3
 global 3:1987–90
 rotaviruses (group A) infections 1:443
 Tanapox virus 3:1972
 transmission 3:1987
 transmission cycle 1:486
 see also individual viruses
Zoonotic agents, limited epidemic potential 1:421
Zoospores
 plant virus transmission 3:1908, 3:1909
 tombusviruses transmission 3:1793
Zoster see Herpes zoster (shingles)
Zoster ophthalmicus see Herpes zoster ophthalmicus
Zovirax see Acyclovir
Zuchini yellow mosaic virus (ZYMV) 3:1374
Zwoegerziekte 3:1962